WITHDRAWN
WRIGHT STATE UNIVERSITY LIBRARIES

D0152720

FIFTH EDITION _____ KISTNER'S GYNECOLOGY
Principles and Practice

FIFTH EDITION _____

Kistner's
Gynecology
Principles and Practice

Kenneth J. Ryan, M.D.
Kate Macy Ladd Professor of Obstetrics and
  Gynecology
Department of Obstetrics, Gynecology, and
  Reproductive Biology
Harvard Medical School
Chairman, Department of Obstetrics and
  Gynecology
Brigham and Women's Hospital
Boston, Massachusetts

Ross Berkowitz, M.D.
Professor of Obstetrics, Gynecology, and
  Reproductive Biology
Harvard Medical School
Chief, Division of Gynecologic Oncology and
  Gynecology
Brigham and Women's Hospital
Boston, Massachusetts

Robert L. Barbieri, M.D.
Associate Professor of Obstetrics, Gynecology, and
  Reproductive Biology
Harvard Medical School
Chief, Division of Fertility and Endocrinology
Department of Obstetrics and Gynecology
Brigham and Women's Hospital
Boston, Massachusetts

YEAR BOOK MEDICAL PUBLISHERS, INC.
CHICAGO • LONDON • BOCA RATON • LITTLETON, MASS.

WP
100
G9973
1990

WRIGHT STATE UNIVERSITY
FORDHAM HEALTH SCIENCES LIBRARY

Copyright © 1986, 1990 by Year Book Medical Publishers, Inc. All rights reserved. No part of this publication may be reproduced, stored in a retrieval system, or transmitted, in any form or by any means—electronic, mechanical, photocopying, recording, or otherwise—without prior written permission from the publisher. Printed in the United States of America.

Permission to photocopy or reproduce solely for internal or personal use is permitted for libraries or other users registered with the Copyright Clearance Center, provided that the base fee of $4.00 per chapter plus $.10 per page is paid directly to the Copyright Clearance Center, 21 Congress Street, Salem, MA 01970. This consent does not extend to other kinds of copying, such as copying for general distribution, for advertising or promotional purposes, for creating new collected works, or for resale.

1 2 3 4 5 6 7 8 9 0 BC 94 93 92 91 90

Library of Congress Cataloging-in-Publication Data
Gynecology (Chicago, Ill.)
    Kistner's gynecology : principles and practice.—5th ed. /
[edited by] Kenneth J. Ryan, Robert Barbieri, Ross Berkowitz.
        p.   cm.
    Rev. ed. of: Gynecology / [edited by] Robert W. Kistner. 4th ed.
c1986.
    Includes bibliographical references.
    ISBN 0-8151-5084-9
    1. Gynecology.   I. Kistner, Robert W. (Robert William), 1917–   .
II. Ryan, Kenneth J., 1926–   .   III. Barbieri, Robert L.
IV. Berkowitz, Ross Stuart.   V. Title.   VI. Title: Gynecology.
    [DNLM: 1. Genital Diseases, Female.   2. Genital Neoplasms, Female.
WP 100 G99715]   89–22538
RG101.G95 1990   CIP
618.1—dc20
DNLM/DLC
for Library of Congress

Sponsoring Editor: Nancy G. Puckett
Associate Managing Editor, Manuscript Services: Deborah Thorp
Production Project Coordinator: Carol Reynolds
Proofroom Supervisor: Barbara M. Kelly

_____ Dedicated to those who inspired us: family, friends, and students.

Robert L. Barbieri, M.D.

Associate Professor of Obstetrics, Gynecology,
and Reproductive Biology
Harvard Medical School
Chief, Division of Fertility and Endocrinology
Department of Obstetrics and Gynecology
Brigham and Women's Hospital
Boston, Massachusetts

Beryl R. Benacerraf, M.D.

Assistant Clinical Professor of Obstetrics,
Gynecology, and Reproductive Biology
Assistant Clinical Professor of Radiology
Harvard Medical School
Consultant in Obstetrical Ultrasound and
Radiology
Brigham and Women's Hospital
Boston, Massachusetts

Joan Bengtson, M.D.

Instructor in Obstetrics, Gynecology, and
Reproductive Biology
Harvard Medical School
Department of Obstetrics and Gynecology
Brigham and Women's Hospital
Boston, Massachusetts

Ross Berkowitz, M.D.

Professor of Obstetrics, Gynecology, and
Reproductive Biology
Harvard Medical School
Chief, Division of Gynecologic Oncology and
Gynecology
Brigham and Women's Hospital
Boston, Massachusetts

Neil J. Finkler, M.D.

Assistant Professor of Obstetrics, Gynecology,
and Reproductive Biology
Harvard Medical School
Department of Obstetrics and Gynecology
Brigham and Women's Hospital
Boston, Massachusetts

Andrew J. Friedman, M.D.

Assistant Professor of Obstetrics, Gynecology,
and Reproductive Biology
Harvard Medical School
Department of Obstetrics and Gynecology
Brigham and Women's Hospital
Boston, Massachusetts

Donald P. Goldstein, M.D.

Assistant Clinical Professor of Obstetrics,
Gynecology, and Reproductive Biology
Harvard Medical School
Department of Obstetrics and Gynecology
Brigham and Women's Hospital
Boston, Massachusetts

Howard M. Goodman, M.D.

Instructor in Obstetrics, Gynecology, and
Reproductive Biology
Harvard Medical School
Department of Obstetrics and Gynecology
Brigham and Women's Hospital
Boston, Massachusetts

Joseph A. Hill, M.D.

Assistant Professor of Obstetrics, Gynecology,
and Reproductive Biology
Harvard Medical School
Department of Obstetrics and Gynecology
Brigham and Women's Hospital
Boston, Massachusetts

Mark D. Hornstein, M.D.

Instructor in Obstetrics, Gynecology, and
Reproductive Biology
Harvard Medical School
Department of Obstetrics and Gynecology
Brigham and Women's Hospital
Boston, Massachusetts

Robert C. Knapp, M.D.

William H. Baker Professor of Gynecology
Harvard Medical School

Department of Obstetrics and Gynecology
Brigham and Women's Hospital
Boston, Massachusetts

Thomas Leavitt, Jr., M.D.

Associate Clinical Professor of Obstetrics,
  Gynecology, and Reproductive Biology
Harvard Medical School
Department of Obstetrics and Gynecology
Brigham and Women's Hospital
Boston, Massachusetts

Patricia M. McShane, M.D.

Medical Director
IVF Australia Program—Boston
Department of Obstetrics and Gynecology
Waltham-Weston Hospital
Waltham, Massachusetts

Wayne A. Miller, M.D.

Clinical Associate Professor in Obstetrics and
  Gynecology
Harvard Medical School
Boston, Massachusetts
Prenatal Diagnostic Center, Inc.
Lexington, Massachusetts

Rapin Osathanondh, M.D.

Associate Professor of Obstetrics, Gynecology,
  and Reproductive Biology
Harvard Medical School
Associate Chief
Ambulatory and Community Obstetrics and
  Gynecology
Brigham and Women's Hospital
Boston, Massachusetts

Veronica A. Ravnikar, M.D.

Assistant Professor of Obstetrics, Gynecology,
  and Reproductive Biology
Harvard Medical School
Department of Gynecology
Massachusetts General Hospital
Boston, Massachusetts

Mitchell S. Rein, M.D.

Instructor in Obstetrics, Gynecology, and
  Reproductive Biology
Harvard Medical School
Department of Obstetrics and Gynecology
Brigham and Women's Hospital
Boston, Massachusetts

Kenneth J. Ryan, M.D.

Kate Macy Ladd Professor of Obstetrics and
  Gynecology
Chairman, Department of Obstetrics,
  Gynecology, and Reproductive Biology
Harvard Medical School
Chairman, Department of Obstetrics and
  Gynecology

Brigham and Women's Hospital
Boston, Massachusetts

Isaac Schiff, M.D.

Joe Vincent Meigs Professor of Gynecology
Harvard Medical School
Chief, Vincent Memorial Gynecology Service
Massachusetts General Hospital
Boston, Massachusetts

Ellen E. Sheets, M.D.

Assistant Professor of Obstetrics, Gynecology,
  and Reproductive Biology
Harvard Medical School
Department of Obstetrics and Gynecology
Brigham and Women's Hospital
Boston, Massachusetts

Robert L. Shirley, M.D.

Assistant Clinical Professor of Obstetrics,
  Gynecology, and Reproductive Biology
Harvard Medical School
Department of Obstetrics and Gynecology
Brigham and Women's Hospital
Boston, Massachusetts

Ruth Tuomala, M.D.

Assistant Professor of Obstetrics, Gynecology,
  and Reproductive Biology
Harvard Medical School
Department of Obstetrics and Gynecology
Brigham and Women's Hospital
Boston, Massachusetts

Brian W. Walsh, M.D.

Instructor in Obstetrics, Gynecology, and
  Reproductive Biology
Harvard Medical School
Department of Obstetrics and Gynecology
Brigham and Women's Hospital
Boston, Massachusetts

Robert M. Wah, M.D.

Adjunct Clinical Instructor
Department of Reproductive Medicine
University of California (San Diego)
Director, Reproductive Endocrinology Division
Department of Obstetrics and Gynecology
Balboa Naval Hospital
San Diego, California

John Yeh, M.D.

Instructor in Obstetrics, Gynecology, and
  Reproductive Biology
Harvard Medical School
Department of Obstetrics and Gynecology
Brigham and Women's Hospital
Boston, Massachusetts

PREFACE TO THE FIFTH EDITION

For over 25 years, *Kistner's Gynecology: Principles and Practice* has been among *the* standard texts in gynecology. Through four editions it has been designed to meet the needs of medical students, interns, and residents in obstetrics and gynecology training as well as established specialists in this field. We are pleased to introduce this new fifth edition continuing the tradition Dr. Robert Kistner began in 1964 with the first edition of *Gynecology: Principles and Practice*. Although this is the first edition which Dr. Kistner has not coordinated, we hope that his original purpose and his vision have been perpetuated.

The field of gynecology is dynamic and important changes and new advances occur continually. Each subsequent edition of *Kistner's Gynecology* has been expanded and revised to include these changes and advances. In the fifth edition, several new chapters have been included.

Estimates vary, but perhaps between 10% and 15% of American couples are involuntarily infertile, and infertility diagnosis and treatment are an increasingly important and growing part of gynecologic practice. Therefore, infertility diagnosis has been expanded to address evaluation of the infertile couple and a new chapter on infertility treatment has also been added. These chapters by Drs. Rein and Schiff and Drs. Wah and Ravnikar, respectively, will be of great interest and value to the reader.

More and more, gynecologic examination demands special techniques and instruments. The role of ultrasonography has grown dramatically and Dr. Beryl Benacerraf has prepared an outstanding chapter on the techniques and applications of pelvic sonography.

Hysteroscopy, laparoscopy, and laser surgery have now become not only an exciting but an indispensable part of modern gynecology. These state-of-the-art technologies allow the contemporary practitioner to obtain direct information in the shortest possible time with minimal risk and cost to the patient. Dr. Andrew Friedman has prepared an all-new chapter on these important advances to our specialty.

The expanded attention to pediatric and adolescent gynecology has also warranted a new chapter and we are fortunate to have the contribution of a leader in this field, Dr. Donald Peter Goldstein. With a growing population of older women, geriatric concerns will also be an important aspect of gynecologic practice. Therefore, issues pertinent to the care of postmenopausal women have been thoroughly discussed and integrated throughout the text. In addition, an entire chapter is now devoted to the menstrual cycle, prepared by editors Drs. Ryan and Barbieri.

Many people must be acknowledged for their support in helping to make this book a reality. The contributors made time in already hectic schedules to ensure that *Kistner's Gynecology: Principles and Practice* continues to make an important contribution to the literature and the practice of gynecology. The contributors join us, too, in thanking our students, family, and friends for their ongoing understanding and support throughout the process of writing this book.

Ms. Mary Ann Murphy and all the support

staff at our institutions are thanked for their unfailing help in preparing the manuscript. Much appreciation must go also to the staff at Year Book Medical Publishers for their enthusiasm and hard work.

Finally, we welcome several new contributors to the fifth edition and also acknowledge our great debt to all the contributors to previous editions. Collectively, they have made this new edition possible. Foremost, of course, sincere thanks must be expressed to Dr. Robert Kistner, who 26 years ago compiled his lecture notes and started a tradition.

KENNETH J. RYAN
ROSS BERKOWITZ
ROBERT L. BARBIERI

PREFACE TO FIRST EDITION

This work is designed both as a textbook and as a general reference book of gynecology to meet the needs of undergraduate medical students, young practitioners of gynecology, and specialists in this field. The format of each chapter is similar, the purpose being to provide a uniform and organized approach to the understanding of multiple disease processes of each organ of the female genital tract. Thus, in each chapter the embryology, anatomy, and histology are correlated with specific malformations. Morphologic variations are correlated with physiologic alterations. Recent advances in the diagnosis and therapy of infectious processes are described in detail. Particular emphasis has been given to the relationship of premalignant to malignant neoplasms, and methods for the prophylaxis of certain tumors are suggested. Because of the importance and increasing incidence of endometriosis a separate chapter on this disease is included. Particular emphasis has been placed on hormonal therapy, and details of management outlined.

Because of my interest in the practical endocrinologic aspects of gynecology, a chapter is devoted to steroid therapy. In this chapter an attempt is made to obviate many of the difficulties of administration associated with the new synthetic preparations. I have included (1) a brief résumé of basic steroid chemistry, (2) a summation of the pharmacology and physiology of androgens, estrogens, and progesterone, together with a similar discussion of the synthetic progestins, and (3) a discussion of proved and proposed indications for the use of these steroids, with specific contraindications and optimum dosage.

The observations and opinions expressed in this text summarize the sum and substance of the teaching and practice at the Free Hospital for Women during the past 15 years. This hospital was opened on November 2, 1875, and has been in continuous operation since that time. It is the only remaining specialty hospital in the United States whose primary objective is the diagnosis and treatment of medical and surgical diseases of the female.

The Free Hospital for Women became internationally known because of the *Textbook of Gynecology* written by Dr. William P. Graves, formerly Professor of Gynecology at Harvard Medical School. Although the fourth and last edition of Graves' textbook appeared in 1928, since that time a multiplicity of original and important contributions has been published by the members of the staff. Outstanding among these have been the innumerable works of Drs. George and Olive Smith concerning the measurement and metabolism of ovarian steroids and gonadotropic hormones during the menstrual cycle, the period of conception, and subsequent pregnancy. During the years 1938 through 1957 Drs. John Rock and Arthur T. Hertig accomplished their monumental studies on the earliest stages of human growth following fertilization. From 1928 through 1958 Dr. Rock directed intensive study and research projects relating to the etiologic factors in infertility. The pathogenesis of carcinoma in situ of the cervix and its relationship to invasive carcinoma have undergone thorough investigation and evaluation by Drs. Paul Younge, Arthur T. Hertig, and Donald G. MacKay. During the past seven years the synthetic progestational agents have been subjected to extensive clinical investigation in specific gynecologic disorders such as endometriosis and endometrial carcinoma.

In preparing a work of this type, material must be gathered not only from the author's personal experience but to a still greater extent from the work of others. I have, therefore, attempted to include the important observations of numerous authors who have published data concerning the clinical material at the Free Hospital for Women. From the great number of publications consulted there have been several to which I have had frequent recourse, both for new material and for corroboration of personal observations. I must, therefore, express a general acknowledgment of indebtedness to Drs. George and Olive Smith, Arthur T. Hertig, Christopher J. Duncan, Paul A. Younge, Donald G. MacKay, and John Rock. I have also drawn on the writings of the late Joe V. Meigs and Langdon Parsons, both former residents at the Free Hospital for Women. In writing the sections on the relationship of endocrinology to gynecology I have received the greatest assistance from the excellent works, *Endocrine and Metabolic Aspects of Gynecology* by Joseph Rogers, *Human Endocrinology* by Herbert S. Kup-

perman, and *The Endocrinology of Reproduction,* edited by Joseph T. Velardo. The reader is referred to these publications for additional and specific details.

I am indebted to Mrs. Edith Tagrin for the excellent illustrations and to Mr. Leo Goodman and Dr. Robert Ehrmann for the photomicrographs. Dr. Arthur T. Hertig and Dr. Hazel M. Gore have also kindly given permission to reproduce many of their excellent photomicrographs previously published in *Tumors of the Female Sex Organs,* published by the Armed Forces Institute of Pathology. The student is advised to refer to these fascicles for a complete survey of the pathology of tumors of the female genital tract.

I also wish to acknowledge a deep indebtedness to the tireless fingers and indefatigable efforts of my secretaries, Mrs. Ann Gregory Metzger, Mrs. Constance M. Rakoske, Mrs. Linda Angelico, and Mrs. Rachel Markiewicz. Valuable assistance has been given to me by the Administrator of the Free Hospital for Women, Miss Lillian Grahn. Finally, the courtesies of the staff of Year Book Medical Publishers have made the final preparation of this manuscript a pleasant task.

ROBERT W. KISTNER

CONTENTS

1

The Nature of Gynecological Practice

Kenneth J. Ryan, M.D.

GYNECOLOGY AND ITS RELATIONSHIP TO OBSTETRICS

Gynecology is that branch of medicine that deals primarily with the health care of women as it relates to the prevention, diagnosis, and treatment of disease of the reproductive system. Gynecology has ancient roots recorded in Egyptian and Greek medical writings; obstetrics as a medical practice evolved much later as physicians supplanted midwives in attending women for labor and delivery. Gynecological practice was consolidated around advances in surgery of the reproductive tract during the 19th century, when the early cases of ovariectomy and hysterectomy and repairs of vesicovaginal fistulas were first described. Obstetrics gradually evolved into a specialty as prenatal care became popular from the beginning of the 20th century and hospital-based births became the rule after World War II in the 1950s. The two disciplines have thus had different origins and emphases in practice—one in surgery, the other in the care of the pregnant woman, parturient, and newborn. Although arguments raged about the differences between obstetrical and gynecological practice to keep the two fields separate, many leaders of the two disciplines recognized commonalities of interest and eventually joined forces into one specialty for both training and practice. In 1930, The American Board of Obstetrics and Gynecology was formed to examine for and certify qualifications in a combined field. Although the German universities had established combined departments of obstetrics and gynecology by the end of the 19th century, many academic programs in England, France, and the United States stubbornly remained divided until the mid-20th century. Medical school and hospital departments, both in the United States and around the world, are now essentially all combined departments of obstetrics and gynecology. Most physicians are now trained in both obstetrics and gynecology, and many still combine both areas in their practice. The tradition has been to emphasize obstetrics as a new practitioner and develop largely a gynecological practice in later years when the unpredictable demands of obstetric practice are borne less easily. In spite of this, most textbooks, including this one, have remained divided because of the sheer volume of material to be covered. Physicians in the real world are more often favoring one field over the other due to the exigencies of modern medical practice or because of further subspecialization. What should not be lost sight of is the way the fields of obstetrics and gynecology and their constituent subspecialties overlap in terms of the interests and needs of patients and the common basic knowledge and clinical skills used by the practitioner in caring for women. The dangers of emphasizing one field over the other can best be illustrated by the classic misadventure in a teaching hospital training program of finding what you are looking for and are led to expect. During the same period of time, residents on the obstetrical service were providing months of prenatal care for an obese supposedly pregnant patient who really had psuedocyesis while other residents on the gynecology service were preparing a patient for surgery for a cul-de-sac mass, which was fortunately recognized in time, before the knife fell, as a pregnancy in a retroflexed uterus. The basic anatomy, physiology, and endocrinology of gynecology share much with that of obstetrics, and clinical problems need the perspective of physicians trained in both fields. The gynecologist must be mindful of the reproductive consequences of gynecological care of the patient, and the obstetrician must be mindful of the impact of pregnancy and its management on the patient's subsequent health and function. When a patient of reproductive age is seen with either bleeding or amenorrhea, a normally implanted or ectopic pregnancy must always be considered in the differential diagnosis, and one must be sensitive to the possibility that gynecological disease may complicate pregnancy.

PRIMARY CARE FOR WOMEN

Although gynecology is a specialty practice, gynecologists often provide primary care for their patients comparable to the services provided by general internists. Obstetricians-gynecologists often provide services comparable to those provided by family practitioners or the now nearly extinct general practitioner. The obstetrician-gynecologist may be the only physician regularly seen by the female patient, not only during pregnancy but also postpartum, especially for routine visits for vaginal cytology, renewal of prescriptions for birth control, and for the very common recurrent problems of cystitis and vaginitis. To these are now added the need for regular screening for breast cancer, blood cholesterol levels, and the health hazards of the postmenopausal years. Women are more apt to go for an annual Papanicolaou test or breast examination than for a general physical checkup, and in the gynecologist's office they can receive all in one visit. The American Board of Obstetricians and Gynecologists recognizes this primary care role as a legitimate part of practice and has emphasized the need for training programs to cover the knowledge and skills required for this broader responsibility. For example, a common basis of malpractice claims against gynecologists has been failure to diagnose or appropriately refer for breast cancer. Some gynecologists shun any broadening of their patient responsibilities beyond a narrow interpretation of the discipline because of limits of time and interest or fear of increased professional liability. It is, however, increasingly difficult to limit one's attention to only problems arising in the pelvis, because of public expectations that a gynecologist will do much more. In addition, the advantage of continuity of one known health care provider for the patient is enormous not only to avoid unnecessary shunting of patients to a different physician

for each complaint but to refer appropriately when it is truly necessary and to act as the patient's ombudsman. Enthusiasm for this broadened role of the gynecologist must be tempered, however, by the limits of practicality when it covers areas in which the individual gynecologist is inadequately trained. Practicing within one's area of competence is a fundamental obligation of the physician whether applied to diagnostics, therapeutics, surgical skills, or counseling. It is also a prudent practice to know one's limitations to avoid liability. One talent for which physicians may mistakenly claim more expertise than they should or, on the other hand, totally neglect is counseling. Providing detailed sound professional advice about genetic testing, sexual behavior, nutrition, or psychological disorders may be more than an individual gynecologist can accomplish, and one should know how to refer such problems when necessary. Although the specialized knowledge and skills for counseling can be learned, they are less well covered during training, and limitations in this area are less well appreciated than for the typical diagnostic and therapeutic skills of gynecology. As with obstetrics, counseling is not detailed in this textbook because of space limitations, but its importance and relevance to practice should be recognized.

RELATIONSHIP OF GYNECOLOGY TO MEDICINE AND SURGERY

Gynecology is neither a wholly medical nor surgical specialty but a combination of both in roughly equal measure, a feature that students often cite as reason for entering the field. There are occasionally internists who limit their practice to gynecological medicine and surgeons who consider gynecology simply a surgical subspecialty, but gynecology practiced separately or with obstetrics requires a combination of medical and surgical skills applied with the uniqueness of female anatomy, endocrinology, and the physiology of reproduction in mind. As science advances, there may be shifts of treatment modalities from surgery to medicine, as in the preference of bromocriptine to surgical extirpation for a pituitary microadenoma and preference for in vitro fertilization and embryo transfer over microsurgical tubal surgery to circumvent infertility caused by some forms of blocked fallopian tubes. Leiomyomas may be managed with gonadotropin-releasing hormone agonists rather than surgical myomectomy, but indications for surgery are being more clearly defined for all these conditions rather than eliminated. It makes no sense to exalt either surgical skills or medical skills as the more important for gynecology since both are indispensible and both must be of high quality.

CHANGES IN GYNECOLOGICAL PRACTICE

Gynecology has changed markedly in both training and practice with the advent of the subspecialty boards of Reproductive Endocrinology (Infertility) and Gynecological Oncology in the 1970s. The technical aspects of medically assisted conception such as in vitro fertilization are so involved as to require a narrower focus of the practitioner of infertility. Radical surgery, chemotherapy, and research into monoclonal antibodies, oncogenes, and growth factors have similarly required a more specialized training in preparation for a more restricted practice limited to gynecological cancer. There has been a fear that what would be left for the field of general gynecology after subspecialization might not be interesting enough to keep it viable as a discipline, but in the past the practitioner of general gynecology could not always compete or provide adequate care in these areas compared with someone who restricted his or her practice and developed specialized expertise. The formation of subspecialty boards simply institutionalized what had been going on for quite some time. In reality, the advances in subspecialty practice have actually expanded the general discipline, because the skills first limited to the subspecialist ultimately become more widely diffused in practice. It is likely that colposcopy, once the exclusive domain of the oncologist, is now utilized widely by the nonspecialist and that much infertility care is provided by generalists utilizing tools developed in subspecialty practice. Many chapters of this textbook are written by subspecialists with the expectation that this knowledge has application in general gynecological practice.

Another change in gynecological practice has been more fundamental and pervasive. This follows the social upheavals of the 1960s and 1970s that protested, among other things, the sexist nature of medicine in general and gynecology in particular. This was the era of disclosures about diethylstilbestrol causing vaginal adenosis and cancer in young women whose mothers had received it during pregnancy to avoid abortion. The fact that this occurred some 14 or more years after birth was particularly distressing and likened to a time bomb. The side effects of the birth control pill (thromboembolic disease) and postmenopausal estrogen replacement therapy (adenocarcinoma of the endometrium) were being uncovered. The intrauterine contraceptive device was found to be associated with infection and occasionally death if combined with a pregnancy while the device remained in place. It was believed that many of these complications of drugs and devices should have been anticipated and that both safety and efficacy would have to be proved in the future before the Food and Drug Administration would release products for clinical use. Excessive numbers of hysterectomies were being discussed as a prime example of unnecessary surgery that helped usher in the requirement of third-party payors for a second opinion. It was noted that women were underrepresented in medicine in general and in gynecology in particular. The gynecologist was often cast as the exploiter rather than the protector of women's health. Although this did little justice to the many dedicated and conscientious gynecologists, it resulted in positive changes in the discipline during the decade of the 1980s. Today about one half of the resident physicians in obstetrics and gynecology (and one third of this text's authors) are women. Food and Drug Administration requirements for drug approvals are now so stringent that they have, unfortunately, discouraged investment in development of new contraceptives and most drug products for use in pregnancy. The use of a second opinion to authorize many operative procedures is now commonplace. The need for adequate clinical trials and technology assessment before the introduction of drugs and medical devices has gained new force. During the same period, medical ethics assumed a more prominent place in the medical school curriculum, and a Patient's Bill of Rights was issued by the American Hospital Association. The next chapter has been fashioned with this recent history in mind.

2   Introduction to the Patient

Kenneth J. Ryan, M.D.

The interaction of the patient with a physician can often be an anxiety-producing event. This is especially true when the physician is a gynecologist, because of the sensitive nature of taking a history about reproductive and sexual function and the need to perform a pelvic examination, which many women find to be unpleasant and embarrassing (Weiss and Meadow, 1979). An agenda item for the feminist movement over the past 20 years has been dissatisfaction with the way gynecological services have been provided and a call for changes in the practice and attitude of the gynecologists, who until recently were essentially all men (Kaiser and Kaiser, 1974). Although the strident rhetoric about the insensitive male gynecologist has now abated somewhat, there are important lessons to be learned from the critics that should be incorporated into the history taking and physical examination practices of gynecologists regardless of their sex.

Patients prefer having their medical history taken in a consultation room fully dressed in their street clothes rather than on the examination table wearing a "johnny." It is expected that physicians will take the time to listen to the patient's story with patience, to carry out the physical examination with some consideration of the patient's feelings, to explain the diagnostic and treatment options thoroughly so the patient can understand them, and finally, to assist the patient to make up her own mind about options in her care. This is fully consonant with our increased preoccupation with the ethical nature of medical practice and the need to make ethics a high priority.

ETHICAL NATURE OF MEDICAL PRACTICE

Three ethical principles are commonly considered basic obligations of the gynecologist to the patient: (1) *respect,* for the patient as an individual human being; (2) *beneficence,* to seek the patient's good and to avoid harm; and (3) *justice,* to treat the patient fairly. These obligations have always been discharged by good physicians as second nature but can best be illustrated by the ways in which they are carried out in practice.

Respect is shown in recognition of the autonomous patient's right to make informed decisions about her health care by providing adequate information and by asking consent for any action recommended by the physician. To many (including most judges making court decisions), this obligation to obtain informed consent takes precedence over all other duties to the patient. The informed consent document for surgery is a "hard copy" of this process, but the obligation transcends specific procedures and encompasses the total physician-patient relationship, which should be one of mutual respect and trust. This supercedes the old-fashioned concept that physician knows best or that medicine is too complex for patients to understand. The obligation of respect also recognizes that when a patient has diminished autonomy (as with a child or mentally disabled person), she must be protected via a legally approved substituted judgment when any procedures are anticipated. Respect is also shown in maintaining the patient's right to privacy and confidentiality and by not calling a patient by her first name (unless you are on a first-name basis) and by certainly asking the physician's staff to refrain from doing so.

Beneficence is discharged in the process of offering "good" medical care. Good is defined by risk-benefit assessments of the various diagnostic or treatment options offered the patient (including no treatment), always seeking the patient's best interests. There are, in most situations, no risk-free options, but the physician has the obligation to make a best judgment on the options available and respect the patient's right to choose for herself. Beneficent acts such as curing a disease or saving a life must be performed with the patient's consent, and hence beneficence under most circumstances cannot take precedence over the respect due an autonomous patient in allowing her to decide on the care she wants to receive.

Justice is rendered when the physician makes access to care, the type of care, the attention provided, and the cost equitable for all of his or her patients, and there is a full disclosure of any economic conflicts in terms of tests, treatments, or facilities in which the physician has an interest. The selection of patients who are offered participation in research or teaching or new forms of therapy would similarly be expected to be nondiscriminatory. Being fair is linked to showing respect, and the two obligations can seldom be in conflict.

HISTORY AND PHYSICAL EXAMINATION

The history and physical examination are the fundamental tools for evaluating the patient for gynecological care. Whether such care is practiced in a clinic setting or a private office, the approach to the patient should be the same. A thorough probing detailed history should be obtained by the physician, preferably in a consultation room before the patient is gowned and prepared for examination. The ensuing physical examination should be comprehensive for the new patient and as detailed as required for subsequent visits.

After the initial history and physical examination, the physician must make decisions about selecting diagnostic tests and procedures. An attempt has been made to introduce quantitative reasoning into the clinical process by subjecting clinical data and diagnostic tests to evaluation for sensitivity, specificity, and accuracy. *Sensitivity* is defined as the number of true positive results for a test divided by the number of all those tested who should have been positive. It is a measure of how often you would make the correct diagnosis and how many cases you might miss by false negative results. *Specificity* is defined as the number of true negative results for a test divided by the number of all those tested who should have been negative. It is a measure of how often you would mistakenly label a person with a problem they do not have by false positive results. *Accuracy* of a test is defined as the number of true positive and true negative results divided by the total number tested, and it more or less defines the general usefulness of a test. It is becoming increasingly common to see such information referred to in evaluation of new diagnostic modalities and should be considered by the physician in the selection of tests. In addition, it is important to recognize that even tests with high sensitivity and specificity may not prove clinically useful if applied to a population of patients in whom the incidence of the disease being tested for is very low. This utility of a test is obtained by application of Bayes' formula, which factors in the prevalence of disease as well as sensitivity and specificity in determining its true predictive value. Decision trees are also becoming popular for outlining the options that might be followed for diagnosis and treatment, using quantitative data when possible at each decision point. This is one way to test the logic and completeness of your clinical analysis of a case (Weinstein and Fineberg, 1980).

The history should follow a systematic format, including the chief complaint, present illness, past medical history, family history, social history, and review of symptoms. The value of seeking the chief complaint in the patient's own words is that it gives a clue to what may be most important to the patient, including the anxieties troubling her. When patients express a list of multiple problems, it is wise to ask them to prioritize the one or ones whose relief would be most welcome in order to focus and arrange the questioning. The taking of the present illness follows from the chief complaint to pursue those avenues of questioning that will best follow up and define the limits of the specific problem. If the complaint is a physical symptom, such as pain, it is important to define its location, its character, and whether it radiates or is associated with the menstrual cycle, bowel or bladder function, or body position and movement. The names of current medications and any concurrent medical care being received are also sought. The date of the last menstrual period should always be recorded.

The past history should encompass all prior obstetrical, surgical, and hospital experiences. Medical records from other physicians and hospitals should always be obtained, especially operative notes and pathology reports. Of special importance is an inquiry regarding possible allergies, medications, smoking, alcohol consumption, and recreational drug use. We now routinely ask for a history of prior mammography reports if the patient is more than 35 years old and prior reports of vaginal cytology. The review of systems adds to the information in the present illness and past history by highlighting those aspects of the patient's present and past health that might otherwise not be remembered if the questioning were not specifically directed to the organ systems and common ailments associated with them. The family history is especially important for determination of risks for cardiovascular disease, diabetes, hypertension, and cancer, all of which are of particular importance when hormones of any kind are prescribed. The social history provides an opportunity to explore the patient's educational and marital status, check an occupational history, and define the extent to which the present complaints may be disruptive to the patient's day-to-day lifestyle.

The physical examination should be a comprehensive examination involving all organ systems and parts of the body when the patient is first seen and at annual examinations. It is especially important for those gynecologists who are in fact, as well as name, the primary physician. Special attention should be directed to blood pressure and thyroid problems so that therapy can be provided when it is needed. Breast examination should be both visual and by palpation with the patient in the erect and supine positions. It is useful to explain to the patient what you are doing as you proceed and reinforce the instruction by giving the patient a booklet on breast self-examination (see Chapter 10).

The gynecologist should include a thorough examination of the breasts not only at the first visit but at subsequent visits (if the interval exceeds 3 months). Inspection of the breasts should be done first with the patient sitting erect with her arms at her sides and then with the arms raised. The maneuver will frequently outline asymmetry or fixation of the nipple or fixed masses under or adjacent to the areola. The supraclavicular areas and the axillae are then palpated with the patient sitting erect. An adequate examination of the axilla can be performed only if the pectoral muscles are relaxed. This is accomplished by supporting the patient's arm in slight abduction and palpating the axilla with the finger tips. Particular attention should be given to the apex of the axilla and the undersurface of the pectoralis major muscle. A systematic examination of the breasts is then performed in both the erect and

supine positions. Masses in the breast are best determined by palpation with the flat surface rather than the tips of the fingers. The whole extent of the breast, as it lies relatively flattened out and balanced on the chest wall, should be systematically palpated. The medial portion is examined first with the patient's arm raised. This flattens the pectoral muscles under the breast, and the examiner's fingers trace a series of transverse lines across the breast from the nipple line to the sternum. Palpation of the lateral portion of the breast is then performed with the patient's arm at her side. The ducts and nipples should be compressed, and if bloody secretion is obtained, it is submitted to cytologic examination. A very common finding is thickening in the upper outer quadrant of the breast; if present, this is noted and repeated observations suggested. It should be borne in mind that the breast normally presents fine nodularity on palpation. During periods of engorgement (especially premenstrually), this nodularity may be accentuated almost to the point of simulating a dominant lump. Differentiation between tumor and such physiologic change is difficult. Usually, with care in palpation and reexamination at a different time in the menstrual cycle, a definite decision can be reached. About 65% of all cancers of the breast occur in this quadrant, and this area should therefore be given particular attention.

The use of a lubricant, glove powder, or soap and water provides a friction-free breast surface for optimum examination. When the patient is in the supine position with her arms above her head, lactiferous duct sinuses and previous biopsy sites are easily palpable, and any questionable areas become more distinct under the friction-free surface.

The examination of the abdomen is begun by inspection, noting the presence of scars, striae, distention, dilated veins, and umbilical eversion. The patient is then asked to lift her head and cough; this will delineate hernias or diastasis recti. Systematic palpation of the viscera is performed to determine abnormalities of liver, gallbladder, spleen, and kidneys. Palpation of the liver is best accomplished with the patient supine, her head and shoulders slightly elevated by pillows. Standing at the patient's right side, the examiner places his or her left hand under the patient's right flank, pressing gently upward with it, and then places the right hand gently but firmly on the abdominal wall. As the patient takes a deep breath, the right hand is moved downward, and as the diaphragm descends, the liver is carried down and its margin and consistency may be noted. An enlarged or tense gallbladder may be similarly palpated. Hydrops of the gallbladder may be confused with acute appendicitis since the tip of the distended gallbladder may extend into the right lower quadrant and since symptoms of nausea and vomiting are frequently associated. The spleen is best palpated by placing the right hand flat with the abdominal wall just at the left costal margin; as the patient inspires, the spleen descends and is palpable if enlarged. The cecum, ascending colon, and sigmoid colon are similarly palpated. The first clue in the diagnosis of diverticulitis of the sigmoid may be obtained at this time if there is tenderness deep in the left lower quadrant. In symmetric midline tumors, regardless of consistency, consideration should be given to the possibility of an intrauterine pregnancy or a distended bladder. Catheterization will reveal the true nature of the latter, but early pregnancy, especially if coincident with other masses such as fibroids or ovarian cysts, is often difficult to diagnose unless constantly kept in mind. Ovarian cysts may usually be differentiated from ascites by percussion, since with large cysts one usually finds areas of dullness over the cyst with tympany in the flanks. With ascites, the small intestine usually floats anteriorly and is tympanitic, whereas the dullness is found laterally.

The costovertebral angles and flanks should also be carefully evaluated in the gynecologic patient since renal and ureteral lesions frequently cause symptoms that the patient interprets as "female trouble." Firm pressure exerted by the index finger in the angle between the spine and the 12th rib will elicit inflammatory kidney processes, which otherwise might go undetected. The procedure for palpating the kidneys is similar to that for palpating the liver.

Both groins are inspected and palpated. Enlargement of the superficial inguinal nodes may be associated with venereal disease (syphilis, granuloma inguinale, chancroid, lymphopathia venereum), and varying degrees of ulceration, so-called buboes, may be revealed.

Cancer of the vulva or lower vagina, acute nongonorrheal vulvitis, tuberculosis, or, occasionally, superficial infections of the skin of the thigh may all cause inguinal lymphadenopathy. Other causes are plantar or lower extremity melanomas, thigh vaccination, and acute bartholinitis. Hodgkin's disease and systemic illnesses characterized by generalized lymphadenopathy should also be considered. In many thin, asthenic female patients, firm, discrete, mobile inguinal nodes are palpable without apparent cause and need no further investigation. The patient should again be asked to raise her head and cough, and careful examination should be performed for detection of inguinal and femoral hernias. Frequently no cause can be found for a complaint of an "aching soreness" in the lower abdomen until the patient is asked to stand and cough or to exert intraabdominal pressure. Examination below Poupart's ligament may often reveal a femoral hernia.

The extremities are examined for edema, ulceration, scars of previous surgery, and varicose veins. Bilateral edema may be caused by increased intrapelvic pressure from a pregnancy, an old phlebitis, or a lymphatic obstruction due to postpartum phlegmasia alba dolens. It may, however, just as well be due to impaired nutrition associated with low serum albumin levels, carcinoma of the ovary with ascites, or cardiac failure or chronic nephritis. Its cause bears investigation. Unilateral edema may follow postpartum or postoperative deep phlebothrombosis. Bilateral edema of the extremities is occasionally congenital and occurs without venous or lymphatic obstruction (Milroy's disease). Ulceration of the legs suggests peripheral vascular disease due to venous stasis or diabetes. Varicose veins or scars of previous vein ligation or stripping should be adequate warning to initiate prophylaxis against thromboembolic disease if surgery is contemplated.

It is well for the gynecologist, as well as the student, to stop at this point and consider the differential diagnosis suggested by the history and the general physical examination. In most gynecological diseases, the history, if accurately given and carefully taken, will narrow down the possibilities to three or four conditions. The general physical examination may further reduce this to two or three, or it may suggest that the original complaint may arise from another organ system. If this is so, appropriate radiographs, endoscopy, and laboratory procedures should be performed. Such procedures will avoid the embarrassment of operating on patients with unsuspected colonic or bladder carcinoma, diverticulitis, renal tumors, pelvic kidneys, and ulcerative colitis.

PELVIC EXAMINATION

Since the pelvic examination is the part of the physician-patient encounter most often dreaded by the patient, it is important to understand why and to work at making it at least more tolerable. Patient's often express feelings of help-lessness, vulnerability, and embarrassment about the pelvic examination, feelings they seldom relate to the examining physician. The dorsal lithotomy position feels awkward to the patient, and the examination is uncomfortable and may be painful. The rectovaginal portion of the examination evoked feelings of disgust and dirtiness when patients were specifically questioned about their reactions (Osofsky, 1967).

Suggestions for improving the experience include having rooms appropriately heated, having comfortable tables, carefully explaining to the patient what the physician will be doing in each part of the examination before performing it, being sensitive to the need for patient "relaxation" and a gentle touch, and using warmed instruments. Although each physician will develop a style that he or she is comfortable with, other suggestions include dispensing with the pelvic drape and maintaining eye contact during the examination and having the nurse unobtrusive. I have continued to use the pelvic drape and try to have the nurse as engaged as possible in a supportive role during the examination. This is especially important with young patients having their first examination. It is always possible to defer the pelvic examination to a second visit if the patient cannot relax sufficiently. It certainly is preferable to proceeding with an uncooperative patient. There have been a disquieting number of instances in which male gynecologists have been accused of an improper examination with sexual overtones such as inappropriate touching or rubbing of the clitoris. Since the nurse should at least always be a chaperone for the male physician, she should be sufficiently attentive to attest to the physician's activities if called on to do so.

The pelvic examination should be carried out with the patient on an examining table with her legs supported and adequately abducted (Fig 2–1). The table should be equipped with a movable backrest so that the head may be raised slightly, permitting better relaxation of abdominal muscles. The buttocks should extend just beyond the end of the table. Good light is essential. The patient is instructed to urinate just before the examination, since a full bladder may be mistaken for a pregnant uterus or an ovarian cyst.

A speculum is inserted without lubrication, and a small amount of secretion is obtained from the cervix by a brush and submitted to cytological examination. Cervical scrapings are also routinely performed.

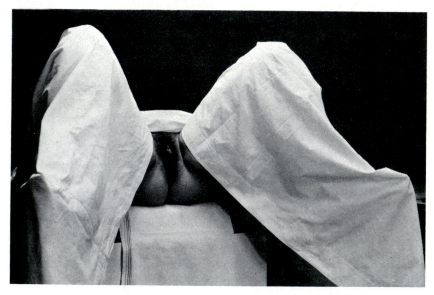

FIG 2–1.
Position for pelvic examination. The patient is placed so that the buttocks extend just beyond the edge of the table. The legs are supported in stirrups and are adequately abducted.

Some mention should be made of the technique of speculum examination. The gynecologist should attempt to use the speculum best adapted for a particular patient, and he or she is aided in this by the variety of instruments available. The one used most commonly is the Graves speculum, which has a posterior blade approximately 11.4 cm long and 3.2 cm wide at its tip. This speculum is available in lengths varying from 8.9 to 12.7 cm and widths from 1.9 to 3.2 cm. The posterior blade of the Graves speculum is usually about 0.6 cm longer than the anterior blade so as to fit into the longer posterior vaginal wall. In some patients, however, when the cervix lies posteriorly or there is a large cystocele, it is advantageous to have a longer anterior blade. The ordinary speculum may then be rotated or a modified Graves speculum with a longer anterior blade used. The Pederson speculum is narrower and flatter and may be used to advantage in nulliparous patients or when the vagina is contracted by senescence, scars, or radiation. In children, a Kelly cystoscope is an ideal instrument for visualization of the vagina (see Chapter 20).

Before insertion, the speculum should be warmed by holding it under warm water, and it should be adequately lubricated unless it is being used for cytological aspiration. Slight pressure is then exerted on the posterior vaginal wall and perineum by the index and middle finger of the left hand, and care is taken to keep the blades away from the sensitive periurethral area. The speculum should be angled when inserted, so that its greatest width is in the anteroposterior diameter of the vagina (Fig 2–2). It is then rotated as it is passed along the posterior vaginal wall, and as the tip reaches the cervix, the anterior blade is elevated by pressure on the lever under the lateral screw. When the proper exposure has been obtained, the lateral set screw is adjusted. If increased vision in the anteroposterior field is desired, the central set screw may be loosened and the blades separated. When the speculum is removed, only the lateral screw should be released, allowing the tips of the blades to fall together. The central screw should not be loosened since, in so doing, vaginal mucosa may be pinched between the lateral aspects of the blades.

Before proceeding to the examination of the vagina and cervix, the examiner should methodically inspect the external genitalia. The general features are illustrated in Figure 2–3. A good sequence is to start with the labia majora and minora, noting the size as well as the presence of edema, inflammation, ulceration, crusting, deformity, discoloration, or atrophy. Dilated veins, nevi, and melanomas are obvious. The thumb and index finger of the right hand separate the labia minora as shown in Figure 2–4, exposing the vestibule with the vaginal and urethral openings as well as those of the periurethral (Skene's) and vulvovaginal (Bartholin's) glands. At this point the patient may be asked to strain down or cough. This will delineate pelvic floor relaxation

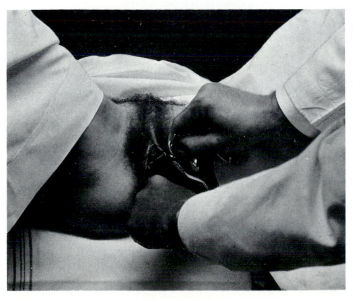

FIG 2–2.
Insertion of speculum. The posterior vaginal wall is depressed by slight pressure with the index finger of the left hand. The speculum is angled to conform to the anteroposterior diameter of the vagina. Care is taken to avoid the periurethral area.

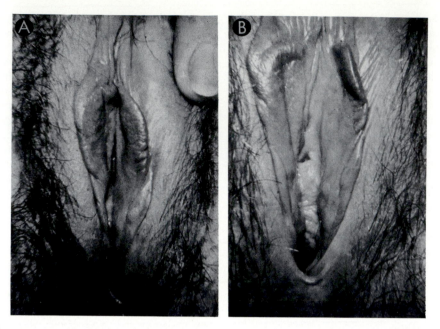

FIG 2–3.
A, normal vulva of multiparous patient. The outer margins of the labia majora are covered with hair, and a slight degree of gaping of the labia minora permits exposure of the introitus. **B,** labia majora are displaced laterally to show clitoris, which labia mi- nora joint anteriorly. The urethral orifice is seen just above a slight relaxation of the anterior vaginal wall. Vaginal orifice is at lowermost portion of labia mi- nora.

FIG 2–4.
Method of beginning the internal examination. The labia majora and minora are held apart with the fingers of the right hand, and first one and then two fingers of the left hand are gently inserted along the posterior vaginal wall.

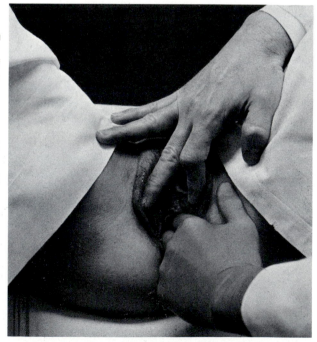

and urinary incontinence. The index finger of the gloved (left) hand is then inserted gently under the urethra, and it is compressed toward the external orifice. A purulent exudate suggests gonorrhea and should be stained and cultured. The urethral orifice should be observed also for polyps, prolapse of the mucosa, ulceration, or caruncle. The index finger may then be rotated and the ducts of the periurethral glands stripped. The vulvovaginal glands should be sought for, placing the index finger in the vagina and the thumb on the perineal skin. Normally they are not palpable, but undue tenderness, swelling, or fluctuation suggests Bartholin's cyst or abscess. At this time the posterior commissure and perineal body may be inspected and palpated. The condition of previous episiotomies should be noted, as should the presence of any small dimples, which indicate the presence of vaginoperineal or vaginorectal fistulas. The integrity of the levator ani muscle may be tested, but it is better done by a later combined rectovaginal examination.

The internal examination is begun by introducing first one and then two fingers of the left hand along the posterior vaginal wall (see Fig 2–4). Specifically then, the fingers elevate and support the uterus and adnexa while the external hand is used to determine the anatomic details of these structures. In addition, any abnormalities of the vagina are noted, and the size, shape, and consistency of the cervix is determined, as is the patency of its external os. The cervix may then be moved laterally; if pain results, it suggests the presence of an inflammatory process.

The vaginal fingers may note at the outset a third-degree uterine retroversion as they advance toward the posterior cul-de-sac, or nodularity and scarring of the uterosacral ligaments may suggest the presence of endometriosis.

The normal position of the uterus is one of anteversion with some anteflexion of the corpus on the cervix. The simplest method to palpate the uterus is to place the two vaginal fingers under the cervix and elevate it and the uterine corpus toward the abdominal wall (Fig 2–5). The external hand is gently placed on the abdomen with the fingers flat and is moved about from below the umbilicus to the symphysis. Intermittent pressure on the uterus between the fingers of both hands will yield information as to size, shape, and con-

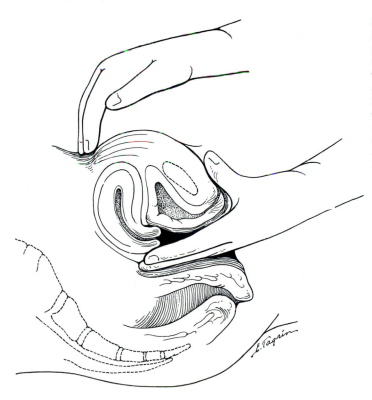

FIG 2–5.
Internal examination. The uterus is palpated by placing two fingers under the cervix, elevating it and the uterine corpus toward the abdominal wall. The external hand is gently placed on the abdomen with the fingers flat and moved about from below the umbilicus to the symphysis. I prefer to stand at the left side of the patient, outside the abducted leg.

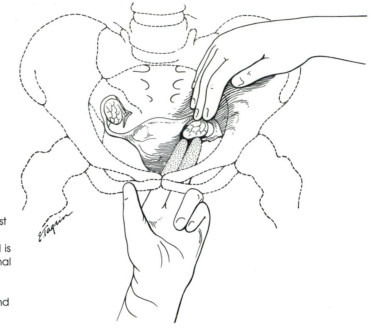

FIG 2–6.
Palpation of adnexal areas. The vaginal fingers are moved to the side of the cervix so that they occupy the lateral and uppermost part of the vagina. By a series of caudad displacements, the hand is brought over the ovary. The vaginal fingers serve only to support the ovary while the external hand is used to determine size, shape, and mobility.

sistency. Ballottement between the two hands yields important information regarding mobility.

The left adnexal area is usually examined next. This is accomplished by moving the vaginal fingers to the left of the cervix so that they occupy the lateral and uppermost part of the vagina (Fig 2–6). On the left side the ovary is frequently underneath the sigmoid colon, so that abdominal palpation must begin rather high. By a series of caudad displacements the hand is brought over the ovary, which can usually be palpated between the two hands. The vaginal fingers usually serve only to support the ovary while the external hand palpates for size, shape, and mobility. The oviduct is usually not palpable in its normal state. The right ovary is palpated in the same fashion; however, if it is not easily felt, the examiner should change hands and place the right hand in the vagina. The natural curvature of the right hand sometimes makes it easier to outline the right adnexa.

When the internal examination is performed, it is important to bear in mind several points:

1. Always begin gently, usually with the insertion of one well-lubricated finger along the posterior wall of the vagina.
2. Gradually insinuate two fingers under the cervix.
3. Apply the abdominal hand easily and slowly.
4. Never apply force or use abrupt motion, since the initial reflex resistance will then actually increase and examination will become impossible.
5. Always examine the painful side last.
6. Employ reassuring discussion with the patient and have her breathe through her mouth during the examination to aid in securing relaxation.

In describing the findings, one must bear in mind that all observers will not interpret the palpatory findings in the same way. Therefore, it is better to give accurate or estimated measurements in centimeters rather than in terms of fruit, eggs, or balls of various sizes. This need not be carried ad absurdum, however, and if both ovaries are normal in all respects, it is simpler to report "sides of the pelvis normal." Abnormal masses should be described as to size, shape, consistency, mobility, position, and whether or not they are tender.

The speculum examination is performed using the technique previously described. The vaginal mucosa is inspected as the speculum is introduced, with observation made of the amount of rugation or the presence of discharge. Primary diseases of the vagina (excluding simple vaginitis)

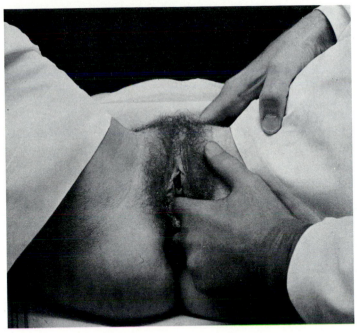

FIG 2–7.
Combined vaginorectal examination enables the examiner to reach almost 2.5 cm higher into the pelvis. Thickening of the rectovaginal septum, cul-de-sac nodules, fixed uterine retroversion, and involvement of the broad ligaments by tumor are more accurately outlined by this method.

are not too common, but one should look for congenital abnormalities such as vaginal septa, double vaginas, double cervixes, and Gartner duct cysts. The cervix is then brought into view and the light adjusted so that the entire portio epithelium is visible.

For the rectovaginal examination, it is now customary to change gloves to avoid cross contamination from the vagina to the rectum of both organisms and blood that might confound the test for occult blood in the stool. The patient should be told what to expect, and with adequate lubrication, the index finger is placed in the vagina and the third finger in the rectum. The rectovaginal septum, cul-de-sac, and posterior aspect of the uterus can be evaluated (Fig 2–7). Frequently a uterus in fixed third-degree retroversion can be outlined only by this method.

This examination is followed by a thorough digital examination of the anus and rectum. The fact that about one half of the malignancies of the rectosigmoid may be palpated by careful digital exploration is adequate reason for making this part of the examination an integral step in the gynecologic survey. A guaiac test for blood in the stool should be routine in every rectal examination.

Several types of office procedures may be appropriate in a given case, such as an endometrial or cervical biopsy. I try to avoid unanticipated procedures on the first patient visit during an initial examination. It is wise to have a friend or husband accompany the patient to the office on the day procedures are performed. For these reasons, it is best not to to discuss such matters with the unprepared patient on the examining table. The consent form should be signed after the patient has been fully informed about the indications, alternatives, and risks and benefits of the procedure.

POSTEXAMINATION CONSULTATION

It is important to leave enough time after the examination for a full discussion of the findings, the need for diagnostic tests, an assessment of the patient's condition, and a plan for therapy and follow-up as appropriate. It is best to do this summation with the patient dressed in her street clothes. This is especially important if one is discussing options for surgery or other involved therapy such as the use of hormones, signing of consent forms, and certainly after the examination of a patient new to the physician. It is important to realize the role the office nurse can play in patient education and in reenforcing the physician's instructions and advice. In addition, there are many patient information pamphlets that can be informative and helpful in making the patient an active participant in her own care.

REFERENCES

Kaiser BL, Kaiser IH: The challenge of the women's movement to American gynecology. *Am J Obstet Gynecol* 1974; 120:652–665.

Osofsky HJ: Women's reactions to pelvic examination. *Obstet Gynecol* 1967; 30:146–151.

Weinstein MC, Fineberg HV: *Clinical Decision Analysis*. Philadelphia, WB Saunders Co, 1980.

Weiss L, Meadow R: Women's attitudes toward gynecologic practices. *Obstet Gynecol* 1979; 54:110–114.

3   The Menstrual Cycle

Kenneth J. Ryan, M.D.

Robert L. Barbieri, M.D.

There are two views of the menstrual cycle: (1) the real world clinical view of cyclic bleeding with all the details of interval, duration, and amount that figure prominantly in the gynecological history; and (2) the more theoretical basic neuroendocrine view of the cycle that underlies the explanation and understanding needed by the gynecologist to optimize diagnosis and treatment. There is a science to both the clinical and basic views of the cycle, and an attempt will be made in this chapter to reconcile and interdigitate the two perspectives.

CLINICAL MENSTRUAL CYCLE

Menstruation is the cyclic uterine bleeding experienced by most women of reproductive age. Normal menstruation represents the cyclic shedding of the uterine secretory endometrium due to a decline in estradiol and progesterone production caused by a regressing corpus luteum.

Duration of the Cycle

The association of menstruation with the lunar cycle is a venerable and romantic notion that has no known basis in reality or causality. Contrary to popular belief, the menstrual cycle of most women does not repeat like "clockwork." The gynecologist routinely asks each patient about menstrual interval, regularity of menstrual intervals, duration of menses, and volume of menstrual flow to establish some sense of normalcy.

Treloar and colleagues (1967) reported on menstrual interval and regularity of menstrual intervals in white women who attended the University of Minnesota. Data were collected prospectively over 30 years, and 275,947 menstural cycles were available for analysis. Table 3–1 summarizes the results of this study. The cycle length usually varies by 1 to 2 days each month, and only 50% of women have a cycle within the 26- to 30-day range that encompasses the so-called typical 28-day interval. For most women, menses starts for the first time at age 13 years (normal range 8–16 years) and stops by age 50 years (normal range 45–55 years). Over the age range of 20 to 40 years, women have the tightest regularity to their cycles, with more variability in the immediate postmenarche and premenopause years. However, the median "normal" cycle length actually declines from 28.87 (±2.75) days at age 20 years to a median of 26.8 (±2) days by age 40 years. Cycle lengths can differ in a population of healthy normal women from 25.4 to 34.7 days at age 20 years and from 24.4 to 30.3 days by age 40 years. By observing a large number of healthy women over 30 years, investigators observed that cycle lengths cluster around a normal biological distribution curve and that individual women tend to vary around a cycle length that is usual for them. During the first few years after menarche and just before menopause, women experience wider deviation from the mean. The concept of "normalcy" has to encompass variations that include 50% of women at age 25 years having cycle lengths either less than 27 days or more than 31 days. Conversely, only 50% of women at this age will have a median cycle length of 28 (±1–3) days in spite of the fact that most women believe that their periods are more regular than they prove to be when carefully monitored. The variation of cycle length included within the normal population be-

TABLE 3−1.

Median and 5% Upper and Lower Bounds on Menstrual Interval in Days From 275,947 Menstrual Cycles*

Chronological Age (yr)	Menstrual Interval (Days)		
	5% Lower Bound	Median	5% Upper Bound
17	22	28	40
25	23	28	37
33	22	27	34
41	22	26	32
49	15	27	>80

*Adapted from Treloar AE, Boynton RE, Behn BG, et al: Variation of human menstrual cycle through reproductive life. *Int J Fert* 1967; 12:77−126.

comes even greater at the extremes of the reproductive life span. By reference to such studies of a large number of women over a considerable period of time, the limits of normalcy have been defined, and in general, cycle lengths less than 24 days are considered polymenorrhea, and those more than 35 days are considered oligomenorrhea (see Table 3−1). The clinical presumption is that most of those cycles that are outside the so-called normal range tend to be anovulatory, and hormone studies have now confirmed this. Careful measurement of cycle interval in a large population of apparently healthy women would not establish whether most of the cycles were ovulatory, but studies combined with daily hormone measurements could look for an association of menstrual interval with whether or not ovulation took place. It is likely that many of the 22- and 23-day cycles reported by Treloar et al. (1967) were anovulatory. It has subsequently been established that known ovulatory cycles (as determined by a luteinizing hormone [LH] surge and normal luteal-phase progesterone) vary from 24 to 35 days and thus the variability of the menstrual cycle within this range is both a common and a normal event from a biological perspective (Landgren et al., 1980).

The average duration of menstruation is between 3 and 7 days, and duration shorter (hypomenorrhea) or longer (hypermenorrhea) than this is considered abnormal.

Amount of Menstrual Flow

The normal duration of menstrual flow ranges from 3 to 7 days, and the amount of total blood loss is generally 80 ml or less. Just as women are poor predictors of the regularity of their cycles, their estimates of blood loss at menses are usually also inaccurate. It has been established that women vary widely from one another in the amount of blood lost at menstruation, but each woman is fairly consistent from month to month in her individual loss when checked by reliable measurements. This pattern has been established for women in several parts of the world in which the average loss and variation are strikingly similar. The method used to measure blood loss involves extracting tampons and pads with a solution of sodium hydroxide to convert heme chromogens to a form that can be measured on a spectrophotometer. When menstrual blood loss exceeded 80 ml in an individual, there was a good correlation with anemia (hemoglobin value less than 12 gm) and with low plasma iron values (Halberg and Nilsson, 1964). Since trying to determine the extent of menstrual blood loss by patient estimates is unreliable, checking for anemia is the only practical way to monitor the extent of menstrual flow.

BIOLOGICAL BASIS OF THE MENSTRUAL CYCLE

To explain why menstrual bleeding occurs at all and why it is cyclical, one must understand the role of hormones and peptide growth factors in controlling cell division and differentiation of the endometrial lining of the uterus and its vasculature. Menstrual bleeding occurs only in higher apes and humans, whereas most mammals do not slough the lining of their uterus at the end of each nonfertile cycle. This striking difference in the reproductive process is probably related to the evolution of viviparity and the unique placentation of primates. In early human pregnancy, there is an extensive invasion by the fetal placenta deep into the endometrial layer so that the fetal cotyledons can be bathed in maternal blood. Each month that pregnancy does not occur, that thick endometrial layer and its spiral blood vessels lose their hormonal support and slough, resulting in menstrual flow. In other mammals, the endometrium is not similarly developed or there is no luteal hormone released unless pregnancy occurs. Although there are no menstural periods in other mammals, some do have cyclic bleeding at the time of ovulation and sexual receptivity (heat).

This is typically seen in the domestic dog. It is interesting to note that scientists and clinicians made the mistaken analogy that human menstrual bleeding was similar to the estrus (ovulatory) bleeding of their pet animals. Prior to the early 20th century, it was taught that human ovulation occurred at the time of menses. This resulted in the development of a rhythm method for family planning that could not have been farther off the mark. It was only after the correct temporal relationships of endometrial changes to menstruation were described (Hitschmann and Adler, 1908) that others over the next 20 years provided the correlation for the dog and the primate of when ovulation takes place in relationship to the secretion of ovarian estradiol and progesterone and their subsequent hormonal effects on the endometrium. This was followed by an understanding of the reciprocal relationships between the pituitary and the gonads in 1932 and isolation of the

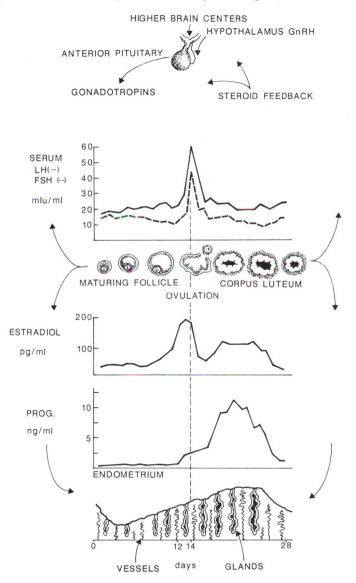

FIG 3–1.

Diagrammatic representation of the menstrual cycle showing the temporal relationships of the pituitary gonadotropins FSH and LH with the ovarian follicular estradiol and luteal progesterone and estradiol and the progressive response of the endometrium to the sequential change in steroids.

pituitary and ovarian hormones. Subsequently, the classic concept of the menstrual cycle evolved. This first included only the interaction of the pituitary, ovary, and endometrium with the release of pituitary follicle-stimulating hormone (FSH) and LH to cause follicular estrogen secretion and endometrial proliferation in the first half of the cycle, followed by an LH surge to cause ovulation with secretion of progesterone and estrogen from the corpus luteum to cause a secretory endometrium in the second half of the cycle (Fig 3–1). The relationship of the pituitary and ovary was characterized as a closed loop negative feedback system, like the relationship of a thermostat to a heating system. The FSH and LH stimulated the secretion of ovarian hormones that, in turn, kept the FSH and LH levels in the right range. When the corpus luteum regressed, the cycle started over (Ryan, 1988; Greep, 1988). This was an oversimplified explanation and was ultimately corrected by the discovery of the role of the hypothalamus in reproduction, the discovery of the positive feedback of estrogen to cause the LH surge and ovulation, and finally the isolation of gonadotropin-releasing hormone (GnRH) in the early 1970s (Sawyer, 1988; McCann, 1988). Our current understanding of the complex neuroendocrine interactions that regulate the menstrual cycle is now sufficiently detailed to be clinically applicable and therefore of practical importance to the gynecologist taking care of patients with menstrual problems.

NEUROENDOCRINE BASIS OF THE MENSTRUAL CYCLE

The menstrual cycle depends on a complex interaction between the brain (of which the hypothalamus is a part), the pituitary, the ovaries, and the endometrium. Generally, input to the system comes from environmental cues (emotion, light, smell, and sound) via the central nervous system (CNS) to the hypothalamus, which transforms neural signals into a neuropeptide (GnRH) output. This, in turn, causes the pituitary to secrete gonadotropins, which stimulate the ovary. The ovary responds by undergoing gametogenesis (developing an oocyte for ovulation) and secreting steroids. The ovarian steroid hormones, estradiol and progesterone, stimulate the endometrial lining for pregnancy and feedback to both the

hypothalamus and pituitary to keep gonadotropins at the right level to control the system. If pregnancy does not occur, the endometrium is sloughed, and the cycle repeats itself (Ryan, 1986).

The complexity of the relationships between the higher brain centers, hypothalamus, pituitary, ovaries, and endometrium can best be illustrated by comparison to the mutiple components of a modern hi-fi stereo system with tuners, tape decks, preamplifiers, amplifiers, and speakers and their ultimate dependence on the radio station transmitter for input signals and the receiving "end-organ" listener who sits with a remote control for feedback to switch stations, adjust the volume, and turn the system on and off. With the hi-fi set, all the components have to be in place and connected for music to be heard, and many things can go wrong when any one of the components malfunctions. This is also true for the neuroendocrine system in its control of the normal ovulatory menstrual cycle. What is required of the gynecologist to "repair" a menstrual dysfunction is similar to that required of the radio repair expert to fix the stereo system when something goes wrong. Both must know all of the components in the system, how each component works, how each is "connected" to the others, how to diagnose malfunctions, and how to correct them. For this reason, we will review the anatomy and function of the neuroendocrine system organ by organ and hormone by hormone.

Hypothalamus and Gonadotropin-Releasing Hormone

The hypothalamus and its pulsatile release of GnRH regulates pituitary gonadotropin secretion and thereby controls ovarian cyclicity and the menstrual cycle. The hypothalamus is an evolutionally ancient part of the brain concerned with regulating the primitive functions needed for survival such as appetite, temperature control, salt and water regulation, growth, and metabolism as well as reproduction. There are two-way neural connections between the hypothalamus and other parts of the nervous system. With all of these activities concentrated in one small area of the brain, it is not surprising that there is an interaction between control of the menstrual cycle, behavior, and other metabolic functions. The hypothalamic nerve cells are derived from the embryonic ventral diencephalon and migrate during early development to form clusters of neurons that constitute the named "nuclei" of the adult hypothalamus, each nucleus composed of neurons devoted to regulation of one or more of the specific functions previously noted. The hypothalamus sits at the base of the brain bounded anteriorly just rostral to the optic chiasm and extending caudad to the mammillary bodies. The dorsal portion of the hypothalamus constitutes the floor of the third ventricle and its lateral walls. The base of the hypothalamus or infundibulum contains the infundibular stalk and hypothalamic-hypophyseal portal vascular system leading into the pituitary gland (Ryan, 1986). Although it was initially thought that the pituitary was the master gland that controlled the reproductive system, it was finally demonstrated by Harris (1972) that the pituitary required a specific anatomic relationship to the hypothalamus to function and to secrete gonadotropins as well as other hypophyseal hormones. The hypothalamus was then demonstrated to produce several releasing and inhibiting hormones that reached the pituitary via the privileged access of the portal vessels and could thereby control pituitary function (McCann, 1988). One of these releasing substances, GnRH, was isolated by Schally et al. (1971) by Guillemin's group (Burgas et al. (1971), for which they subsequently received the Nobel prize. Gonadotropin-releasing hormone is a decapeptide (Fig 3–2), which has now been synthesized (McCann and Rettori, 1987; Friedman and Barbieri 1988). The neurons that produce GnRH are localized to the hypothalamic interstitial and preoptic nuclei

and to the arcuate nucleus located in the ventral hypothalamus just above the median eminence. In classic experiments on the *Rhesus* monkey, Knobil (1980) demonstrated that if the arcuate nucleus is destroyed, the pituitary can no longer secrete gonadotropic hormones. The cycling of ovarian function stops, and in the absence of ovarian hormones, endometrial stimulation and regression cease. However, administration of hourly pulses of GnRH could restart the system. It had been observed previously that FSH and LH are normally secreted in pulses with intervals of 1 hour. If GnRH was given continuously, gonadotropin secretion would stop, or if the interval of administration of GnRH was too short or too long, the response of the pituitary was impaired. Knobil has since identified a pulse-generating signal that normally stimulates the release of pulsatile GnRH from the arcuate nucleus of the hypothalamus, and it is presumed that each such pulse reaches the pituitary to result in the intermittent hourly pulses of LH and FSH measured in the peripheral blood (Crowley et al., 1985). Since it has not been possible to easily measure GnRH levels in peripheral blood, confirmation for pulsatile secretion of GnRH has come from animal studies in which sampling directly from the hypophyseal portal system provides evidence for the pulse.

The hypothalamus acts like a transducer to convert nerve impulses into pulses of neuropeptides such as GnRH to which the pituitary can respond. The neurons of the hypothalamus are highly specialized and not only synthesize and package these neuropeptides but transport them down their axons to be released into the portal vessels that carry the hormones to the pituitary cells where they will act. The signal to these GnRH-secreting neurons comes from other hypothalamic neurons or afferent neural connections via neurotransmitters (Fig 3–3). In addition to the releasing factors, neurotransmitters are produced and released by hypothalamic neurons to influence other neurons and sometimes the pituitary as well. One neurotransmitter that acts this way is dopamine, which can act in the hypothalamus and can also be released into the hypophyseal portal vessels to act in the pituitary to inhibit the secretion of prolactin. Dopamine, norepinephrine, and serotonin are three neurotransmitters that are produced or released in the hypothalamus that can directly or indirectly affect GnRH production and secretion (Moore, 1986). There are

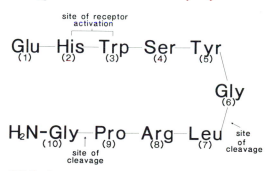

FIG 3–2.
Chemical structure of GnRH with arrows at points critical for receptor binding and cleavage inactivation (From Friedman AJ, Barbieri RL: Leuprolide acetate: Applications gynecology. *Curr Probl Obstet Gynecol Fertil* 1988; 6:209. Reproduced by permission.)

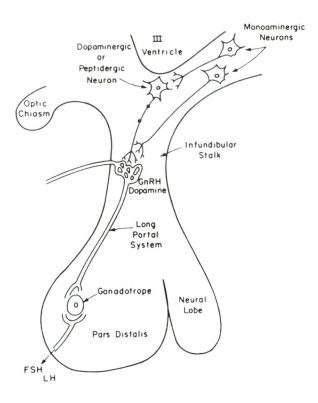

FIG 3–3.

Diagrammatic representation of the relationship of hypothalamic neurons to hypophyseal-portal blood vessels that have privileged access to pituitary gonadotropes (From Ryan KJ: The endocrine pattern and control of the ovulatory cycle, in Insler V, Lunenfeld B (eds): *Infertility: Male and Female.* New York, Churchill Livingstone, 1986, pp 57–72. Reproduced by permission.)

also receptors for the ovarian steroids estradiol and progesterone on hypothalamic neurons, and it is believed that the steroids modulate the menstrual cycle not only by effects on the pituitary but by effects on the hypothalamic nerve cells, which, in turn, regulate the pulse frequency of GnRH release. These effects of the steroids are in addition to their generally accepted feedback actions at the level of the pituitary and are probably achieved via the intermediacy of the neurotransmitters previously described. Finally, endogenously released opioid peptides such as β-endorphin also influence GnRH pulses by action in the hypothalamus, which normally results in a decline in LH pulse frequency during the luteal phase of the cycle (Yen, 1986). This also provides a clue to the heretofore unexplained relationship of emotional problems with menstrual irregularity. It is reasonable to believe that "hypothalamic" amenorrhea and other menstrual problems will prove to be a consequence of defects in GnRH pulse generation (Crowley, 1985).

Pituitary: Major Link of the Brain to Ovarian Function

The pituitary with its pulsatile secretion of gonadotropins is the major link of the brain to ovarian function. During embryonic development, the anterior lobe of the pituitary is derived from a pinching off of a portion of the oral cavity, whereas the posterior lobe is an extension of the neural tissue linked to the hypothalamus. The two lobes come into apposition to form the definitive adenohypophysis attached to the median eminence by the infundibular stalk, which, in turn, is surrounded by some anterior pituitary cells and designated the pars tuberalis. The adult pituitary is 10 by 13 by 6 mm and weighs 0.5 gm. The anterior pituitary composes three fourths of the total gland. The gland sits in the sphenoid bone in a cavity known as the *sella turcica* and is separated from the cranial cavity by the dura, which the pituitary stalk and blood vessels penetrate. The anterior pituitary is comprised of a range of cell types, each type specific for one or more of the pituitary hormones. It is believed that one cell type is specific for both LH and FSH (gonadotropes), and another is specific for prolactin (lactotrope; Ryan, 1986).

The pituitary cells receive signals from the hypothalamus in the form of pulsatile GnRH secretion and, in response, synthesize and secrete FSH and LH in pulses to match the GnRH signal. The secretion of gonadotropins by the pituitary is also modulated by a negative feedback effect of steroid hormones, especially ovarian estradiol, which keeps FSH and LH levels in the 10 to 20 mIU/ml range during most of the cycle. When estradiol is no longer secreted at the menopause or after oophorectomy, gonadotropins are released from negative feedback control and may rise to more than 100 mIU/ml. In addition, estradiol has a direct positive feedback effect on the pituitary. When the estradiol level rises in the serum as secretion from the preovulatory follicle intensifies, it reaches a level (200 to 300 pg/ml for 24 to 48 hours) that triggers a surge of LH from the pituitary, which, in turn, causes ovulation about 12 hours after the peak of gonadotropin is reached. Hence, ovulation is triggered by an LH surge caused only when there is a developed estradiol-secreting follicle that is ready to ovulate in response to the gonadotropin signal.

The gonadotropins are glycoproteins, each composed of two subunits bound together noncovalently. The subunits are designated as alpha and beta. Follicle-stimulating hormone and LH each contain the same alpha subunit containing 89 amino acids (in common with thyroid-stimulating hormone [TSH] and human chorionic gonadotropin [hCG]). It is the beta subunit that is different for each of these four hormones and confers to them their biological and immunological specificity (Catt and Pierce, 1986). The gonadotropins, derived largely from menopausal urine, are now commercially available for use in stimulating ovulation in patients with pituitary or hypothalamic disease.

Ovarian Development

During embryonic development, primitive germ cells migrate from the yolk sac to the mesonephric ridge, where the definitive ovary develops. The primitive germ cells, or oogonia, divide by mitosis and increase their numbers to several million until about 6 months of intrauterine development, when mitotic division stops. Starting at 8 to 13 weeks, oogonia also continually enter meiosis until all are converted to oocytes, which are arrested in the dictyate stage. The process is completed by 6 months postpartum. Oocytes remain arrested in meiotic prophase until stimulated to resume meiosis during the preovulatory period of each ovulatory cycle in response to the LH surge. The number of oocytes continually declines during life, and by puberty only 300,000 remain, from which only a few hundred will be ovulated over the life of the woman.

The earliest stage of follicular development is designated the primordial follicle, which consists of the oocyte surrounded by a basal lamina and some spindle-shaped cells. When the oocyte becomes surrounded by cuboidal granulosa cells, the structure is designated a *primary follicle.* In going from a primordial to a developed follicle, the oocyte grows, becomes invested with a clear band called the *zona pellucida,* and is surrounded by a dividing layer of granulosa cells, all without benefit of gonadotropin stimulation. It is at this point that follicles are recruited for each ovarian cycle during active reproductive life (Ross and Schreiber, 1986).

Follicular Development

Resting follicles are recruited into a cohort of follicles, only one of which will be destined to ovulate, with the remainder undergoing atresia. The follicles each start out with an oocyte surrounded by a band of granulosa cells, which is, in turn, surrounded by a band of modified fibroblast-like cells called *theca interna.* Both FSH and LH are necessary for the follicle to develop. Luteinizing hormone stimulates the thecal cells to divide and produce androgens, which can be converted to estrogens by the granulosa cells. Follicle-stimulating hormone stimulates the granulosa cells to divide and to increase the enzymes necessary to convert thecal androgens to estradiol (aromatization). The granulosa cell numbers increase dramatically to 50 million in the dominant follicle. The follicle increases in volume by forming a fluid-filled cavity, or antrum, of about 5 ml, and its diameter increases some 400-fold to 2.5 cm. The follicle destined to ovulate can be identified by all of these characteristics. It has captured FSH in its antral fluid, it has the optimal number of granulosa cells for its size, and it produces estradiol in preference to androgens. The follicles destined for atresia have not captured enough FSH to accomplish maturation. They have fewer granulosa cells and more androgen than estrogen in their follicular fluid, which, in fact, causes the atresia (McNatty et al., 1979). Most important, oocytes derived from the mature healthy follicle will resume meiosis more often than oocytes derived from follicles destined for atresia. The follicular development of the dominant follicle thus creates an environment in which the oocyte matures and is ready to resume meiosis. Enough estradiol is secreted from its granulosa cells to trigger the LH surge of the pituitary by positive feedback, which will cause the follicle to ovulate at a time when it is "ripe." The estradiol produced by the same follicle induces endometrial proliferation, which prepares the uterus for further development if conception occurs. It has been demonstrated that if the ripe follicle is destroyed, the estradiol level drops quickly, the FSH level rises in response to a transient release from negative feedback, and it takes 2 weeks for another follicle to develop to the same stage. In other words, the 2-week timing of the follicular phase of the cycle depends on the ability of the ovary to respond. The "clock" is in the ovary, even though it depends on the pituitary to make it run (DiZerga and Hodgen, 1981).

Ovulation

In all spontaneously ovulating mammals, estradiol from the developing follicle or follicles triggers an abrupt release of pituitary LH by direct feedback to the pituitary, which induces the ovulatory process. Just prior to ovulation, the intrafollicular FSH and estradiol induce LH receptors on the cell surfaces of the granulosa cells so that when the follicle ruptures, its cells can become "luteinized" in the developing corpus luteum in response to LH. The preovulatory follicle starts secreting a little more progesterone, and as the LH surge increases, the follicular estradiol level declines sharply. How LH induces ovulation is not yet completely understood. There is a thinning and weakening of the portion of the follicular wall (stigma) from which extrusion of the oocyte will take place. The process involves production of prostaglandins and activation of plasmin and takes about 12 hours from the peak of the LH surge.

Luteal Phase of the Cycle

Following ovulation, the follicle collapses and undergoes reorganization. There is an ingrowth of thecal cells and blood vessels, and the granulosa cells luteinize. They increase in size and develop characteristic morphological changes. The lutein cells develop receptors on their cell surface to bind and internalize serum cholesterol bound to low-density lipoprotein (LDL-cholesterol). This cholesterol becomes the major precursor for the production of the increased amounts of progesterone now synthesized by the corpus luteum. This progesterone induces a secretory change in the estrogen-primed endometrium to prepare it for a pregnancy. Estradiol is also produced by the corpus luteum, and the production of both steroid hormones is dependent on continued stimulation by pituitary LH. If pregnancy occurs, the corpus luteum will be stimulated by fetal hCG, which will extend its life span until the placenta can assume its endocrine function at about 7 to 8 weeks of pregnancy. In the absence of pregnancy, the corpus luteum regresses, the lowered level of steroid hormones induces the pituitary to increase gonadotropin secretion, and a new cycle of follicular recruitment begins. The lowered steroid hormone levels also cause collapse of the endometrial vasculature, and menstruation is the result. Why the corpus luteum regresses in the primate at the end of each nonfertile cycle is not completely understood. In many animals, prostaglandin produced in the uterus in response to progesterone reaches the corpus luteum and causes luteolysis in a form of negative feedback. In these animals, simple hysterectomy will prolong the life of the corpus luteum. In the primate, it is believed that prostaglandin produced locally in the corpus luteum itself causes its own destruction.

Ovarian Compartments

It should be apparent from the foregoing description of ovarian function during the menstrual cycle that the ovary is a dynamic organ with cyclic changes in morphology and hormone secretion. The ovary can be thought of in terms of three major compartments: (1) the follicles, (2) the corpora lutea, and (3) the stroma. The follicular compartment contains all the primordial and primary follicles that are hormonally and structurally quiescent until they are recruited into the cohort of growing follicles for a given cycle by pituitary FSH and LH. The follicular compartment also includes the growing follicles that are actively secreting hormones. From the pool of growing follicles, the dominant follicle will be selected for ovulation, and the others will regress in atresia. The estradiol secreted from the ovary during the follicular phase of the cycle is derived predominantly from the cohort of developing follicles. The ovulatory follicle, however, provides the bulk of the estradiol. After the LH surge is released just prior to ovulation, estradiol production declines rapidly, leading up to ovulation itself. Ovarian steroid production is next dominated by the corpus luteum, in turn derived from the ruptured follicle. This compartment makes progesterone and estradiol until it regresses in response to prostaglandin signal. Follicles and corpora lutea in various stages of development are distributed in the stromal compartment of the ovary, which consists of largely dense fibroblast-like cells. The stroma itself produces largely androgens, which become the dominant secretory product of the ovary whenever follicles or corpora lutea are not functional. This can occur in anovulatory states and after the menopause when follicles and oocytes are depleted (Ryan and Smith, 1965; Savard et al., 1965).

Two-Cell Theory

The concept of ovarian compartments evolved from studies on isolated follicles, corpora lutea, and stroma studied in vitro. That the compartments made the steroids attributed to them was established by extracting the steroids from the isolated tissue, demonstrating specific enzymatic biosynthetic pathways in the isolated tissue extracts, and demonstrating that the ovary containing the dominant follicle or corpus luteum secreted the appropriate steroids into its venous effluent, compared with the contralateral ovary. These studies were followed by further manipulation of the cells that make up the follicle. Granulosa and thecal cells could be separated from each other and studied alone and in recombination (Ryan, 1980). From such studies it was discovered that theca cells had LH receptors and could make androstenedione and testosterone and androstenedione de novo. Granulosa cells, on the other hand, had FSH receptors and, when stimu-

lated with FSH, responded by increasing their ability to metabolize androgens to estrogens. This explained the need for both LH and FSH for follicular development (Dorrington and Armstrong, 1979). A theory evolved that the theca makes androgens in response to LH, which is transported to the granulosa cells, which under the effect of FSH converts the androgen to estrogen (Fig 3–4). The dominant preovulatory follicle does this better than follicles destined for atresia, which can make the androgen but, failing adequate conversion to estrogen, undergo degeneration under the influence of their own accumulating androgens (Ross and Schreiber, 1986).

Steroid Structure

The cyclopentenophenanthrene ring structure is the basic carbon skeleton for all steroid hormones. The carbon skeleton consists of a five-carbon cyclopentane ring conjoined to a phenanthrene molecule, which is itself made up of three six-carbon rings configured as shown in Figure 3–5. The carbons are shared where each of the rings meet one another so that carbons 5 through 10, 8, 9, 13, and 14 are common to adjoining rings. The rings are designated A, B, C, and D. The numbering of the carbons of the skeleton is important for indicating where hydroxyl groups, side chains, and other additions are added to the ring to define a specific hormone. The numbering allows precise designation of the steroid structure and hence should be kept in mind to distinguish between the hormones, which are all closely related. Since the ring systems are relatively planar and rigid, stereoisomers that need to be distinguished also occur. In general, molecules or atoms that extend in space above the plane of the ring are designated β, and those below the plane are designated α. Axial and equatorial designations are also used to specify a more exact configuration and relationship of one insertion on the carbon to the other.

There are three physiologically important steroid nuclei: estrane (18 carbon atoms), androstane (19 carbon atoms), and pregnane (21 carbon atoms) (see Fig 3–5). All the important gonadal steroids are derivatives of these three steroid nuclei. Specific suffixes and symbols are used to indicate changes in these basic structures. For example, when the C-4, C-5 carbon bond is unsaturated, and a double bond is present, the suffix

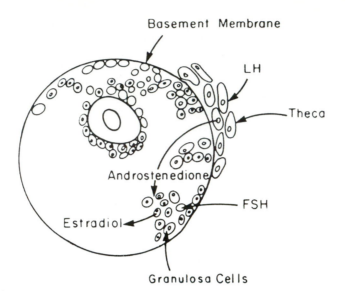

FIG 3–4.

Diagram of relationship of granulosa and thecal cells of the follicle. Note LH-stimulated thecal androstenedione being transported to FSH-stimulated granulosa cell for aromatization to estradiol (From Ryan KJ: The endocrine pattern and control of the ovulatory cycle, in Insler V, Lunenfeld B (eds): *Infertility: Male and Female.* New York, Churchill Livingstone, 1986, pp 57–72. Reproduced by permission.)

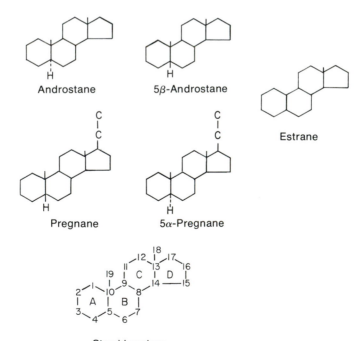

FIG 3–5.

Structural formula showing the basic steroid nucleus with appropriate numbering of the carbon atoms. The basic C-18 steroid estrane, the C-19 steroids, androstane and 5β-androstane, and the basic C-21 steroids, pregnane and 5α-pregnane, are illustrated.

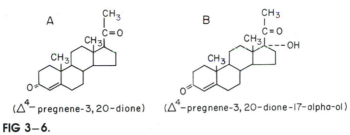

FIG 3–6.

Structural formulas for **A,** progesterone, and **B,** 17α-hydroxyprogesterone.

"ene" replaces the "ane" ending. If a keto (=O) group is substituted for two hydrogens, the suffix "one" is used together with the number of the carbon to which it is attached. The 4-ene-3-one grouping is present in many biologically active steroids (testosterone, progesterone, cortisol). If a hydroxy (OH) group is substituted for a hydrogen, the suffix "ol" is used.

In Figure 3–6, the structural formula for progesterone is shown. Progesterone is a derivative of the C-21 compound pregnane. Since there is a double bond in ring A, the term pregnane is changed to pregnene. The position of the double bond (between carbon atoms 4 and 5) is designated as Δ^4. Two ketone groups are present, one

on the carbon 3 and another on the carbon 20 atom, thus 3,20-dione (meaning two ketone groups). Therefore, the systematic name for progesterone is Δ^4-pregnene-3,20-dione. Figure 3–6 also shows the structure and systematic name for 17-hydroxyprogesterone. Note that the −OH group at the C-17 position is below the plane of the carbon ring and is therefore designated 17-α-ol.

Biochemistry of Steroid Biosynthesis

The quantitatively important sources of steroid production are the ovaries, the testes, and the adrenals. Each of these glands makes hor-

The Core Reactions

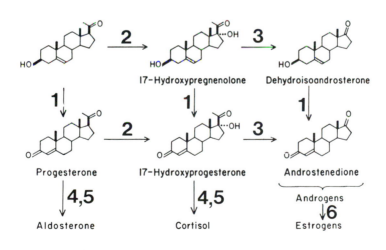

FIG 3–7.

The ovary, the testis, and the adrenal produce six common core steroids. The core Δ^5 steroids are pregnenolone, 17α-hydroxypregnenolone, and dehydroepiandrosterone. The core Δ^4 steroids are progesterone, 17α-hydroxyprogesterone, and androstenedione. The core steroids are the important precursors for the production of all gonadal steroids, glucocorticoids and mineralocorticoids. Progesterone is an important gonadal steroid and is the pre-cursor for all mineralocorticoids. 17α-Hydroxyprogesterone is the precursor for all glucocorticoids. Androstenedione is the precursor for the androgens and estrogens. Enzyme no. 1 is 3β-hydroxysteroid-dehydrogenase-isomerase; enzyme no. 2, 17α-hydroxylase; enzyme no. 3; 17,20-lyase; enzyme no. 4, 21-hydroxylase; enzyme no. 5, 11β-hydroxylase; and enzyme no. 6; aromatase.

mones that are unique to that gland. For example, the ovary secretes large amounts of estradiol. The testis secretes large amounts of testosterone. The adrenal gland is responsible for the production of cortisol and aldosterone. In addition to these unique steroid products, each gland can produce some common "core" steroids: progesterone, 17-hydroxyprogesterone, and androstenedione (Fig 3–7). These core steroids are the important precursors for the production of all gonadal steroids, glucocorticoids, and mineralocorticoids. Discussion of the biosynthesis of these core steroids follows.

Cholesterol is the parent steroid from which all the gonadal steroids, glucocorticoids, and mineralocorticoids are derived. Classical concepts of steroidogenesis state that the steroid-producing glands, such as the ovary, synthesize cholesterol from acetate and then utilize the cholesterol to produce progestins, estrogens, and androgens. However, recent evidence suggests that plasma cholesterol is the precursor for some adrenal and ovarian steroid hormones. In the circulation, cholesterol is carried in lipoprotein packages, which consist of a core of apolar cholesterol and cholesterol esters surrounded by a shell of amphiteric phospholipids and apoproteins. The LDLs and the high-density lipoproteins (HDLs) contain most of the cholesterol present in the circulation. The adrenal and ovarian cells responsible for steroidogenesis have membrane receptors for the LDL lipoprotein package. The circulating LDL binds to these receptors and becomes incorporated into the cell by a process of endocytosis.

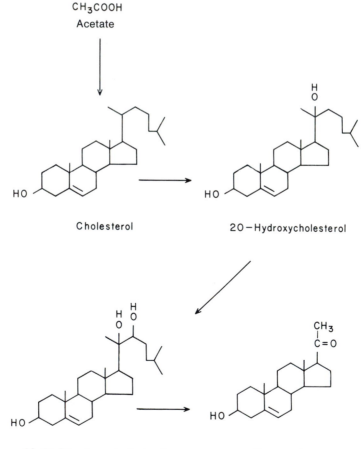

FIG 3–8.
Conversion of acetate to pregnenolone via cholesterol, 20-hydroxycholesterol, and 20,22-dihydroxy-cholesterol.

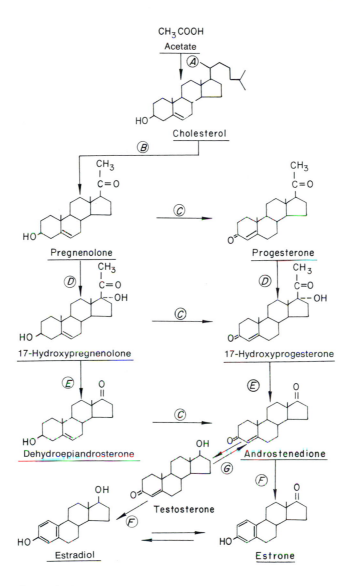

FIG 3–9.

Possible metabolic pathways for the ovarian biogenesis of estrogens. Letters above arrows denote the following metabolic pathways and the enzyme systems involved: *A,* formation of the sterol nucleus; *B,* cleavage of cholesterol side chain with formation of C-21 steroid; *C,* isomerase reaction with changing of double bond from C-5 to C-4, and dehydrogenation at C-3: 3β-ol dehydrogenases; *D,* 17α-hydroxylation (i.e., introduction of hydroxy radical in α position on C-17); *E,* cleavage of side chain, converting C-21 to C-19 steroids; *F,* aromatization (i.e., introduction of double bonds into *ring A* with conversion of C-19 to C-18 steroids); *G,* 17β-ol dehydrogenase reactions (reversible) (i.e., conversion of hydroxy radical in β position on C-17 to ketone group, or vice versa). (From Smith OW, Ryan KJ: *Am J Obstet Gynecol* 1962; 84:141. Reproduced by permission.)

The cholesterol from the LDL is released for utilization by the cell by the action of lysosomal enzymes.

Once cholesterol is released from the lipoprotein package, it must be transported to the mitochondria, where it binds to the cholesterol cleavage enzyme and is metabolized to pregnenolone (Fig 3–8). Pregnenolone is then metabolized to the other core steroids (progesterone, 17-hydroxyprogesterone, and androstenedione) by three enzyme systems (see Fig 3–7). In turn, progesterone can be secreted, or metabolized, to the important mineralocorticoid aldosterone. 17-Hydroxyprogesterone can be secreted, or metabolized, to the important glucocorticoid cortisol. Androstenedione can be secreted, or metabolized, to the gonadal steroids testosterone and estradiol (Fig 3–9).

There are only three types of reactions that all steroids can undergo: (1) removal or addition of hydrogen, as in the conversion of pregnenolone to progesterone (3β-hydroxysteroid dehydrogenase; (2) hydroxylations (addition of −OH), as occurs in the conversion of progesterone to 17-hydroxyprogesterone (17-hydroxylase); and (3) conjugation reactions, such as sulfoconjugates and glucuroconjugates.

The conversion of cholesterol (C-26) to progesterone (C-21), to androstenedione (C-19), and, finally, to estradiol (C-18) requires the sequential removal of different carbon side chains. These cleavage reactions are accomplished by multiple hydroxylations of neighboring carbon bonds. This produces a highly unstable intermediate compound, which reaches a lower-energy state by separation of the carbon side chain from the parent steroid nucleus. For example, in the conversion of cholesterol to pregnenolone, multiple hydroxylations occur at the C-20, C-22 carbon bond, leading to a breakdown of the parent compound to pregnenolone and the isocaproic aldehyde side chain (see Fig 3–8). The following enzymes involve cleavage of carbon side chains from the parent molecule: cholesterol cleavage enzyme, 17,20-lyase, and aromatase (see Figs 3–7 to 3–9).

Steroid hormones are produced in the gonads and adrenals and secreted in the circulation. In the circulation, steroids are transported to peripheral tissues where further chemical transformations can occur. In the liver, multiple hydroxylation, hydration, and conjugation reactions occur, leading to loss of steroid activity. However, in some peripheral tissues, potent steroid agonists can be locally produced from weak precursors. For example, the weak androgen androstenedione can be converted in fat tissue to the important estrogen estrone by the enzyme aromatase. This *peripheral conversion* is of utmost importance in such disease states as polycystic ovarian disease and endometrial hyperplasia.

Another important peripheral conversion is that of androstenedione into the potent androgen testosterone. In women, 50% to 70% of circulating testosterone arises from the peripheral conversions of androstenedione derived from the ovary and adrenal.

Steroid Pathways in the Ovarian Follicle and Corpus Luteum

Steroid biosynthetic pathways were defined for the human ovarian follicle based on enzymatic studies of tissue in vitro and by studies on isolated and recombined granulosa and thecal cells (Ryan and Smith, 1965; Ryan et al., 1968). The pathway involves the steps just described. The 2-carbon acetate molecule can be converted to the 27-carbon cholesterol molecule by a series of complex reactions. There is then loss of part of the cholesterol side chain to form the 21-carbon pregnenolone, which is converted to progesterone, side chain cleavage of the pregnenolone and progesterone to form 19-carbon androgens, and finally, aromatization to the 18-carbon estrogens. Although both theca and granulosa can carry out all of these steps, theca is most facile in taking acetate to androgens and granulosa cells most facile in the last aromatization step to form estrogens from androgens (Ryan and Smith, 1965). In the corpus luteum, a new form of steroid production takes place, the acetate to cholesterol steps are bypassed, and the cell uses preformed cholesterol obtained from the blood stream to make progesterone. This probably accounts for the jump in progesterone production in the transition from the follicle to the corpus luteum. To sequester cholesterol, the luteal cells develop receptors that can bind LDL-cholesterol for internalization and processing (Turek and Strauss, 1982). Estrogens can then be formed in the corpus luteum as a further metabolic step from progesterone.

Regulatory Proteins

Many functions that occur in the follicle and corpus luteum cannot be readily explained by the direct action of gonadotropins or steroids. This includes such phenomena as the life-long meiotic arrest of oocytes until they are to be ovulated, and then resumption of meiosis, or development of the rich blood supply of the dominant follicle, further vascularization of the corpus luteum, and then vascular regression each month. It has long been known that isolated granulosa cells cannot be made to divide in vitro by either steroids or gonadotropins. There was a growth factor in pituitary gonadotropin extracts that made granulosa cells divide in vitro, but it disappeared on purification of the gonadotropins. This led to the discovery of fibroblast growth factor (FGF), isolated first from the pituitary and since known to be made in the ovary. Fibroblast growth factor is not only a potent mitogen for the granulosa cells but also the angiogenic factor that is probably responsible for marked vascular proliferation of folliculogenesis and corpus luteum formation.

Inhibins and activins have also been isolated from the ovary. These proteins may have both local effects on the ovary and distant effects on the pituitary. Inhibin is the long-sought nonsteroidal feedback substance that controls the level of FSH by a direct negative feedback on the pituitary. Although long predicted as important in the male reproductive system, inhibin was isolated first from follicular fluid. Inhibin seems to be secreted by the dominant follicle along with estradiol. Its production is stimulated by FSH action on the granulosa cell.

A host of other regulatory proteins identified in other cells and biological systems have since been shown to also be made in the ovary. These include the epidermal growth factor first isolated from the salivary glands of mice, which is also a potent mitogen for granulosa cells and is believed to be made in the ovarian follicle. Transforming growth factors first found in viral transformed cells are now also known to be made in the ovary. Transforming growth factor beta is believed to have an effect on augmenting resumption of meiosis. Müllerian-inhibiting substance, so important for embryonic male development, has also been found to be synthesized in the ovarian follicle and has been considered as a possible oocyte meiosis inhibitor. The insulin-like growth factors are also synthesized in the follicle and appear to have an effect on granulosa cell function. It is still too early to define the role, if any, that each of these regulatory proteins plays in normal ovarian development and hormonal activity. There are receptors for essentially all of these factors on granulosa cells, and they are synthesized by either granulosa or thecal cells. They therefore function as autocrine (effect on cell of origin) or paracrine (effect on adjoining cells) regulators that have to be considered along with the endocrine steroids and gonadotropins as major players in the complex control of the reproductive cycle. Another fascinating aspect of these regulatory proteins is

that many are related to one another by interesting homologies in their amino acid sequences. Transforming growth factor beta, inhibins, and müllerian-inhibiting substance all share common amino acid sequences. The same is true for epidermal growth factor and transforming growth factor alpha, FGF, interleukin-1, insulin-like growth factor 1, and proinsulin. This will make study more difficult if they bind to one another's receptors and act as agonist or antagonist, making identification of the natural ligand problematical (Ryan and Makris, 1987).

Relaxin, a protein hormone with a long history but no well-defined role in primate reproduction, has now been shown to be made in the ovary and predominantly in the corpus luteum, with greater production in early pregnancy (Weiss et al., 1977). Relaxin shares interesting homologies with insulin, but its role, if any, in the ovary or in the menstrual cycle has not been established. Both renin and angiotensin have also been found in follicular fluid and are believed to be made locally in the ovary (Lightman et al., 1987).

Estrogen and Progesterone Effects on the Endometrium

The bottom line for endocrine function in the menstrual cycle is the mechanism by which hormones cyclically stimulate the endometrial lining in preparation for pregnancy and cause its regression if pregnancy does not occur. Estradiol stimulates proliferation and gland formation as well as vascular growth in the endometrial cells. It increases its own intracellular receptor, which augments its response. In addition, progesterone receptors are developed in the cells in response to estrogen. It is highly likely that estrogen does not directly cause mitosis in the cells but achieves this secondarily via regulatory proteins like those described for the ovary. In humans, estrogen development of the endometrium clearly anticipates being augmented by progesterone after ovulation. If ovulation does not occur and no progesterone is secreted, the endometrium may continue to proliferate under a constant estrogen level into a form of hyperplasia frequently seen in anovulatory states. At a constant estrogen level or if the estrogen level declines or is withdrawn completely, the endometrium cannot be maintained and starts to bleed. This estrogen withdrawal or breakthrough bleeding is typified by being variable in duration and amount depending on the prior level of hyperplasia. It is not menstrual bleeding from a secretory endometrium, and it is the commonest basis of dysfunctional bleeding.

The proliferative phase development of the endometrium under the effect of estrogen is followed sequentially by postovulatory progesterone stimulation of the estradiol-primed endometrium. Spotting at the time of ovulation may represent an endometrial response to the sharp drop in the estrogen level just before the corpus luteum is formed before progesterone can further develop the cells. After ovulation, the endometrium is ready to respond to progesterone, since progesterone receptors were developed by estradiol in the early phase of the cycle. Progesterone causes gland development and decidualization of the stromal cells with a further spiraling and tortuosity of the underlying vasculature. This clearly is a suitable lining for implantation and placentation if pregnancy occurs. In the sterile cycle, both progesterone and estrogen production by the corpus luteum declines as a result of luteolysis, and the collapsing of blood vessels and sloughing with menstrual bleeding occur. This is true menstrual bleeding after progesterone withdrawal of a well-developed secretory endometrium, which is generally more orderly in duration and amount than withdrawal bleeding from estrogen alone as previously noted. This is the basis for treating anovulatory bleeding with progesterone. Much of our knowledge of the effects of the steroid hormones on endometrium has come from the pioneering animal studies of Hisaw and Greep (Ryan, 1988). In addition, Markee studied the changes in the endometrium of the monkey as transplanted to the anterior chamber of the eye, where it could be observed throughout the cycle and in response to specific hormones (Ryan, 1988). Finally, Noyes et al. (1950) from our own institution made the correlation between the histological appearance of human endometrial specimens obtained at surgery with the day of the menstrual cycle when the tissue was obtained. They defined the range of effects that can be observed when the estrogen of the follicular phase of the cycle is followed by progesterone during the luteal phase.

Dating the Endometrium

Specific changes occurring in the stromal and glandular elements of the endometrium during the menstrual cycle have been of interest to both pathologist and clinician. By close scrutiny of these changes, it has been possible to date the endometrium (within a range of about 48 hours), particularly in the postovulatory phase of the cycle. This correlation between the date of the cycle and the histological appearance of the endometrium has particular importance in the study of the infertile patient. For purposes of simplicity, a 28-day cycle, with ovulation occurring on the 14th day, will be described. The first day of the menstrual period will be considered the first day of the cycle, with the menstrual flow lasting 4 days. The *proliferative phase* of the cycle then begins at the termination of the *menstrual phase*. The postovulatory phase, or *secretory phase,* in this cycle extends from day 14 to day 28. It should be remembered that the changes to be described occur only in the functional layers of the endometrium and not in the basal layer or in the lower uterine segment. Biopsies of the endometrium therefore have significance only if an adequate amount of functional endometrium is obtained. It is recognized that all parts of the endometrium do not undergo simultaneous change since the tissue responsiveness may vary, depending on blood supply, adjacent leiomyomas, and so forth. In the normal cycle, however, an approximation of dating within 48 hours is frequently of considerable help.

Proliferative Phase

Under the stimulation of estrogen, the endometrium gradually rebuilds its substance. The early proliferative phase extends from the fourth through the seventh days, the middle proliferative phase extends from day 8 through day 10, and the late proliferative phase lasts from day 11 until the time of ovulation on day 14 (Fig 3–10). Discussion of the characteristic histologic pattern of each phase (modified after Noyes et al., 1950) follows.

Early Proliferative Phase (Fig 3–11).—The glands are short, narrow, with mitotic activity (some glands remaining from menstrual phase may show secretory exhaustion). The surface epithelium is regenerating between openings of glands. The stroma is compact, with few mitoses, stellate or spindle shaped cells with scanty cytoplasm, and large nuclei.

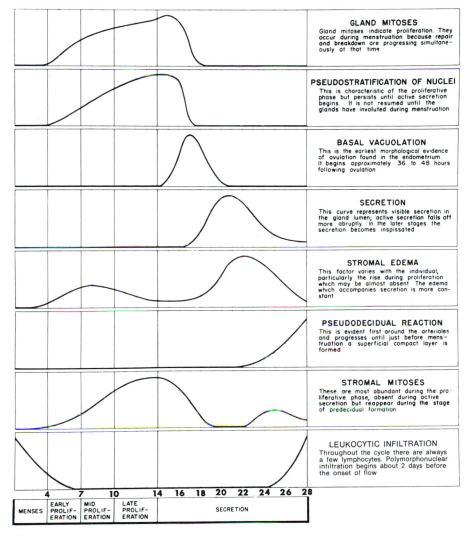

FIG 3–10.
Changes in various morphological features utilized in dating the endometrium; graphs correlate with their appearance and disappearance during the menstrual cycle. (From Noyes RW, Hertig AT, Rock J: Dating the endometrial biopsy. *Fertil Steril* 1950; 1:3. Reproduced by permission.)

Middle Proliferative Phase (Fig 3–12).—The glands are longer with slightly curved effect. There is beginning pseudostratification of nuclei (nuclei appear superimposed in layers, but actually all cells are attached at same level). The stroma has edema of variable degree. There are numerous mitotic figures. Scanty cytoplasm and edema give a "naked nucleus" effect. The surface epithelium is covered with columnar epithelium.

Late Proliferative Phase (Fig 3–13).—The glands are tortuous as a result of active growth.

There are numerous mitoses pseudostratification of nuclei. The stroma is dense with active growth pattern and numerous mitoses.

Secretory Phase

The changes after ovulation are due to the effects of estrogen and progesterone on an endometrium previously stimulated, or "primed," with estrogen. As previously mentioned, this phase lasts about 14 days, the first 7 days of which are characterized by typical changes in the glandular epithelium. During the last 7 days, specific stromal

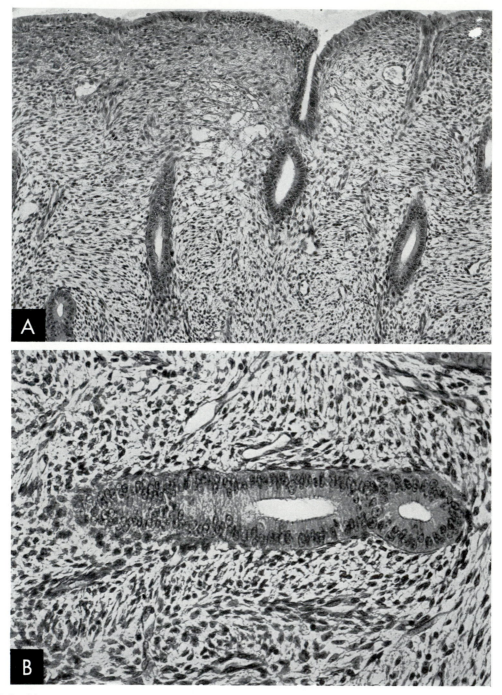

FIG 3–11.

Early proliferative endometrium. **A,** surface epithelium thin; glands sparse, narrow, and straight. (Magnification ×150.) **B,** few mitoses in glands and stroma; little pseudostratification of gland nuclei. (Magnification ×400.) (From Noyes RW, Hertig AT, Rock J: Dating the endometrial biopsy. *Fertil Steril* 1950; 1:3. Reproduced by permission.)

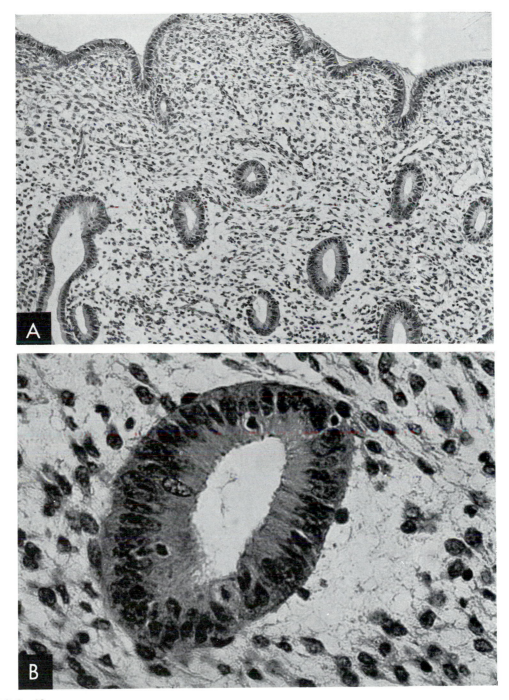

FIG 3–12.
Endometrium showing intermediate degree of proliferation. **A,** glands slightly tortuous; tall columnar surface epithelium. Extracellular fluid is not always as marked as in this section. (Magnification ×150.) **B,** glands show numerous mitoses with pseudostratification becoming marked. Note the "naked nucleus" type of stromal cell with fine anastomosing processes. (Magnification ×400.)

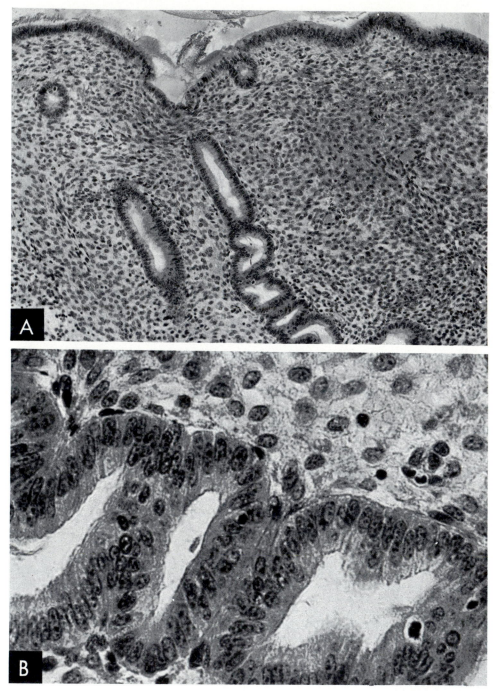

FIG 3–13.
Late proliferative endometrium. **A,** glands tortuous; stroma usually quite dense. (Magnification ×150.) **B,** epithelial nuclei are pseudostratified and oval in shape. (Magnification ×400.) (From Noyes RW, Hertig AT, Rock J: Dating the endometrial biopsy. *Fertil Steril* 1950; 1:3. Reproduced by permission.)

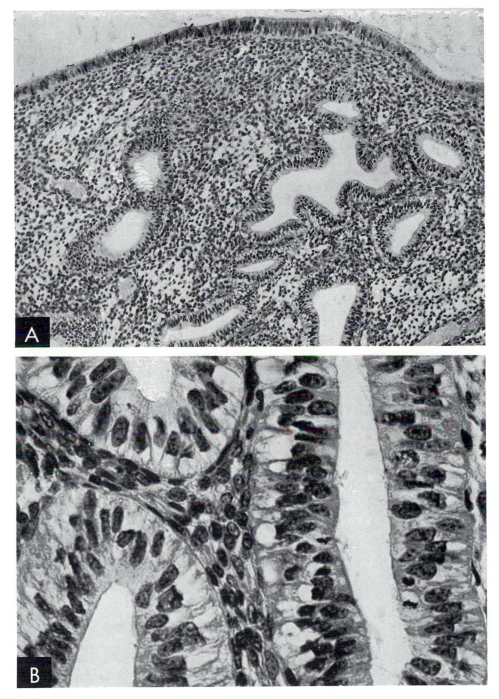

FIG 3–14.
Second postovulatory day. **A,** glands tortuous; stroma dense; cells consist of nearly naked nuclei. (Magnification ×150.) **B,** gland mitoses very numerous; pseudostratification of nuclei exaggerated by subnuclear vacuoles. (Magnification ×40.) (From Noyes RW, Hertig AT, Rock J: Dating the endometrial biopsy. *Fertil Steril* 1950; 1:3. Reproduced by permission.)

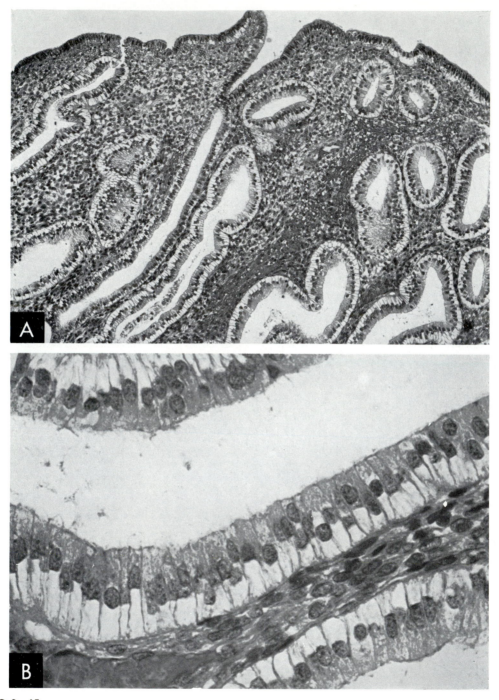

FIG 3—15.
Third postovulatory day. **A,** gland nuclei are pushed to the center of the epithelial cells with cytoplasm above and vacuoles below them. (Magnification ×150.) **B,** gland mitoses rare; pseudostratification de-creasing. (Magnification ×400.) (From Noyes RW, Hertig AT, Rock J: Dating the endometrial biopsy. *Fertil Steril* 1950; 1:3. Reproduced by permission.)

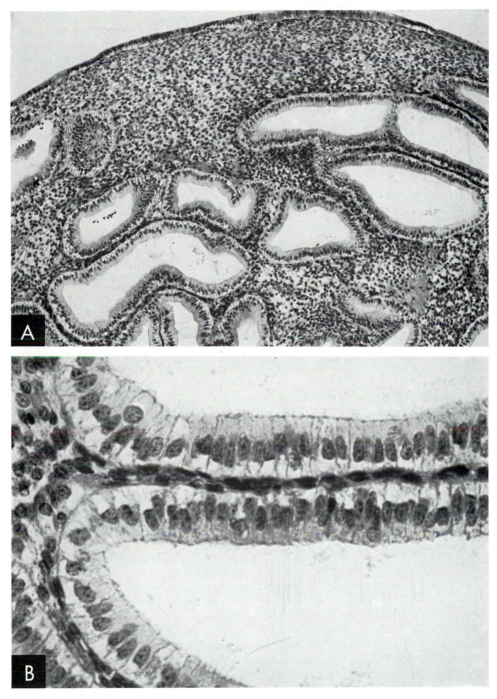

FIG 3–16.
Fourth postovulatory day. **A,** gland nuclei are return-ing to base of cells. Wisps of secretory material are present in lumina. (Magnification ×150.) **B,** some vacuoles are pushed past the nucleus on their way to empty glycogen into the lumen. Mitoses and pseudostratification of nuclei are absent. This is the stage of arrival of ovum in the uterus. (Magnification ×400.) (From Noyes RW, Hertig AT, Rock J: Dating the endometrial biopsy. *Fertil Steril* 1950; 1:3. Repro-duced by permission.)

changes occur that may be used for dating purposes.

Day 15.—Day 15 shows essentially a late proliferative pattern except for occasional vacuoles below the nuclei of the glands.

Day 16 (Fig 3–14).—Basal vacuoles are seen in most glands. It is the last day of pseudostratification. There are mitoses in the glands and stroma.

Day 17 (Fig 3–15).—Characteristic pattern of subnuclear glycogen vacuoles is evident, with homogeneous cytoplasm above the nuclei of the glands. The position of the nuclei rather regular. There is loss of pseudostratification of cells with an increase in diameter and tortuosity. Mitotic figures in glands and stroma rare.

Day 18 (Fig 3–16).—Subnuclear vacuoles appear smaller as the nuclei move back toward the base of the cell. Secretion of glycogen into the lumen of the gland begins. There are no mitoses.

Day 19.—Few subnuclear vacuoles are seen. It resembles day 16 pattern except for secretion in lumen of gland and absence of pseudostratification and mitoses.

Day 20 (Fig 3–17).—Occasionally there are subnuclear vacuoles. Acidophilic secretion is prominent in the gland lumen.

Day 21.—Beginning stromal effects are evident; cells of stroma have dark, dense nuclei with filamentous cytoplasm. Stromal edema is beginning.

Day 22 (Fig 3–18).—Day 22 is the maximum point of stromal edema. Thin-walled spiral arterioles may be seen. Secretion in gland lumen is active but subsiding and undergoing inspissation.

Day 23 (Fig 3–19).—Edema of stroma persists, but a characteristic change is a condensation of the stroma around the spiral arterioles. This is due to an enlargement of stromal nuclei with an increase in cytoplasm and is called *predecidual change*.

Day 24 (Fig 3–20).—Predecidual collections surrounding arterioles are marked. There are active stromal mitoses, but stromal edema is lessening. The endometrium is now beginning to undergo involution unless it is maintained by pregnancy.

Day 25 (Fig 3–21).—Predecidua is forming beneath the surface epithelium, and there is some edema around the arterioles. Lymphocytic infiltration of the stroma is beginning.

Day 26.—Gradual increase in predecidua is seen throughout stroma, with infiltration of polymorphonuclear leukocytes.

Day 27.—Predecidua is prominent around the blood vessels and under surface epithelium. There is marked infiltration of polymorphonuclear leukocytes.

Day 28.—There is beginning focal necrosis of the predecidua with small areas of stromal hemorrhage. Stromal cells are clumped together. There is extensive polymorphonuclear leukocytic infiltration. Tortuous glands appear to have undergone secretory "exhaustion."

Certain specific changes in glands and stroma may be considered to indicate physiologic changes occurring in the endometrium. Thus, *gland mitoses* indicate active proliferation and growth and may be found from day 3 or 4 of the cycle until day 16 or 17. *Pseudostratification* of gland nuclei begins after the postmenstrual involution and usually disappears by day 17. It is an indication of proliferative glandular growth, and its appearance is due to crowding of nuclei when the gland is sectioned transversely. *Basal vacuolation* is the earliest morphologic evidence of ovulation discernible in the endometrium. Although occasionally one may be seen in the absence of progesterone, basal vacuoles are usually identified between day 15 and day 19, the glycogen being pushed into the gland lumen about day 19 or 20. The characteristic lining up of the nuclei above the vacuoles is best seen on day 17 and is an excellent indication of recent ovulation.

The secretory function of the glands is evident from day 18 until day 22 by the appearance of loose, feathery material in the lumina. If the blastocyst implants itself on the surface of the endometrium about 6 days after ovulation, it would appear that morphology and function are well

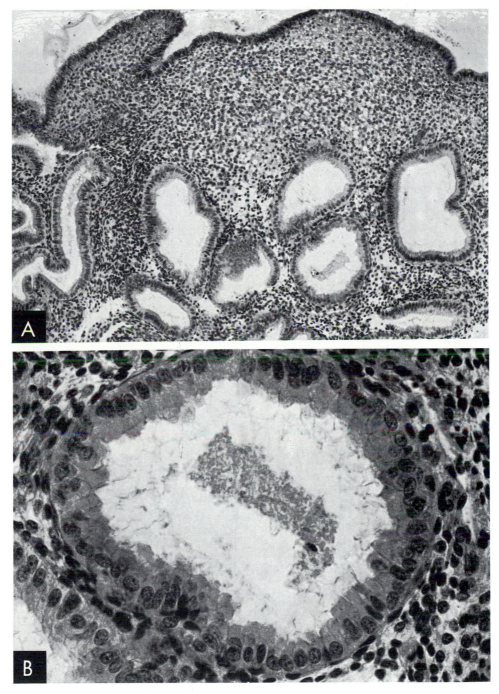

FIG 3–17.
Sixth postovulatory day, corresponding to beginning implantation in fertile cycle. **A,** secretion in gland lumen at peak; beginning of accumulation of extravascular fluid in stroma. (Magnification ×150.) **B,** subnuclear vacuoles rare; nuclei round and basally located. (Magnification ×400.) (From Noyes RW, Hertig AT, Rock J: Dating the endometrial biopsy. *Fertil Steril* 1950; 1:3. Reproduced by permission.)

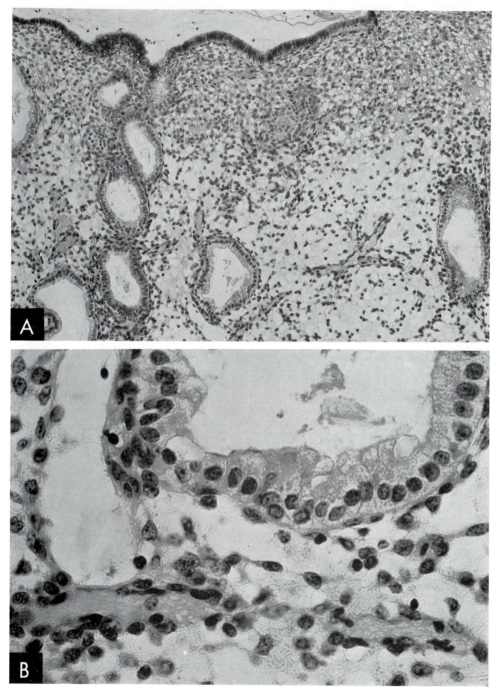

FIG 3–18.
Eighth postovulatory day. **A,** extracellular fluid maximal. Walls of spiral arterioles are not prominent. (Magnification ×150.) **B,** stromal cells still appear as small, dense "naked nuclei" widely separated by extracellular fluid. Glandular secretion still active but subsiding. (Magnification ×400.) (From Noyes RW, Hertig AT, Rock J: Dating the endometrial biopsy. *Fertil Steril* 1950; 1:3. Reproduced by permission.)

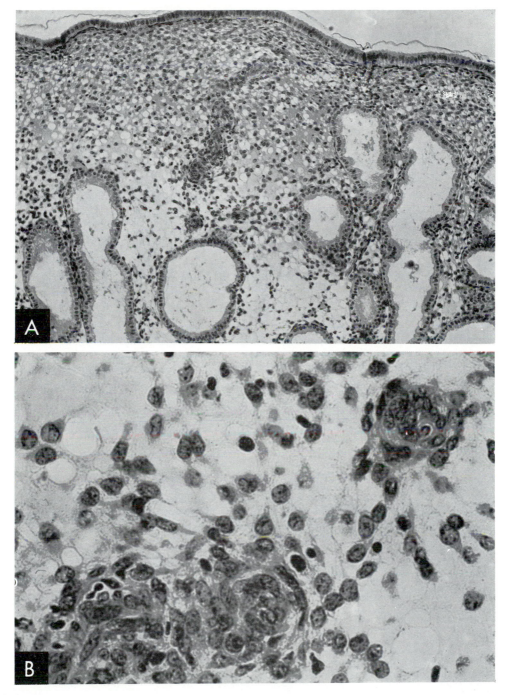

FIG 3–19.

Ninth postovulatory day. **A,** spiral arterioles become prominent because of condensation of surrounding stroma. (Magnification ×150.) **B,** both nuclei and cytoplasm of periarteriolar stromal cells are enlarging. This is the earliest predecidual reaction. (Magnification ×400.) (From Noyes RW, Hertig AT, Rock J: Dating the endometrial biopsy. *Fertil Steril* 1950; 1:3. Reproduced by permission.)

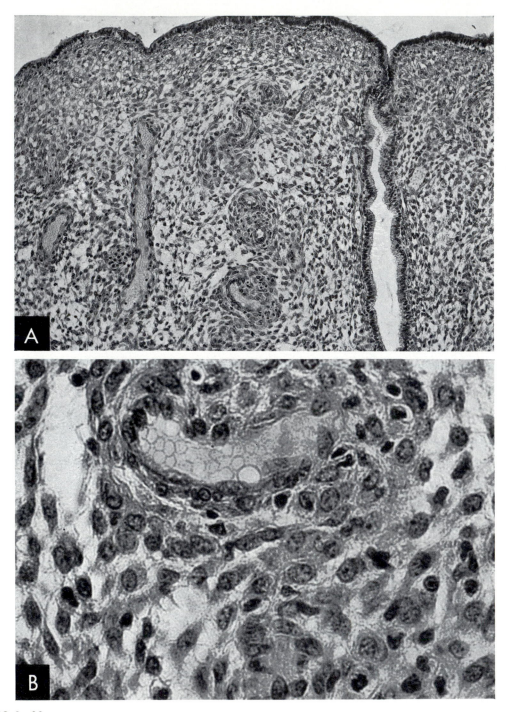

FIG 3–20.
Tenth postovulatory day. **A,** spiral arterioles and surrounding predecidua still more prominent; extracellular fluid subsiding. (Magnification ×150.) **B,** thickening of periarteriolar predecidual cuff; stromal mitosis evident. (Magnification ×400.) (From Noyes RW, Hertig AT, Rock J: Dating the endometrial biopsy. *Fertil Steril* 1950; 1:3. Reproduced by permission.)

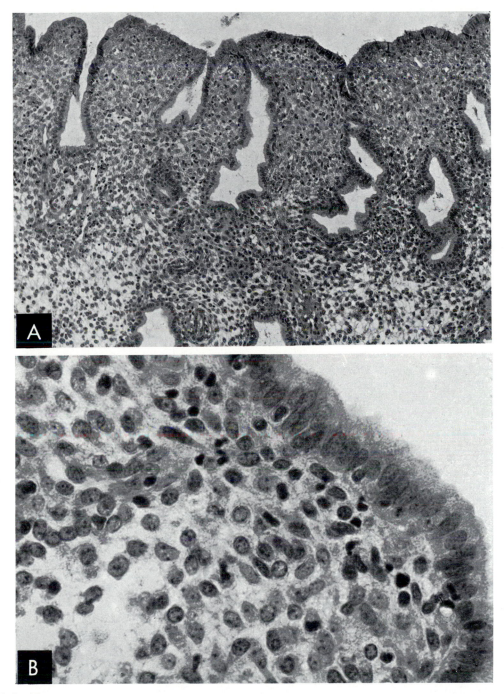

FIG 3–21.
Eleventh postovulatory day. **A,** pseudodecidua begins to differentiate under surface epithelium. Stroma of the stratum spongiosum still contains extracellular fluid except in areas near a spiral arteriole. (Magnification ×150.) **B,** round-cell infiltration accompanies predecidual differentiation. Stromal cells swell to become predecidual in type. (Magnification ×400.) (From Noyes RW, Hertig AT, Rock J: Dating the endometrial biopsy. *Fertil Steril* 1950; 1:3. Reproduced by permission.)

correlated, since days 20 to 22 would be critical ones from the standpoint of nutrient materials. The *edema* of the stroma, most striking between days 22 and 23, may represent an effort of the endometrium to simplify the implantation process by lessening tissue resistance. Periarterial *predecidual reaction* is evident beginning about days 23 and 24 and may represent a protective mechanism against premature vascular disruption. The predecidua is looked on as providing a supporting framework for newly developed blood vessels to aid in their increased load should pregnancy supervene. These changes in morphological features are graphically summarized in Figure 3–10.

MENSTRUAL ABNORMALITIES

Amenorrhea and Oligomenorrhea

Primary vs. Secondary Amenorrhea

Primary amenorrhea is present when the first menses has not occurred by age 16 years. Primary amenorrhea is usually due to a genetic or congenital developmental defect (Joseph and Thomas, 1982). Primary amenorrhea is often associated with disorders of pubertal development (Reindollar, 1981). The differential diagnosis of primary amenorrhea is presented in detail in Chapter 20. Secondary amenorrhea is present when a woman with previously regular, cyclic menses has 3 or more months of amenorrhea. By necessity, this definition is arbitrary. Episodes of physiological amenorrhea (the perimenarchal period, the immediate postpartum state, and lactation) should not prompt an evaluation of secondary amenorrhea. Secondary amenorrhea is usually due to environmental effects (stress, exercise) or acquired (not congenital) disease. Oligomenorrhea is present when the interval between menstrual cycles is routinely greater than 35 days. The etiological mechanisms that cause oligomenorrhea are identical to those that cause secondary amenorrhea. Therefore, the differential diagnosis, evaluation, and therapy of oligomenorrhea are similar to those for secondary amenorrhea. Secondary amenorrhea is at least 10 times commoner than primary amenorrhea.

Secondary Amenorrhea

As noted earlier, secondary amenorrhea is present when a woman with previously regular, cyclic menses has 3 or more months of amenorrhea. The commonest cause of secondary amenor-

rhea is pregnancy. Before a detailed workup of secondary amenorrhea is begun, pregnancy should be ruled out with a sensitive test for β-hCG. Once pregnancy is excluded, the workup of secondary amenorrhea can be organized by systematically evaluating the four major compartments necessary for reproduction: (1) hypothalamus, (2) pituitary, (3) ovary, and (4) uterus. Studies of large numbers of women with secondary amenorrhea demonstrate that the etiologic causes of secondary amenorrhea are usually distributed as follows: (1) 55% of cases are due to hypothalamic causes, (2) 20% of cases are due to pituitary diseases, (3) 20% of cases are due to ovarian dysfunction, and (4) 5% of cases are due to uterine abnormalities (Table 3–2; Reindollar et al., 1986; Hull et al., 1979, Fries, 1974). The workup of secondary amenorrhea is outlined in Figure 3–22.

Hypothalamic Causes.—The arcuate nucleus of the hypothalamus contains neurons that are neuroendocrine transducers. These neurons receive *neural inputs* from many diverse brain areas and integrate these signals into a pusatile *endocrine output* (GnRH secretion). Maintenance of normal ovarian follicular function requires a GnRH pulse frequency of approximately one pulse per hour. Marked decreases in GnRH pulse frequency (or amplitude) will prevent ovarian follicular development and can result in amenorrhea. The congenital absence of GnRH neurons produces primary amenorrhea and is often termed *Kallmann's syndrome*. As noted in Table 3–2, the commonest disorders that produce marked decreases in GnRH pulse frequency (and consequently secondary amenorrhea) are (1) abnormalities of weight, (2) strenuous exercise, (3) environmental stress, and (4) infiltrative diseases of the hypothalamus. Each of these abnormalities is reviewed.

Abnormalities of Weight.—The onset of menarche appears to be determined in part by (1) total body weight and (2) percent of body fat. Normal menarche requires that approximately 17% of body mass be fat. Teleologically, body fat is an important determinant of ovulation because successful pregnancy, birth, and lactation requires a large amount of stored energy. The direct measurement of body fat requires neutron activation analysis of nitrogen or potassium or the assessment of dilution of deuterium oxide in the body

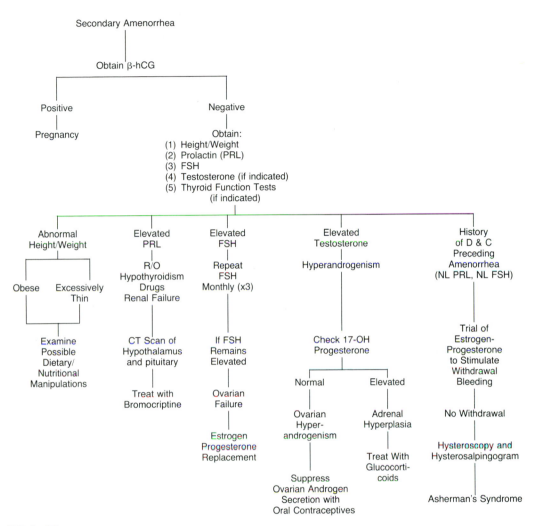

FIG 3–22.
Workup for diagnosis of secondary amenorrhea.

water space. Indirect measurements of body fat such as those made by skinfold calipers, height-weight nomograms, and underwater weighing are often inaccurate. However, in the clinical setting, direct measurement of body fat is difficult to perform. Frisch has published a nomogram relating height and weight that can be clinically useful in the evaluation of secondary amenorrhea (see Fig 3–22). The Frisch nomogram allows the clinician to use the patient's height and weight to make an estimation of the critical mass required to maintain normal menstrual function (Frisch, 1985). For example, a woman who weighs 46 kg and is 157 cm tall is below the critical body mass required to maintain menses. In such a woman, the leanness alone may be causing amenorrhea. Height and weight measurements are easy to obtain and should be carefully made in all women with amenorrhea.

The extremest example of the association between weight loss and amenorrhea is the disease of anorexia nervosa. Anorexia nervosa is a major psychiatric problem present in about 0.5% of young women. The typical diagnostic features of anorexia nervosa include (1) onset between ages 10 and 25 years; (2) weight greater than 15% below normal, (3) distorted body image (the patient believes she is not thin, whereas objective observers are impressed by the patient's emaciation); and (4) amenorrhea, constipation, low blood

TABLE 3–2.

The Commonest Causes of Secondary Amenorrhea (Excluding Pregnancy) and Their Relative Frequency

	Relative Frequency (%)
Hypothalamus	
Abnormalities of weight (and nutrition)	25
Exercise	15
Stress	15
Infiltrative disease (craniopharyngioma, sarcoidosis)	<1
Pituitary	
Prolactin-secreting pituitary tumors	17
Empty sella syndrome	2
Sheehan's syndrome	<1
ACTH-secreting pituitary tumors (Cushing's disease)	<1
Ovary	
Ovarian failure	15
Polycystic ovarian disease	5
Uterine	
Asherman's syndrome	5

pressure, hypercarotenemia, and diabetes insipidus. Anorexia nervosa is associated with numerous endocrine abnormalities; these are summarized in Table 3–3. Some patients with anorexia nervosa develop eating habits that are characterized by episodes of food gorging (bulimia) immediately followed by self-induced vomiting. Anorectic patients with the bulimia-vomiting complex are extremely difficult to treat, and as many as 5% of these women will die (usually from a combination of electrolyte imbalance, prerenal azotemia, malnutrition, and cardiac arrhythmias).

TABLE 3–3.

Neuroendocrine and Endocrine Abnormalities Observed in Women With Anorexia Nervosa

Hormone Deficiencies	Hormone Excess
Vasopressin	Cortisol
GnRH	Growth hormone
LH and FSH	Reverse T_3
Prolactin	
Total thyroxine (T_4)	
Total triiodothyronine (T_3)	
Dehydroepiandrosterone sulfate	
Estradiol	
Progesterone	

Many anorectic individuals surreptitiously use diuretics to control body weight; such use is often associated with severe electrolyte imbalance.

The cause of anorexia nervosa is unknown. Many psychiatrists believe that anorexia nervosa is a psychological manifestation of dysfunctional family relationships. Family environments that stress perfection and overachieving may foster the development of anorexia nervosa. Anorexia nervosa causes exceedingly low GnRH pulse frequencies, which prevents ovarian follicular development and results in amenorrhea. Treatment of women with anorexia nervosa with intravenous pulses of GnRH typically results in ovulatory menstrual cycles.

Mild cases of anorexia nervosa can often be treated with a number of low-risk counseling interventions: (1) explaining the association of weight loss and amenorrhea in a reassuring manner, (2) exploring the patient's distorted body image, (3) discussing problems of adolescent self-esteem in a supportive manner, and (4) exploring dysfunctional family relationships. Many cases of anorexia nervosa will require skilled therapy by psychiatrists and counselors experienced in this problem.

Women with secondary amenorrhea and height and weight measurements that suggest that leanness is the cause of the amenorrhea still need a complete amenorrhea evaluation (e.g., serum prolactin level, FSH level; see Fig 3–22). Many women with pituitary tumors and hyperprolactinemia are also extremely lean. To avoid incorrect diagnoses, one must be sure that the amenorrhea evaluation is as complete as possible. For women with low body fat percentage as the cause of the amenorrhea, dietary changes can often cause the resumption of normal ovulatory menses. Simple dietary changes can include adding bread and butter to two meals per day or adding a dessert to one meal per day.

Strenuous Exercise.—During the last 10 years, there has been a tremendous increase in the number of well-trained women athletes. For the majority of women who exercise at only mild to moderate exertional levels, for 30 to 60 minutes each day, the exercise will not disrupt menstrual function. For the women athlete who exercises at high intensity for 1 hour or more daily, the exercise can often cause a marked decrease in GnRH pulse frequency, which will cause amenorrhea. The mechanisms by which strenuous exercise decreases GnRH pulse frequency are not clear. However, weight loss, low body fat, and stress are contributing factors. Many competitive women athletes have less than 22% total body fat. This low body fat percentage is not always compatible with maintenance of normal menstruation. The stress of athletic competition may also contribute to the loss of menstrual cyclicity.

Regular exercise is an exceedingly effective way of maximizing health. Regular exercise appears to decrease the risk of developing fatal heart disease and certain cancers. Therefore, in general, physicians should not counsel women to abandon their exercise programs. In women of reproductive age, exercise-induced amenorrhea is associated with a decrease in bone density. The severity of the decrease in bone density and its clinical consequences appears to be dependent, in part, on the severity of the hypoestrogenism and the type of exercise. For example, stress fractures are uncommon in heavyweight oarswomen and swimmers. In contrast, stress fractures are common in professional dancers. The dancers are typically very lean, have marked hypoestrogenism, and stress their bones with high-impact training. Given the overwhelmingly positive health effects of exercise, we do not believe that exercise-induced amenorrhea in a woman not seeking immediate fertility requires treatment. These women should be thoroughly evaluated to exclude other causes of secondary amenorrhea, such as pituitary tumor. If osteoporosis is present, treatment with combined estrogen-progestogen contraceptives can increase bone density and may reduce the risk of stress fracture.

Environmental Stress.—A significant percentage of high school girls who leave home to go to college develop secondary amenorrhea. Examinations, sports competition, loss of a spouse, and other stresses can also cause secondary amenorrhea. The mechanisms by which stress causes secondary amenorrhea have not been fully elucidated. However, evidence that corticotropin-releasing factor (CRF) may be involved in stress-related amenorrhea is mounting. Corticotropin-releasing factor is a hypothalamic neuroprotein that stimulates pituitary ACTH and consequently controls adrenal cortisol production. During stress, CRF may be chronically elevated. Interestingly, elevated hypothalamic concentrations of CRF inhibit GnRH pulsation. Recent experiments in primates suggest that hypothalamic opi-

oids, such as endorphin, may mediate the CRF suppression of GnRH pulsatility. The decrease in GnRH pulse frequency results in amenorrhea. In general, stress-related amenorrhea requires no therapy and will spontaneously resolve once the stress ceases. Before deciding that environmental stress is the cause of amenorrhea, the physician must ensure that other diseases that cause amenorrhea (e.g., pituitary tumor, ovarian failure, anorexia nervosa) are not present.

Infiltrative Disease of the Hypothalamus.—Infiltrative disease of the hypothalamus is a rare cause of secondary amenorrhea. Histiocytosis X (infiltration of hypothalamus by lipid-laden histiocytes), sarcoidosis (infiltration of hypothalamus by granulomas) and craniopharyngiomas (tumors of Rathke pouch remnants) all can cause secondary amenorrhea. Although these diseases are rare, failure to diagnose them can have important health implications for the patient.

Pituitary Causes.—As noted in Table 3–2, the commonest pituitary causes of secondary amenorrhea are (1) prolactin-secreting pituitary tumors, (2) empty sella syndrome, (3) Sheehan's syndrome, and (4) ACTH-secreting pituitary tumors (Cushing's disease). Prolactinomas are 10 times commoner than all other pituitary causes of secondary amenorrhea and therefore will be discussed in detail.

Prolactin-Secreting Pituitary Tumors (Prolactinomas).—Hyperprolactinemia is a common finding in women with secondary amenorrhea. The commonest causes of hyperprolactinemia are (1) pregnancy, (2) prolactin-secreting pituitary tumors, (3) psychoactive drugs (e.g., phenothiazines), (4) renal failure, (5) hypothroidism, and (6) infiltrative diseases of the hypothalamus. In a patient with hyperprolactinemia, pregnancy, hypothyroidism, and renal failure should be ruled out by appropriate laboratory tests (β-hCG, T_4, TSH, blood urea nitrogen, and creatinine levels). Drug use can be assessed by a careful history. If the hyperprolactinemia can be documented on two or more occasions, a structural study of the hypothalamus and pituitary needs to be obtained. The two best methods of studying hypothalamic-pituitary structure are magnetic resonance imaging (MRI) or high-resolution x-ray computed tomography (CT) scanning. Magnetic resonance imaging has the advantage of superior resolution

(MRI 1–2 mm; CT scan 3 mm) and no radiation dosage. However, MRI is expensive and not widely available. The resolution of an MRI scan depends, in part, on the strength of the magnetic field. For high-resolution study of the hypothalamic-pituitary area, MRI units with a field strength greater than 1 tesla should be used. Clinicians should be aware that most MRI units do not have a field strength of 1 tesla.

In patients with hyperprolactinemia, the MRI or CT scan usually reveals normal hypothalamic-pituitary anatomy (idiopathic hyperprolactinemia) or a pituitary tumor (prolactinemia). For clinical purposes, pituitary tumors are divided into two broad categories based on tumor size: microademonas (less than 1 cm) or macroadenomas (1 or more cm). Large pituitary tumors are often associated with headache and visual field changes. The mechanisms by which prolactinomas produce amenorrhea are not completely understood. Hyperprolactinemia appears to be associated with abnormalities in catecholamine metabolism in the hypothalamus. Apparently by altering patterns of hypothalamic catecholamine metabolism, hyperprolactinemia causes a decrease in GnRH pulsation.

The four goals of the treatment of patients with prolactinomas are (1) normalization of serum prolactin levels, (2) preservation of anterior pituitary function, (3) decrease in size of the pituitary tumor, and (4) prevention of future recurrences of the tumor. The three therapeutic modalities currently available to achieve these goals are (1) bromocriptine therapy, (2) transphenoidal microsurgical resection of the pituitary tumor, and (3) radiotherapy. Radiotherapy is a poor alternative because it may take many years to produce a beneficial effect, usually results in panhypopituitarism, and can damage normal adjacent structures. Transphenoidal microsurgical resection of small pituitary tumors is successful in approximately 75% of cases. However, in more than 50% of the cases that are apparently "successfully" treated by surgery, recurrence of the tumor will occur within 5 years. Because of these considerations, chronic bromocriptine therapy is the treatment of choice for prolactinomas.

Prolactin is unique among the anterior pituitary hormones because it is under tonic inhibition by hypothalmic dopamine. Normal pituitary lactotrophes and cells in prolactinomas contain high concentrations of cell surface dopamine receptors. Activation of these dopamine receptors suppresses prolactin secretion and decreases overall cellular metabolism. Bromocriptine is a dopamine agonist; it is a synthetic derivative of an ergot alkaloid with a structure resembling dopamine. Bromocriptine binds to pituitary dopamine receptors, inhibits prolactin secretion, and decreases lactotrope cellular metabolism. In patients with prolactinomas, bromocriptine therapy normalizes serum prolactin levels in 85% of cases and decreases pituitary size in 60% of cases. Unfortunately, cessation of bromocriptine therapy is usually accompanied by the return of hyperprolactinemia, return of amenorrhea, and regrowth of the tumor to pretreatment size (Barbieri and Ryan, 1983).

Bromocriptine is the agent of choice for the induction of ovulation in anovulatory, infertile women with hyperprolactinemia. There are virtually no contraindications to bromocriptine except for a previous history of sensitivity to ergot compounds. Before initiation of bromocriptine therapy, the possible adverse effects of a pregnancy in a woman with a prolactin-secreting pituitary tumor need to be assessed. If the prolactin-producing tumor is small (microademona, less than 1 cm in diameter), a pregnancy is usually associated with few (less than 5%) adverse clinical outcomes. However, if the prolactin-producing tumor is large (macroadenoma, more than 1 cm in diameter) a bromocriptine-induced pregnancy is associated with adverse clinical outcomes in approximately 40% of cases. These adverse outcomes include enlargement of the tumor, severe headaches, visual field defects (bitemporal hemianopsia secondary to compression of the optic chiasm, cranial nerve palsies, and intrapituitary hemorrhage). Given these observations, infertile women with microprolactinomas can be treated with bromocriptine with the expectation that few problems will occur in a subsequent pregnancy. However, infertile women with macroprolactinomas should probably have a neurosurgical procedure to "debulk" the tumor prior to attempting pregnancy. If treatment with bromocriptine results in a pregnancy, the bromocriptine should be discontinued (Barbieri and Ryan, 1983).

Initiation of bromocriptine therapy can be associated with nausea, vomiting, postural hypotension, and syncope. Clinical experience suggests that these side effects can best be avoided by prescribing small amounts of bromocriptine, to be taken at bedtime, and gradually increasing the dose. A standard protocol for starting bromocriptine therapy is (1) 1.25 mg (one-half tablet) of bromocriptine each night for 7 days; then (2) 2.5 mg (one tablet) of bromocriptine each night for 7 days; and finally, (3) the standard dose of 2.5 mg of bromocriptine twice daily. In an occasional patient, bromocriptine in doses between 7.5 and 15 mg/day will be required to fully suppress prolactin overproduction. In many cases, bromocriptine in doses as low as 2.5 mg/day will normalize prolactin levels and result in ovulatory menses.

Empty Sella Syndrome.—The roof of the pituitary gland (the diaphragm sella) is perforated by the pituitary stalk, which connects the hypothalamic median eminence to the pituitary. In cases where the perforation in the diaphragm sella is excessively large, the pia and accompanying cerebrospinal fluid can herniate into the pituitary fossa. This herniation of fluid, which can be under reasonably high pressure, can produce compression atrophy of the pituitary gland, resulting in hypopituitarism and amenorrhea. The empty sella syndrome can be documented by high-resolution x-ray CT scanning of the pituitary. Therapy is directed to the specific replacement of documented hormonal abnormalities.

Sheehan's Syndrome.—Sheehan's syndrome is the presence of hypopituitarism caused by acute pituitary necrosis occurring after a postpartum hemorrhage. During pregnancy, the pituitary gland doubles in size due to an increase in size and number of pituitary lactotropes. The enlarged pituitary of pregnancy is especially vulnerable to ischemia from hypotension. Severe postpartum hemorrhage and shock will often lead to acute panhypopituitarism. In milder cases, hormonal reserve of single pituitary hormones (e.g., ACTH) may be lost. In patients with suspected Sheehan's syndrome the physician should carefully search for hypocortisolism and hypothyroidism If gonadotropin reserve is lost, estrogen replacement therapy will be required. For patients with Sheehans' syndrome desiring a future pregnancy, exogenous gonadotropin therapy is the treatment of choice.

Cushing's Disease.—Cushing's disease is the presence of an ACTH-producing pituitary tumor that results in chronic hypercortisolism. The evaluation of Cushing's disease is discussed in Chapter 12.

Ovarian Causes.—*Premature Ovarian Failure.*—Loss of all ovarian follicles results in the cessation of normal ovarian cyclicity (ovarian failure). Ovarian failure prior to age 40 years is termed premature ovarian failure. Loss of all ovarian follicles results in a marked increase in the serum FSH level secondary to a loss of estrogen and inhibin feedback inhibition of FSH. Therefore, the diagnosis of ovarian failure is best made by measuring the serum FSH level. In cases of complete ovarian failure, the FSH level will usually be greater than 40 mIU/ml. In cases of incipient ovarian failure, the FSH level may be between 20 and 40 mIU/ml. In women with incipient ovarian failure, FSH levels can fluctuate markedly. Measurement of FSH and estradiol levels monthly for 3 months will often assist the physician in gauging the permanency of the ovarian failure.

The commonest cause of premature ovarian failure is genetic abnormality in the sex chromosomes. Although most of these patients have ovarian failure prior to puberty, some will have a few years of normal menstrual function and then cease to menstruate. Therefore, any woman with ovarian failure prior to age 30 years should be screened for chromosomal abnormalities by karyotyping.

Ovarian failure can also be caused by autoimmune processes. Women with polyglandular autoimmune endocrine disease (e.g., hypoparathyroidism, Addison's disease, hypothyroidism, diabetes mellitus) can develop antiovarian antibodies and ovarian failure. One of the best studied examples of autoimmune ovarian failure occurs in women with myasthenia gravis. Women with myasthenia gravis produce antiacetylcholine receptor antibodies, which results in neuromotor abnormalities. Women with myasthenia gravis can also produce anti-FSH receptor antibodies, which results in accelerated loss of developing follicles. Thus, accelerated follicular destruction leads to premature ovarian failure.

Ovarian failure can also be caused by chemotherapy (especially the alkalyting agents, e.g., cyclophosphamide), radiotherapy (as little as 500 rad to the ovaries), wedge biopsy of the ovaries, and infections (Koyama, 1977).

Specific therapy for ovarian failure is not available. Women with premature ovarian failure are at high risk of developing osteoporosis and cardiovascular disease due to hypoestrogenism and thus should be offered estrogen replacement therapy unless specific contraindications exist. Advances in assisted reproductive technologies have now made it possible for women with ovarian failure to carry a pregnancy using donor eggs and in utero fertilization. In this procedure, a donor egg is fertilized with sperm from the partner of the woman with ovarian failure. The patient is treated with estrogen and progesterone to prime the uterus to receive the developing embryo. The availability and success of donor egg programs suggests that in young women a conservative approach should be taken toward the removal of a normal uterus at the time of oophorectomy for adnexal pathology. For a full discussion of the benefits of hormone replacement therapy, see Chapter 16.

Ovarian Hyperandrogenism.—Severe cases of ovarian hyperandrogenism can cause secondary amenorrhea. Ovarian hyperandrogenism is discussed in detail in Chapters 9 and 12.

Uterine Causes.—*Asherman's Syndrome.*—Asherman's syndrome is the presence of intrauterine scar tissue that interferes with normal endometrial growth and shedding. In Asherman's syndrome, the intrauterine scar tissue usually develops after vigorous curettage of infected endometrium in a patient who has recently been pregnant. Therefore, the history is an important clue to the presence of Asherman's syndrome. A commonly used endocrine manipulation to test for the presence of Asherman's syndrome is to prescribe 2.5 mg of conjugated estrogens daily for 35 days and medroxyprogesterone for the last 10 days (days 26 to 35). Failure to have a withdrawal bleed after such a challenge strongly suggests the presence of Asherman's syndrome. The diagnosis can be confirmed by a radiologic test (hysterosalpingogram) or direct visualization of the scar tissue (hysteroscopy).

The typical treatment of Asherman's syndrome involves surgical lysis of the intrauterine adhesions (with hysteroscopy or curettage), followed by long-term stimulation of the endometrium with estrogen. Some women who become pregnant after therapy for Asherman's syndrome will develop placentation defects such as placenta accreta.

Laboratory Evaluation.—The goal to the laboratory evaluation of secondary amenorrhea is to ensure that no serious disease process is causing the amenorrhea (e.g., hypothalamic or pituitary tumor, premature ovarian failure). The initial step in this process is to exclude the possibility of a pregnancy. At times this can be accomplished by a history and physical examination, but a measurement of the serum or urine hCG level is a more reliable way to exclude pregnancy. In our practice, all women with amenorrhea have serum prolactin and FSH levels measured. An elevated serum prolactin level can be due to multiple causes (e.g., pregnancy, tumor, pituitary tumor, hypothyroidism, renal failure, or psychoactive drugs), each of which requires further evaluation. An elevated FSH level suggests the presence of ovarian failure. Some authorities recommend a progestin withdrawal test to diagnose ovarian failure. It is our opinion that the sensitivity (less than 50%) and specificity (less than 50%) of the progestin withdrawal test for the diagnosis of ovarian failure are poor (Hull et al., 1979). We do not recommend its use for this purpose. Two tests that may be of value in the diagnosis of secondary amenorrhea are serum testosterone and thyroid function tests. Occasionally, women with ovarian androgen overproduction will present with amenorrhea. Usually signs such as hirsutism and acne will point to this diagnosis. Occasionally, women with hypothyroidism or hyperthyroidism will present with oligomenorrhea or amenorrhea. A good screening test for thyroid disease is the new immunoradiometric assay for TSH. It can be used to screen for both hyperthyroidism and hypothyroidism.

Although the progestin withdrawal test is of little value in diagnosing ovarian failure, it can be of value in evaluating hypothalamic-pituitary function in patients with secondary amenorrhea. The test consists of the administration of a progestin and monitoring the amount of uterine bleeding that occurs in the week after the progestin challenge. Prior to administration of the test, pregnancy must be excluded. The progestin can be administered orally (10 mg of medroxyprogesterone acetate/day for 5 days) or parenterally (100 mg of progesterone in oil). If the uterus is normal, bleeding in the week after the progestin challenge is a sign that significant endogenous estrogen production is present. Failure to bleed in the week after the progestin challenge suggests the presence of very low endogenous estrogen production. This is usually due to severe hypothalamic-pituitary dysfunction with very little GnRH, LH, or FSH output. Women with amenorrhea and an abnormal progestin withdrawal test result need to be evaluated carefully and followed closely. Many clinicians suggest that these women should have a structural study of the hypothalamus and pituitary. Occasionally, these amenorrheic women have a large hypothalamic or pituitary tumor that is endocrinologically silent.

ABNORMAL AND EXCESSIVE UTERINE BLEEDING

Abnormal uterine bleeding is one of the most commonly encountered clinical problems in gynecology. Uterine bleeding is abnormal if the bleeding pattern is *irregular* (polymenorrhea, less than 21 days between cycles; oligomenorrhea, more than 35 days between cycles), abnormal in *duration* (hypermenorrhea, more than 7 days of bleeding) or abnormal in *amount* (menorrhagia, more than 80 ml of blood loss during menses). Menometrorrhagia is an all-encompassing term used to describe irregular or excessive bleeding (or both) during menstruation or between menstrual cycles.

Abnormal uterine bleeding can be caused by a myriad of problems, including (1) pregnancy (e.g., spontaneous abortion, ectopic pregnancy, gestational trophoblastic disease), (2) tumors of the uterus (benign and malignant), (3) infection (e.g., endometritis), (4) hormonal abnormalities (e.g., anovulation and estrogen therapy), (5) intrauterine foreign bodies (e.g., intrauterine device, or IUD), and (6) coagulopathies (Table 3–4). The differential diagnosis of abnormal uterine bleeding is complex, but a systematic approach to the patient with uterine bleeding will usually result in the diagnosis of a treatable disease process.

The endometrium is a remarkably dynamic tissue. During the follicular phase of the menstrual cycle, under the stimulation of estrogen, the endometrium grows from 0.5 to 3.5 mm in height. Histologically, this growth is marked by many *mitoses* in the endometrial glands (proliferative phase). During the luteal phase of the menstrual cycle, the production of large amounts (25 mg/day) of progesterone by the corpus luteum causes the endometrium to stop growing and to differentiate in preparation for implantation of an embryo (secretory phase). At the end of the menstrual cycle, the programmed demise of the corpus luteum results in the withdrawal of progesterone and estrogen, causing sloughing of the endometrium and the initiation of menstrual bleeding.

The initiation and termination of normal menstrual bleeding require the orderly interaction of hormonal and structural events. The luteal-phase endometrium consists of three zones: basalis, stratum spongiosum, and stratum compactum. The inferior-most zone is the basalis, which connects the base of the endometrium to the myometrium. The basalis is the source of endometrial regeneration after menstrual sloughing has occurred. The stratum spongiosum is the midzone of the the endometrium. In the luteal phase, the stratum spongiosum is the largest zone and represents 50% of total endometrial height. The most impressive histological features of the stratum spongiosum is the presence of spiral, or coiled, arteries. These spiral arteries are very vasoactive. Just prior to the onset of menstruation, decreases in estrogen and progesterone levels and increases in prostaglandin levels cause the spiral arteries to undergo intense vasoconstriction. The vasospasm in the spiral arteries causes ischemia in the upper zones of the endometrium and initiates menstrual

TABLE 3–4.

Differential Diagnosis of Abnormal Uterine Bleeding

- I. Pregnancy
  - A. Spontaneous abortion
  - B. Ectopic pregnancy
  - C. Gestational trophoblastic disease
- II. Tumors of the uterus
  - A. Benign
    1. Cervical polyps
    2. Endometrial polyps
    3. Fibroids
  - B. Malignant
    1. Cervical cancer
    2. Endometrial cancer
    3. Fallopian tube cancer
- III. Infection
  - A. Endometritis
  - B. Cervicitis
- IV. Hormonal abnormalities
  - A. Endogenous (anovulation dysfunctional uterine bleeding)
  - B. Exogenous (hormone administration, e.g., estrogens)
- V. Intrauterine foreign body (e.g., IUD)
- VI. Coagulopathies
  - A. Platelet disorders
  - B. Abnormalities

sloughing of the endometrium. The superficial layer of the endometrium is the stratum compactum. The strata spongiosum and compactum comprise the "functional" zones of the endometrium, which participate in the cyclic process of menstruation.

The mechanisms by which pregnancy or tumors of the uterus cause abnormal uterine bleeding are easily understood. Implantation of the embryo involves invasion of the trophoblast into the endometrium and parasitization of the maternal blood supply. If the pregnancy should degenerate, the maternal blood supply becomes directly exposed to the uterine cavity, and bleeding ensues. Tumors of the uterus can cause abnormal bleeding by disrupting the normally continuous endometrial surface. Discontinuity in the endometrial surface results in bleeding. Endometritis produces abnormal uterine bleeding by disrupting the continuity of endometrial glands and blood vessels. The first step in the normal process of clotting is formation of a platelet plug. Any disease that interferes with the formation of a platelet plug (von Willebrand's disease or thrombocytopenia) can be associated with abnormal uterine bleeding. The hormonal abnormality that is the commonest cause of abnormal uterine bleeding is anovulation. Chronic exposure of the endometrium to estrogen without the stabilizing effects of progesterone produces a fragile endometrial surface that is prone to bleeding.

Diagnostic Evaluation

The history should characterize the temporal pattern, the duration, and the amount of bleeding. Contraceptive and sexual practices and the use of hormonal medication need to be explored. Bleeding during previous surgery and a family history of abnormal bleeding require discussion. The physical examination focuses on a determination of intravascular volume status (e.g., orthostatic hypotension, tachycardia), a careful pelvic examination to assess whether the bleeding is vaginal or uterine, and a thorough evaluation of uterine size. (Is it enlarged, irregular, or tender?) Examination of the skin for ecchymoses or petechiae may provide evidence for an underlying coagulopathy.

The laboratory evaluation of abnormal uterine bleeding should include (1) a complete blood cell count (CBC), (2) a Papanicolaou smear; (3) a sensitive blood pregnancy test (β-hCG); and (4) an endometrial biopsy, if necessary. The CBC will provide evidence for the diagnosis of anemia or thrombocytopenia. The Papanicolaou smear provides evidence for the presence of cervical cancer (and in some instances, endometrial cancer). A normal β-hCG test result rules out pregnancy. The endometrial biopsy provides a direct pathological evaluation of endometrial histology (e.g., endometrial cancer, hyperplasia, endometritis). These four tests, and a complete history and physical examination, will result in the diagnosis of a treatable disease in most cases of abnormal uterine bleeding.

Hormonal Abnormalities Causing Abnormal Uterine Bleeding

Normal, cyclic uterine bleeding requires the sequential appearance of estrogen alone (to promote endometrial growth), followed by the appearance of progesterone (to cause differentiation of the endometrium). As noted earlier, the cessation of estrogen and progesterone secretion (demise of the corpus luteum) initiates menstrual sloughing of the endometrium. The key factors that ensure normal menstrual cyclicity are the sequence of estrogen stimulation of the endometrium, followed by progesterone-induced differentiation. Processes that interfere with this normal sequence will often result in abnormal uterine bleeding. The commonest process that interferes with this normal sequence is constant estrogen stimulation in the absence of cyclic progesterone exposure. This can occur due to endogenous hormonal abnormalities (anovulation) or exogenous administration of estrogen.

Dysfunctional uterine bleeding is the term used to describe abnormal bleeding due to hormonal abnormalities. Dysfunctional uterine bleeding is the presence of abnormal uterine bleeding in the absence of pregnancy, tumor, infection, or coagulopathy. Most cases of dysfunctional uterine bleeding are associated with anovulation. For example, elite women athletes often develop anovulation and amenorrhea. In elite women athletes, low levels of GnRH result in very little ovarian estrogen production. Although many elite women athletes are anovulatory, they do not develop abnormal uterine bleeding, because their estrogen levels are too low to stimulate endometrial growth. These considerations also explain why prepubertal girls (less than 9 years old) and menopausal women do not usually develop abnormal uterine bleeding (low estrogen, no progesterone). In contrast, women with the polycystic ovary syndrome have significant amounts of continuous ovarian estrogen production but no ovulation and no progesterone production. These women are at high risk for developing dysfunctional uterine bleeding. In summary, dysfunctional uterine bleeding occurs most often in those anovulatory women who are producing significant amounts of ovarian estrogen. Anovulatory women who are producing no ovarian estrogen do not usually develop dysfunctional uterine bleeding.

Continuous ovarian estrogen production associated with anovulation occurs most commonly in teen-age girls and perimenopausal women. Consequently, the diagnosis of dysfunctional uterine bleeding is made most often for women in these two age groups. In teen-age women, the hypothalamus begins to secrete GnRH once a critical body mass (weight) is achieved. The GnRH secretion stimulates LH and FSH secretion, which causes an increase in ovarian estrogen production, but ovulation may not occur. The continuous estrogen exposure results in endometrial growth. The absence of ovulation and progesterone exposure prevents the proper maturation of the endometrium and may result in abnormal uterine bleeding. In teen-age women who are not pregnant, abnormal uterine bleeding is almost always due to a hormonal abnormality (anovulation) or a coagulopathy.

Like teenage girls, perimenopausal women develop dysfunctional uterine bleeding because of continuous exposure to estrogen without exposure to progesterone. In perimenopausal women, the ovary becomes depleted of healthy follicles and oocytes. Due to the low number of follicles present in the ovary, FSH levels become abnormally elevated. This stimulates estrogen production from the few remaining ovarian follicles. These "aged" follicles are often unable to grow to a size that would initiate ovulation. The hormonal milieu is therefore characterized by continuous estrogen unopposed by progesterone. In contrast to teenage girls, perimenopausal women frequently have endometrial hyperplasia or endometrial cancer as the cause of uterine bleeding. Therefore, all perimenopausal women with abnormal uterine bleeding need to have an endometrial biopsy or dilatation and curettage (D&C) to ensure that endometrial cancer is not present. Perimenopausal women with abnormal uterine bleeding should

never be treated with hormones until the results of the endometrial biopsy are available.

Chronic exposure to estrogen unopposed by progesterone is associated with a high risk of developing dysfunctional uterine bleeding. In most women, the ovary is the major source of estrogen production. However, estrogen can also be produced in fat tissue by the extraovarian aromatization of androstenedione to estrone. In markedly obese women, the excess adipose tissue results in abnormally increased extraovarian estrogen production. Since obesity is also associated with anovulation, obese women are at high risk for developing abnormal uterine bleeding.

The three groups of women who are at the greatest risk of developing dysfunctional uterine bleeding are teenage girls, obese women, and perimenopausal women. Before making a diagnosis of dysfunctional uterine bleeding, the clinician must be sure that pregnancy, tumor, and infection are not the cause of the bleeding. If chronic estrogen exposure unopposed by progesterone is the cause of the bleeding, therapy is directed to replacement of adequate amounts of progesterone. The method of progesterone replacement used to treat dysfunctional uterine bleeding depends on the patient's clinical presentation. For the teenage girl, oral contraceptives provide an excellent means of replacing her progesterone deficiency. For the perimenopausal woman, administration of an oral progestogen for 10 to 14 days each month helps regulate endometrial cyclicity. Many different oral progestins can be used for this purpose. One of the most commonly used oral progestins is medroxyprogesterone acetate (10 mg/day for 10 to 14 days each month). For the woman with anovulation and dysfunctional uterine bleeding who desires fertility, ovulation induction with clomiphene citrate or gonadotropins will cause ovulation, endogenous progesterone production, and possibly pregnancy. Many forms of progesterone replacement are available. The oral administration of "natural" progesterone results in low levels of progesterone in the blood due to intestinal and hepatic metabolism. However, natural progesterone can be given intramuscularly (100 mg each month) or intravaginally (25 mg three times daily for 10 days each month). The progesterone vaginal suppositories are very expensive, which limits the practicality of this dosage form.

Synthetic progestins that are well absorbed via the oral route have been produced. Medroxy-

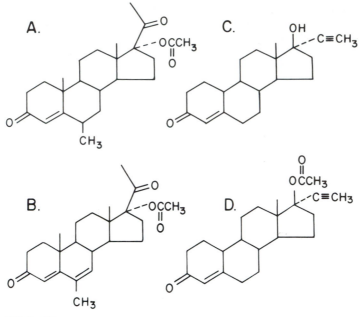

FIG 3–23.
Chemical structures of **(A)** medroxyprogesterone acetate, **(B)** megestrol acetate, **(C)** norethindrone, and **(D)** norethindrone acetate.

progesterone acetate and megestrol acetate are two synthetic progestins that are structurally very similar to progesterone (Fig 3–23, A and B). Typically, medroxyprogesterone is administered at a dose of 10 or 20 mg daily for 10 to 14 days. This duration of therapy is recommended because courses of progestin therapy shorter than 10 days can fail to prevent the appearance of endometrial hyperplasia. Courses of progestin therapy are repeated every month or every other month until the patient begins to ovulate spontaneously.

Norethindrone, norethindrone acetate, and norgestrel are three synthetic progestins that are structurally similar to progesterone and testosterone (Fig 3–23, C and D). Due to the structural similarities between norethindrone, norethindrone acetate, norgestrel, and testosterone, these three synthetic progestins have androgenic actions. All three decrease HDL levels at doses that are commonly used. Decreased HDL levels may be associated with an increased risk of atherosclerosis. In general, medroxyprogesterone acetate and megestrol acetate are the preferred agents for the treatment of abnormal uterine bleeding. If norethindrone or norethindrone acetate is to be used in the treatment of dysfunctional uterine

bleeding, it is usually prescribed at a dose of 5 mg daily for 10 to 14 days.

Occasionally, abnormal uterine bleeding is caused by the administration of hormones. The chronic administration of exogenous estrogen will often result in abnormal uterine bleeding (chronic estrogen unopposed by progesterone). This clinical occurrence is so widely appreciated that it is unusual to find a woman with an intact uterus who is being treated with unopposed estrogen. Approximately 20% of women receiving danazol have irregular uterine bleeding. In these women, endometrial biopsy specimens usually demonstrate atrophic endometrium.

An unusual endocrine cause of dysfunctional uterine bleeding is hyperthyroidism or hypothyroidism. Women with dysfunctional uterine bleeding who fail to respond to the standard therapy should be screened for thyroid disease by a careful history, physical examination, and thyroid function tests.

Abnormal Uterine Bleeding Due to Infections

Infections of the endometrium are characterized grossly by hyperemia and microscopically by edema and white blood cell infiltration. Disruption of vascular integrity by the infection can result in abnormal uterine bleeding. Bleeding caused by endometritis is usually characterized by intermittent spotting, not severe hemorrhage.

When compared with the fallopian tube, the endometrium is relatively resistant to infection. Incomplete spontaneous or therapeutic abortion can often cause endometrial infections. In this setting, causative organisms include *Escherichia coli,* enterococci, *Psedomonas aeruginosa,* and *Bacteroides* species. These infections are best treated by broad-spectrum antibiotic therapy and D&C. Endometritis not associated with a recent pregnancy can be due to *Chlamydia* or *Mycoplasma* species. These patients can be treated with tetracycline (250 mg orally four times daily for 3 weeks) or doxycycline (100 mg orally twice daily for 2 to 3 weeks).

Abnormal Uterine Bleeding Caused by Coagulopathies

The initial step in clot formation is the formation of a platelet plug. Diseases that inhibit platelet aggregation or decrease platelet number can be associated with abnormal uterine bleeding. Thrombocytopenia can be caused by a variety of diseases, including acute and chronic leukemias, lymphomas, and idiopathic thrombocytopenic purpura. Currently, the commonest cause of thrombocytopenia is treatment with high-dose chemotherapeutic agents, such as cyclophosphamide. von Willebrand's disease is a disorder of platelet aggregation and clot formation caused by an abnormal factor VIII. Abnormal uterine bleeding caused by coagulopathies is best treated by correcting the underlying abnormality. However, in many cases this is not possible.

An alternative approach is to produce a quiescent endometrium that is not cycling and that will not undergo withdrawal bleeding. This can be accomplished by chronic GnRH agonist therapy or with combined estrogen-progestogen oral contraceptives. The GnRH agonists produce paradoxical inhibition (downregulation) of pituitary gonadotropin production and cause the cessation of ovarian estrogen production. In a hypoestrogenic environment, the endometrium becomes inactive. Leuprolide acetate is a GnRH agonist that can be used in the treatment of abnormal uterine bleeding. The daily, subcutaneous administration of 0.5 mg of leuprolide acetate will result in a decrease in LH and FSH production and a cessation of ovarian follicular activity. The low estrogen levels associated with leuprolide acetate therapy produce a quiescent endometrium that does not cycle. Another approach is to use combined estrogen-progestin oral contraceptives to prevent a menstrual bleed during an episode of thrombocytopenia. This approach is of special value for women receiving cyclic courses of chemotherapeutic agents, such as cyclophosphamide. In these women, the oral contraceptives can be used to prevent a menstrual bleed during the thrombocytopenic episode that follows the chemotherapy. After the thrombocytopenic episode is past, the oral contraceptives can be stopped, and a "normal" withdrawal bleed will be initiated.

Treatment of Life-Threatening Uterine Bleeding

Occasionally, women will come to the emergency room of a hospital with life-threatening vaginal bleeding. Rapid evaluation and therapy are required to minimize morbidity and mortality. Initial evaluation should include a CBC, coagulation studies (prothrombin time, partial thromboplastin time), a rapid, sensitive pregnancy test, and if indicated, an endometrial curettage. Coagulopathies require correction with the appropriate replacement products (platelets or fresh frozen plasma). If the uterus is structurally normal by physical examination, ultrasound, or both, the pregnancy test result is negative, and the D&C does not slow the bleeding, aggressive hormonal therapy may be required. Conjugated estrogens (25 mg intravenously every 4 hours for three doses) have been used successfully in the treatment of life-threatening uterine hemorrhage that is not due to a pregnancy or tumor. Alternatively, large doses of a combined estrogen-progestin medication may be used. For example, 0.05 mg of ethinyl estradiol plus 0.5 mg of norgestrel (Ovral) given four times daily for up to 7 days may slow the bleeding.

In severe cases of uterine bleeding, where conventional therapy has failed, angiographic embolization of the uterine arteries may help control the bleeding. In some cases, hysterectomy may be required to treat episodes of life-threatening uterine bleeding.

DYSMENORRHEA

Dysmenorrhea, or painful menstruation, is one of the commonest gynecologic problems. Approximately 50% of all women experience dysmenorrhea, and approximately 5% of women of reproductive age are incapacitated for 1 to 3 days each month because of dysmenorrhea. For clinical purposes, dysmenorrhea is often divided into two broad categories: primary and secondary. Primary dysmenorrhea is the presence of painful menstruation in the absence of demonstrable pelvic disease. Secondary dysmenorrhea is the occurrence of painful menstruation due to pelvic pathology, such as endometriosis, chronic pelvic inflammatory disease, or uterine leiomyomas. It is often difficult to differentiate between primary and secondary dysmenorrhea based on the history and physical examination. Trials of empiric drug therapy and diagnostic laparoscopy are often necessary to discover the cause of the dysmenorrhea.

In primary dysmenorrhea, the pain characteristically begins with the onset of menstruation and lasts for 12 to 72 hours. The pain is usually confined to the lower abdomen and is most intense in the midline. The pain is often described as crampy and intermittently intense. In some women, back pain and thigh pain may be severe. The abdominal pain is often accompanied by nausea, diarrhea, fatigue, headache, and a general sense of malaise. The pain is usually most severe on the first day of menstruation and gradually diminishes.

Current evidence suggests that prostaglandin $F_{2\alpha}$ ($PGF_{2\alpha}$) and prostaglandin E_2 (PGE_2) released from the endometrium at the time of menstruation cause primary dysmenorrhea (Ylikorkala and Dawood, 1978). Prostaglandin $F_{2\alpha}$ and PGE_2 are derivatives of the fatty acid arachidonic acid. The sequential stimulation of the endometrium by estrogen, followed by progesterone, results in a dramatic increase in prostaglandin production by the endometrium. At the time of menstruation, the endometrial cells undergo lysis and release $PGF_{2\alpha}$ and PGE_2. Prostaglandins induce smooth muscle contraction (or relaxation) in many diverse tissues. Uterine smooth muscle contractions induced by the prostaglandins produce the colicky, spasmodic, laborlike lower abdominal and back pain characteristic of dysmenorrhea. Prostaglandin-induced uterine contractions can last many minutes and may produce intrauterine pressures greater than 60 mm Hg. When uterine pressure exceeds mean arterial pressure for a prolonged period of time, uterine ischemia will ensue. Uterine ischemia results in the accumulation of anaerobic metabolites that can stimulate the small type C pain neurons. In many ways, primary dysmenorrhea is the manifestation of "angina" of the uterus. Many factors can modulate prostaglandin-induced uterine contractions. For example, strenuous exercise can increase uterine tone (possibly because of decreased uterine blood flow). Many women athletes note that strenuous exercise at the time of menstruation increases the severity of their dysmenorrhea. Other women report that caffeine ingestion can decrease the severity of dysmenorrhea. Caffeine may increase uterine cyclic adenosine monophosphate levels, resulting in decreased uterine tone. In addition to stimulating uterine contractions, $PGF_{2\alpha}$ and PGE_2 can cause contraction of bronchial, bowel, and vascular smooth muscle, producing bronchoconstriction (asthma), diarrhea, and hypertension. As noted earlier, diarrhea is commonly associated with primary dysmenorrhea.

The hypothesis that prostaglandins, released from the endometrium, cause primary dysmenorrhea is supported by the observation that endometrial concentrations of PGE_2 and $PGF_{2\alpha}$ correlate with the severity of dysmenorrhea. In general, women with the highest endometrial concentrations of $PGF_{2\alpha}$ and PGE_2 have the severest dysmenorrhea (Chan et al., 1979). High rates of endometrial prostaglandin production require the sequential stimulation of the endometrium by estrogen followed by progesterone. In general, women who menstruate but do not ovulate (no progesterone) do not have primary dysmenorrhea. In most girls, the menses, which immediately follow menarche (approximately age 12 years), are anovulatory due to immaturity of the hypothalamic-pituitary axis. Since regular, ovulatory, cycles may not begin until 2 to 5 years after menarche, it is not unusual to find that for many teenagers the onset of primary dysmenorrhea occurs a few years after menarche.

Secondary dysmenorrhea is the occurrence of painful menstruation due to pelvic pathology such as endometriosis or chronic pelvic inflammatory disease. The major clinical goal of the evaluation of dysmenorrhea is to identify whether the process is primary or secondary. It is often difficult to differentiate between primary and secondary dysmenorrhea based on history and physical examination. However, many women with secondary dysmenorrhea will report that the dysmenorrhea (1) began after age 20 years, (2) often lasts for 5 to 7 days each month, and (3) has progressively increased in severity. In addition, women with secondary dysmenorrhea usually report the occurrence of pelvic pain at times other than menses. By definition, women with primary dysmenorrhea have a normal pelvic examination. Women with secondary dysmenorrhea may also have a normal pelvic examination if the pelvic pathology cannot be palpated (e.g., stage I endometriosis, adenomyosis, pelvic adhesions). Some women with secondary dysmenorrhea have markedly abnormal pelvic examinations. If the pelvic examination is abnormal, appropriate clinical action should be immediately undertaken (e.g., ultrasound, diagnostic laparoscopy, exploratory laparotomy). For example, a woman with dysmenorrhea and a pelvic examination suggestive of severe endometriosis (cul-de-sac induration, uterosacral ligament nodularity, adnexal masses) should be scheduled for laparoscopy or laparotomy to confirm the diagnosis. In the evaluation of a woman with dysmenorrhea, pelvic ultrasound may be helpful in identifying uterine (fibroids) or adnexal masses (hydrosalpinx) that cannot be palpated on pelvic examination. In women with secondary dysmenorrhea, a CBC and erythrocyte sedimentation rate (ESR) may raise the suspicion of chronic pelvic inflammatory disease (high white blood cell count and high ESR).

In a woman with dysmenorrhea, a history consistent with primary dysmenorrhea, and a normal pelvic examination, it is our policy to treat as for primary dysmenorrhea. If aggressive therapy for primary dysmenorrhea fails to relieve the pain, additional studies (e.g., ultrasound, laparoscopy) should be considered to determine if a cause of secondary dysmenorrhea is present. As previously noted, the cause of primary dysmenorrhea is elevated endometrial prostaglandin production. Therefore, the therapy for primary dysmenorrhea should be directed at reducing endometrial prostaglandin production. Anti-inflammatory agents that directly inhibit prostaglandin production or action (ibuprofen) and agents that suppress ovulation (oral contraceptives) are very effective in reducing endometrial prostaglandin production. Table 3–5 lists inhibitors of prostaglandin production that have been used successfully in the treatment of dysmenorrhea. All of these agents inhibit the cyclooxygenase enzyme. In addition to inhibiting the cyclooxygenase enzyme system, mefenamic acid also directly blocks activation of

TABLE 3–5.

Inhibitors of Prostaglandin Synthesis Commonly Used in the Treatment of Dysmenorrhea

Drug Class	Drug	Standard Dose
Fenamates	Mefenamic acid	500-mg loading dose 250 mg 4 times daily
	Flufenamic acid	100–200 mg 3 times daily
	Tolfenamic acid	133 mg 3 times daily
Phenylpro-pionic acid	Ibuprofen	400 mg 4 times daily
	Naproxen sodium	550-mg loading dose; 275 mg 4 times daily
	Ketoprofen	50 mg 3 times daily

the prostaglandin receptor. The agents listed in Table 3–5 are associated with a very low incidence of serious adverse effects. In fact, ibuprofen is available without a prescription. Side effects of the prostaglandin synthesis inhibitors include gastrointestinal irritation and ulceration, nausea, prolonged bleeding time, renal papillary necrosis, and decreased renal blood flow.

In general, we initiate therapy for dysmenorrhea with ibuprofen at a dose of 400 mg orally four times daily. Therapy is initiated just prior to menses for those women who can accurately predict the onset of menses or at the time of onset of menses. Therapy usually lasts 3 to 4 days. If ibuprofen (an arylpropionic acid derivative) fails to be effective, we usually initiate a trial with a drug in the fenamate class (mefenamic acid). If naproxen is to be used in the treatment of primary dysmenorrhea, we prefer the sodium salt because it is more rapidly absorbed and reaches a higher peak plasma level than the acid.

Oral contraceptives contain a combination of estrogen (ethinyl estradiol) and a progestogen (19-norprogestin). Oral contraceptives suppress endometrial prostaglandin production by inhibiting ovulation (no endogenous progesterone production) and by preventing normal synchronous endometrial growth and differentiation (constant estrogen and progestogen prevents normal endometrial growth).

If 3 to 6 months of therapy fails to produce a significant decrease in dysmenorrhea, the clinician should carefully review the history and physical examination to ensure that a cause of secondary dysmenorrhea has not been overlooked. Pelvic ultrasound and diagnostic laparoscopy should be considered if the patient fails to respond to treatment with prostaglandin synthesis inhibitors. Two studies of chronic pelvic pain, one in a population of adolescent girls (Goldstein et al., 1980) and one in a population of adult women (Kresch et al., 1984) demonstrate the importance of performing diagnostic laparoscopy in women with chronic pelvic pain that fails to respond to supportive therapy. In both studies a significant number (more than 30%) of women with chronic pelvic pain had documented pelvic abnormalities (e.g., adhesions, endometriosis, pelvic inflammatory disease) that accounted for the pain.

PREMENSTRUAL SYNDROME

Premenstrual syndrome (PMS) can be defined as the cyclic recurrence during the luteal phase of the menstrual cycle of a combination of distressing physical, psychological, or behavioral changes that interfere with familial, social, or work-related activities. Approximately 20% of women of reproductive age have PMS. For most of these women, the symptoms are mild or moderate. Approximately 5% of women of reproductive age have such severe PMS that it threatens their work and interpersonal relationships. Premenstrual syndrome is commonest in women 25 to 45 years of age. The symptoms of PMS are diverse but include (1) body pain (headache, cramps, fatigue), (2) water retention (weight gain, swelling, painful breasts), (3) negative affect (depression, crying, loneliness, irritability), (4) autonomic reactions (cold sweats, dizziness, fainting), (5) behavioral changes (decreased efficiency, difficulty concentrating, lowered motor coordination), and (6) somatization (feelings of suffocation, chest pain, ringing in the ears, blind spots, blurry vision, numbness, tingling). To provide order to these diverse symptoms and signs, Abraham (1983) devised a classification schema consisting of four categories (Table 3–6). These categories are not all-inclusive, but they do help the clinician organize history taking for patients with PMS.

The first step in the diagnosis of PMS is to have the patient keep a daily symptom diary for 2 months. If examination of the daily symptom diary reveals that the symptoms are temporally clustered prior to menses (late luteal phase) and disappear 2 or 3 days after the initiation of menses, PMS should be strongly suspected. In addition

TABLE 3–6.

Abraham's (1983) Classification of Premenstrual Syndrome

A—anxiety
Nervous tension
Mood swings
Irritability
Anxiety
C—cravings
Headache
Craving for sweets
Increase appetite
Heart pounding
Fatigue
Dizziness or faintness
D—depression
Depression
Forgetfulness
Crying
Confusion
Insomnia
H—water-related symptoms
Weight gain
Swelling of extremities
Breast tenderness
Abdominal bloating

to late luteal-phase symptoms, an occasional woman with PMS has periovulatory exacerbation of symptoms. If examination of the symptom diary reveals no symptom-free week in the early follicular phase, a chronic psychiatric disorder such as depression or anxiety should be strongly suspected.

Approximately 30% of women who seek treatment for PMS have a chronic psychiatric disorder. As noted above, these women can often be identified by the absence of a symptom-free week in the follicular phase of the menstrual cycle. In addition, some experienced practitioners suggest that all women with symptoms consistent with PMS complete a personality inventory such as the Minnesota Multiphasic Personality Inventory to further screen for individuals with depression or pathological anxiety. Women with symptoms of PMS who also have major depression or severe anxiety are best treated by referral to individuals experienced in supportive psychiatric or psychological counseling. In summary, the diagnosis of PMS is a two-step process. The first step involves obtaining a daily symptom diary to assess the temporal relationship of the symptoms to menses. The second step involves screening for chronic psychiatric problems. Since there is no "blood test" for the diagnosis of PMS, the skills of each clinician are challenged in the evaluation of each woman with this disorder (Freeman et al., 1985).

The etiology of PMS is not understood. Numerous theories have been proposed—estrogen excess, progesterone deficiency, fluid retention, vitamin B_6 deficiency, hyperprolactinemia, hormone allergies, and prostaglandin abnormalities—but none has been proved. Currently, a popular theory is that progesterone or metabolites of progesterone interact with neurotransmitters and ion channels in the brain. Recent experiments suggest that metabolites of progesterone may modulate neural γ-aminobutyric acid receptors (a common neural ion channel). Another hypothesis is that some women develop abnormalities of endogenous neural opioid peptides and demonstrate symptoms of endogenous opioid withdrawal in the late luteal phase of the menstrual cycle. Investigators have demonstrated abnormally low levels of circulating opioid peptides in women with PMS in the late luteal phase of the menstrual cycle. In all likelihood, the symptoms of PMS are due to the complex interaction of ovarian hormones, central neurotransmitters, and the autonomic nervous system (Reid and Yen, 1981).

Therapy for PMS should include a comprehensive program of education, psychological counseling and support, exercise, dietary manipulations, and if necessary, pharmacological interventions. Effective dietary manipulations include minimizing daily intake of alcohol, nicotine, simple sugars, caffeine, and salt. Exercise programs and psychological counseling can help the individual with PMS regain control of her life. Pharmacological therapy of PMS is controversial. At least 10 different pharmacologic agents have been used in the treatment of PMS. These agents include mefanamic acid, alprazolam, bromocriptine, vitamin B_6, γ-linoleic acid, GnRH agonists, progesterone, oral contraceptives, diuretics, and lithium. A major problem with pharmacological trials for the treatment of PMS is that few have been conducted in a randomized, prospective fashion utilizing placebo controls. Since placebo therapy can cause significant improvement in PMS, controlled clinical trials are absolutely necessary before a drug can be accepted as effective for the treatment of PMS (Maddocks et al., 1986). Five agents that have been demonstrated to be of significant clinical value are mefanamic acid,

γ-linoleic acid, GnRH agonists, alprazolam, and diuretics. The use of each agent in the treatment of PMS will be described.

Mefanamic acid is a nonsteroidal agent that inhibits prostaglandin synthesis and competes for binding at the prostaglandin receptor site. In addition to its use in PMS, mefanamic acid is also of value in the treatment of moderate pain. As noted in Table 3–5, for the treatment of PMS, mefanamic acid is usually administered as a 500 mg loading dose, followed by 250 mg four times daily for up to 7 days. Prolonged administration of mefanamic acid is not recommended since it can result in decreased renal blood flow and renal papillary necrosis. Common side effects of mefanamic acid therapy include diarrhea, nausea, vomiting, and drowsiness. Mefanamic acid is especially effective in the treatment of pain symptoms associated with PMS.

γ-Linoleic acid (evening primrose oil) is a dietary supplement especially useful in the treatment of breast symptoms, bloating, weight gain and edema associated with PMS. γ-Linoleic acid is a precursor for prostaglandin E_1 (PGE_1) and may be effective in the treatment of PMS because it alters prostaglandin production and metabolism. A standard dose of γ-linoleic acid is 3 gm/day in the late luteal phase of the cycle. γ-Linoleic acid is available without a prescription in stores specializing in dietary supplements.

Gonadotropin-releasing hormone agonists such as nafarelin and leuprolide are especially useful in the treatment of severe PMS (Muse et al., 1984). Synthetic changes in amino acids 6 and 10 of the hypothalamic decapeptide GnRH produce agents with long half-lives and high affinity for the pituitary GnRH receptor. Chronic administration of these compounds produces a transient stimulation of pituitary LH and FSH secretion and then paradoxically results in the complete suppression of LH and FSH secretion. Therefore, chronic administration of the GnRH agonists produces an anovulatory, amenorrheic state that usually results in complete relief of the symptoms of PMS. The major side effects of the GnRH agonists are attributable to hypoestrogenism (e.g., osteoporosis, hot flashes, dry vagina). Prolonged use of GnRH agonists (greater than 6 months) has not been demonstrated to be safe. Effective doses of the GnRH agonists are 0.5 mg of leuprolide administered subcutaneously daily or 200 μg of nafarelin administered twice daily intranasally.

Alprazolam is a member of the benzodiazepine class of psychoactive agents. The molecular mechanism of action of alprazolam is unknown, but all benzodiazepines cause a dose-related CNS depressant effect. Alprazolam is especially effective in the treatment of anxiety caused by PMS. For the treatment of PMS, alprazolam is recommended at a dose of 0.25 mg three times daily during the late luteal phase of the cycle. The dose can be titrated to the needs of the patient. A major side effect of alprazolam is drowsiness. In some patients, discontinuance of benzodiazepines can produce withdrawal symptoms that include insomnia, dysphoria, abdominal cramps, sweating, tremors, and convulsions. When prescribing alprazolam for the treatment of PMS, the clinician must carefully screen for the occurrence of withdrawal symptoms. If withdrawal symptoms occur, the drug should be permanently discontinued.

In women with significant premenstrual weight gain (more than 1.5 kg), short-term diuretic therapy may help relieve the symptoms of bloating, edema, and breast fullness. Metolazone (2.5 mg/day) or spironolactone (25 mg four times daily) administered during the late luteal phase of the menstrual cycle has been shown to be effective in the treatment of PMS. All diurectics can produce electrolyte imbalance, and women given diurectics for PMS should be evaluated for electrolyte abnormalities.

Three agents that have been reported to be successful in the treatment of PMS in uncontrolled trials are progesterone, oral contraceptives, and lithium. However, controlled clinical trials have failed to consistently demonstrate a beneficial effect of these agents. Until further research is completed, we would not recommend their use in the treatment of PMS.

Vitamin B_6 at doses of 500 mg daily has been demonstrated to be effective in the treatment of PMS. However, at this dose level, vitamin B_6 therapy is associated with the onset of sensorineural deficits. Given the potentially serious side effects of high-dose vitamin B_6 therapy, we do not recommend its use.

Bromocriptine is a dopamine agonist that is extremely effective in the treatment of hyperprolactinemia. The majority of controlled clinical trials do not suggest that it is of significant value in the treatment of PMS. If it is to be used in the treatment of PMS, it should probably be reserved for women with complaints isolated to the breast. It should be emphasized that pharmacological therapy should not be an isolated intervention in the treatment of PMS. Drug therapy should be a part of a comprehensive program of dietary, exercise, and counseling therapy.

REFERENCES

Abraham GE: Nutritional factors in the etiology of the premenstrual tension syndromes. *J Reprod Med* 1983; 28:446.

Barbieri RL, Ryan KJ: Bromocriptine, endocrine pharmacology and therapeutic applications. *Fertil Steril* 1983; 39:727.

Burgas R, Butcher M, Ling N, et al: Structure moleculair du facteur hypothalamique (LRF) d'origine ovine controlant la secretion de l'hormone gonadotrope hypophysaire de luteinisation (LH) *C R Acad Sci* 1971; 273:1611.

Catt KJ, Pierce JG: Gonadotropic hormones of the adenohypophysis, in Yen SSC, Jaffe RB, (Eds): *Reproductive Endocrinology*. WB Saunders Co, Philadelphia 1986, pp 75–114.

Chan WY, Dawood MY, Fuchs F: Relief of dysmenorrhea with the prostaglandin synthetase inhibitor ibuprofen: effect of prostaglandin levels in menstrual fluid. *Am J Obstet Gynecol* 1979; 135:102.

Crowley WF, Filicori M, Spratt DI, et al: The physiology of gonadotropin-releasing hormone (GnRH) secretion in men and women. *Recent Prog Horm Res* 1985; 41:473.

DiZerga GS, Hodgen GD: Folliculogenesis in the primate ovarian cycle. *Endocr Rev* 1981; 2:27.

Dorrington JH, Armstrong DT: Effects of FSH on gonadal functions. *Recent Progr Horm Res* 1979; 35:301.

Freeman EN, Sondheimer S, Weinbaum PJ, et al: Evaluating premenstrual symptoms in medical practice. *Obstet Gynecol* 1985; 65:500.

Friedman AJ, Barbieri RL: Leuprolide acetate: Applications in gynecology. *Curr Probl Obstet Gynecol Fertil* 1988; 6:209.

Fries H: Epidemiology of secondary amenorrhea. *Am J Obstet Gynecol* 1974; 118:473.

Goldstein DP, deCholnoky C, Emans SJ, et al: Laparoscopy in the diagnosis and management of pelvic pain in adolescents. *J Reprod Med* 1980; 24:251.

Greep RO: Gonadotropins, in McCann SM (Ed): *Endocrinology, People and Ideas*. Bethesda, Md, American Physiological Society, 1988, pp 63–85.

Halberg L, Nilsson L: Determination of menstrual blood loss. *Scand J Clin Lab Invest* 1964; 16:244.

Harris GW: Humours and hormones. The Sir Henry Dale Lecture for 1971. *J Endocrinol* 1972; 53:ii.

Hitschmann F, Adler L: Der Bau der Uterusschleimhaut des geschlechtsreifen Weibes, mit besonderer Berücksichtigung der Menstruation. *Mschr Geburtsh Gynak* 1908; 27:1–82.

Hull MGR, Knuth UA, Murray MAF, et al: The practical value of the progesterone challenge test in the assessment of the estrogen state and response to clomiphene in amenorrhea. *Br J Obstet Gynaecol* 1979; 86:799.

Joseph A, Thomas IM: Cytogenetic investigation in 150 cases with complaints of sterility or primary amenorrhea. *Hum Genet* 1982; 61:105.

Knobil E: The neuroendocrine control of the menstrual cycle. *Recent Prog Horm Res* 1980; 36:53.

Koyama H: Cyclophosphamide-induced ovarian failure. *Cancer* 1977; 39:1403.

Kresch AJ, Seifer DB, Sachs LB, et al: Laparoscopy in 100 women with chronic pelvic pain. *Obstet Gynecol* 1984; 64:672.

Landgren BM, Unden AL, Diczfalusy E: Hormonal profile of the cycle in 68 normally menstruating women. *Acta Endocrinol* 1980; 94:89.

Lightman A, Tarlatzis BC, Rzasa PJ, et al: The ovarian renin-angiotensin system. *Am J Obstet Gynecol* 1987; 156:808.

Maddocks S, Hahn P, Moller F, et al: A double-blind placebo-controlled trial of progesterone vaginal suppositories in the treatment of premenstrual syndrome. *Am J Obstet Gynecol* 1986; 154:573.

McCann SM (ed): in *Endocrinology, People and Ideas*. Bethesda, Md, American Physiological Society, 1988, pp 41–62.

McCann SM, Rettori V: Physiology of luteinizing hormone–releasing hormone. *Semin Reprod Endocrinol* 1987; 5:33.

McNatty KP, Smith SM, Makris A, et al: The microenvironment of the human antral follicle. *J Clin Endocrinol Metab* 1979; 49:851.

Moore RY: Neuroendocrine mechanisms: Cells and systems in Yen SSC, Jaffe RB (eds): *Reproductive Endocrinology*. Philadelphia, Saunders Co, 1986, pp 3–31.

Muse KN, Cetel NS, Futterman LA, et al: The premenstrual syndrome: The effects of "medical ovariectomy." *N Engl J Med* 1984; 311:1345.

Noyes RW, Hertig AT, Rock J: Dating the endometrial biopsy. *Fertil Steril* 1950; 1:3.

Reid RL, Yen SSC: Premenstrual syndrome. *Am J Obstet Gynecol* 1981; 139:85.

Reindollar RH: Delayed sexual development: A study of 252 patients. *Am J Obstet Gynecol* 1981; 140:371.

Reindollar RH, Novak M, Tho SPT, et al: Adult-onset amenorrhea: A study of 262 patients. *Am J Obstet Gynecol* 1986; 155:531.

Ross GT, Schreiber JR: The Ovary, in Yen SSC, Jaffe RB (eds): *Reproductive Endocrinology*. Philadelphia, Saunders Co, 1986, pp 115–139.

Ryan KJ: Human ovarian function, in Sakamoto S, Tojo S, Nakayama T (eds): *Gynecology and Obstetrics*. Proceedings of the IX World Congress of Gynecology and Obstetrics. Amsterdam, Excepta Medica, 1980, pp 3–9.

Ryan KJ: The endocrine pattern and control of the ovulatory cycle, in Insler V, Lunenfeld B (eds): *Infertility: Male and Female*. New York, Churchill Livingstone, 1986, pp 57–72.

Ryan KJ: Endocrine function of the ovary, in McCann SM (ed): *Endocrinology, People and Ideas*. Bethesda, Md, American Physiological Society, 1988, pp 201–213.

Ryan KJ, Makris A: Significance of angiogenic and growth factors in ovarian follicular development, in Mahesh VB, Dhindsa, DS, Anderson E, et al (eds): *Regulation of Ovarian and Testicular Function*. New York, Plenum Press, 1987, pp 203–209.

Ryan KJ, Petro Z, Kaiser J: Steroid formation by isolated and recombined ovarian granulosa and thecal cells. *J Clin Endocrinol Metab* 1968; 28:355.

Ryan KJ, Smith OW: Biogenesis of steroid hormones in the human ovary. *Recent Prog Horm Res* 1965; 21:367.

Savard K, Marsh JM, Rice BF: Gonadotropins and ovarian steroidogenesis. *Recent Prog Horm Res* 1965; 21:285.

Sawyer CH: Anterior pituitary neural control concepts, in McCann Sm (ed): *Endocrinology, People and Ideas*. Bethesda Md, American Physiological Society, 1988, pp 23–39.

Schally AV, Arimura A, Kastin AJ, et al: Gonadotropin-releasing hormone: One polypeptide regulates secretion of luteinizing and follicle-stimulating hormones. *Science* 1971; 173:1036.

Treloar AE, Boynton RE, Behn BG, et al: Variations of the human menstrual cycle through reproductive life. *Int J Fertil* 1967; 12:77.

Tureck RW, Strauss JF III: Progesterone synthesis by luteinized human granulosa cells in culture. The role of de novo sterol synthesis and lipoprotein-carried sterol. *J Clin Endocrinol Metab* 1982; 54:367.

Weiss G, O'Byrne EM, Hochman JA, et al: Secretion of progesterone and relaxin by the human corpus luteum in midpregnancy and at term. *Obstet Gynecol* 1977; 50:679.

Yen SSC: Neuroendocrine Control of Hypophyseal function in Yen SSC, Jaffe RB (eds): *Reproductive Endocrinology*. Philadelphia, Saunders Co, 1986, pp 33–74.

Ylikorkala O, Dawood MY: New concepts in dysmenorrhea. *Am J Obstet Gynecol* 1978; 130:833.

4 _____ The Vulva

Thomas Leavitt, Jr., M.D.

GENERAL CONSIDERATIONS

The vulva, or external female genitalia, includes the following structures: labia majora, labia minora, clitoris, vestibule, hymen, vestibular bulbs, mons veneris, urethral meatus, vulvovaginal glands, and periurethral gland ducts. The outer portion of the vulva is covered by somewhat altered skin, which contains hair follicles and sweat and sebaceous glands. This is modified on the inner surface so that the inner portions of the labia minora are moist and do not contain hair follicles. The vulva serves as the entrance to the vagina and, in the normal state, covers and protects the urethral orifice. The labia have specific importance in the process of urination since it has been found that, following vulvectomy, uncontrolled "spraying" is a common complaint.

The anatomic location of the vulva predisposes its structures to unusual and occasionally rare disorders. At the same time, systemic diseases such as diabetes, anemia, Addison's disease, and gout may manifest themselves first by vulvar changes and complaints therefrom. The importance of venereal diseases as a major cause of symptomatology from these structures is obvious, and each will be considered in this chapter. Since a good portion of the vulvar area may be properly classified as skin, it is at once evident that any specific cutaneous disease may occur here, but because of certain variations, diagnosis may be difficult or even impossible. Difficulty in diagnosis is aggravated by the tendency of the patient to procrastinate and to use self-medication when the lesion involves the genitalia. Patient delay is of extreme importance when the disease is malignant, since carcinoma involving these structures has a poor prognosis unless discovered early. Of equal importance in this problem is the responsibility of the physician. Numerous studies have shown that "physician delay" may actually exceed "patient delay" by many months.

Success in the diagnosis and treatment of lesions of the vulva will be forthcoming only if the physician investigates completely all possible etiologic factors and performs a meticulous examination. A thorough interview should determine the exact site and duration of specific complaints as well as generalized symptoms. Inquiry should be made about diarrhea or discharge, applications of lotions, medications or soaps, systemic medications, contraceptives, sexual habits, clothing changes, and, of major importance, events that might be causative in producing mental stress, worry, or anxiety. The examiner should scrutinize closely the oral mucosa, fingernails, scalp, and pubic hair as part of the gynecologic examination. It is not sufficient to allay symptoms, since recurrence is commonplace. Therefore, the cause of the disorder must be found and specific therapy instituted.

EMBRYOLOGY

In the female, as in the male, the external genitalia develop in connection with the genital tubercle, a conical prominence caudal to the umbilical cord. This tubercle appears in the 8-mm embryo (5 weeks)* as a simple protrusion (Fig 4–1) and later is noted to present a groove along its caudal surface—the urethral groove. The urethra is subsequently formed from this groove. The genital tubercle becomes clearly defined as a

*Measurements correspond to values of F.P. Mall, and ages are "ovulation age," or 2 weeks less than menstrual age.

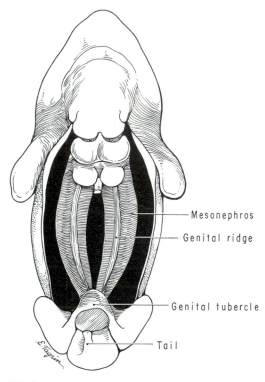

FIG 4–1.
Schematic representation of 9-mm human embryo in frontal section to show anatomic relations of the genital tubercle.

phallus in the 16- to 18-mm embryo (6–7 weeks), whereas the specific external genitalia of either male or female type are formed in the 40-mm embryo (10 weeks).

The cloacal membrane is an epithelial structure located in the ventral portion of the embryo caudal to the genital tubercle. This membrane consists of an inner (cephalic) layer of entodermal cells and an outer (caudal) layer of ectodermal cells. When the cloacal membrane perforates about the 12th week, the openings of the urethra, vagina, and anus are clearly visible. The rudimentary external genitalia appear about the sixth week of embryonic life as swellings on either side of the cloacal membrane. These swellings later project to form the genital folds, which extend cephalad to join the genital tubercle (Fig 4–2). The genital folds become the labia minora, and the clitoris is derived from the genital tubercle. The labia majora develop from swellings at the outer sides of the genital folds (lateral genital folds). These lateral genital folds join cephalad to form the genital eminence or mons veneris, whereas caudad they

curve medially to form the posterior commissure. About the fifth or sixth month a secondary upgrowth of tissue around the clitoris forms a fold, or hood, about it, the preputium clitoridis, or prepuce.

When the cloaca becomes divided into a dorsal and ventral segment by the downgrowth of a septum, which grows mainly from mesoderm, two compartments are formed. The ventral portion constitutes the urogenital sinus and is bounded at its lower end by the cloacal membrane. The wolffian ducts are embedded in this mesoderm of the downgrowing septum on either side and later become implanted in the septum. When division is complete, they open into the urogenital sinus. Above the site of their implantation, the urogenital sinus dilates to become the urinary bladder. The dorsal segment formed by the aforementioned downgrowth of mesoderm (sometimes called the urorectal fold) differentiates into the rectum. Thus, at this stage of development (12- to 14-mm embryo), both rectum and bladder are continuous with the urogenital sinus, which is closed at its lower end by the cloacal membrane (Fig 4–3). Bartholin's glands appear as outgrowths from the walls of the urogenital sinus.

At the site where the solid müllerian ducts join the sinus, the hymen is ultimately formed. As these solid masses of cells at the termination of the müllerian ducts proliferate, vaginal bulbs form, which grow downward along the posterior wall of the sinus. They increase in size and press against the walls of the sinus, invaginating it, so that the upper part of the sinus becomes gradually shortened. In this manner, the openings of the ducts of Bartholin's glands are brought close to the hymenal margin. Later, the solid vagina, thus formed, breaks down in the center and, at the site where its cavity opens into the sinus, the hymenal orifice is formed. The remainder of the urogenital sinus in front of the hymen forms the vestibule. Figure 4–4 illustrates the definitive female genital system.

ANATOMY AND HISTOLOGY

Labia Majora

The skin covering the labia majora is thick, contains many sebaceous and sweat glands, and is covered with hair except along the lower part of the inner aspect. The extent of the glandular de-

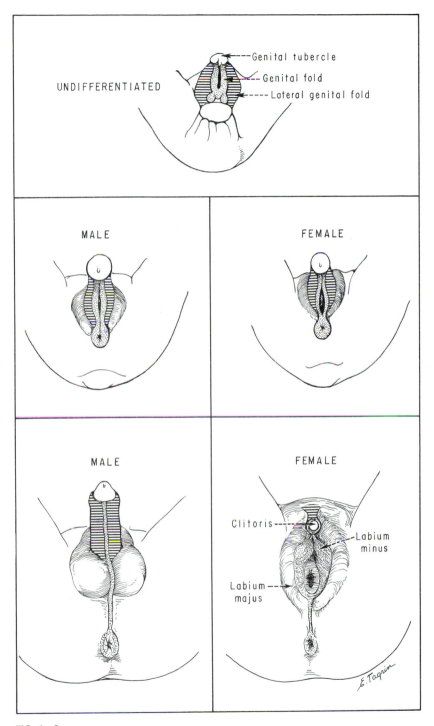

FIG 4–2.
Schematic drawing to show the homologous development of the external genitalia from the undifferentiated state.

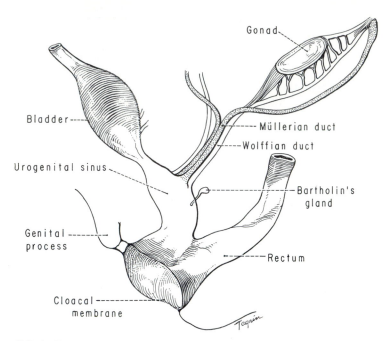

FIG 4–3.
Schematic drawing of the undifferentiated genital system of the 12- to 14-mm embryo.

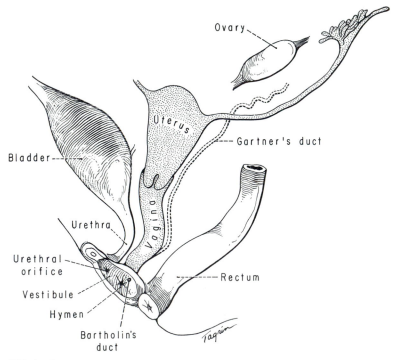

FIG 4–4.
Schematic drawing of the differentiated female genitalia.

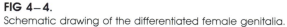

velopment is pronounced and accounts for the frequency of sebaceous retention cysts and hair follicle infections in this region. On the inner aspect of the labia majora, the sebaceous glands empty directly on the skin surface and are less numerous. The skin is made up of typical stratified squamous epithelium with moderate keratosis and a well-vascularized dermis. Involuntary muscle fibers, or dartos, are present but are much less developed than in the corresponding tissue, the scrotum, of the male. A large amount of fatty tissue is usually present, situated in lobules separated by elastic and connective tissue fibers. This elastic connective tissue forms a well-defined sac with an inner opening pointing toward the inguinal region. It is at this point that the round ligament enters the labium from each side, its fibers dispersing and passing into the fibroelastic sac just described.

The labia majora form the lateral extent of the vulva. These folds continue cephalad toward the lower abdomen and fuse in the midline as the anterior commissure, or mons pubis. The union of the labia majora caudally is known as the posterior commissure and is the lowermost extent of the vulva (Fig 4–5).

The blood supply of the labia majora is derived from the internal pudendal artery through the posterior labial branch and also from a small branch of the obturator artery. The veins have approximately the same source but also communicate with the vesicovaginal plexus and the inferior hemorrhoidal veins. The nerve supply is from multiple sources. The pudendal nerve, derived from the second to fourth sacral nerves, gives off the perineal branch from which the posterior labial nerve arises. The latter innervates the labia majora and the lateral portion of the urethral triangle. In addition, adjunctive supply is afforded by the ilioinguinal, internal branch of the geni-

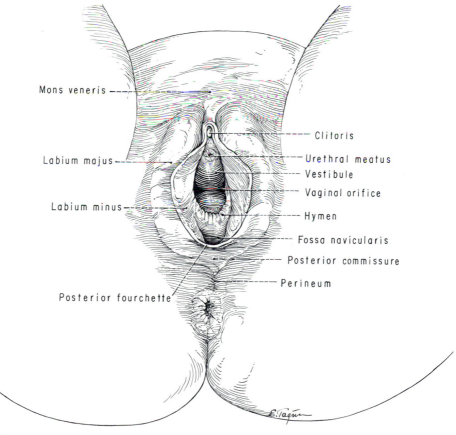

Mons veneris
Clitoris
Labium majus
Urethral meatus
Vestibule
Vaginal orifice
Labium minus
Hymen
Fossa navicularis
Posterior commissure
Perineum
Posterior fourchette

FIG 4–5.
External genitalia of the female.

tocrural and the genital branch of the lesser sciatic (posterior femoral cutaneous). The nerve supply of the perineum and vulva is shown in Figure 4–6.

Labia Minora

The labia minora consist of two cutaneous folds, which are usually concealed by the labia majora. In certain instances they may be greatly hypertrophied and project beyond the labia majora. They lie directly approximate to each other with a convex free border and extend caudad from the prepuce of the clitoris to join the labia majora as they terminate in the posterior fourchette. Between this fourchette and the hymenal ring is a curved depression, the fossa navicu-

laris (see Fig 4–5). The labia minora are reduplications of skin and not mucosa, although some pathologists have classified the labia minora and vagina as "mucous membrane" and the labia majora as skin. Mucus, however, is not secreted from either the vagina or the labia minora.

The skin of the labia minora contains abundant pigment and blood vessels. Microscopically, the stratified squamous epithelium is characterized by minimal keratinization, but the rete ridges are numerous and prominent. The dermis is made up of connective tissue fibers with numerous bundles of elastic tissue and blood vessels but with minimal fatty tissue. Sweat glands and hair follicles are usually absent, but sebaceous glands are abundant. As mentioned, the prepuce of the clitoris is continuous with the labia minora and is his-

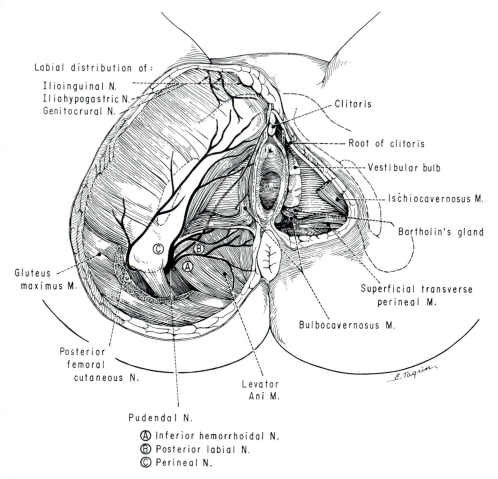

FIG 4–6.

The nerve supply of the vulva is represented at left. At the right, the ischiocavernosus and bulbocavernosus muscles have been reflected to show the anatomy of the clitoris and vestibular bulbs.

tologically similar except for its extreme vascularity. The blood supply is derived from the labial vessels, as previously described, and from the dorsal artery to the clitoris, which is a terminal branch of the internal pudendal artery. The nerve supply is the same as that of the labia majora.

The labia minora may become enlarged so that, even in virginal women, they may project beyond the majora. Immediately preceding and during coitus they become moist and lubricated with secretions from the vulvovaginal and sebaceous glands.

Clitoris

The clitoris is composed of two roots, which traverse the pubic rami to unite beneath the symphysis in the clitoridean body. The body terminates in the upper portion of the vestibule as the glans. The roots and body are covered by overlying muscle, but the glans is exposed. Figure 4–6 illustrates the relationship of the root of the clitoris to the overlying ischiocavernosus muscle. The roots, or crura, are 3 to 4 cm long in the flaccid state but in erection are 4.5 to 5.0 cm long. The body is 2.5 to 3.0 cm long and is surrounded by a connective tissue capsule of fibroelastic tissue termed the clitoridean fascia. The covering of the glans is modified cutaneous tissue, not mucosa. Unlike the penis, the glans clitoridis contains no corpus spongiosum and does not possess as much erectile tissue.

The function of the clitoris seems to be that of a "nerve center" for coitus. Prior to contact, sexual stimulation causes vascular engorgement and enlargement, so that when the penis is inserted, the clitoris becomes particularly sensitive to the to-and-fro motion of the shaft. Orgasm in the female may be brought about by this stimulation even in the absence of the vagina and consists of an interrelated reflex resulting in forceful contractions of both voluntary and involuntary musculature of the pelvis and pelvic viscera. After the process of orgasm has been experienced and a conditioned reflex established, the presence of the clitoris is not absolutely necessary. Women who have had simple or radical vulvectomy with excision of the clitoris are capable of experiencing orgasm.

The arteries of the clitoris arise from the internal pudendal artery. The veins correspond to the arteries, except for the large dorsal vein of the clitoris, which runs beneath the arcuate ligament of the symphysis through a small notch and communicates with the pelvic veins.

Vestibular Bulbs

Vestibular bulbs correspond to the corpus spongiosum of the male and consist of truncated masses of erectile tissue placed on either side of the vaginal orifice. They are situated above the inferior fascia of the pelvic diaphragm and below the bulbocavernosus muscles (see Fig 4–6). The anterior ends taper to join the bulb of the opposite side in the pars intermedia, whereas the posterior surfaces are in contact with Bartholin's glands.

Hymen

The hymen is an irregular, membranous fold of varying thickness that partially occludes the vaginal orifice. It extends from the floor of the urethra to the fossa navicularis and may be complete (imperforate), totally absent, incomplete, or cribriform. The hymen may be avulsed by examination, trauma, surgery, or coitus. Usually irregular remnants persist, forming a fleshy fringe about the vaginal opening (the carunculae myrtiformes) (see Fig 4–5).

Vestibule

The vestibule is an elliptical space that is situated just inside the labia minora and extends from the glans clitoridis to the posterior side of the hymenal ring. The orifices of the urethra, vagina, and vulvovaginal gland ducts open into the vestibule (see Fig 4–5).

The vestibule is the only portion of the genital tract arising from endoderm. The area is bounded by the hymenal ring extending the keratinized skin of the labia minora, extending anteriorly to the frenulum of the clitoris and posteriorly to include the fourchette. Hart's line defines the outer limits. The epithelium differs in that it is not pigmented, is nonkeratinizing squamous, and does not contain skin adnexa. A variable number of mucus-secreting vestibular glands as well as the orifices of Bartholin's gland ducts are present (Woodruff and Friedrich, 1985).

Bartholin's Abscess and Cysts

Plugging of Bartholin's duct may result in indolent, often asymptomatic, growth of a cyst.

Such cysts are capable of being infected by a variety of organisms, ultimately resulting in abscess formation and frequently cellulitis of the surrounding perineal and often perirectal areas. Treatment of the cyst or abscess consists of infiltrating the skin overlying the mass, making an incision distal to the hymenal ring and in the vicinity of the duct orifice. Breaking up trabeculations in the case of the abscess is important. A Word catheter should be left in place, sutured to the skin for 4 to 6 weeks. This allows for epithelialization of a fistula and subsequent return of the gland to normal function. Recurrence rates using incision and drainage are reported at 68% to 75%. Marsupialization recurrence rates are 24%. Fistulization rates are reported at 17%. This technique will fail when the catheter falls out prematurely and the fistula tract does not have time to become properly epithelialized (Yavetz et al., 1987).

Vestibular Gland Adenomas

Vestibular gland adenomas are benign and are frequently associated with prior surgery or a history of chronic inflammation of vestibular tissue. Such adenomas are usually not appreciated until further resection of the vestibular epithelium has been carried out (Axe et al., 1986).

Vulvodynia

Subsets of vulvodynia include dermatoses, lichen sclerosis, dermatitis, eczema, and lichen planus (McKay, 1988). Recurrent exposure to *Candida* may be an underlying cause. Subclinical involvement with human papillomavirus (HPV) may be a subtle cause. Clues may be obtained by application of 5% acetic acid.

Essential vulvodynia may respond to 50 to 75 mg of amitriptyline daily, especially in those patients who note no symptom-free days.

Vulvar Vestibulitis

Diagnostic criteria include severe pain on vestibular touch or attempted entry to vagina, tenderness to Q-tip pressure localized within the vulvar vestibule, and the physical findings of vestibular erythema of various degrees (Friedrich, 1987).

For reasons unknown, this disease has reappeared after a 50-year absence. There is an apparent predilection for white patients, and the syndrome is thought not to be of infectious origin

primarily. Spontaneous remission rates up to 35% have been reported. Vestibulectomy and advancement of vaginal epithelium result in an approximately 60% success rate. Response to drug therapy in small uncontrolled groups using acyclovir and capsaicin has been encouraging (Friedrich, 1988). Treatment by laser is contraindicated.

Mons Veneris

The mons veneris is the most cephalad portion of the vulva (see Fig 4–5) and consists of an accumulation of subcutaneous fat in excess amount in a rounded pad overlying the symphysis pubis. It is covered by pubic hair and the skin is similar to that of the labia majora. The fat pad characteristically remains even after marked inanition and weight loss. The typical female escutcheon of hair over the mons is triangular and usually does not extend upward along the abdomen, although there is much variation in this respect, depending on racial and familial traits.

Urethral Meatus

The urethral meatus, the orifice of the urethra, is situated just caudad to the glans clitoridis and may be visualized by separating the labia minora. It has a cleftlike appearance with slightly raised lateral margins and is the uppermost structure of the vestibule (see Fig 4–5).

Periurethral Gland Ducts

The periurethral gland ducts are the external orifices of the periurethral (Skene's) glands, which are situated beneath the urethral floor. The orifices are extremely small, yet are usually grossly visible crypts just lateral to and somewhat posterior to the urethral orifice. These glands arise, as do the mucous glands that empty into the distal urethra, from the urethral mucosa itself and are histologically similar. They are stated to be the rudimentary homologue of the prostate gland in the male and are commonly invaded by the gonococcus organisms, in which case pus may be expressed from the openings.

Vulvovaginal Glands

The vulvovaginal glands, known commonly as Bartholin's glands, are the homologue of the bulbourethral glands in the male. They are racemose and secrete mucus, particularly during sexual stimulation. Situated at each side of the vaginal orifice, below the hymen, the glands are normally small and can be palpated only in rather thin women or if enlarged by inflammation or tumor. The duct openings are in the posterior introitus. Rapid growth occurs at puberty, and shrinkage occurs after menopause. Microscopically, the glands show a single layer of high columnar epithelium in the alveoli, but the duct is lined by transitional epithelium except for a short invagination of stratified squamous epithelium at the orifice.

MALFORMATIONS

Congenital malformations of the vulva are rare but do occur in association with the stigmata of female hermaphroditism (Young, 1937), hypospadias, or incomplete cloacal separations. Complete absence (aplasia) of the vulva occasionally accompanies rudimentary internal genitalia and resembles the secondary atrophy of senility. The labia majora may show some differentiation but are flattened and contain little fat and practically no hair follicles. The labia minora are present, the clitoris rudimentary, and the perineal body short.

Vulvar atresia may occur but is usually incomplete and consists of partial agglutination of the labia with stenosis of the introitus and occasionally an imperforate hymen. Vulvar duplication may occur along with duplication of the vagina, cervix, and uterus. Vulvar fusion has been described in the newborn following the administration of certain progestational agents to the mother during the first 12 weeks of gestation (see Chapter 20).

A comprehensive classification of abnormal sexual development has recently been devised by Robboy et al. (1987; Table 4–1). Such a classification depends on the basic criteria of genital anatomy, gonadal anatomy, chromosomal make-up, and specific genetic or metabolic defects.

Normal development of the male or female genital tract begins with the influence of sex chromosomes on the indifferent gonad with a resulting ovary or testis, testicular differentiation preceding that of the ovary by 5 weeks. Testicular Sertoli's cells elaborate müllerian inhibiting sub-

TABLE 4–1.

Classification of Intersexual Disorders*†

Disorders associated with normal chromosome constitution
  Female pseudohermaphroditism
    Adrenogenital syndrome (testosterone overproduction due to adrenocorticoid insufficiency)
      21α-Hydroxylase deficiency
      11β-Hydroxylase deficiency
    Maternal ingestion of progestins or androgens
    Maternal virilizing tumors
  Male pseudohermaphroditism
    Gonadal defects
      Testicular regression syndrome (gonadal destruction)
      Leydig's cell agenesis
        Defective hCG-LH receptor
      Defects in testosterone synthesis
        Testosterone and adrenocorticoid insufficiency
        20,22-Demolase deficiency
        3β-Hydroxylase dehydrogenase deficiency
        17α-Hydroxylase deficiency
      Testosterone insufficiency only
        17,20-Desmolase deficiency
        17β-Hydroxysteroid (17-ketosteroid reductase) dehydrogenase deficiency
      Persistent müllerian duct syndrome (defect in müllerian-inhibiting system)
    End-organ defects
      Disordered androgen receptor binding
        Androgen insensitivity syndrome (testicular feminization)
        Incomplete androgen insensitivity syndrome (Reifenstein's syndrome)
      Disordered testosterone metabolism
      5α-Reductase deficiency
Disorders associated with abnormal sex chromosome constitution
  Sexual ambiguity infrequent
    Klinefelter's syndrome
    Turner's syndrome
    XX Male syndrome
    Pure gonadal dysgenesis (some forms)
  Sexual ambiguity frequent
    Mixed gonadal dysgenesis (MGD)
      Pure gonadal dysgenesis (some forms)
      Dysgenetic male pseudohermaphroditism
    True hermaphroditism

*From Robboy SJ, Lombardo JM, Welch WR: Disorders of abnormal sexual development, in Kurman R (ed): *Blaustein's Pathology of the Female Genital Tract*, ed 3. New York, Springer-Verlag, New York, 1987, pp 15–35. Used by permission.
†Idiopathic or unclassified conditions exist within each major category. We assume that each category of male pseudohermaphroditism with defects in specific protein products or receptors has forms where the abnormality is total or partial or where the defect results from a qualitatively abnormal structure.

stance (MIS). Absence of MIS permits development of fallopian tubes, uterus, and upper vagina. Production of MIS from both testes is mandatory since reduced unilateral output results in a streak or ovary with uterus and tube and vagina. Testosterone secretion in adequate amounts originates from Leydig's cells under the stimulus of human chorionic gonadotropin and is necessary for development of the epididymis, vas deferens, and seminal vesicles. On rare occasions, exogenous testosterone or testosterone derived from a maternal source may be responsible for the differentiation of female fetal organs into definitive male organs.

Absence of tissue ability to convert testosterone to dihydrotestosterone (DHT) results in failure of development of the prostate, penis, and scrotum. Therefore, absent development of male genitalia may be secondary to a lack of adequate secretion of testosterone or absent conversion in the end organ to DHT by 5α-reductase or 5α-reductase deficiency. End-organ insensitivity and mild deficiencies of 5α-reductase may result in hypospadias, persistent urogenital sinus, and defects in scrotal fusion.

Finally, internal and external female genitalia may develop and differentiate without any influence from hormones from the fetal ovary unless influenced by the effect of MIS. Elevated levels of androgen prior to 10 to 12 weeks of gestational age will result in ambiguous or normal-appearing external male genitalia with the urethra opening into the vagina. Elevation of androgen levels in the female fetus after 20 weeks' gestational age results only in clitoral hypertrophy. Drugs associated with female pseudohermaphroditism include 17α-ethinyltestosterone, 17αethinyl-19-nortestosterone, and, occasionally, diethylstilbestrol, androgens, and intramuscular progesterone. A variety of maternal ovarian tumors have been associated with virilization of the female infant, the commonest being a persistent luteoma that manifests itself in mild degrees of fusion of the labia and clitoral enlargement.

Determination of such abnormalities early is important for gender identification in childrearing, for alleviation of psychological problems attendant to a wrong gender being assigned, and for prevention of life-threatening situations (e.g., in congenital adrenal hyperplasia) and possible malignancy (e.g., in testicular feminization and mixed gonadal dysgenesis).

Correlation of sex chromosomes, external genital morphology, internal genital morphology, and gonadal histology is essential to the diagnosis of disorders of sexual development.

Adrenogenital Syndrome

Clitoral hypertrophy may signal deficiency of 3β-hydroxysteroid dehydrogenase or 21-hydroxylase, the latter being the commonest finding in the adrenal-genital syndrome. If androgen excess was present prior to the 16th week of gestation, there may be a common urogenital sinus into which vagina and urethra open. More marked changes may result in a misdiagnosis of a cryptorchid male, with or without hypospadias. Associated deficiencies of other enzymes related to glucocorticoid and mineral-corticoid synthesis can be responsible for life-threatening metabolic problems (see Chapter 20).

The treatment of minor changes such as agglutination of labia can be accomplished in the early weeks of life by gentle massage and traction to separate the agglutination. If this fails, more vigorous efforts under anesthesia will be necessary. The use of estrogen cream is helpful in preparing these tissues and allowing them to remain apart once successful lysis of the fusion has been carried out.

Hymen

The hymen is often involved in developmental defects, the commonest types being the (1) imperforate, (2) septate, (3) fenestrate, and (4) cribriform. An imperforate hymen is usually unnoticed until the menarche, at which time menstrual blood accumulates behind the membrane with resultant hematocolpos and hematometra. Blood may rarely be forced into the peritoneal cavity, giving rise to the signs and symptoms of peritonitis. The diagnosis is usually obvious by inspection; there is a bluish, bulging membrane presenting at the introitus (Fig 4–7). Rectal examination will reveal a distended vagina and an enlarged uterus (occasionally the size of a 12- to 14-week gestation). This condition should be treated in the operating room by a generous cruciate incision or by excision of a portion of the hymen. Further surgery or exploration is not warranted at this time.

A rigid hymen is frequently seen as a cause

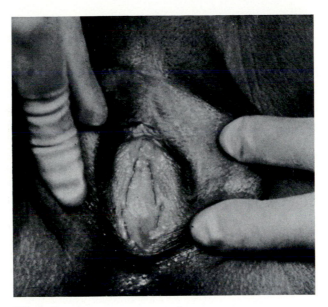

FIG 4–7.
Imperforate hymen.

for dyspareunia. This may be due to the presence of an excess amount of tough, fibrous tissue or to the presence of multiple small orifices, none of which is large enough to admit the penis. Although both of these types may be helped by gradual dilatation, surgical correction is preferable. A hymenectomy is a simple procedure, and the results are immediate and permanent.

Clitoris

The commonest abnormality of the clitoris is not really a malformation but an enlargement seen in association with hermaphroditism. The latter condition may be due to adrenal hyperplasia or tumor, gonadal dysgenesis, or unknown causes. Arrhenoblastoma or hilus cell tumor of the ovary may also cause enlargement of the clitoris.

Urethra

Malformations of the urethra include stenosis, diverticula, and hypospadias. Mild degrees of stenosis are fairly common and usually cause no symptoms. In some patients there may be tenesmus and recurrent cystitis from urinary retention. Urethral dilatation and treatment of the cystitis are attended by marked relief. Diverticula may be regarded as an abnormality resulting from incom-

plete development of the urethrovaginal septum. There may be single or multiple outpouchings of the urethra along its caudal surface but without connection with the vagina. The diagnosis is made by expressing urine or, occasionally, pus by firm pressure on the diverticulum. Treatment should be surgical excision. Hypospadias also results from an incomplete separation of the urethra from the vagina, with a resultant congenital urethrovaginal fistula. It may be looked on embryologically as an arrest in the normal development of the urethra in which the posterior (ventral) aspect is incomplete. Thus, in the female, an opening between the urethra and the vagina persists. (Epispadias is extremely rare and refers to the urethral orifice being anterior, i.e., ventral, to its normal position [e.g., clitoral, subsymphyseal, or complete, as in bladder exstrophy].) Treatment in hypospadias (or epispadias) is surgical.

PHYSIOLOGIC ALTERATIONS

The vulvar skin represents a surface area that is sensitive to many systemic alterations and diseases and may be the site of the first cutaneous manifestation of such conditions. The most commonly encountered diseases are diabetes, uremia, and blood dyscrasias.

Diabetes

Diabetic vulvitis may be the first sign of previously undiagnosed diabetes and may present when known diabetes is out of control. There is marked acute erythema, often with some edema, and the patient will complain of external burning as urine crosses the vulva. Frequently there is an associated monilial vulvovaginitis. Hyperkeratosis ensues with the passage of time. Therefore, the clinical picture may be mixed, with patches appearing opaque and white interspersed with red areas on vulvar skin. Control of diabetes and the use of antifungal agents, both vaginally and topically on the vulva, when combined with the use of topical steroids provide marked improvement over a period varying from 1 week to 10 days.

Uremia

Late-stage renal disease with uremia may result in "uremic frost" of the vulva as well as of the oral mucosa. Labial surfaces are covered with a gray-white-brown membrane containing urea and uric acid deposits. Treatment consists of local cleansing measures and correction of renal failure, if appropriate.

Blood Dyscrasias

Leukemia, aplastic anemia, and agranulocytosis may cause rather typical vulvar ulceration. These ulcers are deep, well-demarcated oval lesions covered usually with a thin, gray membrane. Such lesions have been found following administration of drugs that result in depressed bone marrow function (e.g., methotrexate), and if death does not ensue, they heal spontaneously following cessation of the drug. In pernicious anemia, vulvar ulceration and hyperpigmentation may be part of generalized tissue devitalization and hypovitaminosis so characteristic of that disease.

Vitamin Deficiency

Pellagra may result in acute and, later, chronic hyperkeratotic vulvitis (white) without the presence of monilia. Sitz baths, topical corticosteroids, and vitamin B replacement will reverse this condition.

Aphthous ulcers are nonspecific manifestations of such systemic diseases as immunodeficiency syndromes and will be dealt with elsewhere.

Circulatory Disturbances

Circulatory disturbances are most commonly evident as edema, varicose veins, and simple hypertrophy. Because of the loose connective tissue of the labia majora, marked edema may be found in generalized anasarca, portal obstruction, or pelvic tumors. A severe edema may be associated with inflammatory conditions such as a chancre or may follow prolonged scratching. Varicose veins are especially prominent during the last trimester of pregnancy in association with hemorrhoids and leg varicosities. The patient may complain of burning, itching, and a feeling of heaviness in the vulva. Relief is accomplished by placing pressure against the vulva in the form of a sanitary napkin or foam rubber held in place by a girdle. Rest with the legs and hips elevated should be taken frequently during the day. Occasionally, surgical excision or injection with sclerosing solutions is necessary for relief. During the puerperium, the veins usually become smaller and asymptomatic. Rarely a telangiectatic angioma may produce unilateral vulvar swelling.

Simple hypertrophy of the labia minora is said to occur when they project more than 4 to 5 cm from their attachment. There is usually an associated hypersecretion of the sebaceous glands, giving the surface a moist and glistening appearance.

VULVAR INJURIES

Accidental Injuries

The usual injury is a hematoma, brought about by a blow to the vulvar area, particularly if there are large varices, or by falling astride some object, with resultant damage to the vestibular bulbs or to the veins of the clitoris. Minor contusions may be treated by cold compresses and pressure. A large hematoma should be evacuated and packed, and antibiotics should be administered. Inspection should be done carefully to determine whether the urethra, bladder, or rectum has been injured. Fatal perforations into the peritoneal cavity, intestine, and bladder have been reported. The vascular trauma in vulvar injuries is usually venous, so that hemostasis may usually be secured by evacuation of the hematoma and firm packing. Individual ligation of small vessels is not necessary unless arterial bleeding is encountered. The venous pressure in the vulva may be reduced somewhat by elevating both hips on pillows, and the swelling may be reduced by application of cold compresses or ice.

Recreational pursuits such as waterskiing, use of snowmobiles, and riding of mechanical bucking bulls have been added to the list of conventional sources of vulvar trauma (accidental injuries). An indwelling catheter is indicated when one is dealing with suspected urethral or vesical trauma or in the presence of large retroperitoneal hematomas or otherwise painful vulvar and perineal injuries, regardless of whether hematomas have been drained, packed, or both.

Coital Injuries

Most minor injuries about the hymen are so constantly associated with coitus that they may be termed *physiologic*. They are usually superficial lacerations at either side of the posterior commissure. Injuries following rape, however, may be extensive and occasionally fatal. Profuse hemorrhage may result from tears of the clitoris or posterior fourchette or from hymenal avulsion. If the hymen is thick and nonyielding, lacerations of the perineum into the rectum may occur.

Treatment consists of surgical repair and supportive measures. The clinician should make complete notes of his or her findings at the time of the first examination. Microscopic search for spermatozoa and smears and cultures for gonorrhea should be made and recorded, since such cases are frequently investigated in criminal court. Although bleeding may be severe enough to necessitate transfusion, treatment is simple, and such lacerations usually heal without scarring. The possibility that syphilis and gonorrhea have been contracted at this time must be considered and prophylactic therapy given.

Obstetric Injuries

Physiologic injuries occurring at the time of delivery include obliteration of the hymenal folds by the passage of the fetal head and abrasions and minor tears of the vestibule, periurethral area, and perineum. Occasionally, however, complete perineal lacerations with division of the anal sphincter occur. All such tears should be debrided and repaired by primary suture at the time of delivery.

Vulvar hematomas may occur following rapid spontaneous delivery or difficult forceps rotations. Large varicose veins seem to be a predisposing factor and should be ligated or excised just prior to delivery. If the hematoma is small and not extending, it may be treated by elevation of the hips and application of cold compresses. Large hematomas may extend retroperitoneally and be palpable above Poupart's ligament. These should be widely incised and packed, and a contralateral vaginal pack should be inserted. Blood transfusions and antibiotics are useful as adjunctive therapy. Only rarely can the bleeding vessel be found for ligation, and even if it is, the packing should be placed as described.

Massive vulvar edema following prolonged pushing during the second stage of labor while in the vertical position on the birthing chair may simulate or obscure hematomas of the vulva (Goodlin and Frederick, 1983). Such edema contributes to extension of episiotomies, difficulty in repair, and subsequent poor healing.

X-Ray Injuries

The vulvar structures do not tolerate x-ray therapy well. In certain instances the reaction has been extreme, with marked erythema, edema, ulceration, and scarring. Although x-ray may be used occasionally as a palliative procedure for extensive vulvar carcinoma, its use for benign conditions such as neurodermatitis or lichen sclerosus is not without hazard.

PRURITUS VULVAE

Pruritus vulvae is a symptom and not a diagnosis, the word pruritus being derived from the Latin *prurire* ("to itch"). The cause for this distressing symptom is often obscure and difficult to determine. It has been estimated that in about 10% of patients seen in private gynecologic practice, this is the chief complaint.

The neural mechanisms for the perception of itching are poorly understood, but it has been suggested that these impulses follow somatic pain fibers. The sensation of itching is therefore a subpain response mediated through the lateral spinothalamic tracts. This explains the absence of itching in patients who have had a chordotomy. Psychiatrists have pointed out that the central mediation of anger, resentment, and eroticism may be exhibited in certain areas of the skin, such as the vulva in the female or the perianal area in the male. The persistence of the stimulus leads to scratching, trauma, and visible damage, thus setting up a vicious cycle. Pathologic changes in the skin, such as hyperkeratosis, rete ridge hyperplasia, and inflammatory changes in the dermis, may be produced experimentally in animals simply by scratching the same skin area repeatedly for a sufficiently long period.

The individual response and the choice of location are intimately allied with the patient's intrapsychic problem, leading to the complexity of the itch-scratch reflex. The intolerable, weak "pain" that is called "itch" is frequently so unpleasant that the patient tries to convert it to a strong pain by scratching. Itching disappears when strong pain is substituted, and such pain is often more endurable, at least temporarily, than the unpleasant sensation of itching. Examples of this are commonplace. Frequently women will, after years of vulvar scratching, resort to stiff brushes to convert itch to pain. Such trauma to the skin prevents natural healing and is followed by other effects, which prolong the dermatitis.

Thus, it is often impossible for the clinician to determine whether the gross vulvar changes seen are due to prolonged scratching or the itching is due to primary skin disease. Biopsy is the only method of making an accurate diagnosis.

Etiology

Two general classifications of pruritus vulvae may be employed: (1) local genital tract causes and (2) systemic causes. The first group may include (1) trichomonas vulvovaginitis, (2) fungous vulvovaginitis, (3) nonspecific bacterial vulvovaginitis, (4) atrophic vulvovaginitis, (5) contact or atopic vulvovaginitis, (6) vulvar dystrophies, and (7) carcinoma. The second group includes (1) diabetes mellitus; (2) drug sensitivity and allergy; (3) chemical irritants; (4) skin diseases—herpes, intertrigo, lichen planus, psoriasis, and urticaria; (5) vitamin deficiencies, especially vitamin A and B complex vitamins; (6) diseases due to animal parasites—pediculosis and scabies; (7) systemic diseases—anemia, leukemia, hepati-

tis (with or without jaundice), and tuberculosis; and (8) neurogenic dermatitis.

Diagnosis

Diagnosis will be aided by a meticulous history, careful examination and selected laboratory studies. The important features of the history are the intensity and duration of pruritus, the relationship to menses, associated leukorrhea or bleeding, and previous allergic or dermatologic episodes. Examination should include a careful survey of skin lesions elsewhere as well as inguinal lymphadenopathy. The local lesion should be examined in good light and its general and specific characteristics noted. Fissuring, ulceration, bleeding, scratch marks, thickening, and discoloration are important signs. In addition, inspection of the urethra, periurethral glands, vagina, cervix, anus, and Bartholin's glands should be made.

Selected laboratory tests of importance are (1) a complete blood study for anemia or blood dyscrasia, (2) urinalysis for diabetes, (3) hanging-drop preparations of vaginal discharge for trichomoniasis and fungous diseases, (4) cultures for nonspecific bacterial infections, (5) cytologic studies for cancer, (6) serologic and antigen studies for venereal disease, (7) blood chemistry examinations for uremia and diabetes, and (8) biopsy for dystrophies or any derangement of skin not responding to short courses of local therapy.

ANIMAL PARASITES

Scabies

Scabies is caused by the female itch mite *Sarcoptes (Acarus) scabiei*. Examination will reveal similar lesions in the sides and webs of the fingers, the palms, axillae, wrist flexures, and over the nipples. Pruritus may be intense but is usually nocturnal. The face is almost always uninvolved. Diagnosis is made by obtaining the *Acarus* from a skin burrow with a needle and examining it under the microscope. Either γ-benzene hexachloride (Kwell) ointment or 25% benzyl benzoate in equal parts of tincture of green soap and water may be used to treat the infestation. A severe dermatitis should first be treated with soothing baths and lotions and topical use of an antibiotic if necessary. It is best to have the patient begin treatment with a prolonged soap and water bath, then rub the selected scabicide into the skin, bathe again only after 24 hours, and change the bed linen and clothing.

Pediculosis Pubis

The pubic or crab louse *(Phthirus pubis)* pierces the skin and secretes a noxious substance, which produces severe pubic and vulvar pruritus. The disease is spread by coitus but possibly also by bedding or toilets. The lice may be found attached to the hairs about 1.3 cm above the skin or at the skin-hair junction. Diagnosis is made by removing the hair and examining it under the microscope. γ-Benzene hexachloride ointment or lotion is equally effective therapeutically.

Oxyuriasis

The vulva of girls may be affected by an intestinal focus of *Oxyuris vermicularis* (pinworms). Treatment includes oral administration of piperazine citrate (Antepar).

Gentian violet in enteric-coated tablets is an effective, inexpensive agent for the treatment of enterobiasis. Therapy for 10 consecutive days is effective and relatively well tolerated, although nausea, vomiting, and abdominal pain are not uncommon.

SEXUALLY TRANSMITTED DISEASES

The major venereal diseases, such as syphilis, gonorrhea, and *Herpesvirus hominis* type 2, are dealt with in great detail in Chapter 19 and will therefore not be covered in this particular chapter. That is not to minimize their importance. It must be stressed that any lingering lesion of the vulva must be considered in the light of the major venereal diseases. The differential diagnosis of a multiplicity of vulvar diseases should include both syphilis and gonorrhea. Appropriate measures, including culture of the urethra, cervix, and anus and serologic tests for syphilis, should be undertaken quite routinely and, when in doubt, dark-field examination technique should be utilized. Culturing any vesicular eruption is extremely important, especially in an attempt to isolate herpesvirus. Techniques that allow for easy transport of culture material are now available. Culture techniques themselves are now extremely reliable.

Lymphogranuloma Venereum

Lymphogranuloma venereum is a venereal infection spread by coitus and now thought to be caused by an organism of the *Chlamydia* group. There is a latent period with prodromal symptoms and fever and malaise lasting 1 to 4 weeks. Papules, pustules, or small ulcers are present for only a few days and may be relatively asymptomatic, with spontaneous healing. Suppurative inguinal adenitis may follow quickly, with subsequent necrosis, abscess formation, and, perhaps, ulceration. Fibrosis and scarring are a late manifestation, and obstruction of surrounding lymphatics may result in marked edema of the vulva. Lymphatic extension of the disease is responsible for involvement of other organs, such as rectum and lower colon, and may be productive of strictures of the urethra and rectum and eventual incontinence. The disfigurement and destruction of vulvar structures may raise a question of hidradinitis suppurativa. However, this entity will spare the labia minora, in contrast to lymphogranuloma venereum.

Diagnosis is made by complement fixation and the Frei test. In the absence of a positive Frei test result, a repeat complement-fixation study 3 or more weeks later should confirm the diagnosis. Treatment includes local cleansing and soothing measures. Buboes (suppurating lymph nodes) must be aspirated and never incised for relief of pain.

Treatment

Tetracycline is very effective. Both penicillin and ampicillin have been reported to be beneficial as well. Therapy should be continued for 3 to 4 weeks in the face of early disease. In the chronic state, antibiotics will contribute nothing, and vulvectomy for severe deformity or colostomy for rectal stricture (or both) will at times be necessary. In the presence of multiple, hard, enlarged lymph nodes, it is extremely important to be careful to rule out the presence of carcinoma.

Chancroid (Soft Chancre)

Chancroid is a rare ulcerative vulvar lesion transmitted by coitus and caused by Ducrey's bacillus *(Hemophilus ducreyi)*. The lesion appears initially as a papule or ulcer. It is virtually the only sharply demarcated lesion with induration that is painful. The organisms may be cultured on blood agar plates.

The diagnosis is difficult to confirm by culture and therefore is frequently made on clinical grounds. Treatment consists of an erythromycin base of 500 mg orally four times daily for 7 days or 250 mg of ceftriaxone intramuscularly once (Schmid et al., 1987).

Granuloma Inguinale

Granuloma inguinale is a chronic granulomatous disease found in the tropics or southern sections of the United States and is characterized by a severe ulcerative tendency. The etiologic agent is a large bacillus—*Donovania granulomatis (Calymmatobacterium granulomatis)*. It is described in tissue stains as a Donovan body, and it may be seen best using Wright's stain, Giemsa stain, or ordinary hematoxylin-eosin preparations on scrapings or biopsy specimens of the lesion. Treatment may be with 1 gm of tetracycline daily for 10 days to 2 weeks. The disease initially begins as a small papular lesion on the labia minor or groin, later becoming serpiginous with pseudobubo or manifesting subcutaneous inguinal granulomas. Streptomycin has been extremely effective in the treatment of this disease but because of its ototoxicity should not be used, at least initially. Biopsies of the skin lesions are important to rule out the coexistence of carcinoma. Occasionally, late-stage manifestations with marked edema and distortion of the vulva may necessitate a vulvectomy (Fig 4–8).

Condylomata Acuminata

From 1966 to 1981, the number of consultations for complaints referable to condylomata acuminata increased 459%, or more than three times the number of consultations required for genital herpes (MMWR, 1983). More than 65% of these consultations were in the age group 15 to 29 years. The highest risk group was 20 to 24 years of age, followed by the group aged 25 to 29 years. Although itch and vaginal discharge account for some of the presenting complaints, a large number of patients present with complaints of pain in both the genital and anal areas. The causative agent is an HPV (MMWR, 1983). The epidemiology and complications of these warts are relatively unknown. There is a marked propensity for prolongation of courses of treatment and recurrence. Treatment modalities consist of topical application of 25% podophyllin in tincture of benzoin, freezing, excision, laser, and desiccation. Treatment of vaginal lesions using topical podophyllin is contraindicated due to systemic absorption, which may be toxic. Transmission of the HPV during birth accounts for the presence of laryngeal warts in the newborn. There is early

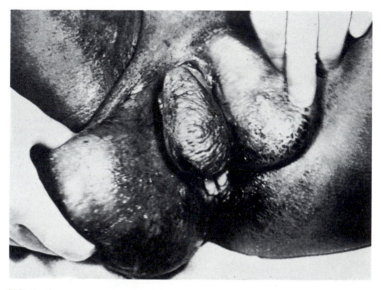

FIG 4–8.
Severe edema and vulvar distortion due to granuloma inguinale.

epidemiologic evidence relating the presence of condyloma to later appearance of cervical carcinoma.

Molluscum Contagiosum

Molluscum contagiosum is a sexually transmitted disease that is on the increase. The etiologic agent is a pox virus that has a long incubation period, resulting in the appearance of new warts 2 to 3 months after treatment of early lesions. This lesion is not thought to be premalignant. The typical wart is dome shaped and papular, with a smooth surface varying from 2 to 6 mm in diameter. It may be skin colored, white, red-purple, or even translucent. The older lesions have a central umbilication. However, only about one third of the lesions display this characteristic. The best treatment is incision and curettement to remove the molluscum body (Fig 4–9). Other therapies include the application of cantharidin, trichloracetic acid, or liquid nitrogen. Cantharidin

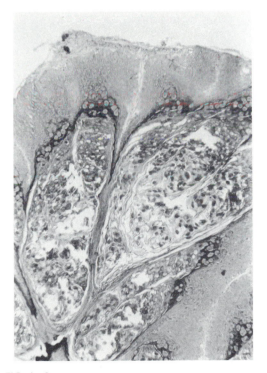

FIG 4–9.
Molluscum contagiosum. A demonstration of the molluscum body, which may be expressed or curetted after nicking the center of the lesion. Touching the cavity with silver nitrate or cryocautery gives good results.

must be used with care, since it will produce vesicles when applied to normal skin. Protection of skin adjacent to the lesion using petrolatum (Vaseline) is recommended. Excision and electrodesiccation are not indicated, since they produce scarring.

Trichomoniasis

Trichomoniasis is usually evidenced as a vaginitis, but the thin, frothy, yellow-green discharge often may cause vulvar itching. The vagina is reddened and inflamed, with a granular or strawberry-like appearance. Diagnosis is made by placing a drop of the discharge on a warm slide to which warm normal saline is added and noting motile *Trichomonas vaginalis.*

Treatment consists of the use of 250 mg of metronidazole (Flagyl) three times daily. Although short courses from 3 to 5 days are now being utilized, many cases are refractory and will need retreatment for 10 days at a time for two to three treatment schedules. Occasionally a patient is intolerant of the drug. Even after retreatment, the disease may persist in some. An old-fashioned remedy consisting of hypertonic saline solution may be extremely beneficial in such instances. A formula for a douche consists of 1 cup of table salt stirred into 4 cups of water (Friedrich, 1983).

FUNGAL DISEASES

Fungous Vulvitis

The vulvar area harbors numerous fungi as saprophytes, and under conditions of lowered general resistance, increased heat, friction, or excessive perspiration, these may become virulent pathogens. Predisposing causes to this transformation are pregnancy and diabetes, and the finding of a fungous vulvitis should be sufficient to alert the clinician to the possibility of the diabetic state. The commonest forms are tinea cruris and candidiasis (moniliasis).

Tinea Cruris

Tinea cruris is characterized by superficial, pale pink to bright red lesions with well-defined scaly borders. By a process of coalescence, the adjacent vulvar skin, thighs, and pubis may become involved. Following periods of scratching or maceration, the process may resemble a weeping type of eczema. Tinea cruris is caused by a specific fungus, *Epidermophyton inguinale,* and the diagnosis may be made by microscopic examination of the scales, by direct Gram stain, or by culture on Sabouraud's maltose agar. Direct mycologic examination of scales, hairs, and scrapings is facilitated by preparing the specimens without heating in an aqueous solution of 0.1% aminolipid and 0.2% basic fuchsin.

In office practice, scrapings planted on dermatophyte test medium (DTM) culture will result in colonies that change color from yellow to red, in contradistinction to *Candida* colonization, in which color change is rare. Examination with Wood's lamp will not demonstrate fluorescence.

Treatment

Clotrimazole (Lotrimin) ointment used three times daily is as specific as it will be for *Candida.* Cool sitz baths relieve the itch. Intermittent use of topical corticosteroid cream and, in the severe case, an oral antihistamine-tranquilizer will provide faster relief of symptoms.

Candidiasis

Nine different yeasts have been identified in the etiology of mycotic vulvitis. Candidiasis (moniliasis) is caused by the commonest saprophyte of the normal vagina and vulva, *Candida (Monilia) albicans.* The lesion begins as a reddish papule, which later becomes vesicular. After these rupture, a moist, red mucous membrane remains. Secondary infection is common, so that the vagina and vulva become markedly edematous and tender. The vulva may be covered with a tenacious, gray-white frosting (Fig 4–10), or there may be marked edema due to recurrent scratching. The commonest symptoms of candidiasis (moniliasis) are intense itching, burning, and swelling. Itching is likely to persist or reappear unless the fungus is completely eliminated by treatment. A whitish, curdlike vaginal discharge, often with a yeasty or disagreeable odor, may develop as the infection becomes more severe. If chafing occurs, a secondary inflammation or dermatitis of the thighs may also be present. Sexual intercourse may be painful or impossible because of the swelling, abrasion, and inflammation. Walking may be uncomfortable because of chafing.

In some patients, these characteristic features of *Candida* infection are so obvious that diagnosis

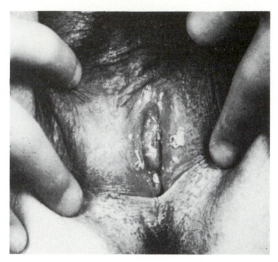

FIG 4–10.
Candidiasis (moniliasis) of vulva.

may be by inspection alone. In others (e.g., older patients), in very early stages of infection, and when secondary bacterial infections are present, diagnosis is more difficult.

Diagnosis, as with tinea cruris, may be made by wet smear, Gram stain, or culture. Nickerson's medium has simplified culturing, since it is available in small vials that may be inoculated and kept in the office at room temperature. A dark brown or black growth occurs on the medium in about 48 hours if *Candida* organisms are present. Colonies growing on DTM culture will show no color. Specific treatment in the form of clotrimazole (Gyne-Lotrimin vaginal tablets and 1% Lotrimin cream and 1% Lotrimin solution), 2% miconazole nitrate (Monistat vaginal cream), nystatin (Mycostatin) vaginal tablets (100,000 units/tablet) and ointment (100,000 units of nystatin/gm) or chlordantoin with benzalkonium (Sporostacin) cream is available.

Nystatin and triamcinolone acetonide (Mycolog) cream applied locally three times daily is also helpful. In severe cases, especially those complicated by gastrointestinal (GI) tract candidiasis, treatment should include the oral administration of two tablets of nystatin (500,000 units/tablet) three times daily for 10 days. Alternative therapeutic agents are 2% aqueous gentian violet (Genapax) suppositories for vaginal placement. In addition, the vulva may be painted with 2% aqueous gentian violet.

Size 0 gelatin capsules containing 600 mg of boric acid powder provide an alternative regimen that is cheaper and less objectionable in terms of vaginal discharge, which is associated with other therapeutic creams and jellies. It may be especially helpful in retreatment of recurring or chronic cases of monilial vaginitis. It is important to use the powder form as opposed to crystals, which may be responsible for male dyspareunia in some cases. One capsule placed high in the vagina at bedtime over a period of 14 days is optimal treatment. However, in some cases it may be necessary to continue to use the capsule on a twice weekly basis for as long as 2 to 3 months, especially in stubborn cases of mixed vaginal infections. Five percent boric acid (Borofax) ointment applied to the vulva is also extremely efficacious. Its effectiveness is unrelated to pH.

Discontinuation of oral contraceptives may be necessary when infection occurs frequently. Phenytoin (Dilantin) may relieve persistent symptoms (i.e., burning, soreness) in patients with neuritis after the skin clears.

OTHER SKIN INFECTIONS

Pyoderma (Impetigo)

Chafing, scratching, abrasion, insect bites, and altered host response provide portals of entry for pathogenic bacteria present in the carrier state in a large portion of otherwise normal individuals. The usual agents are a *Staphylococcus* or β-hemolytic *Streptococcus* (or both). This disease is characterized by thin-walled vesicles that rupture, leaving a reddened weeping spot that soon becomes crusted over and exudes pus from beneath. Clear vesicles and pustules are frequently clustered around the central lesion. Disease is readily spread to or from other parts of the body (Friedrich, 1983).

Ecthyma

Ecthyma resembles impetigo grossly but invades the epidermis to involve the dermis. Because of the depth of penetration of the infection, subsequent scarring is common (Friedrich, 1983).

Folliculitis

Folliculitis occurs with infection of the hair follicles and nearby sebaceous glands and takes on the appearance of a papule, later becoming pustulated. The progression of this lesion to a boil that ultimately becomes fluctuant is not uncommon.

Widespread involvement of tissue produces cellulitis, lymphangitis, or both. The latter entities are accompanied by constitutional symptoms, including fever and chills (Friedrich, 1983).

Erysipelas

Erysipelas is a variant of streptococcal infection, being more superficial than cellulitis but still accompanied by severe systemic symptoms, including headache, fever, and chills. One of the characteristics of this lesion is a very sharp border that is mildly indurated.

Any of these entities requires culturing of free pus to obtain sensitivity studies. While one is awaiting culture reports, penicillin or erythromycin are good agents to start with. Cleaning of the affected areas with antibacterial soap and water is helpful, and reduced activity will help to minimize spread. Instruction in scrupulous hygiene with washing of hands thoroughly after touching the area of infection is most important to minimize spread to other areas of the body. Any streptococcal infection may subsequently be associated with glomerulonephritis. Many types of infections are frequently superimposed on underlying dermatoses. Furthermore, aspects of this disease raise the possibility of syphilis and invasive carcinoma, and failure of such lesions to respond to treatment rather rapidly must ultimately result in a biopsy. Serologic tests for syphilis must be done routinely (Friedrich, 1983).

Erythrasma

Erythrasma is an asymptomatic red lesion, usually symmetric, with distinct margins that are not elevated. The source of this lesion is a gram-positive intracellular bacterium, *Corynebacterium minutissimum*. The organism may be seen under the microscope using scrapings of the skin. It is extremely difficult to culture and requires special media. The lesion itself may fluoresce under Wood's lamp secondary to production of a porphyrin by the bacterium. Cure for this lesion is obtained using oral erythromycin or tetracycline over a 10-day period (Friedrich, 1983).

Necrotizing Fasciitis

Necrotizing fasciitis is a potentially fatal disease known for its ability to develop where there has been no apparent injury and also in areas of minor injury. A similar process known as *progres-*

sive bacterial synergistic gangrene is most frequently associated with wound infection (Meltzer, 1983). Necrotizing fasciitis is frequently seen on a background of diabetes and preexisting vascular disease, and mortality rates as high as 70% have been reported in diabetics with the disease. Likely organisms in both entities belong to the coliform group, and there is also a predominance of enterococci. Patients with progressive bacterial synergistic gangrene are much less ill but are always potential candidates for the development of the more severe necrotizing fasciitis.

Treatment must be very aggressive, with institution of antibiotic therapy and very wide surgical excision of all tissue back to margins that appear grossly normal and bleed easily. Frequently, more than one trip to the operating room for wide surgical excision is necessary, since initial attempts often fall short of what is ultimately required.

The mortality rate exceeds 30%. Early diagnosis and prompt treatment will minimize mortality. In an aging population subject to arteriosclerosis, renal failure, cancer, and malnutrition, the accompanying immunosuppression may lead to more frequent occurrence of this entity (Friedrich, 1983; Roberts, 1987).

AUTOIMMUNE DISEASES

Crohn's Disease

Crohn's disease is found primarily in the colon and small bowel. Early symptoms are low abdominal and pelvic pain, which may mislead the gynecologist into believing that there is a gynecologic pelvic pathologic condition. On the other hand, this disease may present initially on the vulva as draining sinuses or abscesses or deep ulceration seemingly remote from rectum or anus (Levine et al., 1982). Constitutional symptoms are often present, including low-grade fever, diarrhea, fatigue, and weight loss. Differential diagnosis includes Behçet's syndrome, tuberculosis, granuloma inguinale, and lymphogranuloma venereum. Radiographic evidence of bowel pathologic changes coupled with the appearance of communicating sinuses generally confirms the diagnosis. Surgical treatment alone is usually to no avail, and the disease may become progressively more destructive with creation of a cloaca. Treatment of the primary disease is mandatory and usually requires a daily dosage of steroids of up to

60 mg plus antibiotics of a systemic nature. Biopsy specimens of the vulvar lesions will reveal nonspecific granulomatous change. Ulcers should be debrided, and sinus tracts and ulcerated areas cleansed repeatedly with povidone-iodine. The addition of metronidazole to the regimen has been found to be helpful (Lavery et al., 1985). Once healing is under way, wide excision of any sinus tracts usually results in good healing.

Behçet's Syndrome (Triple Symptom Complex)

Manifestation of this syndrome includes the ulceration of buccal mucous membrane, vulvar ulceration, and iritis or iridocyclitis. Biopsy results of vulvar ulcers reveal a nonspecific picture of inflammation and vasculitis. Ulcers are more often small but very deep and tend to come and go almost on a spontaneous basis. Herpes and Stevens-Johnson syndrome should be ruled out. Herpes lesions come and go almost spontaneously in many individuals. The first line of defense is merely careful local cleansing measures and observation. The use of corticosteroids may be helpful, and there have been reports that cyclic oral contraceptives, which are predominantly of an estrogenic nature, may be helpful. Surgery for this lesion is thought to be contraindicated unless the vulvar lesions are extremely destructive, with fenestration and scarring from loss of vulvar tissue.

DISEASE OF SWEAT GLANDS

Hidradenitis Suppurativa (Gordon, 1978)

Hidradenitis suppurativa is an infection resulting from mixtures of *Staphylococcus, Streptococcus,* and, occasionally, coliform organisms. The disease results from plugging of these glands by keratin, subsequent rupture, secondary infection with abscess formation, and ultimately fistulous tracts (Thomas et al., 1985). It is not seen before puberty. This infection is unique in that it involves only the apocrine glands; therefore, the disease affects mainly labia majora, intercrural folds, occasionally the mons, and, extremely rarely, the clitoris or labia minora. A secretory and a suppurative phase may be exhibited simultaneously. Axillary sweat glands may be involved as well. Due to the cyclic nature of the disease, in early stages it may respond favorably to the use of intermittent oral estrogens or cyclic oral contraceptives. Once the disease progresses to the suppurative phase, multiple intercommunicating sinuses develop; it is typical at this stage that when one area is pressed, pus will be seen extruding at a distance from another sinus. In early stages careful cleansing with soap or povidone-iodine solution may be helpful, and institution of intermittent courses of oral antibiotics may also help to diminish the progression of the disease. In spite of these measures, the chronic phase may develop, leading to multiple-abscess formation; these abscesses can be drained periodically but the end result is deep scarring beneath multiple recurrent sinuses. Ultimately, the treatment of choice for this condition is wide surgical excision with sparing of the labia minora, the clitoris, and the prepuce, and subsequent skin grafting (Conway et al., 1952). This approach will provide marked improvement and return a discouraged person to everyday activity within a relatively short time. This entity is frequently confused with folliculitis and also with lymphogranuloma venereum. However, lymphogranuloma results in massive edema and destruction of the labia minora as well as labia majora.

Fox-Fordyce Disease

Fox-Fordyce disease is also limited to the sweat glands and is papular in appearance, secondary to plugging of these glands. It is believed that subsequent extravasation of the contents of the sweat glands into the epidermal tissue results in the intense pruritus that accompanies the lesion. The axilla may be simultaneously involved with the same process, and there appears to be some relationship between the complaint of pruritus and a particular time in the menstrual cycle. Treatment may be successful using cyclic oral contraceptives; occasional relief with topical estrogen is noted.

CONTACT DERMATITIS

Contact dermatitis of the vulva may be caused by true primary irritants or by an underlying immunologic response to an external or, occasionally, internal agent. A detailed history must be taken to elucidate any of the many possible offending agents, including poison ivy, artificial fibers contained in clothing, toilet tissue (especially perfumed or colored), condoms, douches, contra-

ceptives, nail polish, perfumes, deodorants, and sanitary napkins. Common causes of allergic contact sensitivity include *p*-aminobenzoic acid derivatives, azo dyes, chromates, cobalt, formaldehyde, lanolin, mercaptobenzothiazole, neomycin, nickel, oleoresins, phenothiazines, rubber compounds, and sulfa drugs. Common sources of primary irritant dermatitis are fatty acid and detergent molecules that are present in agents used to wash or bleach clothing. Some of these are not only irritants but may be allergens, photoallergens, or both. The lesion takes the form of eczematous dermatitis with erythema, edema, vesicles, oozing, and crusting. In the chronic stage, it may be lichenified with hyperkeratotic scaling and, therefore, appear to be a white lesion. Excoriations and secondary infection are common. Treatment includes elimination of the offending agents, if one can be found, and during the acute phase, application of cool compresses of boric acid solution or saturated solution of aluminum acetate and aluminum subacetate 1%. Cornstarch and baking soda baths are helpful with the patient soaking one hour twice a day. Infection is eradicated with topical and/or systemic antibiotics. Corticosteroid cream and antihistamine or tranquilizers, or both, are very helpful in the acute phase. Additional lesions involved in the vulvar reaction may be purpura, vesicles, and, occasionally, ulceration.

ATROPHIC VULVITIS

Atrophic vulvitis is usually coexistent with a vaginitis of similar nature. Symptoms include vulvar burning, itching, and dyspareunia. Bleeding may occur from ulceration or telangiectasia. This physiologic, atrophic skin change usually starts at the climacteric or after artificial menopause, and the generally accepted cause is estrogen deficiency. The entire process is too complex, however, to be explained on this factor alone. Exogenous estrogen therapy will not reverse or prevent this ultimate change in most individuals. Other hormones and related factors presumably contribute to the general aging phenomenon. The mons pubis becomes less prominent, and the labia majora shrink and flatten as the result of loss of subcutaneous fat. The adjacent skin becomes thin and shiny, the hair becomes sparse, and tissue elasticity is diminished. As a result, the vaginal orifice becomes narrowed or even stenotic, with resultant dyspareunia. A thin, watery discharge may be present. Diagnosis is evident by noting the degree of cornification of vaginal cells in a hanging-drop preparation or Papanicolaou smear. For the vaginal component of the disease, local applications of estrogenic creams or small oral doses of estrogens for short periods are quite effective. Combinations of estrogens with androgens will occasionally give superior results, especially when libido has been diminished. Emolient creams, starch baths, sedatives, and antipruritic lotions should afford relief in most cases.

Simple Kraurosis

Simple kraurosis of the vulva is a primary sclerosing atrophy limited to the labia minora, vestibule, urethra, and clitoris (Woodruff, 1978). It occurs most commonly in postmenopausal women. The labia majora, perineum, and perianal regions are not usually involved. In the early stages, the skin may be red and glistening with isolated patches of dark red or dull purple (kraurosis rouge). In later stages, the skin becomes pale yellow and has a smooth, glistening surface, obliterated labial folds, atrophic mons veneris, and scanty, broken-off pubic hairs. The vaginal orifice is narrowed and barely admits the index finger.

Histologically, there is hyperkeratosis (excess keratin above the epithelium) with flattening of the rete ridges, edema and homogenization of the cutis collagen, separation of the elastic fibers, and mild arteriosclerotic changes in the deeper blood vessels. Simple kraurosis bears no known relationship to carcinoma of the vulva.

WHITE LESIONS

White lesions of the vulva are the result of processes of depigmentation with loss or destruction of the melanocyte's ability to manufacture melanin, sclerosis of vessels that nourish skin, or the production of hyperkeratosis. Because of the occasional coexistence of white lesions of skin proximal with established cancer, it has frequently been assumed that the white change is related to the onset of cancer. Bonney and Berkley have pointed out that malignant potential is more often related to the presence of hyperplastic lesions. Because of the general confusion, previous terminology such as kraurosis and leukoplakia have fallen into disrepute. Following the suggestion of

Jeffcoat 10 years earlier, the International Society for the Study of Vulvar Disease established a nomenclature in 1975 in an attempt to remedy the situation. This classification that is as follows: (1) hyperplastic dystrophy (a) without atypia, (b) with atypia; (2) lichen sclerosus; (3) mixed dystrophy (a) without atypia, (b) with atypia. The terminology for classification of atypia that is currently in use is as follows: VIN I, mild dysplasia; VIN II, moderate dysplasia; and VIN III, severe dysplasia/carcinoma in situ. The exact relationship of atypia to the onset of carcinoma is still unclear, but certainly those with the most marked change are worthy of local surgical attention and follow-up (Soper and Creasman, 1986). Associated intense pruritus with resulting self-inflicted trauma and attendant recurrent chronic healing processes may be related as much to development of atypias as to any other source. Treatment of the itch is conservative, with topical applications of appropriate agents once carcinoma has been ruled out by knife or punch biopsies. Vulvectomy is indicated for marked widespread atypism after failure of conservative therapy.

Lichen Sclerosus

This disease may be seen at any age, involving both the young and old. Neck, trunk, axilla, and extremities may be involved, or the lesion may present primarily on the vulva. The general skin background is pale and parchment-like, peppered with whitish papular-appearing areas over the atrophic background (Fig 4–11). Mild edema and agglutination of the prepuce are not uncommon. Biopsy will reveal a thin epithelium, at times atrophic in appearance and at times with hyperkeratosis. Histologically there is loss of rete ridges, a collagenized subepithelial zone, and, beneath this, a layer of inflammatory cells (Fig 4–12).

Tissue studies using acridine orange and radiolabeled thymidine demonstrate an increase in metabolic activity. Phosphorus 32 study shows no increase in rates of mitosis. Harrington and Dunsmore noted a 34% incidence of clinical autoimmune diseases and an increased frequency of circulating autoantibodies to a variety of tissues. In families studied, a majority have mother-daughter expression of a characteristic HLA pattern. Others have noted increased levels of circulating urogastrone, a GI peptide, with proliferative epidermal effects.

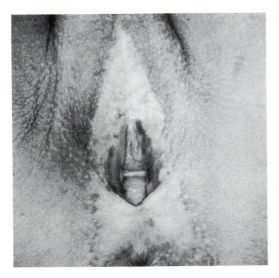

FIG 4–11.
Lichen sclerosus of vulva.

Treatment with laser has been followed with high recurrence rates.

The relationship of lichen sclerosus to carcinoma is controversial. Three percent to 5% of adult women develop superimposed squamous cell carcinoma of the vulva, a frequency 10 times greater than that seen in the general population (Lynch, 1987).

There is recent evidence that many cases of hypertrophic dystrophy should be classified as mixed dystrophy since hyperplasia seems to be complicating the presence of lichen sclerosus rather than the association between the two being a random one (Hewitt, 1986).

Treatment of lichen sclerosus is best accomplished using a 2% testosterone preparation in petrolatum or lanolin base. If itching and burning persist following this regimen, intermittent use of corticosteroid cream may be helpful. Application of testosterone should be done on a daily basis until the symptoms are brought under control; following this, intermittent use throughout the month will tend to keep symptoms under control.

Clinical response to sex hormones (testosterone) is not 100% (Friedrich and Kalra, 1984). The number and the saturation of receptor sites may be more important than the level of circulating hormones.

Vulvectomy with or without grafting cannot be expected to eradicate the process. It will always recur and be accompanied by the same symptoms.

Hyperplastic Dystrophy

This term embraces hyperkeratotic white lesions including lichen simplex chronicus and hypertrophic vulvitis, as well as neurodermatitis. The microscopic picture is nonspecific and characterized by elongation of rete pegs, hyperkeratosis, and the presence of dermal inflammation (Fig 4–13). One cannot assign significance to the lesion without biopsy, since it is what is going on at the depths of the lesion that is important (Fig 4–14) and not the appearance of the lesion. In any event, biopsy is mandatory to establish a diagnosis and assess the presence or absence of any atypia. The treatment of choice for these lesions is the use of topical corticosteroids. Boric acid preparations are soothing and aid in alleviating the in-

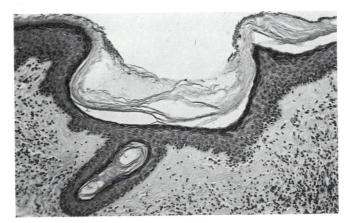

FIG 4–12.
Histologic appearance of lichen sclerosus.

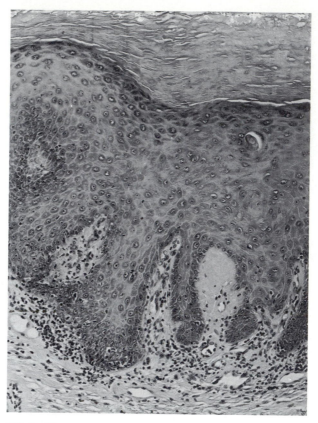

FIG 4–13.
Histologic changes in hyperplastic dystrophy.

tense itch. With proper therapy the lesions should disappear. Failure of the original lesion to disappear or the reappearance of a new lesion warrants repeated biopsy.

Mixed Dystrophy

Mixed dystrophy is defined as the presence of both lichen sclerosus and hyperplastic dystrophy. Multiple biopsies are mandatory to rule out atypia and to determine the extent of atypia present. Aggressive topical therapy with alternating testosterone and corticosteroids usually results in regression of the disease.

OTHER WHITE DISORDERS

Vitiligo

This disease process may be present anywhere on the body and is characterized by a process in which melanocytes are destroyed. Commonly, dark hair may be seen growing from a white patch of skin. The disease is transmitted by dominant genes within families, and its onset may be noted in early life.

Albinism

Here, an enzyme deficiency prevents normal formation of the melanin pigment. A white forelock of hair is characteristic.

Leukoderma

This entity is nonspecific and results from chronic trauma; it often follows inflammatory diseases of the vulva. Ultimately, the area will become repigmented.

Intertrigo

Intertrigo ensues from the presence of a constant moist environment, most often found in the

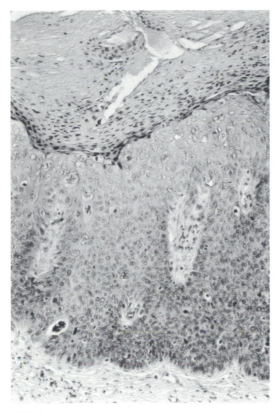

FIG 4–14.
Carcinoma in situ of the vulva beneath a thick hyperkeratotic patch.

depths of the skin folds (i.e., beneath a large panniculus or in the groin). Chronic low-grade dermatitis is almost always present. Good hygiene, use of all-cotton underwear, and the application of drying powders are general aids in clearing the condition. If fungi or bacteria are present and do not respond to conservative measures, specific fungicidal or bactericidal topical agents may be necessary.

CARCINOMA IN SITU— INTRAEPITHELIAL NEOPLASIA

The criteria for the diagnosis of this disease as set forth by the International Society for the Study of Vulvar Disease (ISSVD) include disorientation and loss of epithelial architecture that extends throughout the full thickness of the epithelium, not including keratinized or parakeratotic layers (Fig 4–15). Grossly, lesions may be white, red, or pigmented. They may be unifocal or multifocal and discrete or coalesced. It is important to

note that approximately 20% of all vulvar carcinomas in situ will appear as dark spots. Other terms found in the literature that are basically synonymous include *Bowen's disease, erythroplasia of Queyrat,* and *Paget's disease.*

Recently, multifocal pigmented verrucous lesions have received added attention under the term *bowenoid papulosis* (Kao and Graham, 1982; Wade et al., 1979).

The term is used by some dermatologists when vulvar intraepithelial neoplasia (VIN) occurs in association with papule formation. It is controversial and should not be used.

In contrast to carcinoma in situ of the cervix, carcinoma in situ of the vulva has different histologic criteria (Iversen et al., 1981). The relationship to invasive cancer is not strong. Only 20% of invasive cancers have adjacent carcinoma in situ. The interval between the peak ages for carcinoma in situ of the vulva and invasive carcinoma of the vulva is greater than that for cervical cancer.

Jones and McLean (1986) reported five un-

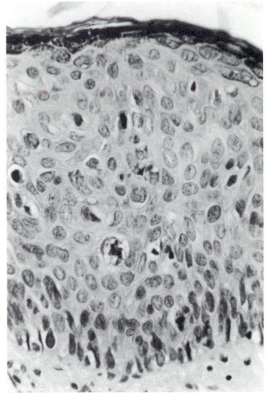

FIG 4–15.
Carcinoma in situ of the vulva with well-keratinized surface epithelium. Note cellular disarray, abnormal mitoses, and dyskeratosis.

treated cases of in situ carcinoma progressing to invasive disease. Four of the five women had previously been treated with pelvic irradiation for other malignant disease. Benedet and Murphy (1982) in a recent review of 81 patients with carcinoma in situ noted that there is an increasing incidence of this disease in young women, with 42% being under the age of 25 years as contrasted to 14% in an earlier time period. The younger age group tended to manifest the disease with more multicentric and more frequent pigmented lesions as opposed to the older age groups, in which unifocal lesions dominated (Wilkinson et al., 1981).

Caglar et al. (1982), reviewing a group of 50 patients, noted the occurrence of carcinoma in situ in 10% of patients who were in a state of immunosuppression. The same phenomenon has been pointed out by Sillman and others (1981). In the series of Caglar et al. (1982), almost one half of the patients were asymptomatic; those with symptoms complained of itch. Sixty-five percent of the lesions were white.

Spontaneous regression of lesions has been noted in patients who were untreated, including some lesions with aneuploidy. There has been an association between this lesion and the previous occurrence of sexually transmitted diseases, including the granulomatous diseases and condylomata acuminata. This tends to suggest some sort of etiologic relationship that still remains to be proved. Studies of nuclear DNA obtained from biopsy specimens of coalesced and unifocal lesions suggest the possible presence of different cell lines, with one possibly undergoing transformation from in situ to invasive cancer. This work needs confirmation by others. The association of other genital malignancies is reported as varying from 20% to 30%. In another series of 65 patients, Bernstein et al. (1983) reported that 84% of patients under the age of 40 years had multifocal disease and 65% of patients older than 40 years had unifocal disease. These authors also charted the site of recurrence of lesions and noted that the area most likely to be involved was the right lower labium majus, which was involved 50% of the time. Kaplan et al. (1981) have reported on 10 patients with intraepithelial carcinoma extending to the anus. Lesions in this area may go unnoticed for some time.

Aggressiveness of VIN cannot be predicted; therefore, treatment should be instituted as soon as the diagnosis is made.

Because of the rising incidence of intraepithelial neoplasia in young women, gynecologic surgeons have radically changed their approach to therapy in an effort to prevent disfigurement at an early age. Several options are available depending on the extent of disease and the patient's preference regarding surgery. Wide local excision with or without skin grafting is preferred therapy for unifocal disease. Partial or total skinning vulvectomy with split thickness grafts provides excellent cosmetic results (DiSaia and Rich, 1981). Meshed grafts extend coverage and are easier to fit inside the rectum.

Use of laser for multifocal disease in non-hair-bearing areas is reported to be useful, but often there is a prolonged uncomfortable convalescence (Bornstein and Kaufman, 1988; Wright and Davies, 1987). This treatment modality will subvert accurate diagnosis where invasive disease is present (DiSaia and Rich, 1981). It may be of value in treatment of clitoral and perianal disease but not anal disease.

Topical fluorouracil alone has not been satisfactory in the hands of many (Krebs, 1987; Lifshitz and Roberts, 1980); however, Sillman et al. (1981) have noted its usefulness as an adjuvant just prior to surgery, since it seems to help in demarcating the areas of epithelial involvement. The use of dinitrochlorobenzene appears to be an effective alternative for some who are unwilling to undergo surgery (Foster and Woodruff, 1982). It might be beneficial as well in patients with multiple lesions. Skin reaction to this treatment, however, is moderate to severe, and it is reported that patients are unwilling subsequently to undergo therapy. With very large lesions occupying most of the vulva, a very careful histologic examination must be performed so as not to overlook a focus of invasive carcinoma. Such lesions are, of course, best dealt with using multiple knife biopsies prior to definitive surgery. However, it is still possible, even after many biopsies, to overlook a focus of invasion. Caglar et al. (1982) and Rettenmaier et al. (1987) noted 6% and 7.1% unexpected early invasion, respectively. Risk of recurrence seems to be unrelated to the status of surgical margins. Recurrence rates after conservative surgery are reported to 30%. Similar rates of recurrence are noted as well in patients treated by vulvectomy. Regardless of what form of therapy is instituted, extremely close follow-up examination over a long period is warranted.

DRY SCALY DERMATOSES

Lichen Planus

Lichen planus is an inflammatory dermatosis of unknown origin that is characterized by multiple, small, flat-topped, polygonal papules that have a peculiar violaceous color and are covered with an often umbilicated horny film, usually associated with lesions elsewhere on the body (wrists, ankles, inner thighs, and oral mucosa). Diagnosis is made by biopsy, which shows acanthosis, hyperkeratosis, absence of parakeratosis, saw-toothed rete ridges, and a bandlike infiltration of chronic inflammatory cells in the upper cutis (Fig 4–16).

There seems to be some relation to an autoimmune cell-mediated response since the disease is common in patients who have had bone marrow transplants with graft-vs.-host reaction. Treatment with steroids and tretinoin benefits oral and cutaneous lesions (Soper et al., 1988). Vulvovaginal lesions are often refractory. Diagnosis is made by biopsy. Vaginal stenosis and atrophy frequently ensue.

Psoriasis

Psoriasis is an inflammatory dermatosis of unknown origin characterized by dry, scaling patches of various sizes covered by silvery white or grayish white scales. It may involve the vulva, although the sites of predilection are the scalp, nails, the extensor surfaces of the limbs, and the sacral area. If vulvar lesions are present, usually there are lesions on these other areas. The disease commonly has periods of exacerbation and remission, which may or may not be associated with subjective symptoms. The diagnosis may be obvious, but biopsy frequently is necessary. Microscopically there are a uniform parakeratosis, thin suprabasal epidermal plates, uniform rete ridge elongation with clubbing, and microabscesses in the stratum corneum. During periods of exacerbation, improvement may be noted with sunbaths, ultraviolet light, or the application of crude tar (2%–5%) or salicylic acid (2%–10%) ointments.

Topical use of fluorinated corticosteroids applied twice daily is helpful. Examples of such compounds include Valisone and Halog. Covering the area with a plastic film such as Saran Wrap may help to achieve a longer-lasting effect. In selected severe cases, the use of methotrexate has been helpful inasmuch as the disease is characterized by rapid cell turnover. Long-term use of topical corticosteroids must be avoided to minimize the likelihood of subepithelial fibrosis. Trauma and emotional stress are to be minimized.

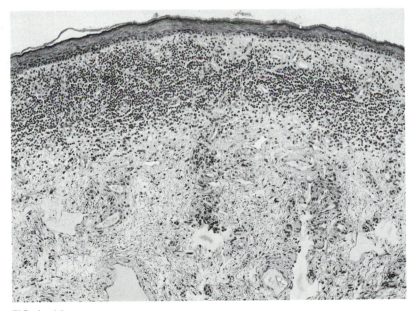

FIG 4–16.
Lichen planus.

Seborrheic Dermatitis

Seborrheic dermatitis is a red rash appearing in areas of skin where there is a high concentration of sebaceous glands. It is not a disease of sebaceous glands per se. However, the skin does appear oily, and whitish-yellow plaques may occur. Common sites of involvement include the scalp (where the term *dandruff* is used), areas behind the ears, over the sternum, between the scapula, crural folds, perianal area, labia majora, mons, and intertriginous areas. With involvement of the vulva, there is severe itching, and the itch-scratch reflex may result in secondary excoriation and infection. The disease is not curable but may be ameliorated by use of tranquilizers, good hygiene, and topical steroids. The treatment of secondary infection is important. Avoidance of psychic stress and use of mild tranquilizers, especially at bedtime, is extremely helpful in moderating symptoms. Asymmetry of this lesion on the vulva is the exception and not the rule and in such cases may be confused with chronic dystrophy or Paget's disease (Friedrich, 1983).

Nonspecific Epithelial Hyperplasia

Nonspecific epithelial hyperplasia includes entities previously described as neurodermatitis, atopic dermatitis, and lichen simplex chronicus. Inflammation, excoriation, and lichenification are present (Lynch, 1987; Fig 4–17, *A*). There is frequently a whitish appearance from absorption of moisture. Hyperpigmentation or lack of pigmentation may be present. The presence of hyperkeratosis (Fig 4–17, *B*) accounts for confusion with other dystrophies. Relief may be obtained by using 0.1% triamcinolone ointment. Cool soaks for 20 to 30 minutes followed by lubrication of the skin using a hand cream immediately thereafter prolong relief of symptoms. Tranquilizers, antihistamines, and sedatives may reduce symptoms in the resulting urge to scratch.

BENIGN NEOPLASMS

The commonest benign neoplasms of the vulva are papillomas, lipomas, fibromas, and hidradenomas. Less common are neurofibromas, lymphangiomas, hemangiomas, and myxomas. In addition, and rarer still, are glomus tumors, granular cell myoblastoma, angiolipoma, sebaceous adenoma, syringoma, and benign lymphoid ha-

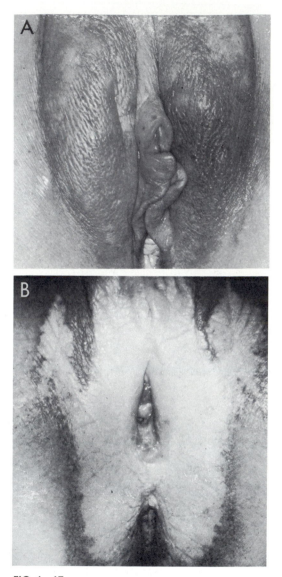

FIG 4–17.
Nonspecific epithelial hyperplasia. **A,** edema and lichenification of early stage. **B,** extensive hyperkeratosis in late stage.

martoma. Excision provides both diagnosis and adequate treatment.

Condylomata acuminata are benign and infectious and have been dealt with earlier in this chapter (Fig 4–18).

Papilloma

The dermal papilloma may occur on the vulva as a benign skin tumor of verrucous type, having a brown color. It may be single or multi-

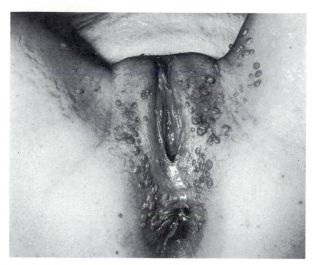

FIG 4–18.
Condylomata acuminata.

ple, and histologically it shows striking hyperkeratosis with acanthosis and elongation of the rete ridges (Fig 4–19). Although the proper name for this lesion is nevus verrucosus, nevus cells are not present in the usual case. It is cured by simple excision.

Lipoma

A lipoma is a benign tumor that arises from the fatty tissue of the labia majora or mons veneris and usually grows slowly and causes no symptoms except when its size is excessive. When this occurs, the mass acquires a pedicle and hangs from the groin or vulva as a pendulum. If the pedicle is wide, it may resemble a hernia. Some lipomas have attained gigantic size, but they usually are not larger than 10 to 12 cm. The histologic appearance is that of normal fat cells with a connective tissue framework and capsule. The incidence of liposarcoma is extremely rare. Nevertheless, the lesion should be excised, since

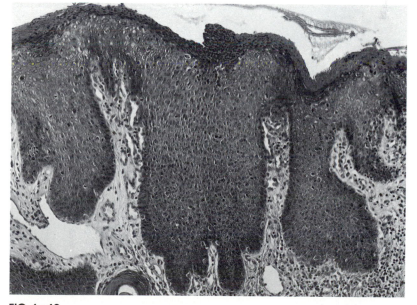

FIG 4–19.
Photomicrograph of vulvar papilloma.

difficulty in walking or in coitus will eventually occur.

Fibroma

A fibroma is a lesion that usually develops as a firm nodule on the labia majora, which then enlarges and develops a pedicle that may hang down for several inches (or feet), so that ulceration and necrosis of the distal portion may occur. The histologic picture is that of any dermatofibroma, with a well-circumscribed lesion made up of intertwined collagen bundles and fibroblasts. In rare cases, the number of nuclei is excessive so that a suspicion of fibrosarcoma is raised. The circumscription of the lesion and absence of mitotic figures and giant cells are usually sufficient to indicate benignancy. These lesions should be surgically removed both for cosmetic effect and for their malignant potential, even though the latter is small.

Hidradenoma

A hidradenoma is a benign, slow-growing, sweat gland tumor, whose histology simulates that of an adenocarcinoma. It is usually about 1 to 2 cm in diameter with a slightly raised, brown surface, which may be umbilicated. As seen in Figure 4–20, the lesion may become quite large, and cystic change may occur. Histologically this is

an adenoma of the vulvar apocrine glands. It is not connected with the epidermis and is usually well encapsulated. The basic pattern is that of a cystlike space in which numerous interlacing villous structures project (Fig 4–21). These structures, as well as the wall of the cyst, are lined by a single layer of high cylindrical cells with eosinophilic cytoplasm and a large, oval, pale-staining nucleus. The cells are regular, and no anaplasia or atypism is evident. A characteristic finding is the layer of myoepithelial cells under the secretory cylindrical cells, a finding similar to that of apocrine tumors in the mammary gland. A rare variant is the clear cell hidradenoma. The lesion is almost always benign, but since a few hidradenocarcinomas have been reported, all should be excised and submitted to pathologic examination (Wick et al., 1985).

MALIGNANT NEOPLASMS

The broad terminology malignant neoplasms includes a variety of lesions of separate structure, the commonest and most important of which are the squamous cell carcinomas of the labia majora, labia minora, and vestibule. Other lesions, fortunately rare, are carcinoma of the clitoris, adenocarcinoma of Bartholin's gland, adenocarcinoma of sweat glands, sarcomas, malignant melanomas, teratomas, and Paget's disease. The entire group

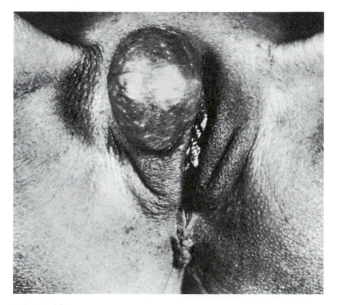

FIG 4–20.
Vulvar hidradenoma.

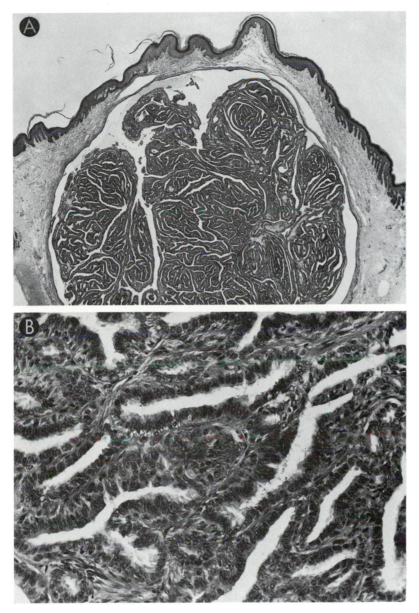

FIG 4–21.
Hidradenoma. **A,** low power; **B,** high power, showing myoepithelial cells under the secretory cylindrical cells.

is said to account for about 1% of all cancers in the female and for 5% to 10% of all cancers involving the female genitalia.

Carcinoma

Vulvar cancer usually occurs in postmenopausal women, about 70% of patients being between 51 and 70 years, with an average age of 61.6 years. Youth does not afford complete protection, however, since Way (1982) has reported 18 patients between 21 and 40 years. Although postmenopausal bleeding will frequently bring the patient to the physician for examination, abnormalities of the vulva go unnoticed or, if discovered, are self-treated for long periods. A dangerous modesty seems to prevail that accounts for serious patient delay. Added to this is the unexplained hesitancy of many physicians to biopsy vulvar lesions when they are first seen and when opportunity for cure is best. Many months are lost, during which time ointments, salves, lotions, and other medications are unsuccessfully tried.

It has become apparent that vulvar carcinoma is not only a disease of the aged but that, as age advances, the incidence of the disease rapidly increases. As the proportion of "old-age" individuals increases in our population, an ever-growing number of vulvar carcinomas will be seen. Thus, the importance of diminishing patient delay is obvious if increased survival is to be realized.

The symptoms complained of most commonly are a localized mass or lump, painful ulcer, discharge, vulvar irritation, dysuria, or bleeding. The duration of symptoms in some series has been as long as 3 or 4 years, but in the cases analyzed at the Brigham and Women's Hospital, it was 13.8 months. Physical examination reveals the lesion to be extremely variable in appearance since in its early form it may merely be an elevated papule or small ulcer. The lesion may be a typical everting, ulcerating mass, or it may be hypertrophic and resemble a papilloma. Another variety is the nonulcerating, superficial type, which produces severe edema and a peau d'orange effect. About two thirds of the lesions are found on the labia majora and the remainder on the labia minora, clitoris, and posterior commissure. The majority of carcinomas are confined to the anterior half of the vulva, including the clitoris, and in most cases the external skin surfaces are far more commonly involved than are the medial surfaces of the labia.

Diagnosis is usually obvious except in very early and nonulcerated lesions. Condylomata acuminata, papillomas, ulcerated chancroid, gummata, and tuberculous ulcers may be confusing, but biopsy, gram stain, and serologic tests will aid in the final diagnosis. The histology is usually that of a moderately well-differentiated, grade 1 or 2

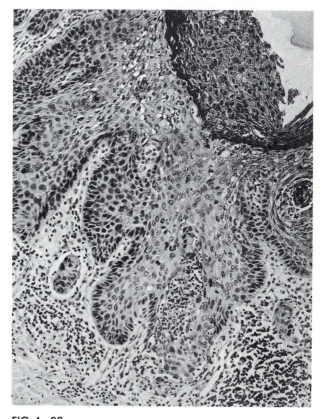

FIG 4–22.
Histologic appearance of early carcinoma of the vulva (low power).

squamous cell carcinoma. Way (1982), however, found a rather large number of his cases to be of the anaplastic type and stated that these lesions are rapidly growing and rapidly metastasizing. In early lesions, the microscopic pattern is that of irregular masses of epidermal cells invading the corium (Fig 4–22). These masses are composed of differentiated squamous and horn cells and dedifferentiated (atypical or dysplastic) squamous cells. Such dysplasia is expressed by variation in size and shape of the cells, hyperplasia and hyperchromasia of nuclei, loss of polarity, absence of prickles, keratinization of certain cells, presence of mitotic figures, and, particularly, atypical and bizarre mitoses. Differentiation is evident as an increased tendency toward keratinization with the formation of "pearls," which are composed of concentric layers of squamous cells with increased cornification toward the center. Extensive "pearl" formation is seen in Figure 4–23. In the Brigham and Women's Hospital series, 21% were classified as grade 1 tumors, 68% as grade 2, and 11% as grade 3.

Clinical staging of carcinoma of the vulva is important, since it refers to the degree of extension of the disease as determined by physical or x-ray examination. It is obvious that survival should be directly correlated with this staging, and this is true not only of carcinoma of the vulva but also of the cervix, breast, and endometrium.

Classification and Staging

The criteria for staging of epidermoid vulvar carcinoma were formulated by the International Federation of Gynecology and Obstetrics (FIGO) in 1967 and were subsequently approved in 1971 (Table 4–2). The rules for classification are similar to those at the other gynecologic sites. Tumors present in the vulva as secondary growths from either a genital or extragenital site should be excluded. Malignant melanoma should be separately reported. The femoral, inguinal, external iliac, and hypogastric nodes are the sites of regional spread.

Franklin evaluated this staging by retrospective application in a review of 164 patients treated

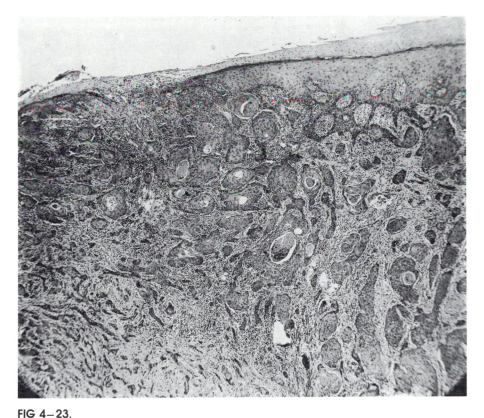

FIG 4–23.
High-power photomicrograph of carcinoma of the vulva. (Courtesy of Armed Forces Institute of Pathology, no. 70121.)

TABLE 4–2.

Clinical Stages of Carcinoma of the Vulva

FIGO nomenclature—1971
  Stage 0
    Carcinoma in situ
  Stage I
    Tumor confined to vulva—2 cm or less in
      diameter. Nodes are not palpable or are
      palpable in either groin, not enlarged,
      mobile (not clinically suspicious of neoplasm).
  Stage II
    Tumor confined to the vulva—more than 2 cm
      in diameter. Nodes are not palpable or are
      palpable in either groin, not enlarged,
      mobile (not clinically suspicious of neoplasm).
  Stage III
    Tumor of any size with (1) adjacent spread to
      the urethra and any or all of the vagina, the
      perineum, and the anus; and/or (2) nodes
      palpable in either or both groins (enlarged,
      firm, and mobile, not fixed but clinically
      suspicious of neoplasm).
  Stage IV
    Tumor of any size (1) infiltrating the bladder
      mucosa or the rectal mucosa or both,
      including the upper part of the urethral
      mucosa; and/or (2) fixed to the bone or other
      distant metastases. Fixed or ulcerated nodes
      in either or both groins.
Tumor-node-metastasis nomenclature
  Primary Tumor (T)
    TIS, T1, T2, T3, T4 See corresponding FIGO stages.
  Nodal Involvement (N)
    NX Not possible to assess the regional nodes.
    N0 No involvement of regional nodes.
    N1 Evidence of regional node involvement.
    N3 Fixed or ulcerated nodes.
    N4 Juxtaregional node involvement.
  Distant metastasis (M)
    MX Not assessed.
    M0 No (known) distant metastasis.
    M1 Distant metastasis present.

at the M.D. Anderson Hospital from 1944 to 1968. His review of factors relating to tumor size, anatomic extent, and clinical evaluation of the possibility of metastatic inguinal lymphadenopathy proved them to be valid criteria for staging. Only minor exceptions to the adequacy of protocol for staging were noted. One was inability to confirm any adverse prognosis associated with perineal involvement by a lesion when it does not encroach on the anus or rectum. Another deficiency was the possibility that stages I and II did not adequately differentiate patient populations of favorable prognosis. Conclusions regarding the

validity of these criteria must await further clinical trials.

Evaluation of accuracy of clinical staging has been addressed by other authors in recent years. Approximately 25% of the time, surgical staging does not agree with clinical staging. Reasons for this include the presence of palpable nodes with no disease, the presence of disease in nonpalpable nodes, and edema surrounding primary lesions, making assessment of lesion size inaccurate. In a recent review from the Mayo Clinic, Podratz et al. (1983) have concluded that clinical staging is of no value. In the same report, a decrease from a 90% 5-year survival rate when lymph nodes are normal to about 45% when they are abnormal is noted. Furthermore, survival fell to 57% for single nodal involvement and to 37% when two or more nodes were involved. Survival for bilateral positive inguinal nodes was 29% at 5 years.

The natural history of vulvar cancer is, in general, that of a slowly growing lesion with spread to groin and pelvic nodes and localization in these areas for long periods. Remote metastases are not common until late in the disease when blood-borne spread may occur. If untreated, there is a subsequent fungating, ulcerative process that destroys the vulva, urethra, and anus, resulting in painful fistulas. Death may occur from ulceration of large blood vessels, from sepsis, or from widespread metastases.

Nodes and Stage.—Frequency of abnormal nodes correlates directly with stage of disease. For stage I disease, recent reports vary from 10% to 15% having abnormal nodes; for stage II disease, 30% to 40%; for stage III disease, up to 80%; and for stage IV disease, 100%.

Tumor Grade.—Histologic grade of tumor now appears to be an independent variable regarding survival. Mayo Clinic experience in this regard is 84% and 83% survival for grades 1 and 2, and 52% for grades 3 or 4.

Lesion Size.—Krupp (1973) has noted that the critical size of the primary lesion is better placed at 3 cm as opposed to 2 cm, therefore confusing classical stage I and II definitions. The Mayo Clinic experience reports 90% 5-year survival for lesions less than 1 cm, 89% for lesions 1 to 2 cm, 83% for lesions 2 to 3 cm, 63% for lesions 3 to 4 cm, and 44% for lesions greater than 4 cm.

Routes of Spread

Dissemination of vulvar carcinoma is usually by way of lymphatic metastases (Plentl and Friedman, 1971), probably by tumor emboli rather than by direct permeation. The commonest route of spread is via the superficial inguinal nodes to the node of Cloquet (the most superior deep femoral node that lies in the upper portion of the femoral canal under the inguinal ligament) and thence to the external iliac nodes. Lesions of the clitoris drain directly to Cloquet's node, and lesions that involve the posterior vulva and lower vagina may also bypass the superficial and deep inguinal nodes and drain directly to the external iliac nodes. It is important to realize that contralateral and bilateral spread may occur with a unilateral lesion.

Treatment

Since Taussig pioneered the radical surgical approach to the treatment of carcinoma of the vulva, there has been little doubt of its efficacy over the last 40 years (Morley, 1976; Way, 1982). Gynecologic surgeons have come to realize that the standard treatment for the disease consists of radical vulvectomy with combined superficial inguinal and femoral lymph node dissection using separate groin incisions (Hacker et al., 1981). The external iliac lymph node dissection (pelvic nodes) has become reserved for those patients in whom Cloquet's node was demonstrated to be positive for tumor. Omission of the deep pelvic node dissection has become acceptable for patients who are poor surgical risks and for those with minimal disease.

Homesley et al. (1986) reported a randomized prospective Gynecologic Oncology Group study wherein 114 patients with abnormal groin nodes received whole pelvis irradiation or pelvic lymphadenectomy. The two major poor prognostic factors were clinically suspicious or fixed ulcerated groin nodes and two or more abnormal groin nodes. The difference in survival was significant ($p = 0.03$). Two-year survival was 68% for radiation and 54% for pelvic node resection. Survival was most dramatic for those being irradiated who had either of the two major poor prognostic factors. The significance of bilaterally involved nodes was contained in the total number of abnormal nodes. Bilaterality was significant as a poor prognostic factor but not independent of the number of abnormal groin nodes. There was no difference in morbidity in the radiation vs. nonirradiated group.

Curry et al. (1980) analyzed the chance of pelvic lymph nodes containing tumor according to the number and area of groin nodes involved. With fewer than four unilateral abnormal nodes, abnormal pelvic nodes were found in 8%. When four or more nodes were abnormal, 50% of pelvic nodes were positive, and when bilateral inguinal or femoral nodes were abnormal, 26% of pelvic nodes were abnormal. With clitoral involvement, 24 of 58 patients (41%) had abnormal nodes. However, there were no abnormal pelvic nodes without abnormal groin nodes.

Hacker et al. (1983) believe that the low incidence of abnormal pelvic nodes in patients with fewer than three abnormal unilateral groin nodes does not justify pelvic lymphadenectomy. Whether or not contralateral groin dissection should be performed for lateral vulvar lesions remains controversial. Morris (1977) suggested that unilateral vulvar lesions may be best treated with groin dissection only on the same side as the lesion.

Macrometastases and Micrometastases

Iversen (1981), reporting on a series of 258 patients, noted metastasis to superficial or deep inguinal lymph nodes (or both) in 38%. Only 64% of these were clinically suspicious. In 15% of the enlarged lymph nodes, no microscopic tumor was found. Five-year survival for patients with lymph node metastasis was 41%. Survival in the face of abnormal nodes depended on whether the metastatic disease was macrometastatic or micrometastatic. Those with micrometastasis had slightly fewer recurrences, 50% vs. 65%, and had a longer survival time and greater overall survival rates than those with macrometastasis, as might be expected. Donaldson et al. (1981) reported on a study of 66 patients noting that patients with regional lymph node metastasis had a 46% survival for three or more years as opposed to 76% survival for patients without nodal involvement. This study, however, highlights the fact that even the best prognostic groups that lacked lymph-space invasion or other unfavorable parameters had a 30% incidence of abnormal nodes.

Early Carcinoma

In 1974, Wharton, Gallagher, and Rutledge reported on a group of 45 patients with invasive carcinoma of the vulva 2 cm or less in diameter. In this group, a subset of 25 patients in whom stromal invasion reached a depth of 5 mm or less was noted. None of these patients had developed abnormal lymph nodes, and subsequently, no lesion recurred and no patient died from vulvar cancer. The authors concluded that their data suggested that patients with early invasion might be better treated with less than full radical surgical therapy.

In 1975, Parker et al. reviewed 60 patients with vulvar squamous cell cancers of less than 2 cm. They noted that 58 of these patients had stromal invasion of 5 mm or less in depth. Three of the 60 patients had pelvic lymph node metastasis. Two of the three had invasion of vascular channels, and the third patient exhibited cellular anaplasia. Subsequent interest in this subject has been intense, with at least 18 articles being published with data suggesting that criteria for lesser surgery were still inexact and that some patients with even 1 mm of invasion were known to have died of their disease.

Hoffman et al., in 1983, pointed out that there is still no widely accepted set of criteria to define the term *microinvasive* when pertaining to carcinoma of the vulva. In their experience with 90 patients with stage I squamous cell carcinoma of the vulva, they noted that anaplasia and lymphovascular invasion were associated with nodal metastasis and that confluence with 3 mm or more of invasion may also be associated with spread to lymph nodes. These authors now recommend wide local excision and hemivulvectomy or total vulvectomy when the depth of invasion is 3 mm or less and nonconfluent. They believe that confluent tumor with less than 2 mm of invasion may also be treated more conservatively.

DiSaia and others (1979, 1981) have treated and prospectively followed up a group of 20 women meeting very rigid criteria, including (1) a primary lesion less than 1 cm in diameter that is confined to the vulva or perineum, and (2) a lesion with invasion limited to 5 mm in depth measuring from the base of the overlying epithelium. Care was taken to evaluate other histologic criteria, including confluency, invasion deeper than 1 mm, vascular-channel invasion, and high degrees of anaplasia. This surgical protocol consisted of careful study of the primary neoplasm after excisional biopsy. Definitive treatment was based on excision of superficial inguinal lymph nodes bilaterally with frozen section at the time. In the absence of metastasis, a wide local excision was carried out at the site of the primary lesion with either primary closure or skin grafting. If nodal disease was present at the time of inguinal dissection, formal superficial and deep inguinal and femoral node dissection was carried out along with standard radical vulvectomy. Subsequent follow-up has failed to reveal any recurrence.

To date, the literature is not in total agreement (Barnes et al., 1980; Buscema et al., 1981; Chu et al., 1981, 1982; DiPaola et al., 1975; Hacker et al., 1983; Jafari and Cartnick, 1976a, 1976b; Kunschner et al., 1978; Magrina et al., 1979; Nakao et al., 1974; Pickel, 1982; Wilkinson et al., 1982; Yazigi et al., 1978). Definitions and terminology employed vary widely. Therefore, great care must be taken in deciding which candidates are best for such a conservative treatment program. DiSaia (1979) now suggests that microinvasive carcinoma should be defined as a well-differentiated keratinizing squamous cell carcinoma, the diameter of the lesion being less than 1 cm, and the depth of the stromal invasion not exceeding 3 mm. There should be no evidence of confluence or lymphatic or vascular invasion. Although evidence is mounting that this is a reasonable approach, since it provides adequate therapy without mutilating anatomy, especially during the reproductive years, it is in no way universally accepted.

In 1987, Sedlis et al. reported 272 cases reviewed by the Gynecologic Oncology Group, noting that the term microinvasive cancer embraces all lesions 5 mm or less in thickness. Since 50% of all vulva cancers are no thicker than 5 mm, and 20% of these metastasize to lymph nodes, the term microinvasive is inappropriate. This study concludes that a statistical model employing several predictors (i.e., tumor thickness, histologic grade, capillary space involvement, clitoral or perineal locations, and clinically suspect nodes) may be more valid in predicting the presence of abnormal inguinal nodes and thus aid in selecting an appropriate form of treatment (Sedlis et al., 1987).

The ISSVD proposes that superficially invasive carcinoma of the vulva be classified as stage 1A vulvar carcinoma and be defined as a single lesion measuring 2 cm or less in diameter with a depth of invasion of 1 mm or less (Wilkinson et al., 1986).

Treatment of Late-Stage Disease

In the Mayo Clinic series, stage III disease did not appear to benefit when radical vulvectomy and inguinal-femoral lymphadenectomy were supplemented with deep pelvic node dissection. No case of pelvic node metastasis was noted without the presence of abnormal inguinal or femoral lymph nodes.

Patients with advanced disease continue to have poor survival in the face of radical surgery and lymphadenectomy. This suggests that the present approach to this disease is not adequate, and therefore the application of adjuvant whole-pelvic radiation therapy, with or without central radiation, may be indicated. More clinicians are initially treating the primary lesion with vulvectomy and superficial and deep femoral and inguinal lymph node dissection but are bringing the patient back at a later date for pelvic exploration and periaortic node biopsy; this will, hopefully, help the clinician to obtain more definitive information about the extent of the disease and be able to make a combined attack on disease that has spread beyond the confines of the vulva and regional nodes. When the disease involves urethra, anus, or vagina, there is increasing likelihood of embolization being present in paravaginal and pararectal lymphatics. This may warrant more aggressive therapy, with selected cases being subjected to exenteration, both total exenteration and posterior exenteration, with or without added radiation therapy.

Recently, Boronow et al. (1987) have dem-onstrated increased survival in stage III and IV disease when combining radical vulvectomy with use of irradiation for vaginal and cervical involvement, thus avoiding removal of bladder and rectum.

Complications

Operative mortality is approximately 2% and is usually related to a cardiovascular complication, including pulmonary emboli. Necrosis of skin flaps, collection of lymph fluid, cellulitis, hematoma formation, urinary tract infection, phlebitis, leg edema, lymphangitis, urinary incontinence, fistula formation, and dyspareunia are occasionally encountered.

Recurrence

When local recurrences occur late following primary therapy, they respond well to local treatment (Podratz et al., 1982). This suggests that the skin of the neovulva subsequently undergoes malignant change, a theory embraced by Taussig.

Verrucous Carcinoma

Verrucous carcinoma (Fig 4–24) is to be distinguished from condylomatous carcinoma, which has a more aggressive course (Crowther et al., 1988). Grossly, it is often mistaken for condy-

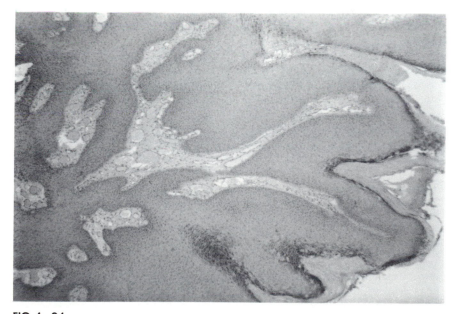

FIG 4–24.
Verrucous carcinoma. A hypercellular infiltrating lesion. Note the uniformly bland-appearing epithelium.

lomata acuminata and treated as such over a period of time. Subsequent biopsy may be misleading unless it is generous and deep. Invasive squamous cell carcinoma and intraepithelial neoplasia may coexist. Microscopically, the features that distinguish it from condyloma include swollen and velamentous rete pegs, absent fibrovascular stocks, and the presence of squamous "pearls" deep in the epithelium. Infiltrating margins are absent, and individual malignant features of the cells throughout the tumor are also lacking, with good cytologic differentiation and uniformity of pattern. On the other hand, condylomatous carcinoma exhibits the hallmarks of invasive squamous carcinoma with infiltrating margins of cellular anaplasia and the presence of keratin "pearls." Treatment of this lesion is by wide local excision or vulvectomy (Japaze et al., 1982). Radiation has been tried and found wanting. Inguinal lymph nodes are frequently enlarged, but in 27 cases reported in the literature, lymph node metastasis has never been demonstrated. Local recurrences are common and should be treated surgically. The etiology of this variant is unknown.

Other Vulvar Malignancies

Carcinoma of Bartholin's Gland

Carcinoma of Bartholin's gland is a rare finding. It may be mistaken for a benign tumor or chronic bartholinitis because of its location. A high degree of malignancy exists because of the rich drainage of the gland lymphatics into the deep as well as the superficial lymphatics.

These lesions may be transitional carcinoma, adenoid cystic tumors, or mucus-secreting tumors, the latter two being less aggressive. Treatment is radical hemivulvectomy, ipsilateral groin node dissection, and irradiation of inguinal and pelvic nodal areas (Copeland et al., 1986).

Basal Cell Carcinoma

Basal cell carcinoma of the vulva is also rather rare, about 75 cases having been reported. It tends to recur locally rather than to spread by lymphatic and blood channels. Breen et al. (1975) recently reviewed the literature on basal cell carcinoma of the vulva and found a ratio of 1 basal cell for every 37 squamous cell carcinomas of the vulva. They added a series of 17 patients to the 96 already reported in the literature. The lesions were described grossly as ulcerations or masses located on the anterior labium majus. Etiologies

were indeterminate, although two patients had previously received vulvar irradiation. Therapy consisted primarily of wide local excision and was effective in that follow-up studies in 16 patients revealed no deaths attributable to basal cell carcinoma. The data of these authors indicate that basal cell carcinoma is a locally invasive, nonmetastasizing tumor (Fig 4–25) best treated by wide local excision, provided the tumor edge does not extend to the margin of excision.

There is some evidence that these tumors do not arise from the basal cells of the epidermis but from hair sheaths or distorted primordia of dermal adnexae. Lever (1956) believes them to be nevoid tumors derived from arrested, embryonal, primary epithelial germ cells. No relationship between leukoplakia and basal cell carcinoma has been demonstrated. Treatment should include a wide and deep local excision.

Sarcoma

This tumor may arise from the connective tissue of the vulva or from a fibroma. Several cases of reticulum cell sarcoma and lymphosar-

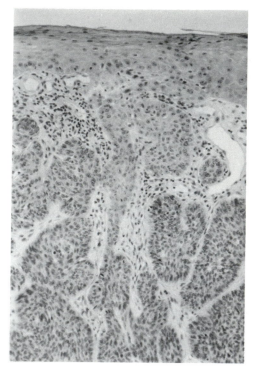

FIG 4–25.
Locally invasive, nonmetastasizing basal cell carcinoma.

coma have recently been added to the literature. The prognosis is poor despite radical surgery.

Melanoma

Melanomas are, by definition, malignant; they account for between 5% and 10% of all vulvar malignancies (Silvers, 1983). They are most often seen in women over the age of 50 years. The lesions may be brown or black. Larger lesions may have associated areas within them that are both red and white. Grossly, this disease cannot be distinguished from many benign lesions; therefore, a diagnosis must be made by biopsy of all pigmented lesions. Ideally, the biopsy should be excisional, with an accompanying 1-cm margin of normal-appearing skin (Day, 1982). When deeply invasive, melanomas metastasize by the lymphatic route and by hematogenous routes as well, the latter being attested to by recurrence at distal sites many years after primary surgery for the vulvar lesion. Depth of tumor invasion is the single best prognostic factor and in general should dictate the kind of surgical therapy to be undertaken. Tumor thickness is measured from the granular layer of the epidermis overlying the tumor to the deepest point of invasion (Breslow, 1970). Tumors invading less than 0.7 cm have the best chance of cure by simple excision only. Tumors invading beyond 3 mm in general have a poor prognosis.

Until now, recommended treatment has always been radical vulvectomy and deep and superficial inguinal and femoral lymphadenectomy combined with deep pelvic node dissection, especially if the tumor involved the anterior vulva or clitoris (Silvers and Halperin, 1978). Such treatment is now considered controversial. Retrospective studies of patients who underwent lymphadenectomy for melanoma at any site failed to show any value to the procedure (Sim et al., 1982). One study has demonstrated possible benefit from lymph node dissection when the lesion invades between 1.5 and 3.0 mm. Critics of these studies say they cannot be considered conclusive due to the retrospective nature of the study (Edington and Monaghan, 1980; Nathanson, 1983). No prospective randomized stratified studies exist. Still, others believe that the radical approach will provide local control of disease with better comfort. It is known that a vast majority of patients with tumor demonstrated in deep nodes will die of the disease. It is also known that most patients with minimal invasive disease will survive

given only local therapy. Hence, critics of the radical surgical approach believe that such treatment is unnecessary in one group and constitutes overtreatment in the other group.

Recent reviews by Wolcott et al. (1988) of the Australian experience as well as recent literature conclude that radical vulvectomy is best reserved only for large central tumors. They believe that optimum treatment should be wide local excision with grafting and bilateral inguinal lymphadenectomy through separate incisions for lesions invading deeper than 0.75 mm. These authors note that regardless of therapy chosen, survival never exceeds 50%, and survival after recurrence is less than 5%.

The classification of invasion according to level was first described by Mihm and Clarke in 1971 and modified by Chung et al. for adaptation to melanoma of the vulva in 1975. Depth of penetration may be correlated with the staging level system in that lesions up to 1.25 mm generally involve epidermis and papillary dermis and have the most favorable prognosis. Lesions extending from 1.25 to 2.25 mm involve the reticular dermis, and lesions extending below that usually involve fat and are designated as level 5 lesions.

Paget's Disease

Paget's disease of the vulva is an intraepithelial carcinoma (Jones et al., 1979). As a disorder of the mammary gland, it is a well-known entity, having been described by James Paget in 1874. It is accepted that mammary Paget's disease is a primary duct cancer that has extended to the epidermis where it causes a cutaneous lesion. Parmley et al. (1975), however, believe that Paget's disease of the vulva is an intraepithelial lesion and that Paget's cells arise de novo in the epithelium or in its appendages. It is entirely possible that this lesion may progress to invasive carcinoma in much the same fashion as Bowen's disease if one accepts the histogenesis as being autochthonous, as suggested by Parmley et al. (1975). Huber, in describing three new cases of vulvar Paget's disease, found a definite adenocarcinoma of the underlying apocrine sweat glands in one. Hart and Millman (1977) reported the first case of intraepithelial disease progressing to invasive carcinoma and lymph node metastasis.

In the vulva, the lesion occurs in women in the later decades of life whose presenting complaint is usually pruritus. Grossly, it is sharply demarcated, florid, red, and moist, with occasional

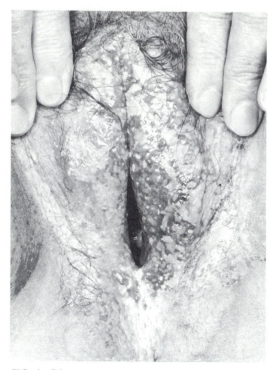

FIG 4–26.
Gross appearance of Paget's disease of the vulva. The dark areas are velvety red, and the white areas are as seen. (From Woodruff JD, Williams TF: *Obstet Gynecol* 1959; 14:86. Reproduced by permission.)

crusting. It may appear eczematoid. Little islands of whitened skin appear between the reddened areas (Fig 4–26). The entire vulva may be involved, with spread to the perineum, mons, and thighs (Gunn and Gallager, 1980). The histologic appearance is characteristic (Fig 4–27). There is acanthosis with elongation and widening of the rete ridges. Paget's cells may be scattered or grouped in clusters, usually in the basalis. They are large cells, lacking prickles, and are surrounded by clear spaces. The cytoplasm is very light and the nuclei are large, round, and pale. Pseudogland formation is common. Treatment should be that of wide and deep excision with careful follow-up despite the long interval that usually elapses before definitive treatment is employed. For invasive disease, radical vulvectomy and bilateral lymph node dissection are mandatory.

Because local recurrences are common, repeated observations and biopsy of suspicious areas are suggested.

Vulvar Paget's disease is an intraepithelial adenocarcinoma that is locally recurrent and has an occasional propensity to invade and metastasize to lymph nodes (Lee and Dahlin, 1981).

Adenocarcinoma of the vulvar apocrine glands is the most commonly associated tumor. Another apocrine adenocarcinoma, carcinoma of

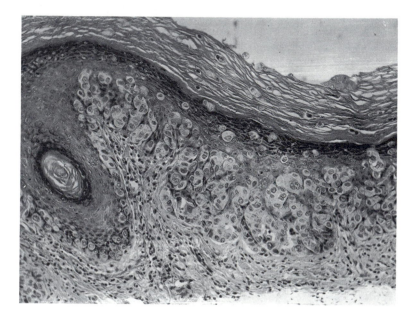

FIG 4–27.
Paget's disease of the vulva showing marked hyperkeratosis and parakeratosis. Large, irregular cells are seen in the basal layer of the epidermis and infiltrating the upper layers as well. The Paget cells contain clear vacuolated cytoplasm and vesicular nuclei, which vary in size, shape, and staining quality.

the breast, either antecedent or concomitant, is the second most frequently associated tumor, having been reported in 14 cases of vulvar Paget's disease. Therefore, preoperative breast screening procedures are indicated in all patients with vulvar Paget's disease.

Metastatic Vulvar Tumors

Metastatic and secondary tumors of the vulva constitute the third largest group of malignant tumors of the vulva. Epidermoid carcinoma of the cervix is the most frequent primary site, followed by the endometrium, kidney, and urethra. Most patients who subsequently develop vulvar metastases have signs of advanced primary tumor when initially diagnosed. Metastatic adenocarcinoma tends to invade the overlying squamous epithelium, whereas epidermoid carcinoma does not. The frequent occurrence of vascular involvement by metastatic tumor incriminates this as the mode of spread to the vulva. The prognosis is poor, and death usually occurs within 1 year of the diagnosis. At the Brigham and Women's Hospital, we have seen two patients with vulvar metastases from adenocarcinoma of the large bowel.

REFERENCES

Anson BI: *An Atlas of Human Anatomy.* Philadelphia, WB Saunders Co, 1950.

Axe S, Parmley T, Woodruff JD, et al: Adenomas in minor vestibular glands. *Obstet Gynecol* 1986; 68:16–18.

Barnes AE, Crissman JD, Schellhas HF, et al: Microinvasive carcinoma of the vulva: A clinical pathologic evaluation. *Obstet Gynecol* 1980; 52:234–238.

Benedet JL, Murphy JJ: Squamous carcinoma in situ of the vulva. *Gynecol Oncol* 1982; 14:213–219.

Bernstein SG, Kovacs BR, Townsend DE, et al: Vulvar carcinoma in situ. *Obstet Gynecol* 1983; 60:304–307.

Bornstein J, Kaufman RH: Combination of surgical excision and carbon dioxide laser vaporization for multifocal vulvar intraepithelial neoplasia. *Am J Obstet Gynecol* 1988; 158:459–464.

Boronow RC, Hickman BT, Reagan MT, et al: Combined therapy as an alternative to exenteration for locally advanced vulvovaginal cancer. *Am J Clin Oncol* 1987; 10:171–181.

Breen JL, Neubecker RD, Greenwald E, et al: Basal cell carcinoma of the vulva. *Obstet Gynecol* 1975; 46:122.

Breslow A: Thickness, cross sectional area and depth of invasion in prognosis of cutaneous melanoma. *Ann Surg* 1970; 172:902.

Buscema J, Stern JL, Woodruff JD: Early invasive carcinoma of the vulva. *Am J Obstet Gynecol* 1981; 140:563–569.

Caglar H, Tamer S, Hreshchyshyn MM: Vulvar intraepithelial neoplasia. *Obstet Gynecol* 1982; 60:346–349.

Chu J, Tamimi HK, Ek M: Stage I vulvar cancer: Criteria for microinvasion. *Obstet Gynecol* 1982; 59:716–719.

Chu J, Tamimi HK, Figge DC: Femoral node metastases with negative superficial inguinal nodes in early vulvar cancer. *Am J Obstet Gynecol* 1981; 140:337–338.

Conway H, Stark RB, Climo S, et al: The surgical treatment of chronic hydradenitis suppurativa. *Surg Gynecol Obstet* 1952; 95:455.

Copeland LJ, Sneige N, Gershenson DM, et al: Bartholin gland carcinoma. *Obstet Gynecol* 1986; 67:794–801.

Crowther ME, Lowe DG, Shepherd JH: Verrucous carcinoma of the female genital tract: A review. *Obstet Gynecol Surv* 1988; 43:263–280.

Curry SL, Wharton JT, Rutledge F: Positive lymph nodes in vulvar squamous carcinoma. *Gynecol Oncol* 1980; 9:63–67.

Day CO Jr, Mihm MC Jr, Sober AJ, et al: Narrower margins for clinical stage I malignant melanoma. *N Engl J Med* 1982; 306:479.

DiPaola GR, Gomez-Rueda N, Arrighi L: Relevance of microinvasion in carcinoma of the vulva. *Obstet Gynecol* 1975; 45:647–648.

DiSaia PJ: A less radical approach to early vulvar cancer. *Contemp Obstet Gynecol* 1981; 18:109–114.

DiSaia PJ, Creasman WT, Rich WM: An alternate approach to early cancer of the vulva. *Am J Obstet Gynecol* 1979; 133:825–832.

DiSaia PJ, Rich WM: Surgical approach to multifocal carcinoma in situ of the vulva. *Am J Obstet Gynecol* 1981; 140:136–145.

Donaldson ES, Powell DE, Hanson MB, et al: Prognostic parameters in invasive vulvar cancers. *Gynecol Oncol* 1981; 12:184–190.

Edington PT, Monaghan JM: Malignant melanoma of the vulva and vagina. *Br J Obstet Gynaecol* 1980; 87:422.

Foster DC, Woodruff JD: The use of dinitrochlorobenzene in the treatment of vulvar carcinoma in situ. *Obstet Gynecol Surv* 1982; 37:55–56.

Friedrich EG Jr: *Vulvar Disease,* ed 2. *Major Problems in Obstetrics and Gynecology,* vol 9. Philadelphia, WB Saunders Co, 1983.

Friedrich EG Jr: Vulvar vestibulitis syndrome. *J Reprod Med* 1987; 22:110–114.

Friedrich EG Jr: Therapeutic studies on vulvar vestibulitis. *J Reprod Med* 1988; 33:514–518.

Friedrich EG Jr, Kalra PS: Serum levels of sex hormones in vulvar lichen sclerosis and the effect of topical testosterone. *N Engl J Med* 1984; 310:488–491.

Goodlin RC, Frederick IB: Postpartum vulva edema associated with the birthing chair. *Am J Obstet Gynecol* 1983; 146:334.

Gordon SW: Hidradenitis suppurativa: A closer look. *J Natl Med Assoc* 1978; 70:239–343.

Gunn RA, Gallager HS: Vulvar Paget's disease: A topographic study. *Cancer* 1980; 46:590–594.

Hacker NF, Nieberg RK, Berek JS, et al: Superficially invasive vulvar cancer with nodal metastasis. *Gynecol Oncol* 1983; 15:65–77.

Hacker NF, Berek JS, Lagasse LD, et al: Management of regional lymph nodes and their prognostic influence in vulvar cancer. *Obstet Gynecol* 1983; 61:408–412.

Hacker NF, Leuchter RS, Berek JS, et al: Radical vulvectomy and bilateral inguinal lymphadenectomy through separate groin incisions. *Obstet Gynecol* 1981; 58:574–579.

Hart WR, Millman JD: Progression of intraepithelial Paget's disease of the vulva to invasive carcinoma. *Cancer* 1977; 40:2333–2337.

Hewitt J: Histologic criteria for lichen sclerosis of the vulva. *J Reprod Med* 1986; 31:781–787.

Hoffman JS, Kumar MB, Molrey GW: Microinvasive squamous carcinoma of the vulva: Search for a definition. *Obstet Gynecol* 1983; 61:615–618.

Homesley HD, Bundy BN, Sedlis A, et al: Radiation therapy versus pelvic node resection for carcinoma of the vulva with positive groin nodes. *Obstet Gynecol* 1986; 68:733–740.

Iversen T: The value of groin palpation in epidermoid carcinoma of the vulva. *Gynecol Oncol* 1981; 12:291–295.

Iversen T, Abler B, Kolstad T: Squamous cell carcinoma in situ of the vulva. A clinical and histopathological study. *Gynecol Oncol* 1981; 11:224–229.

Jafari K, Cartnick EN: Microinvasive squamous cell carcinoma of the vulva. *Am J Obstet Gynecol* 1976a; 125:2, 274.

Jafari K, Cartnick EN: Microinvasive squamous cell carcinoma of the vulva. *Gynecol Oncol* 1976b; 4:158–166.

Japaze N, van Dinh T, Woodruff JB: Verrucous carcinoma of the vulva: A study of 24 cases. *Obstet Gynecol* 1982; 60:462–466.

Jones RE, Austin C, Ackerman AB: Extramammary Paget's disease: A critical re-examination. *Am J Dermatopathol* 1979; 1:101–132.

Jones RW, McLean MR: Carcinoma in situ of the vulva: A review of 31 treated and 5 untreated cases. *Obstet Gynecol* 1986; 68:499–507.

Kaplan AL, Kaufman RH, Birken RA, et al: Intraepithelial carcinoma of the vulva with extension to the anal canal. *Obstet Gynecol* 1981; 58:368–371.

Kao FG, Graham JH: Bowenoid papulosis. *Int J Dermatol* 1982; 21:445–446.

Koff AK: Embryology of the female generative tract, in Curtis AH (ed): *Obstetrics and Gynecology*. Philadelphia, WB Saunders Co, 1933.

Krebs HB: Prophylactic topical 5-fluorouracil following treatment of human papilloma virus-associated lesions of the vulva and vagina. *Obstet Gynecol Surv* 1987; 42:466–467.

Kunschner A, Kanbour AI, David B: Early vulvar carcinoma. *Am J Obstet Gynecol* 1978; 132:599–606.

Kurman RJ, Sha KH, Lancaster WD, et al: Immunoperoxidase localization of papilloma virus antigens in cervical dysplasia and vulvar condylomas. *Am J Obstet Gynecol* 1981; 140:931–935.

Lavery HA, Pinkerton JHM, Sloan J: Crohn's disease of vulva—two further cases. *Br J Dermatol* 1985; 113:359–363.

Leads from the *MMWR* 1983; 32:23, 24, Centers for Disease Control, Atlanta. *JAMA* 1983; 250:336.

Lee RA, Dahlin DC: Paget's disease of the vulva with extension into the urethra, vulva and ureters: A case report. *Am J Obstet Gynecol* 1981; 140:834–836.

Lever WF: *Histopathology of Skin*, ed 2. Philadelphia, JB Lippincott Co, 1954.

Levine EM, Barton JJ, Grier EA: Metastatic Crohn disease of the vulva. *Obstet Gynecol* 1982; 60:395–397.

Lifshitz S, Roberts JA: Treatment of carcinoma in situ of the vulva with topical 5-fluorouracil. *Obstet Gynecol* 1980; 56:242–244.

Lynch PJ: Vulvar dystrophies and intraepithelial neoplasias. *Dermatol Clin* 1987; 5:789–799.

Magrina JF, Webb JJ, Gaffey TA, et al: Stage I squamous cell cancer of the vulva. *Am J Obstet Gynecol* 1979; 134:453–459.

McKay H: Subsets of vulvodynia. *J Reprod Med* 1988; 33:695–698.

Meltzer RM: Necrotizing fasciitis and progressive bacterial synergistic gangrene of the vulva. *Obstet Gynecol* 1983; 51:757–760.

Morley GW: Infiltrative carcinoma of the vulva: Results of surgical treatment. *Am J Obstet Gynecol* 1976; 124:874–884.

Morris J McL: A formula for selective lymphadenectomy; its application to cancer of the vulva. *Obstet Gynecol* 1977; 50:152–158.

Nakao CY, Nolan JF, DiSaia PJ, et al: Microinvasive epidermoid carcinoma of the vulva with an unexpected natural history. *Am J Obstet Gynecol* 1974; 120:1122–1123.

Nathanson L: Update on melanoma. *Clin Cancer Briefs* 1983; 4:3–13.

Nichols DH, Milley PS: *Clinical Anatomy of the Vulva, Vagina, Lower Pelvis and Derneum in Sciarra. Gynecology and Obstetrics*. New York, Harper & Row, Publishers, 1980.

Parker RT, Duncan I, Rampone J, et al: Operative management of early invasive epidermoid carcinoma of the vulva. *Am J Obstet Gynecol* 1975; 1:349–355.

Parmley TH, Woodruff JD, Julian CG: Invasive vulva Paget's disease. *Obstet Gynecol* 1975; 46:341–346.

Patten BM: *Human Embryology,* ed 2. New York, McGraw-Hill Book Co, 1953.

Pickel TH: The early stages of vulvar carcinoma, diagnostic problems. *J Reprod Med* 1982; 27:465–470.

Plentl AA, Friedman EA: *Lymphatic System of the Female Genitalia*. Philadelphia, WB Saunders Co, 1971.

Podratz KC, Symmonds RE, Taylor WF: Carcinoma of the vulva: Analysis of treatment failures. *Am J Obstet Gynecol* 1982; 143:340–351.

Podratz KC, Symmonds RE, Taylor WF: Carcinoma of the vulva: Analysis of treatment and survival. *Obstet Gynecol* 1983; 61:63–74.

Rastkar G, Okagaki T, Twiggs LB, et al: Early invasive and in situ warty carcinoma of the vulva: Clinical, histologic and electron microscopic study with particular reference to viral association. *Am J Obstet Gynecol* 1982; 143:814–820.

Rettenmaier MA, Berman ML, DiSaia PJ: Skinning vulvectomy for the treatment of multifocal vulvar intraepithelial neoplasia. *Obstet Gynecol* 1987; 69:247–250.

Robboy SJ, Lombardo JM, Welch WR: Disorders of abnormal sexual development, in Kurman R (ed): *Blaustein's Pathology of the Female Genital Tract,* ed 3. New York, Springer-Verlag New York, 1987, pp 15–35.

Roberts DB: Necrotizing fasciitis of the vulva. *Am J Obstet Gynecol* 1987; 157:568–571.

Schmid GP, Sanders LL Jr, Blount JH, et al: Chancroid in the United States: Re-establishment of an old disease. *JAMA* 1987; 258:3265–3268.

Scott JC Jr, Smith ML: Benign neoplasms of the vulva, in *Sciarra Gynecology and Obstetrics*. New York, Harper & Row, Publishers, 1980.

Sedlis A, Homesley H, Bundy BN, et al: Positive groin lymph nodes and superficial squamous cell vulvar cancer, a gynecologic oncology group study. *Am J Obstet Gynecol* 1987; 156:1159–1164.

Sillman FH, Boyce JG, Macasaet MA, et al: 5-Fluorouracil/chemosurgery for intraepithelial neoplasia of the lower genital tract. *Obstet Gynecol* 1981; 58:356–360.

Silvers DN: What you need to know about tumors of melanocytes. *Contemp Obstet Gynecol* 1983; 20:140–149.

Silvers DN, Halperin AJ: Cutaneous and vulvar melanoma: An update. *Clin Obstet Gynecol* 1978; 21:1117–1133.

Sim S, Taylor W, Pritchard D, et al: A prospective randomized study of the efficacy of routine elective lymphadenectomy in management of malignant melanoma [abstract]. *Proc Int Cancer Congr* 1982; 13:658.

Soper DE, Patterson JW, Hurt WG, et al: Lichen planus of the vulva. *Obstet Gynecol* 1988; 72:74–76.

Soper JT, Creasman WT: Vulvar dystrophies. *Clin Obstet Gynecol* 1986; 29:431–439.

Thomas R, Barnhill D, Bibro M, et al: Hidradenitis suppurativa: A case presentation and review of the literature. *Obstet Gynecol* 1985; 66:592–595.

van Slyke KK, Michel VP, Rein MF: Treatment of vulvovaginal candidiasis with boric acid powder. *Am J Obstet Gynecol* 1981; 141:145–148.

Wade TR, Rorf AW, Ackerman AB: Bowenoid papulosis of the genitalia. *Arch Dermatol* 1979; 115:306–308.

Way S: *Malignant Disease of the Vulva*. New York, Churchill Livingston, 1982.

Wharton JT, Gallager S, Rutledge FN: Microinvasive carcinoma of the vulva. *Am J Obstet Gynecol* 1974; 118:159–162.

Wick MR, Goellner JR, Wolfe JT, et al: Vulvar sweat gland carcinomas. *Arch Pathol Lab Med* 1985; 109:43–47.

Wilkinson EJ, Friedrich EG Jr, Fu YS: Multicentric nature of vulvar carcinoma in situ. *Obstet Gynecol* 1981; 58:69–74.

Wilkinson EJ, Kneale B, Lynch PJ: Report of the ISSVD terminology committee. *J Reprod Med* 1986; 31:973–974.

Wilkinson EJ, Rice MJ, Pierson KK: Microinvasive carcinoma of the vulva. *Int J Gynecol Pathol* 1982; 1:29–39.

Wilson EE, Malinak LR: Vulvovaginal sequellae of Stevens-Johnson syndrome and their management. *Obstet Gynecol* 1988; 71:478–480.

Woodruff JD: Diagnosis and management of benign lesions of the vulva. *Curr Probl Obstet Gynecol* 1978; vol 1, no 2.

Woodruff JD, Friedrich EG Jr: The vestibule. *Clin Obstet Gynecol* 1985; 28:134–141.

Woolcott RJ, Henry RJW, Houghton CRS: Malignant melanoma of the vulva: Australian experience. *J Reprod Med* 1988; 33:699–702.

Wright VC, Davies V: Laser surgery for vulva intraepithelial neoplasia: Principles and results. *Am J Obstet Gynecol* 1987; 156:374–378.

Yavetz H, Lessing JB, Jaffa AJ, et al: Fistulization: An effective treatment for Bartholin's abscesses and cysts. *Acta Obstet Gynecol Scand* 1987; 66:63–64.

Yazigi R, Piver MS, Tsukada Y: Microinvasive carcinoma of the vulva. *Obstet Gynecol* 1978; 51:368–370.

Young HH: *Genital Abnormalities. Hermaphroditism and Related Adrenal Disease*. Baltimore, Williams & Wilkins Co, 1937.

Zacur H, Genabry R, Woodruff JD: The patient at risk for development of vulvar cancer. *Gynecol Oncol* 1980; 9:199–208.

5 _____ The Vagina and Female Urology

Joan Bengtson, M.D.

The vagina is a tubular, fibromuscular structure that extends from the vestibule to the uterus. It is the interface between the environment and the generative tract. Its functions are to provide an outflow duct for menstrual discharge, to receive the penis during intercourse, and to form the lowermost part of the birth canal.

There is a close association between the structure and function of the vagina and the lower urinary tract. The embryological development of the urinary and reproductive tracts are closely linked, and a congenital anomaly in one often heralds an abnormality in the other. Anatomically the two systems are juxtaposed. Symptoms arising in one may be difficult to distinguish clinically from the other. The physician must be familiar with the fundamental principles of female urology to adequately care for gynecological patients.

EMBRYOLOGY

Vagina

The embryology of the vagina is controversial despite extensive historic interest in the topic and renewed interest stimulated by diethylstilbestrol (DES)–associated pathology in more recent decades. Although certain events are well established, the histogenesis of the vaginal epithelium is uncertain. One theory favors a dual origin such that the upper portion of the vagina derives from the mesodermal müllerian ducts and the lower portion of the vagina from the endodermal urogenital sinus. Another proposes that the entire vagina originates in the urogenital sinus.

Development is identical in male and female fetuses until the seventh week. The indifferent stage ends in boys when the developing testes begin producing androgenic steroids (Wilson et al., 1981). Androgens stimulate development of the mesonephric (wolffian) duct system into the epididymis, vas deferens, and seminal vesicles. In addition, a polypeptide, müllerian-inhibiting factor (MIF) is produced and acts to suppress growth and induce resorption of the müllerian ducts. In girls, the absence of androgens and MIF results in further development of the müllerian structures.

The müllerian ducts develop in the embryos of both sexes during the sixth week (11-mm stage; Koff, 1933). They form as bilateral longitudinal evaginations of the coelomic epithelium into the mesonephric ridge ventrolateral to the mesonephric duct. Tubular structures result as the process of evagination is completed. Each müllerian duct remains open to the coelomic cavity at its cephalic end via an ostium. Caudally, the duct initially runs parallel and lateral to the mesonephric duct. It then crosses ventral to the mesonephric duct to meet the contralateral müllerian duct in the midline (Fig 5–1). The ducts fuse, forming the primordial uterovaginal canal (30-mm embryo). This structure initially contains a longitudinal septum. The septum usually disappears by the 11th week (56-mm embryo). The cranial segment of each müllerian duct ultimately forms a fallopian tube, its ostium becoming the fimbriated extremity. As the midline septum resorbs from the fused middle segment, the uterine corpus and cervix form. The caudal end of the fused müllerian ducts joins the urogenital sinus.

The attachment of the distal, fused müllerian ducts to the urogenital sinus simulates a proliferation of cells in its dorsal wall. A prominence called the *müllerian tubercle* is formed (Koff, 1933). The adjacent urogenital sinus epithelium also proliferates bilaterally, forming the sinovaginal bulbs (63-mm embryo). Further proliferation

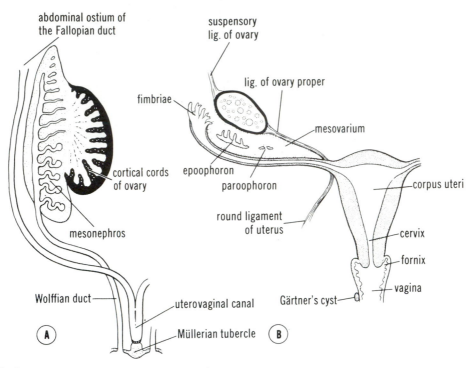

FIG 5–1.
A, schematic drawing of the genital ducts in the female at the end of the second month of development. Note the müllerian tubercle and the formation of the uterovaginal canal. *B,* the genital ducts after descent of the ovary. The only parts remaining of the mesonephric system are the epoophoron, paroophoron, and Gartner's cyst. Note the suspensory ligament of the ovary, the ligament of the ovary proper, and the round ligament of the uterus.

results in the formation of a solid midline cord of cells called the *vaginal plate* (120-mm embryo). Growth and elongation of the vaginal plate increases the distance between the uterocervical canal and the urogenital sinus (Fig 5–2). It also divides the urogenital sinus into an upper portion that develops into the bladder and urethra (the vesicourethral canal) and a lower portion that forms the definitive urogenital sinus and ultimately the vestibule.

Canalization of the vaginal plate occurs as the central cells degenerate beginning at the urogenital sinus and proceeding cranially to form the vault. The process is completed by approximately the fifth month. The lumen of the vagina remains separated from the lumen of the urogenital sinus by the formation of the hymen. The hymen usually develops at least a partial opening sometime later.

The ultimate derivation of the vaginal squamous epithelium is disputed (Forsberg, 1973). Koff (1933) suggests that caudal extension of the müllerian uterovaginal canal results in formation of the upper four fifths of the vagina, whereas the lower one fifth derives from the endodermal urogenital sinus. The hymen demarcates the junction. After canalization occurs, the müllerian columnar epithelium is replaced by upward migration of squamous columnar epithelium from the urogenital sinus (Ulfelder and Robboy, 1976). Bulmer (1957) suggests that the vaginal plate is essentially entirely derived from proliferation of the sinovaginal bulbs, and thus the entire vagina is of urogenital sinus origin. It is likely that a normal interaction of both müllerian and urogenital sinus tissue is necessary for normal vaginal development.

Kidneys and Ureters

The kidneys and ureters are formed through a series of three stages that recapitulate development of the excretory system in primitive vertebrates. During the third week, the mesoderm

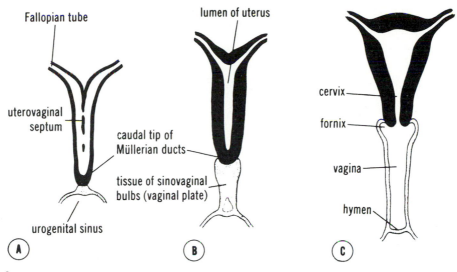

FIG 5–2.
Schematic drawing showing the formation of the uterus and vagina. *A,* at 9 weeks. Note the disappearance of the uterovaginal septum. *B,* at the end of the third month. Note the tissue of the sinovaginal bulbs, extending between the uterus and the urogenital sinus. *C,* newborn. The vagina and the fornices are formed by vacuolization of the tissue of the sinovaginal bulbs.

forming the nephrogenic cord along the dorsal body wall gives rise to several pairs of tubules, the pronephros. This system is transient and nonfunctioning in the human (Crelin, 1978). Formation and degeneration of the pronephros proceed in a cranial to caudal sequence and are complete by the end of the fourth week. The only persistent component of this system is the pronephric duct. Initially it comprises the union of the pronephric tubules, but as they degenerate, it continues to grow caudally to join the cloaca during the fifth week. Subsequently, it is retained as the mesonephric duct.

The second primitive kidney, the mesonephros, develops within the nephrogenic cord caudal to the pronephros beginning in the fourth week. The tubules begin as blind vesicles that grow to join the mesonephric duct laterally. Medially each tubule forms a Bowman's capsule and associates with a vascular glomerulus. The mesonephros probably functions to produce urine in the human fetus during the third and fourth months (deMartino and Zamboni, 1966). In girls, the entire system degenerates, leaving only vestigial remnants. The persistent tubules may be identified in the mesovarium of the adult as the epoophoron and paroophoron, and the mesonephric duct becomes Gartner's duct within the broad ligament and lateral paravaginal tissues. In boys, the mesonephros also degenerates, but the

duct persists and under the influence of androgens forms the male genital duct system.

The third and permanent kidney, the metanephros, arises from the metanephric mesenchyme, the most caudal portion of the mesodermal nephrogenic cord. Its collecting system, the ureter, develops as an outbudding of the mesonephric duct. The ureteric bud arises from the caudal end of the mesonephric duct (Fig 5–3). It grows cranially, pushes into the metanephric mesenchyme, and induces this tissue to differentiate into the permanent nephrons (Grobstein, 1955). Factors originating in the metanephric mesenchyme, in turn, induce a series of dichotomous subdivisions in the cranial portion of the ureter, ultimately forming the calyceal collecting system. The distal portion elongates to form the permanent ureter. Apparent ascent and medial rotation of the metanephros to its permanent position occur as a result of rapid growth of the caudal structures of the embryo over the ensuing weeks. The metanephros functions in urine formation by the fourth month of fetal life. Fetal urine is a major component of amniotic fluid.

Bladder and Urethra

The bladder and urethra derive predominantly from endodermal tissue. The expanded distal portion of the hindgut, the cloaca, is divided

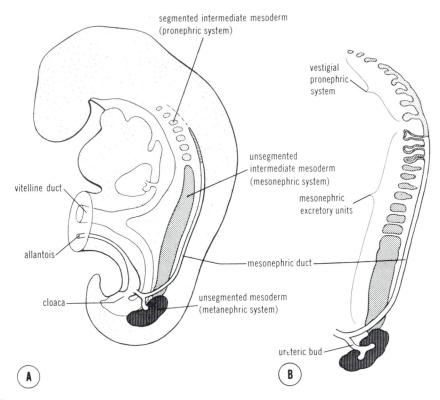

FIG 5–3.

A, schematic diagram showing the relation of the intermediate mesoderm of the pronephric, mesonephric and metanephric systems. In the cervical and upper thoracic regions, the intermediate mesoderm is segmented; in the lower thoracic, lumbar, and sacral regions, it forms a solid, unsegmented mass of tissue, the nephrogenic cord. Note the longitudinal collecting duct, initially formed by the pronephros but later taken over by the mesonephros. *B,* schematic representation of the excretory tubules of the pronephric and mesonephric systems in a 5-week-old embryo. The ureteric bud penetrates the metanephric tissue. Note the remnant of the pronephric excretory tubules and longitudinal collecting duct.

by the urorectal fold into the anterior urogenital sinus and the posterior rectum during the fourth week (Vaughn and Middleton, 1975). The urogenital sinus is further divided into the vesicourethral canal, which forms the bladder and upper urethra, and the definitive urogenital sinus, which forms most of the urethra, the paraurethral glands, and the vestibule. Within the base of the bladder is a specialized structure, the trigone, which derives partly from mesoderm.

The vesicourethral canal receives the allantois cranially. By the fourth month of fetal life, attenuation and elongation of the allantois result in formation of a ligamentous structure, the urachus. This persists in adult life as the median umbilical ligament of the anterior abdominal wall.

Laterally, the vesicourethral canal receives the orifices of the common excretory ducts. They consist of the mesonephric duct distal to its junction with the metanephric duct. Differential growth results in the establishment of an independent orifice between the metanephric duct (the ureter) and the developing bladder (Fig 5–4). The mesonephric duct orifice becomes displaced distally, opening into the upper urethra. In girls, although most of the mesonephric duct undergoes degeneration, the terminal portion ultimately becomes incorporated into the bladder wall, giving rise to a part of the trigone and posterior upper urethra (Tanagho and Smith, 1968). Thus, this segment of the bladder is of mesodermal origin.

Distally, the vesicourethral canal elongates and contributes to the formation of the upper anterior urethra. The majority of the urethra, how-

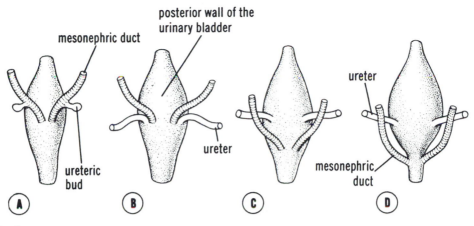

FIG 5–4.
Schematic drawings to show the relationship of the ureters and mesonephric ducts during development. Initially the ureter is formed by an outgrowth of the mesonephric duct, but with time it obtains a separate entrance into the urinary bladder.

ever, derives from the urogenital sinus. The posterior segment of the urogenital sinus further differentiates into the vestibule and the distal vagina.

ANATOMY AND HISTOLOGY

Vagina

The vagina is a compressed but distensible musculomembranous canal extending from the vulva to the uterine cervix (Fig 5–5). It is directed cephalad and posterior from the vestibule toward the sacral promontory. Anteriorly, the vagina is closely related to the bladder and urethra. The trigone lies against the upper third of the vagina. The urethra courses inferiorly opposed to the anterior vaginal wall. The tissue between these structures, the vesicovaginal septum and the urethrovaginal septum, consists of supporting fibrous tissue of the endopelvic fascia and a potential avascular space.

The posterior vaginal wall is related to the peritoneal cul-de-sac of Douglas at its upper third, the ampulla of the rectum at its middle third, and the perineal body at its lower third. The relationship to the cul-de-sac of Douglas is of clinical importance because it provides an easy route of access to the peritoneal cavity through the vagina. The rectovaginal septum, like its anterior counterpart, has a potential avascular plane between supporting layers of endopelvic fascia. Though closely apposed in the region of the septum, the vaginal and rectal orifices become more widely separated by the perineal body. The perineal body is an important structure that provides a central area of insertion for the supporting musculature of the urogenital diaphragm and pelvic floor.

The lateral relations of the vagina include the parametrial tissues at its superior extent. The ureters pass through this tissue 1 to 2 cm lateral to the vagina as they course toward the trigone. At the junction of the middle and lower thirds of the vagina, the pubococcygeus portion of the levator ani muscle forms a hiatus through which the vagina passes. At the introitus, the vagina is related laterally to the bulbocavernosus muscles. Lateral to these muscles is the ischiorectal fossa.

Superiorly the uterine cervix projects into the vagina through its anterior wall. As a result of this arrangement, the posterior wall of the vagina is longer than the anterior wall by approximately 3 cm. The recesses of the vaginal vault above the cervix are called the *fornices*, the deepest being the posterior fornix.

The vaginal length is variable but usually ranges from 8 to 10 cm. The perineal muscles cause a relative constriction of the outlet diameter. The midportion is flattened when relaxed, creating only a potential space, but has a remarkable ability to distend. This is exemplified at the time of delivery when the vault must accommodate passage of the fetus. Stretching is allowed by the presence of multiple circumferential folds, or rugae, in the vaginal wall. The rugae becomes less prominent after menopause.

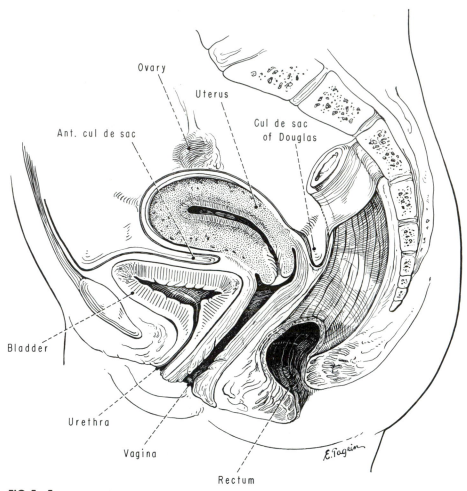

FIG 5–5.

Sagittal section of the human female pelvis showing the anatomical relations of the vagina.

Histologically, three layers can be distinguished in the vagina: (1) mucous membrane, (2) muscularis, and (3) adventitia (Blaustein, 1982). The mucous membrane is composed of a nonkeratinized, stratified squamous epithelium and a lamina propria. The epithelium is continuous onto the cervical portio. Estrogen stimulation in reproductive-age women causes thickening of the epithelium and promotes glycogen storage in the superficial layers (Friedrich, 1983). The lamina propria is a dense layer of fibroelastic tissue generously supplied with blood vessels. It functions as erectile tissue during sexual arousal. Deep to the mucosa is the muscularis, consisting of an inner circular and outer longitudinal layer of smooth muscle. The layers are not distinguished by interposed fascial fibers. The adventitial layer consists of dense connective tissue, nerves, and blood vessels. It is continuous with the endopelvic fascia, the supporting fibrous layer investing all the pelvic viscera and muscles.

Urinary Tract

The ureters are bilateral tubes that function as conduits to convey urine from the kidneys to the urinary bladder. Each ureter is 30 to 34 cm long and 6 to 10 mm in diameter. It is retroperitoneal throughout its course from the renal pelvis to the bladder. The abdominal portion comprises the superior 15 cm and runs caudally anterior to the psoas muscle, crossing the genitofemoral nerve. The right ureter is crossed by the duodenum, the right colic and ileocolic vessels, and the terminal ileum. The left is crossed by the left colic vessels and the sigmoid mesentery and vessels.

The pelvic portion begins near the sacroiliac articulation at the linea terminalis of the iliac bone. As it descends into the true pelvis along the lateral wall, it is crossed by the ovarian vessels coursing within the infundibulopelvic ligament. It crosses the common iliac artery near its bifurcation to lie medial to the visceral branches of the anterior division of the internal iliac artery. As the ureter continues its course into the pelvis, it travels along the superior surface of the levator ani muscle in the most inferior portion of the broad ligament. In this location it is surrounded by the extensive venous plexus of the uterus, and it is crossed by the uterine artery at approximately the level of the internal cervical os, 1 to 1.5 cm lateral to the cervix (Hofmeister, 1982). Each ureter then turns medially, coursing closely to the anterior vaginal fornix to enter the base of the bladder. The interstitial portion of the ureter is approximately 1 cm in length and traverses an oblique course anteromedially to open via a slitlike orifice at the bladder trigone (Woodburne, 1968).

The bladder is a highly distensible organ that changes shape and its superior relations as it fills with urine. The superior surface, or dome of the bladder, is covered with visceral peritoneum, which reflects onto the bladder from the anterior abdominal wall. The inferior surfaces are not covered by peritoneum. Anteriorly it is separated from the pubic bone by a potential, avascular retroperitoneal space called the *space of Retzius*. Posteriorly it is related to the anterior surface of the uterine cervix and anterior fornix of the vagina.

The trigone is a specialized area in the base of the bladder that represents the continuation of the muscular layer of the ureters as they are incorporated into the bladder wall (Woodburne, 1968). The trigone is a triangular area delineated by the ureteral orifices, the interureteric ridge that forms the base, and the internal urethal meatus at the apex. The trigone forms a relatively fixed, unyielding segment of the bladder important in supporting the outlet during storage of urine and in coordinating the funneling effect necessary for efficient emptying of the bladder (Tanagho and Smith, 1968).

The female urethra is approximately 4 cm long. It is positioned behind the pubic symphysis and anterior to the vagina. The external urethral meatus forms a slitlike orifice in the vestibule about 2 cm posterior to the clitoris. Vestigial homologues of the male prostatic ducts form the paraurethral glands of Skene that open into the posterior urethra just behind the meatus.

The histological structure of the urinary tract from the renal calyces to the urethra is consistent, varying only by increasing in thickness. It is well suited to the functions of storage and propulsion of urine. Three component layers are identified: a mucosa, muscularis, and adventitia (Hurt, 1988).

The mucosal lining is transitional epithelium, three to five cells thick in the ureters and up to eight cells thick in the bladder. In the contracted state, the epithelium is thick and the cells round. As the viscus distends to accommodate stored urine, the epithelium becomes thin as the individual cells flatten parallel to the surface. There is no discernible basement membrane. The lamina propria is composed of collagenous and elastic fibers.

The muscularis is comprised of an inner longitudinal and outer circular layer with an additional outer longitudinal layer beginning in the distal ureter and continuing in the bladder. The layered arrangement is less discrete in the urinary tract compared with the gastrointestinal (GI) tract. This results in a more interlaced, anastomosing pattern in the bladder. The inner longitudinal layer of each ureter flattens out as it enters the bladder to form the sheetlike trigone. This layer continues downward into the proximal urethra as well.

The muscularis is surrounded by a loose fibroelastic adventitia. It provides the structural framework through which the blood vessels and nerves course. Its loose attachment allows for the mobility necessary in physiological filling and emptying.

The urethra lacks a discrete circumferential sphincter, and considerable anatomic variation has been observed in the paraurethral structures (DeLancey, 1986). The outer circular layer of the detrusor muscle is continuous onto the urethra and contributes to a smooth muscle sphincter mechanism. Some authors (Woodburne, 1968) have described a condensation of smooth muscle fibers at the proximal urethra into a slinglike structure capable of compressing the lumen and contributing to bladder continence. Additional voluntary sphincter function is provided by decussating striated muscle fibers of the ischiocavernosus and bulbocavernous muscles. There is also abundant elastic tissue in the urethral wall. This participates in the continence mechanism by creating intrinsic resistance along the urethral tube.

MALFORMATIONS

Vagina

Vaginal anomalies are rare. They may be classified as (1) absence, (2) failure of lateral fusion, and (3) failure of canalization.

Congenital absence of the vagina (the Rokitansky-Küster-Hauser syndrome) resulting from müllerian duct agenesis occurs with an incidence of 1 in 4,000 to 5,000 female births (Griffin et al., 1976). The embryological defect affects the development of a variable portion of the fused, caudal end of the müllerian (paramesonephric) duct. The etiology is not known but does not appear to be genetic. It is usually associated with uterine agenesis, but in approximately 8% of patients, a rudimentary bipartite uterus with a functional endometrium is present (Wiser and Bates, 1984).

The clinical presentation depends on the presence or absence of a functioning uterus. Ovarian function is normal and may induce cyclic pain and endometriosis from the endometrium. However, the usual chief complaint is primary amenorrhea. Vaginal agenesis is second only to gonadal dysgenesis in causing this disorder (Reindollar et al., 1981). Patients have a normal female karyotype and normal growth and development of secondary sexual characteristics, important factors that assist in the differential diagnosis. There is a frequent association with renal and skeletal anomalies, and these should be sought (Griffin et al., 1976).

If symptoms arise from a rudimentary uterine anlage, it should be surgically removed. Otherwise, the goal of management is to create a vaginal vault adequate for sexual function. This may be accomplished by surgical or nonsurgical means. The Frank nonsurgical method for formation of a vagina utilizes progressive application of vaginal dilators to the introital region. It requires considerable patient cooperation and diligence but is reported to achieve good results without complications (Rock et al., 1983). Alternatively, the McIndoe vaginoplasty involves surgical dissection of the areolar tissues in the potential vaginal space, followed by placement of a split thickness skin graft to achieve epithelialization. The

possibility of pregnancy exists for those rare women with an intact uterus, so the surgical approach with uterine conservation is preferred in this group (Bates and Wiser, 1985).

Failure of lateral fusion of the paramesonephric ducts results in longitudinal septa. As with agenesis, the extent of the developmental abnormality can be variable. There may be only a partial, distal fibromuscular band in the sagittal plane of the vagina. In the extreme situation, there may be duplication of all the müllerian derivatives such that the patient has two separate uterine horns, cervices, and vaginas. In some cases, the hemivagina created by the septum does not communicate with the introitus (Buttram, 1983). This causes obstruction of the ipsilateral uterine horn and results in painful hematocolpos and hematometra with menstruation. If the contralateral horn continues to discharge its menstrual effluent normally, the diagnosis may not be considered unless the tender mass is appreciated on careful physical examination. Symptomatic women require surgical resection of the septum to relieve the obstruction. Surgery is also indicated for dyspareunia, but asymptomatic septa do not require treatment.

Failure of canalization of the vaginal plate results in transverse septa. They can occur at any level and can be complete or partial (Rock and Azziz, 1987). The incidence is reported as 1 in 30,000 to 80,000 females. The diagnosis usually manifests at menarche when cyclic abdominal pain from retained menstrual blood prompts an evaluation. Preoperative evaluation should include a pelvic ultrasound to delineate the septal thickness and to demonstrate a normal uterus and ovaries. An intravenous (IV) pyelogram is done to exclude renal anomalies and ureteral obstruction. Treatment requires surgical resection of the septum and reanastomosis of the upper and lower vaginal vaults.

The hymen probably forms at the junction of the vaginal plate and the urogenital sinus. It can also fail to develop its normal lumen and result in retained menstrual blood, dyspareunia, or both. Treatment is accomplished by a cruciate incision in the membrane, followed by resection of the triangular membranous flaps.

Urinary Tract

The genital and urinary tracts develop in close association. In girls, normal development of the mesonephric system precedes and is partly responsible for inducing normal development of the paramesonephric ducts. Following fusion of the caudal ends of the müllerian ducts, the downward growth of the müllerian tubercle separates the urogenital sinus into its urinary and vaginal components. A consequence of this interdependence is that abnormalities in one system are commonly associated with abnormalities in the other.

Some important lower urinary tract malformations become manifest during infancy or childhood and thus are diagnosed by the pediatrician. Others, such as ureteral duplication, may remain silent into adulthood and then may be detected as a result of an unrelated surgical procedure.

Urinary tract malformations of special importance to the gynecologist include (1) unilateral renal agenesis, (2) ureteral duplication, (3) ectopic ureteral orifice, and (4) ureterocele.

Unilateral renal agenesis occurs with an incidence of approximately 1 per 1,000 (Magee et al., 1979). Associated genital tract anomalies, usually partial or complete uterine duplication, occur in 35% to 45% of affected women. Several mechanisms have been proposed, including failed differentiation of the nephrogenic ridge, failed differentiation of the mesonephric duct and ureteral bud, and failed development of the metanephric blastema. The earlier in development the urinary tract aberration occurs, the more severe are the associated abnormalities in the genital tract. The diagnosis of unilateral renal agenesis is usually made while evaluating the patient for symptomatic renal disease or at surgery. When it is identified, it should prompt a structural evaluation of the genital tract. There is no renal functional derangement unless there is compromise of the single kidney.

Duplication of the ureter may be partial or total and occurs in approximately 1% of the population (Vaughn and Middleton, 1975). The Y-shaped partial duplication results when the ureteral bud branches before establishing contact with the metanephric blastema. Two complete ureters result from growth of a duplicated ureteral bud arising from the mesonephric duct. The ureters usually cross each other within a common vascular sheath so that the ureter draining the upper renal pole enters the bladder more medial and distal to its mate (the Meyer-Weigert rule). It may occur so inferior, that it is considered an ectopic ureter (see later discussion). The interstitial segment of the distal ureter tends to be shorter,

and thus it may be more prone to vesicoureteral reflux. In addition to possible reflux, the clinical importance of this condition is to recognize its existence so that the duplicated ureter may be avoided during surgery.

An ectopic ureteral orifice may open into the urethra, vestibule, vagina, or uterus (Zornow, 1977). It most often occurs as a ureteral duplication with the ectopic ureter draining the superior renal pole as expected by its more distal position. If the involved ureter opens distal to the urethral sphincter, incontinence results. The usual clinical presentation is with constant dribbling of urine and a concurrent normal voiding pattern. In children, it may be misinterpreted as enuresis. If the ureter opens to the uterus or vagina, signs and symptoms of vaginitis may be most prominent. Symptomatic ectopia is treated surgically usually by ipsilateral ureteroureterostomy or reimplantation into the bladder.

A ureterocele is a cystic dilatation of the distal ureter (Vaughn and Middleton, 1975). It may be congenital or acquired and usually involves the interstitial ureter. It is probably the result of an incomplete perforation of the bladder by the ureter that results in a localized increase in hydrostatic pressure. The usual clinical presentation is recurrent urinary tract infections due to obstruction. Treatment requires surgical resection of the involved segment with reimplantation into the bladder.

PHYSIOLOGIC ALTERATIONS

Vagina

Vaginal physiology depends on an appropriate hormonal and bacteriologic milieu. The vagina is a target organ for ovarian estrogen (Semmens et al., 1985). Estrogen induces proliferation and maturation of the stratified squamous epithelium, enhances glycogen storage in the superficial cells, and increases blood flow through the paravaginal tissues. The increased thickness of the epithelium and good blood supply act to create an effective mechanical barrier between the vagina and the environment. The stored glycogen participates in the formation of a microbiologic barrier.

The vaginal squamous epithelium consists of layers of cells that demonstrate progressive maturation as they are displaced upward by proliferation of the basal stratum germinativum (Blaustein, 1982). Cells desquamate and may be collected for cytological evaluation. The appearance will reflect the influence of estrogen on epithelial growth. Cells should be obtained by scraping with a spatula along the lateral wall of the upper third of the vagina. They are smeared thinly on a slide, fixed, and submitted for cytological study. Three cell types are seen:

1. *Parabasal cells* originate just above the stratum germinativum and are small round cells with a high nuclear/cytoplasmic ratio.
2. *Intermediate cells* are larger and polygonal. The nuclear/cytoplasmic ratio is less than for parabasal cells, but a definite nuclear chromatin pattern is observed.
3. *Superficial cells* are large, polyhedral, flat cells with small, pyknotic nuclei.

Estrogen stimulation results in a predominance of the more mature superficial cells. An absolute absence of estrogen or a hormonal environment marked by a relative decrease in the estrogen/progesterone ratio favors desquamation of parabasal cells. Functionally, this situation results in a less protective mucous membrane subject to traumatic injury. It may manifest clinically with dyspareunia or bleeding.

Glycogen storage in the intermediate and superficial cells is promoted by estrogen. It serves as a substrate for carbohydrate metabolism by the bacterium *Lactobacillus vaginalis*. The product of fermentation is lactic acid, which maintains a low vaginal pH (normal 3.5 to 4.5). The acidity favors continued growth of the nonpathogenic *Lactobacillus* and inhibits colonization by more virulent organisms.

A wide variety of bacteria can be cultured from the normal vagina (Eschenbach, 1983). The number and type depend in part on the culture media used. *Lactobacillus, Staphylococcus epidermidis*, diphtheroids, and aerobic and anaerobic streptococci are most frequently isolated in culture. These organisms are normally present in numbers insufficient to cause clinical infection and do not require treatment.

Estrogen deprivation results in a decrease in blood flow in the paravaginal tissues. This is restored when estrogens are supplied exogenously (Semmens et al., 1985). Tissue turgor and production of vaginal fluids in basal and sexually aroused states are dependent on adequate blood flow. The vaginal mucosa lacks true glands. Vaginal fluids are produced by transudation across the epithelium and are influenced by the hormonal status as well as the presence of erotic stimuli. Decreased vaginal lubrication associated with low-estrogen states can result in trauma and dyspareunia.

Physiology of Micturition

The bladder functions to store urine until conditions are appropriate to completely expel its contents. Its function is controlled by a complex neurologic system involving both central and peripheral components. The micturition reflex occurs involuntarily but is capable of coming under volitional control with maturation of the cerebral cortex pathways.

The bladder wall is innervated by sensory fibers that carry sensations of pain, temperature, and proprioception (stretch) to the spinal cord (Bradley et al., 1976). They synapse in the cord with efferent motor nerves that return to the bladder to complete a reflex arc and with neurons that transmit information about bladder sensation up the cord to the brain stem and cortex. The motor neurons supplying the detrusor muscle originate in the sacral spinal segments S2-4 in an area called the *sacral micturition center*. The activity of this area is modulated by input from bladder afferent nerves as well as from signals originating in detrusor reflex centers in the brain stem and the frontal lobe of the cerebral cortex. After appropriately integrating the information from the bladder with that from higher centers, the motor neurons send signals to both the detrusor and the bladder sphincter to initiate a coordinated micturition event.

The motor neurons are parasympathetic and thus form ganglionic synapses within the wall of the bladder. Postganglionic neurons then carry the information to the smooth muscle cells of the detrusor. Stimulation by release of the neurotransmitter acetylcholine results in a detrusor contraction. The role of the sympathetic nervous system in the control of bladder function is less well established for humans (Gosling et al., 1977). The existence of adrenergic receptor sites in the bladder and sphincter is known. Beta receptors are predominant in the detrusor, and stimulation of these is thought to cause inhibition of detrusor contractility. Alpha receptors are in abundance in the sphincter region, and stimulation causes contraction of these muscle fibers. Thus, a picture emerges of autonomic influence on bladder function such that parasympathetic activation initiates bladder emptying while sympathetic activation relaxes the detrusor and stimulates the sphincter to promote the filling and storage function of the bladder.

Despite intense investigative efforts, the physiology of the bladder sphincter mechanism remains poorly understood. From a simplified point of view, continence is maintained during the bladder storage phase because at all times intraurethral pressure exceeds intravesical pressure. Intravesical pressure remains low during filling due to the high compliance of the detrusor muscle. This allows the bladder to accommodate increasing volumes of urine with only a minimal increase in intravesical pressure. Intraurethral pressure remains high because of a combination of factors that contribute to a sphincterlike effect (Hurt, 1988). The important determinants of intraurethral pressure include (1) paraurethral smooth muscle reflex contraction (the smooth muscle sphincter), (2) striated pelvic muscle contraction (the external sphincter), (3) tissue turgor resulting from blood flow in the paraurethral vascular bed, and (4) the mucosal seal resulting from the elastic properties of the urethral wall. An extremely important aspect of the continence mechanism is the intra-abdominal location of the proximal urethra. It assures that any increase in intra-abdominal pressure that causes extrinsic pressure to be applied to the bladder is applied equally to the proximal urethra. The relative pressure relationship between bladder and the proximal urethra is unchanged. Intraurethral pressure continues to exceed intravesical pressure, and continence is therefore maintained.

Before being brought under voluntary control, bladder emptying occurs as a simple reflex phenomenon. Stretching of the detrusor is detected by proprioceptive endings within the bladder wall, and signals are sent to the sacral micturition center. The parasympathetic motor neurons are activated, and the signals transmitted back to the bladder cause the detrusor to contract. Suppression of the reflex is accomplished by a learned response, through inhibitory signals impinging on the sacral micturition center from the brain stem micturition center and directly from the cerebral cortex. Voluntary control of micturition requires activation of the reflex to accomplish bladder emptying only at appropriate times.

Once activated, a series of events occurs to coordinate bladder and sphincter control. The striated muscle of the pelvic floor and external sphincter relax, the smooth muscle of the urethra relaxes, and simultaneously the detrusor contracts. The coordinated activity allows the bladder to empty through a low-resistance conduit. Thus, emptying is accomplished without the need to generate high intravesical pressures, a situation that could result in reflux into the ureters.

VAGINITIS

Vaginitis is one of the commonest gynecologic diagnoses, accounting for a substantial percentage of ambulatory visits annually. Vaginitis can present with a variety of symptoms and signs depending on the underlying etiology. The usual manifestations occurring singly or in combination are an abnormal vaginal discharge, vaginal discomfort, pruritis, and an abnormal odor. Almost all cases result from an infection involving one of three organisms: *Candida albicans, Trichomonas vaginalis,* and *Gardnerella vaginalis.* Inflammatory vaginitis occurs much less frequently as a result of a localized allergic reaction, a reaction to a foreign body, nonspecific inflammation (desquamative inflammatory vaginitis), or as a result of senescent changes in the vaginal mucosa. Infectious cervicitis or a cervical ectropion can cause a copious discharge that egresses via the vagina but should not be mistaken for a primary pathological process of the vaginal mucosa.

Establishing the correct diagnosis is paramount for successful treatment of vaginitis and requires a logical, comprehensive approach to the patient with the aforementioned complaints. The evaluation should begin with an accurate history. The symptoms should be elucidated in detail. The presence of a discharge and its specific characteristics are important. Associated symptoms of pruritis, pain, and dysuria should be noted. Also, several factors can predispose to vaginitis by altering the normal vaginal physiology. Use of systemic antibiotics for an unrelated condition may suppress the growth of the *Lactobacillus.* This creates an environment favoring growth of pathogens. The estrogenic status of the patient, exposure to sexually transmitted diseases, and the presence of comorbid diseases that may cause a degree of immunocompromise are other important considerations.

The physical examination provides the next

opportunity to gather information leading to an accurate diagnosis. Often vaginitis becomes symptomatic only after it spreads to involve the very sensitive vulvar skin. The vulvar skin should be inspected for evidence of a rash, erythema, excoriation, or edema. The gross appearance of the vaginal mucosa should be assessed. Thin, pale mucosa lacking rugae suggests relative or absolute estrogen deprivation. Erythema, increased vascularity, mucosal ulcerations, or other lesions are noted. The status of the cervical portio is likewise evaluated. If a discharge is present, its specific characteristics will be helpful in establishing the diagnosis. Characteristics that should be assessed are the amount, color, consistency, odor, and pH.

The most useful clinical tool available to establish the diagnosis is the microscopic appearance of the vaginal discharge. Two preparations are used. In one, the vaginal secretions are suspended in isotonic saline solution, and a coverslip is applied. The slide is observed for the presence of the motile protozoan *Trichomonas,* "clue cells," and leukocytes. Clue cells are vaginal mucosal cells with a dense stippled appearance due to attached *G. vaginalis* organisms. The second preparation is a suspension of the vaginal discharge in 10% potassium hydroxide. The cellular elements present on the slide are lysed by the KOH, leaving the mycelia of *C. albicans* unobscured. If the diagnosis remains doubtful, Gram stains and cultures using specific media will help establish the diagnosis.

Candidiasis

Approximately one third of vaginitis cases are caused by fungal infections. The etiologic agent is *C. albicans* in 85% to 95% of patients, with *Candida glabrata* accounting for most of the remaining infections. *Candida albicans* is a ubiquitous saprophyte that may be isolated from the vagina in up to 20% of asymptomatic women (Oriel et al., 1972). Treatment is not indicated unless symptoms are present, which generally requires the presence of large numbers of organisms. It is thought that alterations in host factors allow overgrowth of the fungus, resulting in symptomatic infection.

Factors that are associated with candidiasis include systemic antibiotics, pregnancy, diabetes mellitus, and immunosuppressants. Antibiotic use may predispose to yeast infections by suppressing the vaginal flora that normally inhibit the growth

of *Candida* through competition for nutrients (Fluery, 1981). The effect is seen most commonly with broad-spectrum antibiotics such as the tetracyclines, and probably depends primarily on suppression of growth of the *Lactobacillus.* The mechanism by which pregnancy predisposes to vaginal candidiasis is not known, but the rate of infection may be doubled in gravidas. An alteration in glycogen metabolism and depression of local cell-mediated immunity have been proposed as mechanisms through which other factors may operate (Syverson et al., 1979). It is important to note, however, that most cases of candidiasis occur in patients with no identified risk factors.

The usual clinical presentation for a patient with candidiasis is with the complaint of vulvovaginal pruritis. The itching is usually intense and may be accompanied by dysuria and dyspareunia. The onset of symptoms may coincide with the menses or intercourse. The patient may notice a thick, white discharge, but it is usually not a prominent feature. Candidiasis is not associated with a foul odor.

On physical examination, extensive involvement of the vulva may be apparent. The skin will demonstrate well-demarcated erythematous areas with scaling, edema, and excoriations. Often the crural and labial folds are affected. The vaginal mucosa may also be inflamed and edematous. The classic finding, however, is a white, thick, curdlike discharge forming patches adherent to the vaginal walls. The pH of the discharge is usually less than 4.5.

The diagnosis is confirmed by identifying budding pseudohyphae or spores on a wet preparation of the vaginal discharge suspended in 10% KOH under light microscopy. Occasionally the wet smear proves too insensitive, or resistant yeast forms are suspected, and vaginal cultures on selective media are required to establish the diagnosis. Nickerson's medium or Sabouraud's agar are most often used to isolate fungi in these more difficult cases (Eschenbach, 1983).

Treatment of candidiasis is accomplished by the topical application of antifungal agents. Several preparations are available. Clotrimazole and miconazole offer the advantage of higher initial cure rates and shorter durations of treatment than nystatin (Higton, 1973). Administration is by vaginal suppository or cream applied high in the vaginal vault daily for 7 days. Creams may also be applied directly to affected vulvar skin. There is some evidence in nonpregnant patients that 3 days of therapy with 200-mg suppositories may be sufficient to effect cure. Another effective therapy is boric acid (Van Slyke et al., 1981). A gelatin capsule containing 600 to 650 mg of boric acid powder is applied daily for 14 days. Results compared with nystatin indicate that it is an effective and inexpensive alternative. Boric acid suppositories may be especially useful in managing patients with persistent infections. Patients may establish an intermittent dosing interval that keeps their symptoms controlled. No serious side effects have been reported with its use, but it should be avoided in pregnancy.

Persistent or frequently recurrent vaginal candidiasis is a difficult problem to treat. Approximately 10% of cases will not respond to initial therapy. Prolonging treatment up to 14 days may cure some patients. If predisposing factors such as poor diabetes control can be eliminated, this is done. Cultures may be obtained to exclude infection with a more resistant *Candida* species. Treatment of an affected sexual partner should be accomplished. It has been suggested that some patients may become chronically infected because of GI colonization with *C. albicans* (Miles et al., 1977). Oral therapy directed at eliminating this reservoir has been advocated. Ketoconazole is an effective oral therapy available for treatment of *Candida*. It is well absorbed from the GI tract, so whether its efficacy is due to a systemic or local action is not known. Hepatotoxicity is the main serious side effect. Prophylactic treatment with ketoconazole may be effective in suppressing symptoms in chronic infections, but the recurrence rates remain high when it is discontinued. Adjunctive measures such as avoidance of harsh soaps in the genital area, elimination of restrictive synthetic underwear, and prolonged air drying of the genital area after washing are also recommended to the patient.

Trichomoniasis

Vaginitis is caused by infection with *T. vaginalis* in 10% to 25% of cases (Osborne et al., 1982). The organism is a flagellate protozoan that can be recovered from the urethra and cervix in addition to the vaginal vault. Its growth is enhanced by a moist, anaerobic environment in which the pH is somewhat more alkaline (5.5 to 6.5) than the normal vagina. Trichomonads are not part of the normal vaginal flora, and infection is usually transmitted through sexual contact.

However, viable organisms have been recovered from swimming pools and fomites such as moist towels, suggesting nonsexual transmission is also possible (Rein and Muller, 1984). Trichomoniasis is frequently associated with other sexually transmitted diseases (Osborne et al., 1982). Patients should be screened for gonorrhea when the diagnosis of trichomoniasis is made.

The clinical manifestations of trichomoniasis vary from asymptomatic infection to an intense local inflammatory response. Systemic infection does not occur. Fifty percent of women from whom the organism can be isolated do not complain of symptoms (McLellan et al., 1982). When symptoms exist, the patient complains primarily of a profuse vaginal discharge. The discharge may cause vulvovaginal discomfort and irritation. Pruritus and odor are less common complaints. Dysuria and dyspareunia are occasionally noted, and if severe inflammation is present, vaginal spotting may occur.

The vulvar examination is often normal but may demonstrate erythema and excoriations. Erythema of the vaginal epithelium may also be noted. A classically described finding in the presence of severe inflammation is the "strawberry cervix," consisting of tiny, punctate hemorrhages grossly visible on the mucosa. It is actually seen in only a small minority of cases. The vaginal discharge is the most striking feature of the examination. The discharge is copious, opaque, gray to yellow-green, and malodorous. Occasionally, small bubbles are present, giving the discharge a frothy appearance. The pH of the discharge is usually 5.0 to 6.5, reflecting the growth requirement of the parasite for a more alkaline environment.

Trichomoniasis is diagnosed by direct identification of the motile organism by microscopy. A wet mount is prepared by suspending a small amount of the discharge in a drop of saline on a microscope slide. A coverslip is applied, and the preparation is examined. The organisms are slightly larger than leukocytes, which are usually abundant in the smear due to the inflammatory response. They are somewhat pear shaped with visible flagella and move with a characteristic jittery motion. Cultures with specialized media are available and may improve the diagnostic accuracy if a particular patient presents a diagnostic dilemma (Fouts and Kraus, 1980). The diagnosis can also be made by identifying the parasites on a Papanicolaou smear. However, this should not be relied on since false negative findings are reported to occur in up to 48% of patients (Perl, 1972).

Trichomoniasis is treated with systemic metronidazole, a derivative of 5-nitroimidazole. Topical therapy is not adequate, perhaps because colonization in the bladder and urether will not be affected by vaginal application and is a source of reinfection. Trichomoniasis is usually a sexually transmitted disease, so the sexual partner must also be treated to avoid reinfection. Metronidazole is taken orally either as a 2-gm single dose or as a 250-mg dose three times daily for 7 days. The cure rates for the two regimens are comparable (Landers, 1988). Single-dose therapy offers the advantages of lower cost, lower total drug dose, and increased patient compliance. Patients should be advised to avoid alcohol consumption during and for 48 hours after treatment with metronidazole to prevent severe nausea and vomiting. Other side effects include a metallic aftertaste and headaches, and peripheral neuropathies have occasionally been reported after prolonged therapy. The drug probably should not be given in pregnancy. There are experimental data in animals suggesting the possibility of carcinogenic potential, though no clinical studies have demonstrated this risk (Eschenbach, 1983). Infected pregnant women may obtain symptomatic relief with clotrimazole, but cure is unlikely.

A 5% to 10% failure rate is reported following a single course of therapy with metronidazole. Most often this is due to poor compliance or failure to treat the patient's sexual partner. However, resistant strains of *T. vaginalis* have been reported and may require more intensive systemic therapy combined with topical application (Lossick et al., 1986). No other effective treatments have been reported.

Gardnerella-Associated Vaginitis

Gardnerella vaginalis is an aerobic, pleomorphic coccobacillus. It is probably part of the normal vaginal bacterial flora. However, under certain conditions, the organism proliferates and interacts with any of several anaerobic bacterial species in the vagina to produce infection (Speigel et al., 1980). The term "nonspecific vaginitis" has been applied to this condition in the past. As the role of *G. vaginalis* has become better defined as an etiologic agent, the term is less appropriate. However, the nature of the complex interaction between the various bacterial species that ulti-

mately results in symptoms remains to be completely elucidated. *Gardnerella*-associated vaginitis is the commonest form of this disease, accounting for 40% to 50% of all cases. It occurs almost exclusively in sexually active women.

The predominant symptom is an unpleasant odor usually associated with a vaginal discharge. Irritative symptoms of dysuria and dyspareunia are usually not present. The appearance of the vulva and vagina on physical examination is normal except for the presence of a vaginal discharge. The discharge is homogeneous, thin, gray-white, and present in moderate quantity.

The diagnosis is based on the clinical evaluation of the discharge. The pH is elevated above 4.5 in virtually all cases and is usually between 5.0 and 5.5. The characteristic fishy odor of the discharge may be noticed and is further evidence of infection. If not, it can be demonstrated by adding 10% KOH to 1 drop of the discharge on a microscope slide. Alkalinization volatizes the two main amines, putrescine and cadaverine, to produce the odor and forms the basis of this so-called whiff test (Fleury, 1981). Microscopic evaluation of the discharge is performed on a wet mount in saline. It is notable for a relative lack of neutrophils and the presence of the characteristic clue cells. Clue cells are desquamated epithelial cells covered with clumps of coccobacilli, which give the cells a speckled appearance. Often the cell borders are obscured by the adherent bacterial clusters. Their presence is very suggestive of the diagnosis of *Gardnerella*-associated vaginitis. Bacterial cultures should not be relied on to establish the diagnosis because of a lack of specificity (Kempers, 1985).

The recommended treatment is 500 mg of metronidazole by mouth two times daily for 7 days. The single-dose regimen effective in treating trichomoniasis is associated with a high rate of relapse when used in this disease and is therefore not recommended (Swedberg et al., 1985). Metronidazole has good activity against anaerobes, and this is probably the basis of its efficacy. It also has minimal impact on the normal vaginal flora. A less effective regimen but one that may be used in pregnancy or if metronidazole is otherwise contraindicated is 500 mg of ampicillin by mouth four times daily for 7 days. *Gardnerella*-associated vaginitis is a disease of sexually active women, but it has not been demonstrated that treatment of the male partner reduces the risk of recurrence. It may be helpful, however, in particularly difficult cases, along with the use of intravaginal acidifying agents (Eschenbach, 1983). There is no indication for treatment of asymptomatic female carriers of *G. vaginalis.*

PELVIC RELAXATION

The vagina is a potential space in the pelvic floor through which the pelvic organs may descend under the influence of gravity if they are not properly supported. Normally, the axis of the vaginal lumen assumes a 45-degree angle from the vertical in an erect posture. Therefore, gravitational forces are not applied directly parallel to the vaginal tube toward the introitus but are absorbed along its length by various musculofascial supports. The important muscular structures of the pelvic floor contributing support include the pelvic diaphragm, the urogenital diaphragm, and the perineal body.

The pelvic diaphragm is the most superior layer of the pelvic floor and consists of the components of the levator ani and coccygeus muscles. The levator ani originates at the pubic and ileal bones and sweeps across the hollow of the pelvis to insert into the ischium and coccyx. Laterally to medially, three components are identified by their origins and insertions: the ileococcygeus, the pubococcygeus, and the puborectalis. The puborectalis is interrupted in its course by the lumina of the urethra, vagina, and rectum. As it encircles and invests these organs, it contributes skeletal muscle support. The coccygeus muscle completes the posterolateral aspect of the pelvic diaphragm, originating at the ischial spine and inserting into the sacrum.

Inferior to the pelvic diaphragm and covering the anterior half of the pelvic outlet is the urogenital diaphragm. This layer is also interrupted by the hollow openings of the urethra and vagina. However, because of the angular course of the tubular structures, the defects in this layer are not aligned vertically with the corresponding defects in the pelvic diaphragm. This is an important mechanism of pelvic support.

The urogenital diaphragm is divided into deep and superficial compartments. The muscular components of the deep compartment of the urogenital diaphragm are the deep transverse perineal muscle and the striated sphincter muscle of urethra. These muscles originate along the ischiopubic rami, course medially, and terminate as fibers

blending into the submucosal tissues of the vagina and urethra, respectively. The most posterior fibers of the deep transverse perineal muscles meet their contralateral counterpart in the midline, inserting into the perineal body. A fascial layer separates the deep muscles from the superficial compartment of the urogenital diaphragm. Three paired muscles define this triangular area of the perineum. They are the bulbocavernous muscles, which surround the vaginal introitus and cover the erectile tissue of the vestibular bulbs, the ischiocavernous muscles, which originate at the ischial tuberosities and insert over the crura of the clitoris, and the superficial transverse perineal muscles.

The perineal body comprises the fibrous central point of insertion of the muscles of the pelvic diaphragm, the urogenital diaphragm, and the external rectal sphincter muscle. Thus, fibers from the levator ani, the deep transverse perineal muscles, the superficial transverse perineal muscles, and the bulbocavernous muscles contribute to this structure, forming the major posterior support for the vagina. As the vagina courses posteriorly toward the hollow of the sacrum, it rests on the perineal body.

The arrangement of the muscles of the pelvic floor in relation to the vagina and to each other is maintained by the endopelvic fascia. This layer provides the necessary strength that binds the muscles to each other, to the pelvic viscera, and ultimately to the fixed support of the bony pelvis. Endopelvic fascia envelopes all the muscles just described, covering their superior and inferior surfaces. In addition, it is continuous onto the bladder, vagina, rectum, and uterus, interdigitating and becoming indistinct from their adventitial layers at the points where these organs pierce the pelvic floor.

In certain locations, the fibers of the endopelvic fascia layer condense to form recognizable ligamentous structures that suspend the uterus and vagina in the pelvis (Fig 5–6). The cardinal ligaments extend from the lateral cervix and upper portion of the vagina to the pelvic sidewalls. Posteriorly, the uterosacral ligaments run from the cervix around the rectum to the sacrum. The peritoneal pouch, or cul-de-sac of Douglas, lies between these ligaments. It separates the rectum from the cervix and posterior vaginal fornix and is a potential weak spot in the floor of the pelvis. Anteriorly, less well-defined fibers extend from the pubic bone to support the urethra and vagina.

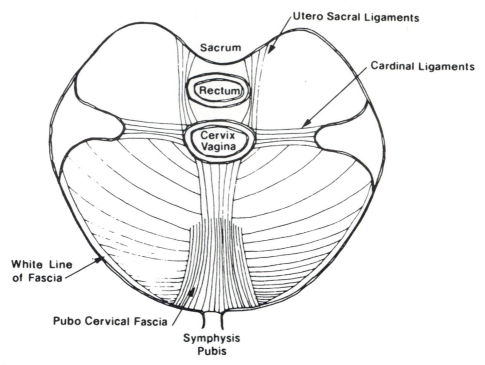

FIG 5–6.
Pelvic fascial supports (plane of midpelvis). Diagrammatic representation of the fascial supports that "suspend" the vaginal vault and cervix in the midpelvic plane. The bladder and urethra are supported by the floor of fascia comprised of the dense midline pubocervical fascia and its extensions to the white line of fascia laterally and the cardinal ligaments posteriorly. This fascia is less dense in its lateral and posterior aspects, as shown.

They are called collectively the *pubocervical fascia*. Extensions of endopelvic fascia along the course of the vagina form part of the vesicovaginal septum anteriorly and the rectovaginal septum posteriorly.

Genital prolapse or pelvic relaxation is the pathological state caused by weakening of the muscular and fascial supporting structures just described. The result is a herniation of one or more of the pelvic viscera through a defect in the pelvic floor. Sometimes the structural alteration results in functional derangements as well. Pelvic relaxation is classified by the organ involved. Usually a combination of various forms of prolapse occur together.

Uterine prolapse exists when the cervix and fundus descend into the vaginal vault as a result of attenuation and lengthening of the uterosacral and cardinal ligaments. The severity is described in degrees of prolapse occurring without traction or straining (Beecham, 1980). If the cervix descends below the ischial spines but remains within the vault, it is called *first-degree prolapse. Second-degree prolapse* refers to descent of the cervix into the vaginal introitus. *Third-degree prolapse,* or procidentia, indicates descent of the cervix and uterus beyond the introitus. Following hysterectomy, it is possible for the apex of the vaginal pouch to undergo similar descent by eversion. This is called a *vaginal vault prolapse.*

A cystocele is a herniation of the bladder base into the anterior vagina (Fig 5–7). It is a bulging of the dilated bladder base through a defect in the endopelvic fascia of the vesicovaginal septum. The term "urethrocele" has been applied when the lower anterior vaginal wall is involved. This is a misnomer, because no dilatation of the urethral wall is demonstrated. Rather, there is a posterior rotational descent of the upper urethra from its normally firm attachment to the posterior surface of the pubic bone. It results from weakening of the fibers of the pubocervical fascia. The herniation of the upper urethra to a position below the pelvic floor is believed to be the main

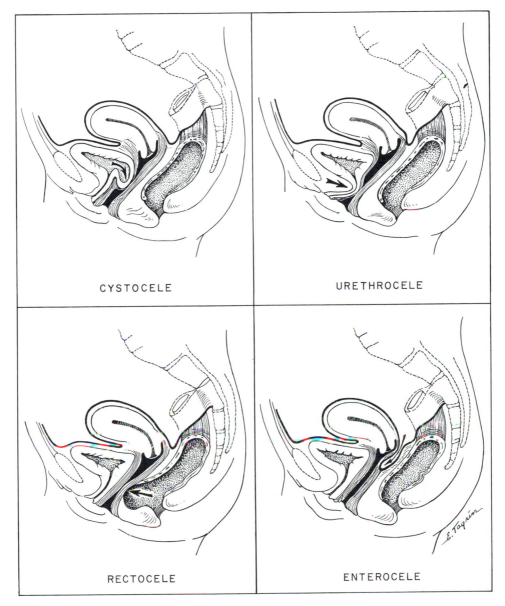

CYSTOCELE

URETHROCELE

RECTOCELE

ENTEROCELE

FIG 5–7.
Diagrammatic representation of the four common-est types of pelvic floor relaxation: cystocele, urethro-cele, rectocele, and enterocele. Arrows depict sites of maximum protrusion.

mechanism by which stress urinary incontinence occurs.

Prolapse involving the posterior vaginal wall may represent either a rectocele or an enterocele. A rectocele is a herniation of the anterior wall of the rectum into the vagina through the weakened endopelvic fascia of the rectovaginal septum. It usually involves the lower half of the vagina. This helps to distinguish it from an enterocele, which usually involves the upper posterior wall of the vagina. An enterocele is a herniation of the poste-rior peritoneal cul-de-sac between the uterosacral ligaments and into the upper posterior wall of the vagina. The herniated peritoneal sac may or may not contain loops of bowel. Even if small bowel is present in the sac, incarceration is very rare. En-teroceles are probably commoner than is generally appreciated due to the inherent weakness of the cul-de-sac as well as its dependent position in the pelvis. Failure to identify and repair a small enterocele is a major cause of failure of surgical procedures to correct pelvic relaxation (Ranney, 1981).

Perineal relaxation refers to weakening of the musculofascial components of the perineal body. It may simply result in a gaping of the introitus at the posterior fourchette. However, if the rectal sphincter is involved, functional aberrations with fecal incontinence may occur.

Etiology

Genital prolapse is a consequence of the bipedal condition. Gravity exerts a constant pull on the pelvic organs through the hollow pelvic outlet and is resisted only by musculofascial supports, not fixed bony structures. However, only a small proportion of women ever develop symptomatic prolapse. Several predisposing factors have been identified among this group. Age is the most important factor associated with prolapse. Pelvic herniation is rarely seen in young women since the effects on the tissues accumulate slowly over time. Menopause may accelerate the process. Estrogen helps to maintain adequate blood flow to the paravaginal tissues, and its deprivation results in atrophic changes that render the tissues more subject to prolapse. Obstetrical trauma is another important factor. Vaginal delivery can result in stretching and tearing of the pelvic tissues, especially the levator ani muscle and the perineal body. It is argued that obstetrical management, including appropriate use of episiotomies with careful anatomic repair, may prevent subsequent prolapse (Pritchard, 1985). Racial and genetic factors that determine the intrinsic strength of the connective tissues may influence the incidence of prolapse. Also, connective tissue diseases such as Marfan syndrome may predispose affected women to these disorders (Stoddard and Myers, 1968). Finally, conditions that result in chronic increases in intra-abdominal pressure are thought to render women more susceptible to pelvic relaxation. Included in this group are chronic coughing, chronic constipation, and heavy lifting.

Signs and Symptoms

Mild degrees of pelvic relaxation may be asymptomatic. More severe forms usually cause the patient to complain of a sagging, or "drop-ping," sensation in the pelvis. Often, it is worse at the end of the day and may be accompanied by a mild lower backache. Some patients will note a bulge or lump protruding from the vagina. The exteriorized mucosa may become irritated and cause discomfort.

In addition to these nonspecific complaints, relaxation of the anterior vaginal wall may disturb the function of the bladder and urethra and result in specific urinary symptoms. A common misconception is that a cystocele causes urinary stress incontinence. In fact, the herniated bladder wall may actually kink the bladder outlet and cause urinary retention (Bump et al., 1988; Richardson et al., 1983). Some patients are able to void only after manually reducing the bulging bladder back to a position superior to the bladder outlet. A cystocele may also prevent complete bladder emptying, and the residual urine may predispose to cystitis. Urinary stress incontinence is a consequence of pelvic relaxation, but it results from a herniation involving the upper urethra, not the bladder.

Posterior vaginal wall relaxation may cause difficulty with defecation. Again, reduction of the bulge by manual pressure may be required to effect a bowel movement. Fecal incontinence occasionally results from severe relaxation involving the rectal sphincter muscle. Usually, this occurs only if the sphincter has been completely avulsed. This symptom is rare and should prompt a search for other causes such as a fistula or a neurological deficit. Perineal relaxation may cause a patient to complain of unsatisfactory sensation with sexual intercourse.

Physical Examination

The diagnosis of pelvic relaxation is established by physical examination. The challenge is to carefully assess each of the various supporting structures, determine which have become lax, and plan effective therapy on that basis. The vaginal introitus and vault are conveniently examined in the lithotomy position. However, prolapse may be prominent only while the patient is standing, and an examination should be performed in this position as well. The mucosa is inspected for evidence of atrophy. Estrogen-deprived epithelium will be thin, friable, pale, and lacking in rugae. Prolonged eversion of the vaginal epithelium may result in traumatic lesions, secondary infection, or hyperkeratosis.

The support of the vaginal walls is assessed

sequentially using a Sims retractor or the disarticulated posterior blade of a Graves speculum. The anterior vaginal wall is evaluated by retracting the posterior wall with the speculum and asking the patient to bear down. The posterior wall is then evaluated by repositioning the speculum to retract the anterior wall. The degree of cervical descent may be further evaluated by applying gentle traction to the cervix with a tenaculum. The rectal examination is essential for differentiating a rectocele from an enterocele. A rectocele is demonstrated by manually pushing the bulging tissues of the weakened rectovaginal septum into the vagina. An enterocele is diagnosed by palpating the slippery herniated peritoneal sac within the rectovaginal septum high in the vaginal vault.

Finally, the degree of descent of the bladder neck may be demonstrated by the "Q-tip test," which is explained in detail in the discussion of urinary incontinence later in the chapter.

Treatment

The approach to treatment of pelvic relaxation depends on the following variables: severity of prolapse, age and general health of the patient, desire for future fertility, sexual activity, and associated pelvic pathology. Mild, asymptomatic prolapse does not require any therapy. Patients at high risk for surgery may benefit from nonoperative management. However, the approach will usually be surgical repair of the lax supporting structures by a plastic procedure.

Nonoperative management includes perineal exercises, treatment of mucosal alterations, and use of vaginal pessaries. The purpose of perineal exercises (also called *Kegel exercises*) is to strengthen the pubococcygeus muscle of the levator ani. The patient is instructed to identify this muscle by stopping the flow of urine during micturition. Once identified, the patient practices tightening the muscle for 3 to 5 seconds in sets of 10 throughout the day. The number of sets is progressively increased until results are appreciated. Perineal exercises are particularly useful to restore vaginal tone in the postpartum state, but they are of limited benefit in cases of severe prolapse.

Restoration of mucosal integrity should precede any contemplated surgery. Healing requires replacement of everted vaginal mucosa to its normal internal position. Often the temporary use of a pessary is required. Pessaries are available in a variety of shapes and sizes. They elevate the vaginal vault and maintain normal anatomic relations by supporting the prolapsing structures against the perineal body or the pubic bone. A pessary may be used temporarily in conjunction with local estrogen therapy to promote healing and restore a good blood supply to the epithelium prior to surgery. Alternatively, some patients are satisfactorily managed over the long run with a pessary and thus never require operative intervention. Such patients do require close follow-up, however. They must be seen at least every 2 to 3 months so the pessary can be removed and cleaned and the mucosa can be inspected for pressure ulcers or infection.

Surgical treatment of genital prolapse is designed to address the specific defects present in an individual patient. The goal is the restoration of normal vaginal anatomy, achieved by repairing the weakened musculofascial supports. Uterine prolapse is best treated by a vaginal hysterectomy. This necessitates completion of childbearing, the absence of pelvic pathology such as ovarian enlargement or large fibroids that are more appropriately managed by laparotomy, and adequate health to tolerate a major surgical procedure. Following removal of the uterus, the stretched uterosacral and cardinal ligaments are foreshortened by plication to suspend the vaginal vault (Cruikshank, 1987). Plication of the uterosacral ligaments also helps to obliterate the cul-de-sac and is important in preventing subsequent enterocele formation, a condition that may contribute to subsequent vaginal vault prolapse (Given, 1985). Older women who are no longer sexually active may be treated for uterine prolapse by a colpocleisis. The uterus is left in situ, but the vaginal space is obliterated surgically by approximating the anterior and posterior walls. It is less satisfying than a procedure that attempts a more anatomically correct repair. However, it is quick and can be performed under local anesthesia, making it applicable to medically frail women for whom a vaginal hysterectomy may be contraindicated.

Prolapse of the vaginal vault following hysterectomy presents a surgical challenge. The normal anatomic supporting structures, the cardinal and uterosacral ligaments, cannot be isolated for repair or relied on to provide adequate support to the vault. Two approaches to this problem have been described. A perineal approach involves dissection of the pararectal space to the level of the sacrospinous ligament (Nichols, 1982). The upper aspect of the vaginal vault is then suspended from the ligament by permanent sutures. Alternatively, an abdominal approach in which the vault is suspended from the periosteum of the sacral promontory by way of an interposed bridge of synthetic mesh may be used (Addison et al., 1985).

Repair of a cystocele is accomplished by an anterior colporrhaphy. The vaginal mucosa is dissected from the bladder, and redundant mucosa is excised. Submucosally, the endopelvic fascia investing the bladder is plicated toward the midline to reduce the bulging bladder tissues and recreate the normal support. The plication may also be carried out near the bladder neck, elevating the vesicourethral angle to its normal anatomic position and correcting bladder neck prolapse. This procedure is called a *Kelly plication* and is applied to correct urinary stress incontinence. Other procedures to restore bladder neck anatomy for the treatment of urinary stress incontinence will be discussed later in the chapter.

A rectocele is repaired by a posterior colporrhaphy. The endopelvic fascia investing the rectum is plicated to reduce the prolapse after dissecting it free from the overlying posterior vaginal mucosa. Usually, it is combined with a perineorrhaphy. A perineorrhaphy approximates the fascia of the perineal muscles (levator ani, deep and superficial transverse perineal, and bulbocavernous muscles) in the midline to recreate a strong perineal body.

An enterocele is a true herniation of a sac of peritoneum along the rectovaginal septum. To effect repair, one must isolate, open, and ligate the sac high on its neck and then excise it. The uterosacral ligaments are plicated in the midline to prevent recurrence (the McCall suture). Alternatively, an enterocele may be repaired abdominally by obliterating the cul-de-sac with concentric pursestring sutures placed in the peritoneum. This approach is called the *Moschcowitz procedure*.

BENIGN CYSTS AND NEOPLASMS

The vagina is an uncommon site for the development of benign cysts and neoplasms. When they occur, they are often asymptomatic and are detected only on pelvic examination. Small, asymptomatic cysts do not require treatment. Larger masses may occlude the vault and cause dyspareunia or pelvic pressure. Surgical excision is

then indicated. Solid tumors should be excised to establish a histological diagnosis and to exclude malignancy.

Vaginal cysts may form from remnants of the mesonephric duct or arise as epithelial inclusion cysts. The mesonephric ducts course laterally to the fused müllerian ducts during vaginal development. Normally, they undergo degeneration due to a lack of androgenic support. When remnants persist, it is called *Gartner's duct*. Foci of cells of Gartner's duct may be located anywhere along the lateral walls of the vagina in the submucosal tissues and also may occur within the leaves of the broad ligament and mesosalpinx. The epithelium may actively secrete a mucinous material that is retained, forming a Gartner's duct cyst. Histologically, the cysts are lined by a single layer of cuboidal or columnar cells. Occasionally a cyst may dissect deeply into the paravaginal tissues, making excision difficult and bloody. Incision, drainage, and marsupialization of the cyst wall is preferred management in this situation.

Epithelial inclusion cysts arise from vaginal epithelium buried under the mucosa during healing from a traumatic injury. Obstetric laceration and episiotomy are common antecedents. The vaginal mucosa is not secretory. However, if the tissue remains viable, cell turnover and desquamation will occur. Subsequent degeneration of the cellular material results in the accumulation of a thick cheesy substance. These cysts are distinguished from Gartner's duct cysts on the basis of their contents, histology (stratified squamous epithelium), and location (Blaustein and Sedlis, 1982). They usually occur in the lower third of the vagina on the posterior or posterolateral wall.

Benign tumors rarely arise from the connective tissue elements of the vagina. Clinically, they present as a firm nontender mass, often within the rectovaginal septum. Histological examination usually reveals smooth muscle elements (leiomyoma), fibrous tissue (fibromyoma), or a mixed pattern. Rarely, skeletal muscle elements (rhabdomyoma) are identified. Surgical excision to exclude malignancy is the indicated management (Tavossoli and Norris, 1979).

The vagina is a relatively common site for extraperitoneal endometriosis, though overall the incidence of vaginal occurrence is low. (Ranney, 1980). Patients may complain of cyclic pain and dyspareunia. The implants often form small cysts that on gross inspection are dark blue. They may be tender to palpation. The diagnosis is established by biopsy. Treatment is by surgical excision or hormonal therapy.

The squamous epithelium of the vagina may become infected with certain types of the human papillomavirus, resulting in condylomas. The soft, verrucous tumors may occur singly, in small clusters, or as confluent growths. Vaginal condylomas may be accompanied by lesions on the cervix, vulva, and perianal skin. Treatment may be difficult. Podophyllin, a cytotoxic agent widely used to treat vulvar condyloma, is not recommended for vaginal therapy. Excessive absorption may occur and result in neurotoxicity. Cryocautery and laser ablation have been applied with some success (Baggish, 1981).

CLEAR CELL ADENOCARCINOMA

In 1971 Herbst and co-workers associated an increased risk of clear cell adenocarcinoma of the vagina in young women with in utero exposure to DES. Diethylstilbestrol, a synthetic estrogen, was administered to some women with high-risk pregnancies to prevent miscarriage, beginning in the mid-1940s. Prior to 1970, only rare cases of clear cell adenocarcinoma had been reported. Following the recognition of the relationship with DES, a registry was established that now contains more than 500 cases of clear cell adenocarcinoma of the vagina and cervix (Melnick et al., 1987). Exposure to DES during gestation has been confirmed in 60% of these cases, and exposure to an unknown medication or hormone occurred in an additional 12%.

The risk of developing clear cell adenocarcinoma among exposed females is approximately 1 in 1,000. The risk increases inversely with gestational age at exposure but is not clearly associated with total dose (Herbst et al., 1979). Occurrence of the cancers appears to be age related. The median age at diagnosis is 19.0 years, and more than 90% of cases have occurred when these women were between 15 and 27 years. The prognosis for survival is related to the extent of disease at the time of diagnosis. Therapeutic modalities used in the treatment of these patients have included surgery, radiation, chemotherapy, and combined approaches.

Clear cell adenocarcinoma of the vagina is not the only DES-related abnormality of the genital tract. Vaginal adenosis and structural anomalies of the genital tract occur more frequently in this group of patients compared with nonexposed controls (Kaufman et al., 1977; Stillman, 1982). Vaginal adenosis is the presence of glandular-columnar epithelium or its mucinous secretory products in the vagina. The prevalence of this condition is more than 90% in DES-exposed women. The lesion is most often encountered on the anterior vaginal wall and may be continuous onto the cervical portio, forming a cervical ectropion. The strong association between adenosis and prenatal DES exposure suggests the drug interferes with normal vaginal development. The precise mechanism is unknown, but perhaps it impedes the replacement of müllerian columnar epithelium by upward growing squamous epithelium from the urogenital sinus (Ulfelder and Robboy, 1976). Adenosis may cause excessive vaginal secretions but is usually asymptomatic. Over time it may regress as the epithelium is converted to a squamous type by metaplasia. Adenosis is usually found in association with the rare adenocarcinomas, but progression of adenosis to cancer has not been documented (Ghosh and Cera, 1983). Adenosis should be followed carefully by cytological and clinical examination but treatment is required only for symptoms.

Diethylstilbestrol-related structural anomalies have been described for the vagina, cervix, uterus, and fallopian tubes. The vagina and cervix may develop a transverse ridge of tissue usually on the anterior portion, but in extreme cases it may be circumferential. They have been variably referred to as hoods, collars, and cockscomb cervices. A pseudopolyp may develop on the exocervix. The polypoid appearance results from a thick constricting stromal groove encircling the exocervix and causing protrusion of the endocervical tissue. The cervix may be hypoplastic, and the vaginal fornices may be absent or poorly developed. Changes in the endometrial cavity that have been described include a small cavity, a T-shaped cavity, and constrictions. They occur more frequently in women with cervical abnormalities (Kaufman et al., 1977). Fallopian tube abnormalities include a withered, foreshortened, and convoluted appearance. The clinical implication of these structural changes is an adverse effect on reproductive potential. Although fertility rates may not be decreased in this group of women, following conception they are at increased risk for spontaneous abortion, ectopic pregnancy, and preterm delivery (Stillman, 1982).

Women with in utero DES exposure may

have an increased risk of cervical intraepithelial neoplasia (CIN) and vaginal intraepithelial neoplasia (VAIN; Robboy et al., 1984). The hypothesized reason for this is the more extensive transformation zone occurring on the cervices of DES-exposed women. The transformation zone is an area of active metaplastic growth and is the site at which CIN develops. Thus far no increase in squamous cell carcinomas has been documented. However, as these patients grow older and approach the age of peak incidence of invasive carcinoma, further close follow-up will be required to exclude a higher risk.

VAGINAL INTRAEPITHELIAL NEOPLASIA

Vaginal intraepithelial neoplasia is an uncommon pathological entity. However, in recent decades it has been diagnosed with increased frequency, probably due to more extensive use of cytological screening even in women who have undergone hysterectomy. The incidence of vaginal carcinoma in situ is approximately 0.2 to 0.3 cases per 100,000 women (Cramer and Cutler, 1974), which is only about one third the rate for invasive lesions. Patients range in age from 25 to 80 years, with a mean age of 50 to 55 years.

A striking association in reported series of patients with VAIN is the occurrence of neoplasia at another genital tract site. Fifty percent to 75% of patients have evidence of another genital tract neoplasm (Lenehan et al., 1986; Benedet and Sanders, 1984; Hernandez-Linares et al., 1980). Most of the prior or concomitant neoplastic lesions are squamous and involve the cervix or vulva. This is cited as support for the hypothesized "field response" of the squamous epithelium of the lower genital tract (Marcus, 1960). According to this theory, tissues with a common embryological origin share susceptibility to common carcinogens. The urogenital sinus is the ultimate source of the epithelium of the vulva, vagina, and cervix. Under appropriate conditions, neoplasms developing in these tissues may arise as multicentric lesions instead of originating with neoplastic transformation of a single cell. This may explain the clinical observation noted. However, there is an alternative explanation. Lower genital tract neoplasms often grow by contiguous spread. Extension of a single lesion to a neighboring tissue may occur without recognition. Incomplete removal or treatment may result. Thus, fail-

ure to initially diagnose the true extent of a single neoplasm might result in a misdiagnosis of independent development of two separate lesions. Regardless of etiology, the important clinical implication is the need for careful evaluation and follow-up of the entire lower genital tract whenever a patient presents with a neoplasm involving the vulva, vagina, or cervix. The carcinogenic agents responsible for squamous cell neoplasms of the lower genital tract are not known. Factors that have been implicated include exposure to radiation and viral infection.

Vaginal intraepithelial neoplasia is asymptomatic except in occasional patients who present with postcoital staining or a vaginal discharge. In some cases, an astute examiner will detect a mucosal lesion on physical examination. However, most patients will have abnormal screening Papanicolaou smears, prompting the clinician to initiate the diagnostic evaluation.

The diagnosis is established by colposcopically directed biopsies. Colposcopic examination of the vagina is difficult and requires diligence. A vaginal speculum is used but must be repositioned repetitively so that the entire mucosal surface is visualized. The lesions of VAIN tend to be multifocal and most commonly occur in the upper third of the vagina. The colposcopic findings are similar to those seen in CIN and include white epithelium, punctation, and mosaicism. White lesions may become more obvious after application of 3% acetic acid solution to the mucosa. An iodine stain such as Schiller's solution may also be used to demonstrate abnormal areas. Normal vaginal epithelial cells stain brown because of the high glycogen content. Dysplastic cells often contain less glycogen and therefore do not take up the dye.

The histological findings of VAIN are similar to those of CIN. The abnormalities are confined to the surface epithelial cells. Neoplastic changes include the presence of abnormal mitotic figures, nuclear pleomorphism, and loss of polarity. The degree of severity is determined by the depth of epithelial involvement. If only the lower third of the cell layers of the squamous epithelium are affected, it is graded VAIN I, or mild; involvement of the middle third yields a grade of VAIN II, or moderate; and of the upper third, VAIN III, or severe. Involvement of the full thickness of the epithelium is called *vaginal carcinoma in situ*.

Vaginal intraepithelial neoplasia is considered a premalignant lesion analogous to CIN.

However, because of its lower incidence, much less information regarding the magnitude of its premalignant potential, transition times, and factors influencing the transition is available. Once it is diagnosed, treatment is indicated to prevent progression. Several treatment options exist. The rationale for all modalities is to excise or destroy the dysplastic cells so that in healing they are replaced by a normal squamous epithelium and to cause minimal damage to the normal epithelium and submucosa in the process. The choice will be dictated by the age of the patient, the desire for future sexual function, and the extent of disease.

Surgical excision has traditionally been the mainstay of therapy. This may involve a wide local excision with primary repair for an isolated lesion or a total vaginectomy if the disease is widespread. Repair following a vaginectomy may be by colpocleisis in a woman no longer sexually active. Otherwise, repair necessitates formation of a neovagina using a split thickness skin graft. Surgical treatment is successful in more than 80% of cases, but recurrences have been reported involving even skin grafts (Gallup et al., 1987a).

Chemotherapy with topical 5-fluorouracil (5-FU) is effective in treating the majority of in situ lesions. It offers the advantage of treating the entire epithelial surface at risk in this potentially multifocal disease. It is a pyrimidine analogue that blocks DNA synthesis, especially in rapidly proliferating tissues. Its effect occurs locally by ulceration and erosion, followed by reepithelialization. Side effects include vulvar irritation and dysuria. A disadvantage compared with surgery is the lack of availability of a histological specimen to exclude concomitant invasive disease. However, a recent review of the reported results with 5-FU suggest remission rates of 85%, a value that compares favorably with those obtained surgically (Sillman et al., 1985).

A more recent approach to the treatment of VAIN utilizes the carbon dioxide laser. Initially it was used to ablate isolated lesions. However, success rates are improved if the entire mucosa is vaporized and are reported to be comparable with those achieved with 5-FU (Jobson and Homesley, 1983). The technique avoids the problem of vulvitis associated with 5-FU, and excellent functional results are reported. As with 5-FU therapy, no histology is available after treatment. Therefore, its use requires an exhaustive pretreatment colposcopic examination to exclude invasive cancer.

Other therapies for VAIN have included radiation therapy and cryocautery. Tissue damage is harder to control with these modalities. As a result, higher failure rates and unacceptable complications due to damage of adjacent organs have occurred, and they are not currently recommended.

MALIGNANT NEOPLASMS

The vagina is a rare site for primary malignant tumors. Only 1% to 2% of genital tract cancers originate in the vaginal tissues. The majority are squamous cell carcinomas. Other primary cancers include melanoma, sarcoma, adenocarcinoma, and endodermal sinus tumors. Most malignant vaginal lesions are secondary. They occur as extensions of cervical or vulvar carcinoma or as metastatic cancers usually arising in the bladder, rectum, uterus, or ovary.

Squamous Cell Carcinoma

Squamous cell carcinomas account for about 90% of primary vaginal cancers. Patients range in age from 30 to 90 years, with an average age at diagnosis of approximately 60 years. The etiology of this tumor is not known. One theory suggests prolonged exposure of the mucosa to irritants has a causative role. This is based on the fact that most cancers are located near the posterior fornix, suggesting a pooling phenomenon. However, no data to substantiate such a relationship are available, nor is there a proved relationship of vaginal cancer to pessary use or prolapse, other potential chronic irritants.

The symptom most often attributed to vaginal cancer is abnormal bleeding or a blood-tinged discharge. Bleeding may occur only with intercourse or douching. Anterior wall lesions may cause urinary symptoms such as frequency, dysuria, and hematuria. Rectal involvement from a posterior wall tumor may manifest as tenesmus, melena, or pain. Most patients report no symptoms, and the diagnosis is then established by pelvic examination. The vaginal vault is highly distensible and can accommodate a relatively large mass lesion before the onset of symptoms. Part of the typical delay in diagnosis is accounted for on this basis. However, many patients delay seeking medical care despite symptoms. This is unfortunate since vaginal cancer occurs in a clinically accessible site, and thus an opportunity for early diagnosis exists (Herbst et al., 1970).

The diagnosis of vaginal carcinoma is made by biopsy of a visible or palpable vaginal lesion. It is essential that the entire muscosal surface be visualized by rotating the speculum blades, and palpated during the pelvic examination. Occasionally small lesions are detected colposcopically in response to an abnormal cytological smear. Gross lesions vary in appearance. They may present as exophytic growths, superficial plaques, or ulcerative lesions. Histologically, neoplastic epidermoid cells are identified invading the submucous tissues as well as the vascular and lymphatic spaces. There is usually an associated inflammatory infiltrate. The histological appearance may be graded based on its degree of differentiation, but this does not give reliable prognostic information (Pride et al., 1979).

Vaginal squamous cell carcinoma spreads by contiguous growth and via the lymphatic vasculature. Local growth occurs initially in the submucous layers, with gradual extension to the paracolpos, bladder, and rectum. Growth may involve the cervix or vulva. However, by convention, a squamous tumor that involves both the vagina and one of the adjacent organs at the time of diagnosis is considered to be a primary cancer of either the cervix or vulva.

Metastatic spread via the lymphatics follows a pattern that depends on the location of the primary lesion. Tumors located in the upper portion of the vagina tend to spread into the pelvic lymph nodes (the iliac, hypogastric, and obturator groups) similar to cervix cancer. Tumors arising in the lower portion of the vagina often metastasize first to the femoral and inguinal lymph nodes, as do vulvar cancers. Lymphatic involvement is present about one fourth of the time at diagnosis (Blaustein and Sedlis, 1982).

Staging is based on a careful history and clinical examination. In addition, a chest x-ray film, IV pyelogram, barium enema, cystoscopy, and proctosigmoidoscopy are performed to determine as accurately as possible evidence for local or distant spread. The staging system is according to the recommendations of the International Federation of Gynecology and Obstetrics (FIGO; Table 5–1). The distribution of patients among the stages varies with the different series reported. Typically 30% to 40% of patients will have stage III or IV disease (Pride et al., 1979; Ball and Ber-

TABLE 5–1.

International Federation of Gynecology and Obstetrics Classification of Vaginal Cancer

Stage 0
  Carcinoma in situ.
Stage I
  Carcinoma limited to the vaginal wall.
Stage II
  Carcinoma involving the subvaginal tissues but
    not extending to the pelvic wall.
Stage III
  Carcinoma extending to the pelvic wall.
Stage IV
  Carcinoma extending beyond the true pelvis or
    involving the mucosa of the bladder or rectum
    (bullous edema alone does not permit
    allotment of a case to stage IV).
Stage IVa
  Involvement of adjacent organs (bladder,
    rectum).
Stage IVb
  Involvement of distant organs.

man, 1982; Herbst et al., 1970; Gallup et al., 1987b).

The treatment of vaginal squamous cell carcinoma has been primarily by radiation therapy, though in some cases surgery may be an option. The therapeutic plan should be individualized. The following factors are considered: the extent of disease, the patient's general health, desire for vaginal function, and childbearing status. In addition, the proximity of the vagina to the bladder and rectum must be recognized to minimize complications.

Surgical excision as primary therapy is applicable only to small localized tumors located in the upper third of the vagina. Tumors arising on the posterior vaginal wall are more easily resected than those occurring anteriorly near the more intimate attachment of the bladder. Treatments reported consist of radical hysterectomy with vaginectomy and excision of the pelvic lymph nodes, radical vaginectomy, and wide local excision (Ball and Berman, 1982). The surgical approach may also be used adjunctively to treat advanced disease or recurrences following radiation therapy.

Radiation therapy has become the main treatment modality for vaginal cancer in most modern series of patients reported (Podczaski and Herbst, 1986). A combined approach using both external radiation therapy and local implants is applied. A dose of 4,000 to 5,000 rad of whole pelvis radiation may be administered first to initiate shrinkage of a large tumor and render local therapy more effective. Radium or cesium implants are then placed intravaginally to deliver an additional 3,000 to 4,000 rad directly to the tumor. This may be impossible to carry out with some very large tumors. In these cases, additional therapy by external beam may be administered.

The normal vaginal mucosa is relatively radioresistant. However, the proximity of the radiosensitive bladder and rectal tissues results in radiation complications in approximately 15% to 25% of patients (Pride et al., 1979; Perez and Camel, 1982; Gallup et al., 1987b). Complications include proctitis, rectovaginal and vesicovaginal fistulas, and strictures. They occur more frequently in patients with advanced disease, who receive higher doses of irradiation.

The prognosis for patients with vaginal squamous cell carcinoma depends primarily on the extent of disease at the time of diagnosis. Stage I disease treated with radiation therapy results in 5-year survival rates of 80% to 90%. Five-year survival rates for higher stages are 45% to 58% for stage II, 25% to 40% for stage III, and up to 10% for stage IV. The overall 5-year survival is approximately 45%.

Recurrences most often occur locally and are commoner in higher stages. Distant metastases occur later and usually involve the lung and bone. Radical surgery may be attempted in selected cases of isolated local recurrence. Chemotherapy is being evaluated for a possible role in cases with systemic recurrence.

Malignant Melanoma

Malignant melanomas may arise from vaginal melanocytes. They are rare tumors, comprising less than 1% of all melanomas in women (Chung et al., 1975). Patients may be asymptomatic or present with a mass, discharge, or vaginal bleeding. The gross appearance of the tumors is variable, ranging from a flat, spreading lesion to a heaped up, polypoid mass. Most lesions are pigmented, but this is not invariable. The diagnosis must be confirmed by histological evaluation of a biopsy specimen.

The prognosis for patients with vaginal melanoma is poor. The disease is often well advanced when diagnosed. The tumors are not responsive to radiation therapy, and effective chemotherapeutic agents have not been identified. Radical

surgical therapy, including lymph node dissection if the primary tumor is more than very superficially invasive, is currently the treatment most often recommended (Liu et al., 1987).

Adenocarcinomas

Adenocarcinoma of the vagina associated with in utero DES exposure has previously been discussed. A much rarer type of vaginal adenocarcinoma is the endodermal sinus tumor. It occurs exclusively in infants, usually less than 2 years of age. The tumor probably arises from extragonadal germ cells. Endodermal sinus tumors occurring in the vagina may secrete α-fetoprotein like their ovarian counterparts. This is a useful marker to monitor disease activity in patients undergoing treatment. Combination therapy consisting of surgery with chemotherapy has resulted in several long-term survivors. The most commonly used chemotherapeutic agents are vincristine, actinomycin D, and cyclophosphamide (Young and Scully, 1984).

Vaginal Sarcomas

Sarcomas are extremely rare, comprising less than 2% of vaginal malignancies. They tend to occur as one of two types based on their age predilection (Davos and Abell, 1975). Sarcoma botryoides (embryonal rhabdomyosarcoma) usually afflicts children less than 2 years of age. The tumors form friable clusters of polypoid masses that protrude from the vagina. They are frequently multicentric and appear to arise from the vaginal subepithelium. Histologically, there is diffuse proliferation of spindled neoplastic cells mixed with embryonic striated muscle cells. Clinically, they are aggressive tumors with a poor prognosis. The traditional therapeutic approach has been radical surgery. However, a multimodal approach combining less radical surgery with chemotherapy or radiation may offer equal efficacy with less morbidity (Friedman et al., 1986).

Vaginal sarcomas in adults are represented by a varied group of histological types. The commonest is the smooth muscle tumor leiomyosarcoma. Others are classified as fibrosarcomas, reticulum cell sarcomas, malignant schwannomas, müllerian stromal sarcomas, and mixed cell types. They are considered to have a poor prognosis. One series reported a 5-year survival of 23% (Davos and Abell, 1975). The extreme rarity of these tumors makes evaluation of treatment regimens difficult. Treatment is usually by radical surgical excision, supplemented by radiation therapy to control local disease.

Secondary Carcinoma

In the vagina, metastatic cancer occurs more frequently than primary disease. Contiguous spread from the uterine cervix accounts for most. Other sites of primary malignancy that may involve the vagina include the vulva, endometrium, ovary, bladder, urethra, rectum, and malignant trophoblastic disease.

URINARY INCONTINENCE

Incontinence is the involuntary loss of urine. It occurs when intravesical pressure exceeds intraurethral pressure at any time except during a voluntary act of micturition. There are several mechanisms by which it can occur and many possible underlying etiologies. The gynecologist is usually called on to manage genuine stress incontinence but must be familiar with the other forms to establish the correct differential diagnosis.

Occasional, mild incontinence is common, occurring in at least one third of all women (Wolin, 1969). It is important to appreciate this and reserve extensive evaluation and treatment for those patients in whom it is clearly indicated. It also suggests that perfect control may not be a necessary goal for therapy. Nevertheless, incontinence is a significant social and medical burden. It is a major reason for institutionalized care, especially among the elderly. It contributes to negative self-esteem and poor quality of life in many of those affected.

Types

The term incontinence may be used to denote a symptom, a sign, or a condition (International Continence Society, 1981). A patient's complaint of involuntary urine loss should always be confirmed by its objective demonstration. However, symptoms and signs alone may not be adequate to establish the mechanism of incontinence in an individual. Further investigation is often required because treatment will depend on the type of incontinence present. Four major types have been described.

Stress incontinence (urinary stress incontinence, genuine stress incontinence) is the involuntary loss of urine occurring when intravesical pressure exceeds intraurethral pressure in the absence of a detrusor contraction. The increase in intravesical pressure results from the passive transmission to the bladder of an increase in intra-abdominal pressure during a contraction of the abdominal wall muscles, diaphragm, or both. The "stress" is the increased intra-abdominal pressure. It is often associated with coughing, sneezing, laughing, straining, or exercise.

Urge incontinence is the involuntary loss of urine associated with a strong desire to void. It is subdivided into two categories. In motor urge incontinence (unstable bladder, detrusor instability), the sensation of urgency arises in association with inappropriate contractions of the detrusor muscle. Normally, detrusor activity is inhibited until the time and place are appropriate for bladder emptying. In sensory urge incontinence (irritable bladder syndrome), there is hypersensitivity of the bladder and urethral receptors, resulting in excessive sensory input and consequent urgency. In some cases, this may prompt an uninhibited detrusor contraction. When a detrusor contraction of sufficient magnitude occurs so that intravesical pressure rises in excess of intraurethral pressure, incontinence results.

Overflow incontinence is the involuntary loss of urine associated with overdistention of the bladder. Intravesical pressure exceeds intraurethral pressure in the absence of a detrusor contraction because of the overfilling of the bladder with excessive volume of urine. Small amounts of urine are lost, but the bladder remains distended.

Extraurethral incontinence (total incontinence) is the involuntary loss of urine through any channel other than the urethra. Urine bypasses the normal continence mechanism in the urethral sphincter. This category includes congenital and acquired lesions.

Clinical Evaluation of the Lower Urinary Tract

The evaluation of the patient with urinary incontinence is crucial because the treatment will vary depending on the underlying pathophysiological mechanism. Some patients may have incontinence resulting from more than one disorder. Treatment options will depend on the severity of incontinence and on associated medical and surgical diseases. Several diagnostic aids are available to assist the clinician. A thorough history and physical examination are essential. Additional urodynamic, endoscopic, and radiological tests are applied as indicated.

The *history* seeks to establish the nature and severity of incontinence. A prepared form such as the Hodgkinson questionnaire is helpful (Table 5–2). Hodgkinson, 1970). Positive responses to questions in group 1 suggest intrinsic urinary tract disease, those in group 2 suggest possible neurologic disorder, and those in group 3 suggest genuine stress incontinence. Other historical data of importance relate to concomitant medical and neurological disease, obstetric history, medications, and assessment of sexual and bowel function.

The *physical examination* is done to exclude pelvic pathology, assess pelvic supports, and evaluate function of the sacral nerve roots. A careful bimanual examination is necessary to exclude a pelvic mass that might exert external compression on the bladder. The mucosal surfaces are inspected carefully for evidence of a fistula and to assess for evidence of atrophy. The vaginal walls are observed for evidence of endopelvic fascia weakening, that is, a cystocele, enterocele, or rectocele. A urethral diverticulum may be demonstrated by palpation of an anterior vaginal mass or by exudation of pus through the urethral meatus on palpation of the anterior vaginal wall.

An evaluation of the ligamentous support of the proximal urethra is essential. Hypermobility resulting in descent of the proximal urethra is believed to be the mechanism of genuine stress incontinence. This assessment may be assisted by the Q-tip test (Fig 5–8; Karram and Bhatia, 1988). A sterile, lubricated cotton swab is placed into the bladder neck. At rest in the lithotomy position, the urethra (and thus the swab) assumes a 0-degree angle to the horizontal plane. The patient is then asked to perform a Valsalva maneuver. If the proximal urethra is normally supported, straining will displace the distal end of the swab only slightly. However, with loss of support, straining will cause the proximal end of the urethra to descend, forcing the distal part of the swab upward to an angle usually exceeding 30 degrees and often approaching 90 degrees.

The sensory function of the sacral nerve roots S2–4 is tested by pin prick and light touch of the vulva, perineum, and buttocks. Motor function is assessed through vaginal and anal sphincter tone. The bulbocavernous, anal sphinc-

ter, and ankle reflexes are elicited. Deficits in sensation or motor function should prompt a more thorough neurological evaluation.

A *urinalysis* and *urine culture* are routinely performed and should precede more invasive testing. Urinary tract infections should be treated and the patient reassessed for resolution of symptoms prior to instrumentation of the lower urinary tract.

Urodynamic studies describe a series of clinical tests available to evaluate the function of the urinary bladder with respect to both the filling-storage phase and the emptying phase. A *frequency-volume* chart or urinary diary may be kept by the patient. She records all fluid intake and urine output in a 24-hour period and notes episodes of incontinence. It provides an objective record of the frequency and timing of voiding and is very helpful in assessing the severity of symptoms (Wyman et al., 1988).

Cystometry is used to evaluate bladder filling and storage. Bladder pressure is measured relative to bladder volume (Fig 5–9). The bladder is filled through a catheter with warm sterile saline while pressures are recorded. Since intravesical pressure is the sum of the detrusor pressure plus intra-abdominal pressure, techniques using multiple pressure transducers to subtract out increases due to contraction of the abdominal wall musculature are used. The parameters determined include (1) bladder compliance ($\Delta P/\Delta V$), (2) bladder capacity, (3) bladder sensation, and (4) detrusor stability. Normally the bladder is compliant, demonstrating pressures of less than 15 cm H_2O throughout filling until capacity is reached. The normal bladder capacity is 350 to 500 ml. Patients usually note a first sensation of filling at 100 to 200 ml but then suppress it until a sensation of maximum filling is noted near capacity. Finally, the detrusor muscle does not normally contract during filling but, rather, remains "stable." Catheterization of the bladder to perform cystometry also provides an opportunity to determine a postvoid residual. Following a spontaneous void, the patient is catheterized. Normally, the urine volume will not exceed 50 ml.

The necessity of performing invasive urodynamic tests in all patients with incontinence is debated. However, the *urinary stress test* should always be done. The patient is examined with a full bladder in both the lithotomy and standing positions. An abnormal test result consists of a discharge of a small amount of urine from the me-

TABLE 5–2.

Urological Questionnaire

Group 1

1.	Have you had treatment for urinary tract disease, such as stones, kidney disease, infections, tumors, or injuries?	Yes	No
2.	Have you had repeated bouts of pyelitis?	Yes	No
3.	Is your urine ever bloody?	Yes	No
4.	Is the volume of urine you usually pass large, average, small, or very small? (circle one)		
5.	When you lose your urine accidentally, are you ever unaware that it is passing?	Yes	No
6.	Do you have a severe sense of urgency before you lose your urine?	Yes	No
7.	Do you lose urine as a constant drip from the vagina?	Yes	No
8.	Did you have difficulty holding urine as a child?	Yes	No
9.	Is it usually painful or difficult to pass your urine?	Yes	No

Group 2

1.	Did you wet the bed as a child?	Yes	No
2.	Do you wet the bed now?	Yes	No
3.	Have you ever had paralysis, polio, multiple sclerosis, a serious injury to your back, a cyst or tumor on your spine, tuberculosis, a stroke, syphilis, diabetes, or pernicious anemia? (If yes, circle proper one.)	Yes	No
4.	Does the sound, sight, or feel of running water cause you to lose your urine?	Yes	No
5.	Is your loss of urine a continual drip, so that you are constantly wet?	Yes	No
6.	Are you ever unaware that you are losing, or are about to lose, control of your urine?	Yes	No
7.	Is your clothing slightly damp, wet, or soaking wet, or do you leave puddles on the floor? (If yes, circle proper one.)	Yes	No
8.	Have you had an operation on your spine, brain, or bladder?	Yes	No
9.	Do you find it necessary to have your urine removed frequently by means of a catheter because you are unable to pass it?	Yes	No

Group 3

1.	Do you lose urine by spurts during coughing, sneezing, laughing, or lifting?	Yes	No
2.	Do you lose urine when you are lying down?	Yes	No
3.	Do you lose urine when you are sitting or standing erect?	Yes	No
4.	When you are urinating, can you usually stop the flow?	Yes	No
5.	Did your urine difficulty start after delivery of an infant?	Yes	No
6.	Did it follow an operation?	Yes	No
7.	Check the type of operation:		
	Hysterectomy, abdominal incision		
	Hysterectomy, removed through the vagina		
	Removal of a tumor, abdominal incision		
	Vaginal repair		
	Suspension of the uterus		
	Cesarean birth		
8	If your menstrual periods have stopped, did the menopause make your condition more severe?	Yes	No
9.	Is your control of urine good unless you cough, sneeze, laugh, lift, or strain?	Yes	No
10.	Do you have difficulty holding urine if you suddenly stand erect from a sitting or lying position?	Yes	No
11.	Do you find it necessary to wear protection because you get wet?	Yes	No

*From Hodgkinson CP: Stress urinary incontinence—1970. *Am J Obstet Gynecol* 1970; 108:1149. Used by permission.

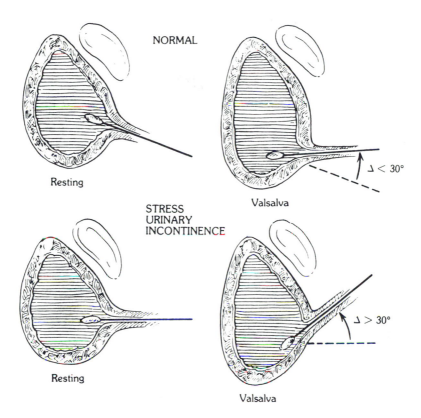

NORMAL

Resting

Valsalva

∡ < 30°

STRESS
URINARY
INCONTINENCE

Resting

Valsalva

∡ > 30°

FIG 5–8.
Diagrammatic representation of the Q-tip test showing mobility of the urethrovesical junction in a continent patient, and a patient with stress urinary incontinence.

atus simultaneously with forceful coughing. The
flow is not delayed in onset and does not continue after the exertion. Demonstration of stress
incontinence should precede virtually all cases of
anticipated surgical repair.

Uroflowmetry assesses the emptying phase of
bladder function by determining the flow rate of
spontaneous micturition. The volume of urine excreted is divided by the length of time of voiding.
Normal rates exceed 15 ml/second. Decreased
rates should prompt further neurological evaluation as well as evaluation for partial obstruction
of the urethra. This is much less common in
women than in men.

Endoscopic techniques allow a visual assessment
of the urethra and bladder mucosa. Although not
done routinely for assessment of incontinence, it
is essential in the workup of persistent hematuria
and may be helpful in syndromes of chronic bladder or urethral pain. Some conditions that may be
diagnosed include fistulas, diverticula, foreign
bodies, tumors, and mucosal inflammation. *Ra-*

diographic techniques such as IV pyelography and
voiding cystourethrography are applied in indicated settings.

Genuine Stress Incontinence

Stress incontinence is considered to be a
manifestation of pelvic relaxation. Weakening of
the fascial supports of the proximal urethra allows
descent or herniation of the bladder neck with
stress. The bladder sphincter mechanism is in the
proximal urethra, and normally this is located
above the urogenital diaphragm in an intra-
abdominal position. When the intra-abdominal
pressure rises, as with coughing or Valsalva's maneuver, the increase is transmitted equally to the
bladder and to the proximal urethra. A constant
pressure relationship is maintained between bladder and urethra, and the patient is continent.
However, if the bladder neck herniates to an extra-abdominal position, an increase in intra-
abdominal pressure is transmitted to the bladder

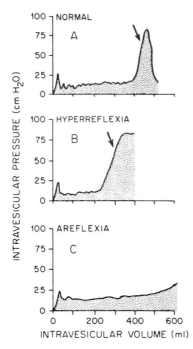

FIG 5–9.
Water cystometrogram in *(A)* a normal patient, *(B)* a patient with detrusor hyperreflexia, and *(C)* a patient with detrusor areflexia (hypotonic bladder).

but not to the proximal urethra. Bladder pressure rises, and when it exceeds intraurethral pressure, incontinence occurs.

The patient will complain of leakage simultaneous with exertion. There is no preceding sense of urgency, and the volume lost is usually small. The symptoms often resolve in the supine position. Several conditions may contribute to pelvic fascia damage. Multiparity, obesity, chronic coughing, and constipation have been associated with stress incontinence, and these may be elicited by history. Other manifestations of pelvic relaxation such as cystocele and uterine prolapse may coexist.

The diagnosis is established by an abnormal stress test result. Demonstrable leakage of urine should be observed with stress if the patient's bladder is adequately filled. Patients with genuine stress incontinence will also demonstrate hypermobility of the bladder neck by the Q-tip test. In addition, other causes of urinary incontinence should be ruled out. A substantial number of patients have a component of both detrusor instability and genuine stress incontinence. It is important to document this prior to treatment. The history alone is often inadequate to separate these

mechanisms since symptoms may overlap. Cystometrics may be necessary to assure detrusor stability. A careful examination will exclude fistulas and neurological abnormalities.

Nonsurgical treatment for stress incontinence should be attempted in mild cases before considering surgical options. The patient should be instructed to empty her bladder in anticipation of vigorous exercise. Pelvic floor exercises (Kegel exercises) may be performed to strengthen the pubococcygeal muscles. Some postmenopausal patients with atrophic changes may improve with estrogen replacement therapy (Hilton and Stanton, 1983). Occasionally, patients will improve with α-adrenergic agonists such as pseudoephedrine or phenylpropanolamine. These drugs increase tone in the smooth muscle of the urethra and thus promote urine storage.

Surgical therapy will often be required to effect relief from symptoms in women with moderate or severe stress incontinence. The goal of surgery is to restore the normal anatomical relations of the urethra by elevating and securing the bladder neck back to an intra-abdominal position. This may be achieved by either an abdominal or vaginal approach. The abdominal approach requires dissection in the extraperitoneal space of Retzius to the level of the paraurethral tissues through an abdominal wall incision. The paraurethral fascia is sutured to the periosteum of the posterior surface of the pubic bone (Marshall-Marchetti-Kranz procedure; Marshall et al., 1949) or to Cooper's ligament (Burch procedure; Burch, 1968).

The traditional vaginal approach is a Kelly plication. The vaginal mucosa is incised and dissected from the underlying endopelvic fascia. The fascia lateral to the proximal urethra is plicated in the midline. This results in elevation of the bladder neck as supporting tissue is secured beneath it. Plication of the endopelvic fascia overlying the bladder is conveniently performed simultaneously to reduce a coexistent cystocele. More recently, transvaginal urethropexy procedures that use long needles to place sutures that suspend the paraurethral tissues from the anterior rectus fascia have been described (Pereyra et al., 1982; Stamey, 1973). The sutures are secured above the fascia via very small (approximately 1 cm) suprapubic incisions. Cystoscopy is performed to assure that the bladder lumen is not traversed by the permanent sutures after placement and before they are tied.

Severe and recurrent cases of stress incontinence have been treated using sling techniques. A strip of fascia, harvested from the anterior rectus sheath or fascia lata, or a synthetic material is used. The sling is passed beneath the bladder neck in the vaginal submucosa and attached to the anterior abdominal wall to elevate the proximal urethra.

Urge Incontinence

Detrusor instability occurs in approximately one third of patients with incontinence and often coexists with genuine stress incontinence (Sand et al., 1987). In some cases an underlying etiology may be identified. Patients with acute inflammation secondary to bacterial cystitis may develop transient detrusor hyperactivity and associated urge incontinence. Neurological conditions affecting upper motor neurons, such as multiple sclerosis, can result in uninihibited detrusor contractions. Most patients, however, do not have a recognizable cause of detrusor instability.

The history of a patient with urge incontinence is usually notable for complaints of frequency, urgency, and nocturia. Episodes of leakage may be associated with stress but occur only after a lag period of several seconds. Other stimuli resulting in incontinence include the sound or feel of running water. The volume of urine lost is greater than with stress incontinence, and positional changes have little effect on symptoms.

A careful neurological evaluation may reveal hyperreflexia in the lower extremities. Often, however, the physical examination is normal. The diagnosis is confirmed by cystometry. During filling, brief increases in bladder pressure in excess of 15 cm H_2O above the baseline pressure indicate inappropriate detrusor contractions. Care must be taken, however, to measure true detrusor pressures and not the passive intravesical transmission of an increase in intra-abdominal pressure.

Several therapeutic modalities are available to treat idiopathic detrusor instability. Pharmacological agents that affect the autonomic innervation of the bladder or directly suppress smooth muscle contractility may be used. The parasympathetic system via the neurotransmitter acetylcholine is the primary neurological stimulus causing detrusor contractions. Anticholinergic drugs have therefore been used to inhibit inappropriate detrusor activity; 15 to 30 mg of propantheline every 4 to 6 hours or 5 mg of oxybutynin chloride every 8 hours are most commonly prescribed. Direct smooth muscle relaxants (flavoxate) and tricy-

clic antidepressants (imipramine [Tofranil]) may also improve bladder storage capabilities.

Nonpharmacological modalities include bladder training drills and biofeedback techniques. The rationale is to enhance cortical suppression of inappropriate detrusor activity similar to that occurring during childhood toilet training. A strict schedule of voiding that seeks to retrain the bladder by progressively increasing the interval between voiding is prescribed (Fantl et al., 1981).

Overflow Incontinence

Overflow incontinence resulting from detrusor atony may be associated with a primary lower motor neuron lesion. Conditions include spinal cord injury, radical pelvic surgery, and diabetic neuropathy. Management is usually by intermittent self-catheterization.

Overflow incontinence may also occur secondary to outflow obstruction. In women this usually occurs in a postpartum or postoperative state in association with urethral edema or pain. Continuous bladder drainage by catheterization for 24 to 48 hours will adequately manage this temporary condition.

Genitourinary Fistulas

Total incontinence usually indicates a fistula that bypasses the normal sphincter mechanism. If the diagnosis is not obvious, small leaks can be demonstrated with the aid of urinary dyes such as oral phenazopyridine (Pyridium). Endoscopic and radiographic studies are required preoperatively to determine the precise extent of the condition.

Successful repair of genitourinary fistulas requires strict adherence to basic surgical principles. The fistulous tract must be identified and excised, including all surrounding scar tissue. Wide mobilization of the tissue layers is necessary to assure reconstruction of normal anatomy without tension on the suture lines. Catheterization to divert the urinary stream and to prevent distention and stress on the suture lines is necessary during healing.

URETHRAL DIVERTICULUM

Urethral diverticula are saclike herniations of the urethral mucosa through a defect in the muscular and adventitial wall. The true incidence of occurrence in the female population is not known. Reported incidences vary between 1% and 4% (Ginsburg and Genadry, 1984). The suggestion has been made that increasing awareness of the condition among physicians increases the frequency with which it is diagnosed (Coddington and Knab, 1983). Diverticula appear to be commonest among women between ages 30 to 50 years and may occur with a higher frequency in blacks (Andersen, 1967).

Urethral diverticula may result from one of several etiologies. A congenital defect in the urethral wall may explain why occasional diverticula are diagnosed in childhood. Alternatively, the congenital defect may not become manifest until later in life. Most diverticula, however, are probably acquired lesions. One theory proposes that traumatic injury, such as occurs in childbirth, may disrupt the integrity of the urethral wall. However, the condition generally is not associated with increasing parity (Pathak and House, 1970). Others have suggested postinflammatory obstruction of the paraurethral glands as an etiology. An abscess cavity forms proximal to the obstruction, and subsequent rupture into the lumen of the urethra results in a diverticulum. It is likely that inflammation is the commonest cause (Ginsburg and Genadry, 1984).

The classic triad of symptoms associated with urethral diverticula consists of dysuria, dyspareunia, and postvoid dribbling. Other symptoms may be related to a urinary tract infection that is often associated. Included in this group are frequency, urgency, and hematuria. Occasionally a patient may complain of the presence of a palpable mass lesion. A significant number of patients are asymptomatic, and the condition is then diagnosed on the basis of physical findings.

A palpable mass in the anterior vaginal wall suggests a urethral diverticulum. The mass is often tender. On palpation of the urethra, pus or urine may be expressed from the meatus. Most diverticula are 1 to 3 cm in diameter and are located in the distal or middle third of the urethra (Andersen, 1967). The ostium almost always occurs on the posterior urethral wall.

Confirmation of the diagnosis is made by radiological or endoscopic methods. A voiding cystourethrogram may demonstrate filling of the diverticulum with dye. If not, the urethra is filled under positive pressure using a special double-ballooned catheter. The balloons obstruct both the external meatus and the urethrovesical junction, allowing dye to be forced even into a narrow-necked diverticular sac. Urethroscopy allows direct visualization of the ostium and occasionally demonstrates more than one opening.

Several surgical procedures have been recommended for the treatment of symptomatic urethral diverticula. In the setting of acute infection with cellulitis, simple incision and drainage are appropriate (Ginsburg and Genadry, 1984). In a subacute situation, excision of the diverticular sac through a vaginal incision is most often performed (Ward et al., 1967). A small probe, a Fogarty balloon catheter, or dye may be placed in the sac to assist the dissection (Moore, 1952). The defect is closed in several layers using fine suture material and without tension on the suture lines. Catheter drainage of the bladder is maintained for several days. If the diverticulum is located in the distal urethra, marsupialization can be performed (Spence and Duckett, 1970). An incision is made from the external meatus to the diverticular sac through the vaginal mucosa and urethral wall. The redundant tissue from the wall of the diverticulum is excised. The urethral mucosa is sewn to the vaginal mucosa to create a new urethral meatus. This procedure can result in iatrogenic incontinence if the incision includes the proximal urethral sphincter mechanism. Other complications of diverticular surgery include urethral strictures, fistula formation, and recurrence of diverticula.

LOWER URINARY TRACT INFECTION

Infections of the lower urinary tract are very common in women, making it essential for gynecologists to be familiar with diagnosis and management. It is estimated that 15% to 20% of women will have at least one urinary tract infection. Several reasons are proposed for the high frequency in women. Included are (1) the relatively short female urethra, allowing ascension of bacteria to the bladder; (2) the proximity of the meatus to the heavily colonized vagina and rectum; (3) inoculation resulting from sexual intercourse; and (4) decreased urethral resistance associated with postmenopausal atrophy. Other special circumstances that predispose to urinary tract infections are pregnancy and urethral catheterization.

The typical manifestation of a urinary tract infection is cystitis, a bladder infection. Patients will almost always complain of a combination of frequency, urgency, dysuria, and hematuria. Some pathogens, however, appear to preferentially infect the mucosa of the urethra, giving rise to urethritis. The commonest cause is *C. trachomatis* (Bowie et al., 1977). Urethral pain, dysuria, and dyspareunia are common complaints. Infection may ascend the ureters and involve the renal parenchyma, causing pyelonephritis. This is usually manifest through systemic signs such as fever and chills as well as costovertebral angle and flank tenderness.

Urinary tract infections are usually defined microbiologically and diagnosed by a urine culture, though in some cases this approach should be modified (Stamm et al., 1982). Significant bacteriuria is defined as the presence of greater than 100,000 (10^5) organisms/ml of urine in a clean-voided midstream specimen. However, some patients will have substantial clinical symptoms from a urinary tract infection and yet fail to meet this criterion, and others will be asymptomatic despite significant bacteriuria. The latter is termed *asymptomatic bacteriuria* and occurs in about 5% of women.

In addition to a quantitative urine culture, the urinalysis is a useful clinical tool that provides immediate data. If the microscopic evaluation of an uncentrifuged drop of urine reveals bacteria, it correlates well with significant bacteriuria on urine culture. A centrifuged specimen is examined for leukocytes. Pyuria exists when five or more white blood cells per high-power field are present. It is virtually always present in bacterial cystitis but may also indicate inflammation secondary to a foreign body, tumor, or trauma. White blood cell or red blood cell casts indicate disease involving the upper urinary tracts.

Most urinary tract infections are caused by *Escherichia coli* (Ronald, 1984). Other organisms isolated are species of *Enterobacter, Klebsiella, Proteus, Pseudomonas, Staphylococcus,* and *Streptococcus. Chlamydia trachomatis* and *T. vaginalis* are other organisms that are capable of infecting the lower urinary tract. They will not be isolated by standard cultures but are frequently associated with pyuria.

The treatment of lower urinary tract infections should be individualized and specifically directed against the responsible organisms. A careful clinical evaluation is necessary to exclude another or more complex cause of the patient's symptoms such as vaginitis or a urethral divertic-

ulum. Quantitative urine cultures and urethral cultures are obtained prior to treatment so that bacterial isolates can be tested in vitro for antibiotic susceptibility. A urinalysis provides confirmatory evidence of the diagnosis and preliminary information regarding the etiology. Treatment can be initiated while awaiting the 24 to 48 hours necessary for culture results but should be reviewed when they are available. Follow-up cultures are always necessary.

Antibiotics effective against common urinary tract pathogens include ampicillin, amoxicillin, timethoprim-sulfamethoxazole, and nitrofurantoin. In uncomplicated infections confined to the lower tract, there is evidence that single-dose regimens are as effective in eradicating the disease as multiple-dose regimens (Souney and Polk, 1982). They offer the advantage of increased compliance, lower cost, and decreased risk of emergence of resistant bacteria. Patients who fail single-dose regimens are likely to have upper urinary tract disease. They will benefit from earlier identification and institution of prolonged regimens and structural studies of the upper urinary tracts. Two common regimens are 3 gm of amoxicillin by mouth or three tablets of double-strength trimethoprim-sulfamethoxazole. Adjuvant measures for patient comfort include adequate hydration and urinary analgesics. A regimen of 200 mg of phenazopyride hydrochloride administered two to three times daily will alleviate dysuria until the inflammation subsides. Infection caused by *Chlamydia* should be treated for 7 to 10 days with oral tetracycline.

REFERENCES

Addison WA, Livengood CH, Sutton GP, et al: Abdominal sacral colpopexy with Mersilene mesh in the retroperitoneal position in the management of post hysterectomy vaginal vault prolapse and enterocele. *Am J Obstet Gynecol* 1985; 153:140–146.

Andersen MJF: The incidence of diverticula in the female urethra. *J Urol* 1967; 98:96–98.

Baggish MS: Carbon dioxide laser treatment for condylomata acuminata venereal infections. *Obstet Gynecol* 1981; 55:711–715.

Ball HG, Berman ML: Management of primary vaginal carcinoma. *Gynecol Oncol* 1982; 14:154–163.

Bates GW, Wiser WL: A technique for uterine conservation in adolescents with vaginal agenesis and a functional uterus. *Obstet Gynecol* 1985; 66:290–294.

Beecham CT: Classification of vaginal relaxation. *Am J Obstet Gynecol* 1980; 136:957–958.

Benedet JL, Sanders BH: Carcinoma in situ of the vagina. *Am J Obstet Gynecol* 1984; 148:695–700.

Blaustein RL: Cytology of the female genital tract, in Blaustein A (ed): *Pathology of the Female Genital Tract,* ed 2. New York, Springer-Verlag New York, 1982, pp 861–866.

Blaustein A, Sedlis A: Diseases of the vagina, in Blaustein A (ed): *Pathology of the Female Genital Tract,* ed 2. New York, Springer-Verlag New York, 1982, pp 59–65, 72–73, 79.

Bowie WR, Wang SP, Alexander ER, et al: Etiology of nongonococcal urethritis: Evidence for *Chlamydia trachomatis* and *Ureaplasma urelyticum. J Clin Invest* 1977; 59:735–742.

Bradley WE, Rockswold GL, Timm GW, et al: Neurology of micturition. *J Urol* 1976; 115:481–486.

Bulmer D: The development of the human vagina. *J Anat* 1957; 91:490–508.

Bump RC, Fantl JA, Hurt WG: The mechanism of urinary continence in women with severe uterovaginal prolapse: Results of barrier studies. *Obstet Gynecol* 1988; 72:291–295.

Burch JC: Cooper's ligament urethrovesical suspension for stress incontinence. *Am J Obstet Gynecol* 1968; 100:764–774.

Buttram VC: Müllerian anomalies and their management. *Fertil Steril* 1983; 40:159–163.

Chung AF, Woodruff JM, Lewis JL Jr: Malignant melanoma of the vulva—a report of 44 cases. *Obstet Gynecol* 1975; 45:638–646.

Coddington CC, Knab DR: Urethral diverticulum: A review. *Obstet Gynecol Surv* 1983; 38:357–364.

Cramer DW, Cutler SJ: Incidence and histopathology of malignancies of the female genital organs in the United States. *Am J Obstet Gynecol* 1974; 118:443–460.

Crelin ES: Normal and abnormal development of ureter. *Urology* 1978; 12:2–7.

Cruickshank SH: Preventing post hysterectomy vaginal vault prolapse and enterocele during vaginal hysterectomy. *Am J Obstet Gynecol* 1987; 156:1433–1440.

Davos I, Abell MR: Sarcomas of the vagina. *Obstet Gynecol* 1975; 47:342–350.

DeLancey JOL: Correlative study of paraurethral anatomy. *Obstet Gynecol* 1986; 68:91–97.

deMartino C, Zamboni L: A morphologic study of the mesonephros of the human embryo. *J Ultrastruct Res* 1966; 16:399–427.

Eschenbach DA: Vaginal infection. *Clin Obstet Gynecol* 1983; 26:186–202.

Fantl JA, Hurt WG, Dunn LJ: Detrusor instability syndrome: The use of bladder retraining drills with and without anticholinergics. *Am J Obstet Gynecol* 1981; 140:885–888.

Fleury FJ: Adult vaginitis. *Clin Obstet Gynecol* 1981; 24:407–438.

Forsberg JG: Cervicovaginal epithelium: Its origin and development. *Am J Obstet Gynecol* 1973; 115:1025–1043.

Fouts AC, Kraus SJ: *Trichomonas vaginalis:* Reevaluation of its clinical presentation and laboratory diagnosis. *J Infect Dis* 1980; 141:137–143.

Friedman M, Peretz BA, Nissenbaum M, et al: Modern treatment of vaginal embryonal rhabdomyosarcoma. *Obstet Gynecol Surv* 1986; 41:614–618.

Friedrich EG: *Vulvar Disease.* Philadelphia, WB Saunders Co, 1983, pp 10–11.

Gallup DG, Castle CA, Stock RJ: Recurrent carcinoma in situ of the vagina following split-thickness skin graft vaginoplasty. *Gynecol Oncol* 1987a; 26:98–102.

Gallup DG, Talledo E, Shah KJ, et al: Invasive squamous cell carcinoma of the vagina: A fourteen year study. *Obstet Gynecol* 1987b; 69:782–785.

Ghosh TK, Cera PJ: Transition of benign vaginal adenosis to clear cell carcinoma. *Obstet Gynecol* 1983; 61:126–130.

Ginsburg DS, Genadry R: Suburethral diverticulum in the female. *Obstet Gynecol Surv* 1984; 39:1–7.

Given FT: Posterior culdoplasty: Revisited. *Am J Obstet Gynecol* 1985; 153:135–139.

Gosling JA, Dixon JS, Lendon RG: The autonomic innervation of the human male and female bladder neck and proximal urethra. *J Urol* 1977; 118:302–305.

Griffin JE, Creighton E, Madden JD, et al: Congenital absence of the vagina: The Mayer-Rokitansky-Kuster-Hauser syndrome. *Ann Intern Med* 1976; 85:224–236.

Grobstein C: Inductive interaction in the development of the mouse metanephros. *J Exp Zool* 1955; 130:319–335.

Herbst AL, Cole P, Norusis MJ, et al: Epidemiologic aspects and factors related to survival in 384 registry cases of clear cell adenocarcinoma of the vagina and cervix. *Am J Obstet Gynecol* 1979; 135:876–886.

Herbst AL, Green TH, Ulfelder H: Primary carcinoma of the vagina. *Am J Obstet Gynecol* 1970; 106:210–218.

Herbst AL, Ulfelder H, Poskanzer DC: Adenocarcinoma of the vagina: Association of maternal stilbestrol therapy with tumor appearance in young women. *N Engl J Med* 1971; 284:878–881.

Hernandez-Linares W, Puthawala A, Nolan JF,

et al: Carcinoma in situ of the vagina: Past and present management. *Obstet Gynecol* 1980; 56:356–360.

Higton BK: A trial of clotrimazole and nystatin in vaginal moniliasis. *Br J Obstet Gynaecol* 1973; 80:992–995.

Hilton P, Stanton SL: The use of intravaginal oestrogen cream in genuine stress incontinence. *Br J Obstet Gynaecol* 1983; 90:940–944.

Hodgkinson CP: Stress urinary incontinence—1970. *Am J Obstet Gynecol* 1970; 108:1141–1698.

Hofmeister FJ: Pelvic anatomy of the ureter in relation to surgery perfomed through the vagina. *Clin Obstet Gynecol* 1982; 25:821–830.

Hurt WG: Histology of the urinary bladder and urethra in the female. *American Uro-Gynecologic Society Quarterly Report*, 1988; 6(1).

International Continence Society: Fourth report on the standardization of terminology of lower urinary tract function: Terminology related to neuromuscular dysfunction of the lower urinary tract. *Br J Urol* 1981; 53:333–335.

Jobson VW, Homesley HD: Treatment of vaginal intraepithelial neoplasia with the carbon dioxide laser. *Obstet Gynecol* 1983; 62:90–93.

Karram MM, Bhatia NN: The Q-tip test: Standardization of the technique and its interpretation in women with urinary incontinence. *Obstet Gynecol* 1988; 71:807–811.

Kaufman RH, Binder GL, Gray PM Jr, et al: Upper genital tract changes associated with exposure in utero to diethylstilbestrol. *Am J Obstet Gynecol* 1977; 128:51–56.

Kempers RD: Vaginitis. *Postgrad Obstet Gynecol* 1985; 5:1–6.

Koff AK: Development of the vagina in the human fetus. *Contrib Embryol* 1933; 24:61–90.

Landers DV: The treatment of vaginitis: *Trichomonas*, yeast, and bacterial vaginosis. *Clin Obstet Gynecol* 1988; 31:473–479.

Lenehan PM, Meffe F, Lickrish GM: Vaginal intraepithelial neoplasia: Biologic aspects and management. *Obstet Gynecol* 1986; 68:333–337.

Liu LY, Hou YJ, Li JZ: Primary malignant melanoma of the vagina: A report of seven cases. *Obstet Gynecol* 1987; 70:569–572.

Lossick JG, Muller M, Gorrell TE: In vitro drug susceptibility and doses of metronidazole required for cure in cases of refractory vaginal trichomoniasis. *J Infect Dis* 1986; 153:948–955.

Magee MC, Lucey DT, Fried FA: A new embryologic classification for urogynecologic malformations: The syndromes of mesonephric duct induced Mullerian deformities. *J Urol* 1979; 121:265–267.

Marcus SL: Multiple squamous cell carcinomas involving the cervix, vagina and vulva: The theory of multicentric origin. *Am J Obstet Gynecol* 1960; 80:802–812.

Marshall VF, Marchetti AA, Krantz KE: The correction of stress incontinence by simple vesicourethral suspension. *Surg Obstet Gynecol* 1949: 88:509–518.

McLellan R, Spence MR, Brockman M, et al: The clinical diagnosis of trichomoniasis. *Obstet Gynecol* 1982; 60:30–34.

Melnick S, Cole P, Anderson D, et al: Rates and risks of diethylstilbestrol-related clear-cell adenocarcinoma of the vagina and cervix. *N Engl J Med* 1987; 316:514–516.

Miles MR, Olsen L, Rogers A: Recurrent vaginal candidiasis: Importance of an intestinal reservoir. *JAMA* 1977; 238:1836–1837.

Moore T: Diverticulum of female urethra: An improved technique of surgical excision. *J Urol* 1952; 68:611–616.

Nichols DH: Sacrospinous fixation for massive eversion of the vagina. *Am J Obstet Gynecol* 1982; 142:901–904.

Oriel JD, Partridge BM, Denny MJ, et al: Genital yeast infections. *Br Med J (Clin Res)* 1972; 4:761–764.

Osborne NG, Grubin L, Pratson L: Vaginitis in sexually active women: Relationship to nine sexually transmitted organisms. *Am J Obstet Gynecol* 1982; 142:962–967.

Pathak U, House M: Diverticulum of the female urethra. *Obstet Gynecol* 1970; 36:789–794.

Perez CA, Camel HM: Long term follow up in radiation therapy of carcinoma of the vagina. *Cancer* 1982; 49:1308–1315.

Pereyra AJ, Lebherz TB, Growdon WA, et al: Pubourethral supports in perspective: Modified Pereyra procedure for urinary incontinence. *Obstet Gynecol* 1982; 59:643–648.

Perl G: Errors in the diagnosis of *Trichomonas vaginalis* infection as observed among 1199 patients. *Obstet Gynecol* 1972; 39:7–9.

Podczaski E, Herbst AL: Cancer of the vagina and fallopian tube, in Knapp RC, Berkowitz RS (eds): *Gynecologic Oncology*. New York, Macmillan Publishing Co, 1986, p 404.

Pride GL, Schultz AE, Chuprevich JW, et al: Primary invasive squamous carcinoma of the vagina. *Obstet Gynecol* 1979; 53:218–225.

Pritchard JA, MacDonald PC, Gant NG: *Williams Obstetrics*, ed 17. New York, Appleton-Century-Crofts, 1985, p 348.

Ranney B: Endometriosis: Pathogenesis, symptoms, and findings. *Clin Obstet Gynecol* 1980; 23:865–874.

Ranney B: Enterocele, vaginal prolapse, pelvic

hernia: Recognition and treatment. *Am J Obstet Gynecol* 1981; 140:53–57.

Rein MF, Muller M: *Trichomonas vaginalis,* in Holmes KK, Måardh P-A, Sparling PF, et al (eds): *Sexually Transmitted Diseases.* New York, McGraw-Hill Book Co, 1984, p 527.

Reindollar RH, Byrd JR, McDonough PG: Delayed sexual development: A study of 252 patients. *Am J Obstet Gynecol* 1981; 140:371–380.

Richardson DA, Bent AE, Ostergard DR: The effect of uterovaginal prolapse on urethrovesical pressure dynamics. *Am J Obstet Gynecol* 1983; 146:901–905.

Robboy SJ, Noller KL, O'Brien P, et al: Increased incidence of cervical and vaginal dysplasia in 3980 diethylstilbestrol-exposed young women. *JAMA* 1984; 252:2979–2983.

Rock JA, Azziz R: Genital anomalies in childhood. *Clin Obstet Gynecol* 1987; 30:682–696.

Rock JA, Reeves LA, Retto H, et al: Success following vaginal creation for Mullerian agenesis. *Fertil Steril* 1983; 39:809–813.

Ronald AR: Current concepts in management of urinary tract infections in adults. *Med Clin North Am* 1984; 68:335–349.

Sand PK, Hill RC, Ostergard DR: Supine urethroscopic and standing cystometry as screening methods for the detection of detrusor instability. *Obstet Gynecol* 1987; 70:57–60.

Semmens JP, Tsai CC, Semmens EC, et al: Effects of estrogen therapy on vaginal physiology during menopause. *Obstet Gynecol* 1985; 66:15–18.

Sillman FM, Sedlis A, Boyce JG: A review of lower genital intraepithelial neoplasia and the use of topical 5-fluorouracil. *Obstet Gynecol Surv* 1985; 40;190–220.

Souney P, Polk BF: Single-dose antibiotic therapy for urinary tract infections in women. *Rev Infect Dis* 1982; 4:29–34.

Spence H, Duckett J: Diverticulum of the female urethra: Clinical aspects and presentation of simple operative technique for cure. *J Urol* 1970; 104:432–437.

Spiegel CA, Amsel R, Eschenbach D, et al: Anaerobic bacteria in nonspecific vaginitis. *N Engl J Med* 1980; 303:601–607.

Stamey TA: Endoscopic suspension of the vesical neck for urinary incontinence. *Surg Obstet Gynecol* 1973; 136:547–554.

Stamm WE, Counts GW, Running KR, et al: Diagnosis of coliform infection in acutely dysuric women. *N Engl J Med* 1982; 307:463–468.

Stillman RJ: In utero exposure to diethylstilbestrol: Adverse effects on the reproductive tract and reproductive performance in male and female offspring. *Am J Obstet Gynecol* 1982; 142:905–921.

Stoddard FJ, Myers RE: Connective tissue disorders in obstetrics and gynecology. *Am J Obstet Gynecol* 1968; 102:240–243.

Swedberg J, Steiner JF, Deiss F: Comparison of single dose vs one week course of metronidazole for symptomatic bacterial vaginosis. *JAMA* 1985; 254:1046–1049.

Syverson RE, Buckley H, Gibian J, et al: Cellular and humoral immune status in women with chronic *Candida* vaginitis. *Am J Obstet Gynecol* 1979; 134:624–627.

Tanagho EA, Smith DR: Mechanism of urinary incontinence: 1. Embryologic, anatomic, and pathologic considerations. *J Urol* 1968; 100:640–646.

Tavossoli FA, Norris HJ: Smooth muscle tumors of the vagina. *Obstet Gynecol* 1979; 53:689–693.

Ulfelder H, Robboy SJ: The embryologic development of the human vagina. *Am J Obstet Gynecol* 1976; 126:769–776.

Van Slyke KT, Michel VP, Rein MF: Treatment of vulvovaginal candidiasis with boric acid powder. *Am J Obstet Gynecol* 1981; 141:145–148.

Vaughn ED, Middleton GW: Pertinent genitourinary embryology: Review for the practicing urologist. *Urology* 1975; 6:139–149.

Ward J, Draper J, Tovell H: Diagnosis and treatment of urethral diverticula in the female. *Surg Gynecol Obstet* 1967; 125:1293–1300.

Wilson JD, George FW, Griffin JE: The hormonal control of sexual development. *Science* 1981; 211:1278–1284.

Wiser WL, Bates GW: Management of agenesis of the vagina. *Surg Obstet Gynecol* 1984; 159:108–112.

Wolin LH: Stress incontinence in young, healthy nulliparous female subjects. *J Urol* 1969; 101:545–549.

Woodburne RT: Anatomy of the bladder and bladder outlet. *J Urol* 1968; 100:474–487.

Wyman JF, Choi SC, Harkins SW, et al: The urinary diary in evaluation of incontinent women: A test-retest analysis. *Obstet Gynecol* 1988; 71:812–817.

Young RH, Scully RE: Endodermal sinus tumor of the vagina: A report of nine cases and review of the literature. *Gynecol Oncol* 1984; 18:380–392.

Zornow DH: Embryology of urinary incontinence. *Urology* 1977; 10:293–300.

6   The Cervix

Ellen E. Sheets, M.D.

Howard M. Goodman, M.D.

Robert C. Knapp, M.D.

EMBRYOLOGY

The cervix as an embryological entity does not begin to develop until the early fetal period at about 12 weeks' gestation, yet its origin is intimately associated with the earlier development of the entire müllerian system. The müllerian (paramesonephric) duct system begins to develop in the fourth week as an invagination of the coelomic epithelium lateral to the wolffian (mesonephric) duct. Initially, these paired ducts run caudally, but they then turn medially to meet in the midline at 6 weeks' gestation, at which point they again run caudally to reach the urogenital sinus at approximately 8 weeks' gestation (Fig 6–1). The point of contact between the now-fused müllerian ducts and the urogenital sinus enlarges to form the müllerian tubercle, with the wolffian ducts entering the sinus immediately lateral to the tubercle.

Evagination of the sinus between the wolffian ducts and the müllerian tubercle produces the sinovaginal bulbs, which proliferate to form the vaginal plate or vaginal cord. This solid plate advances in a caudal-cranial direction, obliterating the fused müllerian ducts (vaginal canal) as the müllerian epithelium degenerates. At 11 weeks' gestation, cavitation commences, again in a caudal-cranial direction, thereby creating the vaginal lumen. At the same time, a constriction appears between the developing corpus and cervix, with the cervix identifiable by a fusiform thickening of the surrounding mesenchyme (Fig 6–2). Cranial proliferation of the vaginal plate around the developing cervix forms the vaginal fornices, which

are well delineated by the 21st week (Ferenczy, 1982; Langman, 1981).

Just prior to the time of proliferation of the vaginal plate, the original müllerian epithelium of the vaginal canal is replaced by a pseudostratified epithelium, still of müllerian origin. Canalization of the vagina results in a stratified squamous epithelium, the origin of which remains in dispute. Koff (1933) suggested that the lower fifth of the vaginal epithelium is derived from the urogenital sinus and the remainder from transformed müllerian epithelium, whereas Bulmer (1957) proposed that sinus and müllerian epithelium are histologically distinct and that the vaginal epithelium is derived completely from sinus epithelium. Forsberg (1965), using histochemical methods, postulated a wolffian origin for the vaginal lining. Forsberg (1972) later showed in animals that inhibiting stratification of the original müllerian epithelium by estrogens caused heterotopic columnar epithelium to form in the adult vagina—a response highly suggestive of the adenosis associated with diethylstilbestrol (DES) exposure. The origin of the adult vaginal epithelium would seem to play no part in this presumed mechanism of stilbestrol teratogenesis.

The origin of the endocervical mucosa is likewise controversial. Fluhmann (1960) postulated that the upward growth of vaginal squamous epithelium, which he believed was of sinus origin, extended into the endocervix, with subsequent columnar transformation. Most authors favor a müllerian origin for the endocervical mucosa.

Abnormalities in the development or fusion of one or both müllerian ducts may result in mal-

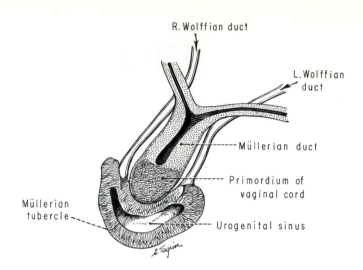

R. Wolffian duct

L. Wolffian duct

Müllerian duct

Primordium of vaginal cord

Müllerian tubercle

Urogenital sinus

E. Tagin

FIG 6–1.

Formation of the lower portion of the vagina. The müllerian tubercle is formed as the terminal ends of the müllerian ducts impinge on the urogenital sinus. Thus, the vagina has a double origin: from the müllerian tubercle and from outgrowths of the urogenital sinus.

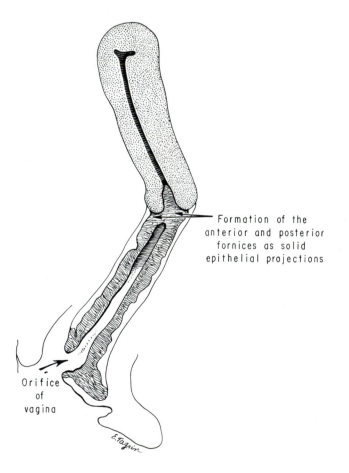

Formation of the anterior and posterior fornices as solid epithelial projections

Orifice of vagina

E. Tagin

FIG 6–2.

Formation of upper portion of the vagina in the 151-mm embryo. At this stage the cranial end of the vagina contains two solid epithelial projections, which become the anterior and posterior fornices.

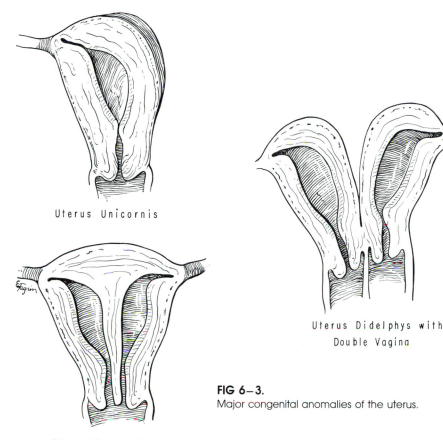

Uterus Unicornis

Uterus Didelphys with
Double Vagina

FIG 6–3.
Major congenital anomalies of the uterus.

Uterus Septus Duplex

formations of the cervix. These include a double cervix with a septate or bicornuate uterus in conjunction with a normal or double vagina; a double cervix with uterus didelphys; or, rarely, complete atresia of the cervix (Fig 6–3).

In any discussion of the embryology of the cervix, mention should be made of the importance of *mesonephric remnants*. Characteristically, these structures are found as minute tubules, or canaliculi, in the lateral cervical wall. They are lined with nonciliated simple columnar or cuboidal cells having translucent cytoplasm and large, round nuclei (Huffman, 1948). Bizarre tumors, both benign and malignant, may arise from these remnants and may prove to be histogenetically confusing if their origin is not appreciated.

ANATOMY

The cervix (Latin, "neck") is the narrowed, most caudad portion of the uterus (Fig 6–4).

Somewhat conical, it has a truncated apex that is directed downward and backward. It measures approximately 2.5 to 3.0 cm in the adult nulligravid and is contiguous with the inferior aspect of the uterine corpus; the point of juncture is known as the isthmus. The vagina is attached obliquely around the center of the cervical periphery, thus dividing the cervix into two segments—an upper, supravaginal portion and a lower, vaginal portion. The cervix enters the vagina at an angle through the anterior vaginal wall and, in most women, its vaginal portion is in contact with the posterior vaginal wall. The supravaginal segment of the cervix is separated anteriorly from the bladder by a layer of endopelvic fascia, the pubovesicocervical fascia. Laterally, at the same level, the cervix is in continuity with the paracervical ligaments or cardinal ligaments of Mackenrodt, which contain the uterine blood vessels. Posteriorly, the supravaginal cervix is covered by peritoneum as it reflects off the uterosacral ligaments downward toward the vaginal apex.

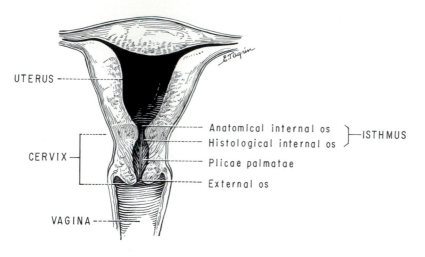

FIG 6—4.
Frontal section of uterine cervix and corpus.

The vaginal portion *(portio vaginalis, exocervix, ectocervix,* or *anatomical portio)* projects into the upper portion of the vagina between the anterior and posterior fornices as a convex prominence of elliptical shape. A small aperture, usually round or slitlike in the nullipara, is in the center of the projection and constitutes the external os. This orifice joins the uterine cavity with the vagina and is surrounded by the anterior and posterior lips. The cervical canal extends from the external os to the anatomical internal os, where it connects with the uterine cavity. It is somewhat fusiform, or spindle shaped, measuring approximately 8 mm at its greatest width.

The isthmus is defined as that area of the uterus between the anatomical internal os above and the histological internal os below. The latter is defined as the area of transition from endometrial to endocervical glands. The isthmic musculature is somewhat thinner than that of the corpus, thereby facilitating effacement and dilation during labor. This area is frequently referred to as the lower uterine segment during pregnancy and labor.

The uterine artery constitutes the major blood supply to the cervix, reaching its lateral walls within the cardinal ligaments (as noted previously). The venous drainage mirrors the arterial system. The cervical lymphatics, which are described in greater detail later, drain primarily laterally to the hypogastric, obturator, and external iliac nodes but also anteriorly to the posterior bladder wall nodes and posteriorly to the presac-

ral nodes. Innervation of the cervix arises from the superior, middle, and inferior hypogastric plexuses and is primarily limited to the endocervix and the deeper areas of the exocervix. This accounts for the relative insensitivity to pain of the exocervix (Ferenczy, 1982).

PHYSIOLOGY

The cervix functions passively as a segment of the birth canal and as a channel for the exit of menstrual discharge. Its primary physiologic function is the secretion of mucus, which facilitates the transport of spermatozoa and subsequently acts as a plug to seal off the gravid uterine cavity from the external environment.

This cervical mucus is subject to profound cyclic changes in relation to the levels of circulating ovarian hormones. In the immediate postmenstrual phase when the circulatory level of estrogen is low, and in the postovulatory period under the influence of progesterone, the cervical mucus is sparse, thick, and viscid. If allowed to dry on a slide, abundant vaginal and cervical cells, leukocytes, and mucous particles can be seen. From the eighth day of the cycle until ovulation, under the stimulation of rising levels of estrogen, the amount of mucus increases, its viscosity decreases, and it becomes highly permeable to spermatozoa. Just prior to ovulation, the mucus is glassy, transparent, and highly elastic. The term *spinnbarkeit* has been applied to this characteristic

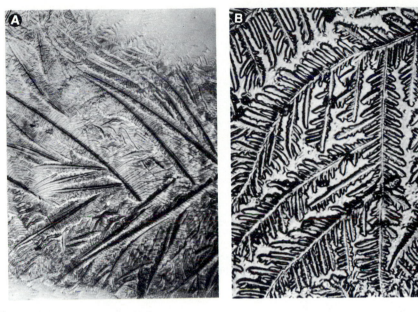

FIG 6–5.
Fern phenomenon in cervical mucus during the normal menstrual cycle between days 12 and 16. **A,** low power; **B,** high power. (Courtesy of Dr. Maxwell Roland.)

elasticity. If allowed to dry on a slide, the mucus assumes the form of fern or palm leaves with few notable cellular elements (Fig 6–5).

Fern Test Technique

The specimen of mucus should be aspirated from the external os after initial dry cleansing. The mucus is permitted to air dry and is then examined under magnification of approximately ×100. False positive fern test results are possible if (1) the aspirating tube is wet, (2) salt solution rather than distilled water has been used for cleaning or sterilizing the tube, or (3) excessive blood is mixed with the mucus.

Mucous secretions and most body fluids show the phenomenon of ferning, or arborization, in the dried state, which seems to represent a special form of crystallization of sodium chloride in the medium of drying cervical mucus. Although ferning per se is a nonspecific process, its occurrence in cervical mucus does depend on adequate estrogenic stimulation.

From a clinical point of view, examination of cervical mucus is a simple test of ovarian function. When no ovarian function occurs, small amounts of exogenous estrogen will cause arborization, whereas progesterone modifies this action of es-

trogen. In amenorrheic patients, a persistently normal fern test result suggests insufficient estrogenic stimulation (Speroff et al., 1985).

PHYSIOLOGICAL ALTERATIONS

Changes in Endocervical Mucosa

With the advent of colposcopy, many of the gross and microscopic variations previously considered to be pathological are now regarded as normal physiological alterations. Prominent among these is the growth of endocervical mucosa onto the anatomical portio, which was believed to be a prolapse of that mucosa. The popular term for this physiological alteration was "cervical erosion," which incorrectly implied that the epithelium was denuded. The proper term now is *eversion,* or *ectropion.* It now appears that this normal physiological growth alteration is related to age, the first pregnancy, and estrogenic stimulation.

During the childbearing years, endocervical glands are found just below the internal os and extend to just below the external os (i.e., onto the anatomical portio), creating this so-called cervical erosion. After age 40 years, as a result of waning ovarian activity, the endocervical mucosa ascends the canal so that during the menopausal years the lowest glands, the original squamocolumnar junction, and the transformation zone are at or above the anatomical external os. Coppleson and Reid (1967) and Song (1964) attribute the downward shift and eversion of the endocervix to an increase in volume of the mucosa during the years when estrogen stimulation was maximal and explains the increase in eversions noted after the first pregnancy (Fig 6–6).

During the latter part of intrauterine development, there is accelerated cervical growth activity, attributed to the high levels of circulating estrogens; such growth is not shared by the corpus.

At birth the cervix/corpus ratio may approach 3 : 1. After birth there is a rapid regression in cervical length, thereby returning to the more normal cervix/corpus ratio seen in the adult. During the third trimester the endocervical cells change from cuboidal to tall columnar with evidence of mucin secretion, and the mucosa deeply infolds into the stroma to form clefts or glands. This excessive *proliferation of endocervical mucosa* after the 28th week produces the congenital eversion seen in 50% of female neonates. In contrast, the endometrium is incompletely developed, usually inactive, and presents only a few tubular glands. Squamous cells of the exocervix in the newborn

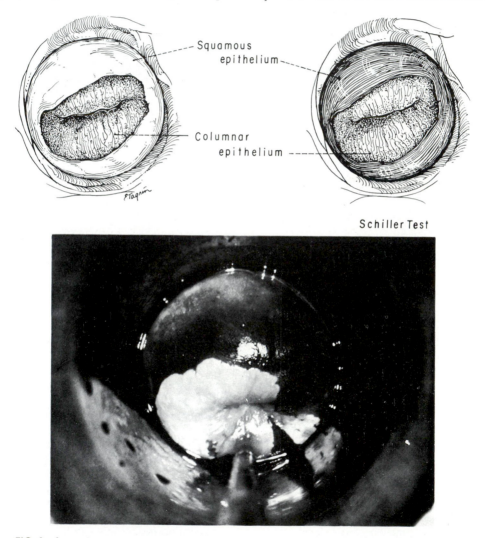

FIG 6–6.
Application of Schiller's solution will stain the normal squamous epithelium dark brown. Endocervical epithelium does not stain.

are likewise affected by maternal estrogens, since they are well stratified and contain abundant glycogen. At puberty, with the stimulation of estrogen from the developing ovarian follicles, these changes presumably occur again, although adequate morphological studies in this age group are lacking (Langman, 1981).

HISTOLOGY

Careful consideration of cervical histology will allow us to understand how and where benign, precancerous, and cancerous lesions of the cervix occur. Although the cervix is essentially composed of two different types of epithelium, squamous and columnar, it is the area of transition between these two epithelial types that gives rise to the three histological zones: (1) the histological portio, (2) the transitional or transformation zone, and (3) the histological endocervix. Further, it is the process of transition from columnar to squamous epithelium that can be altered such that precancerous and cancerous lesions arise.

Histological Portio

The histological portio is defined as cervical stroma devoid of glands and covered by stratified squamous epithelium (Fig 6–7). This epithelium is 15 to 20 cells thick and demonstrates a progressive and orderly maturation from the lower-most basal layer through the prickle cell layer to the su-

perficial zone, where cornification occurs under estrogenic stimulation.

The basal layer (stratum germinativum), which is responsible for epithelial regeneration, consists of a single row of small cylindrical cells with large nuclei and scanty cytoplasm. Mitotic figures may occasionally be seen. Above the basal cells is a layer of larger polyhedral cells, 4 to 10 cells thick, arranged in an irregular mosaic pattern and interconnected by numerous tonofilament-desmosomal complexes. These characteristic intercellular bridges have led to the designation *prickle cells,* and their location has led to the designation *parabasal cells.* The cytoplasmic basophilia seen in these first two cell types is attributed to their RNA content. The beginning of cytoplasmic glycogenization is seen in the parabasal layer.

Above the prickle cells is a layer of larger oval or navicular cells with relatively small nuclei. These cells are involved in ascending maturation, during which nuclear size remains constant while cytoplasmic volume gradually increases. This layer has been called the *intermediate, clear cell,* or *navicular zone.* The most superficial layer, or stratum corneum, consists of flattened, elongated cells with small pyknotic nuclei. These are the cornified cells or squames seen in cytological smears. The superficial and intermediate cells are rich in glycogen but appear clear in histologic sections, since the glycogen is washed out during fixation.

The basal layer is usually quite regular and does not show the rete peg formation seen in the vulva and vagina. The cervical squamous epithelium rests on a basement membrane, which is in-

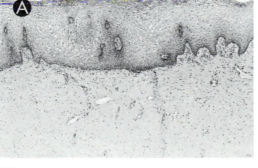
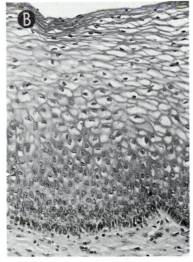

FIG 6–7.
A, normal exocervix (magnification ×50). **B,** high-power magnification (×150) to show process of stratification and cornification.

consistently seen under the light microscope and appears to consist of condensed stromal collagen. The underlying fibrous connective tissue stroma contains a lush capillary network at the epithelial junction, with scattered papillae extending upward into the epithelium (Forsberg, 1965).

Transformation Zone

The transformation zone lies between the histological portio and the endocervical mucosa and consists of endocervical stroma and glands covered by squamous epithelium. The squamous epithelium comes to lie on the endocervical stroma as a result of several physiologic or pathologic processes to be described later. Although these processes cause upward displacement of the squamocolumnar junction, the junction between the histological portio and the transformation zone can be termed the *original squamocolumnar junction*. The anatomical location of the transformation zone is dependent on age, estrogen influence, and previous trauma or surgery on the cervix. With Figure 6–4 as a guide, the transformation zone may be located on the vaginal portion of the cervix, at the external os, or above the external os within the cervical canal. Therefore, one should not equate the location of the histological transformation zone with the location of the anatomical external os. The importance of the location of this zone will become apparent in the section on colposcopy.

Histological Endocervix

The histological endocervix is lined by a single layer of tall columnar epithelial cells characterized by dense, basal nuclei and pale pink-staining cytoplasm in standard hematoxylin-eosin preparations (Fig 6–8). Two cell types are present in this epithelium: the more prevalent mucus-secreting cells and scattered ciliated cells located in patches within the cervical canal and in gland orifices. The slight variation in height of these cells gives the appearance of a picket fence in histological sections. These endocervical glands are actually formed by complex, cleftlike infoldings of the epithelium, which appear as simple glandular units in histological section (Fluhmann, 1960; Ferenczy, 1982). Although this concept renders the term "gland" a misnomer, reference to endocervical "glands" will most likely persist. The cleft arrangement increases the surface area of the endocervical mucosa, thereby permitting increased

production of mucus, the secretion of which is dependent on estrogen. Maximal production and secretion occurs prior to ovulation, and in certain patients true mucorrhea exists.

For some years the location of cervical lesions, particularly those of a neoplastic nature, has been a matter of controversy between clinicians and pathologists. This, again, is a consequence of the erroneous assumption that an anatomical area is synonymous with a histologic zone of the same designation. For example, the clinician defines a lesion of the portio as one existing on that area of the cervix that can be visualized with a speculum; the pathologist, on the other hand, defines a lesion of the portio as one arising in the squamous epithelium of the histological portio. A lesion arising in the transformation zone (overlying endocervical glands) or in the columnar epithelium may thus be classified pathologically as endocervical even though it is located on the anatomic portio. Obviously, the anatomical location of a lesion must be clearly distinguished from its histological location.

It is important that clinicians be aware of the fact that the majority of early neoplastic cervical lesions in women of childbearing age occur on the anatomic portio, where they are readily available for biopsy. Again, it should be emphasized that histopathological reports indicating that the majority of these lesions occur in the endocervix refer only to their histological position.

From the anatomical and histological characteristics described earlier, it is obvious that the cervix differs from the corpus in several important ways:

1. The cervix has only a small surface covered by peritoneum.
2. Approximately 85% of the cervix is made up of fibrous connective tissue.
3. There are no cervical venous sinuses.
4. Cervical mucosa does not undergo marked menstrual change as does the endometrium, although there are some cyclic changes dependent on estrogen and progesterone.
5. The vaginal cervix is covered by stratified squamous epithelium.

Squamous Metaplasia and Epithelialization

After menarche and through the reproductive period, the previously described cervical ectropion essentially disappears, and the squamoco-

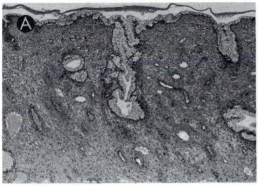
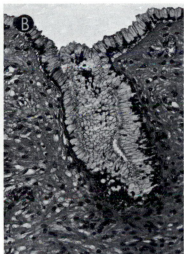

FIG 6–8.
A, normal endocervix (magnification ×50). **B,** high-power magnification (×150) to show typical high columnar epithelium.

lumnar junction moves out of view within the cervical canal. Two mechanisms for replacement of the endocervical eversion by squamous epithelium have been proposed as the histogenesis of the transformation zone. Since virtually all cases of cervical squamous neoplasia originate in the transformation zone, its histogenesis provides insight into the oncogenesis of cervical neoplasia.

The first mechanism is termed squamous metaplasia, which is the result of a process known as subcolumnar "reserve cell" metaplasia. These reserve cells are undifferentiated spherical or polygonal cells with plump, centrally placed, dark-staining nuclei and scant cytoplasm. They come to lie beneath the columnar epithelium, and their origin is controversial. It has been proposed that they are derived from (1) embryonal rests of urogenital sinus epithelium, (2) direct or indirect metaplasia of columnar cells, (3) basal cells of the portio, or (4) stromal cells. Coppleson and Reid (1967) suggest that the metaplastic process is initiated by the exposure of the endocervical mucosa to the lower pH of the vagina and that estrogen plays a crucial role by promoting endocervical hyperplasia and prolapse and acidifying the vaginal environment. In support of this mechanism is work done by Hellman and associates (1954), who found a striking increase in reserve cell hyperplasia and metaplasia after the administration of large doses of estrogen to postmenopausal women.

The probable sequence of events in the metaplastic process may be outlined as follows:

1. Endocervical eversion.
2. Reserve cell hyperplasia (Fig 6–9,A).
3. Reserve cell metaplasia and stratification (Fig 6–9,B).
4. Sloughing of overlying columnar epithelium.
5. Differentiation into a multilayered immature squamous epithelium.
6. Differentiation into a mature stratified squamous epithelium.

The end point of the metaplastic process is differentiation into squamous epithelium that is indistinguishable from native squamous epithelium. The more commonly seen immature metaplastic epithelium is characterized by lack of surface maturation and glycogen and is usually sharply demarcated from the adjacent portio. Particularly active squamous metaplasia filling multiple glands may be confused with carcinoma in situ, although hyperchromatism, nuclear atypia, and abnormal mitotic activity are not present.

The second mechanism by which squamous epithelium comes to overlie endocervical stroma has been termed squamous epithelialization (Johnson et al., 1964). The initiating event may be a true pathological erosion of the distal endocervix followed by an ingrowth or overglide of portio squamous cells.

In the early stages of this process, the squamous epithelium may be seen as a tenuous strand of immature squamous cells gradually decreasing in height as they are stretched over an otherwise denuded and inflamed stroma. Others (Ferenczy, 1982; Johnson et al., 1964) have shown that the squamous epithelium of the portio may grow beneath the adjacent, intact endocervical epithelium, with loss of the overlying co-

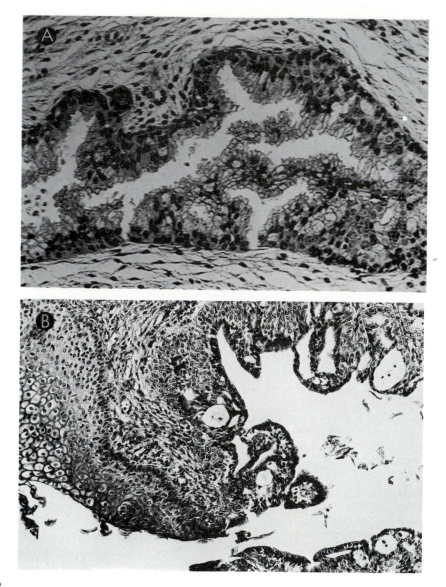

FIG 6–9.
A, hyperplasia of reserve cells in the endocervix. **B,** squamous metaplasia from reserve cells of the endocervix occurring at the histological external os. Normal stratified squamous epithelium is seen at left. (Courtesy of Drs. Louis M. Hellman and Alexander Rosenthal.)

lumnar cells on maturation and stratification of the squamous elements. As with many reparative and regenerative processes, mitotic activity with associated basal cell hyperplasia may be considerable, although the atypia of malignancy is absent. Extension of the new epithelium over the mouth of the endocervical gland may result in occlusion and formation of mucinous retention (nabothian) cysts. These are grossly visible on the portio as spherical elevations or small cysts 2 to 10 mm in diameter (Fig 6–10). Microscopically, the cystic space is seen to be lined with low cuboidal or flattened endocervical cells.

BENIGN CERVICAL LESIONS

Cervical Polyps

Cervical polyps are usually derived from the endocervix as a result of a chronic papillary endo-

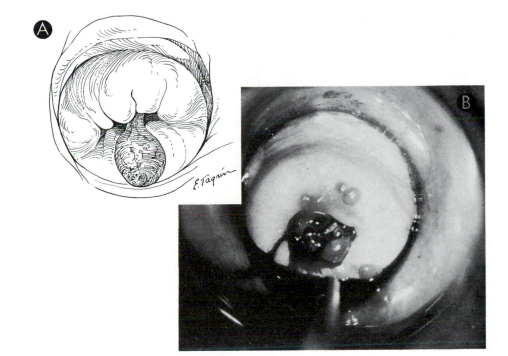

FIG 6–10.
Endocervical polyps. **A,** a solitary polyp protruding through the external os. **B,** several endocervical polyps occluding the exocervix. Several nabothian (mucous) cysts are seen on the portio epithelium.

cervicitis and present as soft, spherical, glistening red masses several millimeters to several centimeters in size (see Fig 6–10). They are frequently quite friable and may be associated with profuse leukorrhea secondary to the underlying endocervicitis. Histologically, they are composed of endocervical epithelium with a fibrovascular stalk. The differential diagnosis includes (1) polypoid fragments of endocervical carcinoma or carcinosarcoma protruding through the os, (2) retained products of conception, (3) the grapelike swellings of sarcoma botryoides that occasionally originate in the cervix, and (4) prolapsing submucous fibroids or endometrial polyps. Most cervical polyps can be grasped with a clamp and twisted free, with the base cauterized for hemostasis. Certainly all cervical polyps should be submitted for pathologic evaluation, although malignant degeneration is extremely rare.

Leiomyomas

Leiomyomas, or fibroids, are the commonest uterine tumors, with cervical involvement occurring in as many as 8% of cases. Cervical leiomyomas are grossly and histologically identical to those found in the corpus. Although they are frequently incidental findings on physical examination, they may cause bowel or bladder symptoms, dyspareunia, or dystocia in labor with excessive growth. Treatment for symptomatic fibroids is either myomectomy or hysterectomy.

Endometriosis

Endometriosis of the cervix presents as red or reddish blue vesicular lesions evident on the exocervix. They are usually asymptomatic but may cause dysmenorrhea or dyspareunia, which is most evident premenstrually. Biopsy specimens are best taken at this time for adequate pathological interpretation. This pattern of endometriosis is frequently seen several months after cervical biopsy, cauterization, or trachelorrhaphy in menstruating women and thus suggests implantation as its etiology. However, areas of decidual reaction may occasionally be seen in the cervices of pregnant women who have not undergone any cervical procedures, suggesting that multipotential cells capable of responding to estrogen and progesterone are present in the cervical stroma. Infertility has been associated with extensive cervical endometriosis and is probably due to destruction of endocervical glands and decreased mucous production. After biopsy confirmation, treatment should consist of deep cauterization, excision, or laser vaporization.

Other less common benign tumors that may involve the cervix include hemangiomas, adenomyomas, fibroadenomas, fibromas, and lipomas.

Keratinization

Since keratinization is not a physiological property of cervical squamous epithelium, any tendency in this direction must be considered abnormal, although some degree of focal keratinization may occasionally be observed in the absence of other abnormalities. Hyperkeratosis and parakeratosis appear as white, raised plaques (leukoplakia), usually grossly visible on the portio. Hyperkeratosis microscopically exhibits a thickened layer of keratin, scant intraepithelial glycogen,

and no cytologic atypia. It is not commonly seen except in cases of procidentia. Parakeratosis, the commonest abnormality presenting as a white cervical lesion, exhibits similar features but with the retention of pyknotic nuclei in the keratin layer (Fig 6–11). There is no evidence to indicate that either hyperkeratosis or parakeratosis is premalignant; however, these histological features may be associated with cervical neoplasia. Therefore, all white lesions of the cervix deserve biopsy for tissue diagnosis.

Chronic Cervicitis

From the time of the earliest clinical and microscopic descriptions of cervical disease, inflammation or, more specifically, chronic cervicitis has been a ubiquitous finding. Either alone or coexisting with other diseases, it has been implicated in the pathogenesis of cervical eversion, squamous metaplasia, basal cell hyperplasia, leukoplakia,

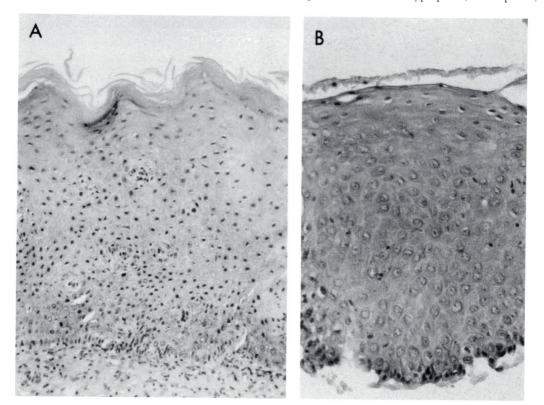

FIG 6–11.
A, hyperkeratosis (magnification ×120). Normal ascending cellular maturation with a thickened keratin layer can be seen. **B,** parakeratosis (magnification ×200). Pyknotic nuclei are evident within the keratin layer. (Courtesy of Dr. Robert Ehrmann and the Division of Women's and Perinatal Pathology, Brigham and Women's Hospital, Boston.)

polyps, and carcinoma. Although Song's (1964) criteria for the diagnosis of chronic cervicitis are the presence of epithelial necrosis and neutrophilic infiltration, leukocytic infiltration was found in 98% of 400 cervices examined by Howard et al. (1951). Chronic cervicitis is noted in nearly every specimen of cervical tissue examined at Brigham and Women's Hospital and has been described in the cervices of newborns and young children. Extensive attempts to confirm bacteriologically that cervical infection is the etiology of chronic cervicitis have rarely revealed pathogenic organisms. Rather, a physiologic role for this infiltrate has been suggested—the removal of dead cells resulting from the metaplastic process.

Clinically, the presenting symptoms of chronic cervicitis are a thick, tenacious yellowish white vaginal discharge with postcoital or postdouche spotting or bleeding. Complaints of pelvic pressure, dyspareunia, or dysmennorrhea suggest that the inflammatory process has extended to the paracervical tissues. Inspection reveals a beefy, friable cervix with a mucopurulent discharge. On culture this may reveal normal commensals or *Staphylococcus, Streptococcus,* or *Escherichia coli,* the clinical significance of which remains in question.

A tentative diagnosis can be made on inspection; however, biopsy and tissue diagnosis are mandatory to rule out cervical neoplasia, which can present with a similar clinical picture. The inflammation and bleeding associated with chronic cervicitis render Papanicolaou smears unreliable in excluding carcinoma. Once carcinoma has been excluded, reassurance is usually all that is needed for the patient with the signs and symptoms of chronic cervicitis. If the symptoms are unacceptable or if this abnormal cervical mucus is believed to play a causative role in infertility, treatment is indicated. Although hot cautery was initially used in a circumferential manner to destroy the abnormal cervical epithelium, its discomfort and scarring have caused it to no longer be the treatment of choice. Now, either cryocautery or laser ablation by vaporization is performed with minimal patient discomfort and a decreased incidence of posttreatment scarring.

Acute Cervicitis

Acute inflammation of the cervix may result from infection by specific microorganisms; as a response to trauma, malignant disease, or radiotherapy; or as one manifestation of a systemic inflammatory disease such as Behçet's syndrome or polyarteritis nodosa. The cervix appears hyperemic and swollen, and an accompanying purulent discharge is usually present. Histologically, stromal edema with a polymorphonuclear infiltrate and mucosal ulceration is seen. Treatment consists of avoiding instrumentation and interdicting coitus, limitation of activity, medicated douches or creams, or specific systemic antibiotic therapy depending on the type and sensitivity of the responsible organism (Dawson, 1981).

The commonest etiology of acute cervicitis is infection with *Neisseria gonorrhoeae*. Stratified squamous epithelium is relatively resistant to gonococcal infection, which is usually limited in uncomplicated cases to involvement of the endocervix, urethra, and rectum. Ascending infection may occur, with extension to the endometrium, fallopian tube, and ovarian and peritoneal surfaces producing pelvic inflammatory disease in approximately 15% of women with cervical infection. Gonococcal endocervicitis may be asymptomatic in as many as 50% of affected women. In the other 50%, the usual symptomatology includes vaginal discharge, dysuria, urinary frequency, labial tenderness, and dyspareunia. Speculum examination reveals an erythematous cervix with a thick, purulent discharge. Diagnosis requires culture techniques, since Gram stain has a sensitivity of only 50% in gonococcal cervicitis. Treatment consists of administration of the appropriate antibiotic (Rein et al., 1976).

During the past decade, the role of *Chlamydia trachomatis* in the pathogenesis of genital tract disease has become well established. As many as 66% of women seen at venereal disease clinics may harbor *Chlamydia* in their cervices. Infection may be asymptomatic, may be limited to the cervix, or may ascend to cause pelvic inflammatory disease. Examination reveals a follicular cervicitis that can be seen histologically to be produced by subepithelial lymphoid follicles. Diagnosis requires culture techniques or the presence of the characteristic intracytoplasmic inclusion bodies seen on Giemsa stains of cervical smears. Of concern is the fourfold increase in cervical neoplasia reported by Paavonen in cervices harboring *Chlamydia*. Although no etiological role for *Chlamydia* in cervical neoplasia has been suggested, this observation merits further study

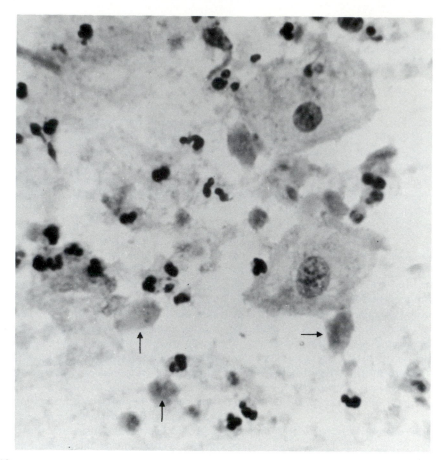

FIG 6– 12.
Papanicolaou smear demonstrating *T. vaginalis* (magnification ×800). The characteristic pear-shaped protozoans with eccentrically placed, spindle-shaped nuclei are shown *(arrows)*. The flagella are usually not well demonstrated on Papanicolaou smears. (Courtesy of Dr. Robert Ehrmann and the Division of Women's and Perinatal Pathology, Brigham and Women's Hospital, Boston.)

(MacDonald-Burns, 1981; Driel et al., 1978; Paavonen, 1982).

Trichomonas vaginalis is a flagellated protozoan that attacks the squamous epithelium of the vagina and cervix, destroying the epithelial cells on contact. In response, there is an outpouring of polymorphonuclear leukocytes and marked proliferation of small blood vessels, yielding the characteristic colposcopic appearance of looped or hairpin capillaries. Although this infection may be asymptomatic, the classic presentation is a profuse greenish gray frothy vaginal discharge with pruritus, dysuria, and, occasionally, vaginal bleeding. Diagnosis is easily made by the presence of the flagellate on microscopic examination of the discharge diluted in normal saline (Fig 6–12). Culture may be required, since wet mounts will miss

approximately 30% of infected women. The pH of the vagina is frequently somewhat alkaline in the presence of *T. vaginalis*. The association of abnormal Papanicolaou smears with trichomonal infections has been well described. Cytological and colposcopic abnormalities revert to normal with appropriate treatment (Borken and Friedman, 1979).

Tuberculous cervicitis is seen in approximately 3% to 5% of all cases of genital tuberculosis. The affected cervix may appear entirely normal, exhibit erythema with a mucopurulent discharge, or be invaded by a fungating mass suggestive of carcinoma. Histologically, caseating or noncaseating granulomas may be seen. Diagnosis requires the demonstration of acid-fast bacilli by suitable staining techniques or by culture. The differential diagnosis of granulomatous cervicitis includes syphilis, lymphogranuloma venereum, granuloma inguinale, chancroid, sarcoid, schistosomiasis, and pinworm.

Viral Cervicitis

Herpes Simplex Virus

Herpesvirus hominis types 1 and 2, the etiologic agents of genital herpes, belong to the large group herpesviruses, which have been found in almost every animal species studied. These are large DNA viruses, with five members associated with disease in humans: herpes simplex virus (HSV) types 1 and 2, varicella-zoster virus, cytomegalovirus, and Epstein-Barr virus. Infection requires direct contact, with an incubation period ranging from 2 to 20 days and averaging 6 days. Clinically, herpes genitalis may be conveniently divided into either primary or recurrent infection, the former reserved for infection resulting from the first exposure to either HSV type 1 or 2 and the latter for any subsequent infection.

Primary infection is not infrequently heralded by a prodromal phase with symptoms of headache, myalgias, malaise, and fever. Multiple painful vesicles, usually 1 to 2 mm, appear on an erythematous background; these rapidly erode and coalesce to form larger ulcers. Cervical involvement occurs in 80% of primary infections and presents as nonspecific inflammation, vesicles, ulcers, or occasionally as a fungating mass indistinguishable from invasive carcinoma. Symptoms include vulvar and pelvic pain, dysuria, and vaginal discharge, the last seen especially with cervical involvement. Complete healing requires several weeks as symptoms and lesions slowly resolve.

Recurrent infection results from reactivation of latent virus thought to reside in sacral ganglia. Some 50% of patients experiencing an initial clinical episode of herpes genitalis will go on to suffer recurrences, with symptoms and signs usually less severe and of shorter duration than in the primary disease.

The clinical impression may be confirmed by culture technique, with characteristic cytopathic

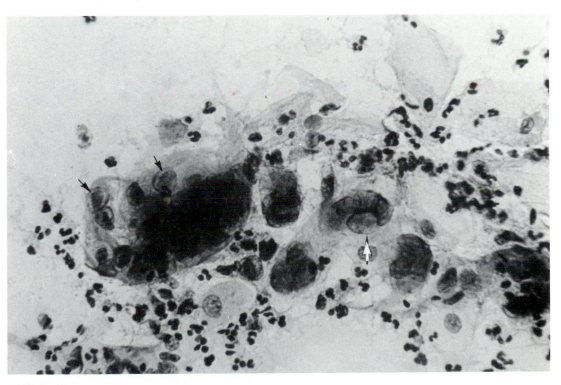

FIG 6–13.
Papanicolaou smear exhibiting the characteristic features of herpesvirus infection (magnification ×530). Intranuclear inclusions *(small arrows)*, which may represent virus particles, and multinucleated giant cells are evident. Enlarged, ground-glass–appearing nuclei can also be seen *(large arrow)*. (Courtesy of Dr. Robert Ehrmann and the Division of Women's and Perinatal Pathology, Brigham and Women's Hospital, Boston.)

effects evident within 1 to 2 days; by serologic conversion following initial infection; or by cytologic methods demonstrating multinucleated giant cells or intranuclear viral inclusion bodies (Fig 6–13).

In addition to the neonatal risk associated with herpetic infection, Nahmias and others (1971) have implicated HSV in spontaneous abortion and premature labor. The association between HSV type 2 and cervical neoplasia will be addressed later.

Human Papillomavirus

The papoviviridae family is composed of two branches: simian virus 40 and polyomavirus make up one side and the papillomaviruses the other. Human papillomaviruses (HPVs) are 8,000-kilobase DNA viruses composed of many different subtypes. Each subtype represents a virus that has less than 50% DNA base sequence homology with other types. Currently, there are greater than 50 types of HPVs, and each type appears to have a preference for a certain epithelial surface. For example, HPV type 1 is involved in plantar warts, whereas HPV types 5 and 14 are involved in a rare external skin disease, epidermodysplasia verruciformis. At this moment, we are concerned mainly with the epithelium of the genital area and HPV types 6, 11, 16, 18, 31, 35, and some types in the 50s, which are found in these epithelial surfaces.

Our understanding of HPV infections has been greatly hampered by the lack of a culture system for the virus. For reasons yet unknown, the mature viral particle for HPV requires the permissive environment of a mature keratinocyte to form and replicate. This has required investigators to use various detection techniques such as antibodies to the viral capsule proteins detected by immunoperoxidase staining, characteristic histological changes, to sophisticated DNA hybridization.

The clinical manifestations of HPV infection have been described since the Roman-Helenistic era and consist of an exophytic, grapelike lesion readily apparent to the naked eye. This classical

FIG 6–14.
Condyloma acuminatum of cervix. (From Kistner RW, Hertig AT: *Obstet Gynecol* 1955; 6:147. Reproduced by permission.)

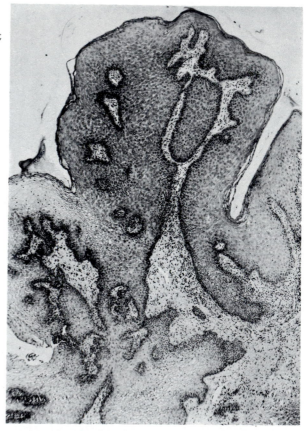

type of venereal wart is rarely found on the cervix (Fig 6–14). Only 254 cases were reported in the literature through 1974 (Syrjanen, 1984).

Microscopically the classic wart is characterized by papillomatosis, acanthosis, lengthening and thickening of the rete pegs, submucosal capillary proliferation, and the presence of koilocytes. Koilocytes were first described by Koss and Durfee in 1956. They exhibit hyperchromasia, multinucleation, and perinuclear cytoplasmic vacuolization (Fig 6–15). Initially, koilocytes were believed to be pathognomonic of HPV infections, but as our understanding of HPV has expanded using DNA hybridization, this constant association has been called into doubt. Further, long-term epidemiological studies with extensive follow-up will be necessary before we can define more clearly the cytological finding of koilocytosis.

In 1977, Meisels et al. described two cervical lesions with koilocytotic atypia and other features suggestive of condylomata but without the typical gross papillary features. The "flat condyloma" is a flattened area of acanthosis with mild accentuation of the rete pegs and koilocytotic changes.

They pointed out the striking contrast between the essentially normal-appearing deeper layers of the epithelium and the superficial areas that exhibit the koilocytosis. The second lesion he described is the endophytic, or inverted, condyloma, which demonstrates gland involvement and may be mistaken for invasive carcinoma. These lesions are usually not visible without the aid of the colposcope, through which they can be seen to exhibit fine punctation on a white background.

Meisels et al. (1977) reviewed 152 cervical smears diagnosed as mild dysplasia and found that 70% were suggestive of HPV infection, leading these authors to consider koilocytotic atypia to be an early phase in the natural history of cervical neoplasia. The relationship between condylomata and cervical carcinoma will be more fully discussed later. Condylomatous cervicitis is a very common disease, with 1% to 2% of all Papanicolaou smears exhibiting koilocytotic changes. When DNA hybridization techniques are used on Papanicolaou smears, the actual incidence of HPV is probably 10-fold higher, representing 10% to 20% of all smears (Bearman et al., 1987; Lorinez et al., 1986). Treatment of cervical

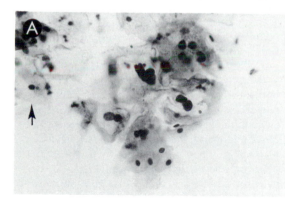

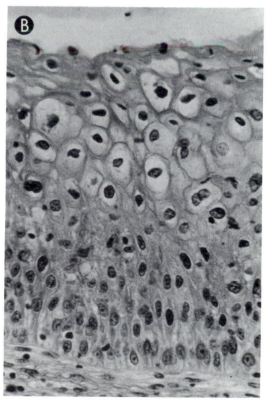

FIG 6–15.
A, koilocytes on a Papanicolaou smear (magnification ×320). The nuclei are hyperchromatic with characteristic perinuclear cytoplasmic vacuolization. Multinucleated forms are evident. A normal superficial cell is shown for comparison *(arrow).* **B,** flat condyloma (magnification ×530). Koilocytotic changes can be seen in the superficial layers. (Courtesy of Dr. Robert Ehrmann and the Division of Women's and Perinatal Pathology, Brigham and Women's Hospital, Boston.)

condylomata depends on several factors, the most important of which are histology and patient preference. If the histology is consistent with only condylomata and contains no cytologic atypia or dysplasia, the lesion can be closely observed or treated with either trichloroacetic acid, cryocautery, or laser. If cytological atypia or dysplasia is present, surgical treatment such as cryocautery or laser should be strongly recommended. Since treatment of a single clinical lesion will not necessarily eradicate the patient's viral infection with HPV, she should be well informed of the potential risks and benefits of treatment and the need for careful, long-term screening. Treatment methods will be more thoroughly discussed in the section under cervical intraepithelial neoplasia.

CERVICAL NEOPLASIA

Fifty years ago, carcinoma of the cervix was the leading cause of death from malignant disease in American women. Since 1940, however, the mortality rate from cervical carcinoma has declined by more than 50%, yet it still ranks sixth in cancer mortality, with estimates of 7,000 deaths each year in the United States. There are 16,000 new cases of invasive cervical carcinoma, with the peak in incidence between ages 45 to 55 years, and more than 44,000 new cases of in situ cervical carcinoma discovered each year in the United States, accounting for more than 60,000 women who require major and potentially morbid treatment annually. Despite the recognition of a significant preinvasive phase and availability of screening methods, cervical neoplasia remains a major health problem.

Epidemiology

Perhaps the earliest epidemiological studies of cervical neoplasia were conducted in 1842 by Rigoni-Stern (1976) who showed that the incidence of cervical carcinoma was higher in married and widowed women and lower in never-married women and among nuns in certain religious orders. Since then, numerous epidemiological studies looking at the association between cancer of the cervix and certain social factors have been reported. In terms of greatest risk, the final common denominator seems to be related to *coitus* and more specifically to onset of regular sexual activity at an early age, and perhaps to multiplicity of sexual partners. The higher incidence of cervical carcinoma in nonwhites compared with that in whites appears to be related to socioeconomic class, which may further be a function of early marriage and early childbearing. The interdependence of prostitution, sexually transmitted diseases, and coitus needs no clarification. Strongly supporting this concept is the rarity of cervical cancer in nuns, as noted by Rigoni-Stern and later by Gagnon (1950). However, it should be stressed that when all proposed factors associated with cervical cancer are evaluated by multivariate analysis, age of first intercourse and number of sexual partners stand alone as risk factors.

The virtual absence of penile carcinoma among Jewish men suggested a relationship between *circumcision* and genital carcinoma, which was first studied in relation to cervical carcinoma by Handley in 1936. He demonstrated a lower incidence of this disease in one ethnic group of Fiji Islanders who practiced ritual circumcision compared with members of another ethnic group who did not. Support for this relationship came from work by Wahi in India, where, again, the incidence of this disease was significantly lower among ethnic groups practicing circumcision. The extremely low frequency of cervical carcinoma among Jewish women lends further support to the proposed protective effect of circumcision. It has been thought that the absence of smegma might account for this protective effect in that early studies indicated smegma to be carcinogenic in animals; however, later work has failed to confirm these findings. These epidemiological observations have not as yet been adequately explained.

The role of the high-risk male was investigated by Kessler (1976, 1981) who found a several-fold increase in risk for the development of cervical carcinoma among women whose husbands had previously been married to women with cervical carcinoma compared with a control population. Again, in reference to undefined social factors, wives of men of lower socioeconomic classes are several times more likely to be diagnosed as having cervical carcinoma than are women married to men in a higher socioeconomic class.

These epidemiological studies clearly implicate a venereal transmission in cervical carcinoma. The recent interest in viral oncogenesis has suggested viruses as possible etiological agents in cervical neoplasia.

The relationship between *HSV infections* and cervical cancer was noted by Rawls et al. (1968) and Josey et al. (1968) and has been examined intensively since then in an attempt to prove that HSV is an etiological agent for cervical neoplasia. Numerous seroepidemiological studies performed worldwide have revealed a significantly higher frequency and titer of HSV type 2 antibodies in patients with cervical carcinoma compared with "controls." Criticisms of these studies included the lack of suitable controls adequately matched for sexual history and the technical difficulty in differentiating exposure to HSV type 1 from HSV type 2, given the serological techniques then available and the extent of antigenic cross-reactivity between these two viruses.

Despite the controversy that arose from these serological data, an intensive search was made to locate HSV DNA or RNA or related proteins within cervical cancer biopsy specimens. Essentially, no constant relationship was found between cervical cancer and HSV on this molecular level, and the data gave rise to further controversy as to HSV's role in cervical cancer.

Some of this controversy was answered when it became apparent that HSV may be oncogenic. Multiple investigators demonstrated that HSV infection can induce chromosomal breaks in the host cell DNA. This and other data such as HSV's ability to mutate certain genes support the fact that HSV is oncogenic. In fact, some investigators believe that these properties of HSV are consistent with an initiator's role in the two-step theory of the development of cancer, and therefore, HSV DNA or RNA does not have to be present to support the role of HSV in the development of cervical cancer (zurHausen et al., 1984; Galloway and MacDougall, 1983; Nahmias and Sawanabani, 1978).

As the evaluation of HSV was progressing, it became increasingly obvious that HPV-related lesions were also present in these cervical lesions. Advancement of HPV understanding took a giant step forward with the isolation in 1980 by Gissman and zurHausen of the DNA from a genital condyloma. This HPV DNA was designated to be HPV type 6. With the use of elegant DNA hybridization techniques, and HPV type 6 as the initial probe, our understanding of HPV's intimate role in the development of intraepithelial neoplasia and invasive cancers of the cervix exploded.

An in-depth discussion of HPV and cervical cancer is beyond the scope of this text, and interested readers are referred to Syrjanen (1984). The strong casual association of HPV and cervical neoplasia, however, does warrant discussion. Since the isolation of HPV type 6 in 1980, more than 50 HPV types have been identified. Using the isolated DNA as a probe, investigators have evaluated precancerous and cancerous lesions of the cervix for the presence of HPV DNA. Many have shown that HPV types 6 and 11 are generally found in classical, exophytic condylomata no matter whether they are found on the vulva, vagina, or cervix. Respiratory papillomas in children also contain HPV type 11 (Mounts and Shah, 1984). The development of more serious lesions such as precancerous (i.e., intraepithelial) neoplasias or cancers of the cervix are associated with HPV types 16, 18, 31, 35, and some of the 50s. Although the vast majority of these lesions seem to stick to one type and follow these general trends, that is not an absolute, so that cancerous lesions can have more than one HPV type present or could be associated with HPV type 6 or 11 and vice versa (Bergeron et al., 1987). This ability of HPV types to be present in all facets of clinical lesions leads to difficulty in predicting which patient will be at risk for a serious clinical problem when one relies solely on HPV type. Add to this dilemma the well-known fact that HPV can remain dormant in normal-appearing skin (Ferenczy et al., 1985), further decreasing the predictive value of screening women for HPV types (Grunebaum et al., 1983).

Now that the actual genetic sequences are known for the vast majority of HPV DNA, investigators are hard at work trying to understand how this virus' casual association with cervical neoplasia can become a causal role. Anecdotal stories regarding malignant transformation of long-standing vulvar, vaginal, and rectal condylomatous lesions into invasive disease abound, but they are at least equaled by those lesions that do not progress. The question then arises of the role of HPV as a promoter that requires some other factor to be present as an initiator, such as HSV or other carcinogens (zurHausen et al., 1984; Galloway and McDougall, 1983).

To summarize the epidemiology of cervical carcinogenesis in broader terms, the causative agent may be transmitted by or be associated with sexual intercourse, and the risk is inversely related to age and duration of exposure. According to the most popular theory, cervical carcinogenesis is thought to commence with an initiating event, such as exposure to an oncogenic virus, during the period of active squamous metaplasia. This is followed by promotion, which may represent continued exposure to the initiating factor or to a second carcinogen, yielding neoplasia. This theory would certainly explain why the vast majority of cervical neoplastic lesions are found in the transformation zone and correlates with the epidemiological risk factors described.

Cervical Intraepithelial Neoplasia

Carcinoma in situ (CIS) may be defined as an intraepithelial lesion with cytological atypia similar to that seen in invasive carcinoma but without evidence of invasion into the stroma (Fig 6–16). These atypical cells extend through the entire thickness of the epithelium and have enlarged, pleomorphic nuclei with dense, coarse chromatin and scant cytoplasm. The polarity of the cells as

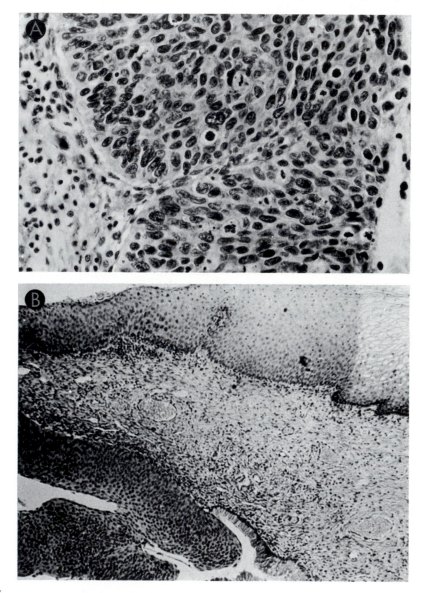

FIG 6–16.
A, carcinoma in situ (CIS) of cervix. (From Hertig AT, Gore HM: Tumors of the female sex organs, fasc 33, *Atlas of Tumor Pathology.* Washington, DC, Armed Forces Institute of Pathology, 1960. Reproduced by permission.) **B,** CIS of cervix with gland involvement. An area of parakeratosis is seen at the upper right.

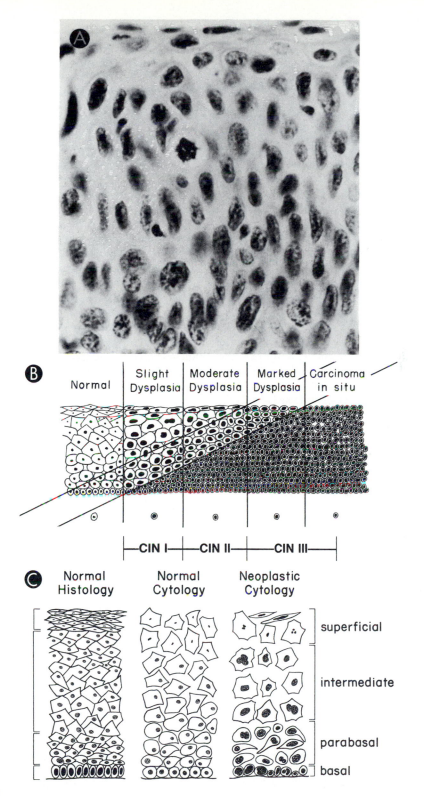

FIG 6–17.
A, high-power magnification of CIS of cervix. **B,** diagrammatic representation of changes in cellular morphology from slight dysplasia to CIS. Nuclear/cytoplasmic ratios are shown at the bottom. **C,** diagrammatic representation of exfoliated cells from the normal cervix compared with variations of exfoliated cells from the neoplastic cervix. (**B** and **C** courtesy of Dr. Paul A. Younge.)

well as the polarity of the epithelium (i.e., the normal surface maturation and differentiation) are lost. Various degrees of parakeratosis may be seen.

Lesions composed of similar atypical cells but that retain some degree of surface maturation have been referred to as "dysplasias" by Reagan et al. (1969). Dysplastic epithelium spans a range of severity, from mild loss of polarity, a high degree of cellular differentiation, and few mitoses (mild dysplasia), to a lesion resembling carcinoma in situ in its marked cytological and nuclear atypia and increased mitotic activity but retaining some degree of epithelial polarization (severe dysplasia) (Fig 6–17). In many cases, pathological differentiation of carcinoma in situ from severe dysplasia may be very difficult and may hinge on minimal cellular flattening in the most superficial cell layers of the epithelium.

The major significance of CIS lies in its role as a precursor to invasive cancer. Multiple series (Kolstad and Klem, 1976; Spriggs and Boddington, 1980) of untreated patients with CIS diagnosed on biopsy have been followed conservatively, with progression to invasive carcinoma, occurring in as many as 70% of cases. More controversial is the ultimate fate of cervical dysplasia and the question as to whether these lesions should be considered premalignant. Observed progression of dysplasia to CIS has been reported in 5% to 60% of cases, and this variation in percentages appears to result from differences in the criteria used to define each lesion and varying periods of follow-up (Richart, 1966; Christopherson and Gray, 1982).

These reports also suggest that dysplastic lesions regress in as many as 50% of cases. It has been shown that biopsy may remove the dysplastic lesion entirely or that the inflammatory process accompanying repair at the biopsy site may destroy remaining areas of atypicality, thereby falsely giving the clinical impression of regression. More recent studies in which patients were diagnosed cytologically and then followed cytologically and colposcopically, thereby eliminating the "biopsy effect," confirm progression of dysplasia to CIS in 40% to 60% of cases and spontaneous regression rates as high as 30% for mild or moderate dysplasia. The more severe the dysplasia, the higher the rate and speed of progression toward CIS and the lower the rate of regression. The average age of patients with dysplasia is consistently 5 to 10 years lower than that of patients with CIS, which runs 10 to 15 years behind the average age of patients with invasive squamous cell carcinoma.

The suggestion that these lesions represent a continuum of change that begins with mild dysplasia and advances through CIS led Richart (1966) to introduce the concept of cervical intraepithelial neoplasia (CIN), with the following classifications: CIN I indicates mild dysplasia, CIN II indicates moderate dysplasia, and CIN III indicates severe dysplasia and carcinoma in situ. Evidence in support of Richart's classification of these lesions as a spectrum of one disease entity comes from the finding of aneuploid changes in the nuclei of dysplastic cells—the same chromosomal changes usually found associated with malignant tumors but not with benign tumors. Autoradiographic studies (Richart, 1963) have demonstrated a steady increase in the mitotic activity of these lesions that corresponds exactly to the degree of histological dedifferentiation and maturation present; this observation is consistent with the postulate that CIN represents stages in a continuum of disease.

Histological and colposcopic observations have established the transformation zone as the site of origin of virtually all CIN. These lesions are thought to arise from the basal cell of the transformation zone and, if progression occurs, to result in large-cell nonkeratinizing squamous cell carcinoma. Small-cell carcinoma is thought to arise from the subcolumnar reserve cells of the endocervical canal, whereas large-cell keratinizing carcinoma is thought to arise from the basal cells of the native squamous epithelium. Large-cell nonkeratinizing squamous carcinoma is by far the commonest histological type seen, supporting the observation that the majority of CIN originates in the transformation zone.

Although a small percentage of cases of CIN will regress spontaneously or after biopsy, a finite percentage will progress to invasion. Until we can predict a priori instances in which CIN will progress, regress, or remain stable, these lesions must be considered premalignant, and the patient must be evaluated, treated, and followed up appropriately. At the same time, each case must be individualized to take into account age, desire for fertility, and the presence or absence of other pelvic disease.

Recently, pathologists have been calling for the concept for CIN to be taken one step farther and for the grades within CIN to be eliminated (Buckley et al., 1982; Koss, 1987). The rationale is based on the premise that significant difference

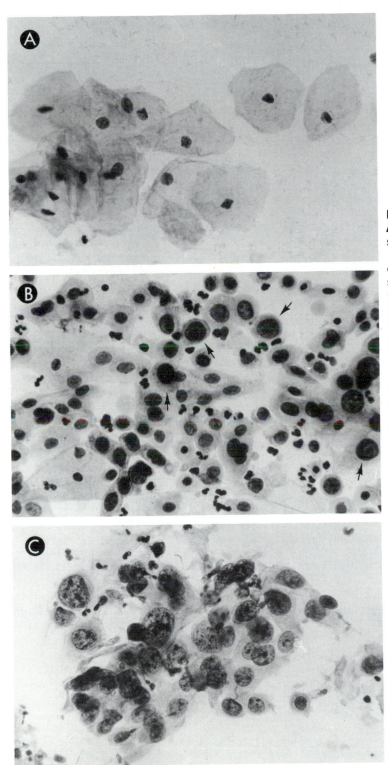

FIG 6–18.
A, class I Papanicolaou smear, benign (magnification ×320). Normal superficial cell, polygonal in shape, with small pyknotic nuclei, **B,** class IV Papanicolaou smear, CIS (magnification ×320). Neoplastic cells are large and uniform in size, with hyperplastic nuclei and an increased nuclear/cytoplasmic ratio *(arrows)*. **C,** class V Papanicolaou smear, invasive cancer (magnification ×320). The nuclei exhibit coarse, clumped chromatin and may contain multiple nucleoli. Marked pleomorphism and atypical mitotic figures may be seen. (Courtesy of Dr. Robert Ehrmann and the Division of Women's and Perinatal Pathology, Brigham and Women's Hospital, Boston.)

of opinion exists among pathologists when it comes to establishing the grade of a CIN lesion and therefore, the individual patient grade does not have any predictive value. They, and others, believe that the designation of well-defined CIN should be enough information for the clinician to establish a treatment and follow-up plan. These opinions remain controversial and bear further discussion before being implemented.

Diagnosis of Cervical Neoplasia

Cytology

The outstanding contribution of recent decades to the field of cancer detection is that of the late George Papanicolaou. In studying cells exfoliated from the female genital tract, Papanicolaou, in the late 1920s, noted characteristic cellular changes associated with cervical carcinoma. These cellular abnormalities include anomalies of staining reaction, pleomorphism, nuclear irregularity, hyperchromasia, the presence of multiple nucleoli, and an increased nuclear/cytoplasmic ratio (Fig 6–18). As with so many important discoveries, fully 20 years elapsed before Papanicolaou's cytological technique (the *Papanicolaou test)* was accepted as a cancer screening measure.

Papanicolaou's classification of the cytological findings consisted of five grades:

    I. Benign
   II. Atypical benign
  III. Suspect
  IV. Probably positive
   V. Positive

Although this classification applied to invasive cancer, it soon became apparent that it was possible to detect and identify specific abnormalities associated with CIS and dysplasia/CIN by means of cytological examination. It is the practice in many laboratories to equate dysplasia/CIN and CIS with the class III and IV designations, respectively.

An appreciation of both qualitative and quantitative variations in cell types found in abnormal smears has enabled cytopathologists to make reasonably accurate diagnostic interpretations. This appreciation has led many centers, Brigham and Women's Hospital included, to drop the classification of the five grades of Papanicolaou smear and to move to a descriptive report. This allows the cytopathologist to deliver a more informative report to the clinician as to the type of histology he or she may be expected to find on biopsy. Hopefully, changing the Papanicolaou smear report will enable the clinician to more closely define those women who require further evaluation and treatment based on cytology rather than reacting only to the grade of the Papanicolaou smear report.

The earliest technique used for collecting cytological material was aspiration from the posterior vaginal fornix via a glass pipette. Although various series reported failure rates of up to 60% in detecting documented CIN and 45% in identifying CIS using this technique, some practitioners continue to employ it. In 1947, Ayre devised a wooden spatula with which a "scrape biopsy" of the cervical epithelial cells could be carried out. He quoted 95% accuracy in screening for cervical neoplasms when this technique was used in conjunction with endocervical sampling.

Despite the overall success of exfoliative cytology, the significant incidence of *false negative smears* has gradually become apparent. The practice of routinely performing a biopsy for every patient with an abnormal cervix was established at the Boston Hospital for Women by Younge in 1936, providing a controlled series from which the relative accuracy of cytology could be determined. If we consider the cases of CIS diagnosed between 1962 and 1968, cytological findings were normal in 16 of 113 cases, or 14.2% (Table 6–1). If we can presume that seven patients with CIS diagnosed at a repeated examination 1 year later also had false negative smears, the cumulative false negative rate rises to 19.2%. The false negative rate for dysplasia is shown to be 26%. Although numerous subsequent reports in the literature confirm the false negative rate for cervical cytological diagnosis to be 15% to 20%, one must keep in mind that increasing the frequency of screening (i.e., decreasing the interval between smears) will have impact on the rate of diagnostic failure to the individual patient (Bearman et al., 1987).

Technique of Obtaining Vaginal and Cervical Smears.—The following equipment is needed:

1. Clean glass (microscope) slides. Those with frosted ends permit easy labeling in pencil with the patient's name and also identify the "right side," or smeared side of the slide.

TABLE 6–1.

Correlations of Initial Cytodiagnosis With Final Diagnosis at the Boston Hospital for Women, 1962 to 1968

Smear	Preclinical Cancer	Carcinoma In Situ With Early Stromal Invasion	Carcinoma In Situ*	CIS* Dysplasia*
Normal	2	0	16 (23)	60 (96)
Atypical	0	1	3	19
Dysplasia	0	1	40	133
Carcinoma in situ	3	5	45	12
Invasive	5	2	9	1
TOTAL	10	9	113 (120)	225 (261)

*Figures in parentheses include cases detected at the first-year repeated examination.

2. A cotton swab moistened with normal saline solution, or an endocervical brush.

3. Spatula to be used for cervical scrapings and to prepare smear.

4. A fixative; any one of several dehydrating agents can be used:
    a. Half-and-half mixture of 95% ethyl alcohol and ether.
    b. Plain 95% alcohol or lesser dilutions to 75%.
    c. Seventy-five percent to 95% methyl alcohol.
    d. Seventy-five percent to 95% isopropyl alcohol or commercially available cytologic fixatives.

Smears are obtained prior to digital examination with the patient in the lithotomy position and without lubricants, which spoil the staining characteristics of the cells. Douches dilute and wet the cells; therefore, a satisfactory smear cannot be obtained within 12 to 24 hours after douching. The moistened swab or endocervical brush is used to sample the endocervix. Some authors (Weitzman et al., 1988; Taylor, 1987) believe that a greater yield of endocervical cells is obtained by the brush over the swab; thus decreasing the number of Papanicolaou smears that are inadequate due to lack of endocervical cells. We have noted an increased incidence of trauma resulting in oozing of the endocervix, which can make subsequent colposcopy after brush usage difficult. One should keep this in mind in those patients scheduled for colposcopy.

The slide is immediately fixed by immersion into a small stoppered bottle containing fixative or sprayed with commercially available fixative.

The spatula is then used to scrape the portio circumferentially at the area of the transformation zone, and a slide is rapidly smeared and fixed.

If one wishes to use a one-slide technique, the endocervix should be sampled and smeared before the cervical scrape is taken. The moisture inherent in the endocervical sample is believed to keep the drying artifact to a minimum prior to fixation of the one slide. Fixation is complete in 15 to 30 minutes if an immersion dehydrating agent is used or immediately if a cytological fixative is used. In either case, air-drying artifact is the commonest error in a Papanicolaou smear technique and should be kept in mind when fixation is performed.

The importance of endocervical sampling cannot be stressed too strongly. This was shown dramatically by Garite and Feldman (1978), who randomized 710 patients into three groups to compare sampling techniques. The first group underwent sampling with a cervical smear only; the second group with an exocervical smear and endocervical sampling with a moistened cotton swab; and the third group with a method chosen based on the location of the squamocolumnar junction, as determined by the patient's physician. The addition of endocervical sampling doubled the detection rate of abnormal cytology. Rubio (1977) demonstrated that the cotton swab traps atypical cells, making the data of Garite and Feldman (1978) even more impressive.

The diagnosis rendered by the cytopathologist can be no better than an accurate interpretation of the cytological abnormality present on the slide. Certainly the clinician can help to limit the number of false negative smears by obtaining a proper smear from the area of the transformation zone as well as by obtaining an adequate endocervical sample and assuring rapid fixation to give the examiner the best chance to provide an accurate diagnosis.

The effectiveness of *mass cervical screening programs* remains somewhat controversial with regard to their ability to decrease the incidence of and mortality from cervical cancer. Epidemiologists have described decreasing incidence and mortality rates of cervical carcinoma in countries where mass screening programs are not operating, suggesting that a change in the natural history of the disease might account for the benefits attributed to cervical cytological screening. Excellent work done by Boyes et al. (1978) in British Columbia, Canada, where a screening program has been in operation since 1949, confirms the marked fall in the incidence and mortality rates of this disease (Table 6–2). They also show a rather dramatic increase in the incidence of cervical can-

cer among a group of unscreened women compared with women undergoing routine cytological screening. Using data obtained from the other provinces, they directly related the decrease in mortality rate of cervical cancer to the level of screening activity. These observations seemingly establish a definite role for the Papanicolaou smear in contributing to the reduction in incidence and mortality rates for cervical cancer.

In 1988, the American College of Obstetrics and Gynecology in conjunction with the American Cancer Society and several other cancer organizations agreed on recommendations for Papanicolaou smear screening intervals. They believe that every woman should have a Papanicolaou smear annually after age 18 years or after the onset of sexual activity. If three consecutive Papanicolaou smears and pelvic examinations 1 year apart are entirely normal, the screening interval can be lengthened at the discretion of the physi-

TABLE 6–2.

Cervical Screening in British Columbia*

Yr	Women Screened Annually	Total Cases of Invasive Cervical Cancer	Incidence per 100,000 Women	Mortality Rate From Cervical Cancer per 100,000 Women
1952	4,140	—	—	—
1953	5,504	—	—	—
1954	8,848	—	—	—
1955	11,707	120	28.4	—
1956	15,106	119	27.2	—
1957	18,719	120	26.0	—
1958	29,869	112	23.7	—
1959	38,849	108	22.6	11.4
1960	54,844	96	19.7	10.6
1961	81,614	115	23.2	9.9
1962	106,176	78	15.5	10.3
1963	119,292	98	19.1	12.9
1964	138,700	86	16.3	11.0
1965	161,556	80	14.7	10.6
1966	182,375	77	13.6	7.7
1967	209,425	85	14.3	7.8
1968	236,234	80	13.0	6.4
1969	266,036	89	13.9	8.8
1970	297,407	82	12.3	7.1
1971	322,436	73	10.6	6.9
1972	336,351	66	9.2	8.0
1973	377,397	71	9.5	6.0
1974	385,303	67	8.6	5.6
1975	—	70	8.7	4.8
1976	—	69	8.4	5.2
1977	—	64	7.6	3.8

*Adapted from Boyes DA, et al: Experience with cervical screening in British Columbia. *Gynecol Oncol* 1981; 12S:143.

cian. They do not recommend lengthening the interval if the patient or her sexual partner has had more than one other sexual partner. These recommendations do not apply to women being followed for abnormal Papanicolaou smears or after treatment of such. All clinicians need to stress the importance of screening and pelvic examinations since detection of other reproductive tract cancers can be found on such examinations.

Biopsy and Histological Diagnosis.— Clinicians have depended on the Papanicolaou smear as a screening method for detection of cervical neoplasia. Serial sampling over time provides a longitudinal look at the cervix, decreasing the impact of isolated false negative smears. The Papanicolaou smear, however, must remain a *screening* technique. Biopsy and histological diagnosis remain the cornerstones in the management of CIN.

A biopsy must be performed on every abnormal, visible cervical lesion. The literature is replete with cases in which a gross cervical abnormality was followed conservatively because multiple Papanicolaou smears were falsely negative or exhibited inflammatory changes only.

Random cervical biopsies were first used to obtain histological material from cervices determined to be abnormal by Papanicolaou's smear in an attempt to obviate conization in all patients with abnormal smears. It has been shown that CINs occur most frequently at the 6 and 12 o'clock positions in the transformation zone and less frequently toward the lateral angles on each side. Biopsy specimens taken at these two positions and then randomly from the remaining cervix may miss 15% of the invasive lesions present as determined by correlation with the subsequent cone or hysterectomy specimen.

A targeting technique developed by Schiller in 1938 (now known as the *Schiller test*) may be used to highlight cervical abnormalities, making them visible for biopsy (see Fig 6–6). A solution of sodium iodide and iodine is painted onto the cervix. The iodine reacts with glycogen to stain the normal squamous epithelium of the cervix and vagina dark brown. Nonstaining or Schiller-positive areas stand out from the dark background and represent surfaces lacking glycogen; these include columnar epithelium, true pathological erosions, immature metaplastic epithelium, and neoplastic lesions. Due to the relatively nonspecific staining patterns, this test is generally

reserved for usage at the time of cervical conization.

Colposcopy has superseded Schiller's technique as the initial step in evaluating abnormal Papanicolaou smears (Wagner and McElin, 1983). Hinselman developed the colposcope in 1925 in an attempt to localize small ulcerations that he theorized represented small cervical neoplasms. He found, however, that the low-power magnification of the colposcope ($\times 6$ to $\times 40$) revealed not the neoplastic cervical epithelium but alterations of the underlying stromal vasculature resulting from the neoplastic process, which could then be visualized through the thin epithelial layer. The degree of alteration in vascular pattern, in intercapillary distance, and in surface color and texture was found to correlate well with the severity of the neoplastic process. These patterns are enhanced by applications of 3% acetic acid to the cervical epithelium. Usage of 3% acetic acid not only cleanses the epithelium but tends to precipitate out nucleic proteins in the superficial layers, giving rise to the classic aceto-white epithelium that is one of the features of abnormal epithelium. (For a detailed review of colposcopy, the reader is referred to a standard colposcopic atlas.)

Adequate colposcopic evaluation requires complete visualization of the transformation zone and the lesion in question as well as correlation between the cytological and histological diagnoses and the clinical impression of the colposcopist. Endocervical curettage should be performed as part of every colposcopic examination. Almost 90% of women with abnormal cytological findings may be adequately evaluated with colposcopy.

Cervical Biopsy

Cervical biopsy is perhaps the most frequent minor surgical procedure performed by the gynecologist. Simple and relatively painless, it may be performed as part of the routine office examination. Contraindications to cervical biopsy are limited to acute pelvic inflammatory disease and acute cervicitis. Certainly patients with coagulopathies should be managed in a hospital setting. Pregnancy is not a contraindication to biopsy.

Technique

The cervix is visualized with a speculum and adequately illuminated. A Papanicolaou smear is repeated at the start of the examination for later correlation with the histology obtained on biopsy. Then the cervix is carefully cleaned and soaked with 3% acetic acid. It is generally believed that the commonest error in colposcopy is not keeping the cervix adequately soaked with acetic acid, such that the abnormal areas are missed. The endocervical curettage is obtained prior to biopsies on the cervical portio to reduce the number of curettages that are contaminated by detached fragments of cervical epithelium. A rectangular biopsy specimen is obtained using a Kevorkian or Younge biopsy punch and is then immediately fixed in Bouin's solution. Postbiopsy bleeding may be controlled by pressure, cauterization with silver nitrate or ferrous subsulfate (Monsel's solution), packing with oxidized regenerated cellulose (Oxycel or Surgicel), or suturing as required. The patient is instructed to avoid douching, use of tampons, and intercourse for 2 weeks after biopsy. Although the procedure is essentially painless, a paracervical block with lidocaine or chloroprocaine (Nesacaine) may be performed.

Cervical Conization

Cervical conization remains the gold standard against which all outpatient evaluation techniques must be weighed. A properly performed conization removes the entire transformation zone and virtually the entire endocervical canal, providing the pathologist with the maximum amount of tissue to rule out invasive carcinoma absolutely. Drawbacks of this procedure include the need for anesthesia, a complication rate approaching 10% in most series (primarily postoperative hemorrhage), and possible adverse effects on future fertility.

The vast majority of patients may be completely and adequately evaluated for CIN on an outpatient basis; however, the clinician must be assured that invasive cancer has been ruled out before consideration can be given to outpatient therapy. If the following conditions are not met, conization is required to rule out invasion:

1. Lesions identified colposcopically must be seen entirely. If they extend to the endocervical canal, their uppermost extent must be seen.
2. The entire transformation zone must be visualized.
3. Results of endocervical curettage must be negative for neoplasia.

4. Biopsies and cytological examination must reveal intraepithelial disease only.
5. Cytological and histological diagnoses must correlate.

Technique

Under adequate general or regional anesthesia, the patient is placed in the dorsal lithotomy position, and the vagina and perineum are gently prepared with povidone-iodine (Betadine) to avoid traumatizing the delicate cervical mucosa. After the bladder has been catheterized, an examination is performed to rule out existing pelvic disease. A weighted retractor is placed in the posterior fornix, a Sims retractor is placed anteriorly, and the cervix is visualized. Colposcopy or Schiller's test is performed to delineate the extent of disease on the portio. A tenaculum is placed on the portio anteriorly, above the planned limit of the cone biopsy. Lateral-angle sutures are placed into the stroma of the cervix at the 3 and 9 o'clock positions to ligate the descending branches of the uterine artery. These sutures are left long (for tying at the end of the procedure). Some clinicians infiltrate the cervix with dilute solutions of 20 units of vasopressin in 20 ml of normal saline or bupivacaine (Marcaine) hydrochloride with epinephrine 1:200,000 to aid hemostasis.

The mucosa is incised circumferentially, maintaining a margin of 2 to 3 mm beyond the lesions (as delineated via colposcopy or Schiller's staining). A cone-shaped specimen to a length of 1.5 to 1.8 cm is carefully excised encircling the endocervical canal. Care is taken to avoid prematurely entering the canal, since neoplastic tissue might then be left behind. A uterine sound may be placed within the canal to aid in the dissection. Manipulation of the mucosa of the specimen should be avoided. Traction may be attained by placing sutures within the stroma of the cone specimen or by grasping this area with forceps. A suture is placed at the 12 o'clock position in the stroma of the specimen to aid in pathologic orientation. The uterus is then sounded and dilated, and an endometrial sample is taken as desired.

Bleeding is usually minimal with this technique. Bleeding points may be electrocauterized or ligated with size 0 chromic sutures in a figure-of-eight pattern. The canal is then packed with Surgicel, which is gently tied into place with the long ends of the lateral sutures. Generally, conization is an outpatient surgery, with the patient observed until the anesthetic has reversed, and then discharged with instructions to avoid douching, use of tampons, and intercourse for 3 weeks.

Therapy for Cervical Intraepithelial Neoplasia

The approach to treatment of CIN has undergone dramatic changes over the past several decades as the pathogenesis of cervical neoplasia has become better understood. In the past, extensive and potentially morbid procedures such as radical hysterectomy and pelvic irradiation were commonly employed to treat the high-grade dysplasias that are now treated on an outpatient basis at little cost and essentially without risk. Earlier lesions were occasionally ignored. The concept of cervical neoplasia as a continuum, as advanced by Richart (1966), implies that these lesions may be treated in a similar manner, with the understanding that progression to invasive cancer is the natural history of a certain unpredictable percentage.

Treatment of CIN III (severe dysplasia and CIS) perhaps remains most controversial. With the realization that radical surgery and irradiation were not necessary, simple hysterectomy became the treatment of choice throughout the United States. Cone biopsy, as primary therapy, was limited to those patients desirous of retaining fertility. Several studies have been done comparing the results obtained from conization compared with hysterectomy. In general, conization approaches hysterectomy for subsequent cure rate in large series for CIN III. The problem arises when the margins of conization are positive for residual disease. Several series have now shown that even in this setting, careful follow-up with Papanicolaou smear, colposcopy, and endocervical curettage will allow the clinician to detect those patients who truly have residual disease. This type of follow-up should be reserved for those patients who wish to avoid hysterectomy for fertility reasons. For those patients who do not wish to retain fertility, hysterectomy either abdominally or vaginally is indicated. Overall, the rates of recurrence of CIN after conization for CIN III range from 2% to 6%, whereas with hysterectomy, the incidence is from 1% to 2% (Abdul-Krim and Nunez, 1985; Buxton et al., 1987; Lubicz et al., 1984). Those patients found to have invasive disease at conization need to receive further therapy. If invasive disease is found in the hysterectomy specimen, additional radiation therapy is generally the treatment of choice, although radical upper vaginectomy with lymph node dissection has achieved excellent results as well (Orr et al., 1986; Heller et al., 1986).

Recently, in the setting of adequate colposcopy and a normal endocervical curettage, some clinicians have used ablative procedures such as cryocautery or laser vaporization. These series recommend usage of these outpatient procedures when the lesion is not extensive (i.e., not greater than 50% of exocervix) and the desire to retain fertility is present. Overall, recurrence rates for both modalities appear to be between 10% and 17% (Burke, 1982; Popkin, 1983).

Conization for any degree of CIN, whether performed as part of the diagnostic evaluation or as primary therapy subsequent to outpatient evaluation, has a cure rate of 98% when surgical margins are normal, thus requiring no further therapy. Close follow-up is suggested, including Papanicolaou smears every 3 months for 1 year and every 6 months thereafter. Given the 70% to 80% cure rate reported after conization with abnormal margins, conservative management with serial endocervical sampling, colposcopy, and cytology is acceptable if patient compliance can be expected. Otherwise, reconization or hysterectomy is indicated. The latter may be relied on as primary management of CIN when the pregnancy is undesired or when pelvic disease coexists. When the upper vagina is shown to be normal preoperatively on colposcopy or Schiller's staining, there is no need for a wide vaginal cuff. Certainly no procedure more extensive than simple hysterectomy is required for treatment of CIN.

Perhaps 85% to 90% of all patients with CIN may have lesions limited to the portio and at the same time fulfill all the criteria obviating conization. These patients are then candidates for outpatient therapeutic modalities, including electrocauterization, cryocauterization, and laser vaporization, which eradicate both the neoplastic lesion and the remainder of the transformation zone, allowing normal squamous epithelium to replace the epithelium that has been removed or destroyed.

Electrocauterization

This technique was at one time widely used, with cure rates approaching 90%. A complication rate of almost 10% (including bleeding, cervical stenosis, and pelvic inflammatory disease) as well as the degree of patient discomfort have detracted from its use, and other safer and virtually painless techniques have been developed.

Cryocauterization

This technique appears to be the simplest and safest outpatient modality developed. This technique employs a cryoprobe, cooled by carbon dioxide or freon, to necrose the surface epithelium that it contacts. Probes of various shapes are available for different cervices. For large lesions, multiple applications may be required. After treatment, a watery discharge is common but resolves in several weeks. Reepithelialization begins immediately and is virtually complete in 6 weeks (Creasman et al., 1981).

Creasman et al. (1981) reviewed the efficacy of cryocautery in CIN and reported failure rates of 6% in CIN I, 7% in CIN II, and 14% in CIN III. Townsend (1974) found the failure rate in his study to be related to lesion size rather than histological grade, with a 96% cure rate in lesions 1 cm or less in diameter, but a 58% cure rate in lesions greater than 1 cm in diameter. This may be a function of the inability to necrose the entire lesion with overlapping applications of the cryoprobe. Savage et al. (1982) showed an 18% increase in the failure rate when the glands were involved, suggesting that the depth of cryonecrosis is limited. Anderson and Hartley (1980) examined 343 cone specimens and found glands to a maximum depth of 7.83 mm and involved glands to a maximum depth of 5.22 mm. More than 99% of the glands, however, were located within 4 mm of the epithelial surface. It has been well shown that when properly performed, cryocautery produces necrosis to a depth of 5 to 6 mm, which should theoretically destroy well more than 99% of the involved glands. The relative cryoresistance in the cases reported by Savage et al. (1982) remains unclear but suggests that gland involvement may be a relative contraindication to this technique.

Criticism of cryocauterization has resulted from reports of invasive carcinoma developing after the procedure, implying that residual neoplasia had been buried during the reparative process and had progressed to invasion while undetectable by cytologic or colposcopic techniques. Sevin et al. (1979) reviewed eight such cases and found that seven of these patients had not undergone a pretreatment endocervical curettage, five had not undergone biopsy, one biopsy was misinterpreted and actually represented invasive carcinoma, and only three patients underwent colposcopic examination, implying that these failures were due to inadequate initial evaluation rather than a consequence of cryocauterization.

Laser Therapy

The most recent addition to the outpatient armamentarium against CIN is the *carbon dioxide laser*. This device produces a coherent, or in-phase, parallel beam of light of very high energy that is capable of instantaneously boiling water and, thus, vaporizing cells. Originally the laser was used to eradicate the lesion itself, thereby sparing the remaining cervix. However, failure rates averaged 10% to 30%, and it became clear that the entire transformation zone could be vaporized safely to a depth of 5 to 7 mm to yield cure rates exceeding 90% (Townsend and Richart, 1983). The major drawbacks of this technique are the cost of the laser apparatus and the greater skill required when compared with cryocauterization. Its proponents site less cervical scarring with laser use compared with cryocauterization. The major benefit from less scarring is the ability to achieve adequate colposcopic evaluation after laser. In younger women, in whom childbearing is an issue, being able to repeat colposcopy in the future should an abnormal cytological smear be obtained, reduces the need to proceed with conization.

An acceptable clinical approach to evaluation of the abnormal Papanicolaou smear and subsequent management is shown in Figure 6–19.

INVASIVE CANCER

Pathology

The gross clinical appearance of invasive cervical lesions is generally of two types: *exophytic* (proliferative) and *endophytic* (ulcerating). The exophytic lesion may involve the cervix totally and have a cauliflower-like appearance, whereas the endophytic lesion has a predilection to invade upward into the endocervical canal, often expanding the lower uterine segment and giving rise to the so-called barrel-shaped cervix. Although an endophytic lesion may infiltrate the tissue adjacent to the cervix earlier than would an exophytic tumor, either type may extend into the parametrium and involve the uterosacral ligaments or may spread onto the vaginal mucosa and down the vaginal canal. This spread causes the tissues to feel firm and nodular. The rectum and bladder may likewise be infiltrated by tumor. Spread toward the bladder usually involves the vesicovaginal septum, with the formation of bullous edema of the bladder prior to actual involvement of the bladder mucosa. Posterior spread involves the rectovaginal

Evaluation and Management of the Abnormal Papanicolaou Smear

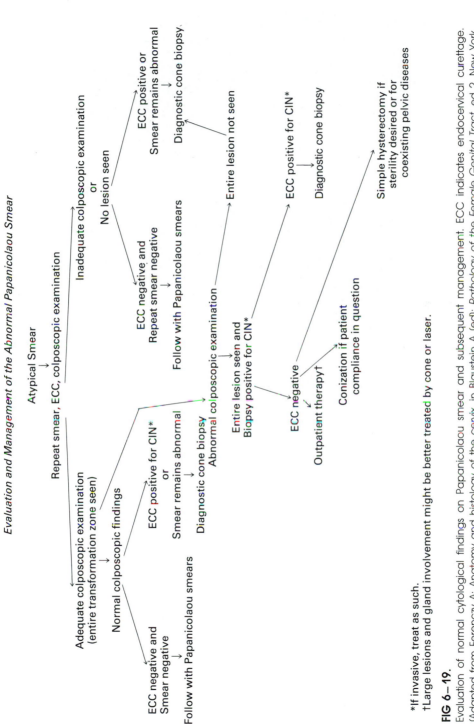

*If invasive, treat as such.
†Large lesions and gland involvement might be better treated by cone or laser.

FIG 6–19.

Evaluation of normal cytological findings on Papanicolaou smear and subsequent management. ECC indicates endocervical curettage. (Adapted from Ferenczy A: Anatomy and histology of the cervix, in Blaustein A (ed): *Pathology of the Female Genital Tract*, ed 2. New York, Springer-Verlag New York, 1982, p 174.)

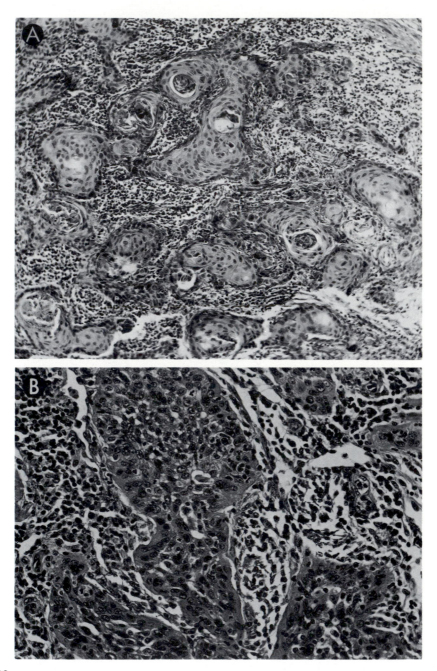

FIG 6–20.
A, typical grade 1 squamous cell carcinoma of the cervix. There is extensive keratinization with "pearl" formation and lymphocytic infiltration of the stroma. (From Hertig AT, Gore HM: Tumors of the female sex organs, fasc 33, *Atlas of Tumor Pathology.* Washing-ton, DC, Armed Forces Institute of Pathology, 1960.) **B,** grade 2 squamous cell carcinoma of the cervix. Several nests of malignant cells show pleomorphism, nuclear hyperchromatism, and atypical mitotic fig-ures.

septum, and only late in the course of the disease is there involvement of the rectal mucosa.

Microscopic Appearance

Squamous cell carcinoma accounts for 80% of invasive cervical cancer. *Adenocarcinoma* accounts for approximately 10% to 15%, and the remainder are sarcomas and primary or secondary lymphomas. Recently the incidence of adenocarcinoma has been reported to be as high as 25% in women younger than 35 years.

Wentz and Reagan (1959) have divided squamous cell carcinoma into three types: keratinizing, nonkeratinizing, and small-cell type. Keratinizing cells show foci of keratinization with cornified "pearls." Nonkeratinizing cells have well-demarcated tumor-stromal borders but no evidence of keratinization or cornified pearls. The small-cell type consists of small, round, or spindle-shaped cells with poorly defined tumor-stromal borders. Although they account for only 1% to 2% of all cervical cancers, small-cell type of cervical cancers should be recognized as a group that covers a wide variety of subtle histologically different cancers that manifest markedly different clinical outcomes.

The significant features differentiating invasive cancer from CIS are the breakdown of the basement membrane and involvement of the stroma. Nests and clusters of epithelial cells can be seen scattered in an irregular pattern within a stroma infiltrated by inflammatory cells (Fig 6–20,A). Individual cells of invasive squamous cell carcinoma show the same characteristics described for in situ cancer, namely, loss of stratification and polarity with numerous atypical mitotic figures, pleomorphism, nuclear hyperchromatism (Fig 6–20,B), and dyskaryosis. Tumor giant cells may be found along with areas of necrosis and cellular degeneration.

The typical appearance of cervical adenocarcinoma is shown in Figure 6–21. Adenocarcinoma arises from the columnar cells lining the endocervical canal and glands. The number of glandular elements is greatly increased, with marked variation in size and shape. Cellular pleomorphism, nuclear enlargement and hyperchromatism, and increased mitotic activity with areas of necrosis and degeneration are seen.

Adenosquamous carcinoma consists of intermingled malignant epithelial cell cores and malignant glandular structures. If the squamous component appears benign, the tumor is referred to as an *adenocanthoma*. The *glassy cell carcinoma* is a mixed carcinoma consisting of a poorly differentiated adenocarcinoma and squamous carcinoma. It is such a rare entity that Maier and Norris (1982) question whether it indeed represents a distinct clinical and pathologic entity. Although this tumor is believed to be poorly responsive to therapy, the number of reported cases is too small to allow any conclusions about survival to be drawn.

Histological Grading of Cervical Cancer

The degree of differentiation of a cancer cell as viewed under high power determines its histological grade. This should not be confused with stage, which defines the extent of disease as deter-

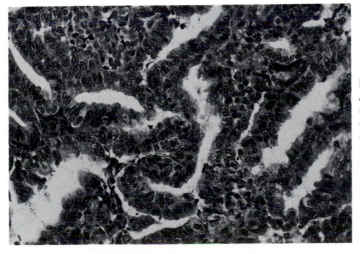

FIG 6–21.
Adenocarcinoma of the cervix. The malignant cells are arranged in a glandular pattern. The typical columnar appearance of the cell has been lost, and numerous cells show atypical mitoses.

mined by physical and radiological examinations. The grade classification most generally accepted is that of Broders, who in 1926 divided tumors into differentiated and undifferentiated groups and then assigned one of three grades depending on the relative amount of cellular differentiation present, with keratinization used as an index of differentiation. By this scheme, grade 1 would be the most differentiated and grade 3 the least differentiated, or most anaplastic. Since this original report, numerous publications concerning histological grading and survival have appeared. Most of these reviews do not consider risk factors other than histological grading that may influence prognosis. However, when Chung et al. (1981) evaluated histological grade and prognosis, they noted that the more undifferentiated the primary tumor and the more bulky the primary tumor and the more bulky the primary lesion, the higher the incidence of pelvic node metastases. Poor prognosis may, in fact, relate more to the size and, ultimately, the stage of the lesion than to the degree of histological differentiation (Goodman et al., in press).

Clinical Staging of Cervical Cancer

Clinical staging remains the most important prognostic criterion in determining the patient's response to therapy. In the early stages of cervical cancer, which are now being seen more often as a result of cytological screening, it is important in any program in which clinical trials are carried out that information be obtained concerning size of lesion, depth of invasion, lymphatic or vascular permeation, and cellular characteristics to allow useful comparisons of treatment protocols to be made. Contiguous spread of cervical cancer into the vagina, adjacent parametrium, and pelvic organs is a rather characteristic course in the natural history of this disease and forms the basis for clinical staging.

Clinical staging of carcinoma of the cervix by the International Federation of Gynecologists and Obstetricians (FIGO) is described in Table 6–3. The gynecologist and radiation therapist should jointly evaluate and stage the tumor while the patient is under anesthesia by means of speculum and bimanual pelvic and rectal examinations. The cervix and vagina must be carefully visualized and biopsy specimens taken of any suspicious areas. Excretory urography is integral to the staging process, since ureteral obstruction almost always

TABLE 6–3.

International Federation of Gynecologists and Obstetricians Clinical Staging of Invasive Cervical Cancer

Stage 0
  CIS, intraepithelial carcinoma.
Stage I
  Carcinoma is confined to the cervix.
Stage Ia
  Preclinical carcinoma; those diagnosed only by microscopy.
Stage Ia1
  Minimal microscopically evident stromal invasion.
Stage Ia2
  Lesions detected microscopically that can be measured. Depth of invasion from the base of epithelium not more than 5 mm, horizontal spread not greater than 7 mm.
Stage Ib
  All other stage I lesions. Occult cancer should be marked "occ."
Stage II
  Carcinoma extends beyond the cervix but has not extended to the pelvic wall. It involves the vagina, but not the lower third.
Stage IIa
  No obvious parametrial involvement.
Stage IIb
  Obvious parametrial involvement.
Stage III
  Carcinoma has extended to the pelvic wall. On rectal examination, there is no cancer-free space between the tumor and the pelvic wall. The tumor involves the lower third of the vagina. All cases with hydronephrosis or nonfunctioning kidney.
Stage IV
  Carcinoma has extended beyond the true pelvis or has clinically involved the mucosa of the bladder or rectum. A bullous edema is not classified as stage IV.
Stage IVa
  Spread of the growth to adjacent organs.
Stage IVb
  Spread to distant organs.

reflects extension of the tumor. Computed tomography can be used in place of excretory urography to evaluate the ureteral status and to provide information regarding pelvic and periaortic nodal status. This information concerning nodal involvement, however, is not part of the clinical staging.

Cystoscopy and proctosigmoidoscopy are recommended for advanced stages and if radiation therapy is planned; for stage I disease, however, the cost effectiveness of these diagnostic procedures is questionable. These findings are recorded, and the stage is determined. *Final staging cannot be changed once therapy has begun.*

Lymphangiography has been used to determine aortic lymph node metastases but has recently been superseded by computed tomography (CT). This latter technique is particularly helpful in evaluating nodal enlargement. A percutaneous biopsy may then be performed to provide histological evidence of metastatic spread. Results of these studies may not be used to change the final staging (as described previously). Because the staging system for cervical cancer is international, all of the diagnostic tests that are employed in staging must be generally available worldwide. Although cervical cancer rarely involves the colon, barium enema may be helpful in ruling out benign disease, particularly if the patient is to receive radiation therapy.

Certain difficulties and misinterpretations are unavoidable in clinical staging. Frequently the examiner interprets pelvic inflammatory processes or scarring due to endometriosis as tumor and "overstages" the disease. Conversely, the lateral pelvis may be soft when palpated, but at surgery, abnormal lymph nodes may be found. Staging will thus vary somewhat with the experience and tactile prowess of the examiner. Discrepancy between the clinical staging and the surgical pathological findings has been reported in as many as 25% to 40% of cases (Piver and Barlow, 1974). It is for this reason that many investigators have elected to perform laparotomy prior to instituting therapy to determine the presence of metastases to the aortic nodes or other sites beyond the pelvis.

Mode of Spread of Cervical Cancer

Carcinoma of the cervix spreads principally by direct local invasion and via lymphatics. The number of tumors with a biological propensity for hematogenous spread totals no more than 5%, but this may result in distant extrapelvic metastatic foci in spite of limited pelvic disease. Tumor growth commonly occurs by contiguous spread to the vagina, uterine cavity, and laterally through the cardinal and uterosacral ligaments. Lateral spread may occur within the substance of the ligaments or in the areolar tissue adjacent to them. Laterally extending carcinoma may encom-

pass and obstruct the ureters as they traverse the paracervical region, causing hydroureter, hydronephrosis, and eventual loss of kidney function that may lead to uremia and, ultimately, death. The cancer may traverse the paravaginal fascia, with extension into the bladder or bowel, resulting in vesicovaginal or rectovaginal fistulas.

Plentl and Friedman (1971) evaluated pelvic node metastases in cervical cancer by stage and found 15.4% abnormal nodes in stage I, 28.6% abnormal in stage II, and 47% abnormal in stage III. They further noted that the preferential metastatic spread is to the external iliac, hypogastric, and obturator lymph nodes. The next most commonly involved groups of nodes are common iliac, parametrial, and paracervical. Therefore, the lymphatic trunks leaving the cervix within the base of the broad ligament tend to be the preferred channels for lymphatic embolization. The posterior channels that drain to the sacral and then periaortic nodes are less frequently used pathways for tumor dissemination. It appears that the parametrial and paracervical nodes are frequently skipped in the transit of tumor emboli to the more preferred distal sites.

Widespread use of pretreatment laparotomy has afforded increased awareness of the spread of cervical carcinoma beyond the pelvis. The incidence of periaortic node metastases is about 5% in stage Ib, 10% in stage IIa, 18% in stage IIb, and 35% in stage IIIb. Buchsbaum (1979) reported 23 patients with abnormal aortic nodes who underwent left scalene node biopsies, of which 8 (34.8%) were abnormal. The distribution sites of distant organ metastases in order of frequency are lung, liver, and bone.

Symptoms and Diagnosis

There are no specific symptoms that characterize cervical cancer, especially in its early stages. Frequently there are no symptoms whatever. Irregular vaginal bleeding, postcoital bleeding, or both may be noted, or there may be only a pink discharge, occasionally odorous. Abnormal vaginal bleeding may first be noted as a prolonged menstrual period or as profuse flow at the time of a normal period. As the disease progresses and more blood vessels are eroded, an initially scant serosanguineous discharge may become grossly hemorrhagic. A common complaint is the daily appearance of a little blood, usually noted just after voiding and seen on the toilet tissue. In advanced cancer a characteristic bloody, malodorous discharge together with pain from either fistula formation or nerve irritation may be present. Pain is a late symptom and is typically of sciatic distribution, with radiation down the back of the buttock, thigh, and knee. Endophytic tumors may cause little or no bleeding or discharge; however, the cancer may spread rapidly to the sacral plexus and produce severe pain.

These symptoms, if due to cervical cancer, will become manifest when lesions are of moderate size. The patient should be advised to visit her physician for proper diagnostic procedures at least once yearly. As noted earlier, CIS presents no characteristic gross lesion and is detectable only by the judicious use of cervical cytological studies and adequate biopsies. Similarly, in early invasive carcinoma, the cervix may appear normal or may exhibit what seems to be an erosion. A biopsy of any suspect lesion on the cervix should always be taken. It should not be necessary to emphasize the importance of a digital and speculum examination in women in all age groups. No patient should be advised to take douches for abnormal discharges or bleeding without having a pelvic examination.

Differential Diagnosis

The lesions most commonly confused with cervical cancer are eversions, polyps, papillary endocervicitis, and papillomas. Tuberculosis, syphilitic chancres, and granuloma inguinale rarely involve the cervix, although it may be impossible to differentiate these benign lesions from early invasive cancer by any method other than biopsy. In many cases repeat or multiple biopsies are necessary before a final diagnosis can be made. This has been particularly true in papillomas of the cervix, which are frequently difficult to distinguish from low-grade papillary carcinomas.

Secondary carcinoma of the cervix may occur by direct extension from the corpus or vagina. Metastatic ovarian, bladder, and breast carcinomas have also been reported, although the breast cancer may first spread to the ovary and secondarily involve the cervix. Lymphomas, particularly histiocytic lymphoma, may present as a cervical tumor.

Treatment

Radiation therapy is the basic treatment modality in the management of cervical cancer. However, surgery may be used to an advantage in early-stage malignancy and should be combined with radiation therapy in special situations.

Staging laparotomy, as noted earlier, has been used in several centers prior to radiation therapy to evaluate metastases outside the pelvis, particularly to periaortic lymph nodes. Although lymphangiography and particularly CT scans have been helpful for delineating periaortic nodes enlarged with metastatic cancer, these techniques have not been of value when microscopic metastases are present. This latter situation must be determined surgically and is the one in which radiation therapy offers the greatest potential for cure. It is hoped that extending the standard pelvic portals to include those nodal groups with documented metastases will improve survival. However, pretreatment laparotomy has not yet been shown to increase the survival of these patients. Also, complications have been reported when periaortic node dissections have been carried out in patients subsequently treated with definitive radiation therapy.

Radiation Therapy

Radiation therapy is administered in most clinics in two forms: external beam whole pelvic radiation and transvaginal intracavitary cesium, with considerable variation as to types of applicators and sequence of administration. In the past, the measurement of radium dosage was expressed in terms of milligram-hours, which was simply a computation of the amount of radium applied (in milligrams) times the number of hours it was in position. However, unless this figure is qualified by a statement of distance factors, filtration, arrangement of sources, and the volume of tissue irradiated, the term is quite meaningless for clinical therapy. A more logical method of expressing radium dosage is similar to that used in calculating x-ray dosage, namely, in terms of the amount of ionization it produces.

Numerous intracavitary applicators have been devised, and practically every major clinic has made some change in their basic construction. The better known ones are the Stockholm, Fletcher, Paris, Manchester, Ernst, and Neary designs. In addition, cervical cancer may be treated by intravaginal cone (x-ray), interstitial needles, interstitial radon seeds, interstitial colloidal gold, or radioactive cobalt. All of these methods strive to deliver a cancericidal dose throughout the tumor-bearing area without causing irreversible damage to normal tissues. This can be accomplished only if an understanding of pelvic anatomy and pathology is combined with a knowledge of the essentials of radiation physics and radiobiology.

Radiation therapy is not without a moderate incidence of *complications* due either to inherent sensitivity or to improper application. The commonest difficulties following radiation treatment are cystitis and proctitis. Cystitis is usually delayed 1 year or more after treatment and is characterized by marked frequency, urgency with occasional incontinence, nocturia, dysuria, and, occasionally, hematuria. Results of urine specimens and cultures are usually normal, but the cystoscopic examination is diagnostic. The bladder mucosa is pale and smooth, blood vessels appear constricted, and there is a loss of normal elasticity, resulting in diminished bladder capacity. The entire process is due to the late effects of radiation, namely, a gradual obliteration of capillaries and scarring of supportive tissues. Treatment is frequently unsatisfactory and protracted, but some relief may be obtained with antispasmodics and with bladder irrigations using dilute silver nitrate or analgesic oily solutions.

Proctitis usually occurs shortly after radium administration but is transient in most cases. Symptoms include diarrhea, tenesmus, and painful defecation. Relief is obtained with a preparation of diphenoxylate hydrochloride and atropine sulfate (Lomotil) or with paregoric. Analgesic rectal suppositories are useful if tenesmus persists, and some patients benefit from steroid enemas. In a few patients the radiation reaction may be delayed 1 year or more, and in these cases there may be constipation, diarrhea, and rectal bleeding. Extensive fibrosis may seriously diminish the caliber of the rectosigmoid region so that colostomy is occasionally necessary. This condition is due to a combined effect of intracavitary treatment and x-rays.

Vesicovaginal and rectovaginal fistulas are only rarely a result of radiation therapy per se. Usually these are due to tumor or the destruction of tumor areas by irradiation. However, poor positioning of the intracavitary applicator or overdosage may result in a fistula in the absence of cancer. This is not the fault of the methods but of the technique (Stryker et al., 1988).

Pelvic inflammatory disease is a contraindication to the use of either intracavitary cesium or x-rays, since it may be markedly activated or aggravated and lead to tubo-ovarian abscesses, septicemia, and, occasionally, death. If pyometra is found at the time of uterine curettage, it should be drained and antibiotics given until evidence of infection has subsided. If inflammatory tubo-ovarian masses are present, a preliminary salpingo-oophorectomy should be carried out prior to radiation therapy.

Vaginal stenosis may develop after radiation treatment. This may be prevented in younger women by frequent examinations and by breaking up the thin synechiae as they develop. Coitus will aid in keeping the vagina of normal size, and local application of an estrogen cream will prevent bleeding due to the changes that are inevitable with senescence. In older women the vagina usually closes off so that the cervix is no longer available for inspection or cytological examination. Although this causes the patient no difficulty, it prevents adequate follow-up by means of vaginal smears.

The use of x-rays may cause nausea and vomiting (radiation sickness) and depression of the bone marrow, with subsequent mild leukopenia. It is our practice to have a complete blood count performed once weekly during the period of x-ray therapy. Similarly, if severe nausea or vomiting develops during treatment, hospitalization is recommended, and phenothiazines and intravenous fluids are given. Skin hyperemia is an occasional result of x-ray therapy, and in some individuals with fair skin, blistering and ulceration may develop. Cessation of treatment for a few days and the use of a soothing ointment will usually permit adequate healing. The skin in these areas remains "tanned" for months, after which there is a gradual whitening with dilatation of capillaries, so that extensive telangiectasia may be evident. Use of the supervoltage technique has minimized this complication.

Other effects of radiation therapy include late small bowel obstruction and perforation, loss of libido, and menopausal symptoms. Bowel obstruction or perforation may occur as late as 10 years after therapy. More often the patient may note vague lower abdominal crampy pain, irregular bowel habits, and blood in the stool. Roentgenograms may give entirely normal findings, but exploration will reveal multiple loops of small bowel adherent to each other and to adjacent structures. In the more severe forms, arteriolar occlusion may result in localized areas of necrosis with perforation. It is well to remember this possible complication of radiation therapy in the differential diagnosis of an acute abdomen.

Loss of libido is not uncommon and may be prevented by a frank discussion of the problem

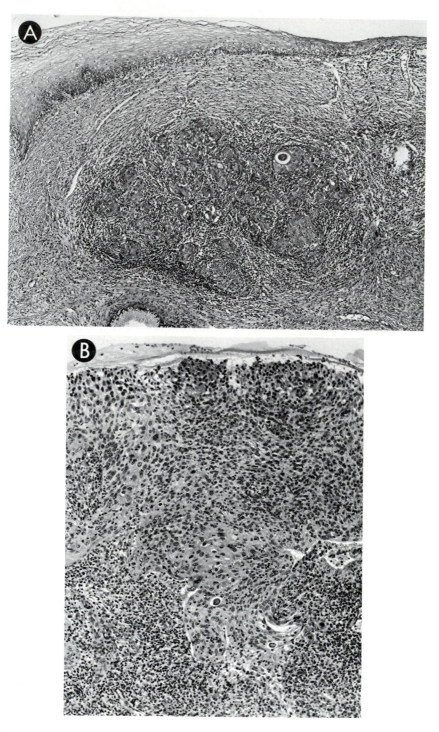

FIG 6–22.

A, microinvasive carcinoma underlying normal portio epithelium. No other areas of invasion could be found in this cervix. Carcinoma in situ from which this miniature cancer must have arisen was found in the endocervix. **B,** late stromal invasion characterized by a confluence of invasive buds into an inflamed stroma. The surface epithelium is absent on the right but overlying CIS is visible on the left.

with the patient during or at the conclusion of treatment. The use of estrogen creams to keep the vaginal mucosa soft and pliable has been mentioned. In addition, androgenic hormones in subvirilizing doses are frequently helpful. Hot flashes and sweats typical of the artificially induced menopause may be troublesome in some patients. Small doses of conjugated estrogens (Premarin, 0.625 mg) will relieve these symptoms and aid in the maintenance of a more normal extragenital endocrine balance. There is no evidence that such estrogenic therapy will bring about a recurrence of cervical cancer.

Appropriate Therapy Based on Clinical Staging

Stage Ia

Considerable controversy continues to surround microinvasive squamous carcinoma of the cervix, not only regarding the implication of the term microinvasion, but also as to what constitutes appropriate treatment. Microinvasive carcinoma has been defined by some as invasion to 3 to 5 mm below the basement membrane (Fig 6–22), whereas others state that microinvasion applies to lesions no greater than 1 mm in depth and that all other lesions should be considered frank invasion. The Society of Gynecologic Oncologists has proposed the following definition: A microinvasive lesion should be defined as one in which neoplastic epithelium invades the stroma in one or more places to a depth of 3 mm or less below the base of the epithelium and in which lymphatic or vascular involvement is not demonstrated. When this definition is used, the risk of lymph node involvement is less than 1%. Therefore, a total extrafascial abdominal hysterectomy without lymph node dissection may be considered adequate treatment for stage Ia disease (Seski et al., 1977).

Although the Oncology Committee of FIGO in 1985 redefined stage Ia cervical cancer (see Table 6–3), no extended clinical follow-up of this definition is available, relating treatment and subsequent outcome. Therefore, most clinicians are still using the cutoff of 3 mm as a deciding point for radical vs. nonradical treatment. Furthermore, preliminary data indicate that cone biopsy may be sufficient therapy when invasive squamous cell carcinoma is limited to less than 3 mm; however, core biopsy is not yet viewed as established therapy for stage Ia disease. Microinvasion can also be treated with intracavitary radioactive sources alone (7,000 to 9,000 rad in one or two insertions). However, since many of these patients are young, surgical treatment is preferable to allow normal ovarian function to be maintained.

Stages Ib and IIa

In these stages either irradiation or radical surgery can be elected, since equally good results are obtained with either modality. Surgery has been preferred in young women because it allows ovarian conservation (the tumor rarely metastasizes to the ovaries) and causes less dyspareunia than does radiation therapy. Survival using either technique is about 85% to 90% for stage Ib and about 75% for stage IIa. The general medical status of the patient must be carefully evaluated before radical surgery is undertaken. Obesity is a major selection factor in that it renders dissection deep in the pelvis extremely difficult.

Bulky endocervical carcinoma (barrel-shaped cervix) has a high incidence of central recurrence, pelvic and periaortic metastases, and distant dissemination. Intracavitary radiation is unable to encompass all the cancer within a tumoricidal dose volume, and despite the use of external radiation, central recurrence is not uncommon. Therefore, an extrafascial total abdominal hysterectomy should be combined with external radiation in this setting (Piver and Chung, 1975).

Invasive cervical carcinoma, stage Ib, that is larger than 3 cm is associated with a high incidence of pelvic node involvement and poor prognosis. It is equally important to note the size of the cervical lesion within a given stage, since this has also been shown to be of prognostic value. Van Nagell et al. (1979) found that for stage I lesions more than 2 to 5 cm in diameter, the failure rate was 24% for surgery but only 11% for radiation. In one large series of women treated by radical hysterectomy, Piver and Chung (1975) reported a 5-year survival of 85% for stage Ib lesions up to 3 cm in diameter but only a 66% survival for tumors 4 to 5 cm in diameter. These studies would suggest that stage I lesions larger than 3 cm are best treated with radiation therapy.

Radical hysterectomy for stages Ib and IIa is an extensive operation. It involves wide resection of the paracervical and vaginal tissues to the lateral pelvic side walls and to the floor of the pelvis. This requires dissection of the ureters to their insertion in the bladder, mobilization of the bladder neck as well as of the rectum to allow for extensive parametrial excision, and bilateral pelvic lymphadenectomy. Operative mortality is less than 1% in most series, but the morbidity rate approaches 35% to 45%. The commonest complication is temporary paralysis of the urinary bladder, and it has become evident that the more radical the surgery, the more serious will be the impairment of bladder function. Although usually not permanent, the urinary stasis often results in chronic cystitis, ureteritis, and pyelonephritis. Some patients have permanent bladder paralysis but learn to control micturition by developing a semiautomatic bladder that will empty itself with the aid of voluntary abdominal pressure. Another serious complication is the development of urinary fistulas, usually of the ureterovaginal type. These occurred in 7% of the patients operated on by Meigs (1944) and in 19% in the series of Barber and Brunschwig (1966). With better patient selection, improved surgical techniques, and the addition of suction drainage, the incidence of these complications has been reduced to less than 2% in most series.

The policy of treatment for invasive carcinoma of the cervix (stages I and IIa) at the Joint Center of Radiation Therapy at the Harvard Medical School combines intracavitary and external radiation. Intracavitary radium giving 8,000 rad divided in two applications is either followed or preceded by 3,500 to 4,000 rad of external parametrial irradiation. A 15 by 15 cm portal is sufficient for stages Ib and IIa. A variety of applicators may be used for radium insertion, but we have found the Fletcher-Suit afterloading applicator particularly helpful.

Stages IIb, III, and IVa

Patients with these stages of cervical carcinoma are best treated with radiation therapy techniques, since adequate dissection beyond the boundaries of tumor is not technically possible. An 18 by 15 cm portal for external radiation encompassing the common iliac nodes and the cephalad half of the vagina is employed. Stage IIb is treated with 3,500 to 4,000 rad of whole-pelvis irradiation along with 1,000 rad of additional parametrial irradiation followed in 2 weeks by one or two intracavitary radium insertions to 5,000 to 6,000 rad. The 5-year survival rate for stage IIb is 60% to 65%.

Stage III is treated with 4,000 to 5,000 rad of whole-pelvis irradiation plus 1,000 to 1,500 rad to one or both pelvic walls followed by intra-cavitary radium to 5,500 to 6,500 mg-hour. The 5-year survival rate for stage III ranges from 25% to 40%.

Patients with stage IVa (bladder or rectal invasion) can be treated with either high-dose whole-pelvis external irradiation and intracavitary sources or with pelvic exenteration.

Recurrent Cervical Carcinoma

Cancer of the cervix, when it recurs, usually does so within 2 to 3 years of primary treatment. Symptoms may include vaginal bleeding, bloody discharge, hematuria, dysuria, constipation, melena, pelvic and leg pain, and fistulas. If sacral backache or pain of sciatic distribution occurs, it is invariably due to invasion of the sacral plexus by tumor. Costovertebral angle and flank pain may herald the development of ureteral obstruction and pyelonephritis. There is usually associated lassitude, anorexia, weight loss, and anemia.

Diagnosis may be simplified by routine cytologic studies on follow-up examination, since tumor cells may be detected before symptoms develop. This, of course, is applicable to recurrence in the vagina and cervix only, since tumor in the pelvic nodes or broad ligament will not exfoliate tumor cells. In most cases the diagnosis depends on an evaluation of symptoms and a careful pelvic examination. Progressive firm nodularity in the paracervical and uterosacral area, felt best on rectal examination, is usually pathognomonic of viable tumor. The anatomical sites of treatment failure in carcinoma of the cervix correlate closely with tumor stage. Cervical or vaginal vault (central) recurrences should always be confirmed by biopsy. Computed axial tomography is useful for defining tumor in enlarged lymph nodes and distant metastases. Abnormalities on the excretory urogram, such as the development of hydroureter and hydronephrosis, suggest periureteral compression by tumor—although radiation fibrosis may on occasion produce the same condition—and may be amenable to surgical correction by means of ureteral implantation or urinary diversion.

Central recurrences are extremely rare in stages Ib and IIa. The usual cause of failure in patients with stage IIIb is parametrial infiltration that could not be controlled with external irradiation. In recent years, better local control has been achieved than in the past as a result of improved radiation technique. However, because of the high incidence of distant metastases in patients with stage III and IV cervical carcinoma, the development of adequate adjuvant therapy is needed to improve their prognosis. Local vault recurrence after radical surgery can be treated with radiation therapy with a salvage rate of about 50% (Deutsch and Parsons, 1974). Usually recurrences after either surgery or radiation are too extensive to be treated with radiation alone. The usual type of recurrence includes spread to the vesicovaginal septum, bladder, rectum, and pelvic and central portion of the parametrium. Surgical therapy for this type of spread requires a multivisceral pelvic resection, commonly known as an exenteration. Before performing exenteration, one must explore carefully to determine the status of disease beyond the pelvis, including aortic and pelvic lymph nodes. If the tumor has spread to the lymph nodes or involves the parametrium with extension to the side walls, the cancer is considered inoperable. Morley (1984) reported on the use of pelvic exenteration for treating recurrent cervical cancer. Of more than 90 patients, 75% were treated with total pelvic exenteration; the remainder were treated with either resection of the bladder anteriorly or excision of the bowel posteriorly, depending on the location of the tumor. The 5-year survival rate for recurrent carcinoma of the cervix in his series was 63%.

Ureteral compression either in the pelvis or near the kidney, with uremia, pyelonephritis, or both, is a major cause of death and is found in about 50% of patients. Other causes of death are infection (peritonitis, pelvic abscess, septicemia), uncontrolled hemorrhage, and extrapelvic metastases. Patients treated for cardiac failure will sometimes have severe pulmonary edema together with edema of the arms and neck. Usually, there is a plethora of the face and neck. This entity is due to superior vena caval obstruction from metastatic cervical cancer.

In 13% of deaths from cancer of the cervix the cause was gastrointestinal tract involvement, usually manifesting itself as large bowel obstruction, particularly at the rectosigmoid level. Occasionally, perforation of the large or small bowel results in fatal peritonitis. Jaundice caused by extensive hepatic metastases may be noted terminally.

Chemotherapy

A variety of single agents have been employed in the treatment of women with recurrent cervical carcinoma, with cisplatin yielding the highest response rates. In general, the response rates obtained with combination chemotherapy have been higher (Jobson et al., 1981), with a similarly increased risk of toxicity. Several combinations that have included cisplatin have demonstrated response rates in excess of 75%. Unfortunately, the durations of response have been dismally short, 4 to 6 months in most series. Since many of the patients have undergone radiation therapy, which compromises bone marrow function, or have impaired renal function, the ability to deliver adequate chemotherapy is often diminished.

Chemotherapy has also been used as a radiosensitizer to enhance the effect of radiation therapy. Piver et al. (1974) reported significantly improved survival among patients with stage IIb and IIIb disease when hydroxyurea was used along with radiation therapy compared with a placebo and radiation therapy alone.

The excellent response rates achieved with combination chemotherapy in women with recurrent disease and the clear relationship between tumor volume and survival have suggested the potential role of upfront chemotherapy to achieve chemocytoreduction prior to conventional radiation therapy or radical surgery. Virtually all investigators reporting their experiences with this neoadjuvant approach have noted dramatic shrinkage of tumor and a high incidence of pathological complete responses in those women undergoing radical surgery following chemotherapy. Whether this neoadjuvant technique will result in improved long-term survival is still unclear (Benedetti et al., 1988).

CARCINOMA OF THE CERVIX IN PREGNANCY

Carcinoma of the cervix complicates pregnancy in approximately 0.01% of patients. Therapeutic decisions are based on the stage of the cancer, the duration of the pregnancy, and the wishes of the mother. Although pregnancy does not appear to have a detrimental effect on the course of the disease, it is essential that the diagnosis be made promptly, since delay in treatment can alter prognosis.

Prior to the third trimester, treatment for the malignancy is carried out according to the stage of disease. For stage I and IIa lesions, radical hysterectomy with pelvic lymph node dissection is acceptable therapy. If radiation therapy is planned, the uterus may be evacuated at the time of the first radium application, or whole-pelvis irradiation may be started. If abortion does not occur, surgical evacuation of the uterus follows the completion of external irradiation at the time of radium application.

For patients in the late second trimester, therapy may be delayed until fetal viability is assured. For stage I and IIa lesions, a classic cesarean section is performed, followed immediately by radical hysterectomy and pelvic lymph node dissection. In more advanced stages, external radiation is delivered after cesarean section. This usually requires a delay of 7 to 10 days until the abdominal incision has healed. After completion of the radiation therapy, intracavitary radiation is employed as outlined earlier for the appropriate stage.

CLEAR CELL ADENOCARCINOMA OF THE CERVIX

Adenocarcinoma of both the cervix and the vagina in women with a median age of 19 years has been found to be associated with maternal ingestion of diethylstilbestrol (DES). As of June 30, 1985, 519 cases of clear cell carcinoma of the cervix or vagina have been identified by the Registry for Research on Hormonal Transplacental Carcinogenesis of the University of Chicago (Senekjian and Herbst, 1987).

Treatment for cervical adenocarcinoma is similar to that outlined for squamous cell carcinoma of the cervix. However, because of the young age of these women, the preferred therapy is radical hysterectomy and pelvic lymph node dissection in patients with stage I and IIa disease. Ovarian conservation is maintained, and if the vagina is involved, vaginectomy followed by reconstruction is performed and provides excellent functional results.

The overall survival for women with DES-associated clear cell carcinoma is 80%. In cases of stage I disease, the 5-year survival exceeds 90%.

Most recurrences of clear cell carcinoma are within 3 years of the initial treatment. Pulmonary and supraclavicular nodal metastases are more frequent when compared with squamous cell carcinoma of either the cervix or the vagina. If there is local recurrence without side wall involvement,

pelvic exenteration may be considered. If either aortic or pelvic nodes are involved, exenteration is contraindicated (Knapp, 1984).

REFERENCES

Abdul-Krim FW, Nunez C: Cervical intraepithelial neoplasia after conization: A study of 522 consecutive cervical cones. *Obstet Gynecol* 1985; 65:77.

American Cancer Society: *Cancer Facts and Figures, 1988*. New York, American Cancer Society, 1988.

Am Coll Obstet Gynecol Newslett 1988; 32(2):1.

Anderson MD, Hartley RB: Cervical crypt involvement by intra-epithelial neoplasia. *Obstet Gynecol* 1980; 55:546.

Ayre JE: Selective cytology smear for diagnosis of cancer. *Am J Obstet Gynecol* 1947; 53:604.

Barber HRK, Brunschwig A: Results of the surgical treatment of recurrent cancer of the endometrium, in Lewis GC Jr, Wentz WB, Jaffe RM (eds): *New Concepts in Gynecological Oncology*. Philadelphia, FA Davis Co, 1966.

Bearman DM, et al: Papanicolaou smear history of patients developing cervical cancer: An assessment of screening protocols. *Obstet Gynecol* 1987; 69:151.

Benedetti PP, Scambia G, Greggi S, et al: Neoadjuvant chemotherapy and radical surgery in locally advanced cervical carcinoma: A pilot study. *Obstet Gynecol* 1988; 71:344.

Bergeron C, et al: Multicentric human papillomavirus infections of the female genital tract: Correlation of viral types with abnormal mitotic figures, colposcopic presentation and location. *Obstet Gynecol* 1987; 69:736.

Blaustein A (ed): *Pathology of the Female Genital Tract*, ed 2. New York, Springer-Verlag New York, 1982.

Borken M, Friedman EA: Duration of colposcopic changes associated with *Trichomonas vaginitis*. *Obstet Gynecol* 1979; 51:111.

Boyes DA, et al: The results of treatment of 4,389 cases of preclinical cervical squamous carcinoma. *J Obstet Gynaecol Br Comm* 1978; 77:769.

Broders AC: Carcinoma grading and practical application. *Arch Pathol* 1926; 2:376.

Buchsbaum HJ: Extrapelvic lymph node metastases in cervical carcinoma. *Am J Obstet Gynecol* 1979; 133:814.

Buckley CH, et al: Cervical intraepithelial neoplasia. *J Clin Pathol* 1982; 35:1.

Bulmer D: The development of the human vagina. *J Anat* 1957; 91:490.

Burke L: The use of the carbon dioxide laser in

the therapy of cervical intrepithelial neoplasia. *Am J Obstet Gynecol* 1982; 144:337.

Buxton EJ, et al: Residual disease after cone biopsy: Completeness of excision and follow-up cytology as predictive factors. *Obstet Gynecol* 1987; 70:529.

Christopherson WM, Gray LA: Dysplasia and preclinical carcinoma of the uterine cervix: Diagnosis and management. *Semin Oncol* 1982; 9:265.

Chung CK, et al: Histologic grade and prognosis of carcinoma of the cervix. *Obstet Gynecol* 1981; 57:636.

Coppleson M, Reid BL: *Preclinical Carcinoma of the Cervix Uteri*. New York, Pergamon Press, 1967.

Creasman WT, et al: Results of outpatient therapy of cervical intraepithelial neoplasia. *Obstet Gynecol* 1981; 12:5306.

Dawson ME: Cervicitis. *Clin Obstet Gynecol* 1981; 8:201.

Deutsch M, Parsons JA: Radiotherapy for carcinoma of the cervix recurrent after surgery. *Cancer* 1974; 34:205.

Ferenczy A: Anatomy and histology of the cervix, in Blaustein A (ed): *Pathology of the Female Genital Tract*, ed 2. New York, Springer-Verlag New York, 1982.

Ferenczy A, et al: Latent papillomavirus and recurring genital warts. *N Engl J Med* 1985; 313:784.

Fluhmann CF: Developmental anatomy of the cervix uteri. *Obstet Gynecol* 1960; 15:62.

Fluhmann CF: *The Cervix Uteri and Its Diseases*. Philadelphia, WB Saunders Co, 1961.

Forsberg JG: Origin of vaginal epithelium. *Obstet Gynecol* 1965; 25:787.

Forsberg JG: Estrogen, vaginal cancer, and vaginal development, *Am J Obstet Gynecol* 1972; 113:83.

Forsberg JG: Cervicovaginal epithelium: Its origin and development. *Am J Obstet Gynecol* 1973; 115:1025.

Gagnon F: Contribution to the study of the etiology and prevention of cancer of the cervix and of the uterus. *Am J Obstet Gynecol* 1950; 60:516.

Galloway DA, McDougall JK: The oncogenic potential of herpes simplex viruses: Evidence for a "hit and run" mechanism. *Nature* 1983; 302:22.

Garite TJ, Feldman MJ: An evaluation of cytologic sampling techniques: A comparative study. *Acta Cytol* 1978; 22:13.

Gissmann L, zurHausen H: Partial characterization of viral DNA from human genital warts (condylomata acuminata). *Int J Cancer* 1980; 25:605.

Goodman HM, Butlar CA, Niloff JM, et al: Adenocarcinoma of the uterine cervix: prognostic factors and patterns of recurrence. *Gynecol Oncol* (in press).

Grunebaum AN, et al: Association of human papillomavirus infection with cervical intraepithelial neoplasia. *Obstet Gynecol* 1983; 62:448.

Handley WS: The prevention of cancer. *Lancet* 1936; 1:987.

Heller PB, et al: Cervical carcinoma found incidentally in a uterus removed for benign indications. *Obstet Gynecol* 1986; 67:187.

Hellman LM, et al: Some factors influencing the proliferation of the reserve cells in the human cervix. *Am J Obstet Gynecol* 1954; 67:899.

Howard L, et al: A study of the incidence and histogenesis of endocervical metaplasia and intraepithelial carcinoma. *Cancer* 1951; 4:1210.

Huffman J: Mesonephric remnants in the cervix. *Am J Obstet Gynecol* 1948; 56:233.

Jobson VW, et al: Chemotherapy of advanced carcinoma of the cervix with cyclophosphamide and cis-platinum. *Proc Am Soc Clin Oncol* 1981; 22:475.

Johnson LD, et al: The histogenesis of carcinoma in situ of the uterine cervix: A preliminary report of the origin of carcinoma in situ in subcylindrical cell anaplasia. *Cancer* 1964; 17:213.

Josey WE, et al: Genital infection with type II herpesvirus hominis. *Am J Obstet Gynecol* 1968; 101:718.

Kessler II: Human cervical cancer as a venereal disease. *Cancer Res* 1976; 36:783.

Kessler II: Etiological concepts in cervical carcinogenesis. *Gynecol Oncol* 1981; 12:57.

Knapp RC: Clear cell carcinoma of the vagina, in Heintz APM, Griffiths CT, Trimbos JB (eds): *Surgery in Gynecological Oncology*. The Hague, Martinus Nijhoff Co, 1984, p 30.

Koff AK: Development of the vagina in the human fetus. *Contrib Embryol Carnegie Inst* 1933; 24:54.

Kolstad P, Klem V: Long term followup of 1,121 cases of carcinoma in situ. *Obstet Gynecol* 1976; 48:125.

Koss LG, Durfee GR: Unusual patterns of squamous epithelium of uterine cervix: Cytologic and pathologic study of koilocytotic atypia. *Ann NY Acad Sci* 1956; 63:1235.

Koss LG: Current concepts of intraepithelial neoplasia in the uterine cervix (CIN). *Appl Pathol* 1987; 5:7.

Langman J: *Medical Embryology*. Baltimore, Williams & Wilkins Co, 1981.

Lorinez AT, Lancaster WD, Kurman RJ, et al: Characterization of human papillomaviruses in cervical neoplasias and their detection in routine clinical screening, in Peto R, zurHausen H (eds): *Viral Etiology of Cervical Cancer.* Banbury Report 21, New York, Cold Spring Harbor Laboratory, 1986.

Lubicz S, et al: Significance of cone biopsy margins and the management of patients with cervical neoplasia. *J Reprod Med* 1984; 29:179.

MacDonald-Burns DC: *Chlamydia* and other genital pathogens. *Clin Obstet Gynecol* 1981; 8:215.

Maier RC, Norris HJ: Glassy cell carcinoma of the cervix. *Obstet Gynecol* 1982; 60:219.

Meigs JV: Carcinoma of the cervix: The Wertheim operation. *Surg Gynecol Obstet* 1944; 78:1.

Meisels A, et al: Condylomatous lesions of the cervix: II. Cytologic, colposcopic, and histopathologic study. *Acta Cytol* 1977; 21:379.

Morley GW: Pelvic exenteration in the treatment of recurrent cervical cancer, in Heintz APM, Griffiths CT, Trimbos JB (eds): *Surgery in Gynecological Oncology.* The Hague, Martinus Nijhoff Co, 1984, p 174.

Mounts P, Shah KB: Respiratory papillomatosis: Etiological relation to genital tract papillomavirus. *Prog Med Virol* 1984; 29:90.

Nahmias AJ, Sawanabani S: The genital herpescervical cancer hypothesis—10 years later. *Prog Exp Tumor Res* 1978; 21:117.

Nahmias AJ, et al: Perinatal risk associated with maternal genital herpes simplex infection. *Am J Obstet Gynecol* 1971; 110:325.

Oriel JD, et al: Infection of the uterine cervix with *Chlamydia trachomatis. J Infect Dis* 1978; 37:443.

Orr JW, et al: Surgical treatment of women found to have invasive cervical cancer at the time of total hysterectomy. *Obstet Gynecol* 1986; 68:353.

Paavonen J: Colposcopic and histologic findings in cervical chlamydial infection. *Obstet Gynecol* 1982; 59:712.

Piver MS, Chung WS: Prognostic significance of cervical lesion size and pelvic node metastases in cervical carcinoma. *Obstet Gynecol* 1975; 46:507.

Piver MS, et al: Hydroxyurea and radiation therapy in advanced cervical cancer. *Am J Obstet Gynecol* 1974; 120:969.

Piver MS, Barlow JJ: Para-aortic lymphadenectomy in staging patients with advanced local cervical cancer. *Obstet Gynecol* 1974; 43:544.

Plentl AA, Friedman EA: Clinical significance of cervical lymphatics, in *Lymphatic Systems of the Female Genitalia.* Philadelphia, WB Saunders Co, 1971, p 98.

Popkin DR: Treatment of cervical intraepithelial

neoplasia with CO_2 laser. *Am J Obstet Gynecol* 1983; 145:177.

Rawls WE, et al: Herpes virus type II: Association with carcinoma of the cervix. *Science* 1968; 161:1255.

Reagan JW, et al: Concepts of genesis and development in early cervical neoplasia. *Obstet Gynecol Surv* 1969; 24:860.

Rein M, Hart G: Gonococcal infection, in Top FH, Wehrle PF (eds): *Communicable and Infectious Diseases.* St Louis, CV Mosby Co, 1976, p 299.

Richart RM: A radioautographic analysis of cellular proliferation in dysplasia and carcinoma in situ of the uterine cervix. *Am J Obstet Gynecol* 1963; 86:925.

Richart RM: Influence of diagnostic and therapeutic procedures in the distribution of cervical intraepithelial neoplasia. *Cancer* 1966; 19:1635.

Rigoni-Stern in The Walton Report. *Can Med Assoc J* 1976; 114:2.

Rubio CA: A trap for atypical cells. *Am J Obstet Gynecol* 1977; 128:687.

Savage EW, et al: The effect of endocervical gland involvement on the cure rates of patients with cervical intraepithelial neoplasia undergoing cryosurgery. *Gynecol Oncol* 1982; 14:194.

Senekjian EK, Herbst AL: Update on DES exposure. *Contemp Obstet Gynecol,* February 1987.

Seski JC, et al: Microinvasive squamous carcinoma of the cervix. *Obstet Gynecol* 1977; 50:410.

Sevin BU, et al: Invasive cancer of the cervix after cryosurgery: Pitfalls of conservative management. *Obstet Gynecol* 1979; 53:465.

Song J: *The Human Uterus: Morphogenesis and Embryological Basis for Cancer.* Springfield, Ill, Charles C Thomas, Publisher, 1964.

Speroff L, Glass RH, Kase N: *Clinical Gynecologic Endocrinology and Infertility.* Baltimore, Williams & Wilkins Co, 1985.

Spriggs AI, Boddington MM: Progression and regression of cervical lesions: Review of smears from women followed without initial biopsy or treatment. *J Clin Pathol* 1980; 33:517.

Stryker JA, Bartholomew M, Velkley DE, et al: Bladder and rectal complications following radiotherapy for cervix cancer. *Gynecol Oncol* 1988; 29:1.

Syrjanen KJ: Current concepts of human papillomavirus infections in the genital tract and the relationship to intraepithelial neoplasia and squamous cell carcinoma. *Obstet Gynecol Surv* 1984; 39:252.

Taylor PT, et al: The screening Papanicolaou

smear: Contribution of the endocervical brush. *Obstet Gynecol* 1987; 70:734.

Townsend DE: Cryosurgery for cervical intraepithelial neoplasia. *Obstet Gynecol Surv* 1974; 34:828.

Townsend DE, Richart RM: Cryotherapy and carbon dioxide laser management of cervical intraepithelial neoplasia: A controlled comparison. *Obstet Gynecol* 1983; 61:75.

Van Nagell JR, et al: Therapeutic implications for patterns of recurrence in cancer of the uterine cervix. *Cancer* 1979; 44:2354.

Wagner AC, McElin TW: Colposcopy, in Sciarra JT (ed): *Gynecology and Obstetrics*. New York, Harper & Row, Publishers, 1984, vol 1, chapter 30.

Weitzman GA, et al: Endocervical brush cytology, an alternative to endocervical curettage? *J Reprod Med* 1988; 33:677.

Wentz WB, Reagan JW: Survival in cervical cancer with respect to cell type. *Cancer* 1959; 12:384.

Wentz WB, et al: Induction of uterine cancer with inactivated herpes simplex virus types I and II. *Cancer* 1981; 48:1783.

zurHausen H, et al: Viruses and the etiology of human genital cancer. *Prog Med Virol* 1984; 30:170.

7 The Uterine Corpus

Neil J. Finkler, M.D.

Andrew J. Friedman, M.D.

GENERAL CONSIDERATIONS

The noun uterus is of Latin derivation and is synonymous with the lay term womb. The Greek word hysteria, however, has come to have wide acceptance, especially with regard to surgical terminology, and the word hysterectomy is well known to nonmedical as well as medical personnel. Hysteria was, at one time, believed to be of uterine origin since this organ was considered the anatomic site of the human mind. As far as is known at present, however, the uterus serves one function: childbearing. Menstruation occurs only when the process of ovulation is not followed by successful fertilization and should not be regarded as a primary function.

The position and physiological characteristics of the uterus lead to the development of numerous irregularities, mostly in the form of abnormal bleeding. The uterine cavity is readily available for thorough investigation by dilatation and curettage (D&C), and this has become the commonest of all gynecological operations. Because of the facility for early and complete diagnosis, together with the intrinsic physical characteristics of the uterus, malignant disease of this organ is attended by a 5-year survival rate of at least 60%, a figure much superior to those for malignancy of the vulva, vagina, cervix, oviduct, and ovary.

The uterus consists of two portions: the corpus and the cervix. Attention will be given in this chapter to disease and physiological aberrations of the uterine corpus.

ANATOMY

The uterus (Fig 7–1) is a muscular, hollow organ that lies in the true pelvis between the bladder and rectum. Its measurements are usually stated to be 7 to 7.5 cm long, 4.5 to 5 cm wide, and 2.5 to 3 cm thick. The cephalic portion of the corpus is known as the fundus and is characterized by lateral flarings known as *horns,* or *cornua.* The oviducts enter the fundus in the region of these cornua and demarcate the fundus from the main body of the uterus. As the corpus approaches the cervix, it becomes narrowed, giving a somewhat triangular appearance when viewed from both the front and the side. This constricted area separates the corpus from the cervix and is known as the *isthmus.* The cavity of the corpus is continuous with that of the endocervix and vagina and has an average depth of about 6 cm and a capacity of 3 to 8 ml. When the cavity is viewed in frontal section, it appears triangular, with the base at the fundus and the two corners extending toward the orifices of the oviducts. In sagittal section the uterine cavity appears as a narrow cleft, whereas in transverse section it has the outline of a flattened ellipse.

The corpus possesses anterior and posterior surfaces, both of which are covered by visceral peritoneum. The anterior surface is slightly convex and, in the normally situated uterus, lies in contact with the most cephalad portion of the urinary bladder. As the uterine peritoneum approaches the region of the isthmus on the anterior uterine wall, it is reflected ventrally onto the bladder and then continues as the parietal layer. The narrow space between these layers of reflected peritoneum is known as the anterior cul-de-sac. A sagittal section through the normal female pelvis (Fig 7–2) will show that the anterior surface of the uterine isthmus is not covered by peritoneum. The posterior surface of the corpus is slightly convex and is completely invested with a peritoneal covering. Caudally this peritoneal envelope is

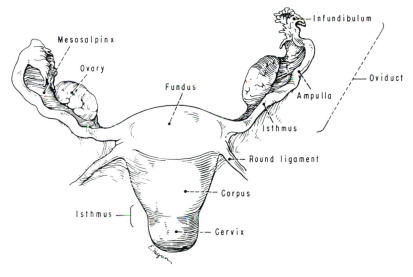

FIG 7–1.
Anterior view of uterus.

continued over the uterosacral ligaments, cervix, and upper portion of the posterior vaginal wall and is then reflected dorsally and cephalad over the rectum and lower sigmoid colon. The space between the reflected layers of peritoneum is known as the *pouch of Douglas,* or *posterior cul-de-sac.* It is of importance to the gynecologist because it is the most dependent portion of the pelvis. Blood or pus may be obtained by culdocentesis or drained through the vagina by incising the posterior cul-de-sac.

The anterior and posterior peritoneal coverings of the corpus join at the lateral uterine margin and form the leaves of the broad ligament (Fig 7–3). The peritoneal surfaces are in close proximity except where they diverge slightly to invest the round and infundibulopelvic ligaments. The broad ligament is, therefore, a double layer of peritoneum that extends from the lateral surface of the uterus outward to the pelvic wall. Its upper border consists of the peritoneal fold over the oviduct and the lateral extension from the

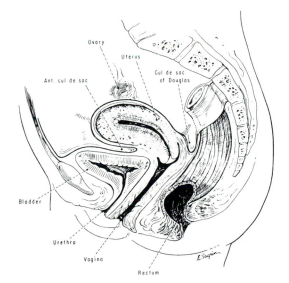

FIG 7–2.
Saggital section through pelvis.

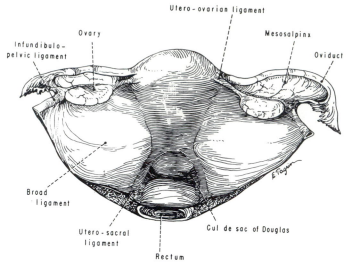

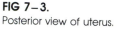

FIG 7–3.
Posterior view of uterus.

ovary encircling the infundibulopelvic vessels. The midportion encompasses the round ligament, and the most inferior portion is thickened and contains a condensation of connective tissue and muscle fibers called the *cardinal ligament* or *transverse cervical ligament of Mackenrodt*. The uterine vessels approach the lateral aspect of the cervix in the cardinal ligament, an anatomical point of importance in total hysterectomy.

The portion of the broad ligament between the ovary and the oviduct contains many small blood vessels and is termed the *mesosalpinx* or *tubal mesentery*. The vestigial remnants of the mesonephric tubules and duct are located within the leaves of the mesentery and are known as the *epoophoron* (lateral portion of the tubules) and the *paraoophoron* (medial portion of the tubules). All of these vestigial tubules are connected with the remnant of the mesonephric duct (Gartner's duct). The blind upper extremity of the duct is occasionally dilated into one or more cystic structures known as *hydatids of Morgagni*. Cysts may develop from the main duct or from one of the smaller tubules and may be confused with ovarian cysts at the time of pelvic examination.

The round ligaments consist principally of bands of muscle tissue that extend laterally from the anterolateral aspect of the fundus. They leave the peritoneal cavity through the internal inguinal ring, traverse the inguinal canal to the labia majora, and terminate by dissemination of fibers into the surrounding tissue. Although the round liga-

ments consist primarily of muscle fibers prolonged from the uterus, there is also an admixture of fibrous and areolar tissue, blood vessels, lymphatics, and nerves. The round ligaments are about 10 to 12 cm long and 0.5 to 0.75 cm thick and are covered by the anterior and posterior leaves of the broad ligament as far as the internal abdominal ring. In the fetus this duplication of peritoneum is prolonged as a short tubular process into the inguinal canal (canal of Nuck). It is generally obliterated in the adult, but occasionally it may persist and be the source of benign cystic structures that are frequently mistaken for hernias. Rarely, endometriosis occurs in this peritoneal projection.

The ligaments were formerly believed to play a major part in uterine support, particularly the maintenance of the normal anterior position. Numerous operations were devised that shortened these ligaments with the hope that this shortening would hold the fundus forward. The round ligaments may have some effect in returning the anterior uterus to its normal position after displacement by a full bladder or after pregnancy. They hypertrophy greatly during pregnancy and may be the source of localized lower quadrant pain, which may simulate that of acute appendicitis. The lymphatics that traverse the ligaments are occasionally the route of metastases to the groin from endometrial carcinoma.

The uterosacral ligaments arise from the posterior wall of the uterus at the level of the internal cervical os. They are made up of connective tissue and involuntary muscle and contain blood vessels, lymphatics, and nerve filaments of the parasympathetic and sympathetic systems. Each ligament describes a posterior arc, passing dorsally around the rectosigmoid inserting on the sacral wall at the level of the second and third sacral vertebrae. The peritoneum over the posterior uterine wall and cul-de-sac is reflected over the uterosacral ligaments throughout their course. The function of these ligaments is to exert tension on the cervix in a dorsal direction, in effect keeping the corpus anterior and the axis of the corpus and cervix at a right angle to the vagina. This prevents the uterus from assuming a position that would be in the axis of, and in direct line with, the vagina—a situation that is almost always associated with uterine prolapse.

The cardinal or transverse cervical ligaments (of Mackenrodt) have been mentioned as forming the inferior aspect or base of the broad ligament. They offer the chief support for the cervix and upper portion of the vagina and do so by integrating posteriorly with the uterosacral ligaments and anteriorly with the cervicovaginal portion of the endopelvic fascia. The cardinal ligaments are composed of muscle fibers and connective tissue that ensheath the uterine vessels, nerve fibers, and lymphatics. As they fan out laterally, the tissues of the ligaments insert into the fascia overlying the obturator muscles and the muscles of the pelvic diaphragm and, as pointed out by Anson and Curtis (1946), follow the course of the major vessels as a supporting framework. Careful dissection has shown that the effective dorsal fixation of the ligaments is provided by the perivascular fibrous tissue of the hypogastric and iliac vessels.

The utero-ovarian ligament (suspensory ligament of the ovary) extends from the lateral aspect of the uterus (between the round ligament and oviduct) to the inferior pole of the ovary. It consists of connective tissue and smooth muscle in a rounded cord and is ensheathed between layers of the broad ligament.

Uterine Structure

The uterus is composed of three separate and distinct layers: (1) the serosa, an outer peritoneal covering; (2) the myometrium, an inner layer of smooth muscle; and (3) the endometrium, the mucous membrane lining the cavity (Fig 7–4). The uterine serosa is continued laterally as the leaves of the broad ligament and is continued anteriorly and posteriorly as bladder and rectal reflections. The myometrium is composed of three rather indistinct layers of smooth muscle fibers. In each layer there is an interlacing and intermixture of the nonstriated muscle cells, which are held in juxtaposition by a connective tissue rich in elastic fibers. The outer muscular layer (stratum supravasculare) is chiefly longitudinal and is continuous with fibers entering the broad and round ligaments, whereas the middle layer is thicker and presents fibers in circular arrangement. The middle layer makes up the major portion of the myometrium and contains many blood vessels located between muscle bands (stratum vasculare). The inner layer represents an exaggerated muscularis mucosae and is composed of thin muscle strands

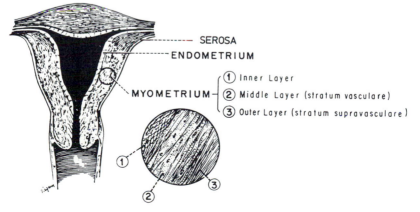

SEROSA
ENDOMETRIUM
① Inner Layer
MYOMETRIUM— ② Middle Layer (stratum vasculare)
③ Outer Layer (stratum supravasculare)

FIG 7–4.
Structure of uterus.

arranged obliquely and longitudinally. The arrangement of the blood vessels between muscle bundles affords an ideal method for hemostasis following delivery. This is borne out clinically by patients whose uteri are atonic following parturition and in whom hemorrhage often results.

The endometrium is a soft inner layer of variable thickness made up of simple tubular glands, a stroma of resting cells in fine connective tissue mesh, and a sensitive vasculature. The histology and physiological variations of this layer are considered in Chapter 3.

Blood Supply

Uterus

To understand the blood supply to the uterus, one must appreciate the blood supply and collateral circulation in the pelvis.

The abdominal aorta bifurcates at the L-4 level directly beneath the umbilicus. Before bifurcating, however, the aorta gives off two major branches: the ovarian arteries and the inferior mesenteric artery. Although the course of the right and left ovarian arteries differ somewhat, they both enter the infundibulopelvic ligament to supply the ovary and communicate with an arcade that anastamoses with uterine artery branches.

The common iliac arteries bifurcate into external and hypogastric (internal iliac) arteries. The hypogastric artery provides the major blood supply to the pelvis and continues through the ischiorectal fossa as the internal pudendal artery. The hypogastric artery is usually divided into an anterior and posterior trunk. The posterior division divides to give off the iliolumbar, lateral sacral, and superior gluteal arteries. The anterior trunk provides both visceral and parietal branches (Table 7–1). The uterus possesses a dual blood supply, receiving branches from both the uterine and ovarian arteries. The uterine artery is derived from the hypogastric anterior trunk (Fig 7–5). It crosses over the ureter at the level of the internal os of the cervix and divides into ascending and descending limbs. The former runs tortuously upward between the leaves of the broad ligament, giving horizontal anterior and posterior branches to the cervix and corpus. As it reaches the cornu, a branch is sent to the round ligament (artery of Samson) and then is projected along the oviduct to anastomose with the ovarian vessels in the mesosalpinx. The descending branch of the uterine artery turns inferiorly and supplies the vagina

TABLE 7–1.

Branches of the Hypogastric Artery

Anterior Division	Posterior Division
Visceral	Iliolumbar
Uterine	Lateral sacral
Superior vesical	Superior gluteal
Middle vesical	
Inferior vesical	
Middle hemorrhoidal	
Inferior hemorrhoidal	
Vaginal	
Parietal	
Obturator	
Inferior gluteal	
Internal pudendal	

from the lateral aspect. It anastomoses freely with the vaginal artery along its course.

The collecting veins from the corpus flow into two longitudinal trunks, which are usually distinct. The anterior surface is drained by the anterior uterine vein situated anterior to the ureter and lateral to the uterine artery. This vein empties into the hypogastric vein. The posterior uterine surfaces, however, drain into a short and long trunk that pass posterior to the uterus and inferior to the uterine artery before joining either the hypogastric or obturator vein.

As previously mentioned, the collateral circulation of the pelvis is luxurious. During hysterectomy, this collateral circulation may lead to difficulty obtaining hemostasis.

The collateral circulation of the pelvis includes arterial supply from the aorta, femoral artery, and external iliac artery communicating with branches of the hypogastric artery (Table 7–2). Ligation of the hypogastric artery has been employed to control pelvic hemorrhage. The main effect is to reduce the arterial pulse pressure to the anterior division of the hypogastric artery. Three major structures need be identified before proceeding with hypogastric artery ligation: the external iliac artery, ureter, and posterior division of the hypogastric artery. The ligation should take place distal to the posterior division takeoff and as close as possible to the origin of the uterine artery.

Endometrium

The processes of menstruation and pregnancy give singular importance to an understanding of the anatomical vascular pattern of the en-

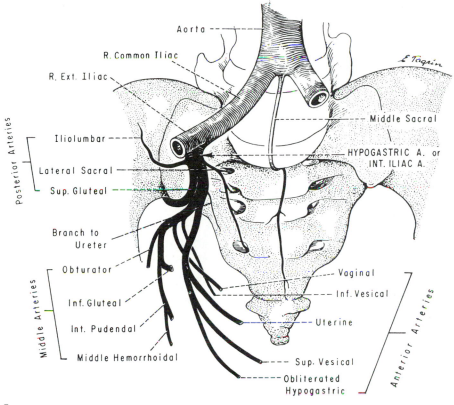

Aorta

R. Common Iliac

R. Ext. Iliac

L. Tagrin

Middle Sacral

Posterior Arteries

Iliolumbar

HYPOGASTRIC A. or INT. ILIAC A.

Lateral Sacral

Sup. Gluteal

Branch to Ureter

Middle Arteries

Obturator

Vaginal

Inf. Vesical

Inf. Gluteal

Uterine

Int. Pudendal

Anterior Arteries

Middle Hemorrhoidal

Sup. Vesical

Obliterated Hypogastric

FIG 7–5.
Divisions of the hypogastric artery.

dometrium. As previously mentioned, a series of radial arteries are given off at right angles from the uterine artery as it courses along the corpus (Fig 7–6). These radial arteries branch in the inner third of the myometrium into straight and spiral (coiled) vessels. The straight arteries pass

TABLE 7–2.
Collateral Circulation of Pelvis

Extrapelvic Source	Hypogastric Branch
Aorta	Uterine artery
Ovarian artery	Middle and inferior
Inferior mesenteric	hemorrhoidal arteries
artery (superior	Iliolumbar artery
hemorrhoidal)	
Lumbar and vertebral	
arteries	
Middle sacral artery	Lateral sacral artery
External iliac artery	Iliolumbar and superior
Iliac circumflex artery	gluteal arteries
Inferior epigastric gives	
rise to obturator in 25%	

only as far as the basal layer of the endometrium and terminate in capillaries in that region. The spiral arteries, however, follow a coiled course throughout the thickness of the endometrium, give off a few branches in the endometrium, then fork and give rise to superficial capillaries just below the surface epithelium. These capillaries form plexuses in the stroma and a meshwork around the glands. In the superficial layer of the endometrium, the capillaries form sinus-like dilatations known as *lakes*. The blood is returned via small veins, which drain these vascular lakes and capillary plexuses. It should be remembered that the vascular pattern is a dynamic one, with constant proliferation and regression. The specific morphological details are considered in the section on menstruation.

Although the prime function of the straight arteries is to supply the basal endometrium, they may also function to support regeneration of the lower portion of the functional layer. The coiled arteries alone supply blood to the superficial third of the endometrium and most of the blood to the

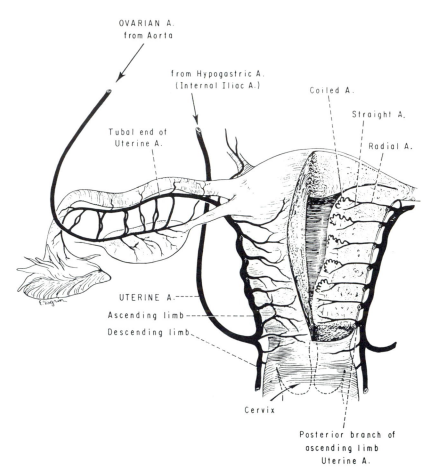

FIG 7–6.
Blood supply to the uterus.

middle third. Some straight arteries may be converted into coiled ones and then later to the straight type. Thus, it is possible that the blood supply of the endometrium could regenerate and develop specificity of function even after complete curettage.

The importance of the coiled arteries is not completely known. It should be pointed out, however, that they are absent or not fully developed in areas where extensive cyclic variations do not occur. Thus, in the lower uterine segment and lateral recesses of the endometrium, the vascular supply is mostly through straight arteries.

Nerve Supply

The uterine extrinsic nerve supply is derived from three sources (Fig 7–7):

1. Motor fibers from the upper sympathetic thoracic ganglia course through the aortic plexus and the celiac ganglion to the superior hypogastric plexus. Fibers then diverge as they pass caudally to form the inferior hypogastric plexus, then forward over the lateral surface of the rectal ampulla to join the pelvic plexus or cervical ganglion of Frankenhauser. From this plexus, fibers pass along the uterosacral ligament to the smooth muscle of the uterus. Clinical evidence indicates that the motor fibers to the uterus leave the spinal cord at levels higher than the 10th thoracic nerve.

2. Sensory fibers are special visceral afferents that run through the hypogastric and aortic plexuses, through the 11th and 12th sympathetic ganglia without synapse, into the dorsal spinal root ganglia of these segments, then up the dorsolateral fasciculus to the thalamus. The sensory sup-

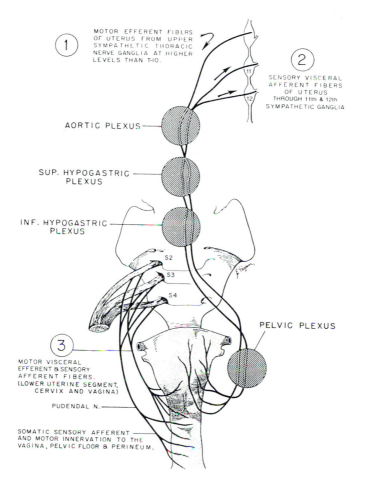

MOTOR EFFERENT FIBERS OF UTERUS FROM UPPER SYMPATHETIC THORACIC NERVE GANGLIA AT HIGHER LEVELS THAN T-10.

SENSORY VISCERAL AFFERENT FIBERS OF UTERUS THROUGH 11th & 12th SYMPATHETIC GANGLIA

AORTIC PLEXUS

SUP. HYPOGASTRIC PLEXUS

INF. HYPOGASTRIC PLEXUS

PELVIC PLEXUS

MOTOR VISCERAL EFFERENT & SENSORY AFFERENT FIBERS. (LOWER UTERINE SEGMENT, CERVIX AND VAGINA)

PUDENDAL N.

SOMATIC SENSORY AFFERENT AND MOTOR INNERVATION TO THE VAGINA, PELVIC FLOOR & PERINEUM.

FIG 7–7.
Nerve supply to the uterus.

ply to the cervix travels through the sacral parasympathetic chain communicating with the second, third, and fourth sacral nerves.

3. Sensory and motor fibers to the lower uterine segment and cervix are found in the sympathetic and parasympathetic plexuses, communicating with the second, third, and fourth sacral nerves. Visceral efferent fibers believed to be motor to the longitudinal muscle of the lower uterine segment and the circular fibers of the cervix and possibly inhibitory to the uterine fundus travel in the parasympathetic chain.

It should be remembered that although the sensory nerve fibers course through pelvic, hypogastric, and aortic plexuses before reaching the 11th and 12th thoracic nerves, they are functionally independent of the autonomic system. The

sensory supply to the cervix, although traversing the sacral parasympathetics, is also functionally independent of the autonomic system.

Lymphatic Supply

The lymphatics of the uterine corpus proceed in four or five channels through the broad ligament just below the oviducts, then upward along the ovarian vessels. In the course of their passage through the parametrium and ovarian ligament, they communicate with the ovarian lymphatics to terminate in the lumbar lymph nodes found in front of the aorta from its bifurcation to the diaphragm. The lymphatics from the lower uterine segment anastomose with adjacent lymph channels from the cervix and drain to the obturator, iliac, hypogastric, and sacral nodes. A third route of lymphatic drainage, especially from the fundal area, is via the round ligament to the superficial inguinal nodes.

UTERINE ANOMALIES

Congenital Anomalies

Müllerian anomalies result from defective fusion or absorption of the female reproductive system during embryonic life. Estimates of the incidence of müllerian anomalies are difficult to establish because the majority of patients with congenital anomalies do not exhibit clinical manifestations (Rock and Jones, 1977). Patients with symptomatic müllerian anomalies will usually have signs of obstruction or reproductive failure. Diagnostic methods of determining the exact nature of a müllerian anomaly have evolved from bimanual examination, postpartum manual exploration, and D&C to more sophisticated techniques of hysterography, laparoscopy, hysteroscopy, ultrasound, and magnetic resonance imaging (MRI). The increased ability of these latter techniques to obtain complete information will undoubtedly increase the reported incidence of the more subtle anomalies.

When reviewing the literature on reproduc-

tive tract anomalies, the clinician is often confused and frustrated by the lack of uniformity in the classification and reporting of müllerian anomalies. Many classification schemes have been proposed, some of which are too simple, some too complex. A useful classification system based on the degree of failure of normal development was proposed by Buttram and Gibbons in 1979. Figures 7–8 to 7–13 depict the six müllerian anomalies according to this classification. This section will discuss the effects of each of these anomalies on reproductive outcome and the treatment of each. For a discussion on the treatment of obstructing congenital anomalies, the reader is referred to Chapter 20.

In a review of 554 patients with class I müllerian anomalies, 8% had isolated vaginal agenesis (class I-A), 83% demonstrated vaginal-cervical-fundal agenesis (class I-E, often referred to as the Mayer-Rokitansky-Kuster-Hauser syndrome), and 9% exhibited androgen insensitivity syndrome (often referred to as testicular feminization syndrome; Buttram, 1983). Estimates of the incidences of the class I-A anomaly and androgen insensitivity syndrome are 1 of 75,000 and 1 of 50,000 phenotypic-appearing females, respectively.

Although rare, patients with class I-A anom-

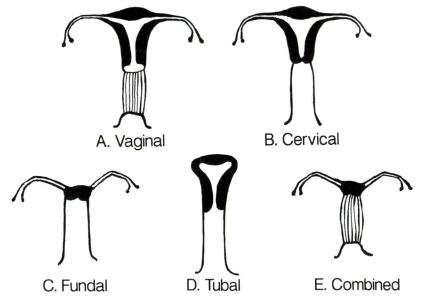

A. Vaginal   B. Cervical

C. Fundal   D. Tubal   E. Combined

FIG 7–8.
A–E, congenital uterine anomalies. Class I: müllerian agenesis or hypoplasia. (From Buttram VC Jr, Gibbons WE: Mullerian anomalies: A proposed classification (an analysis of 144 cases). *Fertil Steril* 1979; 32:40. Reproduced by permission.)

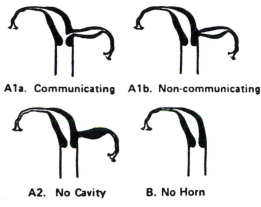

A1a. Communicating   **A1b. Non-communicating**

A2. No Cavity   **B. No Horn**

FIG 7 – 9.
Congenital uterine anomalies. Class II: unicornuate uterus. (From Buttram VC Jr, Gibbons WE: Mullerian anomalies: A proposed classification (an analysis of 144 cases). *Fertil Steril* 1979; 32:40. Reproduced by permission.)

alies may be treated by creation of an artificial vagina (i.e., McIndoe procedure) with good success in restoring menses and achievement of pregnancy. However, most patients with suspected class I-A anomalies will have associated uterine or cervical abnormalities.

Patients with class I-E anomalies comprise the second largest subpopulation of patients presenting with primary amenorrhea (gonadal dysgenesis is the commonest etiology). Although fertility is not possible in this group of patients, sexual intercourse may be possible by creation of an artificial vagina by dilator therapy (Frank, 1938), vaginal reconstruction (McIndoe procedure; McIndoe, 1950), or the Williams vulvovagino-

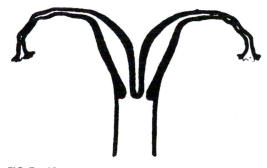

FIG 7 – 10.
Congenital uterine anomalies. Class III: Uterus didelphys. (From Buttram VC Jr, Gibbons WE: Mullerian anomalies: A proposed classification (an analysis of 144 cases). *Fertil Steril* 1979; 32:40. Reproduced by permission.)

plasty (Capraro and Gallego, 1976). Pure cases of cervical agenesis (class I-B), fundal agenesis (class I-C), and tubal agenesis (class I-D) are exceedingly rare.

In a review of the literature published since 1959 on class II anomalies (i.e., unicornuate uterus), Buttram (1983) reported a 33% spontaneous abortion rate, a premature delivery rate of 29%, with a live birth rate of 66%. However, many patients in these reviewed series may actually have had class III anomalies (i.e., uterus didelphys). In a review of 31 patients with true class II anomalies experiencing 60 pregnancies, there were 40% live births, 17% premature deliveries, and 48% spontaneous pregnancy losses occurring in the first and second trimesters (Buttram, 1983).

Resection of a noncommunicating horn-containing endometrium (i.e., class II-A1b) is recommended to prevent the development or spread of endometriosis. Patients with communicating horns (i.e., class II-A1a) may benefit from uterine unification (i.e., Strassmann procedure; Strassmann, 1961), excision of the horn, or expectant management depending on the size of horn and associated symptoms. Ectopic pregnancies in patients with noncommunicating uterine horns (i.e., classes II-A1b and II-A2) due to transperitoneal migration of sperm or fertilized ova have been reported and frequently result in catastrophic rupture of the rudimentary uterine horn (O'Leary and O'Leary, 1963).

Although limited data are available, it appears as though reproductive outcome in patients with uterus didelphys (class III) is similar to that noted in patients with unicornuate uteri (class II). In a series of 124 pregnancies, 55% resulted in a live birth, with a 43% abortion rate and 45% premature deliveries (Buttram, 1983). Because of the "acceptable" fetal salvage rate and the difficulty of a uteroplasty, surgical therapy is rarely performed. Suggested therapeutic modalities for this anomaly, without documented efficacy, include a modified Strassmann procedure and cervical cerclage (Gros et al., 1974; Strassmann, 1966). Of note is that sagittal vaginal septa appear concurrently with uterus didelphys approximately 75% of the time.

The bicornuate uterus (classes IV-A and IV-B) is impossible to distinguish from the septate uterus (classes V-A and V-B) by hysterography. Unless two distinct horns can be palpated at pelvic examination, laparoscopy or, occasionally, ul-

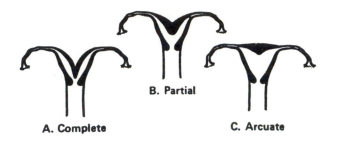

B. Partial

A. Complete   C. Arcuate

FIG 7–11.
A–C, congenital uterine anomalies. Class IV: bicornuate uterus. (From Buttram VC Jr, Gibbons WE: Mullerian anomalies: A proposed classification (an analysis of 144 cases). *Fertil Steril* 1979; 32:40. Reproduced by permission.)

trasound (Worthen and Gonzalez, 1984) is necessary to distinguish these two classes of müllerian anomalies. Unfortunately, many older series group both bicornuate and septate uteri together when discussing reproductive outcome. In a review of 110 patients with known bicornuate uteri, 57% of pregnancies resulted in live births, 35% ended in spontaneous abortion, and 23% delivered prematurely. The Strassmann procedure is appropriate treatment for symptomatic patients with bicornuate uteri. Vaginal septa are seen in less than 5% of patients with bicornuate uteri.

The arcuate uterus (class IV-C), defined as a small convex indentation of the upper uterine cavity with or without an indented external uterine contour, is considered a variant of a normal uterus. The true arcuate uterus is not associated with infertility or pregnancy loss and, thus, should not be treated surgically.

Except for anomalies associated with in utero diethylstilbestrol (DES) exposure, septate uteri (class V) are the commonest müllerian anomalies. The rate of pregnancy loss is extremely high in this group and is approximately double that for class IV patients. In combined series, approximately two third of conceptions terminated in abortion, one third delivered prematurely, and 28% resulted in live births (Buttram, 1983). It has been hypothesized that poor blood supply to the uterine septum may be the cause of such a high abortion rate. Accordingly, the chance of reproductive failure is higher the more complete the septum. Approximately 25% of patients with septate uteri have associated sagittal vaginal septa.

Fortunately, fetal salvage rates range between 70% and 90% in patients treated surgically (Buttram, 1983; McShane et al., 1983). The Tompkins metroplasty, Jones wedge procedure, and, more recently, hysteroscopic division of the uterine septum (Daly et al., 1983; DeCherney et al., 1986; Perino et al., 1987; Valle and Sciarra, 1986) are appropriate surgical treatments for patients with symptomatic septate uteri. In properly selected patients, hysteroscopic metroplasty is a shorter, simpler operation with less trauma, lower morbidity, and decreased recovery time and cost and has an increased opportunity for a vaginal delivery than abdominal metroplasty (i.e., Tompkins or Jones procedures; Fayez, 1986).

In patients with müllerian anomalies in

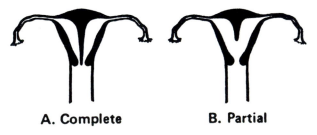

A. Complete   B. Partial

FIG 7–12.
A and **B,** congenital uterine anomalies. Class V: septate uterus. (From Buttram VC Jr, Gibbons WE: Mullerian anomalies: A proposed classification (an analysis of 144 cases). *Fertil Steril* 1979; 32:40. Reproduced by permission.)

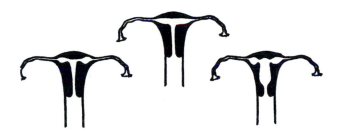

FIG 7–13.
Congenital uterine anomalies. Class VI: DES anomalies. (From Buttram VC Jr, Gibbons WE: Mullerian anomalies: A proposed classification (an analysis of 144 cases). *Fertil Steril* 1979; 32:40. Reproduced by permission.)

classes I-V, 31% demonstrated abnormalities on intravenous pyelograms (IVPs; Buttram and Gibbons, 1979). The commonest abnormality was unilateral renal agenesis, usually found on the ipsilateral side of the associated müllerian agenesis or hypoplasia. There appears to be no increase in structural urological abnormalities on IVP examination in patients with septate uteri.

Between the late 1940s and 1970, approximately 2 to 3 million women received DES during pregnancy, exposing 1 to 1.5 million female offspring in utero (Stillman, 1982). The degree of reproductive failure in in utero–exposed females is directly correlated with the dosage of DES used during pregnancy (Barnes et al., 1980). In a series of 267 DES-exposed women undergoing hysterosalpingography (HSG; Kaufman et al., 1980), 69% demonstrated upper genital tract abnormalities. A significant relationship was found between abnormal HSG findings and structural abnormalities of the cervix and vaginal epithelium. Of all women with abnormalities in uterine contour, 31% demonstrated small T-shaped cavities, 19% had normal-sized T-shaped cavities, 13% exhibited small cavities ("hypoplastic uterus"), 6% showed T-shaped cavities with constriction, 5% demonstrated small cavities with constriction, 4% had constriction alone, and 8% had other assorted anomalies (Kaufman et al., 1980).

Of all DES-exposed women, viable birth rate was significantly lower in women demonstrating abnormal uterine contours by HSG when compared with those with normal-appearing uterine cavities (Kaufman et al., 1980). In addition, women with abnormal HSGs had a higher incidence of ectopic pregnancies, spontaneous abortions, and premature deliveries than women with normal x-ray findings. In combined series totaling 579 pregnancies in DES-exposed women, the ectopic pregnancy rate was 5.4%, the spontaneous abortion rate 27%, the premature delivery rate 28%, and the viable birth rate 63%. In addition to an increased incidence of poor pregnancy outcome, considerable debate exists as to whether or not DES-exposed women have a higher rate of both primary and secondary infertility when compared with unexposed controls.

The incidence of second trimester abortions is higher in DES-exposed women than in those with other müllerian anomalies. Kaufman et al. (1980) reported a 19% first trimester abortion rate and a 12% second trimester pregnancy loss rate in DES-exposed patients. Such rates suggest that if prophylactic cervical cerclage is efficacious in any patient exhibiting a müllerian anomaly, it should be most effective in those with DES changes. Currently, no surgical procedure will restore normal uterine contour in DES-exposed women demonstrating abnormal uterine shape.

Acquired Anomalies

Asherman's Syndrome

Asherman's syndrome is the partial or complete obliteration of the uterine cavity by adherence of the uterine walls due to scarring. It is associated with menstrual abnormalities, particularly amenorrhea or hypomenorrhea, infertility, and recurrent abortion. Although first described in 1894 by Heinrich Fritsch in a patient who developed secondary amenorrhea after curettage for delayed postpartum hemorrhage, the syndrome acquired worldwide attention following Asherman's original publication in 1948.

The incidence of Asherman's syndrome is difficult to determine. It has been estimated to comprise 1.7% of all women experiencing secondary amenorrhea (Jones, 1964). The diagnosis is frequently made by HSG findings (Fig 7–14), but hysteroscopy is the most accurate method of detection (March et al., 1978).

Curettage performed on a gravid or recently gravid uterus is the commonest cause of Asherman's syndrome. In combined series evaluating predisposing factors in patients with intrauterine adhesions, 91% of cases were associated with pregnancy-related curettage. In 67% of cases, Asherman's syndrome developed after postabortion curettage, in 22% after postpartum curettage, in 2% after cesarean section, and in less than 1% following molar evacuation (Schenker and Margalioth, 1982). Many investigators have hypothesized that gestational changes bring about softening of the uterus, making it more difficult to gauge the depth of curettage. The resultant denudation of the basalis layer favors adhesion formation over endometrial regeneration. Other rare causes of Asherman's syndrome include infection (i.e., genital tuberculosis), myomectomy, metroplasty, and curettage performed on a nonpregnant uterus.

Symptoms of Asherman's syndrome include menstrual and fertility dysfunction. Amenorrhea, present in 37% of patients (Schenker and Margalioth, 1982), may result when adhesions oc-

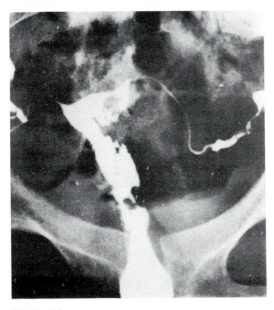

FIG 7–14.
Severe Asherman's syndrome noted on hysterosalpingogram. (From Toaff R, Ballas S: Traumatic hypomenorrhea-amenorrhea (Asherman's syndrome). *Fertil Steril* 1978; 30:379. Reproduced by permission.)

clude the cervix or obliterate the entire uterine cavity. Hypomenorrhea, seen in 31% of patients (Schenker and Margalioth, 1982), may occur with partial cervical or cavitary obliteration. Dysmenorrhea and menometrorrhagia are also occasionally present. Only 6% of patients with diagnosed Asherman's syndrome had normal menses.

Infertility is the commonest presenting symptom in patients with Asherman's syndrome and is seen in 43% of cases of intrauterine synechiae (Schenker and Margalioth, 1982). Infertility secondary to Asherman's syndrome is frequently accompanied by menstrual abnormalities. The two most commonly theorized reasons for infertility due to intrauterine adhesions include interference with sperm transport and embryo implantation.

Approximately 14% of patients with Asherman's syndrome present with recurrent pregnancy losses (Schenker and Margalioth, 1982). Repeated abortions have been attributed to defective endometrial vascularization and growth near the site of nidation and to decreased uterine cavity size.

In patients with Asherman's syndrome who conceive, there is a high incidence of complications. Premature labor, placenta accreta, placenta previa, and postpartum hemorrhage are not uncommon, especially in patients who have undergone treatment for intrauterine synechiae (Friedman et al., 1986; Jewelewicz et al., 1976). Placenta accreta is thought to occur when defective basalis, due to the original endometrial insult as well as the treatment, allows abnormal trophoblastic penetration. The incidence of gravid hysterectomies is high in patients who exhibit abnormal placentation and postpartum hemorrhage.

Asherman's syndrome may be diagnosed by hysterography or hysteroscopy (see Fig 7–14). Many investigators believe that hysterography can only suggest the diagnosis and that hysteroscopy must be performed for confirmation.

Treatment of Asherman's syndrome requires surgical removal of intrauterine adhesions with simultaneous prevention of new adhesion formation. Methods of adhesion removal include abdominal hysterotomy, hysteroscopic lysis of adhesions, and D&C. Where possible, hysteroscopic treatment is preferable because of its associated lower morbidity and cost when compared with the abdominal approach. Because of the high risk of uterine perforation when a vaginal procedure is performed, it is recommended to perform concurrent laparoscopy.

Following removal of intrauterine adhesions, many surgeons insert an intrauterine stent, such as an intrauterine device or Foley catheter to separate the uterine walls in an effort to prevent new adhesion formation. Postoperative treatment with high-dose estrogen therapy, followed by progestin withdrawal, is also often used to facilitate endometrial proliferation over previously scarred areas. The use of antibiotics and steroids are less consistently employed in the prevention of postoperative intrauterine synechiae. To date, no randomized series has been performed evaluating the efficacy of these postoperative adjuvant measures.

Results of surgical therapy are excellent in the restoration of normal menstrual function and good in patients presenting with fertility problems. In combined series totaling 1,586 patients treated for Asherman's syndrome, 84% had restoration of normal menses, 11% had hypomenorrhea, and 5% suffered from amenorrhea (Schenker and Margalioth, 1982). In patients presenting with infertility, 51% conceived, resulting in 55% term births, 9% premature deliveries, 25% abortions, and 9% ongoing at the time of the reports (Schenker and Margalioth, 1982). Placenta accreta occurred in 9% of deliveries, with other severe complications occurring in 3% of treated patients. The prognosis of patients with Asherman's syndrome is related to the degree of endometrial obliteration. In patients with extensive intrauterine synechiae, restoration of fertility and normal menstrual function is more difficult to achieve.

LEIOMYOMAS

Uterine leiomyomas, commonly known as fibroids, are well-circumscribed, nonencapsulated benign tumors. They are composed mainly of smooth muscle and contain varying amounts of fibrous tissue. Other synonyms for these tumors include fibromyoma, fibroma, myofibroma, and myoma.

Incidence and Etiology

Leiomyomas are the commonest solid pelvic tumors in women, occurring in 20% to 25% of women in their reproductive years (Novak and Woodruff, 1979; Robbins and Cotran, 1979). It is currently accepted that leiomyomata are unicellular in origin (Townsend et al., 1970). Although factors responsible for the initial neoplastic transformation of a myometrial cell are not well understood, clinical observations and animal data suggest that an estrogenic milieu may be necessary. In humans, leiomyomas arise only during the reproductive years; de novo formation of these tumors is seldom, if ever, seen prior to puberty or following menopause. In a guinea pig model, multiple leiomyomas may be produced following prolonged estrogenic stimulation (Lipshultz, 1942; Nelson, 1937).

Once leiomyomatous neoplastic change has occurred, it appears as though various hormones may impact on their growth. Estrogenic effects on leiomyoma growth have been most extensively studied. It is not uncommon to note growth of these tumors during pregnancy and regression following menopause. Several investigators have demonstrated a higher intramyoma estrogen environment when compared to myometrium of the same uterus (Farber et al., 1972; Otubu et al., 1982; Pollow et al., 1978; Soules and McCarty, 1982; Wilson et al., 1980). Treatment of premenopausal women with leiomyomas with gonadotropin-releasing hormone (GnRH) agonists induces a hypoestrogenemic pseudomenopausal state and consistently causes shrinkage of both uterine and leiomyoma volumes (Friedman et al., 1987; Maheux et al., 1985). Data on the relationship of other hormones (progesterone, growth hormone, human placental lactogen, androgens) to leiomyoma pathogenesis are scant and inconclusive. It is likely that hormonal stimulation of leiomyoma growth involves growth factors (i.e., epidermal growth factor, insulin-like growth factor I), although more research is needed to clarify this point.

Leiomyomas are characterized by their location in the uterus (Fig 7–15). Subserosal leiomyomas are located just under the uterine serosa and may attach to the corpus by a narrow or broad base. Intramural leiomyomas are found predominantly within the thick myometrium but may distort the cavity or cause an irregular external uterine contour. Subserosal and intramural leiomyomas comprise the majority of all leiomyomas. Submucous leiomyomas comprise 5% of all leiomyomas (Novak and Woodruff, 1979) and are located just under the uterine mucosa (endometrium). These may also attach to the uterine corpus by a narrow or broad base. Other types of lei-

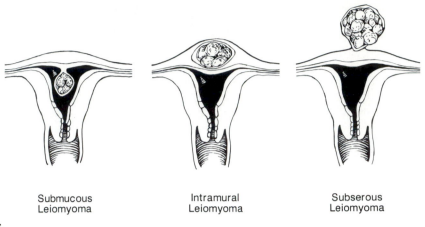

Submucous
Leiomyoma
Intramural
Leiomyoma
Subserous
Leiomyoma

FIG 7–15.
Leiomyomas classified according to their location in the uterus.

omyomas include "parasitic" myomas, which receive their blood supply from structures other than the uterus (i.e., omentum), and seedling myomas, which are smaller than 4 mm in greatest diameter.

Pathology

The gross appearance of a leiomyoma is somewhat variable, but in general the tumor is circumscribed and well demarcated from the surrounding muscle. A pseudocapsule, which is merely flattened uterine muscle that has become compressed as the size of the tumor increases, is present. The consistency is usually firm or actually hard, except in cases in which degeneration or hemorrhage has occurred. The color is light gray or pinkish white, depending on the degree of vascularity. When the leiomyoma is cut across, the tissue will usually project above the level of the surrounding myometrium. When viewed in the fresh state, the smooth muscle bundles can usually be identified in a pattern of intertwining or whorl-like arrangement.

The microscopic appearance of a leiomyoma is usually rather characteristic, in that the nonstriated muscle fibers are arranged in bundles of varying sizes running in multiple directions (Fig 7–16), giving the pattern noted grossly. High-power examination reveals the spindle-shaped cells to have elongated nuclei, which are, for the most part, of uniform size and staining quality. Connective tissue elements of varying amounts may be noted between the muscle cells. In certain tumors the amount of the connective tissue element may be excessive, in which case the term *fibromyoma* may be more descriptive.

Degenerative changes may occur, the commonest being hyalinization and cyst formation. These changes are due to diminished vascularity of the connective tissue element, so that the detail of connective tissue fibers is lost. The hyalin material presents no cellular detail, stains deeply with eosin, and may show remnants of muscle bundles interspersed between the homogeneous matrix. If the hyalinized connective tissue undergoes liquefaction necrosis, cystic degeneration then occurs. The cysts may then become filled with a gelatinous material that oozes forth when the tumor is cut across. This may be followed, especially in long-standing cases, by focal areas of calcification. In postmenopausal women, these calcified leiomyomas may be evident on x-ray examination. Another type of degeneration is that known as *acute red degeneration,* occasionally seen as a complication of pregnancy. In this situation, the cut surface simulates raw meat, this carneous change being due to hemorrhage into a partially hyalinized leiomyoma. This hemorrhagic complication is the result of accumulation of blood in the tumor because of venous obstruction and may occur during the rapid growth associated with pregnancy or immediately postpartum, when the venous drainage is occluded. Acute red degeneration of leiomyomas has also been reported in association with the use of massive medroxyprogesterone acetate (Depo-Provera) therapy in the treatment of endometriosis.

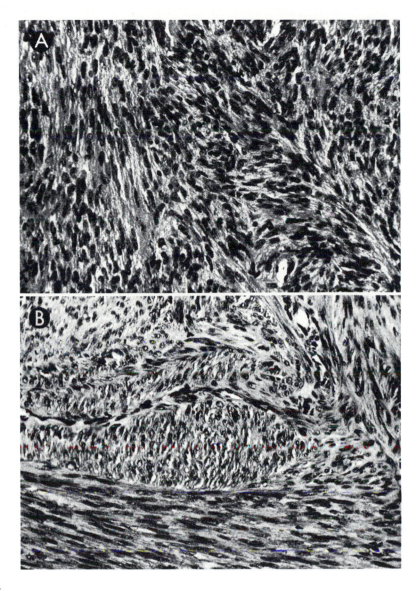

FIG 7–16.
A, high-power view of leiomyomas, showing typical structure. The tumor is composed of groups of smooth muscle cells arranged in twists and whorls in an interlacing pattern. It is relatively avascular. **B,** higher power shows cellular detail. The smooth muscle fibers in the central portion have been cut across their long axes. Note uniform appearance and lack of mitoses.

Symptoms

It is estimated that between 20% and 50% of women with leiomyomas experience tumor-related symptoms (Babknia et al., 1978; Hunt and Wallach, 1974; Ingersoll, 1963). Menorrhagia is a common symptom, occurring in approximately 30% of women undergoing myomectomy (Buttram and Reiter, 1981). Although the incidence of menorrhagia may not be affected by the presence of submucous leiomyomas, the severity of bleeding may be increased when submucous fibroids are present (Malone and Ingersoll, 1975; Rubin and Ford, 1974).

Approximately 34% of patients in combined series evaluating preoperative symptoms of patients undergoing myomectomy experienced pelvic pain or pressure (Brown et al., 1967; Counseller and Bedard, 1937; Finn and Muller, 1950; Loeffler and Noble, 1970; McCormick, 1958; Miller and Tyrone, 1933; Munnell and Martin, 1951; Ranney and Frederick, 1979). Most patients with leiomyomas who experience pelvic pain have some other pelvic disease such as salpingitis, endometriosis, diverticulosis, or ovarian carcinoma. In pregnancy, pelvic pain may occur if leiomyomas undergo degeneration. Pelvic pressure may also be accompanied by urinary frequency and, less commonly, constipation.

A review of reported cases of myomectomy, in which preoperative abortion rates were recorded, revealed that 441 (41%) of 1,063 pregnancies ended in spontaneous abortion (Buttram and Reiter, 1981). Although these statistics describe a selected population, it is likely that leiomyomas are associated with a significantly increased risk of abortion.

A number of other symptoms associated with leiomyomas are infrequently encountered. Uterine leiomyomas alone are an infrequent cause of infertility. Polycythemia has been reported in a patient with fibroids with autonomous production of erythropoietin by a leiomyoma (Weiss et al., 1975). Ascites, hydronephrosis, and bowel obstruction due to leiomyoma impingement on pelvic and abdominal structures have also been reported (Buttram and Reiter, 1981).

Sarcomatous transformation of leiomyomas is a rare but potentially lethal complication of uterine fibroids. It is estimated to occur in approximately 0.1% of women with leiomyomas (Buttram and Reiter, 1981) and is more frequently seen in large or rapidly growing myomas (Baggish, 1974; Hannigan and Gomez, 1979; Novak and Woodruff, 1979).

Diagnosis

The diagnosis of leiomyomas is usually easily made by bimanual examination. The uterus is enlarged, is often irregular, and may be palpated abdominally above the symphysis. Ultrasound, magnetic resonance imaging (MRI) and computed tomography (CT) may be useful in confirming the diagnosis, although these modalities may not distinguish between leiomyomas and adenomyomas. In patients experiencing menorrhagia or recurrent pregnancy losses, hysterography, with both anteroposterior and cross-table lateral views, may be useful. Finally, laparoscopy and hysteroscopy can aid in definitive diagnosis.

Treatment

The primary therapeutic approach in patients with large or symptomatic leiomyomas is surgical. Hysterectomy is the commonest operative technique used to treat this disorder. In the United States, approximately 175,000 hysterectomies are performed yearly for leiomyomas, making this diagnosis the commonest indication for hysterectomy (Easterday et al., 1983). Hysterectomy, the only true "cure" for leiomyomas, is often recommended in patients presenting with a uterus greater than 12-week gestational size, although it is important to individualize the choice of therapy.

In women wishing to preserve childbearing potential, a myomectomy may be performed. Approximately 18,000 myomectomies are performed yearly in the United States (National Center for Health Statistics, 1987). Myomectomy may diminish menorrhagia in roughly 80% of patients presenting with this symptom (Buttram and Reiter, 1981). It is essential to inform a patient undergoing myomectomy that there is a significant risk of recurrence of leiomyomas following myomectomy. In combined series, it is estimated that 15% of patients will develop symptomatic fibroids following myomectomy and that 10% will require a second major operative procedure (i.e., second myomectomy or hysterectomy; Buttram and Reiter, 1981). Approximately 18% of women undergoing myomectomy will require blood transfusion, and the need for transfusion is greater in women with large fibroids.

Gonadotropin-releasing hormone agonists induce a hypoestrogenic pseudomenopausal state and are a recent development in the medical approach to the treatment of leiomyomas. Because fibroids are dependent on estrogen for their development and growth, induction of a hypoestrogenic state will cause shrinkage of these tumors and myometrial mass. Uterine volume has been shown to decrease by 50%, on average, after 3 months of GnRH agonist therapy (Friedman et al., 1987, 1988). In addition, treatment with a GnRH agonist will induce amenorrhea, allowing women with menorrhagia-induced anemia to increase iron stores and hemoglobin concentrations significantly (Friedman et al., 1988). However, cessation of GnRH agonist treatment results in an increase in leiomyomas and uterine size to pretreatment volume within 3 to 6 months in the majority of women (Friedman et al., 1987). Currently, it is not recommended to treat with GnRH agonists for more than 6 months because of the potential development of osteoporosis in treated women. Thus, GnRH agonists may be useful as a preoperative treatment when decreasing uterine and fibroid size and inducing amenorrhea are important goals of therapy. By increasing hemoglobin concentrations in previously anemic women, this therapy may allow some women to donate autologous blood should the need for transfusion arise intraoperatively or postoperatively.

Androgenic agents (e.g., danazol, gestrinone) and progestins (e.g., medroxyprogesterone acetate, depo-medroxyprogesterone acetate, norethindrone) have also been used to control menorrhagia in women with leiomyomas. These medications do not consistently decrease uterine or fibroid volume, however. The combination of a medical and surgical approach to women with leiomyomata is still relatively new and requires further study.

ADENOMYOSIS

Adenomyosis is a benign uterine disease in which endometrial glands and stroma are found within the myometrium. This invasion by the endometrium induces hypertrophy and hyperplasia of the myometrium, producing a diffusely enlarged uterus.

Incidence and Etiology

The diagnosis of adenomyosis can be made only on microscopic examination of a hysterectomy specimen. For this reason, the exact incidence is not known. It is generally estimated that 20% of women have adenomyosis. However, when careful analysis of multiple myometrial sections is performed, the incidence may be as high as 65% (McElin and Bird, 1974).

Adenomyosis is associated with childbearing. It is estimated that at least 80% of women with this disorder are parous (Israel and Woutersz,

1959; McElin and Bird, 1974; Molitor, 1971; Wee and Bryan, 1963). However, the incidence of adenomyosis is not correlated with increasing parity. Adenomyosis most commonly produces symptoms in women between the ages of 40 and 50 years (McElin and Bird, 1974).

Although the exact etiology is unknown, the most accepted theory of histogenesis was proposed by Meyer in 1900. Meyer postulated that the normal barrier between the endometrium and myometrium that prevents intrusion of endometrial glands and stroma is somehow attenuated. Following alteration of this barrier, invasion of the endometrium occurs under the influence of estrogen stimulation.

Adenomyosis is commonly found in the same uterus in which other pathology is discovered. More than 80% of women with adenomyosis will have another pathologic process in their uteri. Fifty percent of patients with adenomyosis had associated leiomyomas. Approximately 11% of patients with adenomyosis will also have endometriosis, and 7% will have endometrial polyps (Bird and McElin, 1981). Often, the symptoms of the associated condition will obscure the diagnosis of adenomyosis.

Pathology

The typical uterus with adenomyosis is boggy and uniformly enlarged. Approximately 80% of uteri with adenomyosis weigh more than 80 gm, but it is unusual for a uterus containing only adenomyosis to exceed 200 gm.

When incised, the uterus containing adenomyosis bulges and assumes a convex configuration. The thickening of the uterine wall is seen to be made up of coarsely trabeculated areas, stippled or granular in appearance, with small yellow or darker cystic points, which may contain serous fluid or old blood. Close inspection of the cut surface will frequently reveal an irregularity of the endomyometrial junction with foci of down-dipping basalis. Although the pathologist usually has no difficulty in making a diagnosis of adenomyosis by gross examination of the cut specimen, the surgeon cannot approach this degree of accuracy with the uterus in situ. He may, however, suspect the disease if a focal area of adenomyosis is mistaken for a leiomyoma and a myomectomy attempted. Areas of adenomyosis do not shell out or lend themselves to easy excision.

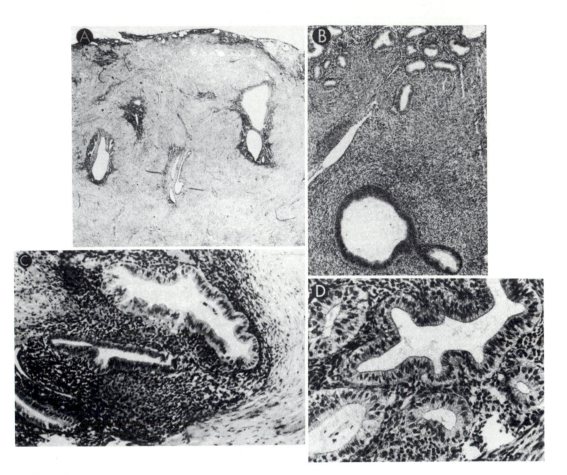

FIG 7–17.
A, typical adenomyosis in the wall of the uterus. Foci of basal type endometrium are located deep in the myometrium. The myometrium surrounding the areas of adenomyosis shows a whorled appearance similar to that seen in leiomyoma. (From Hertig AT, Gore HM: Tumors of the vulva, vagina and uterus, in *Tumors of the female sex organs:* part 2; section 9, fasc 33, *Atlas of Tumor Pathology.* Washington, DC, Armed Forces Institute of Pathology, 1960. Reproduced by permission.) **B,** higher power of an area of adenomyosis showing cystic dilatation. The basal endometrium is at the top. **C,** adenomyosis in which the glandular element at the top right has undergone anaplasia. The glands are surrounded by typical endometrial stroma. **D,** adenomyosis showing secretory effect.

Microscopic Appearance

The pathognomonic feature of this disease is the occurrence of endometrial tissue, glands, and stroma within the myometrium (Fig 7–17), at least one low-power field (some authors demand two) from the endomyometrial junction. The misplaced endometrial tissue is similar to that of the basalis of the endometrial cavity and therefore does not always respond to hormonal stimulation. Occasionally, however, secretory change may be noted, or there may be cystic or adenomatous hyperplasia. In several studies, a functional response in the aberrant endometrium was found in only about 50% of the cases in which the normally located endometrium was functional. Decidual changes in the stroma of adenomyotic areas have been noted during pregnancy and spontaneous ruptures of these areas have been reported. Symptoms of dysmenorrhea or constant pelvic pain might be anticipated if areas of adenomyosis demonstrated functional capacity, with edema and bleeding. The cause of symptoms in patients whose uteri do not show functioning areas of adenomyosis is unknown.

Malignant neoplasia may rarely occur in the glands, stroma, or both, about 30 malignant adenomyomas having been reported. These may be in the form of adenocarcinoma, sarcoma, or carcinosarcoma.

The myometrium is usually altered in uteri with extensive adenomyosis so that a surrounding zone of hypertrophy-hyperplasia is usually recognizable. Phagocytized hemosiderin may be seen deep in the myometrium, indicating previous extravasation of blood.

If the process of adenomyosis has extended into the cornua of the uterus and then laterally into the isthmic portion of the oviduct, a process indistinguishable from salpingitis isthmica nodosa (except that inflammatory cells are usually present in the latter condition) may develop.

Symptoms

Adenomyosis most commonly produces symptoms in women between the ages of 40 and 50 years. Approximately 60% of women experience abnormal uterine bleeding, with 50% demonstrating hypermenorrhea and 25% manifesting metrorrhagia. The depth of penetration of endometrial glands and stroma into the myometrium is not correlated with the occurrence of hypermenorrhea (Bird et al., 1972). However, hypermenorrhea is more commonly seen in women with increased density of endometrial elements within the myometrium noted on microscopic examination.

Dysmenorrhea is the second commonest symptom in patients with adenomyosis, occurring in 25% of women (Bird and McElin, 1981). The incidence of dysmenorrhea is correlated with the depth of penetration and density of endometrial elements within the myometrium.

Diagnosis

A review of the literature demonstrates that only 15% of instances of adenomyosis are correctly diagnosed preoperatively. The reasons for this low percentage are twofold: (1) many, if not most patients with adenomyosis only are asymptomatic; and (2) the presence of adenomyosis is often overshadowed by associated pathology (i.e., leiomyomas, endometriosis).

Dilatation and curettage does not aid in diagnosis. Pelvic ultrasound may be suggestive but is not definitive. The role of nuclear MRI is not defined at this time.

Treatment

The only definitive treatment for adenomyosis is total hysterectomy, with or without ovarian conservation. Synthetic progestins are not helpful and may actually increase pelvic pain in some patients. The use of GnRH agonists has been used in a small number of cases, resulting in a decrease in uterine size and amenorrhea. Unfortunately, this treatment is only temporary; regrowth of the uterus and return of symptoms usually occur within 6 months of cessation of therapy.

ENDOMETRIAL POLYPS

Endometrial polyps are hyperplastic overgrowths of glands and stroma of rather localized extent that form a projection above the surface. Such polyps may be sessile or pedunculated and rarely show foci of neoplastic growth.

The prevalence of polyps has been estimated between 10% and 24% of women undergoing endometrial biopsy or hysterectomy (Van Bogaert, 1988). Endometrial polyps are rarely seen in women less than age 20 years. The incidence of these polyps rises steadily with increasing age, peaks in the fifth decade of life, then gradually declines following the menopause.

The commonest symptom noted in women with endometrial polyps is metrorrhagia, occurring in 50% of symptomatic women. In addition, postmenstrual spotting is not uncommon. Less commonly noted symptoms include menorrhagia, postmenopausal bleeding, and breakthrough bleeding while on hormonal therapy. Overall, endometrial polyps account for 25% of abnormal bleeding in both premenopausal and postmenopausal women (Van Bogaert, 1988).

The diagnosis is often made on microscopic examination of a specimen obtained after thorough D&C. Hysterography is rarely helpful when polyps are small but may be suggestive as a smooth space occupying lesion when the polyp is large. Hysteroscopy with directed biopsy is particularly helpful in the diagnosis of small intracavitary polyps.

The commonest histological finding in endometrial polyps is proliferative endometrium, which is seen in 44% of women (Van Bogaert, 1988). Secretory endometrium, when present, is frequently out of phase. The incidence of adenomatous hyperplasia and adenocarcinoma has been reported in 0.6% of endometrial polyps (Van Bogaert, 1988).

The majority of patients with endometrial polyps are cured by thorough curettage. This is especially true in the postmenopausal age group. Therapy must be guided by the histological pattern of the polyp itself and of the endometrium. Hysterectomy must be performed if adenocarcinoma is noted, but progestin therapy may be useful in patients with adenomatous hyperplasia or proliferative endometrium. Finally, the use of estrogen-progestin combinations is often successful and may be the treatment of choice in younger women.

INFECTIONS

Infections of the uterine corpus are, for the most part, infections of the endometrium and are encompassed in the broad term *endometritis.* The commonest etiologic factors are infected abortions, parturition, gonorrhea, *Mycoplasma,* and *Chlamydia.* Certain office gynecological procedures may occasionally be followed by endometrial infection. These include biopsy and cauterization of the cervix, endometrial biopsy, hysterosalpingography, and tubal insufflation. Cervical stenosis subsequent to conization, cauterization, or irradiation may diminish or prohibit uterine drainage and be a predisposing factor in the etiology of pyometra.

Postabortal Infection

A most serious type of endometrial infection is that associated with septic abortions. This entity results from the introduction of pathogenic bacteria into the uterine cavity by a catheter, sound, curet, or pack. The conceptus and its membranes provide an ideal culture for growth of organisms, and the increased vascularity brought about by pregnancy permits rapid and widespread dissemination. The commonest bacteria identified from cultures are the nonhemolytic, anaerobic streptococci, enterococci *(Escherichia coli, Pseudomonas aeruginosa, Bacterium aerogenes)* and *Clostridium perfringens.* An increasing number of pathogenic staphylococci have also been identified. The pathological process usually begins as a necrotizing endometritis and deciduitis at the placental site with spread along the decidua and into the myometrium. Microscopically, there is an acute inflammatory exudate, the decidua contains leukocytes and plasma cells, and there is extensive necrosis and thrombosis of small vessels. The inflammatory process may extend into the myometrium, forming multiple small abscesses, and dissemination into small veins and lymphatics may be extensive. The myometrium appears pale and flabby and microscopically shows cytolysis and edema.

The signs and symptoms of an infected abortion are pelvic pain, vaginal bleeding, fever, and chills. A history of recent dilatation and evacuating usually aids in the diagnosis. Examination may reveal evidence of pelvic peritonitis with lower abdominal rigidity and rebound tenderness. The abdomen is usually distended because of ileus, and bowel sounds are hypoactive. Pelvic examination may disclose a cervical os that is soft and acutely tender, and the broad ligaments feel thickened in the acute phase and ligneous in later phases of the process. The temperature is elevated, usually more than 38.4° C, and there is tachycardia and leukocytosis.

Treatment

Treatment of endometritis must be individualized and based on history, clinical presentation, and laboratory findings. In general, the primary treatment of endometritis is medical management.

The workup of such patients should include pelvic ultrasound to rule out significant tubo-ovarian abscesses and retained products of conception. An ultrasound suggesting retained products of contraception requires formal D&C with evacuation of uterine contents.

Patients with elevated temperature and elevated white blood cell count or erythrocyte sedimentation rate or severe symptoms require IV hydration and IV antibiotics. Antimicrobial therapy is often begun on an empiric basis while results of initial blood cultures and cervical cultures for *Neisseria gonorrhoeae* are pending. The choice of antibiotic depends on clinical presentation, specific toxicities and allergies, and individual preferences. In general, broad-spectrum antibiotics should be initiated and tailored to culture reports. Multiple drug therapies are preferred over simple-drug therapies. The antibiotic experience with treating endometritis has followed the experience with pelvic inflammatory disease and tubo-ovarian abscesses (see the discussion of antibiotic therapy in pelvic inflammatory disease).

The timing and extent of surgical procedures

in patients with septic abortions were initially investigated by Neuwirth and Friedman (1963). In this early study, patients treated by antibiotics and IV hydration for the first 12 to 24 hours, followed by uterine evacuation, experienced less septic sequalae than patients treated by D&C first, followed by antibiotics. If retained products of conception are seen on ultrasound or are clinically suspected, evacuation of uterine contents will often improve symptoms and hasten the recovery.

Hysterectomy for septic complications of endometritis is generally reserved for patients who fail to improve after D&C and patients who clinically deteriorate on therapy.

Sequelae of inadequately treated endometritis include continued infection and lateral spread. Tubes and ovaries may become secondarily involved. Long-standing, untreated endometritis may lead to the development of septic pelvic vein thrombophlebitis. Prior to the days of legal abortion, septic abortions frequently went untreated for long periods of time. Development of septic emboli was common and often a cause of death.

Historically, bacteremia resulting from severe infection of the female reproductive tract was lethal. Although the use of modern antibiotics has made this occurrence less common, it remains a possible sequelae of septic abortion.

Septic shock may result from endotoxin or exotoxin, more frequently the former. Gram-negative endotoxic shock most commonly is found in association with *E. coli, Proteus, Klebsiella,* and *P. aeruginosa.* The pathophysiology and metabolic effects have been well described (Godsoe et al., 1988; Skowranski, 1988; Vadas et al., 1988).

Clinically, patients with septic shock may first demonstrate anxiety and slight disorientation. As the disease becomes manifest, shaking chills and hypotension may result. Patients appear cold and clammy, and nausea, vomiting, and oliguria or anuria may be present.

The treatment of septic shock is aimed at (1) maintaining volume and central venous pressure, (2) applying effective antibiotic therapy, and (3) identifying and removing the source of sepsis.

The use of intensive care units and invasive monitoring has greatly aided the treatment of septic shock. Widespread use of pressor support, vasodilators, and ionotropic agents has helped reduce mortality from septic shock. Controversy as to the use of naloxone (Nishijima et al., 1988; Roberts et al., 1988) or high-dose corticosteroids

(Schumer, 1976) in the management of septic shock still exists.

The clinician treating women in the reproductive years must be aware of the possible sequelae of septic abortions and must be able to recognize early signs of septic shock. The most important feature in successfully treating patients with septic abortion is early recognition and prompt, aggressive, treatment.

Tuberculosis

Tuberculosis of the female genital tract is uncommon in the United States and is usually an incidental finding at laparotomy for pelvic inflammatory disease or infertility. The diagnosis may be made by endometrial biopsy (Padubidri et al., 1980) and has also been reported on vaginal smears (Misch et al., 1976) and at laparoscopy (Sutherland, 1979).

Genital tuberculosis is said to occur in 3% to 8% of patients with pulmonary disease. Pelvic tuberculosis rarely occurs in infertile patients in the United States, although incidences as high as 5% to 10% in infertile patients have been reported in patients from Europe, Asia, and South America.

Sutherland (1985) reported a personal series of 710 women with pelvic tuberculosis between 1951 and 1985. The overall success rate in eradicating infection following treatment with isoniazid, rifampin, and ethambutol approached 90%. Surgical intervention was restricted to those patients who failed to respond to conservative management. Surgical treatment of choice is hysterectomy and bilateral salpingo-oophorectomy, although the adnexa may be spared in the young woman. Successful pregnancy outcome has occurred following treatment for pelvic tuberculosis (Sutherland, 1985).

ENDOMETRIAL HYPERPLASIA

The endometrium is remarkably prolific tissue with the potential for hyperplastic changes. Although the relationship between hyperplasia and the development of carcinoma of the endometrium is not firmly established, histological evidence suggests that some hyperplasias are premalignant lesions.

The majority of patients with endometrial hyperplasias present with abnormal uterine bleeding. A history of abnormal bleeding prompting endometrial biopsy is probably sufficient for diagnosis except for the perimenopausal and postmenopausal patient where a fractional D&C should be performed to rule out a coexisting carcinoma. Hyperplastic lesions usually are associated with the same risk factors as for carcinomas. Prolonged periods of unopposed estrogen is the presumptive stimulus for the development of hyperplasia. Obese women have increased conversion of androstenedione to estrone, thus accounting for the estrogen stimulus. Younger women with anovulatory cycles have continuous estrogen because of the anovulation.

Malignant Potential

Although the transition from endometrial hyperplasia to invasive carcinoma of the endometrium is not firmly established, several observations suggest that hyperplasias may be premalignant lesions. Hysterectomy specimens containing endometrial carcinoma often contain adjacent areas of hyperplasia. Prospective studies have suggested that 10% to 30% of women with biopsy-proved hyperplasias develop carcinoma (Wentz, 1974).

The classic description of hyperplasias into the terms cystic and adenomatous hyperplasias made dilineation of the risk factors for the development of endometrial cancer difficult to assess. Cystic hyperplasia appears to have a low neoplastic potential. Adenomatous hyperplasia has a greater malignant potential and appears to be more closely related to the degree of cytological atypia (Welch and Scully, 1977). More recently, women with hyperplasias classified by degree of cytologic atypia were examined for the risk of developing endometrial cancers (Kurman et al., 1985). The results demonstrate that 23% of women with untreated cytologically atypical hyperplasia developed endometrial cancer compared with 1.6% of women with endometrial hyperplasia without atypia.

Pathology

The classic histological description of endometrial hyperplasia into the one term adenomatous hyperplasia should be replaced by more accurate cytological descriptions because of differences in natural history among this heterogeneous lesion. More specifically, the degree of architec-

tural abnormalities and cytological atypia should be stated. Some hyperplasias present with marked architectural abnormalities with minimal cytological changes, whereas often lesions contain marked cytological atypia only (Fig 7–18).

The histological criteria separating severe hyperplasia and well-differentiated carcinoma may be difficult. In general, lesions not demonstrating back-to-back glands or cribriform patterns should be considered hyperplasia and not carcinoma.

Treatment

The treatment of endometrial hyperplasia should be based on the patient's age, desire for childbearing, and the histology of the lesion. Adolescents with hyperplasia should take a combination estrogen-progesterone pill for 6 months. Endometrial sampling should be performed at completion of therapy. Most important, an etiology of the hyperplasias should be sought and appropriately treated.

Women in the reproductive age group should also be treated with a combination pill and the endometrium sampled at completion of therapy. Patients desiring pregnancy should seek ovulation induction at completion of therapy of the hyperplasia.

Treatment of the postmenopausal patient with hyperplasia should be individualized. Patients with hypermenorrhea or high degrees of cytologic atypia should undergo hysterectomy. High-dose progestin therapy and follow-up endometrial sampling are recommended for the remaining patients. Should the patient not respond to hormonal therapy, hysterectomy is recommended. If the hyperestrogenic state is due to obesity, the menopausal patient will need to remain on progestins indefinitely or until she loses weight. Approximately 90% of endometrial hyperplasias will be successfully managed by progestins.

ENDOMETRIAL CANCER

Endometrial cancer is the commonest gynecologic malignancy in the United States, with approximately 37,000 cases annually and 3,000 deaths (Silverberg and Lubera, 1988). Historically, cancer of the uterine cervix had been commoner than corpus cancer. In recent years, how-

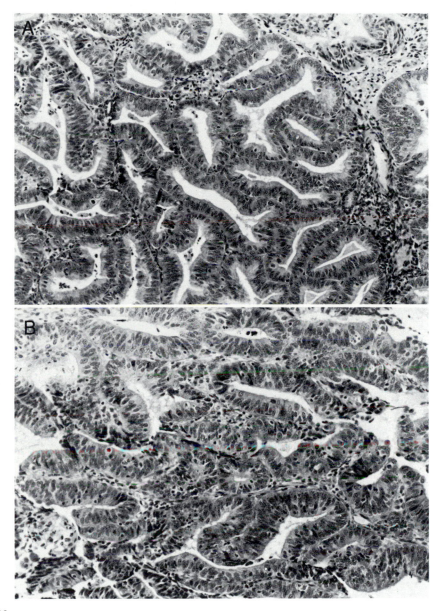

FIG 7–18.
A, endometrial hyperplasia demonstrating architectural abnormalities without cytological atypia. **B,** endometrial hyperplasia with both architectural and cytological atypia. (Courtesy of Drs. W. Welch and J. Semple.)

ever, this trend has reversed because of the decline in invasive cervical cancer and an increase in endometrial cancer (Cramer et al., 1974). The incidence of endometrial cancer peaks in the sixth decade (Cramer and Knapp, 1979), with a steady rise between 45 and 55 years (Cramer et al., 1974).

Risk Factors

The most important risk factor associated with the development of endometrial cancer is obesity (Davies et al., 1981). Epidemiologic studies have concluded that the risk for developing endometrial cancer increases with the degree of obesity; women up to 22.7 kg overweight have a threefold increased risk, whereas women greater than 22.7 kg overweight have a ninefold increased risk.

Obesity appears to increase the risk for endometrial cancer by increasing estrogen production and bioavailability. In postmenopausal women, the ovaries and adrenals secrete negligible amounts of estrogen. The majority of estrogen is in the form of estrone as a result of aromatization of adrenal androstendione to estrone in fatty tissue and muscle. Increased production of estrone has been documented in obese women (Judd et al., 1980; Lucas and Yen, 1979) and is a result of obesity and not the presence of endometrial cancer.

Similarly, obese women have decreased levels of sex hormone–binding globulin, accounting for increased bioavailability of circulating estrogen (Gambone et al., 1982).

Other factors said to increase risk for the development of endometrial carcinoma are diabetes, hypertension, and late menopause. Hypertension is often associated with obesity, and when controlled for weight, hypertension does not appear to increase the risk. Diabetes mellitus, however has been reported to increase the risk of developing endometrial cancer even if controlled for weight and age (MacMahon, 1974).

The risk of developing endometrial cancer is increased in patients with polycystic ovaries (Coulan et al., 1983). The increased risk is probably a result of chronic estrogen stimulation secondary to anovulation. Similarly, patients with estrogen-secreting ovarian tumors are at increased risk for developing endometrial cancer.

Exogenous estrogen has been clearly established as a risk factor for endometrial cancer. Initially, epidemiological studies did not correlate estrogen use with endometrial cancer, but a number of case control studies and cohort studies have documented the association (Antunes et al., 1979; Jick et al., 1979; Smith et al., 1975). The risk increases with estrogen dosage and duration of use.

A number of factors may reduce the risk of endometrial carcinoma. Exogenous estrogen is now clearly established as a risk, but this increased risk may be prevented by progestin therapy (Gambrell, 1978). Progesterone acts as an antiestrogen by decreasing estrogen and progesterone receptor synthesis. In addition, progesterone activates estradiol 17β-dehydrogenase, an enzyme that converts estradiol to the less potent estrogen estrone. Menopausal women who take both estrogen and progestin have a lower risk of developing endometrial cancer than women who take no hormonal replacement. Estrogen replacement therapy should be administered with progestin only if the uterus is present.

The use of combination contraceptive pills also reduces the risk of endometrial cancer (Hulka et al., 1982; Weiss and Sayvetz, 1980). The protective benefit increases with duration of use and appears to be related to the protective benefit of the progestin component.

Endometrial cancer developing in an estrogen user appears to have a better prognosis than endometrial cancer arising in a nonuser (Chu et al., 1982; Underwood et al., 1979). The fact probably is a result of detection of early lesions and not a result of estrogen use. When corrected for stage, depth of invasion, and grade, estrogen user survival was similar to nonuser survival (Elwood and Boyes, 1980).

Diagnosis

The majority of patients with endometrial carcinoma present with abnormal bleeding. Patients with postmenopausal bleeding require endometrial sampling to rule out the presence of an endometrial cancer. Menopausal patients taking estrogen and progestin should also undergo endometrial sampling for any abnormal or irregular bleeding.

The papanicolaou smear is a poor test for screening patients for endometrial cancer. If a papanicolaou smear from a postmenopausal patient shows endometrial cells, however, endometrial sampling is necessary because of the possibility of endometrial hyperplasia or cancer (Ng et al., 1974).

A number of techniques are available for endometrial sampling, including methods to obtain cytological and histological specimens. We prefer techniques that provide histological specimens because it provides easier interpretation and less unsatisfactory specimens. Suction curettage has provided a safe, reliable method for obtaining office endometrial sampling. Formal D&C for endometrial sampling is reserved for patients who cannot tolerate the office procedure. If endometrial carcinoma is detected on office biopsy, a formal fractional D&C with endocervical curettage is performed.

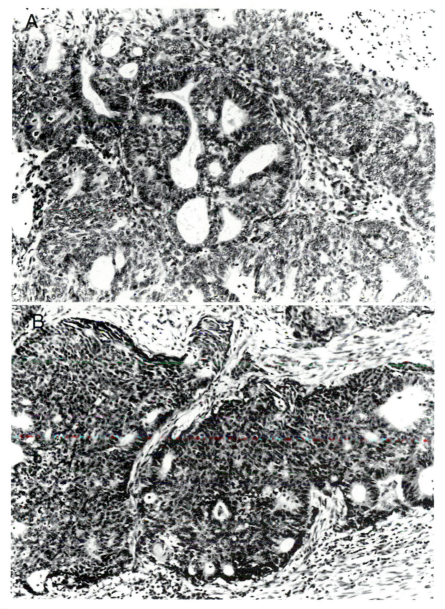

FIG 7–19.
A, endometrial adenocarcinoma, well differentiated (grade 1). **B,** endometrial adenocarcinoma, poorly differentiated (grade 3), demonstrating sheets of malignant cells without identifiable gland formation. (Courtesy of Drs. W. Welch and J. Semple.)

Pathology

The histology of endometrial cancer is adenocarcinoma in approximately 90% of the cases. Similar to endometrial hyperplasias, the lesions may be focal or diffuse. An enlarged uterus may indicate extensive involvement, although such involvement may be seen even with small uteri.

Histologically, endometrial carcinomas contain back-to-back glands or a cribriform pattern, indicating gland within gland formation (Fig 7–19). Cytologically, mitoses are almost always present. Epithelial stratification is present, and connective tissue between glands is absent. The cells are characterized by prominent nucleoli and eosinophilic, granular cytoplasm. The degree of architectural abnormalities are used to grade the tumors according to the International Federation of Gynecology and Obstetrics (FIGO). Tumors are graded 1 to 3 based on the degree of glandular and solid tumor elements. Grade 1 tumors are well-differentiated neoplasms composed predominantly of glandular elements. Grade 2 tumors are moderately differentiated with mixed gland and solid components. Grade 3 lesions are poorly differentiated with a predominantly solid component.

Squamous differentiation is sometimes seen in association with endometrial adenocarcinoma. The term adenoacanthoma is used for endometrial adenocarcinoma with benign squamous differentiation and adenosquamous carcinoma reserved for adenocarcinoma with malignant squamous epithelium. The influence of squamous differentiation on the prognosis of the disease has been controversial. It is generally accepted that the squamous component does not influence the aggressiveness of the lesion (Hendrickson et al., 1982).

It should be noted that approximately 10% of endometrial carcinomas are associated with the production of mucus, a feature commonly seen in adenocarcinomas of the cervix. Mucous production does not appear to influence prognosis. Endometrial biopsy showing mucus-producing adenocarcinoma requires the clinician and pathologist to determine whether the primary tumor is endometrial or endocervical in origin.

Evaluation of Patients

Once a diagnosis of endometrial cancer is made on endometrial biopsy, a thorough history and physical examination must be performed. Fractional D&C is the definitive diagnostic and staging procedure. The endocervical canal should be curetted before the corpus is sounded. The endocervical canal is then dilated and the endometrial cavity curetted.

Initial laboratory evaluation should include a complete blood cell count, blood chemistry, including liver function test, and chest radiograph. The hysteroscope has been recommended to evaluate endometrial carcinomas for endocervical involvement and depth of invasion (DeVore et al., 1982). Although tumor spill through the fallopian tube has not been a problem, the same information may be easily obtained at D&C or by in-

specting the uterine cavity at the time of hysterectomy (Malviya et al., 1989).

Abdominal and pelvic CT scans may be of use to detect gross disease. The use of high-resolution ultrasound and MRI may prove to be of benefit in the preoperative evaluation of endometrial cancer patients, although the efficacy of such procedures has not yet been established.

Cystoscopy, proctoscopy, and gastrointestinal radiographs should be performed only when bladder or bowel involvement is suspected. Similarly, bone scan and liver scan should not be performed unless blood chemistries suggest possible metastatic disease.

The production of the tumor-associated antigen CA-125 is associated with nonmucinous epithelial ovarian carcinomas. Recent investigations suggest that elevated CA-125 levels in patients with endometrial cancers are predictive of metastatic disease (Pastner and Mann, 1988). Large-scale studies are underway to confirm these results before recommending routine preoperative CA-125 in patients with known endometrial cancer.

Staging

Endometrial carcinoma is staged according to the FIGO staging system, as shown in Table 7–3. The staging system is based on clinical information obtained from presurgical evaluation and diagnostic fractional D&C.

The staging system fails to recognize important prognostic variables and is not based on surgical or pathological correlation. Microscopic ovarian metastases, for example, would place a patient in stage III but can be detected only on histological grounds. In addition, the staging system fails to recognize differences in cell types and makes no allowance for histologically well-organized tumors with highly aggressive clinical behavior, such as papillary serous carcinoma or clear cell carcinoma. Similarly, the staging system does not allow upstaging of patients with tumors believed to be confined to the uterus but found to have intraperitoneal or nodal disease at the time of surgery.

Despite inadequacies in the staging system, it does allow for an estimate of prognosis at least based on stage. The overall survival of patients is shown in Table 7–4. The survival for stage I disease is greater than 90% but decreases to 54% in stage III disease and 9% in patients with stage IV disease.

TABLE 7—3.

International Federation of Gynecologists and Obstetricians Staging System for Endometrial Cancer*

Stage I
  Carcinoma confined to the corpus.
Stage Ia
  Length of uterine cavity ≤ 8 cm.
Stage Ib
  Length of uterine cavity > 8 cm.
Stage I adenocarcinoma subgroups
  Grade 1
    Highly differentiated.
  Grade 2
    Moderately differentiated with partly solid
      areas.
  Grade 3
    Poorly differentiated with predominantly solid
      areas.
Stage II
  Carcinoma involving the corpus and the cervix.
Stage III
  Carcinoma extending outside the uterus but not
    outside the true pelvis.
Stage IV
  Carcinoma extending outside the true pelvis or
    involving the mucosa of the bladder or rectum.
Stage IVa
  Spread to adjacent organs.
Stage IVb
  Spread to distant organs.

*Adapted from FIGO report: Classification and staging of malignant tumors in the female pelvis. *Int J Gynaecol Obstet* 1971; 9:172—179.

Treatment

Hysterectomy and adnexectomy are the cornerstone of management for patients with endometrial cancer. Radiotherapy or chemotherapy may be indicated based on surgical and pathological findings.

At laparotomy, a complete abdominal and retroperitoneal exploration is warranted. Peritoneal washings for cytological examination should be obtained on entry into the abdomen. The prognostic significance of abnormal washings, however, remains controversial. Creasman et al. (1981) reported a higher incidence of recurrence in patients with abnormal washings, with a majority of patients recurring intra-abdominally. A report in 1983, however, found no prognostic significance of abnormal washings in stage I disease (Yazigi et al., 1983). More recently, abnormal peritoneal cytology was found to negatively

TABLE 7—4.

Survival and International Federation of Gynecologists and Obstetricians Stage*

Stage	5-Yr Survival (%)
I	90
II	83
III	54
IV	9

*Adapted from Niloff JM, Eifel PJ, Bloomer WD, et al: Malignancy of the uterine corpus, in Knapp RC, Berkowitz RS (eds): *Gynecologic Oncology.* New York, Macmillan Publishing Co, 1986, p 293.

impact the 2-year survival rates, although the majority of patients (64%) with abnormal peritoneal cytology had tumor outside the uterus (Imachi et al., 1988). The role of peritoneal cytology in dictating management of this disease awaits future prospective studies controlling for other prognostic variables.

At laparotomy, biopsy of the omentum may be indicated if one suspects involvement. The pelvic and para-aortic nodes should be palpated and any suspicious nodes excised. Para-aortic node dissection is a potentially morbid procedure and may be technically difficult in an obese patient undergoing hysterectomy. Because of the potential morbidity, nodal dissection should be conducted in the presence of suspiciously enlarged nodes or in patients at risk for nodal involvement.

The risk of aortic nodal involvement is correlated with both the grade of tumor (Burrell et al., 1982; Cheon, 1969; Piver et al., 1982) and degree of myometrial invasion (Piver et al., 1982). The overall incidence of abnormal aortic nodes in stage I disease ranges from 10% to 15%. In a study by Piver et al. (1982), however, no patients with stage I disease and superficial invasion of grade 1 tumors had aortic nodal involvement. The incidence of nodal involvement increased to 38% in patients with stage I disease and grade 3 lesions and 45% in patients with stage I disease and myometrial invasion greater than one half of the myometrial thickness. Stage also bears influence on aortic nodal involvement, with increasing stage associated with a higher percentage of aortic nodal involvement. Aortic nodal sampling may therefore be performed in patients with stage I, grade 3 lesions or deep myometrial invasion. In addition, patients with stage II and III disease should have aortic node sampling.

When the extrafascial hysterectomy is performed, the fallopian tubes should be occluded before uterine manipulation. Adnexectomy should be performed because of the 8% to 10% incidence of ovarian or tubal metastases (Plentl and Friedman, 1971). The role of vaginal hysterectomy should not be underestimated, particularly for selected patients believed to be poor risks for an abdominal approach. The vaginal approach carries significant disadvantages, however, including the inability to perform abdominal exploration and palpate pelvic and aortic lymph nodes. In addition, the adnexa may be difficult to remove using a vaginal approach.

Treatment by Stage

Stage I.—Patients with stage I endometrial cancer should be treated by total abdominal hysterectomy and bilateral salpingo-oophorectomy. Radiation therapy alone may control disease although local control and survival are improved with surgery.

The indications for lymph node sampling have been discussed previously. The role of preoperative or postoperative radiation therapy has been the subject of many studies (Davis, 1964; Eifel et al., 1983; Hendrickson et al., 1982; Shah and Gree, 1972). We prefer the use of postoperative radiation because it allows treatment planning based on surgical and pathological findings and carries no increased risk of complications (Bean et al., 1978). Patients receiving postoperative radiotherapy are those with grade 3 lesions or deep myometrial invasion.

Stage II.—Approximately 10% to 15% of endometrial carcinomas involve the endocervix and are designated stage II lesions. Two different approaches have been implemented in treating stage II disease. The first approach utilizes radical hysterectomy and pelvic lymphadenectomy, whereas the other approach employs combination of radiation therapy and simple hysterectomy. Most data suggest that the latter approach results in improved survival and local control. Using preoperative external beam and intracavity radiation and extrafascial hysterectomy and bilateral salpingo-oophorectomy, Kinsella et al. (1980) reported a 10-year disease-free survival of 83%. Patients with gross cervical involvement, however, did worse than patients with microscopic cervical involvement only.

Stage III.—Because data may be reported using either clinical or surgico pathological stag-

ing, one must be careful when analyzing data related to patients with stage III endometrial carcinoma. Surgico pathological stage III patients with microscopic involvement of the ovaries or tubes have 80%, 5-year relapse-free survival when treated with combination surgery and radiation therapy. Patients with gross disease in the pelvis, however, have 5-year relapse-free survival of 15% treated in the same manner (Bruckman et al., 1980). Treatment failures are commonly upper abdominal, and such patients may benefit from whole abdomen radiation or systemic therapy.

Stage IV.—Patients with stage IV disease require individualized treatment, consisting mostly of radiotherapy and systemic agents. Patients with bladder or rectal involvement may be treated by pelvic exenteration when the tumor is confined to the central pelvis.

Recurrences

Endometrial carcinomas may metastasize intra-abdominally, hematogenously, or via lymphatics. The commonest site of local recurrence is the vagina, with distant recurrences seen in the abdomen, lung, liver, and bone. Most recurrences develop within 3 years of initial diagnosis, and patients with early recurrence do poorly (Liebel and Wharam, 1980).

The treatment of recurrences depends on site of relapse and previous therapy. In general, vaginal recurrences may be treated with radiation therapy or systemic therapy consisting of hormonal manipulation or cytotoxic chemotherapy.

Hormonal Therapy

Hormonal manipulation with progestin therapy produces overall response rates of approximately 30%. Receptor-rich neoplasms generally have higher response rates (Creasman et al., 1980; Ehrlich et al., 1988), and well-differentiated tumors are generally more receptor rich than anaplastic neoplasms. Differentiation, however, is not an adequate predictor of receptor content (Gurpide, 1981).

Studies examining steroid receptor content and clinical outcome in patients with endometrial carcinomas indicate that patients with stage I disease and progesterone-negative receptors have higher recurrence rates than patients with receptor-rich tumors (Ehrlich et al., 1988). In recurrent disease, progesterone receptor–positive tumors respond much more frequently to progesterone therapy than receptor-negative tumors (85% vs. 15%).

The use of tamoxifen has also undergone investigation. Tamoxifen may induce progesterone receptors, thus making tumors previously unresponsive now respond to progestin therapy (Mortel et al., 1983). The exact role of this agent remains to be elucidated.

Cytotoxic Chemotherapy

Many therapeutic trials have been undertaken to establish an effective chemotherapeutic regimen for recurrent or locally advanced endometrial cancer. Single-agent trials have reported responses to doxorubicin (Adriamycin), cyclophosphamide, cisplatin, 5-fluorouracil, and hexamethylmelamine (Deppe et al., 1981; Thigpen et al., 1979).

Overall, the ideal combination of drugs has not yet been established and awaits prospective trials.

OTHER UTERINE MALIGNANCIES

Whereas 90% of endometrial malignancies are adenocarcinomas, the remaining malignant tumors are biologically unique. The two main cell types are papillary serous carcinomas and the sarcomas.

Uterine Papillary Serous Carcinomas

Uterine papillary serous carcinomas histologically resemble ovarian papillary serous carcinomas. These tumors contain tufts of stratified anaplastic cells, frequent mitotic figures, and, occasionally, psammoma bodies (Fig 7–20).

Biologically, these tumors are aggressive, with poor 5-year survivals. Although clinically believed to be confined to the uterus, many of these tumors are found to have widespread intraabdominal disease at time of laparotomy (Chambers et al., 1987). The pattern of spread and aggressive nature of these lesions resembles ovarian carcinoma, and therapies under investigation consist of ovarian-type chemotherapy and whole abdominal radiation therapy.

Uterine Sarcomas

Sarcomas are unusual gynecological malignancies but are commonest in the uterus (Forney and Buchsbaum, 1981). The only known risk factor for the development of gynecological sarcomas is prior radiation therapy (Antman, 1986; Meredith et al., 1986). There presently remains no evidence to link uterine sarcomas with viral infection.

Controversy exists as to the proper classification of uterine sarcomas (Norris and Taylor,

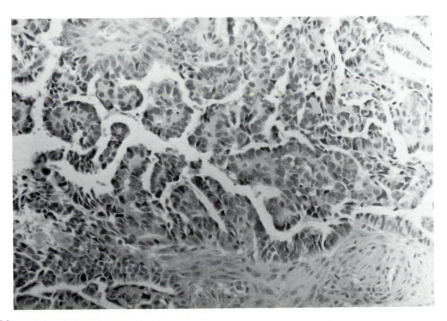

FIG 7–20.
Papillary serous carcinoma of the endometrium displaying papillary tufts of stratified, malignant epithelium histologically similar to ovarian papillary carcinoma. (Courtesy of Dr. D. Genest.)

TABLE 7–5.

Classification of Uterine Sarcomas*

Pure homologous
   Leiomyosarcoma
   Endometrial stromal sarcoma
   Endolymphatic stromal meiosis
   Angiosarcoma
   Fibrosarcoma
Pure heterologous
   Rhabdomyosarcoma
   Chondrosarcoma
   Osteosarcoma
   Liposarcoma
Mixed sarcomas
   Mixed homologous
   Mixed heterologous
Malignant mixed müllerian tumors
   Homologous type
   Heterologous type

*Adapted from Antman KH: Malignancy of the uterine corpus, in Knapp RC, Berkowitz RS (eds): *Gynecologic Oncology.* New York, Macmillan Publishing Co, 1986, p 299.

1966). Table 7–5 displays an accepted classification schema. These tumors are generally divided into pure sarcomas, mixed sarcomas, and malignant mixed müllerian tumors. Within each group, subdivisions are made for homologous elements (tumors containing cell types normally seen in the uterus) or heterologous elements (cell types not normally seen in the uterus). Overall, mixed müllerian sarcomas predominate, followed by leiomyosarcoma and endometrial stromal sarcoma (Salazar et al., 1978). The remaining tumors are exceedingly rare.

Leiomyosarcoma

Leiomyosarcomas usually occur in the presence of other leiomyomas. The incidence of malignant degeneration of uterine leiomyomas is reported to be approximately 0.1%.

Classification of leiomyosarcoma requires high mitotic count (more than 10 mitoses/10 high-power fields [HPF]; Kempson and Bari, 1970) or histologically invasive or metastatic disease. Microscopically, leiomyosarcomas have a characteristic appearance with spindle, round, or giant cell types. Pleiomorphism and multinucleated giant cells may be seen (Fig 7–21).

No effective therapy for metastatic disease has been reported, and patients who do well have tumors confined to the uterus. Prognosis for pa-

tients with tumors outside the uterus is extremely poor (Hannigan and Gomez, 1979).

Other lesions that must be distinguished from leiomyosarcomas include leiomyoma of uncertain malignant potential, benign metastasizing leiomyoma, intravenous leiomyomatosis, and cellular leiomyomas. Intravenous leiomyomatosis is an interesting benign tumor with potentially fatal outcomes. These tumors arise in the uterus or its blood vessels. Tumor may extend into the vena cava and right atrium and has been reported to obstruct venous return (Tierney et al., 1980).

Endometrial Stromal Sarcomas

Stromal tumors of the endometrium are divided into endometrial (endolymphatic) stromal myosis, and endometrial stromal sarcomas.

Endometrial stromal myosis is an indolent-behaving sarcoma, occurring in younger women. Recurrences or metastases are infrequent and may occur many years after primary therapy. The lesion may be hormonally dependent; oophorectomy and progestin therapy have been reported to cause tumor responses (Gloor et al., 1982). It has less than 10 mitoses/10 HPF.

Endometrial stromal sarcoma, however, is a biologically virulent tumor that metastasizes quickly and is commonly fatal with high mitotic counts (more than 10 mitoses/10 HPF) (Norris et al., 1969). Grossly, these tumors may be polypoid and fleshy. Microscopically, they are composed of spindle-shaped cells with varying amounts of cytoplasm. Tumor giant cells may be seen (Fig 7–22).

Mixed Müllerian Sarcomas

Mixed müllerian sarcoma is the commonest uterine sarcoma and appears to arise from the endometrial stroma or from undifferentiated cell rests. Survival is related to degree of invasion with few, if any, survivors if tumor is deeply invading the uterus or outside the uterus (Antman, 1986).

Microscopically, these tumors are made up of carcinomatous and sarcomatous elements of either heterologous or homologous type (Fig 7–23). The only proved therapy for the lesion is hysterectomy and bilateral salpingo-oophorectomy.

Treatment of Sarcoma

The optimal treatment for uterine sarcomas depends on the stage of disease. In general, pa-

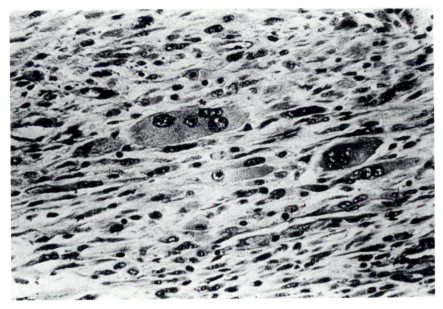

FIG 7—21.
Leiomyosarcoma demonstrating pleomorphism of muscle cells and multinucleated giant cells.

tients with tumors confined to the uterus with minimal invasion do well with hysterectomy and bilateral salpingo-oophorectomy.

The role of adjuvant radiotherapy and chemotherapy is difficult to establish. Radiation ther-

apy offers no improvement in survival to surgery alone in patients with stage I disease (Salazar et al., 1978). However, pelvic irradiation reduces the incidence of pelvic recurrence.

The most active chemotherapy agent is doxo-

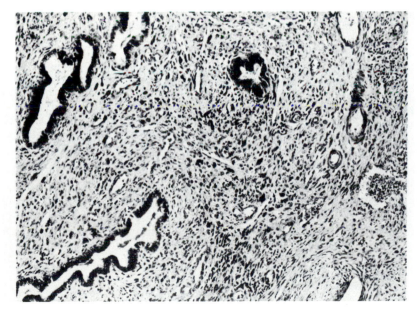

FIG 7—22.
Endometrial stromal sarcoma with neoplastic endometrial stroma and pleomorphic, giant cells scattered about normal proliferative glands.

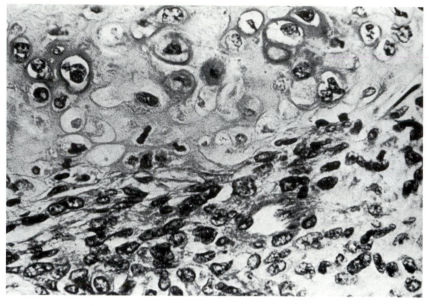

FIG 7–23.
Mixed mesodermal sarcoma of the uterus showing tendency of the tumor to form cartilage.

rubicin. Doxorubicin-containing regimens in an adjunctive setting did not improve survival in patients with sarcomas (Antman et al., 1984). One recent report suggested that combination chemotherapy with vincristine, dactinomycin, and cyclophosphamide may improve survival in patients with stage I uterine sarcomas when compared with historical controls (van Nagell et al., 1986). This latter study, however, was based on only seven patients without a prospective control group.

Natural History

Sarcomas may recur locally or at distant sites, and patients should be carefully followed. Uterine sarcomas tend to progress rapidly, with 90% of recurrences occurring within the first 2 years. More than 90% of recurrences appear outside the pelvis.

The treatment of metastatic sarcoma should be palliative, with doxorubicin the most effective single agent. The use of progestational agents should be considered, particularly if the sarcoma has measurable steroid receptor content. However, despite earlier enthusiasm over hormonal manipulation of sarcomas, recent studies suggest that receptor status does not correlate with prognosis or disease-free survival in patients with uterine sarcomas (Soper et al., 1984).

REFERENCES

Anson BJ, Curtis AH: Anatomy of the female pelvis and perineum, in Curtis AH (ed): *Textbook of Gynecology.* Philadelphia, WB Saunders Co, 1946.

Antman KH: Uterine sarcomas, in Knapp RC, Berkowitz RS (eds): *Gynecologic Oncology.* MacMillan Publishing Co, 1986, pp 297–310.

Antman KH, Surit H, Amato D, et al: Preliminary results of a randomized trial of adjuvant Adriamycin for sarcomas. *J Clin Oncol* 1984; 2:601–608.

Antunes CMF, Stolley PD, Rosenshein NB, et al: Endometrial cancer and estrogen use. *N Engl J Med* 1979; 300:9–13.

Asherman JG: Amenorrhoea traumatica (atretica). *J Obstet Gynaecol Br Emp* 1948; 55:23–25.

Babknia A, Rock JA, Jones HW: Pregnancy success following abdominal myomectomy for infertility. *Fertil Steril* 1978; 30:644–648.

Baggish MS: Mesenchymal tumors of the uterus. *Clin Obstet Gynecol* 1974; 17:51–59.

Barnes AB, Colton, T, Gunderson J, et al: Fertility and outcome of pregnancy in women exposed in utero to diethylstilbestrol. *N Engl J Med* 1980; 302:609–615.

Bean HA, Bryant AJS, Carmichael JA, et al: Carcinoma of the endometrium in Saskatchewan: 1966–1971. *Gynecol Oncol* 1978; 6:503–514.

Bird CC, McElin TW: Adenomyosis and other benign diffuse enlargements of the uterus, in Sciarra JJ (ed): *Gynecology and Obstetrics.* New York, Harper & Row, Publishers, vol 1, 1981, pp 1–13.

Bird CC, McElin TW, Manalo-Estrella P: The elusive adenomyosis of the uterus—revisited. *Am J Obstet Gynecol* 1972; 112:583–589.

Brown JM, Malkasian GD, Symmonds RE: Abdominal myomectomy. *Am J Obstet Gynecol* 1967; 90:126–130.

Bruckman JE, Bloomer WD, Marck A, et al: Stage III adenocarcinoma of the endometrium. Two prognostic groups. *Gynecol Oncol* 1980; 9:12–12.

Burrell MD, Franklin EW, Powell JL: Endometrial cancer: Evaluation of spread and follow-up in one hundred eighty nine patients with stage I or stage II disease. *Am J Obstet Gynecol* 1982; 144:181–185.

Buttram VC: Müllerian anomalies and their management. *Fertil Steril* 1983; 40:159–163.

Buttram VC, Gibbons WE: Mullerian anomalies: A proposed classification (an analysis of 144 cases). *Fertil Steril* 1979; 32:40–46.

Buttram VC, Reiter RC: Uterine leiomyomata: Etiology, symptomatology and management. *Fertil Steril* 1981; 36:433–445.

Capraro VJ, Gallego MB: Vaginal agenesis. *Am J Obstet Gynecol* 1976; 124:98–106.

Chambers JT, Merino M, Kohorn EI, et al: Uterine papillary serous carcinoma. *Obstet Gynecol* 1987; 69:109–113.

Cheon HK: Prognosis of endometrial carcinoma. *Obstet Gynecol* 1969; 34:680–684.

Chu J, Schweid AI, Weiss NS: Survival among women with endometrial cancer: A comparison of estrogen users and nonusers. *Am J Obstet Gynecol* 1982; 143:569–573.

Coulan CB, Annegers JF, Krantz JS: Chronic anovulation syndrome and associated neoplasia. *Obstet Gynecol* 1983; 61:403–407.

Counseller VS, Bedard RE: Uterine myomectomy. *JAMA* 1937; 111:675–678.

Cramer DW, Cutler SJ, Christine B: Trends in the incidence of endometrial cancer in the United States. *Gynecol Oncol* 1974; 2:130–134.

Cramer DW, Knapp RC: Review of epidemiologic studies of endometrial cancer and exogenous estrogen. *Obstet Gynecol* 1979; 54:521–526.

Creasman WT, DiSaia PJ, Blessing J, et al: Prognostic significance of peritoneal cytology in patients with endometrial cancer and preliminary data concerning therapy with intraperitoneal radiopharmaceuticals. *Am J Obstet Gynecol* 1981; 141:921–927.

Creasman WT, McCarty KS, Barton TK, et al: Clinical correlates of estrogen and progesterone-binding proteins in human endometrial adenocarcinoma. *Obstet Gynecol* 1980; 55:363–370.

Daly DC, Walters CA, Soto-Albors CE, et al: Hysteroscopic metroplasty: Surgical technique and obstetric outcome. *Fertil Steril* 1983; 39:623–678.

Davies JL, Rosenshein NB, Antunes CMF, et al: A review of the risk factors for endometrial carcinoma. *Obstet Gynecol Surv* 1981; 36:107–116.

Davis EW: Carcinoma of the corpus uteri: A study of 525 cases at the New York Hospital (1932–1961). *Am J Obstet Gynecol* 1964; 88:163–170.

DeCherney AH, Russell JB, Graebe RA, et al: Resectoscopic management of mullerian fusion defects. *Fertil Steril* 1986; 45:726–728.

Deppe G, Jacobs AJ, Bruckner H, et al: Chemotherapy of advanced and recurrent endometrial carcinoma with cyclophosphamide, doxorubicin, 5-fluorouracil and megestrol acetate. *Am J Obstet Gynecol* 1981; 140:313–316.

DeVore GR, Schwartz PE, Morris JMcL: Hysterography: A five year follow-up in patients with endometrial carcinoma. *Obstet Gynecol* 1982; 60:369–372.

Easterday CL, Grimes DA, Riggs JA: Hysterectomy in the United States. *Obstet Gynecol* 1983; 62:203–212.

Ehrlich CE, Young PC, Stehman FB, et al: Steroid receptors and clinical outcome in patients with adenocarcinoma of the endometrium. *Am J Obstet Gynecol* 1988; 158:796–807.

Eifel PJ, Ross JC, Hendrickson MR, et al: Adenocarcinoma of the endometrium: Analysis of 256 cases with disease limited to the uterine corpus: Treatment comparisons. *Cancer* 1983; 52:1026–1031.

Elwood JM, Boyes DA: Clinical and pathologic features and survival of endometrial cancer patients in relation to prior use of estrogens. *Gynecol Oncol* 1980; 10:173–183.

Farber M, Conrad S, Heinrichs NL, et al: Estradiol binding by fibroid tumors and normal myometrium. *Obstet Gynecol* 1972; 40:479.

Fayez JA: Comparison between abdominal and hysteroscopic metroplasty. *Obstet Gyncol* 1986; 68:399–403.

Finn WF, Muller PF: Abdominal myomectomy: Special reference to subsequent pregnancy and to the reappearance of fibromyomas of the uterus. *Am J Obstet Gyncol* 1950; 60:109–114.

Forney JP, Buchsbaum HJ: Classifying, staging

and treating uterine sarcomas. *Contemp Obstet Gynecol* 1981; 18:47–69.

Frank RT: The formation of an artificial vagina without operation. *Am J Obstet Gynecol* 1938; 35:1053–1059.

Friedman A, DeFazio J, DeCherney A: Severe obstetric complications after aggressive treatment of Asherman syndrome. *Obstet Gynecol* 1986; 67:864–867.

Friedman AJ, Barbieri RL, Benacerraf BR, et al: Treatment of leiomyomata with intranasal or subcutaneous leuprolide, a gonadotropin-releasing hormone agonist. *Fertil Steril* 1987; 48:560.

Friedman AJ, Barbieri RL, Doubilet PM, et al: A randomized, double-blind trial of a gonadotropin releasing-hormone agonist (leuprolide) with or without medroxyprogesterone acetate in the treatment of leiomyomata uteri. *Fertil Steril* 1988; 49:404–409.

Fritsch H: Ein Fall von volligem Schwund der Gebarmutterhohle nach Auskratzung. *Zentralbl Gynaekol* 1894; 18:1337–1341.

Gambone JC, Pardridge WM, Lagasse LD, et al: In vivo availability of circulating estradiol in postmenopausal women with and without endometrial cancer. *Obstet Gynecol* 1982; 59:416–421.

Gambrell RD Jr: The prevention of endometrial cancer in postmenopausal women with progestogens. *Maturitas* 1978; 1:107–112.

Gloor E, Schnyder P, Cikes M, et al: Endolymphatic stromal meiosis. *Cancer* 1982; 50:1888–1893.

Godsoe A, Kimura R, Herndon D, et al: Cardiopulmonary changes with intermittent endotoxin administration in sheep. *Circ Shock* 1988; 25:61–74.

Gros A, David A, Serr DM: Management of congenital malformations of the uterus: Fetal salvage. *Acta Eur Fertil* 1974; 5:301–309.

Gurpide E: Hormone receptors in endometrial cancer. *Cancer* 1981; 48:638–641.

Hannigan EV, Gomez LG: Uterine leiomyosarcoma. *Am J Obstet Gynecol* 1979; 134:557–564.

Hendrickson MR, Ross JC, Eifel PJ, et al: Adenocarcinoma of the endometrium. Analysis of 256 cases with carcinoma limited to the uterine corpus: Pathology review and analysis of prognostic variables. *Gynecol Oncol* 1982; 13:373–392.

Hulka BS, Chambless LE, Kaufman DG, et al: Protection against endometrial carcinoma by combination product oral contraceptive. *JAMA* 1982; 147:475–477.

Hunt, JE, Wallach EE: Uterine factors in infertility—an overview. *Clin Obstet Gynecol* 1974; 17:44–53.

Imachi M, Tsukamoto T, et al: Peritoneal cytology in patients with endometrial carcinoma. *Gynecol Oncol* 1988; 30:76–86.

Ingersoll FM: Fertility following myomectomy. *Fertil Steril* 1963; 14:596–601.

Israel SL, Woutersz, TB: Adenomyosis: A neglected diagnosis. *Obstet Gynecol* 1959; 14:168–174.

Jewelewicz R, Khalaf S, Neuwirth RS, et al: Obstetric complications after treatment of intrauterine synechiae (Asherman's syndrome). *Obstet Gynecol* 1976; 47:701–705.

Jick H, Watkins RN, Hunter JR, et al: Replacement estrogens and endometrial cancer. *N Engl J Med* 1979; 300:218–222.

Jones WE: Traumatic intrauterine adhesions: A report of 8 cases with emphasis on therapy. *Am J Obstet Gynecol* 1964; 89:304–309.

Judd HL, Davidson BJ, Frumar AM, et al: Serum androgens and estrogens in postmenopausal women with and without endometrial cancer. *Am J Obstet Gynecol* 1980; 136:859–871.

Kaufman RH, Adam E, Binder GL, et al: Upper genital tract changes and pregnancy outcome in offspring exposed in utero to diethylstilbestrol. *Am J Obstet Gynecol* 1980; 137:299–307.

Kempson RL, Bari W: Uterine sarcomas. Classification, diagnosis and prognosis. *Hum Pathol* 1970; 1:331–349.

Kinsella TJ, Bloomer WD, Lavin PT, et al: Stage II endometrial carcinoma: 10 year follow-up of combined radiation and surgical treatment. *Gynecol Oncol* 1980; 10:290–297.

Kurman RJ, Kaminski PF, Norris HJ: The behavior of endometrial hyperplasia. A long term study of "untreated" hyperplasia in 170 patients. *Cancer* 1985; 56:403–412.

Leibel SA, Wharam MD: Vaginal and paraaortic lymph node metastases in carcinoma of the endometrium. *Int J Radiat Oncol Biol Phys* 1980; 6:893–896.

Lipshultz A: Experimental fibroids and the antifibromatogenic action of steroid hormones. *JAMA* 1942; 120:173.

Loeffler FE, Noble AD: Myomectomy at the Chelsea Hospital for Women. *J Obstet Gynaecol Br Commonw* 1970; 77:167–171.

Lucas WE, Yen SC: A study of endocrine and metabolic variables in postmenopausal women with endometrial carcinoma. *Am J Obstet Gynecol* 1979; 134:180–186.

MacMahon B: Risk factors for endometrial cancer. *Gynecol Oncol* 1974; 2:122–129.

Maheux R, Guilloteau C, Lemay A, et al: Luteinizing hormone-releasing hormones agonist and uterine leiomyoma: A pilot study. *Am J Obstet Gynecol* 1985; 152:1034.

Malone LJ, Ingersoll FM: Myomectomy in infertility, in Behrman SJ, Kistner RW (eds): *Progress in Infertility*. Boston, Little, Brown & Co, 1975, p 85.

Malviya VK, Depp G, Malone JM, et al: Reliability of frozen section examination in identifying poor prognostic indicators in stage I endometrial adenocarcinoma. *Gynecol Oncol* 1989; 32:120.

March CM, Israel R, March AD: Hysteroscopic management of intrauterine adhesions. *Am J Obstet Gynecol* 1978; 130:633–637.

McCormick TA: Myomectomy with subsequent pregnancy. *Am J Obstet Gynecol* 1958; 75:1128–1133.

McElin TW, Bird CC: Adenomyosis of the uterus. *Obstet Gynecol Annu* 1974; 3:425–437.

McIndoe AH: The treatment of congenital absence and obliterative conditions of the vagina. *Br J Plastic Surg* 1950; 2:254–263.

McShane PM, Reilly RJ, Schiff I: Pregnancy outcomes following Tompkins metroplasty. *Fertil Steril* 1983; 40:190–194.

Meredith RF, Eisert DR, Kaka Z, et al: An excess of uterine sarcomas after pelvic irradiation. *Cancer* 1986; 55:2003–2007.

Meyer R: Uber Drusen, Cyste und Adenom in Myometrium bei er Wachsen. *Z Geburtshilfe Gynakol* 1900; 43:130–138.

Miller H, Tyrone C: A survey of a series of myomectomies with a follow-up. *Am J Obstet Gynecol* 1933; 26:575–581.

Misch KA, Smithies A, Twomey D, et al: Tuberculosis of the cervix; cytology as an aid to diagnosis. *J Clin Pathol* 1976; 29:313–316.

Molitor JJ: Adenomyosis: A Clinical and pathologic appraisal. *Am J Obstet Gynecol* 1971; 110:275–281.

Mortel R, Zaino R, Satyaswaroop PG: Modulation of growth and sex steroid receptor concentrations by tamoxifen in human endometrial carcinoma transplanted into nude mice. *Proc Soc Gynecol Oncol* 1983; 19:23.

Munnell EW, Martin FW: Abdominal myomectomy, advantages and disadvantages. *Am J Obstet Gynecol* 1951; 62:109–114.

National Center for Health Statistics: *Hysterectomies in the United States 1965–84*. Vital and Health Statistics Series 13, no 92, publication no 88–1753, 1987.

Nelson WO: Endometrial and myometrial changes including fibromyomatous nodules induced in the guinea pig by oestrogen. *Anat Rec* 1937; 68:99.

Neuwirth RS, Friedman EA: Septic abortion: Changing concept of management. *Am J Obstet Gynecol* 1963; 85:24.

Ng ABP, Reagan JW, Hawliczek CT, et al: Significance of endometrial cells in the detection of endometrial carcinoma and its precursors. *Acta Cytol* 1974; 18:356–361.

Nishijima MK, Breslow MJ, Miller CF, et al: Effect of naloxone and ibuprofen on organ blood flow during endotoxic shock in pig. *Am J Phys* 1988; 255:H177–H184.

Norris HJ, Taylor HB: Mesenchymal tumors of the uterus. *Cancer* 1966; 19:1459–1466.

Norris HJ, Taylor HB: Meschymal tumors of the uterus: I. A clinical and pathological study of 53 endometrial stromal tumors. *Cancer* 1969; 19:755–766.

Novak ER, Woodruff JD: Myoma and other benign tumors of the uterus, in *Gynecologic and Obstetric Pathology*, ed 8. Philadelphia, WB Saunders Co, 1979, p 260.

O'Leary JL, O'Leary JA: Rudimentary horn pregnancy. *Obstet Gynecol* 1963; 22:371–377.

Otubu JA, Buttram VC, Besch NF, et al: Unconjugated steroids in leiomyomas and tumor bearing myometrium. *Am J Obstet Gynecol* 1982; 43:130–133.

Padubidri V, Baijal L, Prakash P, et al: The detection of endometrial tuberculosis in cases of infertility by uterine aspiration cytology. *Acta Cytol* 1980; 24:319–324.

Pastner B, Mann WJ: Use of CA125 in monitoring patients with uterine sarcoma. A preliminary report. *Cancer* 1988; 62:1355–1381.

Perino A, Mencaglia L, Hamou J, et al: Hysteroscopy for metroplasty of uterine septa: Report of 24 cases. *Fertil Steril* 1987; 48:321–323.

Piver MS, Lele SB, Barlow JJ, et al: Paraaortic lymph node evaluation in stage I endometrial carcinoma. *Obstet Gynecol* 1982; 59:97–100.

Plentl AA, Friedman EA: Lymphatic system of the female genitalia, in *The Morphologic Basis of Oncologic Diagnosis and Therapy*, Philadelphia, WB Sanders Co, 1971; pp 123–130.

Pollow K, Sinnecker G, Boquoi E, et al: In vitro conversion of estradiol-17-beta into estrone in normal human myometrium and leiomyoma. *J Clin Chem Clin Biochem* 1978; 16:493.

Ranney B, Frederick I: The occasional need for myomectomy. *Obstet Gynecol* 1979; 53:437–441.

Robbins SL, Cotran RS: Leiomyoma (fibromyoma), in *The Pathogenic Basis of Disease,* ed 2. Philadelphia, WB Saunders Co, 1979, p 1271.

Roberts DE, Dobson KE, Hall KW, et al: Effects of prolonged Naloxone infusion in septic shock. *Lancet* 1988; 2:699–702.

Rock JA, Jones HW Jr: The clinical management of the double uterus. *Fertil Steril* 1977; 28:798–806.

Rubin A, Ford JA: Uterine fibromyomata in urban blacks. *S Afr Med J* 1974; 48:2060–2063.

Salazar OM, Bonfiglio TA, Patten SF, et al: Uterine sarcomas. Natural history, treatment and prognosis. *Cancer* 1978; 42:1152–1160.

Schenker JG, Margalioth EJ: Intrauterine adhesions: An updated appraisal. *Fertil Steril* 1982; 37:593–610.

Schumer W: Steroids in the treatment of clinical septic shock. *Ann Surg* 1976; 184:333–341.

Shah CA, Gree TH: Evaluation of current management of endometrial carcinoma. *Obstet Gynecol* 1972; 39:500–509.

Silverberg E, Lubera JA: *Cancer statistics, 1988. CA* 1988; 38:5–22.

Skowranski GA: The pathophysiology of shock. *Med J Aust* 1988; 148:576–579.

Smith DC, Prentice R, Thompson DJ, et al: Association of exogenous estrogen and endometrial carcinoma. *N Engl J Med* 1975; 293:1164–1167.

Soper JT, McCarty KS Jr, Hinshaw W, et al: Cytoplasmic estrogen and progesterone receptor content of uterine sarcomas. *Am J Obstet Gynecol* 1984; 150:342–348.

Soules MR, McCarty KS Jr: Leiomyomas: Steroid receptor content: Variations within normal menstrual cycles. *Am J Obstet Gynecol* 1982; 143:6.

Stillman RJ: In utero exposure to diethylstilbestrol: Adverse effects on the reproductive tract and reproductive performance in male and female offspring. *Am J Obstet Gynecol* 1982; 142:905–921.

Strassmann EO: Operations for double uterus and endometrial atresia. *Clin Obstet Gynecol* 1961; 4:240–251.

Strassmann EO: Fertility and unification of double uterus. *Fertil Steril* 1966; 17:165–171.

Sutherland AM: Laparoscopy in diagnosis of pelvic tuberculosis. *Lancet* 1979; 2:95.

Sutherland AM: Gynecologic tuberculosis: An analysis of a personal series of 710 cases. *Aust NZ J Obstet Gynecol* 1985; 25:203–207.

Thigpen JT, Bushsbaum HJ, Mongan C, et al: Phase II trial of Adriamycin in the treatment of advanced or recurrent endometrial carcinoma. *Cancer Treat Rep* 1979; 63:21–27.

Tierney W, Ehrlich CE, Barley JC, et al: Intravenous leiomyomatosis of the uterus with extension into the heart. *Am J Med* 1980; 306:745–746.

Townsend DE, Sparks RS, Baluda MC, et al: Unicellular histogenesis of uterine leiomyomas as determined by electrophoresis of glucose-6-phosphate dehydrogenase. *Am J Obstet Gynecol* 1970; 107:1168.

Underwood PB JR, Miller MC III, Kreutner A, et al: Endometrial carcinoma: The effect of estrogens. *Gynecol Oncol* 1979; 8:60–73.

Vadas P, Pruzanski W, Stefanski E, et al: Pathogenesis of hypotension in septic shock. *Crit Care Med* 1988; 16:1–7.

Valle RF, Sciarra JJ: Hysteroscopic treatment of the septate uterus. *Obstet Gynecol* 1986; 67:253–257.

Van Bogaert L-J: Clinicopathologic findings in endometiral polyps. *Obstet Gynecol* 1988; 71:771–773.

van Nagell JR Jr, Henson MB, Donaldson ES, et al: Adjuvant vincristine, dactinomycin and cyclophosphamide therapy in stage I uterine sarcomas. *Cancer* 1986; 57:1451–1457.

Wee JC, Bryan AC: Adenomyosis: Twenty years' experience. *J Med Assoc State Ala* 1963; 32:317–324.

Weiss DB, Aldor A, Aboulafia Y: Erythrocytosis due to erythropoietin-producing uterine fibromyoma. *Am J Obstet Gynecol* 1975; 12:358–363.

Weiss NS, Sayvetz TA: Incidence of endometrial cancer in relation to the use of oral contraceptives. *N Engl J Med* 1980; 302:551–554.

Welch WW, Scully RE: Precancerous lesions of the endometrium. *Hum Pathol* 1977; 8:503–512.

Wentz WB: Progestin therapy in endometrial hyperplasia. *Gynecol Oncol* 1974; 2:362–367.

Wilson EA, Yong F, Rees ED: Estradiol and progesterone binding in uterine leiomyomata and in normal uterine tissues. *Obstet Gynecol* 1980; 55:20–25.

Worthen NJ, Gonzalez F: Septate uterus: Sonographic diagnosis and obstetric complications. *Obstet Gynecol* 1984; 64:34S–37S.

Yazigi R, Piver MS, Blumenson L: Malignant peritoneal cytology as prognostic indication in stage I endometrial cancer. *Obstet Gynecol* 1983; 62:359–362.

8 The Oviduct and Ectopic Pregnancy

Patricia M. McShane, M.D.

John Yeh, M.D.

ANATOMY AND HISTOLOGY

The oviducts (fallopian tubes) are paired muscular canals that extend from the uterus to the ovaries, each measuring about 12 cm. These structures transport the ova into the uterine cavity, but in humans, as in most mammalian species, the oviduct is not in continuity with the ovary—it is only in apposition with it. Both tubes are covered with peritoneum and lined with epithelium and, except for a short intrauterine portion, are enveloped in the free margin of the broad ligament known as the mesosalpinx.

The oviduct emerges from the uterine wall at the junction of the corpus and fundus. The proximal segment arches laterally and posteriorly, adjacent to the lower pole of the ovary, then assumes a tortuous course along the mesovarial border of the ovary to the fimbriated end. At this point the tube is in direct relation to the medial ovarian surface. Normal variations from this description are common, especially if there is a marked uterine retroversion. In disease states such as gonococcal salpingitis, both tubes may be displaced behind the uterus into the posterior cul-de-sac, whereas with adhesions due to a ruptured appendix, the oviduct may be displaced laterally and fixed to the lateral pelvic wall or cecum. In endometriosis the fimbriae are usually patent, but the rest of the oviduct may be densely adherent to the ovary or to the posterior peritoneum.

Four subdivisions of the oviduct are described (Fig 8–1):

1. The *interstitial* portion is short and begins at the superior angle of the uterine cavity, communicating with the latter by a minute ostium. It extends through the thickness of the myometrium, angulating through the fundus to exit at the uterine cornu just superior to the attachments of the round and utero-ovarian ligaments. It may have a tortuous course (Merchant et al., 1983).

2. The *isthmic* portion is a relatively straight, narrow but thick-walled segment. It gradually increases in luminal diameter and shows a diminution in thickness of the wall as it progresses laterally.

3. The *ampullar* portion is the longest segment of the oviduct (approximately 6 cm). In its normal state it is slightly convoluted and has a relatively thin, dilatable muscular wall.

4. The *infundibular* portion is the trumpet-shaped terminal portion of the oviduct. It is divided into numerous delicate folds or fimbriae, which give a fringed appearance. One of these folds is prolonged and is attached to the mesosalpinx (fimbria ovarica). Frequently it lies in apposition to the tubal pole of the ovary.

The wall of the oviduct consists of three layers, an external or serous, an intermediate muscular, and an internal mucous layer. The serous covering is an extension of the broad ligament peritoneum and invests the tube completely except for the attachment of the mesosalpinx and the intrauterine portion. Beneath the mesothelial cells of the serosa is a connective tissue layer containing mostly blood vessels and nerves, which intermingle with the subjacent muscular layer. The outer

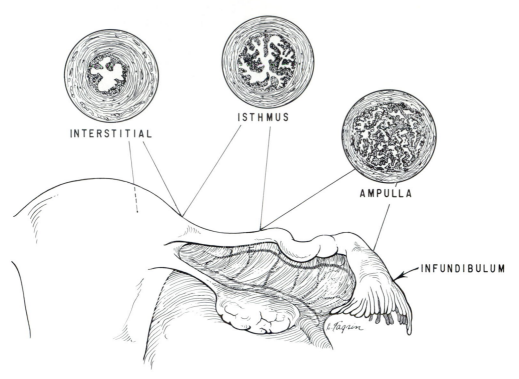

FIG 8–1.
Anatomical divisions of the oviduct.

layer of the muscularis is arranged longitudinally, whereas the inner layer is arranged circularly. The mucous membrane lining presents a characteristic folded, somewhat arborescent pattern, which is most pronounced toward the fimbriated portion (plicae tubariae). These longitudinal folds begin as four duplications of the mucosa in the interstitial portion of the tube enclosing a small lumen. The lumen of the oviduct becomes larger as it approaches the fimbriated portion and thus affords added space for increased mucosal folding. As the ampullary portion of the tube is reached, the plicae are extremely complicated and present numerous reduplications and outpouchings (Fig 8–2). The mucosa is lined with a columnar epithelium containing ciliated and nonciliated or "secretory" cells. Intercalary or "peg" cells are most easily identified in the premenstrual and menstrual period. The endosalpinx, like the endometrium, exhibits a cyclic morphological variation depending on hormonal stimulation (Donnez et al., 1985; Jansen, 1980). During the proliferative phase of estrogen stimulation, the epithelium is uniformly tall with prominent ciliated cells and narrow nonciliated cells. During the

late secretory phase, the ciliated cells are much lower, and the secretory cells are quite prominent, giving a rather uneven surface to the mucosa. During the menstrual phase, the epithelium is rather low, since the secretory cells have now been depleted of their cytoplasm. Intercalary cells are numerous during the menstrual phase, and their appearance at this time suggests that they may merely be remnants of emptied secretory cells. The immediate postmenstrual phase presents a low epithelial surface in the oviduct, but regeneration is rapid during the proliferative phase. It is likely that estrogen is responsible for ciliogenesis and that progesterone causes deciliation under some conditions (Jansen, 1984).

During the postmenopausal period, the epithelium is low and flat, the tubal folds become rounded and fibrous and their cilia disappear, but these may be restored by estrogen replacement.

The tubal epithelium in patients with endometrial hyperplasia is usually high, with uniform, narrow cells, most of which are ciliated. This represents the effects of persistent estrogen stimulation without the normal cyclic intervention of progesterone. The hormonal effect is even more evident during pregnancy when a decidual reaction in the stromal cells may be extensive. Tubal infections cause morphological changes in tubal epithelium, especially loss of ciliated cells (Fig 8–3).

The arterial blood supply to the fallopian tube is generous, anastomosing from two sources. A tubal branch of the uterine artery passes through the mesosalpinx to join branches of the ovarian artery. The venous drainage similarly occurs through branches of the uterine and ovarian veins.

Lymphatic drainage follows the ovarian vessels, thereby draining into lumbar or para-aortic nodes in the area of the renal vein and inferior vena cava on the right and into the nodes between the ovarian vein and renal vein on the left.

Both sympathetic and parasympathetic nerve fibers are found. Sympathetic fibers arise from T-10 through L-2 and synapse in numerous plexuses, ultimately providing adrenergic innervation to the tubal musculature. Parasympathetic nerves arises from the vagus nerve and from S2–4 through the pelvic nerve. Sensory fibers end in T-10 and T-4, and referred pain may be experienced in these dermatomes.

EMBRYOLOGY

The oviducts are formed by differentiation of the unfused paramesonephric ducts. (The fused portions form the uterus and a significant portion of the vagina.) The paramesonephric (müllerian) ducts arise early in the seventh week, lateral and parallel to the mesonephric duct, by a process of invagination of the coelomic epithelium opposite the cranial end of the mesonephros. The solid portions of the ducts extend caudally through primitive mesenchyme and cross the mesonephric duct anteriorly at the level of the caudal end of the mesonephros.

The commonest type of congenital anomaly of the oviduct is the absence of the ampullary portion (or a rudimentary one), which probably occurs because of torsion and subsequent ischemic atrophy. Supernumerary oviducts are rare, but duplication of the ampullary region and accessory tubal ostia are relatively common (Daw, 1973). Accessory tubes that arise along the course of the oviduct never communicate with the lumen but the accessory ostia located near the main ostium always do. Unilateral absence of the oviduct

is uncommon, but when it does occur, it is associated with ureteral and renal abnormalities on the involved side (Zaitoon and Florentin, 1982). Bilateral tubal absence is rare and is usually associated with uterine and vaginal agenesis. In such cases, there may be normal ovaries that are attached laterally to the free edge of the empty broad ligament. Absence of one or both tubes may be secondary to autoamputation. Segmental atresia and persistence of the coiled fetal pattern are rare anomalies but may be seen occasionally when large numbers of laparotomies are done for so-called idiopathic infertility.

Women exposed to diethylstilbestrol (DES) prenatally are known to have a variety of malformations of their müllerian structures, including the oviduct. DeCherney and colleagues performed laparoscopies on 16 infertile women with DES exposure (DeCherney et al., 1981). The patients were found to have "withered" tubes that were foreshortened, sacculated, and convoluted with pinpoint fimbrial openings or distal tubal occlusion. Mice experimentally exposed to DES were also seen to exhibit oviductal structural abnormalities at doses similar to those given to women therapeutically (McLachlan et al., 1982).

TUBAL PHYSIOLOGY

The major physiological functions of the tube are reproductive: passage of spermatozoa, ovum pickup, provision of an adequate site for fertilization and early embryonic development, and transport of the conceptus to the uterus. Whether the oviduct has significant immunological or antibacterial function is not well established, although immunologically competent cells are present in the tube.

The mechanism of capture of the oocyte by the fallopian tube varies among mammalian species, with some species exhibiting a periovarian sac isolating the ovary from the peritoneal cavity and presumably assuring capture by the oviduct (Beyth, 1986). In the human, there is no anatomically isolated site, but the well-developed fimbriae are able to reach almost any point on the ovary, apparently allowing efficient capture. Anatomical features such as the multitude of epithelial folds with their predominance of ciliated cells beating in the direction of the uterus are undoubtedly important (Blandau, 1969). It is also known that the ligaments surrounding the tube

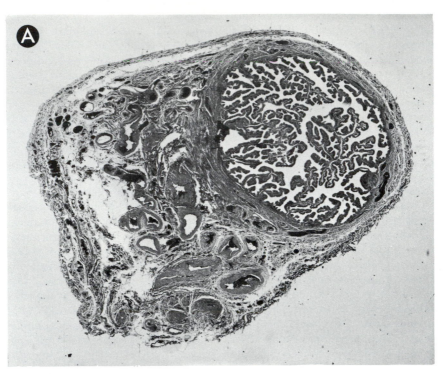

FIG 8—2.
A, normal oviduct. *(Continued.)*

and the ovaries exhibit contractions that may be influenced by epinephrine, norepinephrine, prostaglandins, and other substances (Jansen, 1984).

The relative importance of the fimbriae, ligamentous movements, and ciliary mechanisms are unclear. It seems likely that there may be redundancy in the ovum pickup mechanism, since fertility can be demonstrated in the absence of fimbria (Kamrava et al., 1982; Metz, 1977), or following surgical reversal of fimbriectomy (Novy, 1980), in women with abnormal tubo-ovarian anatomical relationships and with disorders of ciliary motion such as Kartagener's syndrome (McComb et al., 1986; Bleau et al., 1978).

The cumulus mass of the oocyte itself is probably critical for both ovum pickup and transport, since rabbits eggs denuded of their covering of sticky granulosa cells are not transported normally (Blandau, 1969).

Ovum transport within the oviduct has been extensively studied in animals, but only a few thorough investigations have been accomplished in women. At least three factors seem to be involved in tubal transport: ciliary action, muscle contractions, and changes in viscosity of tubal fluid. Ciliary activity in the human oviduct can be demonstrated to actively transport particles, even in the absence of muscle contraction (Gaddum-Rosse et al., 1973). Larger particles (e.g., the ovum) are permanently in contact with the mucosal cells, a steady movement toward the ampullary-isthmic junction being effected. An increase in muscular activity has been noted at the ovulatory phase of the menstrual cycle as well as slower, more uniform contractions during the premenstrual phase (Talo and Pulkkinen, 1982). These muscular contractions begin at the ampulla and proceed to the isthmus. Further, the frequency of the ampullary contractions is higher than those found in the isthmus. In all probability the action of the cilia provides the primary mechanism for ovum transport within the tube, aided and abetted by the muscular contractions.

It is known from the pioneering studies of Croxatto et al. (1978) that the fertilized ovum resides within the oviduct for approximately 3 days. The ovum remains in the ampulla for approximately 72 hours and then rapidly traverses the isthmus (Croxatto et at., 1978). The reason for this delay in transit is presently unknown. Al-

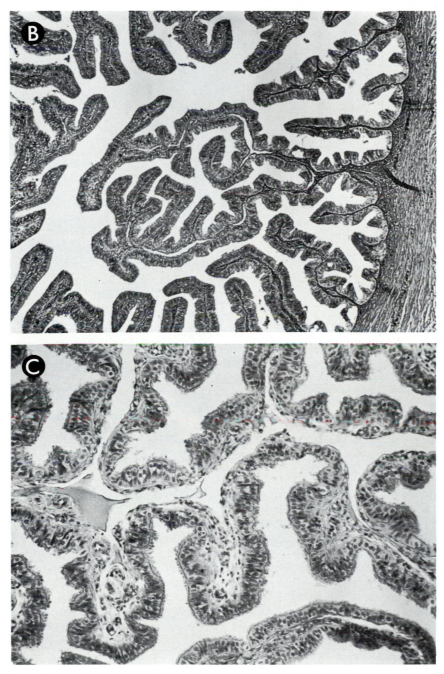

FIG 8−2. (cont.).
B, higher power to show epithelium in proliferative phase. **C,** higher power to show epithelium in secretory phase. (From Hall JE: *Applied Gynecologic Pathology.* New York, Appleton-Century-Crofts, 1963, p 197. Reproduced by permission.)

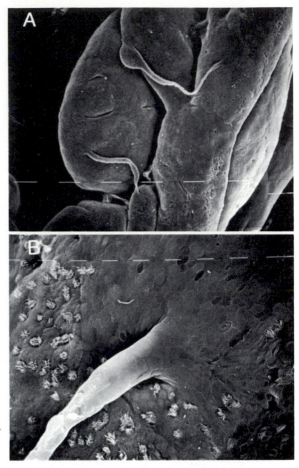

FIG 8–3.
A, scanning electron micrograph of tubal epithelium following tubal infection with distortion of endosalpingeal folds and "microadhesions" (approximately 50 ×).
B, higher power view demonstrating loss of ciliated cells and microadhesion (approximately 640 ×). (Courtesy of James E. Wheeler, M.D., Hospital of the University of Pennsylvania, Philadelphia.)

though fertilized ova are retained in the ampullary portion of the tube in the rabbit, this is accomplished by a physiological closure of the isthmus. There is no evidence of a similar mechanism in the human female.

One possible mechanism of the delay of the oocyte or conceptus at the ampullary isthmic junction is the presence of a tenacious column of mucus in the isthmus at the time of ovulation (Jansen, 1984). A decrease in this secretion and an apparent increase in cilia by scanning electron microscopy becomes evident several days after ovulation. Tubal secretion appears to be under endocrine control (Leese, 1988).

Attempts to alter ovum transport in women through excision or transposition of tubal segments and with gonadal steroids or neuroactive drugs have failed to completely elucidate the mechanisms of passage (Hoffman, 1980). It is conceivable that failure of precision in the process of ovum transport is a cause of infertility in some individuals.

The delay in the oviduct is probably related to maturation of the ovum. Chang (1950) demonstrated a definite relation between the age of the ovum and the ability to implant. Thus, if rabbit ova were transferred from the oviduct to the uterus within 24 hours of fertilization, implantation did not occur. After 48 hours a small number of implantations occur, but the majority implanted when transfer was effected after 3 days. This important observation has implications that may influence the practice of in vitro fertilization (IVF) in the future, since current practice is to replace the embryos into the uterine cavity at 48 hours.

The role of the oviduct in sperm transport in speculative. It has been known for many years that sperm can be found in the ampulla of the fallopian tube within minutes of insemination (Settlage et al., 1973). Although intrinsic sperm motility and uterine contractions due to intercourse and seminal plasma may play a role, inert particles deposited at the cervix have also been observed to gain entry to the peritoneal cavity via the uterus and oviducts, seemingly contrary to the prevailing ciliary and muscular transport activity (Stone et al., 1985).

A concentration gradient of sperm has been observed in the female reproductive tract. The cervix probably acts as both a barrier and a reservoir of sperm. The next significant anatomic barrier is thought to be the isthmus of the tube, possibly effected by its tenacious mucus. Screening out of abnormal forms is thought to occur at each site.

The role of the oviductal fluid in sperm capacitation is not known, although in experimental animals sperm must reside within reproductive tract fluids for a number of hours for fertilization to occur. Capacitation is the process of membrane changes necessary for fertilization.

Tubal fluid results from transudation and secretion (Leese, 1988). Tubal fluid volume increases with estrogen stimulation and decreases with progesterone stimulation. Principal components include electrolytes, including a high concentration of potassium, metabolic substrates, and bicarbonate. Albumin and immunoglobin G are the most abundant proteins. At the time of ovulation and for several days thereafter, unique proteins can be demonstrated in the fluid (Lippe et al., 1981), suggesting a role in fertilization and early zygote development. The ability to accomplish IVF and pregnancy in the absence of these unique proteins suggests that they might enhance the efficiency of this process but may not be required for the early events.

Present evidence strongly suggests that the oviduct functions in more than just a passive nature and serves as more than a simple conduit for ova and sperm. The changes in tubal morphology and fluid accumulation are obviously under hormonal regulation. The formation and elaboration of specific substances needed for growth and development of the ovum are similarly controlled by estrogen and progesterone.

Physiological Salpingitis

In the course of routine examination of fallopian tubes removed at the time of hysterectomy at the Brigham and Women's Hospital, numerous cases of salpingitis associated with menstrual endometrium have been encountered. Although the inflammatory reaction was of the acute variety and was associated with an infiltration of polymorphonuclear leukocytes, it did not have the precise pathological appearance of acute salpingitis due to bacterial infection. Nassberg et al. (1954) described this inflammatory process in 43 of 69 patients who had hysterectomy and salpingectomy at the time of menstruation. The inflammatory reaction was characterized by polymorphonuclear leukocytes within the lumen of the tube, in the stroma of the tubal plicae, but only rarely in the muscularis. The plicae showed edema, stasis of leukocytes within their capillaries and dilatation of the lymphatics. The inflammatory process was confined to the mucosal part of the oviduct, and the muscle walls were seldom involved. There was no associated evidence of healed follicular salpingitis as characterized by infiltration of lymphocytes, plasma cells, or fusion of the tips of the plicae. No bacteria were demonstrated, and the patients showed no evidence of infection clinically. Since the inflammation was superficial and submucosal and since endometrial debris as well as leukocytes and red blood cell debris were found in the lumina, it was suggested that the cause of this reaction was related to the regurgitation of menstrual blood into the oviducts during the menstrual period. Although this inflammatory reaction appears to be quite severe, there is no evidence that residual damage to the tube occurs. Even during the acute phase, neither necrosis nor destruction of any portion of the tubal structure is noted.

Nontuberculous Granulomatous Salpingitis

Nontuberculous granulomatous salpingitis is a rather common type of salpingitis, which may be a sequela of salpingograms performed with iodine-oil preparations. The granulomatous lesion produced by the deposition of this oil in the tubal mucosa may simulate tuberculosis. The tubercle, however, is atypical, organisms are not identified by proper staining, and cultures are negative. Furthermore, caseation necrosis is not seen.

Deposition of talc granules into the peritoneal cavity at the time of surgery may lead to a similar granulomatous salpingitis. Apparently the talc granules are ingested by the fimbriated portion of the oviduct and become embedded in the endosalpinx. These are most commonly seen in the fimbriated and ampullary portion of the tube. Systemic diseases, including Crohn's disease and infections such as actinomycosis and schistosomiasis, may occasionally give rise to a granulomatous salpingitis, which may be confused with that of tuberculosis.

TUBAL ECTOPIC PREGNANCY

Ectopic pregnancy continues to be a major diagnostic problem and is responsible for approximately 15% of all obstetrically caused maternal deaths in the United States each year (Atrash et al., 1987). The declining case fatality rate has been offset by the fourfold increase in incidence since 1970. Most maternal deaths are due to hemorrhage and are thought to be preventable (Dorfman et al., 1984). The incidence of ectopic pregnancy is variable, depending on the type of hospital reporting the data, but is around 1 in 120 pregnancies in the United States.

The use of antibiotics and conservative treatment of pelvic inflammation has undoubtedly increased the incidence of tubal gestation (Westrom et al., 1981), although no evidence of salpingitis can be found in 50% to 75% of cases (Pauerstein et al., 1986; Walters et al., 1987). Studies in Sweden and the United States found serological evidence of prior chlamydial infection in more than 50% of women with ectopic pregnancies, whereas only 20% of matched controls had antibodies positive for *Chlamydia* (Svensson et al., 1985; Brunham et al., 1986). A history of clinical pelvic inflammatory disease (PID) is known to be a risk factor (Brunham et al., 1986; Marchbanks et al., 1988). Both the gross anatomical alterations such as adherence of mucosal folds and the ultrastructural events of deciliation and denuding of epithelium related to chronic salpingitis may be implicated (see Fig 8–3). Infertility itself is associated with an increased risk of ectopic pregnancy even after controlling for PID (Marchbanks et al., 1988; Yang et al., 1987). Clomiphene citrate and other hormonal therapies may be etiologic (Yang et al., 1987; Marchbanks et al., 1985). The first IVF pregnancy was tubal, and ectopic pregnancies continue to number approximately 5% of pregnancies following IVF and GIFT (gamete intrafallopian transfer) (Australian in Vitro Fertilization Group, 1985).

Current intrauterine device use is a strong risk factor (Marchbanks et al., 1988), as is a prior tubal sterilization, especially with coagulation (McCausland, 1980, 1982; Stock and Nelson, 1984). Tubal reconstructive surgery carries a risk of ectopic pregnancy ranging from 3% to 10%, depending priniciplally on the degree of intrinsic tubal damage (Lavy et al., 1987). Whereas women with one prior ectopic have a risk of about 10% of a repeat ectopic pregnancy, whether or not the tube was removed (Lavy et al., 1987), DES daughters experience approximately 5% ectopic pregnancies (Corson and Batzer, 1986).

Clinicians caring for patients with any of these risk factors should inform their patients of the increased risk. Early surveillance of pregnancies may lead to prompt diagnosis and intervention, reducing the scope of intervention required in some cases and perhaps reducing mortality.

Other practices such as smoking (Chow et al., 1988) and douching (Chow et al., 1985) are associated with an increased risk of tubal pregnancy. Fortunately, induced abortion has not shown to increase the risk in recent studies (Daling et al., 1985; Marchbanks et al., 1988).

Diagnosis

Presenting Signs and Symptoms

Pain.—Pain is the commonest and most consistent symptom associated with ectopic pregnancy (Newton, 1988), but the type is variable depending on the duration of the gestation and the extent of hemorrhage. Most of the patients with ectopic pregnancy complain of cramplike pelvic or lower abdominal pain on the affected side early in the gestation. This pain may be due to uterine contractions and distention of the tubal serosa.

Lancinating pelvic pain associated with fainting is frequently seen in patients with acute rupture of an ectopic pregnancy, whereas dull, aching pain occurs in those having an organized hematoma around an unruptured ectopic pregnancy. About 10% of the patients have shoulder pain in addition to pelvic pain, an almost certain indication of intraperitoneal spill of blood and diaphragmatic irritation.

Abnormal Vaginal Bleeding.—A careful, accurate history of the recent menstural periods is of extreme importance in diagnosis. The exact dates of the previous three bleeding episodes together with the character and duration of flow should be ascertained. Frequently, it will be discovered that the most recent bleeding did not occur at the expected time in the cycle and that it was slightly diminished in amount. In approximately 50% of patients, the menstrual history will be normal. Most of these patients, however, will have noted spotting or intermittent slight vaginal bleeding since the last normal menstrual period, and in about 10% of patients the bleeding begins simultaneously with the onset of pain. Profuse bleeding with passage of large clots is not a common symptom unless the patient has associated leiomyomas. Continued diminished bleeding and the absence of large clots is more characteristic of ectopic pregnancy than threatened or incomplete abortion.

Amenorrhea of 2 or 3 months' duration may be associated with an ectopic pregnancy occurring in the interstitial portion of the oviduct or in a rudimentary uterine horn, since rupture in these areas is delayed.

Pregnancy Signs and Symptoms.—Nausea, vomiting, and breast engorgement are not usually seen because of the early termination of the gestation. They may be present in pregnancies occurring in the uterine cornua or interstitial portion of the oviduct.

Physical Examination

The condition of the patient may vary from normal to one of extreme shock with pallor, clammy skin, sweating, tachycardia, and hypotension. The majority of patients, however, do not present this typical textbook picture, which is associated with acute loss of blood into the peritoneal cavity. An exception to this is seen in rupture of a rudimentary horn or interstitial pregnancy. The intraperitoneal hemorrhage in these patients is massive because of the vascularity of the area and its double blood supply.

Temperature.—A ruptured ectopic pregnancy, even with a large pelvic hematoma, will cause only a slight elevation in temperature. In patients having acute rupture the temperature is frequently found to be subnormal, and it is uncommon to find it exceeding 38.3° C. This characteristic of the temperature to remain subnormal or only slightly elevated is a valuable sign in differentiating PID and septic abortion.

Pulse Rate.—The pulse rate is characteristically rapid when the ectopic pregnancy has ruptured but otherwise is normal.

Blood Pressure.—The blood pressure reflects both the acuteness of the process and the degree of blood loss. In patients with unruptured ectopic pregnancies as well as those with slowly leaking ruptures with hematoma formation, the blood pressure is normal. Systolic pressures less than 80 mm Hg are seen in only about 10% of patients. Pulse and blood pressure should be taken with the patient in the recumbent position and then immediately after sitting up. Significant increases in pulse and decrease in blood pressure with this maneuver indicate substantial compensated hemorrhage.

Abdomen.—Examination of the abdomen usually yields negative findings in patients with an unruptured or locally confined process. There may be lower quadrant tenderness if a large peritubal hematoma has formed. In the presence of massive intraperitoneal bleeding, the abdomen is diffusely tender and presents typical muscular rigidity. If the intraperitoneal bleeding is of several days' duration, abdominal distention due to small bowel ileus may be noted. Occasionally a periumbilical blue discoloration is noted in patients with massive intraperitoneal bleeding (Cullen's sign).

Pelvic Examination.—Findings are extremely variable, depending on the duration of pregnancy and the amount of intraperitoneal bleeding. The cervix and uterus are usually of normal size and consistency, but manipulation of the cervix causes pelvic pain in most patients if there is leakage of blood or rupture of the tube. In early unruptued tubal pregnancy, the tubal enlargement may be too slight to be detected by bimanual examination and is frequently missed. If the adnexa on the opposite side are normal to palpation, the chances of tubal pregnancy are greater. Since chronic salpingitis is a predisposing factor to the development of ectopic pregnancy, the finding of contralateral disease does not eliminate the possibility.

After tubal abortion or rupture, the adnexal area is exquisitely tender. If the tube has ruptured, it is apt to be less markedly enlarged than when tubal abortion has taken place. Liquid blood in the cul-de-sac produces a doughy or full feeling, although frequently both adnexal areas will be thought to be normal even when bathed in liquid blood. After the blood has clotted, it is easily felt as a soft, somewhat indefinite, tender mass in the cul-de-sac or adnexal region.

The importance of limiting bimanual examinations and observing extreme gentleness in doing this procedure must be emphasized. Examination under anesthesia is frequently desirable since the pain associated with manipulation of the internal genitalia limits the examiner considerably. Shock following a pelvic examination under anesthesia is suggestive of a ruptured ectopic pregnancy but may also occur subsequent to rupture of a tubo-ovarian abscess.

Laboratory and Other Diagnostic Procedures

Pregnancy Testing and Ultrasound.—Conventional pregnancy tests with low sensitivity are helpful only if positive, since a large number of potentially life-threatening tubal pregnancies may present with low human chorionic gonadotropin (hCG) values. Conversely, even high hCG levels may not be reassuring, since advanced interstitial pregnancies may have normal levels of hCG until rupture. It is imperative to combine pregnancy testing with other diagnostic modalities and to maintain a high index of suspicion (Newton, 1988).

A positive pregnancy test result effectively excludes many other causes of abdominal symptomatology such as appendicitis, degenerating fibroids, salpingitis, adnexal masses or torsion, or a ruptured corpus luteum. However, an abnormal hCG test result does not distinguish a normal intrauterine pregnancy from threatened abortion or ectopic pregnancy. In a clinically stable patient, the hCG levels may be used to distinguish among these possibilities when the patient has risk factors for tubal pregnancy, such as prior tubal surgery, or has mild symptoms such as early pregnancy bleeding.

Although the absolute level of hCG is not predictive of outcome in early pregnancy, serial hCG levels can distinguish normal pregnancies from abnormal gestations with a high degree of sensitivity, since abnormal gestations produce less hCG (Batzer and Corson, 1986). In early pregnancy, prior to detectability by ultrasound, the hCG level should double approximately every 2 days. Fritz and Guo (1987) have published a nomogram that predicts the change in hCG levels over 2- to 4-day sampling intervals at various hCG levels. If the second hCG value falls below confidence limits, it virtually excludes a normal intrauterine pregnancy and would normally dictate that an ultrasound test be used to ascertain the presence of an intrauterine sac or adnexal mass. If no mass is present, performance of a uterine curettage should demonstrate placental tissue. If no tissue is obtained, laparoscopy should be performed to evaluate the site of pregnancy. Clinically stable reliable patients may occasionally be prudently managed in a more conservative fashion, since some normal pregnancies may have slow progression of hCG levels.

With the transabdominal ultrasound technique, a uterine sac is detectable in experienced hands when the hCG level is approximately 6,500 mIU/ml, or about 2 weeks after missed menses (Romero et al., 1985b). The newer transvaginal probe is better able to detect early pregnancies because of higher resolution and anatomic proximity; intrauterine pregnancy can be detected at about 3,600 mIU/ml. Vaginal ultrasound has a much enhanced ability to image adnexal masses (Shapiro et al., 1988), often including demonstration of an empty uterus and an adnexal sac with a positive fetal heart motion (Fig 8–4).

Future work may confirm the study of Yeko and colleagues (1987), which suggests that a single progesterone value may differentiate normal from ectopic gestations.

Blood Examination.—Determination of the leukocyte count is not of particular assistance. Approximately 50% of the patients with ectopic pregnancy have a white blood cell count less than 10,000/cu mm, and in 75% it is less than 15,000/cu mm. A leukocytosis exceeding 20,000/cu mm has been noted in only about 10% of patients, and a persistent leukocytosis of this degree favors a diagnosis of PID. There is an initial leukocytosis immediately following tubal rupture, but this usually returns to normal within 24 hours unless there is recurrent bleeding.

The erythrocyte count and hematocrit reflect the extent of bleeding, but the initial determination is modified by preexisting anemia and the state of hydration. In hospitals having a large indigent population, about 50% of the patients have an erythrocyte count less than 3 million/cu mm prior to bleeding from ruptured ectopic pregnancy. Of more importance than the initial count are *sequential* determinations of the hemato-

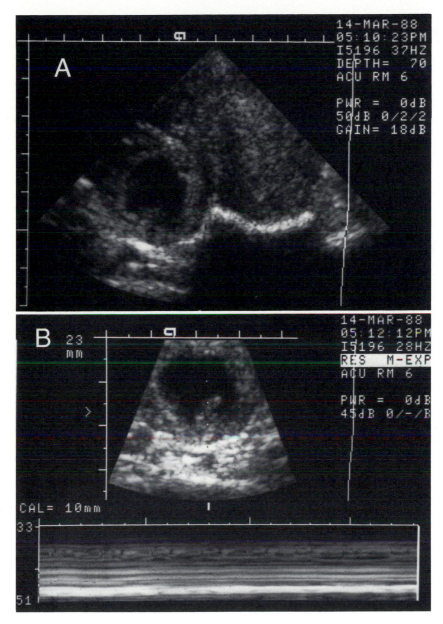

FIG 8–4.
A, tubal ectopic pregnancy by vaginal ultrasound scan. Gestational sac with fetal pole, situated next to empty uterus. **B,** fetal heart beat demonstrated by M-mode vaginal ultrasound. (Courtesy of Dr. Peter M. Doubilet, Director of Ultrasound, Brigham and Women's Hospital, Harvard Medical School, Boston.)

crit and erythrocytes. A gradual decrease is frequently associated with persistent leakage of blood into a peritubal hematoma.

In patients with a chronically leaking ectopic pregnancy and gradual absorption of blood, the serum bilirubin level and icteric index may be elevated.

Culdocentesis.—Culdocentesis is of particular value if the cul-de-sac is bulging. It may be done without general anesthesia using a long 15- to 18-gauge needle on a 10- or 20-ml syringe. A dry tap is unusual and should warrant another attempt. The fluid obtained may suggest (1) if clear, serous, and straw colored—a normal pelvis;

(2) if turbid but serous—PID; (3) if blood tinged and serous—ruptured ovarian cysts, ovulation bleeding, or occasionally, PID; (4) if bright red and grossly bloody—recently bleeding corpus luteum, recently ruptured ectopic pregnancy with fresh bleeding, or a traumatic cul-de-sac aspiration; (5) if *old, brownish blood*—ectopic pregnancy with intraperitoneal bleeding over a few days or weeks. *Blood does not clot,* or at times tiny clots may be aspirated.

Romero et al. (1985a) studied 158 women with nonclotting blood on culdocentesis; 84% had ectopic pregnancies, of which more than one half were unruptured. A normal culdocentesis with a normal hCG test result was 99% predictive of not having an ectopic pregnancy. Sixteen percent of women with ectopic pregnancy had a nondiagnostic culdocentesis, however.

Laparoscopy.—Laparoscopy is the optimum diagnostic procedure in patients with a suspected unruptured ectopic pregnancy. In the future, laparoscopic resection of the gestation may frequently be practiced. Occasionally, the pregnancy may be too small to be seen by laparoscopy, or other adnexal pathology may make proper inspection of the adnexal impossible (Kim et al., 1987). It should also be remembered that the level of hCG correlates poorly with the size of the pregnancy (Cartwright et al., 1987).

Uterine Curettage.—If chorionic tissue is found either grossly or microscopically, the presence of an intrauterine pregnancy is obvious. The rare combination of intrauterine and extrauterine pregnancy (heterotopic pregnancy), however, is still a possibility. If the curettings show only decidua, a diagnosis of ectopic pregnancy must be considered. It is possible, however, to curet a pregnant uterus and miss the ovum so that only decidual tissue is obtained. Similarly, a decidual reaction in the endometrial stroma may be brought about by a corpus luteum cyst, a luteinized follicular cyst, or granulosa cell tumor or by the administration of potent synthetic progestational agents.

In general, it may be concluded that when decidua without chorionic tissue is found by curettage, there is a good possibility of an ectopic pregnancy, but the absence of decidua does not exclude tubal pregnancy, especially if the bleeding is of several weeks' duration. The endometrium in such patients may be secretory, proliferative, or menstrual.

Specific morphological changes in the epithelium of the endometrium have been described in association with either intrauterine or extrauterine pregnancy. This *Arias-Stella reaction* has been called an anaplasia of pregnancy and, if found, should alert the clinician to the possibility of an ectopic pregnancy. This morphological pattern has not been described in the endometrium of patients receiving synthetic progestational agents for pseudopregnancy.

Since the findings from curettage are equivocal in so many patients and since a normal intrauterine pregnancy may be interrupted, this procedure is not advised as a routine diagnostic procedure.

Treatment

The optimum treatment for ectopic pregnancy is surgical removal. It should be performed as rapidly as possible after diagnosis has been made, and supportive therapy, if necessary, should be administered in the operating room.

It is known that many ectopic gestations abort or spontaneously resolve and expectant treatment has been advocated (Fernandez et al., 1988; Garcia et al., 1987). Expectant treatment of ectopic pregnancy is nevertheless hazardous since the gestational sac and adjacent oviduct may rupture without warning, and the patient may die from massive hemorrhage. Furthermore, chorionic tissue may persist, and tubal function is by no means guaranteed (Gomel and Filmar, 1987).

Despite inconvenience, it has been advised that "the sun never set on a possible ectopic pregnancy." Transfusions of whole blood should be given to patients who are in shock, the patient transferred to the operating room as soon as possible, and transfusion continued throughout the procedure.

The management of ectopic pregnancy demands that hemorrhage be prevented or arrested. Therefore, treatment usually consists of excision of the involved tube. If the patient has been in shock or if there is massive intraperitoneal hemorrhage, operation should be limited to removal of the ectopic pregnancy and control of hemorrhage. In some patients who are operated on for ectopic pregnancy and whose condition is good, a hysterectomy may be indicated. It is the usual treatment for interstitial pregnancy. It may also be advisable if one oviduct has been previously removed, if one oviduct is irreparably damaged, or in the presence of other indications. Since the development of IVF, hysterectomy is usually not performed for patients desiring preservation of reproductive potential.

When the ectopic gestation involves the fimbriated portion of the tube or even the ampulla (Fig 8–5), and particularly in a patient who has been infertile, conservative procedures may help preserve the childbearing potential (Hallatt, 1986; Strangel, 1986; Strangel and Gomel, 1980). Both lateral incisions of the tubes and salpingostomy with or without primary closure have been suggested as methods of tubal preservation.

"Milking," or fimbrial expression, of a distal ampullary pregnancy appears to be safe and effective if it is easily accomplished without undue force or bleeding (Sherman et al., 1987). The optimal conservative therapy for isthmic gestation is segmental resection with either immediate or delayed anastamosis (DeCherney and Boyers, 1985). Perhaps because ectopic pregnancies may invade and destroy the musculature of the narrow isthmic segment (Pauerstein et al., 1986), linear salpingostomy appears to lead to tubal obstruction or recurrent ectopic gestation in a number of cases.

Laparoscopic treatment of small unruptured ectopic pregnancies has now become commonplace (Bruhat et al., 1980; DeCherney and Diamond, 1987; Dubuisson et al., 1987). Most proponents of the technique require that the gestation be less than 4 cm and ampullary (Cartwright et al., 1986), but others report excellent results with most hemodynamically stable women (Reich et al., 1988; Silva, 1988). Although standard laparoscopy instrumentation can be used, use of an endocoagulator or laser and several specialized instruments optimizes the procedure. Salpingostomy with a scissors, cautery or laser is the standard technique, although salpingectomy or segmental resection can be performed through the laparoscope (Dubuisson et al., 1987; Reich et al., 1988).

If a patient has had conservative treatment, either by laparotomy or laparoscopy, it is imperative that the hCG titer be followed to determine completeness of the procedure (Kamrava et al., 1983), since a significant minority of patients have evidence of persistent trophoblast (DiMarchi et al., 1987; Vermesh et al., 1988). Recurrent ectopic pregnancy in a blind ampullary segment is another potential complication of conservative therapy (Cartwright and Entman, 1984).

Methotrexate has been used successfully in small series of women with small unruptured tubal gestations (Sauer et al., 1987). Current protocols include visualization of the pregnancy with laparoscopy and inpatient parenteral methotrexate injections followed by folinic acid rescue (Sauer et al., 1987). Treatment courses can last as long as 8 days if hCG levels do not fall and are sometimes limited by hepatic toxicity and other side effects. This approach would seem to be of limited value for routine tubal pregnancy when laparoscopic treatment is available. Successful treatment of cervical (Oyer et al., 1988) and interstitial (Tanaka et al., 1982) pregnancies has been reported, thereby avoiding hysterectomy. Intra-amniotic injection of methotrexate under ultrasound visual-

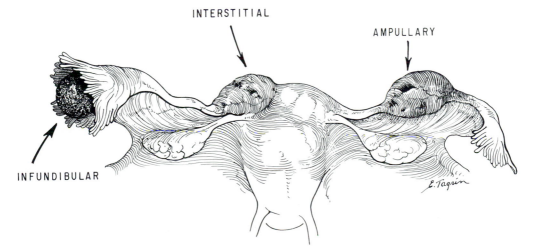

FIG 8–5.
Anatomic sites of tubal ectopic pregnancies.

ization may make the therapy more acceptable (Leeton and Davison, 1988).

Other ancillary surgical procedures may be performed without increasing morbidity if the patient's general condition is good and if massive intraperitoneal hemorrhage has not occurred. Appendectomy has been performed in many patients in this group, and abdominal myomectomy has been carried out in a few nulliparous patients who desire to have children (Cromartie and Kovalcik, 1980).

Fertility After Ectopic Pregnancy

There is no doubt that the occurrence of an ectopic pregnancy is a major accident for a patient who wishes subsequently to become pregnant. It has been estimated that only about one third of such patients will ever succeed in delivering a living child, although recent estimates have been higher (Nagamani et al., 1984; Thorburn et al., 1988; Tuomivaara and Kauppila, 1988).

More than one third will become pregnant, but many will lose the gestation by either miscarriage or recurrent ectopic pregnancy. It has been estimated that such patients are seven to eight times more likely to have a subsequent misplaced pregnancy than are women who have not had ectopic gestations. Many studies have shown similar fertility rates and recurrent ectopic pregnancy rate whether tubal conservation is achieved (Tuomivaara and Kauppila, 1988), but selection bias may be important. Previous infertility is a risk factor for poor reproductive performance subsequent to the occurrence of a tubal gestation (McComb et al., 1986; Sherman et al., 1982; Thorburn et al., 1988). Older and nulliparous women, as well as those with contralateral tubal damage, have poorer subsequent outcomes (Langer at al., 1982).

Women experiencing a second ectopic pregnancy have approximately a 30% chance of a third ectopic pregnancy but also a 50% chance of a term delivery, so that a conservative approach is warranted (DeCherney et al., 1985; Tulandi, 1988). Tubal conservation is also warranted when a pregnancy occurs in the woman's only remaining tube, since about 50% of these patients will successfully deliver, although at least 20% can be expected to have another ectopic pregnancy (DeCherney et al., 1982; Oelsner et al., 1986).

Previously, it had been suggested that removal of the ovary on the side of a salpingectomy for ectopic pregnancy might improve the pregnancy rate by "putting all the eggs in one basket." This approach, never proved conclusively, would seem to be unjustified in the current era of assisted reproductive techniques such as IVF.

COMBINED INTRAUTERINE AND EXTRAUTERINE PREGNANCIES

Until recently, it had been estimated that the incidence of heterotopic pregnancy was only about 1 in 30,000. However, recent increased use of ovarian hyperstimulation may be responsible for a dramatic increase in this incidence.

The diagnosis of combined pregnancy should be considered if the patient gives a history of ectopic pregnancy or has unilateral lower abdominal tenderness with concomitant evidence of an intrauterine pregnancy. If the uterus is enlarged, the cervix is closed, and there is minimal vaginal bleeding, the physician should always be suspicious of this combination. The persistence of lower abdominal pain following spontaneous abortion of an early uterine pregnancy should suggest that an ectopic pregnancy may coexist. Sonographic examination will usually show both intrauterine and extrauterine pregnancies. The treatment for combined pregnancy should be removal of the extrauterine pregnancy. Postoperative attention should be directed toward the preservation of the intrauterine gestation. Routine curettage in extrauterine pregnancy is not advised because of the possibility of interruption of an intrauterine pregnancy.

SALPINGITIS ISTHMICA NODOSA

Salpingitis isthmica nodosa is a disease process of unknown etiology, characterized by nodular thickenings in the intramural and isthmic portions of the oviduct. Microscopically, the nodules are noted to be in the muscular wall of the tube and to contain nests of glandlike tissue. Frequently the lumina of these glands are connected to the central tubal lumen. This disease process is also known variously as diverticulosis adenomyosis of the tube, adenosalpingitis, and endosalpingiosis. The incidence is variable and depends on the detailed examination of the pathologist and on the number of microscopic sections taken through this portion of the oviduct. The disease occurs most commonly between the ages of 25 and 50 years, with an average age of 35 years. It is commoner among blacks than among whites.

The pathogenesis of this disease is controversial, but several theories have been advanced as to its origin. One theory suggests that this disease is the sequel of inflammation of either gonorrheal or tuberculous type. The support for the inflammatory origin is provided chiefly by the fact that associated inflammation is found in 75% to 80% of cases. Bilateral lesions are also quite common.

It has been suggested that the islands of glandular tissue are formed as a result of an extension of the mucosa during the acute inflammatory process. Thus, minute intraluminal abscesses may rupture or dissect into the softened muscularis. Against this theory is evidence that salpingitis isthmica nodosa is often contralateral to the classic inflammatory process (Benjamin and Beaver, 1951).

In several reports of patients with salpingitis isthmica nodosa, fewer than 50% had an associated inflammatory process. In such patients the lesion was thought to be of noninflammatory origin, and it was suggested that the process arose from a proliferation or hyperplasia of the epithelial lining cells of the isthmus or possibly by a contiguous spread of uterine adenomyosis (Wrork and Broders, 1942).

The congenital origin of salpingitis isthmica nodosa was championed by numerous authors at the turn of the century. Since the condition is found only in the woman and not in the fetus, this theory has been disputed.

The gross appearance of salpingitis isthmica nodosa (Fig 8−6) is usually characteristic. The le-sions are bilateral in about 35% of patients. Usually the nodules are multiple and irregularly distributed, presenting a somewhat beaded appearance. The nodules vary from a few millimeters to 2.5 cm in diameter and frequently are sharply circumscribed, firm, irregular but with a smooth surface.

The microscopic appearance of salpingitis isthmica nodosa (Fig 8−7) is variable, depending on the duration of the lesion. In its earliest form there is a simple outpocketing of the tubal mucosa into the musculature. In its fully developed state, glandlike spaces are scattered throughout the myosalpinx and are associated with hyperplasia and hypertrophy of the muscle fibers. In cystically dilated glands there is flattening of the epithelium, whereas in the smaller glandular spaces the epithelium is a mixture of that seen in the tube and endometrium. There is a surrounding stroma of collagenous fibrous connective tissue, which is usually infiltrated with plasma cells, leukocytes, or eosinophils.

Diagnosis and Treatment

The diagnosis of salpingitis isthmica nodosa is usually made at the time of laparoscopy or laparotomy for infertility or PID. In 1951, Bunster demonstrated that this lesion, which he called *tubal diverticulosis,* could be diagnosed by means of salpingography and he published hysterosalpingograms revealing such diverticula. Siegler, in 1955, was able to diagnose tubal diverticulosis in 1.6% of 1,160 hysterosalpingograms performed on patients whose primary complaint was infertility. He suggested that the diagnosis should be sus-

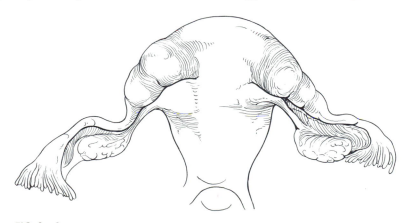

FIG 8−6.
Salpingitis isthmica nodosa.

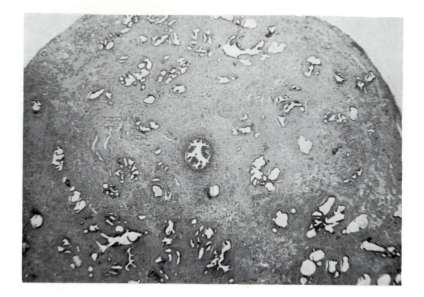

FIG 8–7.
Salpingitis isthmica nodosa. Photomicrograph shows multiple islands of epithelium in tubal isthmus. The tubal lumen is evident in the center of the section.

pected in a woman in the fourth decade of life who has had a history of unexplained involuntary sterility for 5 years or more and in whom no previous PID had occurred. Siegler further cautioned that the radiograph of tubal diverticulosis must be differentiated from that of tubal tuberculosis. In the latter condition, the oviducts are usually rigid, devoid of peristalsis, and are often occluded at the proximal end of the ampulla.

Except for a possible association with ectopic pregnancy (Dubuissen et al., 1986; Homm et al., 1987), the lesions per se are innocuous and require no specific treatment. The lesion is not considered to be premalignant. If tubal diverticulosis is discovered as an incidental finding at laparotomy and the tubes are grossly normal, nothing need be done. A patient with a long-standing history of infertility, however, who has bilateral isthmic occlusion due to diverticulosis could be considered a candidate for reconstructive surgery.

MICROSURGERY OF THE FALLOPIAN TUBES

The use of the microscope to assist in operations of the pelvis has been in practice for only the last 20 years. In gynecology, microscopic surgery has become important because of the recent increase in the incidence of PID, with its conse-

quent pelvic adhesion formation, and because of the desire of a number of women who have had tubal ligations to reverse their surgery. In addition, there is a subgroup of infertile women in whom properly selected and performed microsurgery would result in a pregnancy rate that is higher than is currently available with IVF. In this section, we describe the principles of microsurgery techniques, the adjuvants used with microsurgical techniques to try to prevent postoperative adhesions, and the indications and the reported outcomes of the gynecological procedures in which microsurgical techniques are used.

Techniques

Proper adherence to the principles of microsurgical techniques is probably the paramount surgical factor that contributes to successful outcome of the surgery. Adequate magnification of the surgical field is significant, but adherence to microsurgical principles is what the surgeon can do to help the patient the most.

Principles

The key principles of microsurgical technique include gentle handling of tissue, precise hemostasis, meticulous tissue dissection, and careful approximation of tissue (Gomel, 1983; Winston, 1980). Gomel (1983) counsels that successful microsurgery is the result of the adherence to these principles. Gentle handling of tissue is required to minimize intraperitoneal trauma and to decrease postoperative adhesions. Precise hemostasis allows improved visualization of the operating area and should be achieved by microdiathermy needle to cauterize the exact area of bleeding. Dessication of exposed tissue should be avoided, and this is done by keeping the operative field constantly irrigated with heparinized Ringer's lactate solution. The heparin is intended to help prevent fibrin deposition and, thus, may help prevent adhesion formation. Meticulous dissection allows complete removal of the abnormal tissues. In addition, meticulous dissection decreases the potential damage from the surgery and allows the careful reapproximation of tissue at the end of surgery. Fine, nonabsorbable suture material should be used. Catgut should be avoided because it could cause significant inflammatory reactions. Finally, care should be taken to avoid the contamination of the pelvis with foreign material, such as talc from gloves, because these materials may provoke an inflammatory response.

The skill and experience of the surgeon also appear to contribute to the successful outcome of microsurgery. Using rabbits, Oelsner et al. (1985) showed a correlation between the number of reanastomoses the surgeon has performed and outcome such as pregnancy rate. This finding suggests that microscopic surgery should be performed by those who have been adequately exposed to its principles.

Microscope

Swolin (1967) was the first to report the use of the operating microscope for surgery of the pelvis. In a study by Hedon et al. (1980), comparison was made between the use of loupes and microscope for tubal anastomosis in rabbits. Though (1) the time needed for the procedure was similar with both instruments, (2) the surgeon's assessment of the anastomosis after the procedure was similar in both groups, and (3) the patency assessment after the surgery was similar in the two groups; the number of rabbits achieving pregnancy was nearly 30% higher in the group in which the operating microscope was used. Thus, it appears that the operating microscope provides better results than with loupes in the most important outcome criterion.

The operating microscope that we are presently using is Model OPMi-1 from Carl Zeiss,

Inc. This is a surgical stereomicroscope with eyepiece magnification ×10 to ×20. We find that this operating microscope has several advantages. Our microscope has fiberoptic coaxial illumination, which provides clear visualization of the operating field. There are two microscope heads so that the surgeon and the assistant can see the same operating field at the same time. Finally, the zoom and focusing can be performed by footpedals operated by the surgeon, freeing the surgeon's hands for other functions.

Surgical Adjuvants

The most important factor determining successful outcome from microsurgery is good microsurgical technique. However, surgical adjuvants are commonly used to attempt to improve postoperative pregnancy rates. In particular, surgical adjuvants are used to try to decrease the postoperative incidence of adhesion formation and postoperative infections. As pointed out by Diamond et al. (1987), when a second-look laparoscopy is performed after surgery for lysis of adhesions, pelvic adhesions are again observed, and, moreover, new adhesions develop in a majority of the women who had the original surgery. The laser has been considered as an alternative technique to decrease the rate of postoperative adhesions. However, as has been shown by Barbot et al. (1987) and Tulandi (1987), the use of laser in lysis of adhesions is no more efficacious than standard techniques in decreasing postoperative adhesions. Thus, a strong need exists to identify the most effective methods to prevent the postoperative adhesion formation.

Antibiotics

In a survey by Holtz (1985) of the charter members of the Society of Reproductive Surgeons of the American Fertility Society (AFS), the most commonly used surgical adjuvant by pelvic surgeons is antibiotic prophylaxis. He found that 73% of his respondents used antibiotics in all surgical cases, whereas 18% used antibiotics only in cases of distal tubal disease. Thus, 91% of the gynecological surgeons used some form of antibiotic prophylaxis. The commonest antibiotics used were first-generation cephalosporins, doxycycline, and second- or third-generation cephhalosporins, in descending order. We routinely use 100 mg of doxycycline intravenously starting from the immediate preoperative period; we are concerned about prophylatic coverage for *Chlamydia,* in addition to the other organisms.

Dextran 70

Dextran 70 is a branched polysaccharide of glucose made from sugar beets, hydrolyzed to an average molecular weight of 70 kilodaltons (kD). It comes as a clear and viscous fluid with the dextran dissolved in 10% dextrose. The presumed benefits of this agent, when instilled intraperitoneally, are that it creates an osmotically induced transudate intraperitoneally and that it covers all intraperitoneal surfaces with a thin film, both of which may prevent adhesion formation. Using female rabbits, Holtz et al. (1980) studied the prevention of adhesion formation and reformation by dextran 70. They reported a reduction in adhesion formation in the animals in which dextran 70 was used after the initial injury. However, there was no decrease in reformation of adhesions in those animals in which dextran 70 was used after lysis of adhesions was performed. Even in animal studies, therefore, dextran 70 may be beneficial only in circumstances in which pelvic insult occurs for the first time.

In our practice, we use 100 ml of dextran 70 intraperitoneally for our microsurgical cases. The instillation is done immediately prior to the closure of the abdominal peritoneum. The commonest reported side effects from the use of this agent include labial edema, fever, ileus, and anaphylaxis (Holtz, 1985). As prophylaxis against anaphylactic reactions, we administer to the patient IV dextran 1, dextran that is hydrolyzed to an average molecular weight of 1 kD, which eliminates the large immune complexes required for anaphylaxis (Ljungstrom et al., 1988).

Steroids

In the past, steroid regimens after surgery were popular with pelvic surgeons because of potential anti-inflammatory effects by the steroids. In animal studies, the anti-inflammatory effects appear to be due to antagonistic reactions to histamine. However, Pfeffer et al. (1980) showed, in microsurgical anastomosis in rabbits, the use of steroids was of no benefit in reducing adhesions. Steroid use involves risks to the patient, including psychiatric disturbance, musculoskeletal pain, edema, and infection. We do not use steroids routinely.

Hydrotubation

In a survey by Holtz (1985), 33% of pelvic surgeons used hydrotubation postoperatively. Hydrotubation is a technique in which lactated Ringer's solution is instilled into the cervix in the immediate postoperative period to try to keep the tubes patent. In a large, prospective, randomized multicenter study, this procedure immediately following surgery did not result in a statistically significant increase in the pregnancy rate (Rock et al., 1984). We do not use hydrotubation at our institution.

Other Adjuvants

Recently, new techniques have been proposed to reduce the rate of postoperative pelvic adhesions. Among them is the study of Boyers et al. (1988), who tested Gore-Tex surgical membrane in rabbits. By their criteria of the extent, type, and tenacity of adhesions found after a second look of the pelvis, the Gore-Tex membrane reduced the experimental adhesion score by more than one half. Another reported modality for the reduction of adhesions is the use of calcium channel blockers. Steinleitner et al. (1988) measured the effects of subcutaneous injections of nifedipine, a calcium channel blocker, on postoperative adhesion formation in golden hamsters. The calcium channel blocker apparently decreased adhesion formation. More research is needed to determine the best ways of decreasing postoperative adhesions in microsurgical operations.

Classification and Outcomes of Microsurgical Procedures

Since the sole purpose of pelvic microsurgery is to help the patient to have a successful pregnancy, it is important to determine which surgical regimens are the most effective for the patient. In other words, what are the rates of spontaneous abortions, ectopic pregnancies, and live births associated with the surgical procedures? In published studies, the most important criteria determining the potential pregnancy rate include the length of follow-up, the severity of disease, the use of adjuvants, and the expression of data (Bateman et al., 1987). Because of this potential for variation in the reporting of the surgical data, it is not surprising that major differences in results are published, along with differences in methods for classifying the surgical procedures.

In 1988, the AFS made a major advance in tubal microsurgery by publishing staging systems for adnexal adhesions, distal tubal occlusion, and tubal occlusion secondary to tubal ligation (American Fertility Society, 1988). The classification schemes for these problems are important because (1) they allow the results of different studies to be compared on a similar basis, (2) they allow the proper documentation of the severity of the disease, and (3) they allow the formulation of an adequate prognosis for the patient.

Adnexal Adhesions

The AFS classification (Fig 8−8) divides adnexal adhesions in four categories: minimal, mild, moderate, and severe. The classification scheme emphasizes that the prognosis for the patient is based on the side with the least adhesions, that the fimbriated end is of critical importance for the patient's prognosis, and that there is a difference between filmy and dense adhesions in future outcome.

Salpingolysis involves the lysis of adhesions in the peritubal regions (Fig 8−9). Though the published results are for surgery done under a variety of circumstances, the results are encouraging. As shown in Table 8−1, of the studies published since 1980, the average rate of pregnancy after salpingolysis is 56%. For this procedure, therefore, the potential for successful outcome is excellent and should be offered as a potential treatment for patients with only adnexal adhesions.

Distal Tube Disease

The AFS scheme for distal tubal occlusion is based on the International Federation of Fertility and Sterility classification on salpingostomy and is presented in Figure 8−10. As Gomel (1983) has pointed out, the most important factors determining outcome after surgical correction are condition of endosalpinx, amount of ampullary dilatation, condition of tubal wall and presence and type of pelvic adhesions. The AFS classification scheme is based on these prognostic factors.

Salpingostomy is the term used to describe the procedure in which the terminal end of the oviduct is reconstructed. The commonest reason for performing this procedure is hydrosalpinx due to PID. Another cause of pelvic adhesions is appendicitis in the past. Occasionally, the obstructed distal tube is completely adherent to the ovary. The advantages of microsurgery in salpingostomy, as delineated by Gomel (1983), are that precise dissection could be performed to separate the tube from the ovary, that the whole tube could be conserved, that ampullary folds could be reconstructed in its physiologic position, and that a more complete hemostasis could be achieved. As shown in Table 8−2, eight papers published since 1980 have enough patients for adequate review. Of the studies, the average pregnancy rate after salpingostomy is 26%. For those patients who have had previous salpingostomies, the success rate after repeat salpingostomies is very low (Lauritsen et al., 1982). We refer these patients for IVF.

TABLE 8−1.

Results of Lysis of Adhesions by Microsurgical Techniques Published Since 1980

Author(s)	Yr	Patients (n)	Pregnancies (n) (%)
Betz et al. (1980)	1980	29	20 (69%)
Patton (1982)	1982	35	22 (63%)
Frantzen and Schlosser (1982)	1982	49	20 (41%)
Donnez and Casanas-Roux (1986)	1986	42	27 (64%)
Tulandi (1986)	1986	33	17 (52%)
	TOTAL	188	106 (56%)

TABLE 8−2.

Results of Salpingostomy by Microsurgical Techniques Published Since 1980

Author(s)	Yr	Patients (n)	Pregnances (n) (%)
DeCherney and Kase (1981)	1981	54	14 (26%)
Frantzen and Schlosser (1982)	1982	85	12 (14%)
Larrson (1982)	1982	54	21 (39%)
Mage and Bruhat (1983)	1983	30	5 (17%)
Verhoeven et al. (1983)	1983	82	28 (34%)
Boer-Meisel et al. (1986)	1986	108	22 (20%)
Donnez and Casanas-Roux (1986)	1986	83	26 (31%)
Kitchin et al. (1986)	1986	102	26 (25%)
	TOTAL	598	154 (26%)

THE AMERICAN FERTILITY SOCIETY CLASSIFICATION OF ADNEXAL ADHESIONS

Patient's Name _____ Date _____ Chart # _____

Age _____ G _____ P _____ Sp Ab _____ VTP _____ Ectopic _____ Infertile Yes _____ No _____

Other Significant History (i.e. surgery, infection, etc.) _____

_____

HSG _____ Sonography _____ Photography _____ Laparoscopy _____ Laparotomy _____

<table>
<tr><td colspan="2">ADHESIONS</td><td><1/3 Enclosure</td><td>1/3 - 2/3 Enclosure</td><td>>2/3 Enclosure</td></tr>
<tr><td rowspan="4">OVARY</td><td>R Filmy</td><td>1</td><td>2</td><td>4</td></tr>
<tr><td>Dense</td><td>4</td><td>8</td><td>16</td></tr>
<tr><td>L Filmy</td><td>1</td><td>2</td><td>4</td></tr>
<tr><td>Dense</td><td>4</td><td>8</td><td>16</td></tr>
<tr><td rowspan="4">TUBE</td><td>R Filmy</td><td>1</td><td>2</td><td>4</td></tr>
<tr><td>Dense</td><td>4*</td><td>8*</td><td>16</td></tr>
<tr><td>L Filmy</td><td>1</td><td>2</td><td>4</td></tr>
<tr><td>Dense</td><td>4*</td><td>8*</td><td>16</td></tr>
</table>

* If the fimbriated end of the fallopian tube is completely enclosed, change the point assignment to 16.

Prognostic Classification for Adnexal Adhesions

	LEFT		RIGHT
A. Minimal	_____	0-5	_____
B. Mild	_____	6-10	_____
C. Moderate	_____	11-20	_____
D. Severe	_____	21-32	_____

Treatment (Surgical Procedures): _____

_____

_____

_____

_____

Prognosis for Conception & Subsequent Viable Infant

_____ Excellent (> 75%)

_____ Good (50-75%)

_____ Fair (25%-50%)

_____ Poor (< 25%)

**Physician's judgment based upon adnexa with least amount of pathology.

Recommended Followup Treatment: _____

_____

_____

Additional Findings: _____

_____

_____

_____

_____

_____

_____

```
            DRAWING
L                                R
```

Property of
The American Fertility Society

For additional supply write to:
The American Fertility Society
2140 11th Avenue, South
Suite 200
Birmingham, Alabama 35205

FIG 8–8.
The AFS classification of adnexal adhesions. (From American Fertility Society: The American Fertility Society classifications of adnexal adhesions, distal tubal occlusion, tubal pregnancis, müllerian anomalies and intrauterine adhesions. *Fertil Steril* 1988; 49:944. Reproduced by permission.)

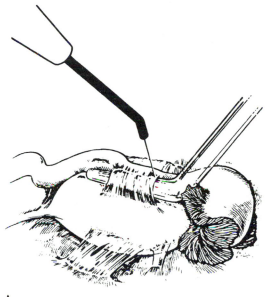

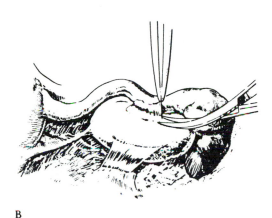

A

B

FIG 8–9.

A and **B,** lysis of peritubal adhesions with microsurgical instruments. (From Patton GW Jr: Microsurgical reconstruction of the oviduct, in Behrman SJ, Kistner RW, Patton GW Jr (eds): *Progress in Infertility,* ed 3. Reproduced by permission.)

Midsegment Reconstruction

Midsection reconstruction of the oviduct is most commonly performed for reversal of sterilization and reanastomosis of a partial salpingectomy performed for a tubal ectopic pregnancy. The AFS scheme for classification of tubal obstruction after tubal ligation are for the purposes of comparing the results of different studies and to give patients a more precise prognosis. According to the AFS scheme, the factors considered to be most important for surgical prognosis are the segmental lengths after repair and the type of anastomosis that is performed. Table 8–3 is a review of the studies published since 1980 of the success rates of microsurgical tubal anastomosis. This table is a summary of the results of different populations and different types of procedures. The average success rate in terms of pregnancy is 56%. The overall success rate of midsegment reconstruction is high enough so that it should be offered to tubal ligation patients as a firstline treatment.

Proximal Tubal Disease

For proximal tubal disease, the available operations could be divided into three categories: cornual implantation, noncornual implantation, and microsurgical anastomosis (Musich and Behrman, 1983). Microsurgical tubocornual anastomosis is associated with an acceptable success rate. McComb (1986) published a series of patients who had microsurgical tubocornual anastomosis for proximal tubal disease. He had a 57% pregnancy rate in these patients. In a study by Patton et al. (1987a) of the patients who had primary anastomosis performed for proximal tubal occlusion and with minimal or no distal disease, the pregnancy rate for the microsurgical anastomosis was 69% after 3 years. It appears that treatment of proximal disease with anastomosis could be as successful as for those patients who undergo midsegment reconstruction. However, if the patient has combined proximal and distal disease, the prognosis is so poor that the patient should be referred for IVF (Patton et al., 1987b).

Alternative Procedures

In patients with severe pelvic adhesions, missing fimbria, poor semen characteristics, or other poor prognostic factors, IVF could be considered as the first choice treatment for the infertile couple. However, alternative procedures are being developed to treat selected patients.

THE AMERICAN FERTILITY SOCIETY CLASSIFICATION OF DISTAL TUBAL OCCLUSION

Patient's Name _____ Date _____ Chart # _____

Age _____ G _____ P _____ Sp Ab _____ VTP _____ Ectopic _____ Infertile Yes _____ No _____

Other Significant History (i.e. surgery, infection, etc.) _____

HSG _____ Sonography _____ Photography _____ Laparoscopy _____ Laparotomy _____

Distal ampullary diameter	<3 cm	3-5 cm	>5 cm
L	1	4	6
R	1	4	6
Tubal wall thickness	Normal/Thin	Moderately Thickened or Edematous	Thick & Rigid
L	1	4	6
R	1	4	6
Mucosal folds at neostomy site	Normal/ > 75% Preserved	35% to 75% Preserved	<35% Preserved Adherent Mucosal Fold
L	1	4	6
R	1	4	6
Extent of adhesions	None/Minimal/Mild	Moderate	Extensive
L	1	3	6
R	1	3	6
Type of adhesions	None/Filmy	Moderately Dense (or Vascular)	Dense
L	1	2	4
R	1	2	4

Prognostic Classification for Terminal Salpingostomy (Salpingoneostomy)

	LEFT		RIGHT
A. Mild	_____	1-3	_____
B. Moderate	_____	9-10	_____
C. Severe	_____	>10	_____

Treatment (Surgical Procedures):

Salpingostomy	L	R
A. Terminal	_____	_____
B. Ampullary	_____	_____

Other: _____
_____
_____
_____
_____

Prognosis for Conception & Subsequent Viable Infant*

_____ Excellent   (> 75%)

_____ Good   (50 - 75%)

_____ Fair   (25%-50%)

_____ Poor   (< 25%)

*Physician's judgment based upon adnexa with least amount of pathology.

Recommended Followup Treatment: _____
_____

Additional Findings: _____
_____
_____
_____
_____

DRAWING

L   R

For additional supply write to:
The American Fertility Society
2140 11th Avenue, South
Suite 200
Birmingham, Alabama 35205

Property of
The American Fertility Society

TABLE 8–3.

Results of Tubal Reanastomosis by Microsurgical Techniques Published Since 1980

Author(s)	Yr	Patients (n)	Pregnancies (n) (%)
Gomel (1980)	1980	118	76 (64%)
Meldrum (1980)	1980	32	16 (50%)
Diamond et al. (1982)	1982	46	25 (54%)
Frantzen and Schlosser (1982)	1982	28	12 (43%)
DeCherney et al. (1983)	1983	129	73 (57%)
Donnez and Casanas-Roux (1986)	1986	82	36 (44%)
Lavy et al (1986)	1986	25	9 (36%)
Rock et al (1987)	1987	80	58 (73%)
	TOTAL	540	305 (56%)

Recently, Novy et al. (1988) reviewed a series of 28 patients who had interstitial fallopian tube obstruction diagnosed at hysterosalpingogram or diagnostic laparoscopy in whom transcervical cannulation of the proximal oviduct was performed. In the patients in whom hysteroscopic cannulation was performed, 92% of the tubes became patent. When the cannulation was performed under fluoroscopic guidance, 84% of the obstructed tubes became patent. Thus, this technique offers hope to those patients in whom interstitial tubal disease is diagnosed and in whom it was believed previously that the prognosis was poor. These results should be considered in light of the interesting findings by Sulak et al. (1987), who showed that in 11 of 18 patients who had tubal resection for presumed proximal tubal disease, there was no histological evidence for proximal disease.

As a final note, what is the incidence of ectopic pregnancy after pelvic microsurgery, a complication that may lead to the loss of the fallopian tube and even threaten the life of the patient? Lavy et al. (1987) reviewed the literature con-

cerning the ectopic pregnancy rate after microscopic tubal surgery. As would be expected, the rate of ectopic pregnancy depended on the type of surgery performed: for patients who have had lysis of adhesions, the ectopic pregnancy rate was 3.5% of the subsequent pregnancies; for salpingostomy, the rate of ectopic pregnancy was 28%; and for midsegment tubal anastomosis, the ectopic pregnancy rate was 3.7% of the pregnancies. Thus, the rate of ectopic pregnancies is dependent on the type of procedure and needs to be kept in mind when one is counseling the patient about the proposed operation.

BENIGN NEOPLASMS

Benign tumors of the oviduct are rare entities, yet a large variety of neoplasms have been reported as having originated in the fallopian tube. Tumors may be located in the wall or within the lumen or occasionally may be pedunculated and project from the fimbriated portion of the tube. In a consideration of benign tumors of the oviduct, lesions such as salpingitis isthmica nodosa, endometriosis, and adenomyosis should be excluded. Similarly, the hydatids of Morgagni are so commonplace that they should not be considered as a tumor mass. The following benign tumors have been reported in the literature: cystic and solid teratomas, papilloma, fibroadenoma, fibroma, leiomyoma, lipoma, hemangioma, lymphangioma, mesothelioma, and mesonephroma.

Somewhat commoner is the adenomatoid tumor (Fig 8–11), sometimes called an angiomyoma, mesothelioma, or a reticuloendothelioma. This is a small circumscribed tumor of the tube usually confined to the muscle wall and found incidentally at the time of laparotomy. It has a characteristic microscopic appearance, being composed of small glandlike spaces lined by cells of mesothelial, endothelial, or even epithelial appearance. Grossly, the tumors appear as gray, gray-white, or yellow discrete nodules occupying the muscularis and rarely exceeding 3 cm in diameter. Because of the glandular arrangements of the cells, the microscopic picture has occasionally been confused with a low-grade adenocarcinoma. The histogenesis of these tumors is not clearly defined, but electron microscopic studies support its origin from mesothelial cells (Taxy et al., 1974). It is not believed that these adenomatoid tumors possess malignant potential.

FIG 8–10.

The AFS classification of distal tubal occlusion. (From American Fertility Society: The American Fertility Society classifications of adnexal adhesions, distal tubal occlusion, tubal pregnancies, müllerian anomalies and intrauterine adhesions. *Fertil Steril* 1988; 49:944. Reproduced by permission.)

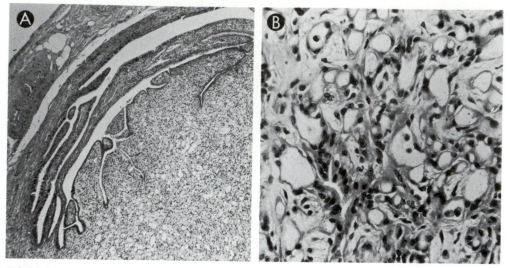

FIG 8–11.
Adenomatoid tumor. **A,** low power. **B,** higher power.

Leiomyomas of the tube are usually asymptomatic lesions that are discovered at laparotomy performed for another indication. Approximately 50 cases have been reported in the literature, but since these tumors are usually solitary and small, it is entirely probable that many have been unreported. Occasionally they have enlarged and produced acute torsion of the oviduct, and degenerative changes similar to those occurring in uterine leiomyomas have been reported.

MALIGNANT NEOPLASMS

Primary Carcinoma

The rarest carcinoma of the female genital tract is primary carcinoma of the oviduct. Since the report of the first patient in 1888, approximately 1,100 cases of this entity have been documented (Podczaski and Herbst, 1986). The incidence of tubal carcinoma varies from 0.1% to 0.5% of all female genital cancers. Metastatic disease is much commoner, accounting for 80% to 90% of fallopian tube malignancies.

The age incidence has varied from 18 to 80 years, but most patients have been between 40 and 65 years, with the mean age in the sixth decade.

Infertility has been a common finding in patients with tubal carcinoma. Salpingitis may be a causative factor accounting for the infertility in these patients. However, it must be remembered that salpingitis is so common and malignancy so rare. In all probability, the tumor itself produces a chronic inflammatory reaction, which eventually seals off the fimbriated portion of the tube and actually may simulate a hydrosalpinx.

Diagnosis

Since it is a rare disease with sometimes subtle or nonspecific symptoms, the diagnosis of primary carcinoma is rarely made before surgery. Although there are no distinctive symptoms that might be called pathognomonic, the most consistent sign is a watery and frequently blood-tinged vaginal discharge. Intermittent or colicky, low abdominal pain associated with abnormal bleeding may also be present. The latter may be manifested as irregular bleeding or spotting during the postmenopausal era and as menstrual irregularities during the childbearing period. Occasionally the discharge may be profuse, although the occurrence of *hydrops tubae profluens* as a characteristic symptom is quite rare. The latter may occur with the release of a watery or blood-tinged fluid from a hydrosalpinx through the uterus and vagina, regardless of whether or not tubal carcinoma is associated.

The physical findings include abdominal enlargement, if ascites is present, and a palpable abdominal mass or, more commonly, a palpable, firm mass found during pelvic examination. The finding of a tubal carcinoma is so rare that it is only occasionally listed as the primary preoperative diagnosis.

In postmenopausal patients the usual diagnosis is ovarian tumor, and in premenopausal patients the commonest diagnoses are leiomyomas and PID. If, however, there is recurrent bleeding, or, particularly, a bloody, watery discharge, in a postmenopausal patient in whom biopsies of the cervix and endometrial curettage have given normal findings, the suspicion of tubal cancer should be strongly entertained. Vaginal smears may disclose neoplastic cells characteristic of tubal cancer, particularly when there is a loss of fluid from the uterus, but only a minority of patients will have abnormal cytology results.

Culdocentesis may also reveal suspicious or definite malignant elements. Occasionally hysterosalpingography has suggested a cancer of the tube, and endoscopy or culdotomy may verify the diagnosis. A dilatation and curettage may reveal tubal cancer metastatic to the endometrial cavity.

Pathology

The lesion is usually unilateral, only about 30% of the patients having had bilateral tumors. If the fimbriated portion of the tube is closed, the gross appearance (Fig 8–12) of the mass may simulate that of a hydrosalpinx or pyosalpinx. If a tube with this appearance is removed during surgery, it should be opened intraoperatively to assure that the necessary surgical staging and treatment be performed.

The serosal surface is frequently roughened and adherent to the large and small intestines. Lesions have been described as large as 17 cm in diameter, although the association of a hydrosalpinx or pyosalpinx may make the gross appearance much larger. Cross-section of the tumor reveals granular tissue that is gray or yellow-tan, with a marked tendency to friability. The lesion is usually situated in the distal third of the tube, from where it may extend through the fimbriated portion. The tubal lumen is usually distended with fluid, and a papillary mass of friable or hemorrhagic tumor lines the mucosal surface.

The pathological diagnosis of primary carcinoma of the oviduct is based on proof that the tumor arises from the endosalpinx. The criteria suggested by Hu et al. (1950) for differentiating between primary and metastatic tumors are as follows:

1. Grossly, the main tumor is in the tube.
2. Microscopically, the mucosa should be chiefly involved and should show a papillary pattern.
3. If the tubal wall is involved to a great extent, the transition between benign and malignant tubal epithelium should be demonstrated.

The microscopic appearance of tubal carcinomas includes papillary medullary growth patterns, varying from well to poorly differentiated (Fig 8–13).

The usual method of spread of tubal carcinoma is via the lymphatics, but tumor growth may occur via the tubal lumen along the mucosal surface. Generalized peritoneal implants are uncommon, due in all probability to closure of the fimbriated portion of the tube.

Metastases are found in about one third of patients (Sedlis, 1978). The iliac, lumbar, and preaortic nodes may be involved by lymphatic permeation, and occasionally dissemination via the round ligament to the inguinal nodes may occur. Hematogenous spread accounts for me-

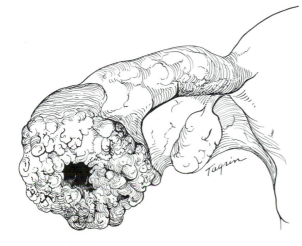

FIG 8–12.
Typical gross appearance of carcinoma of the oviduct.

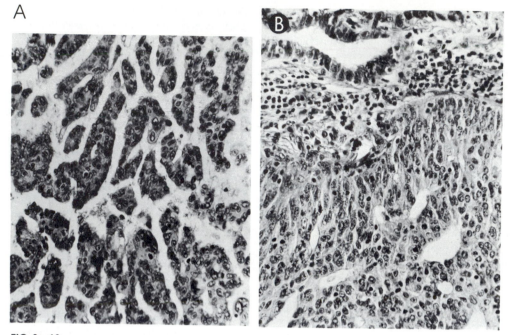

FIG 8—13.
Typical papillary carcinoma of oviduct. **A,** low power. **B,** higher power.

tastases to the liver, lungs, stomach, and supra-clavicular lymph nodes. The ovary, uterine corpus, and vagina may be involved by direct extension.

The clinical staging of carcinoma of the tube is as follows: listed in table 8—4.

Treatment

The initial method of treatment is total hysterectomy with bilateral salpingo-oophorectomy. If there is extension to the endocervix or upper portion of the vagina, a radical hysterectomy and pelvic lymphadenectomy is advisable.

Dubulking should be performed for disease outside the extirpated pelvic organs. Intraoperative staging is important and includes omental biopsy, peritoneal cytology, and para-aortic node sampling.

Additional therapy should be considered if the disease has spread beyond the tubal serosa. Although external radiation therapy has been used in more than one half of the reported cases, a variety of different treatment protocols were used, and the value of the treatment is difficult to prove (Podczaski and Herbst, 1986).

Intraperitoneal chromic phosphate (phosphorus 32) has been used in cases with no gross residual disease after surgery in an attempt to control peritoneal dissemination. Thus far, the experience has been too limited to establish efficacy (Benedet et al., 1977). Various forms of chemotherapy have also been tried, with some dramatic reports of regression of advanced disease, especially with alkylating agents (Podczaski and

TABLE 8—4.

Clinical Staging for Fallopian Tube Carcinoma*

Stage I: Growth limited to the tube.
Stage Ia: Growth limited to one tube, no ascites.
Stage Ib: Growth limited in two tubes, no ascites.
Stage Ic: Growth limited to one or both tubes, ascites present with malignant cells in fluid.
Stage II: Growth involving one or both tubes with pelvic extension.
Stage IIa: Extension and/or metastases to the uterus or ovary.
Stage IIb: Extension to other pelvic tissues.
Stage III: Growth involving one or both tubes with widespread intraperitoneal metastases to abdomen.
Stage IV: Growth involving one or both tubes with distant metastases extraperitoneally.

*Adapted from Turunen A: Carcinoma of fallopian tube. *Int J Obstet* 1969; 7:24.

Herbst, 1986). Cisplatin in combination with other agents has resulted in impressive 5-year survivals in some series (Maxson et al., 1987).

Prognosis is based primarily on stage rather than tumor grade. If a primary cancer of the tube is discovered early and removed promptly, the prognosis is good. The prognosis in general is considered to be poor, although the 5-year survival rate is directly related to the extent of the disease.

Prior to 1926, only three 5-year survivals were reported in the first 200 cases in the literature. More recently, the 5-year survival rate has been reported as 38% (Sedlis, 1978), although some patients are alive with disease. Alertness to the possibility of tubal cancer, prompt intervention, and adequate treatment will improve this discouragingly low "cure rate."

Sarcoma

Sarcomas are extremely rare tumors, less than 30 cases have been reported in the literature (Podczaski and Herbst, 1986). The age incidence and clinical picture are similar to those in carcinoma of the tube. If the disease is extensive, the commonest symptoms are pelvic pain, abdominal enlargement, and malaise. Physical examination may reveal abdominal distention, a pelvic mass, and emaciation. The tubal tumor varies from 2 to 20 cm in diameter, and the cross-section reveals a soft, papillary or pultaceous intraluminal mass. Microscopically, the sarcoma is most commonly of the spindle-cell type, but other variations such as round cell, myosarcoma, myxosarcoma, perithelioma, and endothelioma have been described.

This most malignant tumor may spread via the bloodstream, via the lymphatics, or by direct extension to adjacent pelvic organs. The optimum method of treatment is total hysterectomy with bilateral salpingo-oophorectomy followed by radiation therapy or chemotherapy. The prognosis is poor, and it is doubtful whether therapy of any type retards the eventual outcome in advanced cases.

Carcinoma Metastatic to the Oviduct

As might be expected, the two organs responsible for most metastatic lesions in the oviduct are the ovary and the endometrium. The method of spread may be either by direct extension or via the lymphatics. Carcinoma of the stomach and pancreas may also metastasize to the tube. The lesions may be unilateral or bilateral, and there is no characteristic gross appearance. Histologically, the tumors are identical with the primary tumor and, in contrast to primary carcinoma of the tube, the serosa of the oviducts as well as the lymphatics of the muscularis and of the mesosalpinx are usually involved. The treatment is that of the primary disease, usually complete hysterectomy and bilateral salpingo-oophorectomy. Postoperative radiation therapy is advisable, but the prognosis for 5-year survival is poor.

REFERENCES

American Fertility Society: The American Fertility Society classifications of adnexal adhesions, distal tubal occlusion, tubal pregnancies, Müllerian anomalies and intrauterine adhesions. *Fertil Steril* 1988; 49:944.

Atrash HK, Friede A, Hogue CJR: Ectopic pregnancy mortality in the United States, 1970–1983. *Obstet Gynecol* 1987; 70:817–822.

Australian in Vitro Fertilization Group: High incidence of preterm birth and early losses in pregnancy after in vitro fertilization. *Br Med J (Clin Res)* 1985; 291:1160.

Barbot J, Parent B, Dubuisson JB, et al: A clinical study of the CO_2 laser and electrosurgery for adhesiolysis in 172 cases followed by early second-look laparoscopy. *Fertil Steril* 1987; 48:140.

Bateman BG, Nunley WC, Kitchin JD: Surgical management of distal tubal obstructions—are we making progress? *Fertil Steril* 1987; 48:523.

Batzer FR, Corson SL: Diagnostic techniques used for ectopic pregnancy. *J Reprod Med* 1986; 31:86–93.

Benedet JL, White GW, Fairey RW, et al: Adenocarcinoma of the fallopian tube. *Obstet Gynecol* 1977; 50:654–657.

Benjamin CL, Beaver DC: Pathogenesis of salpingitis isthmica nodosa. *Am J Clin Pathol* 1951; 21:212.

Betz G, Engel T, Penny LL: Tuboplasty—comparison of the methodology. *Fertil Steril* 1980; 34:534.

Blandau RJ: Gamete transport; comparative aspects, in Hafey ESE, Blandau RJ (eds): *The Mammalian Oviduct*. Chicago, University of Chicago Press, 1969, pp 129–162.

Bleau G, Richer CL, Bousquet D: Absence of dynein arms in cilia of endocervical cells in a fertile woman. *Fertil Steril* 1978; 30:362.

Boer-Meisel ME, te Velde ER, Habbema JDF, et al: Predicting the pregnancy outcome in patients treated for hydrosalpinx: A prospective study. *Fertil Steril* 1986; 45:23.

Boyers SP, Diamond MP, DeCherney AH: Reduction of postoperative pelvic adhesions in the rabbit with Gore-Tex surgical membrane. *Fertil Steril* 1988; 49:1066.

Bruhat MA, Manhes H, Mage G, et al: Treatment of ectopic pregnancy by means of laparoscopy. *Fertil Steril* 1980; 33:411–414.

Brunham RC, Binns B, McDowell J, et al: Chlamydia trachomatis infection in women with ectopic pregnancy. *Obstet Gynecol* 1986; 67:722–726.

Beyth Y: Ovum pick up mechanism, a reappraisal. *Curr Probl Obstet Gynecol Fertil* 1986; 9:83–122.

Cartwright PS, Entman SS: Repeat ipsilateral tubal pregnancy allowing partial salpingectomy: A case report. *Fertil Steril* 1984; 42:647–648.

Cartwright PS, Herbert CM, Maxson WS: Operative laparoscopy for the management of tubal pregnancy. *J Reprod Med* 1986; 31:589–592.

Cartwright PS, Moore RA, Dao AH, et al: Serum β-human chorionic gonadotropin levels relate poorly with the size of a tubal pregnancy. *Fertil Steril* 1987; 48:679–680.

Chang MC: Development and fate of transferred rabbit ova or blastocysts in relation to the ovulation time of recipients. *J Exp Zool* 1950 114:197.

Chow W, Daling JR, Weiss NS, et al: Vaginal douching as a potential risk factor for tubal ectopic pregnancy. *Am J Obstet Gynecol* 1985; 153:727–729.

Chow W, Daling JR, Weiss NS, et al: Maternal cigarette smoking and tubal pregnancy. *Obstet Gynecol* 1988; 71:167–170.

Corson SL, Batzer FR: Ectopic pregnancy. A review of the etiologic factors. *J Reprod Med* 1986 31:78–85.

Cromartie AD, Kovalcik PJ: Incidental appendectomy at the time of surgery for ectopic pregnancy. *Am J Surg* 1980; 139:244–246.

Croxatto HB, Ortiz MES, Diaz S, et al: Studies on the duration of egg transport by the human oviduct: Ovum location at various intervals following LH peak. *Am J Obstet Gynecol* 1978; 132:7.

Daling JR, Chow WH, Weiss NS, et al: Ectopic pregnancy in relation to previous induced abortion. *JAMA* 1985; 253:1005–1008.

Daw E: Duplication of the uterine tube. *Obstet Gynecol* 1973; 42:137–138.

DeCherney AH, Boyers SP: Isthmic ectopic pregnancy: Segmental resection as the treatment of choice. *Fertil Steril* 1985; 44:307–312.

DeCherney AH, Cholst I, Naftolin F: Structure and function of the fallopian tubes following exposure to diethylstilbestrol (DES) during gestation. *Fertil Steril* 1981; 36:741–745.

DeCherney AH, Diamond MP: Laparoscopic salpingostomy for ectopic pregnancy. *Obstet Gynecol* 1987; 70:948–950.

DeCherney AH, Kase N: A comparison of treatment for bilateral fimbrial occlusion. *Fertil Steril* 1981; 35:162.

DeCherney AH, Maheaux R, Naftolin F: Salpingostomy for ectopic pregnancy in the sole patent oviduct: Reproductive outcome. *Fertil Steril* 1982; 37:617–622.

DeCherney AH, Mezer HC, Naftolin F: Analysis of failure of microsurgical anastomosis after midsegment, non-coagulation tubal ligation. *Fertil Steril* 1983; 39:618.

DeCherney AH, Silidker JS, Mezer HC, et al: Reproductive outcome following two ectopic pregnancies. *Fertil Steril* 1985; 43:82–86.

Diamond MP, Christianson CD, Daniell JF: Microsurgical reanastomosis of the fallopian tube: Increasingly successful outcome for reversal of previous sterilization procedures. *South Med J* 1982; 75:443.

Diamond MP, Daniell JF, Feste J, et al: Adhesion reformation and de novo adhesion formation after reproductive pelvic surgery. *Fertil Steril* 1987; 47:864.

DiMarchi JM, Kosasa TS, Kobara TY, et al: Persistent ectopic pregnancy. *Obstet Gynecol* 1987; 70:555–558.

Donnez J, Casanas-Roux F: Prognostic factors of fimbrial microsurgery. *Fertil Steril* 1986; 46:200.

Donnez J, Casanas-Roux F, Caprasse J, et al: Cyclic changes in ciliation, cell height, and mitotic activity in human tubal epithelium during reproductive life. *Fertil Steril* 1985; 43:554–558.

Dorfman SF, Grimes DA, Cates W, et al: Ectopic pregnancy mortality, United States, 1979 to 1980: Clinical aspects. *Obstet Gynecol* 1984; 64:386–390.

Dubuisson JB, Aubriot FX, Cardone V: Laparoscopic salpingectomy for tubal pregnancy. *Fertil Steril* 1987; 47:225–228.

Dubuisson JB, Aubriot FX, Cardone V, et al: Tubal causes of ectopic pregnancy. *Fertil Steril* 1986; 46:970–972.

Fernandez H, Rainhorn JD, Papiernik E, et al: Spontaneous resolution of ectopic pregnancy. *Obstet Gynecol* 1988; 71:171–174.

Frantzen C, Schlösser H-W: Microsurgery and postinfectious tubal infertility. *Fertil Steril* 1982; 38:397.

Fritz MA, Guo S: Doubling time of human chorionic gonadotropin (hCG) in early normal pregnancy: Relationship to hCG concentration and gestational age. *Fertil Steril* 1987; 47:584–589.

Gaddum-Rosse P, Blandau RJ, Thiersch JB: Ciliary activity in the human and Macaca nemestrina oviduct. *Am J Anat* 1973; 138:269–175.

Garcia AJ, Aubert JM, Sama J, et al: Expectant management of presumed ectopic pregnancies. *Fertil Steril* 1987; 48:395–400.

Gomel V: Microsurgical reversal of female sterilization: A reappraisal. *Fertil Steril* 1980; 33:587.

Gomel V: An odyssey through the oviduct. *Fertil Steril* 1983; 39:144.

Gomel V, Filmar S: Arrested tubal pregnancy. *Fertil Steril* 1987; 48:1043–1046.

Hallatt JG: Tubal conservation in ectopic pregnancy: A study of 200 cases. *Obstet Gynecol* 1986; 154:1216–1221.

Hedon B, Wineman M, Winston RML: Loupes or microscope for tubal anastomosis? An experimental study. *Fertil Steril* 1980; 34:264.

Hoffman JJ: The fallopian tube: An upsurge of interest. *Curr Probl Obstet Gynecol* 1980; 3:5–52.

Holtz G: Current use of ancillary modalities for adhesion prevention. *Fertil Steril* 1985; 44:174.

Holtz G, Baker E, Tsai C: Effect of thirty-two per cent dextran 70 on peritoneal adhesion formation and re-formation after lysis. *Fertil Steril* 1980; 33:660.

Homm RJ, Holtz G, Garvin AJ: Isthmic ectopic pregnancy and salpingitis isthmica nodosa. *Fertil Steril* 1987; 48:756–758.

Hu CY, Taymor ML, Hertig AT: Primary carcinoma of the fallopian tube. *Am J Obstet Gynecol* 1950; 59:58.

Jansen RPS: Cyclic changes in the human fallopian tube isthmus and their functional importance. *Am J Obstet Gynecol* 1980; 136:292–308.

Jansen RPS: Endocrine response in the fallopian tube. *Endocr Rev (Baltimore)* 1984; 5:525–542.

Kamrava M, Seibel MM, Thompson IE, et al: Intrauterine pregnancy following transperitoneal migration of the ovum. *Obstet Gynecol* 1982; 60:391–393.

Kamrava MM, Tymor ML, Berger MJ, et al: Disappearance of human chorionic gonadotropin following removal of ectopic pregnancy. *Obstet Gynecol* 1983; 62:486–487.

Kim DS, Chung SR, Moon IP, et al: Comparative review of diagnostic accuracy in tubal pregnancy: A 14-year survey of 1040 cases. *Obstet Gynecol* 1987; 70:547–554.

Kitchin JD III, Nunley WC, Bateman BG: Surgical management of distal tubal occlusion. *Am J Obstet Gynecol* 1986; 155:524.

Langer R, Bukovsky I, Herman A, et al: Conservative surgery for tubal pregnancy. *Fertil Steril* 1982; 38:427–430.

Larsson B: Late results of salpingostomy combined with salpingolysis and ovariolysis by electromicrosurgery in 54 women. *Fertil Steril* 1982; 37:156.

Lauritsen JG, Pagel JD, Vangsted P, et al: Results of repeated tuboplasties. *Fertil Steril* 1982; 37:68.

Lavy G, Diamond MP, DeCherney AH: Pregnancy following tubocornual anastomosis. *Fertil Steril* 1986; 46:21

Lavy G, Diamond MP, DeCherney AH: Ectopic pregnancy: Its relationship to tubal reconstructive surgery. *Fertil Steril* 1987; 47:543–556

Leese H: The formation and function of oviduct fluid. *J Reprod Fert* 1988; 82:843–856.

Leeton J, Davison G: Nonsurgical management of unruptured tubal pregnancy with intra-amniotic methotrexate: Preliminary report of two cases. *Fertil Steril* 1988; 50:167–169.

Lippe J, Krasner J, Alfonso LA, et al: Human oviductal fluid proteins. *Fertil Steril* 1981; 36:623–629.

Ljungstrom KG, Renck H, Hedin H, et al: Hapten inhibition and dextran anaphylaxis. *Anaesthesia* 1988; 43:729.

Mage G, Bruhat M-A: Pregnancy following salpingostomy: Comparison between CO_2 laser and electrosurgery procedures. *Fertil Steril* 1983; 40:472.

Marchbanks PA, Annegers JF, Coulam CB, et al: Risk factors for ectopic pregnancy. *JAMA* 1988; 259:1823–1833.

Marchbanks PA, Coulam CB, Annegers JF: An association between clomiphene citrate and ectopic pregnancy: A preliminary report. *Fertil Steril* 1985; 44:268–270.

Maxson WZ, Stehman FB, Ulbright TM, et al: Primary carcinoma of the fallopian tube: Evidence for activity of cisplatin combination therapy. *Gynecol Oncol* 1987; 26:305–313.

McCausland A: High rate of ectopic pregnancy following laparoscopic tubal coagulation failures. *Obstet Gynecol* 1980; 136:97–100.

McCausland A: Endosalpingosis ("endosalpingo-blastosis") following laparoscopic tubal coagulation as an etiologic factor of ectopic pregnancy. *Obstet Gynecol* 1982; 143:12–24.

McComb P: Microsurgical tubocornual anastomosis for occlusive cornual disease: Reproducible results without the need for tubouterine implantation. *Fertil Steril* 1986; 46:571.

McComb P, Langley L, Villalon M, et al: The oviductal cilia and Kartagener's syndrome. *Fertil Steril* 1986; 46:412–416.

McLachlan J, Newbold R, Shah H, et al: Reduced fertility in female mice exposed transplacentally to diethylstilbestrol (DES). *Fertil Steril* 1982; 38:364–371.

Meldrum DR: Microsurgical tubal reanastomosis—the role of splints. *Obstet Gynecol* 1981; 57:613.

Merchant RN, Prabhu SR, Chougale A: Uterotubal junction—morphology and clinical aspects. *Int J Fertil* 1983; 28:199–205.

Metz KGP: Failures following fimbriectomy. *Fertil Steril* 1977; 28:66–71.

Musich JR, Behrman SJ: Surgical management of tubal obstruction at the uterotubal junction. *Fertil Steril* 1983; 40:423.

Nagamani M, London S, St Amand P: Factors influencing fertility after ectopic pregnancy. *Obstet Gynecol* 1984; 149:533–536.

Nassberg S, McKay DG, Hertig AT: Physiological salpingitis. *Am J Obstet Gynecol* 1954; 67:130.

Newton J: Ectopic pregnancy. *Br Med J (Clin Res)* 1988; 297:633–634.

Novy MJ: Reversal of Kroener fimbriectomy sterilization. *J Obstet Gynecol* 1980; 137:198–204.

Novy MJ, Thurmond AS, Patton P, et al: Diagnosis of cornual obstruction by transcervical fallopian tube cannulation. *Fertil Steril* 1988; 50:434.

Oelsner G, Boeckx W, Verhoeven H, et al: The effect of training in microsurgery. *Am J Obstet Gynecol* 1985; 152:1054.

Oelsner G, Rabinovitch O, Morad J, et al: Reproductive outcome after microsurgical treatment of tubal pregnancy in women with a single fallopian tube. *J Reprod Med* 1986; 31:483–486.

Oyer R, Tarakjian D, Lev-Toaff A, et al: Treatment of cervical pregnancy with methotrexate. *Obstet Gynecol* 1988; 71:469–474.

Patton GW Jr: Pregnancy outcome following microsurgical fimbrioplasty. *Fertil Steril* 1982; 37:150.

Patton PE, Williams TJ, Coulam CB: Microsurgical reconstruction of the proximal oviduct. *Fertil Steril* 1987a; 47:35.

Patton PE, Williams TJ, Coulam CB: Results of microsurgical reconstruction in patients with combined proximal and distal tubal occlusion: Double obstruction. *Fertil Steril* 1987b; 48:670.

Pauerstein CJ, Croxatto HB, Eddy CA, et al: Anatomy and pathology of tubal pregnancy. *Obstet Gynecol* 1986; 67:301–308.

Pfeffer WH, Wheeler JE, Tschoepe RL, et al: The effect of dexamethasone and promethazine administration on adhesion formation, tubal function, and ultrastructure following microsurgical anastomosis of rabbit oviducts. *Fertil Steril* 1980; 34:162.

Podczaski E, Herbst AL: Cancer of the vagina and fallopian tube, in Knapp RC, Berkowitz RS (eds): *Gynecologic Oncology*. New York, Macmillan Publishing Co, 1986, pp 399–424.

Reich H, Johns DA, DeCaprio J, et al: Laparoscopic treatment of 109 consecutive ectopic pregnancies. *J Reprod Med* 1988; 33:885–890.

Rock JA, Guzick DS, Katz E, et al: Tubal anastomosis: Pregnancy success following reversal of Falope ring or monopolar cautery sterilization. *Fertil Steril* 1987; 48:13.

Rock JA, Siegler AM, Meisel MB, et al: The efficacy of postoperative hydrotubation: A randomized prospective multicenter clinical trial. *Fertil Steril* 1984; 42:373.

Romero R, Copel JA, Kadar N, et al: Value of culdocentesis in the diagnosis of ectopic pregnancy. *Obstet Gynecol* 1985a; 65:519–522.

Romero R, Kadar N, Jeanty P, et al: Diagnosis of ectopic pregnancy: Value of the discriminatory human chorionic gonadotropin zone. *Obstet Gynecol* 1985b; 66:357–360.

Sauer MV, Gorrill MJ, Rodi IA, et al: Nonsurgical management of unruptured ectopic pregnancy: An extended clinical trial. *Fertil Steril* 1987; 48:752–754.

Sedlis A: Primary carcinoma of the fallopian tube. *Obstet Gynecol Surv* 1961; 16:209–226.

Sedlis A: A carcinoma of the fallopian tube. *Surg Clin North Am* 1978; 58:121–129.

Settlage DSF, Motoshima M, Tredway DR: Sperm transport from the external cervical as to the fallopian tubes in women: A time and quantitation study. *Fertil Steril* 1973; 24:655.

Shapiro BS, Cullen M, Taylor KJW, et al: Transvaginal ultrasonography for the diagnosis of ectopic pregnancy. *Fertil Steril* 1988; 50:425–429.

Sherman D, Langer R, Herman A, et al: Reproductive outcome after fimbrial evacuation of tubal·pregnancy. *Fertil Steril* 1987; 47:420–424.

Sherman D, Langer R, Sadovsky G, et al: Improved fertility following ectopic pregnancy. *Fertil Steril* 1982; 37:497–502.

Silva PD: A laparoscopic approach can be applied to most cases of ectopic pregnancy. *Obstet Gynecol* 1988; 72:944–946.

Stangel J: Conservative surgical procedures for tubal pregnancy. *J Reprod Med* 1986; 31:103–115.

Stangel J, Gomel V: Techniques in conservative surgery for tubal gestation. *Clin Obstet Gynecol* 1980; 23:1221–1228.

Steinleitner A, Lambert H, Montoro L, et al: The use of calcium channel blockade for the prevention of postoperative adhesion formation. *Fertil Steril* 1988; 50:818.

Stock RJ, Nelson KJ: Ectopic pregnancy subsequent to sterilization: Histologic evaluation and clinical implications. *Fertil Steril* 1984; 42:211–216.

Stone SC, McCalley M, Braunstein P, et al: Radionuclide evaluation of tubal function. *Fertil Steril* 1985; 43:757–760.

Sulak PJ, Letterie GS, Coddington CC, et al: Histology of proximal tubal occlusion. *Fertil Steril* 1987; 48:437.

Svensson L, Mardh PA, Ahlgren M, et al: Ectopic pregnancy and antibodies to Chlamydia trachomatis. *Fertil Steril* 1985; 44:313–316.

Swolin K: Fifty fertility operations: Literature and methods. *Acta Obstet Gynecol Scand* 1967; 46:234.

Talo A, Pulkkinen MO: Electrical activity in the human oviduct during menstrual cycle. *Am J Obstet Gynecol* 1982; 142:135–152.

Tanaka T, Hayashi H, Kutsuzawa T, et al: Treatment of interstitial ectopic pregnancy with methotrexate: Report of a successful case. *Fertil Steril* 1982; 37:851–852.

Taxy JB, Battifora H, Oyasu R: Adenomatoid tumors: A light microscopic, histochemical and ultrastructural study. *Cancer* 1974; 34:306.

Thorburn J, Philipson M, Lindblom B: Fertility after ectopic pregnancy in relation to background factors and surgical treatment. *Fertil Steril* 1988; 49:595–600.

Tulandi T: Salpingo-ovariolysis: A comparison between laser surgery and electrosurgery. *Fertil Steril* 1986; 45:489.

Tulandi T: Adhesion reformation after reproductive surgery with and without the carbon dioxide laser. *Fertil Steril* 1987; 47:704.

Tulandi T: Reproductive performance of women after two tubal ectopic pregnancies. *Fertil Steril* 1988; 50:164–166.

Tuomivaara L, Kauppila A: Radical or conservative surgery for ectopic pregnancy? A follow-up study of fertility of 323 patients. *Fertil Steril* 1988; 50:580–583.

Verhoeven HC, Berry H, et al: Surgical treatment of distal tubal occlusion: A review of 167 cases. *J Reprod Med* 1983; 28:293.

Vermesh M, Silva P, Sauer M: Persistent tubal ectopic gestation: Patterns of circulating B-human chorionic gonadotropin and progesterone, and management options. *Fertil Steril* 1988; 50:584–588.

Walters MD, Carlton E, Pauerstein CJ: The contralateral corpus luteum and tubal pregnancy. *Obstet Gynecol* 1987; 70:823–826.

Westrom L, Bengtsson LPH, Mardh PA: Incidence, trends, and risks of ectopic pregnancy in a population of women. *Br Med J (Clin Res)* 1981; 282:15–18.

Winston RML: Microsurgery of the fallopian tube: From fantasy to reality. *Fertil Steril* 1980; 34:521.

Wrork DH, Broders AC: Adenomyosis of the fallopian tube. *Am J Obstet Gynecol* 1942; 44:412.

Yang C, Chow W, Daling JR, et al: Does prior infertility increase the risk of tubal pregnancy? *Fertil Steril* 1987; 48:62–66.

Yeko TR, Gorrill MJ, Hughes LH, et al: Timely diagnosis of early ectopic pregnancy using a single blood progesterone measurement. *Fertil Steril* 1987; 48:1048–1050.

Zaitoon MM, Florentin H: Crossed renal ectopia with unilateral agenesis of fallopian tube and ovary. *J Urol* 1982; 128:111.

9 _____ The Ovary

Ross Berkowitz, M.D.

Robert Barbieri, M.D.

The ovary is a complex organ that combines both gametogenic and endocrine functions. The estradiol and progesterone produced by the adult ovary are the primary hormonal regulators of the breast, uterus, and fallopian tubes. As such, the ovary is the master gland in gynecology. In the adult ovary, the gametogenic and endocrine functions of this organ are integrated to produce the repetitive process of follicular development, ovulation, corpus luteum formation, and, if pregnancy does not occur, corpus luteum regression. The repetitive growth and regression of intraovarian structures appears to predispose this major organ of reproduction to the development of multiple abnormalities of structure and function.

EMBRYOLOGY

The development of the ovary requires the coordinated assembly of three distinct embryonic tissues: (1) the primordial germ cells, (2) the coelomic epithelium of the urogenital ridge, and (3) the ovarian mesenchyme. The primordial germ cells will differentiate into oocytes. The granulosa cells and surface epithelium of the ovary will develop from the coelomic epithelium. The ovarian mesenchyme will give rise to the stroma and theca.

Four weeks after conception, a genital ridge develops medial to the mesonephric ridge. The initial ridge consists of an inner core of ovarian mesenchyme and a thick outer layer of proliferating coelomic epithelium. In the mesenchyme are cellular condensations lying at right angles to the coelomic epithelium called the *primitive sex cords*.

At this stage of development, the male and female gonad cannot be distinguished by histologic appearance, and the gonad is referred to as the *indifferent gonad*. If the indifferent gonad becomes a testis, the primitive sex cords will develop into the seminiferous tubules. If the indifferent gonad becomes an ovary, the primitive sex cords will regress and become the rete testis. Differentiation of the indifferent male gonad into a testis begins 6 weeks after conception. Differentiation of the indifferent female gonad into an ovary usually begins approximately 12 weeks after conception. At this time the cortical or secondary sex cords develop. The cortical cords arise by the invagination of the coelomic epithelium into the ovarian mesenchyme. Entry of primordial germ cells into these cortical cords will give rise to the primordial follicles.

These germ cells, now termed *oogonia*, are incorporated into the cortical sex cords. Mitosis ceases, and the oogonium differentiates into a primary oocyte. The primary oocyte progresses into the prophase of the first meiotic division and then becomes dormant, entering a period of cellular hibernation, which will last until puberty. The primary oocyte is surrounded by flattened follicular cells derived from the secondary sex cords and destined to become granulosa cells. The oocyte and the surrounding granulosa cells form a unit called the *primordial follicle*. During fetal life, the ovary is relatively quiescent. This contrasts with the fetal testis, which makes large amounts of testosterone.

Six weeks after conception, the male and female gonads are indistinguishable. A gene on the distal arm of the Y chromosome, termed the *testis-*

determining factor (TDF), is responsible for causing the indifferent gonad to become a testis. In the presence of TDF, the indifferent gonad becomes a testis. In the absence of the TDF, the indifferent gonad will become an ovary. In rare cases, the TDF gene can cross over from the Y to the X chromosome in a developing spermatogonia. If a sperm bearing the Y copy of TDF on an X chromosome fertilizes an oocyte, the resulting 46 XX individual will develop testes, not ovaries (Page and de la Chapelle, 1984). The TDF gene appears to code for a zinc finger protein. This class of proteins plays an important role in regulating transcription of DNA.

ANATOMY

The ovary has three major anatomical connections. The inferior pole of the ovary is attached to the uterus by a fibromuscular cord, the utero-ovarian ligament. The upper pole of the ovary is attached to the distal portion of the oviduct and is supported by the infundibulopelvic ligament. The infundibulopelvic ligament represents the upper margin of the broad ligament lateral to the tubal ostium and contains the ovarian vessels. The lateral portion of the ovary is attached to the posterior surface of the broad ligament by the mesovarium, a thin fold of tissue by which blood vessels and nerves enter the hilus of the ovary.

The arterial supply of the ovary is provided by both the ovarian artery and branches of the uterine artery. The ovarian artery arises from the aorta opposite the second and third lumbar vertebrae and crosses the psoas muscle in its descent to the pelvic brim. The ovarian artery enters the infundibulopelvic ligament and divides to give off small branches to the oviduct. The main ovarian artery enters the ovary through the hilus and divides into two medullary branches, which supply the opposite poles of the ovary. The main trunk of the ovarian artery also anastomoses with the ascending division of the uterine artery. The venous drainage of the ovary is similar to the arterial arrangement, except that the right ovarian vein terminates in the inferior vena cava, whereas the left ovarian vein empties into the left renal vein.

The nerve supply of the ovary is derived from branches of the renal and aortic sympathetic plexuses as well as from the celiac and mesenteric ganglia.

OVARIAN FOLLICLE

The functional unit of the lung is the alveolus. The functional unit of the kidney is the nephron. The functional unit of the ovary is the follicle. All gametogenic and most endocrine functions of the ovary are controlled by the ovarian follicle.

The ovarian follicle consists of three key components: (1) the oocyte, (2) the granulosa cells, and (3) the thecal cells. An understanding of the development and interrelationships of these three components is best obtained by tracing the development of a primordial follicle (Fig 9–1).

The *primordial follicle* consists of an oocyte, arrested in the diplotene stage of meiotic prophase, surrounded by a single layer of flattened granulosa cells. The primordial follicle is in a state of cellular hibernation until it is recruited to enter a growth phase. The factors that stimulate the primordial follicle to enter a growth phase have not been identified, but it is known that this process is independent of gonadotropin secretion. The number of primordial follicles that enter a growth phase each cycle appears to be a fixed proportion of the primordial follicles remaining in the ovary. This is a critical characteristic of the regulation of the ovarian follicular pool. Growth in the primordial follicle is characterized by an increase in the size of the oocyte, a change in shape of the granulosa cells from flattened to cuboidal, and an increase in the number of gap junctions between the granulosa cells and oocytes.

Growth of a primordial follicle into a healthy *preantral follicle* is dependent on gonadotropin stimulation, especially follicle-stimulating hormone (FSH). The preantral follicle is characterized by (1) an enlarged oocyte; (2) the development of a membrane that surrounds the oocyte, the zona pellucida; (3) a multilayer proliferation of granulosa cells; and (4) the development of an outer layer of theca cells derived from the ovarian stroma (see Fig 9–1). The key to the growth of the preantral follicle is stimulation of granulosa cell growth by FSH and estradiol. Multiple "positive" feedback loops help propel the growth of the preantral follicle. For example, FSH stimulates the production of FSH receptors, thereby increasing granulosa cell sensitivity to FSH, resulting in a magnification of FSH stimulation.

High local concentrations of estradiol and FSH stimulate the production of fluid in the in-

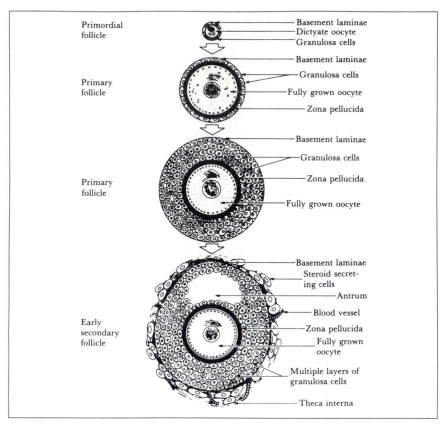

Primordial follicle
— Basement laminae
— Dictyate oocyte
— Granulosa cells

— Basement laminae
— Granulosa cells
Primary follicle
— Fully grown oocyte
— Zona pellucida

— Basement laminae
— Granulosa cells
Primary follicle
— Zona pellucida
— Fully grown oocyte

— Basement laminae
— Steroid secreting cells
— Antrum
Early secondary follicle
— Blood vessel
— Zona pellucida
— Fully grown oocyte
— Multiple layers of granulosa cells
— Theca interna

FIG 9–1.
Structure of the ovarian follicle.

terstices of the granulosa cells (Call-Exner bodies). Eventually the fluid coalesces to give rise to the *antral follicle*. It is likely that the follicle with the greatest blood flow and the highest intrafollicular concentration of FSH and estradiol will be selected to ovulate. Estradiol production in the antral follicle is controlled by both the thecal and granulosa cells, the two-cell theory of follicular estrogen production (Fig 9–2).

The basic components of the two-cell theory of follicular estrogen production are as follows: (1) the theca cells contain luteinizing hormone (LH) receptors but not FSH receptors; (2) stimulation of the theca by LH results in the production of androstenedione (the theca does not contain the enzyme aromatase and cannot convert the androstenedione to estrogen); (3) the granulosa cells contain FSH receptors, and FSH stimulates the production of the enzyme aromatase, which can convert thecal androstenedione to estrone; and (4) the granulosa cell contains large amounts

of an estrogen-specific 17-ketosteroid reductase enzyme, which can convert the estrone to estradiol but not androstenedione to testosterone (Barbieri et al., 1988a). The antral follicle accounts for 95% of the estradiol production during the reproductive life of a woman. The remaining 5% of the estradiol arises from the extraovarian aromatization of androgens in such tissues as fat and muscles.

Experiments in nonhuman primates have documented that the large antral follicle controls the timing of ovulation. The ovary, not the hypothalamic-pituitary unit, is the time keeper (Zeitgeber) of the menstrual cycle. The preovulatory antral follicle contains a large number of granulosa and thecal cells contributing to estradiol production. When the antral follicle reaches a diameter of 18 to 25 mm, it contains approximately 40 to 60 million granulosa cells. A follicle of this size can secrete approximately 400 μg of estradiol/day, which results in circulating estradiol concen-

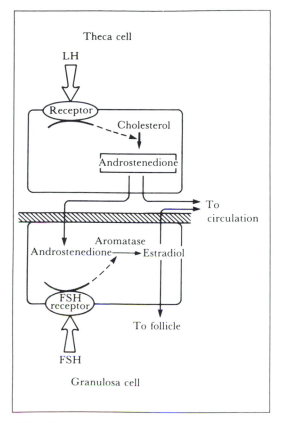

FIG 9–2.
Two-cell, two-gonadotropin theory of follicular estrogen production.

trations of 200 to 300 pg/ml. When circulating estradiol is maintained in the range of 200 to 300 pg/ml for 48 hours, an LH surge is triggered. The LH surge produces a large number of changes in the antral follicle: (1) a marked increase in granulosa cell cyclic adenosine monophosphate, leading to an increase in progesterone production and a decrease in estradiol production; (2) accelerated maturation of the oocyte, leading to dissolution of nuclear membrane (germinal vesicle breakdown) and completion of meiosis I (extrusion of the first polar body); and (3) an increase in production of follicular prostaglandins, collagenase, and plasmin, resulting in dissolution of the follicle wall and extrusion of the oocyte. Ovulation occurs approximately 36 to 42 hours after the initiation of the LH surge.

After ovulation, the basement membrane of the follicle dissolves, blood vessels grow into the follicle, luteinization of the thecal and granulosa cells is completed, and the follicle is transformed

in a corpus luteum (Latin for "yellow body"). The corpus luteum is 20 to 30 mm in diameter. The most important endocrine feature of the luteal phase of the menstrual cycle is the large amount of progesterone (25 mg/day) secreted by the corpus luteum. During the luteal phase of the cycle, progesterone is secreted as pulses in response to pulses by pituitary LH. The peak steroidogenic activity of the corpus luteum is reached 7 to 8 days after the LH surge, and the functional demise of the corpus luteum begins 2 to 3 days before the onset of menses. The life span of the corpus luteum is programmed to be 12 to 14 days unless pregnancy occurs, and the human chorionic gonadotropin (hCG) secreted by the trophoblast rescues the corpus luteum. The precise mechanisms that govern luteolysis are not known, but an increase in prostaglandin production by the corpus luteum appears to precede luteolysis. With completion of luteolysis, progesterone and estradiol concentrations fall, resulting in the onset of menses.

Recruitment, Selection, and Dominance

At puberty, the ovary contains approximately 200,000 follicles. From this follicular pool, less than 500 follicles will be selected to ovulate. The remaining 199,500 follicles will die without expressing their gametogenic potential. The concepts of recruitment, selection, and dominance help to explain the process by which only 1 of every 400 follicles is chosen for ovulation (Goodman and Hodgen, 1983).

As noted earlier, during each cycle a large number of primordial follicles leave the resting pool of follicles and enter a growth phase. The process regulating the entry of follicles into a growth phase is called recruitment. The factors governing the process of recruitment are poorly characterized. It appears that the initial phase of recruitment is independent of gonadotropin concentrations. As previously noted, of every 400 follicles recruited only 1 follicle will ovulate. The process by which the initial pool of recruited, growing follicles is winnowed to the species-specific ovulatory quota is termed selection. The status of the follicular microenvironment is crucial to the process of selection. The inner portion of each follicle is enclosed by a basement membrane of extracellular matrix. No blood vessels cross the basement membrane. Therefore, each follicle can create its own unique microenvironment. The small antral follicles that can create a microenvironment most conducive to growth will continue on a favorable growth trajectory, whereas other follicles will undergo atresia. Experimental evidence suggests that the follicles that can capture the greatest share of ovarian blood flow and create an intrafollicular microenvironment characterized by high concentrations of FSH and estradiol have the best growth potential.

At the beginning of the follicular phase of the menstrual cycle (day 1 of menses), there are four to six antral follicles 4 mm in diameter in the ovaries. By day 8 of the cycle, one of these follicles has been selected, and the remaining follicles will become atretic. From day 8 of the cycle until the onset of the next menses (day 28 of the cycle), the one selected follicle is dominant and suppresses the growth of all the remaining follicles. The dominant follicle prevents the growth of other follicles by secreting sufficient estradiol and inhibin to suppress pituitary FSH production, the key hormone governing follicular growth. Surgical removal of the dominant follicle is followed by the growth of a new cohort of small antral follicles that compete to become dominant. The processes of selection and dominance help ensure that, on average, only one egg is ovulated each cycle.

Ovarian Follicular Pool

The peak number of ovarian follicles is 6×10^6 and occurs in fetal life at approximately 20 weeks of gestation (Block, 1952; Baker, 1971). During the late second trimester, and throughout the third trimester of fetal life, a marked loss of germ cells occurs, resulting in approximately 2×10^6 ovarian follicles at birth. By the first menses (median age 12.8 years), the number of remaining follicles is approximately 200,000. By 52 years of age, most women have loss all functional ovarian follicles, and menopause has begun (Fig 9–3).

Careful analysis of the rate of loss of follicles in humans and rodents suggests that the loss of ovarian follicles is best described by an exponential function (Faddy et al., 1983). This means that during each time period t, a fixed percentage of the total number of remaining follicles in the ovaries are lost. Over the life of the ovary, fewer follicles are lost during each succeeding time period t because fewer follicles are present at the beginning of each succeeding time period t.

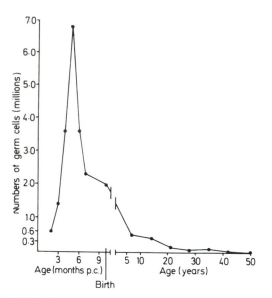

FIG 9–3.
Number of follicles present in the human ovary throughout life.

The fact that most follicular loss is governed by an exponential function has important clinical implications. The surgical removal of one ovary or the removal of 50% of each ovary (50% loss of all follicles) will not significantly change the age of menopause, because the remaining follicles redistribute the entry into a growth phase. Experimental studies in rodents suggest that more than 90% of all follicles must be surgically removed from the ovaries before a significant impact on the age of menopause is apparent.

Prepubertal and Menopausal Ovary

The prepubertal ovary is a small elongated structure measuring 1 to 2 cm in length. Between birth and age 4 years, the hypothalamic-pituitary unit secretes both LH and FSH, and ovarian follicles will grow and secrete small amounts of estradiol. Between 4 and 8 years of age, the hypothalamic-pituitary unit secretes very little LH or FSH, and the ovary is quiescent. Starting at age 8 years, the peripubertal increase in LH and FSH will lead to ever increasing levels of follicular activity and estradiol secretion. The increase in ovarian follicular activity will ultimately result in menarche (mean age 12.8 years), and the first ovulation will occur approximately 1 year after menarche. Because the prepubertal ovary is relatively quiescent, cystic or solid structures on the ovary greater than 2 cm in diameter need investigation.

At menopause, the ovary becomes devoid of functional follicles, and estradiol production ceases, resulting in amenorrhea and hot flashes. In normal women, the menopausal ovary, stimulated by high concentrations of LH, secretes testosterone from the stroma. Testosterone secretion from the ovary accounts for at least one half of total testosterone production in the menopausal woman (Judd et al., 1974). This ovarian testosterone may play a role in regulating libido and bone density. In postmenopausal women with normal body weight, the ovary does not secrete estradiol. In obese menopausal women, the ovary may secrete small amounts of estradiol. Since the menopausal ovary consists of stroma but no follicles, it is small (less than 2.0 by 2.0 by 1.5 cm) and is usually not palpable as a distinct structure on bimanual examination. In a menopausal woman, an ovary that is palpable on bimanual examination is cause for concern and requires clinical evaluation (Barber and Graber, 1971).

Functional Disorders of the Ovary

Corpus Luteum Defect

In 1949, Jones reported that in a study of 255 menstrual cycles in 98 infertile women, a significant percentage of the cycles were characterized by short luteal-phase length as determined by basal body temperature charts, diminished urinary pregnanediol excretion, and an out-of-phase endometrial biopsy. Subsequent studies confirmed that corpus luteum defect, or luteal-phase deficiency, is a common disorder, occurring in as many as 5% of menstrual cycles in normal fertile women and infertile women. The causes of corpus luteum defect are not completely characterized. Most investigators believe that abnormalities in the follicular phase of the menstrual cycle that cause suboptimal follicular growth prior to ovulation are associated with subsequent suboptimal corpus luteum performance. Endocrine abnormalities that can result in corpus luteum defect include hyperprolactinemia and abnormally elevated LH pulse frequency. Corpus luteum defect is best diagnosed by obtaining an endometrial biopsy specimen in the late luteal phase and examining the biopsy specimen for evidence of a delay in endometrial maturation. In infertile women with endometrial biopsy specimens demonstrating maturational delay of 4 days or greater, treatment of the corpus luteum defect will often be associated with subsequent pregnancy.

Luteinized Unruptured Follicle

In 1978, Marik and Hulka and Koninckx and colleagues reported the absence of ovulatory stigmata on the ovaries of a number of infertile women during the periovulatory phase of the menstrual cycle. They postulated that in some infertile women experiencing regular cyclic menses and apparently normal ovulatory cycles, failure of the oocyte to escape the follicle might be the cause of the infertility. Subsequent studies suggest that in fertile women, as many as 5% of all menstrual cycles are associated with luteinized unruptured follicle (LUF). In infertile women, the frequency of cycles with LUF may be greater than 5%, but LUF rarely occurs in repetitive cycles in the same woman. This suggests that LUF may not be a major cause of infertility. Interestingly, recent studies suggest that the administration of antiprostaglandins such as indomethacin to preovulatory women can cause LUF (Killick and Elstein, 1987). This suggests that infertile women should refrain from using antiprostaglandins during the preovulatory phase of the menstrual cycle.

Ovarian Hyperandrogenism

In as many as 5% of women of reproductive age, the ovary produces excess quantities of the androgens androstenedione and testosterone. Excessive ovarian production of androgens results in hirsutism, oligo-ovulation or anovulation, and menstrual dysfunction such as amenorrhea or menometrorrhagia. The causes of functional ovarian hyperandrogenism are incompletely characterized but include excess pituitary secretion of LH and elevated production of insulin.

In a subgroup of women with functional ovarian hyperandrogenism, LH pulse frequency and pulse amplitude are markedly elevated. Since the LH pulse frequency is elevated, it is likely that gonadotropin-releasing hormone (GnRH) pulse frequency is elevated (Waldstreicher et al., 1988). The mechanisms responsible for this increase in GnRH pulse frequency are unclear. However, increases in hypothalamic norepinephrine levels or decreases in hypothalamic dopamine or opioid levels may account, in part, for the changes in LH pulse frequency. The elevated LH level stimulates ovarian thecal and stromal tissues to produce excessive quantities of androstenedione and testosterone. In addition, the elevated LH level may produce premature luteinization of granulosa cells in 2- to 8-mm antral follicles, causing the termination of follicular growth. The accumulation of antral follicles 2 to 8 mm causes the ovaries to develop a polycystic appearance, hence the descriptive term *polycystic ovary syndrome*. The premature termination of follicular growth prevents any follicle from reaching a size necessary to trigger an LH surge and ovulation. Consequently, oligo-ovulation or anovulation develops.

The elevated ovarian secretion of androstenedione and testosterone produces numerous biochemical changes, including (1) a decrease in sex hormone–binding globulin production from the liver, leading to an increase in free testosterone levels; and (2) an increase in 5α-reductase activity in the hair follicles, resulting in an increase in local dihydrostestosterone production. These changes can result in hirsutism and acne.

A unique opportunity to identify a specific molecular and genetic cause of ovarian hyperandrogenism is provided by the recent observation that abnormalities in the insulin receptor gene are often associated with ovarian hyperandrogenism (Barbieri et al., 1988b; Barbieri and Ryan, 1983). In Kahn type A diabetes, a gene defect results in an inability to produce adequate numbers of functional insulin receptors. This genetic abnormality decreases glucose utilization in muscle and liver, is associated with an increase in circulating glucose levels, and results in a marked increase in pancreatic insulin production. In normal women, circulating insulin concentrations seldom exceed 150 μU/ml after a carbohydrate challenge. In women with Kahn type A diabetes, insulin concentrations often exceed 1,000 μU/ml after a carbohydrate challenge. Insulin, at high concentrations, is able to bind to insulin-like growth factor 1 (IGF-1) receptors and stimulate the tyrosine kinase activity of this receptor system. Human ovarian stroma and theca contain IGF-1 receptors, and IGF-1 and LH synergize to stimulate androstenedione and testosterone production. In patients with Kahn type A diabetes, we believe that the marked hyperinsulinemia synergizes with normal concentrations of LH to stimulate excessive androgen production from the ovary. The association between hyperinsulinemia and hyperandrogenism may also explain the observation that obesity is commonly associated with hyperandrogenism.

Treatment of functional ovarian hyperandrogenism is best directed at normalizing LH and insulin concentrations. The production of LH can be normalized by administering combined estrogen-progestogen preparations or GnRH agonists. Insulin concentrations can often be lowered in obese individuals by weight loss. Spironolactone, an inhibitor of the androgen receptor, can be used as an adjuvant to estrogen-progestogen preparations to help decrease facial hair growth (Lobo, 1988). In women with ovarian hyperandrogenism, anovulation, and infertility, ovulation induction with clomiphene citrate or human menopausal gonadotropins is often successful. Women with hyperandrogenism and anovulation are at risk for the development of endometrial hyperplasia and endometrial adenocarcinoma. These women should be treated at regular intervals with a 12- to 14-day course of a progestogen to inhibit the development of endometrial hyperplasia and cancer.

McCune-Albright Syndrome

The McCune-Albright syndrome afflicts girls less than 8 years of age and consists of the triad of café au lait spots, fibrous cysts of the bones, and precocious puberty due to the premature activation of ovarian follicular function. Recent studies suggest that in the McCune-Albright syndrome, cyclic follicular growth and estradiol production occurs in the absence of pituitary gonadotropin secretion. Ketoconazole and testolactone, two drugs that directly inhibit steroidogenic enzymes involved in estrogen production, are often used to treat this disorder (Feuillan et al., 1988).

OVARIAN NEOPLASMS

Of all gynecological cancers, malignant disease of the ovary ranks first as a cause of death in the United States. Nearly 11,000 American women die from ovarian cancer annually, and more than 8 to 10 times that number undergo operative procedures for both benign and malignant ovarian neoplasms each year. Despite its frequency, early diagnosis of ovarian cancer is the exception. In the United States, fully 72% of ovarian carcinomas have metastasized by the time of diagnosis. For this reason, the early recognition and management of abnormal ovarian enlargement is imperative. Proper concern for malignancy, however, must be tempered by an attitude of conservatism toward reproductive function in the younger patient. In this regard, a planned period of observation or noninvasive diagnostic procedures may constitute optimal management.

A consideration of ovarian neoplasms must encompass not only the wide range of benign and malignant tumors but also those tumor-like conditions of the ovary that are actually non-neoplastic. Familiarity with physiological and pathological conditions of other pelvic and lower abdominal organs that may simulate ovarian enlargement obviously is essential to the logical formulation of a differential diagnosis.

Classification

A formidable number of histological tumor types derived from the various cellular components of the ovary have both fascinated pathologists and confounded clinicians. Numerous classifications of ovarian tumors have been proposed, each having certain advantages and disadvantages. Classifications based on presumed histological origin allow broad grouping into similar clinical and histological types from which more specific subgroups may be derived.

The usefulness of histogenetic classifications in predicting survival has been limited by a substantial group of unclassifiable tumors, the frequent heterogeneity of cell types, and the variability in the malignant behavior within these histological types.

For many years pathologists and gynecologists have been aware of a specific group of papillary ovarian tumors with atypical proliferative activity but without the other histological hallmarks of malignancy. The clinical course is compatible with the histological appearance of a tumor of low-grade malignancy despite the occasional occurrence of superficial peritoneal metastases. This group with low potential malignancy has also been termed *borderline* and *grade 0*. Although the International Federation of Gynecology and Obstetrics (FIGO) histological classification includes a low potential malignancy category for each of the epithelial tumors, the designation is applicable primarily to the serous and mucinous cell types. Aure et al. (1971) found that whereas 21% of serous and 39% of mucinous carcinomas were considered to be of low malignant potential, only 3% of endometrioid carcinomas and none of the clear cell carcinomas were noninvasive.

The World Health Organization (WHO)

Committee on Ovarian Neoplasms under the leadership of Serov and Scully (1973) have proposed an extremely detailed histogenetic classification that allows both for variability within cell types by adding additional subtypes and for the frequent admixture of cell types (Table 9–1). It is hoped that this classification will be universally adopted and replace the multiplicity of classifications that have been shrouded in controversy and confusion.

Approximately 1.5% of American women develop ovarian cancer. Based on a number of published series, several general comments regarding the relationship of benign to malignant ovarian neoplasms may be made. Approximately 20% of all ovarian tumors are malignant, but the ratio of benign/malignant tumors declines after age 40 years. In the series reported by Bennington et al. (1968), only 6% of ovarian tumors were malignant in women less than age 45 years, whereas 33% were malignant in women between the ages of 45 and 74 years. The relative frequency of the commoner malignant tumors is given in Table 9–2.

About 4% of ovarian neoplasms are discovered in children less than 10 years old, and approximately 50% of these are malignant. These are usually solid teratomas or carcinomas, but occasionally a dysgerminoma or granulosa cell tumor may be found. The benign varieties are usually dermoid or epithelial cysts.

Diagnosis

Symptoms

Ovarian neoplasms are frequently asymptomatic. Unfortunately, subjective complaints are likely to occur only after complications arise, after the tumor has reached considerable size, or, in the case of malignancy, after dissemination has taken place. A recent nationwide survey indicated that 72% of ovarian cancers have disseminated by the time of diagnosis (Cutler et al., 1976).

Specific symptoms depend on the size, location, and type of the tumor, as well as on the presence of complicating factors such as torsion, hemorrhage, infection, or rupture. The usual presenting complaints include lower abdominal pain or pressure or concern for a mass or abdominal enlargement (Table 9–3). Unfortunately, these symptoms are related to either the accumulation of ascites, the size and weight of the tumor, or ad-

TABLE 9–1.

World Health Organization Histological Classification
of Ovarian Tumors*

I. Common "epithelial" tumors
   A. Serous tumors
      1. Benign
         a. Cystadenoma and papillary cystadenoma
         b. Surface papilloma
         c. Adenofibroma and cystadenofibroma
      2. Of borderline malignancy (carcinoma of low malignant potential)
         a. Cystadenoma and papillary cystadenoma
         b. Surface papilloma
         c. Adenofibroma and cystadenofibroma
      3. Malignant
         a. Adenocarcinoma, papillary adenocarcinoma, and papillary
            cystadenocarcinoma
         b. Surface papillary carcinoma
         c. Malignant adenofibroma and cystadenofibroma
   B. Mucinous tumors
      1. Benign
         a. Cystadenoma
         b. Adenofibroma and cystadenofibroma
      2. Of borderline malignancy (carcinoma of low malignant potential)
         a. Cystadenoma
         b. Adenofibroma and cystadenofibroma
      3. Malignant
         a. Adenocarcinoma and cystadenocarcinoma
         b. Malignant adenofibroma and cystadenofibroma
   C. Endometrioid tumors
      1. Benign
         a. Adenoma and cystadenoma
         b. Adenofibroma and cystadenofibroma
      2. Of borderline malignancy (carcinoma of low malignant potential)
         a. Adenoma and cystadenoma
         b. Adenofibroma and cystadenofibroma
      3. Malignant
         a. Carcinoma
            i. Adenocarcinoma
            ii. Adenoacanthoma
            iii Malignant adenofibroma
         b. Endometrioid stromal sarcomas
         c. Mesodermal (müllerian) mixed tumors, homologous, and
            heterologous
   D. Clear cell (mesonephroid) tumors
      1. Benign: adenofibroma
      2. Of borderline malignancy (carcinomas of low malignant potential)
      3. Malignant: carcinoma and adenocarcinoma
   E. Brenner tumors
      1. Benign
      2. Of borderline malignancy (proliferating)
      3. Malignant
   F. Mixed epithelial tumors
      1. Benign
      2. Of borderline malignancy
      3. Malignant
   G. Undifferentiated carcinoma
   H. Unclassified epithelial tumors
II. Sex cord stromal tumors
   A. Granulosa-stromal tumors
      1. Granulosa cell tumor

(Continued.)

TABLE 9–1. (cont.)

       2. Tumors in the thecoma-fibroma group
         a. Thecoma
         b. Fibroma
         c. Unclassified
     B.. Androblastomas: Sertoli-Leydig cell tumors
       1. Well differentiated
         a. Tubular androblastoma; Sertoli's cell tumor (tubular adenoma of Pick)
         b. Tubular androblastoma with lipid storage; Sertoli's cell tumor with lipid storage (folliculome lipidique of Lecene)
         c. Sertoli-Leydig cell tumor (tubular adenoma with Leydig's cells)
         d. Leydig's cell tumor; hilus cell tumor
       2. Of intermediate differentiation
       3. Poorly differentiated (sarcomatoid)
       4. With heterologous elements
     C. Gynandroblastoma
     D. Unclassified
  III. Lipid (lipoid) cell tumors
  IV. Germ cell tumors
     A. Dysgerminoma
     B. Endodermal sinus tumor
     C. Embryonal carcinoma
     D. Polyembryoma
     E. Choriocarcinoma
     F. Teratomas
       1. Immature
       2. Mature
         a. Solid
         b. Cystic
           i. Dermoid cyst (mature cystic teratoma)
           ii. Dermoid cyst with malignant transformation
       3. Monodermal and highly specialized
         a. Struma ovarii
         b. Carcinoid
         c. Struma ovarii and carcinoid
         d. Others
     G. Mixed forms
  V. Gonadoblastoma
     A. Pure
     B. Mixed with dysgerminoma or other form of germ cell tumor
  VI. Soft tissue tumors not specific to ovary
  VII. Unclassified tumors
  VIII. Secondary (metastatic) tumors
  IX. Tumor-like conditions
     A. Pregnancy luteomna
     B. Hyperplasia of ovarian stroma and hyperthecosis
     C. Massive edema
     D. Solitary follicle cyst and corpus luteum cyst
     E. Multiple follicle cysts (polycystic ovaries)
     F. Multiple luteinized follicle cysts, corpora lutea, or both
     G. Endometriosis
     H. Surface-epithelial inclusion cysts (germinal inclusion cysts)
     I. Simple cysts
     J. Inflammatory lesions
     K. Parovarian cysts

*From Serov SF, Scully RE: *Histological Typing of Ovarian Tumors.* International Histological Typing of Tumors, no 9. Geneva, World Health Organization, 1973.

TABLE 9–2.

Ovarian Cancer: Common Cell Types and Relative Frequency

Cell Types	%
Serous cystadenocarcinoma	40
Mucinous cystadenocarcinoma	12
Endometrioid carcinoma	15
Undifferentiated adenocarcinoma	15
Clear cell carcinoma (mesonephroma)	6
Granulosa-theca cell tumor	3
Dysgerminoma	1
Malignant teratoma	1
Metastatic carcinoma*	5
Others	2

*Undetected primary cancers mostly of the Krukenberg type.

TABLE 9–3.

Symptoms of Ovarian Neoplasms

Symptom	Cases	
	No.	%
Pain or discomfort	198	56.7
Distention or mass	177	50.7
Abnormal uterine bleeding	120	34.4
Urinary	59	16.9
Gastrointestinal	57	16.3

herence to surrounding structures with resultant traction or pressure. In other words, the usual symptoms are those of advanced growth. In some instances, particularly with benign tumors, the diagnosis is made during a routine pelvic examination. When pain is present, it is usually not severe and may be described as a mild discomfort in the lower abdomen. Vague digestive disturbances such as flatulence, eructations, and abdominal discomfort may precede other symptoms by many months. The combination of moderate anorexia or indigestion and slight abdominal enlargement should alert the physician to the possibility of ovarian cancer even if a pelvic mass is not readily apparent.

Abnormal uterine bleeding was noted in 34% of patients with ovarian tumors reported from the Boston Hospital for Women (Kent and McKay, 1960), and a similar incidence has been reported in other series (see Table 9–3). In a few instances, endometrial metastases and coexistent lesions such as leiomyomas, polyps, and even primary endometrial carcinomas are responsible, but the cause of bleeding is often obscure. Uterine bleeding associated with gonadal stromal tumors known to be hormonally active is easily explained on the basis of endometrial stimulation. It now appears that a number of benign and malignant tumors considered hormonally inactive may also be associated with increased sex steroid production. The origin of these sex steroids has been at-

tributed to the stimulation of normal thecal tissue to produce androstenedione (MacDonald et al., 1976) by adjacent tumor.

Other specific complaints may relate to the location, size, and weight of the primary tumor or its metastases. Tumors expanding in the anterior pelvis can exert pressure sufficient to compromise bladder capacity or provide some degree of outflow obstruction. Pressure at the pelvic brim may produce ureteral obstruction and secondary pyelonephritis. In addition to vague digestive complaints, compression of the rectosigmoid by an expanding posterior pelvic mass can cause significant constipation or even partial large bowel obstruction. Similarly, adhesion formation between the tumor and sigmoid colon or terminal ileum may result in torsion and intermittent obstruction.

Severe pain of sudden onset is indicative of an acute complication. The commonest of these is torsion of the ovarian pedicle. Tumors with a narrow or elongated pedicle are most prone to this complication. Benign cystic teratomas (dermoid cysts) are particularly susceptible since they are freely mobile with a slender pedicle and are disproportionately heavy. Twisted ovarian cysts cause severe, localized pain often accompanied by nausea and vomiting. If the torsion is incomplete, partial occlusion of the blood supply results in venous stasis with extravasation of serum and blood into the cyst cavity. The mass rapidly enlarges, becomes exquisitely tender, and is susceptible to rupture or hemorrhage. On physical examination, there may be abdominal rigidity with local and rebound tenderness. Pelvic examination discloses a firm, tender mass, but the findings may be variable, depending on the size and location of the cyst. If torsion is sufficient to produce obstruction of the arterial supply, infarction and necrosis of the cyst wall may result in perforation and peritonitis. It is generally recommended that ovarian cysts with a twisted pedicle not be unwound prior to removal because of the possibility of venous embolization by thrombi or necrotic debris. Thin-walled cysts of the follicular or corpus luteum type may rupture into the peritoneal cavity, and if accompanied by significant bleeding, symptoms of intraperitoneal hemorrhage and shock may ensue. The release of old blood and debris promptly causes a severe local peritonitis.

Hemorrhage into an ovarian cyst is a common complication and may occur spontaneously or as the result of physical trauma. Bleeding can be profuse, filling and enlarging the cystic cavity in the manner of a hemorrhagic corpus luteum. Intermittent hemorrhage with slow growth and thickening of the capsule is common with an endometrioma. Soft, pultaceous tumors such as granulosa cell tumors are particularly prone to vessel rupture and hemorrhage within their substance.

Physical Signs

The diagnosis of an ovarian neoplasm is usually made on bimanual pelvic examination. To clearly outline adnexal masses, the bladder and lower bowel should be empty and the abdominal musculature relaxed. Rectovaginal examination is essential and allows palpation of the surface of a mass in the posterior cul-de-sac. By displacing the cervix anteriorly, nodularity of the uterosacral ligaments may be detected, suggesting endometriosis or local metastases. A precise preoperative diagnosis of an ovarian neoplasm may be difficult. In our patients with ovarian carcinoma, a pelvic mass was noted in 86% and an abdominal mass in 76%. Huge cysts that fill the abdomen are usually mucinous or serous cystadenomas. Thin-walled physiological cysts of the corpus luteum or follicle range from 3 to 6 cm in diameter and because of their mobility may be difficult to palpate. It is generally agreed that these cysts rarely exceed 6 cm in diameter.

A number of palpable characteristics are helpful in differentiating benign from malignant ovarian masses. A smooth, regular surface suggests a benign cyst, whereas an irregular or nodular surface is indicative of malignancy. If there is fixation, the examiner should suspect malignancy, endometriosis, inflammatory process, or adhesions secondary to necrosis. Otherwise, benign tumors tend not to form adhesions, and unless they reach gigantic proportions, they are quite

mobile on manipulation. A soft cystic mass is likely to be a physiological cyst in the premenopausal woman or a simple cyst in the postmenopausal woman. Malignant epithelial tumors often contain cystic areas interspersed with hard nodules, or they have a solid consistency. The presence of firm nodules in the cul-de-sac or nodularity along the uterosacral ligaments in association with an ovarian mass strongly suggests either endometriosis or carcinoma with cul-de-sac metastases.

Most ovarian neoplasms are in a position lateral or posterior to the uterus. The benign cystic teratoma (dermoid cyst) is a notable exception and is usually found anterior to the broad ligament.

Bilateral involvement is indicative of malignancy. In the series reported by Bennington et al. (1968), 9% of benign tumors and 42% of malignant tumors were bilateral. Regarding the benign and malignant tumors as a whole, 16% were bilateral, and of these 53% were malignant.

Clinically evident ascites is present in 25% of patients with malignant ovarian tumors. The aspiration of ascitic fluid for cytological examination may provide useful information prior to laparotomy. Rarely, benign ovarian tumors, particularly fibromas and serous cystadenomas, are associated with nonmalignant ascites and right pleural effusions. This clinical picture is known as Meigs' syndrome, and the mechanism by which the serous effusions form is unknown. A pleural effusion does not necessarily connote inoperability and should always be tapped for cytological examination. Occasionally, malignant ovarian tumors are associated with nonmalignant serous effusions (pseudo-Meigs' syndrome).

Differential Diagnosis

Before we proceed to the various lesions that may be confused with ovarian neoplasms, it should be emphasized that common midline "tumors" that on occasion may simulate an ovarian cyst are a distended urinary bladder and enlargement of the uterus due to an intrauterine pregnancy. All patients should void before pelvic examination. During the first 8 to 12 weeks of pregnancy, the uterine corpus is smooth, soft, cystic, and freely mobile. Since the lower uterine segment is particularly soft, the corpus may be palpated as a separate mass unless particular care is taken during examination.

Several conditions involving the colon frequently simulate ovarian neoplasms. These include a low-lying, distended cecum, a redundant sigmoid colon, an appendiceal abscess, impacted feces in the rectosigmoid, carcinoma of the sigmoid, and diverticulitis.

A localized appendiceal abscess may be confused with an ovarian neoplasm undergoing hemorrhage, rupture, or torsion. A previous history of upper abdominal or periumbilical pain associated with nausea, vomiting, and subsequent localization of the pain in the right lower quadrant together with local peritoneal signs will aid in diagnosis. Occasionally, however, the initial symptoms of acute appendicitis are obscure, and the abscess develops gradually with the formation of a thick, adherent capsule.

A firm, fixed mass in the left side of the pelvis of women more than age 50 years strongly suggests carcinoma of the ovary or rectosigmoid. A history of altered bowel habits, colicky pain, blood or melena, or diminution in the caliber of the stool suggests sigmoid cancer. The diagnosis is confirmed by barium enema or sigmoidoscopy and biopsy of the tumor mass. In some cases, however, the sigmoid colon and left ovary are so intimately adherent in a carcinomatous process than even the pathologist finds it impossible to determine the primary site.

Diverticulitis of the sigmoid colon is a frequent cause of erroneous gynecologic diagnoses. Although many women more than age 40 years have asymptomatic diverticulosis, a mass in the left side of the pelvis following rupture of a diverticulum may be difficult to distinguish from ovarian cancer. A typical attack of diverticulitis is manifested by intermittent cramplike abdominal pain, usually in the left lower quadrant, associated with diarrhea, and small amounts of blood and mucus in the stool. Evidence of peritoneal irritation together with leukocytosis and fever aid in the differential diagnosis. Pelvic examination will elicit localized tenderness but otherwise is not of great value since perforation results in a firm mass that lodges in the left side of the pelvis or iliac fossa. Diagnosis will depend on a barium enema, which should be done during a quiescent period of the disease and should reveal diverticula, an irritable colon, and areas of stenosis.

The oviduct or mesosalpinx may also give rise to cystic structures, which must be differentiated from those arising in the ovary. A parovarian cyst may arise from the rudimentary structures in the mesosalpinx and develop between the leaves of the broad ligament. These cysts are usually unilateral, somewhat fixed, ovoid, and thin walled. A tubal ectopic pregnancy may closely simulate an acute accident arising in an ovarian tumor, such as torsion or hemorrhage. Symptoms suggesting pregnancy and a chorionic gonadotropin level by β-subunit assay will aid in the correct diagnosis. Perhaps the lesion most commonly mistaken for an ovarian tumor is a pedunculated uterine leiomyoma, particularly if the tumor is solitary and somewhat soft. Such leiomyomas ("fibroids") are usually freely mobile, but careful examination may reveal an area of attachment to the uterus. It is impossible to delineate adequately a parasitic or intraligamentous fibroid since these lesions are relatively fixed and may be situated in areas directly adjacent to the ovary. If the pedicle of a pedunculated fibroid undergoes torsion and infarction, the presenting signs and symptoms will be indistinguishable from those of a twisted ovarian cyst.

Ultrasound examination of the abdomen and pelvis has become a standard diagnostic test for evaluating pelvic masses. Ultrasound may determine the origin of the pelvic mass, delineate the internal appearance of the mass, and define associated abdominal findings. The presence of septations, papillary structures, solid tissue, and bilaterality suggests malignancy in an ovarian mass. Furthermore, ascites and omental, nodal or hepatic metastases are strongly indicative of malignancy. However, the sensitivity of ultrasound in diagnosing ovarian cancer in premenopausal and postmenopausal women with adnexal masses was only 50% and 78%, respectively (Finkler et al., 1988).

Tumor-associated antigens have been recently identified in ovarian cancer and have been successfully employed in monitoring patients. Approximately 80% of patients with advanced epithelial ovarian cancer have elevated serum levels of CA-125 (Bast et al., 1981). Studies have been performed to assess the value of CA-125 levels in discriminating benign from malignant pelvic masses. In postmenopausal patients with pelvic masses, the predictive value of an elevated CA-125 level for ovarian cancer was 98% (Malkasian et al., 1988). However, in premenopausal patients, the predictive value of an abnormal test result was only 49%, whereas the predictive value for a normal test result was 93%. CA-125 values may be elevated in benign gynecological conditions, including endometriosis, adenomyosis, and pelvic inflammatory disease (Barbieri et al.,

1986). The predictive value of an elevated CA-125 level in a premenopausal patient is therefore limited. CA-125 measurement may also contribute to the accuracy of ultrasound in assessing pelvic masses (Finkler et al., 1988). Other tumor-associated antigens may also prove to be useful in the evaluation of pelvic masses.

Non-neoplastic Cysts of Graafian Follicle Origin

In any consideration of ovarian neoplasms, the student and clinician must be familiar with the physiological variations of the ovulatory cycle that occasionally result in a nonneoplastic cyst. The normal ovary from a fertile patient usually has as many as 8 to 10 follicles visible on midsagittal section, which vary from 3 to 5 mm in diameter. Since all follicles are cystic to some degree, we have arbitrarily adopted a diameter of 2.5 cm as the dividing line between a cystic follicle and an actual follicle cyst.

Follicle cysts may occur at any age before the menopause and on occasion reach a diameter of 7 to 8 cm. An ovary containing a single large follicle cyst is usually asymptomatic but may give rise to a sense of pelvic discomfort or heaviness on the affected side. Because of associated hormonal activity, the patient may have noted irregularity of the menstrual cycle such as delayed flow followed by irregular and intermittent spotting. The latter symptoms are likely to induce the patient to seek medical consultation, at which time the cyst is discovered. Occasionally, spontaneous rupture and subsequent bleeding, which is usually self-limited, produces acute pelvic pain.

Grossly, follicle cysts are thin-walled and translucent, although occasionally intracystic bleeding may impart a dark brown appearance. Granulosa and theca-interna cells show varying degrees of luteinization.

On pelvic examination follicle cysts are mobile and somewhat soft on compression. Occasionally, they are inadvertently ruptured during examination. Treatment of a follicle cyst should be conservative unless rupture and hemorrhage warrant surgical intervention. If the cyst is less than 6 cm in diameter, the patient should have a pelvic examination in 6 weeks. Functional ovarian cysts normally regress within 6 weeks. If examination is performed after the next menstrual period, the cyst will often have disappeared. For cysts 6 cm or larger or those that persist through two or more menstrual cycles, laparoscopy may clarify the diagnosis. When doubt exists, laparotomy is indicated. Since follicle cysts are dependent on pituitary gonadotropic stimulation, we have used oral contraceptives to hasten their disappearance.

Cystic Structures Derived From the Normally Ruptured Follicle

Corpus Luteum Cyst

The mature corpus luteum has a central core filled with blood. After resorption, the cavity normally may be distended with hemorrhagic or clear fluid, making the corpus luteum itself a cystic structure. A corpus luteum cyst results from an abnormal persistence or exaggeration of this physiological process. A *corpus luteum hematoma* may cause local pain, amenorrhea, and signs closely resembling a tubal ectopic pregnancy. Although most hematomas of the corpus luteum do not exceed 7 or 8 cm, several as large as 11 cm in diameter have been described. Following the resorption of the blood, a typical corpus luteum cyst may evolve.

The diagnosis of a corpus luteum cyst cannot be made with exact precision but should be suspected in a patient who has noted delayed menses followed by irregular staining and a constant discomfort or sense of heaviness in one side of the pelvis. A positive diagnosis of a corpus luteum cyst or hematoma can usually be made by laparoscopy.

A ruptured hemorrhagic corpus luteum may result in all the signs and symptoms of intraperitoneal bleeding. The clinical picture includes lower abdominal pain, nausea, and vomiting, rectus muscle spasm, and rebound tenderness. Pelvic examination will reveal an enlarged, tender ovary or, if bleeding has been extensive, a doughy or fluctuant cul-de-sac. The temperature may be elevated to 38°C, and moderate leukocytosis is usually present. The blood loss occasionally is severe, exceeding 1,000 ml.

Gross examination of a corpus luteum cyst or hematoma reveals the yellowish color in the thin wall of the cyst. Both granulosa and theca-lutein cells will be found in the wall, together with organizing fibrous connective tissue and erythrocytes.

Large physiological ovarian cysts may be associated with hydatidiform mole or choriocarcinoma. They result from the stimulus of excessive hCG hormone secreted by these trophoblastic tumors. Bilateral lutein cysts occur in about one third of these patients. Surgical extirpation of the ovaries is not necessary, however, since lutein cysts gradually regress, and the ovaries return to normal size and function after removal of the trophoblastic tissue. These cysts may reach rather large proportions, filling the pelvic cavity on both sides. Each large cyst is made up of multiple locules varying from 1 to 2 cm in diameter. Each locule contains a clear yellow fluid, and each cystic cavity is lined by luteinized theca-interna cells, which resemble the lutein cells of the corpus luteum.

Luteoma of Pregnancy

Luteoma of pregnancy consists of hyperplastic nodules of luteinized theca cells, which are multiple in 50% of reported cases and involve both ovaries in 30% of cases. In contrast to the theca-lutein cyst, which is a physiological response to elevated levels of chorionic gonadotropin, the luteoma represents an exaggerated response to normal levels of hCG. Although the pregnancy luteoma may attain a diameter of 16 cm, most have been discovered at cesarean section. Spontaneous regression of the nodules has been noted consistently during the postpartum period. The most dramatic feature of the pregnancy luteoma has been the frequent association with maternal and fetal virilization. In 22 of the 74 reported cases, maternal virilization was evident; among these, 7 of 11 female neonates were also virilized. In all instances, virilizing signs regressed post partum.

Simple Cyst

The simple cyst rarely arouses the interest of pathologists but is of considerable importance to clinicians in light of its frequent occurrence during the menopausal years. These cysts are translucent, thin-walled structures that contain a thin serous fluid and are somewhat soft to palpation. They rarely exceed 10 cm in diameter. Their internal surface is impeccably smooth and free of papillary projections. Although simple cysts are almost always unilateral, the opposite ovary usually contains a number of germinal inclusion cysts.

Microscopically, the internal surface is lined by flattened mesothelial cells resembling peritoneum, but areas of cuboidal cells consistent with coelomic metaplasia are often present. Simple cysts are most likely derived from germinal inclusion cysts in which the coelomic epithelium has

undergone complete or partial regression after cystic enlargement. In the event of differentiation rather than regression, cysts of identical gross appearance are lined by tubal-type epithelium. These serous cystomas are usually categorized with the serous cystadenomas despite their lack of proliferative activity.

Simple cysts are surprisingly persistent, and since they occur in postmenopausal women, early laparotomy is required to exclude a malignant process. Both ovaries should be removed because of the possibility that a second simple cyst or cystadenoma will arise in the contralateral ovary.

Cystomas of Germinal Epithelial Origin (Common Epithelial Tumors)

Most clinically important ovarian neoplasms fall into the category of cystomas of germinal epithelial origin. These tumors include the serous and mucinous cystadenomas and cystadenocarcinomas, benign and malignant endometrioid tumors, the clear cell carcinomas, and the rarely malignant Brenner tumor. With progressive epithelial proliferation, all of the cystomas, particularly endometrioid and clear cell carcinomas, tend to become solid. Those epithelial tumors in which the stroma predominates, such as cystadenofibromas and Brenner tumors, have a solid morphology from the outset.

The histogenesis of the ovarian cystomas represents one of the more curious phenomena in human biology. McKay (1962) and Lauchlan (1972) have described graphically the process whereby germinal epithelium recapitulates the embryogenesis of the müllerian duct, with which it shares a common derivation from the coelomic epithelium of the urogenital ridge. The germinal epithelium of the adult ovary consists of a flattened layer of mesothelial cells indistinguishable from other visceral peritoneum. Although the mechanism is unclear, the surface of the aging ovary becomes progressively convoluted, forming irregular gyri and sulci. In most instances the surface continuity of deep mesothelial invaginations is closed off by intervening stroma, thereby forming germinal inclusion cysts, or "cortical glands," a common finding in the postmenopausal ovary.

In the event of neoplastic transformation, the new coelomic epithelium undergoes proliferation, and concurrent cellular differentiation to specific cell types completes the embryologic recapitulation of the müllerian duct lumen. Consequently, the tumor epithelium may resemble endosalpinx (serous cystoma), endocervix (mucinous cystoma), or endometrium (endometrioid cystoma) (Fig 9–4). Scully (1970b) has suggested that the clear cell carcinoma is an endometrial variant, although benign and malignant aggregates of the component cells may be found at other locations in the female genital tract. Despite a probable derivation from germinal epithelium, the Brenner tumor is not a convincing example of müllerian differentiation since its characteristic cell resembles urinary bladder epithelium. Nevertheless, the epithelial elements of Brenner tumors and mucinous tumors are frequently mixed. It is apparent that müllerian differentiation from coelomic epithelium may proceed in several directions simultaneously since a number of tumors containing various mixtures of serous, mucinous, endometrioid, and clear cell components within a single cyst have been described.

The stages of cystoma histogenesis may be summarized as (1) invagination, (2) coelomic metaplasia, (3) occlusion and cyst formation, (4) proliferation, and (5) differentiation. These steps may not always follow the sequence, and they may not all take place. Without deep invagination or isolation from the surface, cyst formation fails, and the result is a papillary epithelial tumor on the surface of the ovary. Should proliferation not take place, a unilocular cyst lined by a single cell layer is formed—the simple serous cyst. The end result of proliferation without differentiation is the highly anaplastic undifferentiated carcinoma.

Both misunderstanding and controversy have resulted from frequent reference to the "müllerian origin" of the common epithelial tumors. This concept is clearly incorrect since these tumors do not arise from the müllerian duct but, rather, represent metaplastic müllerian epithelium at ectopic sites. Woodruff and Telinde (1976) have pointed out that the ovarian cystomas arise from mesothelium and that histologically identical tumors occasionally arise from extragonadal pelvic peritoneum. As pointed out by Hertig and Gore (1961), the peritoneal mesothelium of the pelvis has the potential for coelomic metaplasia and müllerian differentiation. In an excellent review of the subject, Lauchlan (1972) has suggested that the term *secondary müllerian epithelium* be used to

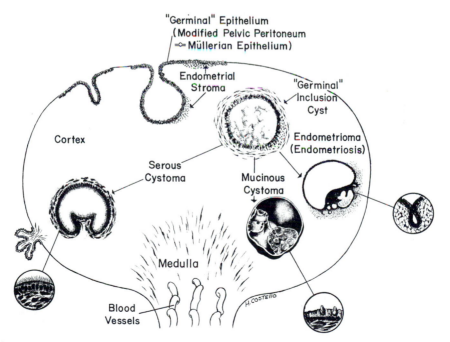

FIG 9–4.

Schematic diagram of origin of ovarian cystomas from surface or "germinal" epithelium. On the surface are a papillary outgrowth of germinal epithelium, an early infolding, a later stage of infolding, and a small focus of endometrial-type stroma lying beneath the germinal epithelium. A germinal inclusion cyst is lying within the cortex and is surrounded mainly by ovarian cortical stroma and partly by endometrial stroma. The three main derivatives are shown. (From Hertig AT, Gore H: *Rocky Mt Med J* 1958; 55:47–50. Reproduced by permission.)

denote any epithelium derived from peritoneum that closely resembles one of the cell types lining the müllerian duct. These cell types include the endosalpinx, endometrium, and endocervix, but not the squamous epithelium of the exocervix. The propensity of peritoneum for secondary müllerian differentiation is greatest overlying the ovary and is decremental as the distance from the ovary increases. Consequently, small serous inclusion cysts are most frequently found on the ovary, tube, uterine serosa, anterior and posterior cul-de-sac, and lateral pelvic peritoneum, in that order. As a rule, these cysts are barely visible, and this condition, known as *endosalpingiosis,* is usually an independent finding of the pathologist. In summary, the ovarian cystomas and their peritoneal counterparts consist of secondary müllerian epithelium derived by metaplasia from certain areas of mesothelium that have retained a specific embryonic potential.

Serous Cystadenomas and Cystadenocarcinoma

The serous cystomas are the commonest of all benign and malignant ovarian neoplasms. They are characterized by an epithelium that closely resembles that of the oviduct, although the degree of resemblance is dependent on differentiation of the tumor epithelium. Variations within this cell type, however, depend on the architectural pattern of tumor growth as well as the degree of epithelial differentiation.

Serous cystadenomas constitute about 25% of benign ovarian tumors. They may be unilocular or multilocular and are bilateral in 15% of cases. They usually do not exceed 10 cm in diameter; rarely, they may become enormous, filling the entire abdomen. The surface is smooth and tends to be grayish white with multiple fine blood vessels visible beneath the serosal surface. In its most simple form, the inner surface is lined by epithelium indistinguishable from that of the fallopian tube (Fig 9–5). Multiple small papillary structures that barely project above the cyst wall give the internal surface a roughened or velvety appearance. The cyst fluid is usually thin and serous, but it may be slightly mucoid, indicating that some mucinous epithelium is present. Although tumor enlargement occurs by fluid accumulation, intracystic proliferation may proceed with the formation of larger and more complex papillary structures. It is at this point that the potentially malignant nature of a serous cystadenoma may for the first time become apparent. In

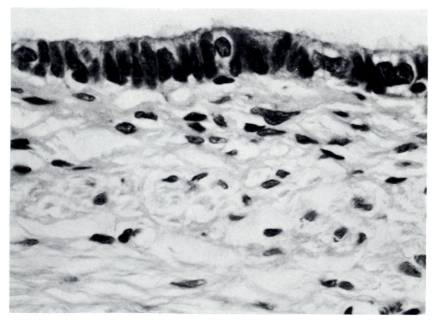

FIG 9–5.
Epithelium lining a serous cyst. (From McKay DG: The origins of ovarian tumors. *Clin Obstet Gynecol* 1962; 5:1189. Reproduced by permission.)

those tumors destined to remain benign, the papillary structure is simple and consists of a broad, dense fibrous stroma covered by a single layer of columnar cells (Fig 9–6). At the time of operation, a serous cystadenoma rarely arouses suspicion of malignancy. The operative procedure performed depends on the age of the patient and her preference regarding ovarian conservation. In women more than 40 years of age, a complete hysterectomy and bilateral salpingo-oophorectomy are indicated. In younger patients, the cyst should be enucleated and opened by the pathologist. Gross inspection should reveal the papillary nature of the cyst, although on occasion a rapid histological section is required. After the diagnosis of a papillary tumor has been established, the remainder of the ovary should be removed. The opposite ovary has a 15% chance of containing a similar, though inapparent, cyst and therefore should be bisected and carefully inspected. Other than complete abdominal exploration, any further treatment should await examination of the permanent histological sections and discussion with the patient. The prognosis is excellent following surgical extirpation of these lesions, and even the threat of a retained contralateral ovary appears minimal.

The malignant potential of a serous cystadenoma is first manifested by a proliferation of the epithelium of the small papillae. The epithelium lining the cyst wall usually retains its original appearance, whereas the papillary epithelium becomes pseudostratified or stratified with a loss of differentiation (Fig 9–7,A). With progressive growth, cellular pleomorphism and increased numbers of mitotic figures become prominent. As the epithelial growth exceeds that of the stroma, tufts of malignant-appearing cells become detached from the papillae and float freely in the cyst fluid (Fig 9–7,B). Rapid proliferation of serous epithelium is often accompanied by the formation of microscopic calcospherites known as *psammoma bodies*. These tiny spherical laminated structures are usually found in areas of cellular degeneration. Most important, there is no evidence of infiltrative growth into the tumor stroma. The justification for this intermediate category is based on clinical outcome. In the series reported by Santesson (1968), the 10-year survival rate in cases of borderline serous cystadenoma was 76%, whereas the corresponding figure for serous cystadenocarcinomas was only 13%. Aure et al. (1971) found that 21% of the proliferating serous tumors were of the borderline category and that more than one half of these women were less than age 45 years. The relative frequency of borderline serous tumors during the childbearing years has been noted by others who have demonstrated that

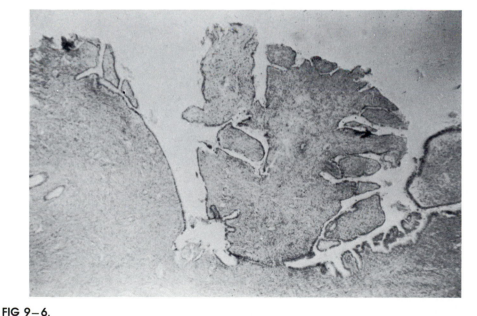

FIG 9–6.
Papillary serous cystadenoma. Broad papillae are covered by a single layer of columnar epithelium.

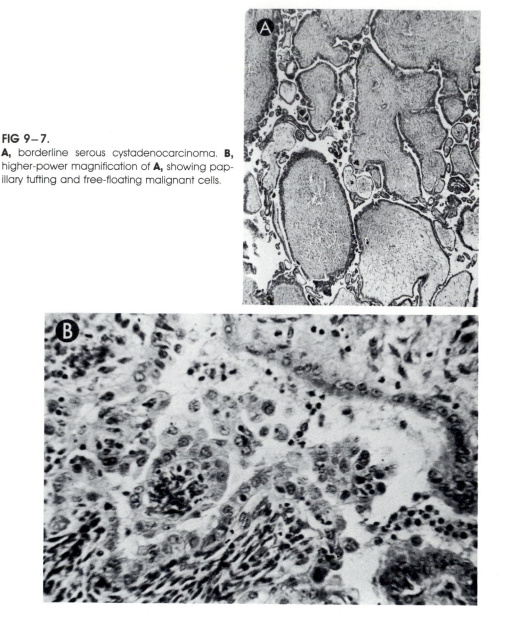

FIG 9–7.
A, borderline serous cystadenocarcinoma. **B,** higher-power magnification of **A,** showing papillary tufting and free-floating malignant cells.

removal of the involved ovary has provided adequate therapy if the tumor was confined to that ovary. Approximately one third of borderline serous cystadenomas are bilateral; thus, wedge biopsy of the contralateral ovary should also be considered.

In the case of serous cystadenocarcinomas, the papillary growth pattern, though similar to that just described, is more extensive. Invasion of the papillary stroma or the tumor capsule may occur even when the cystic tumor is small (Fig 9–8,A). The stroma itself is diminished by rapid epithelial proliferation, and long, thin branching papillae tend to coalesce and form friable, cauliflower-like masses. Papillary growth on the external surface of the cyst usually follows perforation of the capsule by invasive tumor. In the well-differentiated tumors, the epithelium continues to resemble the oviduct, and ciliated cells may occasionally be found. In addition, the architecture consists of well-formed, frondlike papillary structures. The coalescence of the papillae and forma-

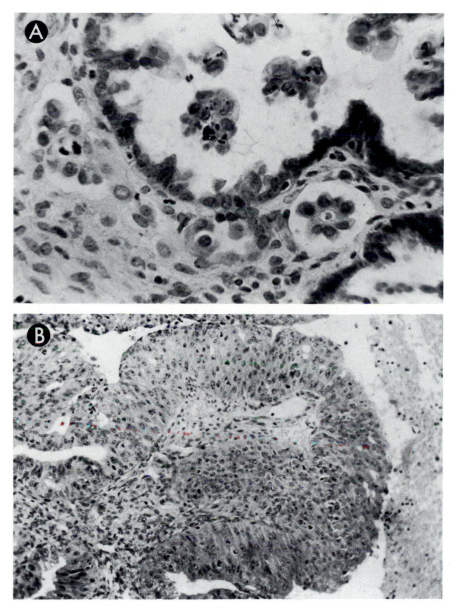

FIG 9–8.
A, early stromal invasion in a well-differentiated serous cystadenocarcinoma. **B,** massive stromal invasion in a poorly differentiated serous cystadenocarcinoma.

tion of solid areas are accompanied by a loss of epithelial differentiation (Fig 9–8,B). The cellular layer increases in thickness with increasing mitotic activity, and the resemblance to tubal epithelium diminishes. In the poorly differentiated tumors, the papillary architecture may be barely evident within large solid areas, and the diagnosis of a serous tumor can be made only by a thorough search for better differentiated epithelium. Approximately 25% of serous cystadenocarcinomas are well differentiated (grade 1), 35% are moderately well differentiated (grade 2), and 40% are poorly differentiated (grade 3). The prognosis of patients with epithelial ovarian cancer is related to the degree of differentiation. This relationship and the treatment of serous cystadenocarcinomas are discussed in the section on carcinoma of the ovary.

Serous Cystadenofibroma.—A cystadenofibroma is usually defined as a cystadenoma in which at least one fourth of the tumor mass consists of fibrous stroma. The epithelial component is almost always tubal in character, and the connective tissue orginates from the cortical stroma, the tunica albuginea, or both. These tumors vary considerably in size but may reach 20 cm in diameter. They are bilateral in 15% of cases and are rarely malignant.

Mucinous Cystadenoma and Cystadenocarcinoma

Mucinous cell types constitute 12% of the common epithelial tumors, and 12% of these are malignant. Although a germinal epithelial origin with endocervical differentiation has been generally accepted, considerable doubt has been cast on the concept of a uniform histogenetic pathway. Nevertheless, the frequent admixture of mucinous epithelium with serous, endometrioid, and clear cell elements within individual cystomas supports a germinal epithelial origin.

Grossly, the outer surface is generally smooth, lobulated, and gray-white. Seventy percent of the benign and malignant mucinous cystadenomas are multilocular. Although mucinous tumors range from microscopic size to 50 cm in diameter, most are between 15 and 30 cm and weigh between 2,000 and 4,000 gm. The serosal surface of the malignant form may show extracystic papillary growth, which becomes densely adherent to adjacent structures, particularly the bowel and bladder. When invasion of the capsule is extensive, rupture of the tumor may occur. Benign tumors are usually not fixed to adjacent structures and are therefore susceptible to torsion. This complication has been reported in as high as 20% of cases.

On section, the number and size of the cystic cavities vary with the amount of stroma. The internal surface of the mucinous cystadenoma is smooth or velvety and does not contain solid or nodular areas. Almost 25% of benign tumors and the greater proportion of malignant tumors will contain intracystic papillary projections, which arouse the suspicion of malignancy. Solid areas and firm nodules are found in about 50% of borderline mucinous tumors and in about 75% of obviously malignant tumors.

Microscopically, the mucinous cystadenomas contain cysts lined by a single layer of well-differentiated mucinous epithelium which closely resembles that of the endocervix except for the absence of ciliated cells (Fig 9–9). The presence of papillary processes does not connote malignancy, provided there is neither nuclear atypism nor stratification of the epithelium.

When the borderline and malignant muci-

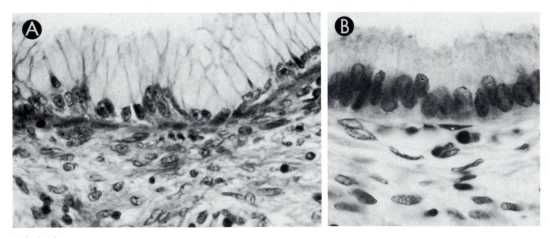

FIG 9–9.
A, mucinous cystoma. The tall columnar "picket" cells resemble the secretory cells of the endocervix. The intracytoplasmic mucin and basal location of the nuclei are characteristic features. **B,** endocervical epithelium. The cellular arrangement is slightly more orderly than in **A,** and occasional cells are ciliated. (From McKay DG: The origins of ovarian tumors. *Clin Obstet Gynecol* 1962; 5:1186. Reproduced by permission.)

nous tumors are considered as a whole, the borderline group constituted 39% in the series reported by Aure et al. (1971) and 71% of the stage I cystadenocarcinomas in Hart and Norris' (1973) series. Microscopically, the borderline tumors contain secondary cysts and short papillary infoldings. The papillary projections tend to be fine and branching and are supported by a delicate connective tissue stroma (Fig 9–10). The cysts are lined by atypical cells, which are stratified into two or three layers and contain variable amounts of intracytoplasmic mucin. The nuclei are irregular and hyperchromatic, and mitotic figures may be abundant. Papillary formation is somewhat greater in the mucinous cystadenocarcinomas, and the marked proliferation of epithelial cells results in a thick, stratified epithelium composed of atypical cells (Fig 9–11). Because a glandular pattern within the stroma is common, invasion has been difficult to determine without reservation. Hart and Norris (1973) have suggested that even though invasion is not demonstrable, stratification of atypical epithelium exceeding three cells in thickness should indicate that the lesion is, in fact, malignant. In their series of 27 patients with stage I cystadenocarcinomas, stromal invasion was identified in only 56%, but the 5-year survival rate was 65%. In contrast, the 5- and 10-year survival rates for patients with borderline tumors were 98% and 96%, respectively.

As a group, the mucinous cystadenocarcinomas are less aggressive than their serous counterparts. In the series reported by Decker and associates (1975) from the Mayo Clinic, only 25% of mucinous cystadenocarcinomas had spread beyond the ovary at the time of diagnosis, and only 6% were poorly differentiated histologically. In contrast, 73% of serous cystadenocarcinomas had disseminated, and 52% were poorly differentiated.

The treatment of mucinous tumors is identical to that of serous tumors. Since mucinous tumors are bilateral in only 8% of cases, conservation of childbearing capacity in younger women is possible with greater frequency.

Pseudomyxoma Peritonei.—Pseudomyxoma peritonei refers to the process of mucinous ascites secondary to mucinous tumors of intraabdominal organs. Although this condition has been associated with primary mucinous carcinomas of the urachus, bowel, and common bile duct, the ovary and the appendix have been the sites of origin in nearly all reported cases, with the ovary predominating. Although pseudomyxoma may arise, rarely, from apparently benign mucinous tumors of the ovary and appendix, there is general agreement that the process is, indeed, malignant. Confusion has resulted from the fact that the primary tumors are highly differentiated and the mucinous ascites itself contains strips of ac-

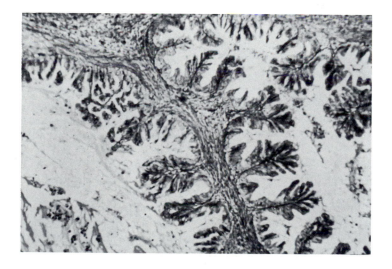

FIG 9–10.
Borderline mucinous cystadenocarcinoma. The papillary projections are fine and branching. In many areas the epithelial layer is two or three cells thick. (From McKay DG: The origin of ovarian tumors. *Clin Obstet Gynecol* 1962; 5:1190. Reproduced by permission.)

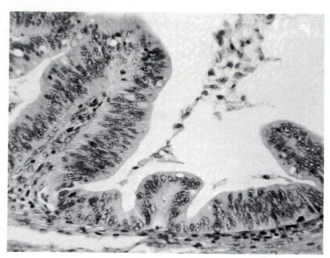

FIG 9–11.
Mucinous cystadenocarcinoma. The epithelial layer is greater than three cells in thickness. Although a suggestion of the mucinous character is present, the cells are anaplastic, with increased mitotic activity.

tively secreting, but benign-appearing, epithelium. In the report of 10 cases by Limber and associates (1973), all 6 of the ovarian tumors contained areas of stromal invasion. The ascites form of the tumor, however, is rarely invasive, and a protracted clinical course is characterized by progressive mechanical interference with GI function frequently resulting in partial bowel obstruction.

The treatment of ovarian pseudomyxoma peritonei consists of surgical excision of the primary tumor (both ovaries are usually involved) and evacuation of as much of the mucinous material as possible. Recurrence within 18 months is frequent, but an aggressive initial operation as well as repeated surgical evacuation has resulted in an overall 5-year survival rate of 45%. The highly differentiated epithelium portends not only slow growth but also relative resistance to adjuvant radiotherapy and chemotherapy.

Endometrioid Carcinoma

In August 1961, a conference of the Cancer Committee of FIGO was held in Stockholm for the purpose of standardizing a histological classification of the common epithelial ovarian tumors. Santesson (1968) presented 616 histologically reviewed primary ovarian cancers of which endometrioid tumors constituted 24.4%. For inclusion in this category, Santesson (1968) did not require evidence of origin from endometriosis but only that the tumors resemble endometrial adenocarcinoma or adenoacanthoma. Since that time, endometrioid carcinomas have been reported to constitute 15% to 20% of all ovarian cancers. A major problem in diagnosis has resulted from the

fact that 25% of endometrioid carcinomas are associated with a histologically similar carcinoma of the endometrium. In this instance, Scully (1970a) has suggested that if the endometrial carcinoma is less than 2 cm in diameter, is well differentiated, and only minimally invades the myometrium, the assumption of synchronous primary tumors in the ovary and endometrium can safely be made.

Grossly, endometrioid carcinomas may be cystic with a velvety inner surface and resemble the benign "chocolate" cyst with an intrinsic tumor mass. More commonly they are semicystic, but they may be entirely solid. About 30% are bilateral, a figure exceeded only by serous cystomas.

Microscopically, endometrioid carcinomas have a glandular pattern that closely resembles that of endometrial carcinoma (Fig 9–12). Areas of squamous metaplasia are common. A mixed papillary pattern is observed frequently, but the papillae are blunt and short in contrast to the fine-branching papillarity of serous cystadenocarcinomas. In the series reported from the Boston Hospital for Women by Kurman and Craig (1972), 13 of the 37 endometrioid carcinomas contained other secondary müllerian elements, and in 11% endometriosis was demonstrated in the same ovary.

The prognosis associated with endometrioid carcinoma is better than that of serous cystadenocarcinomas because of an increased percentage of localized and well-differentiated tumors in the former group. In the Boston Hospital for Women series, 47% of patients had stage I tumors; 28%, stage II; and 26%, stage III and stage IV. The overall 5- and 10-year survival rates were 46%

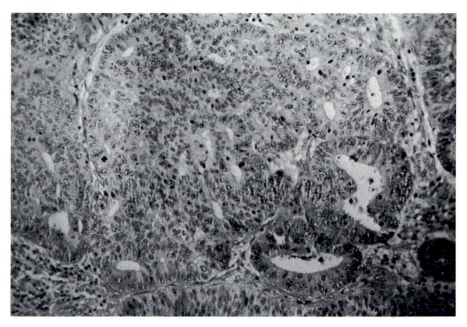

FIG 9–12.
Endometrioid carcinoma of the ovary indistinguishable from a primary carcinoma of the endometrium. The tumor was unilateral, and the uterine cavity was uninvolved.

and 37%, respectively. For stage I tumors the 5- and 10-year survival rates were 69% and 63%, and the corresponding figures for stage II disease were 50% and 30%. Kurman and Craig (1972) found that the influence of histological grade was significant.

The treatment of endometrioid carcinoma of the ovary is the same as for the other malignant cystomas. Preservation of childbearing capacity is less feasible in light of the 30% bilaterality, but these tumors tend to be commoner in older women. The mean age in the Boston Hospital for Women series was 57 years, with a range of 36 to 86 years.

Clear Cell Carcinoma

Clear cell carcinoma of the ovary has been proposed to arise from müllerian differentiation of the germinal epithelium. Kurman and Craig (1972) at the Boston Hospital for Women have added credence to this thesis by demonstrating endometrioid, serous, and mucinous elements in 5 of their 12 cases of clear cell carcinoma. As a corollary, these authors found clear cell elements within seven endometrioid carcinomas, eight serous carcinomas, and one undifferentiated carcinoma.

On gross examination, clear cell carcinomas vary from a predominantly cystic to a predominantly solid architecture. The cystic spaces usually are filled with chocolate-like fluid and contain pale brown polypoid masses. Clear cell carcinomas are bilateral in less than 10% of cases. Microscopically, they are made up of masses of large polyhedral epithelial cells, which contain a small nucleus and abundant clear cytoplasm (Fig 9–13,A). Cystic spaces or tubules are lined by clear cells and by "hobnail" cells (Fig 9–13,B).

Clear cell carcinomas constitute approximately 5% of the malignant ovarian tumors. Although a number of clinical reports have been published, the largest representative series consists of 95 cases reported from the Emil Novak Ovarian Tumor Registry (OTR) by Rogers et al. (1972). The ages ranged from 10 to 79 years, but 78% of patients were between the ages of 40 and 70 years. In 63% the tumor was confined to one ovary, and 68.2% of patients fell into the stage I category. In 19% of cases the tumor had spread to the pelvic peritoneum (stage II), and in 11.6% the upper abdomen was involved (stage III). The tumor had disseminated beyond the abdominal cavity in only one instance (stage IV). Whereas a 5-year survival rate of 63% was obtained with

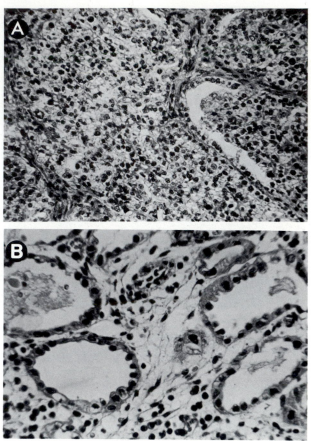

FIG 9–13.
A, clear cell carcinoma. Solid masses of large clear cells are interspersed with tubular structures. **B,** hobnail cells, a characteristic of clear cell tumors throughout the female genital tract.

stage I tumors, only 17% of patients with stage II and none of the patients with stage III and stage IV disease survived. These figures are consistent with smaller reported series and indicate that (1) a greater number of clear cell carcinomas are confined to the ovaries at the time of diagnosis than with the other malignant cystomas; (2) the 5-year survival rate for stage I clear cell carcinomas is similar to that of other malignant cystomas; and (3) once the tumor has disseminated beyond the ovary, the survival rates are lower than with the other malignant cystomas. The initial surgical procedure should be the same for clear cell carcinomas as for the other epithelial tumors, but aggressive postoperative adjuvant therapy must be instituted in any case of extraovarian spread.

Brenner Tumor

The Brenner tumor consists of multiple nests of benign transitional-type epithelium (urothelium) distributed throughout a dense fibrous stroma (Fig 9–14). Brenner tumors are relatively uncommon, accounting for no more than 0.5% of ovarian tumors. Although several histogenetic theories have been advanced, an origin from germinal epithelium has now been generally accepted. Arey (1961) demonstrated by three-dimensional reconstructions that the epithelial component consists of intricately branching cords, which radiate from a common stalk, which, in turn, arises from an epithelial plaque at the ovarian surface. Even a müllerian connection is retained since 20% of Brenner tumors coexist with mucinous cystadenomas.

The finding of a Brenner tumor is usually incidental to hysterectomy for other indications in premenopausal women in their late 30s and 40s. As a consequence of their slow growth rate, larger and symptomatic Brenner tumors tend to be discovered after the menopause. Symptoms are related to the size of the tumor and are those characteristic of any benign ovarian neoplasm. Several cases of Meigs' syndrome have been reported.

Although usually small (3 to 8 cm in diame-

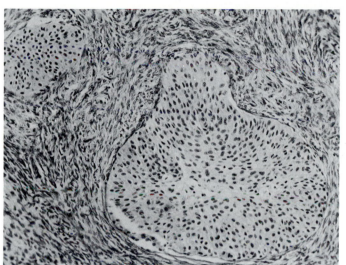

FIG 9–14.
Brenner tumor. Nests of epithelial cells resembling urothelium surrounded by a fibromatous connective tissue matrix.

ter), Brenner tumors may reach large proportions. They are bilateral in only 8% of cases. On gross examination, these tumors are smooth, slightly lobulated, and quite firm, though cystic areas may be palpated.

More than 35 malignant Brenner tumors have been reported, and a potentially malignant or proliferating group has been identified. In contrast to the usual benign form, the proliferating tumors tend to be cystic. Because of more rapid growth, they are larger and more frequently symptomatic. The microscopic picture is one of multiple cystic spaces lined by well-differentiated but proliferating urothelium which forms papillary projections into the cyst cavities. Stromal invasion is absent, and metastases have not been observed. Miles and Norris (1972) compare the proliferating Brenner tumor with a low-grade papillary transitional cell carcinoma of the bladder.

Malignant Brenner tumors are characterized by foci of papillary transitional cell carcinoma intermixed with benign and proliferating urothelium. Marked cellular pleomorphism and stromal invasion are obvious. Metastatic disease and death have been reported.

In light of the rarity of malignant change, particularly in younger women, and the infrequency of bilaterality, unilateral oophorectomy is adequate treatment in the younger age group. Perimenopausal and postmenopausal women, however, should undergo hysterectomy and bilateral salpingo-oophorectomy. The relative frequency of mucinous cystadenomas in the opposite ovary as well as the possibility of a metachronous Brenner tumor militates against ovarian conservation without good cause.

Gonadal Stromal Tumors

The designation gonadal stromal tumor is applied to all tumors that arise from the ovarian stroma without regard to the embryonic origin of specific precursor cells. Although the term *mesenchymal tumors* has been proposed, the WHO designation *sex cord-stromal tumors* maintains the connotation of embryonic precursors while avoiding the controversial assumption that the sex cords are derived from the mesenchyme.

Most gonadal stromal tumors contain recognizable ovarian cell types and are termed *granulosa-theca cell tumors*. A smaller proportion consists of testicular cell types and these are called *Sertoli-Leydig cell tumors*. It must be emphasized that testicular-type cells in the ovary are sex chromatin positive. A very small percentage of tumors, classified as lipid cell tumors, consist of several clinically and histologically similar subtypes. Ten percent of gonadal stromal tumors cannot be classified because of intermixtures of poorly differentiated cellular elements.

For the most part, granulosa-theca cell tumors secrete estrogens, whereas Sertoli-Leydig cell and lipid cell tumors produce androgens. At least 15% of gonadal stromal tumors are said to be hormonally inert, but this estimate is based on clinical interpretations rather than on laboratory evidence. The type of hormonal production is also variable. A small percentage of granulosa-theca cell tumors cause virilization, whereas a few Sertoli-Leydig cell tumors secrete estrogen. In some instances both estrogen and androgen are produced by the same tumor. These variations probably relate not only to the functional tissue type but also to the extraglandular conversion of an estrogen and androgen precursor, namely, androstenedione.

Granulosa-Theca Cell Tumors

Granulosa-theca cell tumors are composed of the cellular constituents of the graafian follicle wall in varying proportion. Approximately 20% are predominantly granulosa cell tumors, 20% are mixed granulosa-theca cell tumors, and 60% are relatively pure thecomas. Granulosa-theca cell tumors constitute 4% to 9% of all ovarian tumors, and about 3% of ovarian cancers are malignant granulosa cell tumors.

These tumors have been observed at all ages from birth to 90 years. Fifty percent are found in postmenopausal women, whereas fewer than 5% are discovered before puberty. In most series the median age is early in the sixth decade. The initial symptoms are usually related to the endocrine activity of the tumor and vary with the amount of hormonal secretion as well as with the age of the patient. Perhaps the most dramatic effect is the development of precocious pseudopuberty in the prepubertal child. During the reproductive years, the clinical picture is less striking, but irregular menses and even amenorrhea are common. In the postmenopausal era the characteristic symptoms are a resumption of uterine bleeding and occasional enlargement of the breasts. Virilization has been described in 1% to 3% of patients with granulosa cell tumors. As the tumor becomes progressively larger, symptoms of pelvic pressure and pain supervene. An unusual characteristic is the propensity of granulosa cell tumors to rupture spontaneously and result in intraperitoneal hemorrhage. As many as 15% of women with this tumor during their reproductive years present with the picture of an acute abdominal catastrophe, which may mimic that of a ruptured ectopic pregnancy.

Granulosa-theca cell tumors are nearly always unilateral, and most series report bilaterality in only 2% to 6%. Grossly, they are mobile, oval, and encapsulated, with a smooth, lobulated surface and a soft, solid, or semicystic consistency. On section, 90% have cystic cavities and more than one half of these contain old blood.

Microscopic examination may reveal a variable architectural structure, but the granulosa cells have a characteristic and monotonously uniform appearance. They are rounded or polygonal with a slightly granular eosinophilic cytoplasm and poorly defined cytoplasmic borders. Nuclei are small and round and are often folded, resulting in the longitudinal groove characteristic of ovarian stromal cells. Interspersed theca cells are spindle shaped with ovoid nuclei and contain cytoplasmic lipid droplets or are occasionally luteinized. Multiple architectural patterns of granulosa cell tumors have been described and have been termed folliculoid, adenomatoid, cylindroid, sarcomatoid, and trabeculoid (Fig 9–15). These patterns have borne no relationship to malignant behavior and ultimate prognosis, and, as pointed out by Norris and Taylor (1968), have led to imprecision in the definition of a distinct clinicopathological entity. The commonest pattern, which has been called folliculoid or microfolliculoid, is characterized by the arrangement of granulosa cells in a rosette fashion with the nuclei at right angles to a central area of pink inspissated material. These structures are termed *Call-Exner bodies* and are pathognomonic of granulosa cell tumors (see Fig 9–15).

Since histological appearance has not been predictive of malignant behavior, estimates of malignant potential have been based on the observed incidence of metastases or mortality from the disease. These observations have varied markedly as exemplified by the survival rates from five recent series listed in Table 9–4. In the OTR series reported by Novak et al. (1971), 25% of tumors were malignant by virtue of primary metastases or recurrence. The corresponding figure reported by Fox et al. (1975) in Manchester, England was

TABLE 9–4.

Granulosa-Theca Cell Tumor Survival Rates*

Series	No. of Patients	Survival Rates (%)	
		5 Yr	10 Yr
Norris and Taylor (1968)†	68	97	93
Novak et al. (1971)	86	64	—
Fox et al. (1975)†	74	68	59
Stenwig et al. (1979)	118	95	88
Björkholm and Silfverswärd (1981)	197	96	89

*Excluding unrelated deaths.
†Actuarial survival rates.

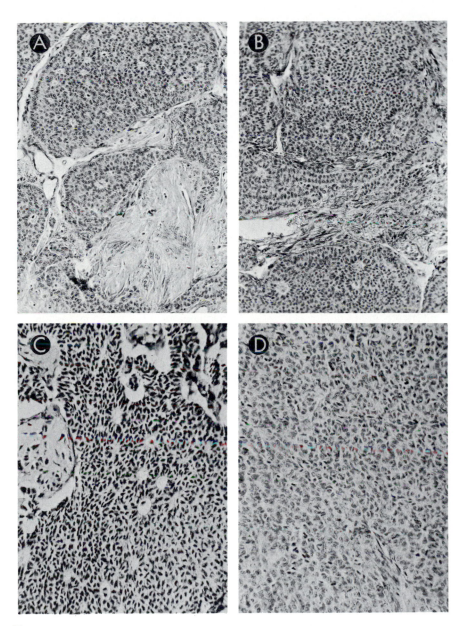

FIG 9–15.

A, granulosa-theca cell tumor showing folliculoid pattern of granulosa cells and collagenous hyaliniza- tion of the thecal stroma. **B,** granulosa-theca cell tu- mor showing a diffuse pattern *(above),* cylindroid pattern *(center)* and folliculoid pattern *(below).* (**A** and **B** from Hertig AT, Gore H: Tumors of the female sex organs: part 3. Tumors of the ovary and fallopian tube, section 9, fasc 33, *Atlas of Tumor Pathology.* Washington, DC, Armed Forces Instutite of Pathology, 1961. Reproduced by permission.) **C,** granulosa- theca cell tumor showing typical Call-Exner bodies in a folliculoid pattern. **D,** poorly differentiated granu- losa-theca cell tumor showing pleomorphism and numerous mitoses in upper right. This tumor was ma- lignant, and death occurred 2 years after surgical excision.

30%, whereas only 10% of patients with granulosa-theca cell tumors reported by Norris and Taylor (1968) from the Armed Forces Institute of Pathology (AFIP) were demonstrably malignant. Norris and Taylor (1968) proposed that the marked variability in reported rates of malignancy and mortality stemmed from (1) the inadvertent inclusion of malignant tumors not meeting the criteria for granulosa cell tumors (Fig 9–15,D), (2) the inclusion in some series of the rarely malignant thecomas, (3) the use of crude mortality rates in a population of aging women prone to die of other causes, and (4) failure in some series to report long-term follow-up of a disease in which most tumor-related deaths occur after 5 years. In an attempt to explain the relatively low 5-year survival rate among the OTR patients, Novak et al. (1971) suggested that either more anaplastic or bizarre cases were registered with the OTR, or undifferentiated carcinomas and sarcomas were inadvertently included.

The diagnosis of granulosa-theca cell tumors is often made at laparotomy indicated by reason of a palpable mass or an acute complication. When signs and symptoms of inappropriate estrogen secretion are unaccompanied by a palpable adnexal mass, the diagnosis may be obscure. In the postmenopause, endometrial hyperplasia is an associated finding in 25% to 50% of patients, and endometrial carcinoma has been described in 3% to 21%. Endometrial hyperplasia in the presence of other estrogen effects such as breast tenderness and vaginal cornification in a postmenopausal woman strongly suggests a granulosa-theca tumor, provided an exogenous source of estrogen has been excluded.

The treatment of granulosa-theca cell tumors usually consists of a hysterectomy and bilateral salpingo-oophorectomy. In light of the relative benignity of these tumors—particularly in those less than 40 years of age—and the infrequency of bilaterality, excision of the tumor and involved ovary is sufficient treatment for young women. In the event of disseminated or recurrent disease, metastases should be excised when possible. Since granulosa-theca cell tumors have been relatively radioresponsive, pelvic or abdominal irradiation may have a beneficial effect. Complete clinical remission has been recently reported in two patients with metastatic granulosa cell tumors treated with cisplatin and doxorubicin (Jacobs et al., 1982). This combination regimen shows promise and deserves further evaluation.

Thecoma.—Although included in the granulosa-theca cell group, thecomas are set apart by possible differences in histogenesis and their almost invariable benignity. The prevalence of thecomas varies widely, depending on histologic criteria. A granulosa-theca cell tumor composed predominantly of theca cells may be considered a thecoma by some, whereas others reserve that diagnosis for tumors composed purely of theca cells. Even in the latter instance, a granulosa cell component is usually found if sufficient histologic sections are examined. At the other end of the spectrum, thecomas may be indistinguishable from fibromas, and many pathologists include thecomas and fibromas in a single category.

Thecomas have been reported in females from 1 to 90 years of age, but most are found in postmenopausal women. The presenting symptoms, hormonal activity, and the association with endometrial carcinoma are similar to those of the granulosa-theca cell group as a whole. Thecomas have been as frequently associated with Meigs' syndrome as have fibromas. Thecomas have been rarely documented to be malignant. In contrast to the granulosa-theca cell tumors, they are more likely to be solid than cystic, and internal hemorrhage is infrequent. The cut surface is firm and white, but yellow areas representing luteinization are visible. Microscopically, the tumor is composed of plump, oval or spindle-shaped cells arranged in a whorled or trabecular pattern. Although thecomas resemble fibromas, they may be distinguished by areas of luteinized granulosa or theca cells.

Fibromas

The incidence of fibromas varies considerably, depending on the care with which ovaries are studied histologically and whether microscopic fibromas are included. The relative frequency reported in the literature varies from 1.5% to 5.0%. Fibromas are most commonly seen during the late childbearing period, the median age being 48 years.

They are bilateral in 10% of cases, and multiple tumors are occasionally discovered within the same ovary. A fibroma is hard and homogeneous in consistency, but on occasion it may feel cystic because of marked edema. Although the cut surface is typically white with a whorled appearance, intrinsic hemorrhage may impart a multicolored appearance.

The symptoms associated with ovarian fibromas are related to their size and are identical to those produced by the other benign ovarian tumors. The weight of the tumor tends to elongate a pedicle, and torsion is a relatively frequent complication. Ovarian fibromas in conjunction with ascites and right hydrothorax constitute Meigs' syndrome. Although the etiology of the serous effusions has not been well explained, partial torsion and occlusion of venous drainage may result in a large, edematous, weeping tumor.

Simple excision is adequate therapy for an ovarian fibroma. If the patient is postmenopausal, the opposite ovary also should be removed to avoid a second fibroma. In this instance, hysterectomy is advisable but by no means mandatory.

Sertoli-Leydig Cell Tumors

The Sertoli-Leydig cell tumor is the commonest virilizing tumor of the ovary, although its prevalence is only 10% that of the granulosa-theca cell tumor. Sertoli-Leydig cell tumors are also known as arrhenoblastomas and androblastomas.

Sertoli-Leydig cell tumors are most frequently found during the childbearing era; 75% occur between the ages of 15 and 45 years, with a median age of 32 years. More than 95% of Sertoli-Leydig tumors are unilateral, and they vary from 0.5 to 10.0 cm in diameter. Both the external and cut surfaces resemble those of the granulosa cell tumors, but cystic and hemorrhagic areas are somewhat less common. The Sertoli cells are represented by cuboidal or columnar cells arranged in cordlike or tubular structures reminiscent of the sex cords or seminiferous tubules of the fetal testis. In its commonest form, the tumor consists of tubules within a stroma containing stromal cells and large polygonal cells (Fig 9–16). These polygonal cells strongly resemble testicular Leydig's cells and may contain crystals of Reinke. These intracytoplasmic bodies are characteristic of Leydig's cells and are visible as eosinophilic rodlike structures.

Although the histological appearance of 10% to 15% of Sertoli-Leydig cell tumors suggests malignancy, reports indicate that less than 5% manifest malignant behavior by metastases or recurrence (Norris and Chorlton, 1974; Ireland and Woodruff, 1976). The diagnosis of a Sertoli-Leydig cell tumor must be made with caution in patients with bilateral tumors or primary metastases unless the histological diagnosis is unequivocal.

Approximately 75% of Sertoli-Leydig cell tumors are associated with androgen production. The endocrinological effect usually begins as a gradual process of defeminization. Some women, however, continue to have ovulatory cycles despite marked virilism. Gradually the feminine sex characteristics regress, and excessive androgen production is manifested by a male habitus, marked hirsutism, acne, temporal balding, voice deepening, and clitoromegaly. Sertoli-Leydig cell tumors are accompanied by normal or only slightly elevated levels of 17-ketosteroids, since the primary hormone secreted is testosterone. When initially elevated, levels of plasma testosterone consistently return to normal following treatment of patients with Sertoli-Leydig cell tumors.

Since less than 5% of Sertoli-Leydig cell tu-

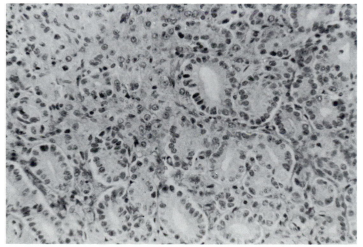

FIG 9–16.
Sertoli-Leydig cell tumor with simple tubular structures lined by columnar cells at the right and a stroma containing large polygonal cells with round central nuclei in the upper left.

mors are bilateral, unilateral oophorectomy appears to be adequate treatment for this tumor, which afflicts predominantly younger women. On the other hand, nearly 10% of tumors are either bilateral or malignant, and hysterectomy and bilateral salpingo-oophorectomy is optimal therapy for women in their 30s no longer desiring pregnancy. Insufficient experience has accumulated to comment on the efficacy of radiotherapy or chemotherapy in advanced or recurrent cases.

Gynandroblastomas

Gynandroblastomas are rare tumors that demonstrate a biphasic differentiation toward both ovarian and testicular structures and thus contain histological elements of both the granulosa cell and the Sertoli-Leydig cell tumor. The histological criteria for diagnosis of a gynandroblastoma must include aggregates of granulosa cells forming Call-Exner bodies and either well-defined tubules or Leydig's cells identifiable by Reinke crystals.

These rare tumors are usually found during the childbearing years, and a disruption of the normal menstrual pattern may precede the diagnosis by several years. Despite the presence of ovarian elements, virilism is the dominant effect of these tumors. In general, the gross appearance, biological behavior, and optimal therapeutic approach are identical to those of the Sertoli-Leydig cell tumors.

Gonadoblastomas

The gonadoblastoma is a rare neoplasm that contains both gonadal stromal and germ cell ele-

ments. The tumor is composed of discrete aggregates of primordial germ cells intermixed with, or surrounded by, immature Sertoli's cells and granulosa cells. The germ cells exhibit mitotic activity in 85% of tumors and overgrow the stromal elements in about 50%. In most instances, the germinomatous component is indistinguishable from the usual dysgerminoma. In nearly 20% of the cases reported by Scully (1970a), however, more malignant germ cell types, including the endodermal sinus tumor, were present. Calcification is present in 80% of tumors and is frequently visible on pelvic roentgenograms (Fig 9–17).

In Scully's (1970a) series of 74 cases, 22% of gonadoblastomas originated in a gonadal streak, 18% originated in a cryptorchid dysgenetic testis, and the remainder originated in gonads of indeterminate type. They were bilateral in one third of the cases. Eighty percent of patients were phenotypic female, and more than one half of these were virilized. Chromosomal analysis carried out in 30 patients revealed 46 XY karyotypes in 57%, 45 XX/46 XY mosaicism in 30%, and a 45 X karyotype in 1 patient.

At the very least, gonadoblastomas represent a germ cell malignancy in situ. Since they are frequently bilateral, treatment should include removal of all gonadal tissue.

Germ Cell Tumors

Dysgerminomas

Dysgerminomas make up less than 2% of primary ovarian cancers, but they are the commonest ovarian malignancy found in postpubertal

FIG 9–17.
Gonadoblastoma showing a central aggregate of germ cells with abundant clear cytoplasm and round, centrally placed nuclei. Granulosa cells are seen in the crescent-shaped area to the left. The Call-Exner bodies tend to contain more than the usual amount of central secretion, and the dark-staining psammoma bodies are intermixed.

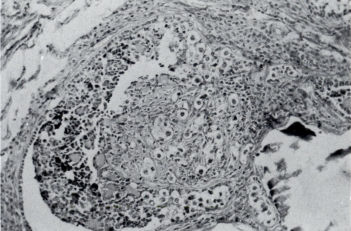

girls and young women. Although the ages range from 2 to 78 years, 85% of these tumors occur before age 30 years.

The dysgerminoma is morphologically identical to its homologue, the testicular seminoma, and both are believed to arise from the primordial germ cells of the indifferent stage of gonadogenesis.

Approximately 10% are bilateral. The tumor cells are uniformly large and polygonal with abundant clear cytoplasm and are morphologically identical to primordial germ cells. The nucleus tends to be centrally placed and contains clumped chromatin and one or two prominent nucleoli. Aggregates of tumor cells are arranged in an alveolar pattern separated by strands of connective tissue that are infiltrated by lymphocytes (Fig 9–18). Isolated syncytiotrophoblastic giant cells are occasionally seen and account for the excretion of hCG in the absence of choriocarcinomatous elements.

The most important microscopic determinant of survival is the presence of other germ cell elements. In Asadourian and Taylor's (1969) study, the 5-year survival rate of 98 patients with pure dysgerminomas was 90%, whereas all 12 patients with admixtures of other cell types were dead within 2 years. Nine of the 30 mixed germ cell tumors analyzed by Kurman and Norris (1976c) were predominantly dysgerminomas.

The authors concluded from their entire series that if more than one third of a stage I neoplasm was composed of endodermal sinus tumor, choriocarcinoma, or grade 3 immature teratoma, the prognosis was poor.

By the time of diagnosis, the tumor has extended beyond the ovaries in 15% to 30% of cases. Metastases may occur by local tumor implantation similar to epithelial tumors, but dysgerminomas also have a propensity for lymphatic dissemination. Pelvic and aortic nodes have been the only sites of metastatic disease in nearly 50% of patients with extraovarian spread.

Attention has been focused on the preservation of childbearing capacity and the corresponding risk of conservative treatment. Malkasian and Symmonds in 1964 reported an 80% 5-year survival rate among 21 patients with unilateral encapsulated dysgerminomas treated by unilateral salpingo-oophorectomy alone. The tumor recurred in 11 patients (52%), but 7 of these were salvaged by radiation therapy. The results reported by Asadourian and Taylor in 1969 are even more encouraging. Unilateral oophorectomy was the primary treatment in 46 of 71 patients with dysgerminomas confined to one ovary. The tumor recurred in 10 of these (22%) but was successfully controlled in 6, resulting in a 5-year survival rate of 91%. Three recurrences were observed among 25 patients who underwent bilateral oophorec-

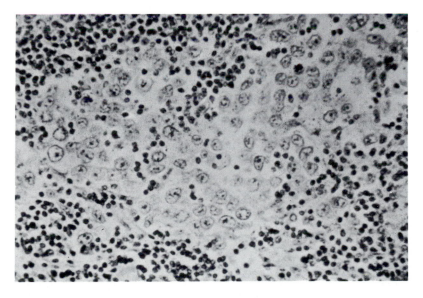

FIG 9–18.
Dysgerminoma showing groups of large, round cells with clear cytoplasm and nuclei containing several nucleoli. Marked lymphocytic infiltration is present.

tomy with and without irradiation (12%), but since these 3 patients died, the survival rate was 88% for this group. Gordon et al. (1981) have also reported 5-year survival in 67 of 72 patients (94%) with dysgerminoma confined to one ovary and treated by unilateral adnexectomy. The marked radiosensitivity of dysgerminomas was demonstrated by Afridi et al. (1976), who successfully treated metastatic tumor even at distant sites in six of seven patients. Radiation doses of only 2,000 to 3,000 rad were required. Krepart et al. (1978) have also reported 3-year survival in 10 of 13 patients (77%) with dysgerminoma and aortic nodal metastases treated with radiation therapy.

Unilateral salpingo-oophorectomy is adequate therapy for most unilateral dysgerminomas, but a number of recurrences must be anticipated. In the young nullipara, this procedure should be performed in conjunction with intraperitoneal saline irrigation for cytological study, wedge biopsy of the contralateral ovary, distal omental biopsy, and pelvic and aortic nodal sampling. Any palpable aortic or pelvic lymph nodes should be removed. The final decision to elect conservative therapy must await thorough histological examination of the tissue and discussions with the patient and her family. An intensive program of surveillance must be designed to cover the first 2 years during which most dysgerminomas recur. In all cases, β-hCG and α-fetoprotein determinations should be carried out immediately after operation, if not before. Not only may the presence of endodermal sinus tumor or choriocarcinomatous elements be revealed, but a useful serum marker may be provided for assessment of therapeutic effect and detection of early recurrence.

When dysgerminoma metastasizes beyond the ovary, standard therapy has been bilateral salpingo-oophorectomy and hysterectomy followed by pelvic and abdominal irradiation. Dysgerminoma is exquisitely radiosensitive, and modest doses of radiation are therefore effective in eradicating even bulky tumor. However, it is becoming increasingly apparent that dysgerminoma, like seminoma, is also very responsive to chemotherapy. Gershenson et al. (1986) reported complete remission in two patients with bulky metastatic dysgerminoma with etoposide, bleomycin, and cisplatin. Patients with advanced or recurrent disease may be able to preserve fertility without compromising cure. In patients with advanced or recurrent dysgerminoma, conservative surgery consisting of unilateral oophorectomy followed by combination chemotherapy may be accepted as an alternative to radiotherapy (Thomas et al., 1987). The majority of women who receive combination chemotherapy for malignant ovarian germ cell tumors can anticipate maintaining normal menstrual and reproductive function (Gershenson, 1988).

Immature (Malignant) Teratomas

The immature teratoma is composed of both embryonal and adult tissues derived from all three germ layers. The largest series of "pure" immature teratomas has been reported from the AFIP by Norris and associates (1976). The ages ranged from 14 months to 40 years, with a median of 19 years. Eighty percent of patients had a palpable abdominal or pelvic mass.

The tumors were all unilateral except one that had metastasized to the opposite ovary. Sixty percent were confined to one ovary (stage I), 15.5% involved other pelvic structures (stage II), and 15.5% involved extrapelvic abdominal structures (stage III). The mode of spread is by implantation on serosal surfaces, and aortic nodal involvement at the level of the renal vessels has been noted. Hematogenous metastases are rare.

The histological picture is variable, but mesodermal elements often predominate. The degree of malignancy is closely correlated with the proportion of immature tissue. Robboy and Scully (1970) and the AFIP workers (Norris et al., 1976) have adopted similar grading systems that are predictive of malignant behavior and eventual outcome. Grade 0 tumors are constituted of mature tissue only, whereas grades 1 through 3 are characterized by an increasing proportion of poorly differentiated embryonal tissue. Mitotic activity increases with the tumor grade.

Both the stage of the disease and the tumor grade are important and independent determinants of prognosis. The influence of these factors on survival in the AFIP series is demonstrated in Table 9–5.

The histological grade of metastases may differ from that of the primary tumor; it also bears a relationship to prognosis. Robboy and Scully (1970) have reported 12 patients with immature teratomas and peritoneal implants composed entirely or predominantly of mature glial tissue. None of these patients died, although persistent tumor was presumed or palpated in seven asymptomatic patients followed for 5 to 38 years after primary operation.

Piver et al. (1976) described the transition of

TABLE 9–5.

Influence of Stage and Grade on Actuarial Survival*

Grade	Stage I		Stage II		Stage III		Total % Survival
	No. of Patients	% Survival	No. of Patients	% Survival	No. of Patients	% Survival	
1	14	100	4	50	4	50	82
2	20	70	2	50	2	0	62
3	6	33	2	0	2	50	30
TOTAL	40	74	8	38	8	38	64

*From Norris HJ, Zirkin HJ, Benson WL: Immature (malignant) teratoma of the ovary: A clinical and pathologic study of 58 cases. *Cancer* 1976; 37:2359. Used by permission.

immature teratomatous metastases to mature teratomas in two patients during chemotherapy (cyclophosphamide and vincristine). These authors suggest that the drugs either selectively destroyed the immature elements, induced maturation, or were unrelated to the maturation phenomenon.

For stage I immature teratomas, surgical treatment consists only of unilateral salpingo-oophorectomy. Combination chemotherapy consisting of vincristine, dactinomycin (actinomycin D), and cyclophosphamide (VAC) has been effective in some cases and should be administered for stage I, grade 2 and 3 lesions. Rupture of the tumor capsule before or during operation has carried an 80% risk of tumor recurrence, and adjuvant chemotherapy is advisable under this circumstance. Patients with stage I, grade 1 tumors require close observation during the first 12 to 18 months. Patients with stage II or III disease or recurrence are best managed by excision of tumor masses when feasible, followed by combination chemotherapy. Two-year disease-free survival was achieved in 6 of 11 patients (55%) with stage III immature teratoma treated with combination chemotherapy (Curry et al., 1978). In the absence of tumor involvement, extirpation of the uterus and contralateral adnexa is needless and should be avoided. Normal full-term pregnancy has been reported following successful combination chemotherapy for ovarian immature teratoma (Jahaveri et al., 1983). Radiation therapy has been ineffective in the management of this disease.

Mature (Benign) Teratomas

The benign cystic teratoma, which is often called a *dermoid cyst* because of a preponderance of epidermal elements, is the second or third commonest ovarian neoplasm. Although cystic teratomas have been found in neonates and octogenarians, they occur predominantly during the repro-

ductive years. The benign cystic teratoma is the most commonly encountered ovarian neoplasm during adolescence and during pregnancy.

The theory of a parthenogenetic origin has been in and out of favor for more than 100 years, but the contribution of Linder and associates (1975) appears to have settled the question once and for all. The only possible explanation for the findings of Linder et al. (1975) is that cystic teratomas arise by parthenogenesis from secondary oocytes.

Benign cystic teratomas have varied widely in size and only 12% are bilateral. The cyst wall tends to be thick and pearly gray, but the color varies, depending on the thickness of the capsule and the hue of the contents. The cystic cavity is usually unilocular and contains a thick, greasy fluid made up of sebum and desquamated cells. Tangled masses of hair are often present, and teeth have been reported in 10% to 30% of tumors. When the contents of a cyst have been emptied, a discrete nodule that projects into the cavity can be found attached to the cyst wall. This structure is known either as *Rokitansky's protuberance* or as the *dermoid process*.

Microscopically, a wide variety of tissues has been found. The cyst wall is lined by stratified squamous epithelium with irregular clusters of underlying dermal elements (Fig 9–19). Although dermal structures are the commonest component of Rokitansky's protuberance, all three germ layers are often represented.

Complications of dermoid cysts include torsion, rupture, and malignant transformation. Torsion is the most frequent of these and has been discussed previously (see the discussion of the diagnosis).

Rupture of benign cystic teratomas is a rare phenomenon. When released into the peritoneal cavity, the cystic contents produce a chemical

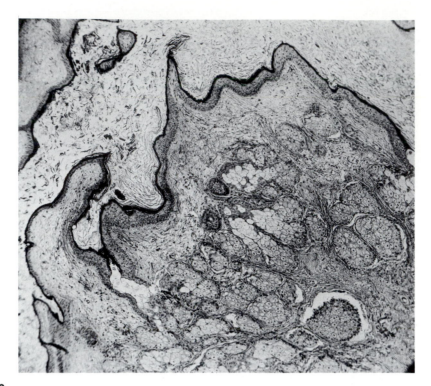

FIG 9–19.
Lining of cystic teratoma, showing desquamation of keratin, normal skin, and sebaceous glands. (From Hertig AT, Gore H: Tumors of the female sex organs: part 3. Tumors of the ovary and fallopian tube, sec- tion 9, fasc 33, *Atlas of Tumor Pathology.* Washington, DC, Armed Forces Institute of Pathology, 1961. Repro- duced by permission.)

peritonitis; although sudden widespread perito- neal contamination is a catastrophic event, the clinical picture varies with the degree and rate of spillage. Consequently, slow leakage through a small defect in the cyst wall often causes chronic abdominal pain, which may be intermittent and diagnostically obscure.

The percentage of benign cystic teratomas containing a malignant tissue component has been generally accepted as 2%. As might be ex- pected, squamous cell carcinomas constitute the majority of these, and transitions from dysplasia and carcinoma in situ have been described. In re- viewing 272 reported cases, Climie and Heath (1968) found that 75% were squamous cell carci- nomas, 6% adenocarcinomas, 6% carcinoid tu- mors, 1.5% malignant melanomas, and 7% sarco- mas. Squamous cell carcinomas usually arise from the skin covering Rokitansky's protuberance. The prognosis is relatively good for all of these if the cyst wall is intact and no gross extraovarian dis- semination has occurred. Climie and Heath

(1968) reported only 2 deaths among 13 patients in whom the tumors met these criteria.

The treatment of benign cystic teratomas is surgical extirpation. Since a clear tissue plane ex- ists between the cyst wall and normal ovary, ova- rian conservation is readily accomplished. Because of the possibility of bilateral tumors, the con- tralateral ovary should be carefully scrutinized. If childbearing function is not a consideration, most gynecologists as well as their patients prefer hys- terectomy and either unilateral or bilateral sal- pingo-oophorectomy, depending on the proxim- ity of anticipated menopause.

Struma Ovarii.—On microscopic examina- tion, 5% to 10% of benign cystic teratomas con- tain clusters of typical thyroid acini. Occasionally, the thyroid tissue occupies all or most of the tu- mor, which is then designated a struma ovarii. The external surface is smooth and rounded, and the cut surface has the glistening amber appear- ance of thyroid tissue. Microscopically, the tissue resembles that of the normal thyroid gland, with rounded follicles that are lined by cuboidal epithelium.

Six percent of patients with struma ovarii are thyrotoxic, but only about one half of these have a disappearance of symptoms after excision of the neoplasm. Papillary or follicular thyroid carcinoma has developed in 5% of strumas, but only 17 of 45 reported cases have been associated with metastases.

Endodermal Sinus Tumor

Among the malignant neoplasms of the ovary occurring before the age of 20 years, the endodermal sinus tumor ranks second in frequency to the dysgerminoma and is equally prevalent before the age of 15 years (Norris and Jenson, 1972). Furthermore, an associated fatality rate of 90% had placed the endodermal sinus tumor first as a cause of death from ovarian cancer in childhood and adolescence.

The largest series published is that of the AFIP (Kurman and Norris, 1976b). The ages of the 71 patients ranged from 14 months to 45 years, with a median of 19 years. The commonest presenting symptoms were abdominal pain in 77%, an abdominal mass in 27%, and fever in 24%. The virulence of this tumor was manifested by a brief interval from onset of symptoms to diagnosis, less than 2 weeks in two thirds of the patients. An acute onset of symptoms resulted from torsion or intraperitoneal rupture in seven patients.

The size of endodermal sinus tumors ranges from 6 to 30 cm in diameter, but the usual size is between 10 and 20 cm. These tumors are consistently unilateral unless gross metastases are apparent. Microscopically, the classic pattern has been termed *reticular* and consists of a network of sinusoidal spaces lined by cuboidal cells with scanty cytoplasm (Fig 9–20). Schiller-Duval bodies, which consist of a mantle of yolk sac endoderm surrounding a capillary, are prominent. Although Schiller-Duval bodies are diagnostic, they were present in only 75% of the AFIP tumors. Kurman and Norris (1976b) point out the ubiquity of intracellular and intercellular hyaline droplets, which were present in 100%. Using an immunoperoxidase reaction, the authors showed that α-fetoprotein was present in all 15 tumors in which the histochemical analysis was carried out and appeared to be concentrated in the hyaline droplets.

In the manner of most malignant ovarian neoplasms, endodermal sinus tumors disseminate by implantation on peritoneal surfaces. Lymph node metastases are also common in autopsy series.

Only 5 of the 71 patients (13%) in the AFIP series survived, and the survival rate was little better when the tumor was confined to the ovary (16%). As noted by others, all deaths occurred during the 30-month interval from diagnosis.

The surgical treatment of endodermal sinus tumors is unilateral salpingo-oophorectomy. No benefit is derived from hysterectomy and bilateral salpingo-oophorectomy unless this procedure is an integral part of a planned operation prior to chemotherapy. Irradiation has been totally ineffective both as a surgical adjuvant with localized tumors and as palliation for advanced or recurrent

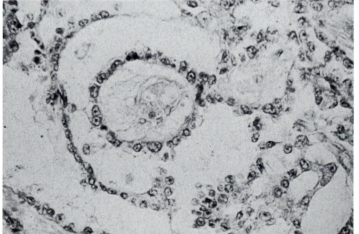

FIG 9–20.
Endodermal sinus tumor. Reticular pattern with a Schiller-Duval body in the center.

disease. One of the more gratifying accomplishments of chemotherapy has been the combined effect of VAC on endodermal sinus tumors. Three of the four stage I patients in the AFIP series who received this drug combination survived. Similarly, Smith and Rutledge (1975) at the M.D. Anderson Hospital and Tumor Institute have reported a disease-free survival rate of 100% among seven stage I patients for periods of 4 to 47 months. More remarkably, 8 of 13 patients with disseminated tumor were free of disease at the time of their report. Subsequent studies by Cangir et al. (1978), Creasman et al. (1979), and Gershenson et al. (1983) have confirmed the dramatic effectiveness of combination chemotherapy with endodermal sinus tumors. Newer combination regimens such as vinblastine, bleomycin, and cisplatin may also prove to be superior to VAC (Gershenson et al., 1986). Clearly, all patients with endodermal sinus tumor should receive adjuvant chemotherapy, although the optimal duration of therapy is not yet defined. The presence of measurable serum levels of α-fetoprotein uniformly associated with yolk sac tumors provides a sensitive marker for assessment of therapeutic results and detection of early recurrence (Romero and Schwartz, 1981).

Choriocarcinoma

The choriocarcinoma is an extremely rare, but highly malignant, tumor that may be primary in the ovary. Almost all primary choriocarcinomas are a component of mixed germ cell tumors. Six of the 30 mixed germ cell tumors reported by Kurman and Norris (1976c) contained choriocarcinomatous elements, and in two this tissue predominated. Although choriocarcinomas rarely obliterate the other germ cell components, the hemorrhagic tendency of choriocarcinomas may obscure their identity.

Ovarian choriocarcinomas are always unilateral. The tumor is extremely friable, consisting of spongy tissue infiltrated by blood. The microscopic appearance is similar to that of the primary uterine choriocarcinoma. There are masses of syncytiotrophoblastic and cytotrophoblastic cells admixed in a plexiform pattern. The opposite ovary is frequently enlarged by theca-lutein cysts or shows marked stromal luteinization as a result of the hCG secretion.

Primary choriocarcinoma usually is a tumor of childhood and early adolescence. The symptoms are those of a rapidly enlarging tumor mass and are often aggravated by ascites. Rupture of the tumor with intraperitoneal hemorrhage is a common complication and represents an acute surgical emergency. The high gonadotropin level stimulates the ovarian stroma and induces precocious puberty in children. Similarly, irregular uterine bleeding and breast enlargement are common symptoms in the postpubertal woman.

Ovarian choriocarcinomas were uniformly fatal until the advent of adjuvant chemotherapy. However, patients with ovarian choriocarcinoma can now achieve complete remission with intensive combination chemotherapy.

Embryonal Carcinoma

Embryonal carcinoma is a rare tumor that was first described in 1976 by Kurman and Norris (1976a). As extraembryonic tumors, they are homologous to the testicular embryonal carcinomas but have previously been classified as endodermal sinus tumors or choriocarcinomas, to which they are closely related. The ages of the 15 patients reported by Kurman and Norris ranged from 4 to 28 years, with a median of 14 years. Although the symptoms were similar to those associated with endodermal sinus tumors, abnormal hormonal manifestations were noted in 60% of patients. These consisted of precocious puberty and irregular bleeding or amenorrhea in the postpubertal patients. Pregnancy test results were positive in all nine patients in whom they were performed.

The tumors were unilateral and ranged from 10 to 25 cm in diameter. Syncytiotrophoblastic giant cells, identified by the immunoperoxidase reaction for hCG, were scattered at the periphery or throughout the stroma. Hyaline droplets characteristic of endodermal sinus tumors were found in 12 of the 15 tumors, and α-fetoprotein was demonstrated in these and in the mononuclear embryonal cells by the immunoperoxidase reaction.

The actuarial 5-year survival rate was 39% for the entire group and 50% for those with localized tumors. Treatment should consist of unilateral salpingo-oophorectomy and adjuvant chemotherapy. Taylor et al. (1985) reported complete remission in three patients with metastatic embryonal carcinoma treated with vinblastine, bleomycin, and cisplatin. Human chorionic gonadotropin and α-fetoprotein may serve as sensitive tumor markers to evaluate response to chemotherapy and allow early detection of recurrence.

Krukenberg's Tumor

The term Krukenberg's tumor should be reserved for those metastatic ovarian tumors with the characteristic histological picture of mucin-laden, signet-ring cells infiltrating a hyperplastic ovarian stroma of spindle-shaped cells. Krukenberg in his original description in 1896 called this tumor a "fibrosarcoma mucocellulare carcinomatodes" and believed it to be a primary ovarian neoplasm. Subsequent studies revealed that it was metastatic, usually from carcinoma of the stomach (Holtz and Hart, 1982). Although colon, breast, and pancreatic carcinomas have produced the same histologic picture, most ovarian metastases from these sites do not.

These tumors are usually bilateral and of moderate size, and, curiously, the normal shape of the ovary is retained. The cut surface typically exhibits gelatinous necrosis and mucin-filled cystic cavities of variable size.

Symptoms of the primary tumor are often absent or unrecognized, and the typical symptoms of a large pelvic mass supervene. With increasing size, ascites and peritoneal implants are often found. Since the ovarian tumor tends to grow more rapidly than the primary tumor, the surgeon may be confronted with an anatomical picture indistinguishable from primary ovarian carcinoma. Rapid histologic section may provide an intraoperative diagnosis and permit a more thorough abdominal exploration if the primary tumor had been overlooked initially. Since many patients have survived for several years after diagnosis, the ovaries as well as the uterus should be removed.

Carcinoma of the Ovary

Epidemiology

Carcinoma of the ovary is the fourth leading cause of cancer deaths among American women, following cancer of the breast, colon, and lung. Approximately 14,000 new cases are diagnosed each year, from which, as mentioned earlier, 11,000 deaths occur annually. According to current estimates, 1 of every 100 women in the United States is destined to die from this disease. Although the age-adjusted mortality rate from ovarian cancer more than doubled between 1930 and 1955, the incidence of the disease did not change significantly during the 22 years between the Second National Cancer Survey, 1947 and the Third National Cancer Survey, 1969 to 1971

(Cramer and Cutler, 1974). Age-specific mortality curves rise sharply after age 40 years and do not decline until after ages 65 and 80 years in nonwhites and whites, respectively. Consequently, it seems safe to conclude that increased longevity unmet by improvement in disease control is responsible for the continuing rise in crude mortality. Despite improvement in therapeutic modalities since 1950, only a minimal gain has been made in nationwide 5-year survival rates—from 29% to 32% (Cutler et al., 1975).

There are wide demographic differences in age-adjusted mortality rates ranging from a low of 1.69 in Japan to 11.02 in Denmark. Parallel differences in breast cancer mortality suggest a common endocrine background, and women with previously treated carcinomas of the breast or endometrium are more likely to develop second primary cancer in the ovary than at other sites. An environmental etiology may be inferred from the observation that Japanese women after immigrating to the United States incur a significantly greater risk of dying from ovarian cancer, which during middle life approaches that of white Americans (Wynder et al., 1969). High dietary intake of animal fat may be associated with an increased risk for ovarian cancer (Cramer et al., 1984). An increased prevalence of ovarian cancer noted in nuns, other single women, and nulliparous married women suggests that incessant ovulation uninterrupted by pregnancy may also be a predisposing factor. (It is of some interest that ovarian carcinoma is the commonest epithelial tumor in the best known of incessant ovulators, the domestic fowl. In addition, the incidence of ovarian carcinoma in hens is greatly enhanced by constant environments designed to promote egg production [Fathalla, 1972].) Also, women who used oral contraceptives have a reduced risk of later developing epithelial ovarian cancer (Cramer et al., 1982a).

Exposure to take (asbestos) may also be related to the development of epithelial ovarian cancer. Graham and Graham (1967) were able to induce ovarian neoplasms with asbestos in guinea pigs. Cramer et al. (1982b) observed that women who regularly dusted their perineum with talc and used talc on sanitary napkins had a threefold increased risk of developing ovarian cancer.

Several studies have reported families in which more than one member developed ovarian cancer (Piver et al., 1984). Cramer et al. (1983) observed an 11-fold increase in risk for ovarian malignancy in women with a history of ovarian cancer among mothers or sisters.

Prevention

Between 4% and 20% of patients with cancer of the ovary previously have undergone pelvic operations with conservation of one or both ovaries. These percentages have led many surgeons to advocate the prophylactic removal of normal ovaries at the time of hysterectomy. Proponents of ovarian salvage argue that the risk of developing cancer in a residual ovary is negligible and is outweighed by the evils of early castration. There is no indication that the risk of ovarian cancer in women with residual ovaries differs from that of the general population or is reduced by removing only one ovary. Prophylactic oophorectomy may be considered in women with increased risk for ovarian cancer such as those with a positive family history. However, following bilateral oophorectomy, an ovarian-like epithelial carcinoma may still develop in the pelvic peritoneum (Tobachman et al., 1982).

Early Detection

The meager overall survival rate for all cases of ovarian cancer can be attributed to failure in early diagnosis. Between 1945 and 1949, only 27% of ovarian cancers were localized at diagnosis, and the corresponding figure for the years 1965 through 1969 was 28% (Cutler et al., 1976). The total failure to achieve earlier detection over a 20-year span reflects both the asymptomatic character of early ovarian cancer and the lack of a means whereby asymptomatic women can be screened for this disease. Despite earlier hopes, the increasingly prevalent annual pelvic examination and cervical cytological smear have failed to increase the proportion of localized cases. In 1964, Graham and co-workers reported on the preclinical detection of ovarian cancer by the cytological examination of peritoneal fluid obtained by transvaginal aspiration of the cul-de-sac. The value of a screening measure, however, is dependent on the prevalence of the disease as well as on the sensitivity of the technique employed. Despite its lethality, the incidence of ovarian cancer is sufficiently low that the detection of a single case would require screening of more than 5,000 women. The demonstration of tumor-associated antigens unique to epithelial ovarian cancers has raised the question of detecting immunoreactivity in women with these tumors. Knauf and Urbach (1980) have measured an ovarian tumor–associated antigen (OCA) in the serum of 78% of women with stage I epithelial ovarian cancer. Bast and co-workers (1981) have developed a monoclonal antibody to human epithelial ovarian carcinoma (CA-125). CA-125 levels were elevated in 50% of women with stage I epithelial ovarian cancer (Zurawski et al., 1988). The development of radioimmunoassays for OCAs may facilitate the early diagnosis of ovarian malignancy as well as monitoring the response to therapy.

Natural History

The primary mode of tumor dissemination consists of penetration of the tumor capsule by proliferating epithelium and subsequent implantation of clonogenic cells on peritoneal surfaces. Intraperitoneal spread follows the usual pathways by which peritoneal fluid and particulate matter are cleared from the cavity. The major route from the pelvis is cephalad along the right paracolic gutter to the undersurface of the right hemidiaphragm and then into the network of diaphragmatic lymphatics. Isolated diaphragmatic involvement has been noted with otherwise localized tumors, and obstruction of diaphragmatic lymphatics by tumor emboli may result in the early onset of ascites. The proximity to the pelvis of omentum, cecum, terminal ileum, and sigmoid colon makes these organs frequent sites of early implantation. In some instances, particularly in the presence of ascites, the surgeon may encounter widespread, 2- to 3-mm visceral and parietal peritoneal implantations. Para-aortic lymph nodes are frequently involved, even early in the course of the disease. Knapp and Friedman (1974) found abnormal aortic nodes in 4 of 22 women with stage I epithelial cancers who underwent para-aortic node dissections. In two patients, involved nodes were not palpably enlarged, but all four women had poorly differentiated tumors. Extra-abdominal dissemination by the lymphatic route is slow, and hematogenous spread is usually a late manifestation. As a group, the epithelial carcinomas are relatively noninvasive, and destruction of vital organs is infrequent. With increasing tumor growth, however, there is a progressive mechanical interference with the function of abdominal organs. Disordered small bowel motility secondary to adhesions and interference with neural transmission through the myenteric plexus is a prominent feature and may simulate small-bowel obstruction. Actual bowel obstruction is not uncommon but usually occurs at multiple sites. The overall effect of interference with GI function, the production of serous effusions, and the metabolic demands of an enlarging bulk of tumor tissue, leads to progressive inanition.

The clinical stage or anatomical extent of tumor growth is considered the best indicator of prognosis. The staging classification proposed by FIGO has been adopted by WHO and the U.S. End Results Group and is now the only acceptable staging system (Table 9–6). Correlation between stage and 5-year survival rates is demonstrated in Table 9–7 for a collected series of patients. Stage I substages relating to the status of the tumor capsule have only recently been added. In a study from the Mayo Clinic reported by Webb et al. (1973), the 5-year survival rate of 111 patients in whom the tumor capsules were intact was 90%, whereas only 57% of 108 patients with capsular penetration or rupture survived.

Variation in survival within the major stages is in part determined by the histological grade that operates independently as a prognostic factor. Of particular importance is the group of tumors variously termed borderline, low-potential malignancy, or grade 0. If frank malignancy is evident, there is further correlation of tumor grade with survival. Thus, the 5-year survival rate with grade 1 tumors may be two to four times that of grade 3 tumors within a given stage. The influence of histological grade on the survival of patients with stage Ia and Ib epithelial carcinomas at the Mayo Clinic is illustrated in Figure 9–21 (Decker et al., 1975). Borderline tumors were not separately considered, and one must assume that they are included in the grade I group, thereby influencing survival favorably. Although there is some interdependence of grade and histological cell type, the latter appears to have little influence on prognosis independent of stage and histological grade.

Treatment

Surgical Treatment.—The initial abdominal operation is the keystone of ovarian cancer management, whatever the stage of disease. Implicit in this statement is the importance of a meticulous abdominal exploration and immediate annotation of the findings. Since 5% of malignant ovarian tumors are metastatic from occult primary cancers of the digestive tract, the stomach, colon, and pancreas must be carefully palpated.

At the time of laparotomy, gross criteria suggesting malignancy include hemorrhagic or solid areas within an ovarian cyst, tumor adherence to

TABLE 9–6.

Inernational Federation of Gynecology and Obstetrics Staging of Ovarian Carcinoma

Stage I
  Growth limited to the ovaries.
Stage Ia
  Growth limited to one ovary; no ascites. No tumor on the external surface; capsule intact.
Stage Ib
  Growth limited to both ovaries; no ascites. No tumor on the external surface; capsules intact.
Stage Ic
  Tumor either stage Ia or Ib but with tumor on the surface of one or both ovaries; or with capsule ruptured; or with ascites present containing malignant cells; or with abnormal peritoneal washings.
Stage II
  Growth involving one or both ovaries with pelvic extension.
Stage IIc
  Tumor either stage IIa or IIb but with tumor on the surface of one or both ovaries; or with capsule or capsules ruptured; or with ascites present containing malignant cells; or with abnormal washings.
Stage III
  Tumor involving one or both ovaries, with peritoneal implants outside the pelvis and/or abnormal retroperitoneal or inguinal nodes. Superficial liver metastasis qualifies as stage III.
Stage IIIa
  Tumor grossly limited to the true pelvis with normal nodes but with histologically confirmed microscopic seeding of abdominal peritoneal surfaces.
Stage IIIb
  Tumor of one or both ovaries with histologically confirmed implants of abdominal peritoneal surfaces, none exceeding 2 cm in diameter; nodes normal.
Stage IIIc
  Abdominal implants greater than 2 cm in diameter and/or abnormal retroperitoneal or inguinal nodes.
Stage IV
  Growth involving one or both ovaries with distant metastases. If pleural effusion is present, there must be abnormal cytology to allot a case to stage IV. Parenchymal liver metastases equals stage IV.

adjacent structures, papillary excrescences on the tumor surface, and the presence of ascites or peritoneal implantation. Despite the presence of one or more of these characteristics, the malignant nature of a tumor cannot be determined with cer-

TABLE 9–7.

Relation of Stage to Prognosis*

Stage	No. of Patients	5-Yr Survival (%)
I	751	61
Ia	528	65
Ib	130	52
Ic	80	52
II	401	40
IIa	40	60
IIb	205	38
III	539	5
IV	101	3

*Collected series.

tainty without excision and microscopic examination. Irrevocable surgical decisions in the young nullipara must await an unequivocal histological diagnosis of malignancy. Fertility may be preserved in young women with stage Ia well-differentiated epithelial ovarian carcinomas. However, careful exploration must be performed to exclude occult extraovarian spread.

When the tumor appears localized to one or both ovaries, greater accuracy in staging will be achieved by thorough palpation of the diaphragm and biopsies of the distal omentum and aortic lymph nodes. The risk for aortic nodal involvement is increased in germ cell and poorly differentiated epithelial ovarian cancers. Cytologic study of saline irrigated through the peritoneal cavity is necessary for the current staging system. Hysterectomy and bilateral salpingo-oophorectomy are usually performed because of the frequency of synchronous or metachronous carcinomas in the contralateral ovary and endometrium as well as the possibility of occult metastases at these sites or on the uterine serosa.

When tumor spread to the pelvic peritoneum has occurred (stage II), hysterectomy, bilateral salpingo-oophorectomy, and excision of all gross tumor is indicated. Rarely, segmental resection of bladder or rectum is necessary.

For more than 30 years, expert opinion has favored the excision of as much tumor tissue as possible even when abdominal dissemination is encountered at primary operation. Although the removal of large masses may afford palliation, there is little firm evidence that "debulking" procedures improve survival unless all or nearly all of the tumor is excised (Aure et al. 1971; Griffiths, 1975). Apparently most important is the reduction in mass size to a point where subsequent chemotherapy or irradiation will exert a maximal effect. In retrospective studies, improved survival of patients who received chemotherapy was evident only with minimal residual disease (Griffiths et al., 1972). Chemotherapy induced complete responses in 45% of patients with residual masses less than 2 cm in diameter, whereas only 23% of patients with larger masses had complete responses (Young et al., 1978). Although these effects are clearly related to a small tumor volume, it can be argued that attainment of the latter depends more on limited or less invasive tumor growth than on extended surgical resection. In an attempt to answer this question, Griffiths (1975) at the Brigham and Women's Hospital used a multiple linear regression equation with survival

FIG 9–21.

Actuarial survival curves by grade for 260 patients with stages Ia and Ib ovarian carcinoma. (From Decker DG, Malkasian GD, Taylor WF: Prognostic importance of histologic grading in ovarian carcinoma. et al: *Natl Cancer Inst Monogr* 1975; 42:9. Reproduced by permission.)

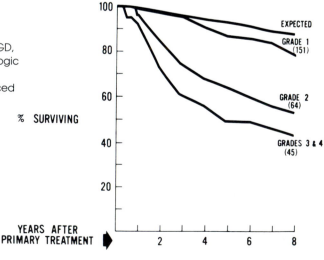

as the dependent variable to control simultaneously for multiple therapeutic and biological variables. Regardless of other prognostic factors, survival was uniformly poor if the diameter of the largest residual tumor mass exceeded 1.0 ± 0.5 cm but increased in proportion to decrements in mass size below 1.5 cm (Table 9–8). Analysis of a subset of patients in whom a residual mass size of 1.5 cm or less was achieved by surgical excision of larger metastatic lesions indicated that this group fared as well as those whose largest metastatic lesions were less than this size limit at the outset (Fig 9–22). The effectiveness of cytoreductive surgery may be limited in patients with clinical ascites or large (more than 10 cm) metastases; median survival in these patients is only 12 months despite successful cytoreduction (Hacker et al., 1983). Despite misconceptions to the contrary, tumor masses need not be transected since lines of cleavage between tumor-bearing peritoneum and normal tissue are usually found. Although limited bowel resection may be necessary, ovarian cancer masses can often be freed from the bowel muscularis by sharp dissection. The omentum, frequently laden with tumor, is removed from the greater curvature of the stomach following ligation of the gastroepiploic vessels. Whatever procedures are necessary, an optimal operation is one that is carefully planned after thorough abdominal exploration, and it cannot be supplanted by the indiscriminate excision of tumor bulk.

TABLE 9–8.

Survival by Diameter of Largest Residual Mass

Size (cm)	No. of Patients	Median Survival (mo)
0	29	39
0.3 (± 0.2)	28	29
1.0 (± 0.5)	16	18
> 1.5	29	11*

*Mean survival 12.7 mo. (SE = 1.56 mo.).

Radiation Therapy.—The merit of postoperative external beam irradiation in stage II disease has been generally accepted, but the supporting data must be interpreted with caution. The apparent advantage conferred by irradiation (Table 9–9) is dampened by the variability of results and small numbers in the control groups. Survival appeared to be dramatically improved by irradiation in some series, but the comparison was historical, and less extensive surgical procedures in the nonirradiated groups were implied. The adverse effect of residual tumor masses larger than 2 cm in diameter was evident in Delclos and Smith's (1973) series.

Currently, pelvic irradiation for stage I and II tumors usually consists of 4,000 to 5,000 rad delivered to the midcoronal plane. For stage II and III disease, the upper abdomen is also irradiated, usually as a separate field, to 3,000 rad. The danger of radiation nephritis and hepatitis when dos-

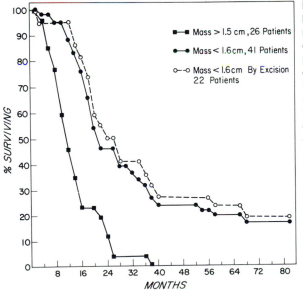

FIG 9–22.

Relationship of survival to size of largest residual metastasis after primary operation for stage III ovarian carcinoma. The survival curve of patients whose mass size was reduced to 1.5 cm or less by excision of larger metastases was identical to that of all patients with a residual mass size below this limit. (From Griffiths CT, Fuller AF Jr: Intensive surgical and chemotherapeutic management of advanced ovarian cancer. *Surg Clin North Am* 1978; 58:131–142. Reproduced by permission.)

TABLE 9–9.

Five-Year Survival Rates*

	Operation Only			Operation and Radiation		
	No.	Range (%)	Mean (%)	No.	Range (%)	Mean (%)
Stage I	319	49–91	66	333	53–80	59
Stage II	89	0–33	24	363	28–69	39
Stage III	268	0–11	5	811	2–17	10

*Collected series.

age exceeds 2,000 and 3,000 rad, respectively, has necessitated corresponding dose limitations to these organs. Consequently, "sanctuary" areas are provided at anatomic sites where metastatic tumor is most likely to lodge. Nevertheless, the importance of upper abdominal irradiation in controlling stage II cancers seems well established (Perez et al., 1975; Delclos and Smith, 1973).

The efficacy of irradiation in the therapy of ovarian cancer was evaluated in a prospective, randomized study of 190 patients with stages Ib, II, and III disease at the Princess Margaret Hospital (Dembo et al., 1979). Patients were randomized to receive either pelvic irradiation alone, pelvic irradiation and chlorambucil, or pelvic and abdominal irradiation. Patients with extensive tumor burdens had a poor prognosis regardless of the treatment strategy. The relapse-free survival in stage II patients with minimal residual disease was 79% in patients treated with pelvic and abdominal irradiation and only 46% in patients treated with pelvic irradiation alone. Pelvic and abdominal irradiation with no diaphragmatic shielding significantly improved patient survival and long-term control of occult or minimal upper abdominal disease. Furthermore, patients tolerated whole abdominal irradiation with minimal morbidity. Therefore, in patients with stage II or III ovarian cancer with minimal residual disease, pelvic and abdominal irradiation appears to be an appropriate therapeutic option with curative potential. Radiation therapy appears to be particularly effective in patients with well-differentiated epithelial ovarian cancer (Dembo, 1985; Schray et al., 1983).

Interest has been reawakened in the intraperitoneal instillation of colloidal radioactive isotopes as a surgical adjuvant for stage I ovarian carcinoma. These agents, particularly gold 138, were used extensively in the 1950s, but results were variable and complications significant. The superficial penetration of alpha and beta particles does not significantly affect tumor masses, but a lethal effect on superficial tumor cell aggregates might be anticipated. In two studies, one employing ^{138}Au and the other phosphorus 32 chromic phosphate, 5-year survival rates of 83% and 93%, respectively, were obtained in stage Ia cases (Clark et al., 1973). In a review by Decker et al. (1973) of experience at the Mayo Clinic with intraperitoneal ^{138}Au, only those patients with stage I disease in whom a malignant cyst had ruptured intraoperatively appeared to benefit from the treatment. Recently, ^{32}P chromic phosphate, a pure beta emitter with a half-life of 14.2 days, has been favored over ^{138}Au (10% gamma emission, half-life 2.7 days) because of a near absence of intestinal complications.

Chemotherapy.—The observation in the early 1950s that nitrogen mustard could induce significant regression in the size of ovarian tumor masses has led to the widespread use of alkylating agents in the management of this disease. The term *alkylating* refers to the ability of this class of drugs to bind a highly reactive alkyl group to metabolically important sites within the cell, rendering them incapable of functioning in their usual manner. The primary antitumor action is related to the ability to cross-link the helical strands of the DNA molecule in the manner of a grappling hook. This mechanism impedes DNA replication and explains the inability of the cell to undergo mitosis. Since these compounds directly attack the DNA molecule, they are equally effective during any phase of the mitotic cycle and may inflict lethal chromosomal damage on noncycling cells. Successful cancer chemotherapy is dependent on the ability of normal host tissue to recover more rapidly than tumor tissue. This differential in cell recovery time, which permits continuation of therapy prior to tumor regrowth, is essential to the achievement of a stepwise fractional reduction in tumor volume.

A variety of alkylating agents have been developed and successfully employed in the treatment of ovarian cancer (Table 9–10). An objective response is defined as a reduction in tumor size by 50% or more, and a complete response signifies a complete disappearance of palpable tumor or tumor demonstrable on roentgenograms. Alkylating agents have the same mechanism of cytotoxic action and about the same spectrum of an-

TABLE 9–10.

Collected Responses of Ovarian Carcinoma to Alkylating-Agent Chemotherapy

Drug	Total No. of Patients	% Responses
Nitrogen mustard	25	36
Chlorambucil	388	51
Melphalan	541	47
Cyclophosphamide	371	45
Thiotepa	337	48

titumor activity. Certainly none of these drugs has demonstrated therapeutic superiority over the others in ovarian cancer. In general, tumors with de novo or acquired resistance to one alkylating agent have been resistant to other alkylating agents.

Cisplatin (*cis*-diamminedichloroplatinum) is not an alkylating agent but cross-links DNA and is cell cycle nonspecific. Importantly, Wiltshaw and Kroner (1976) reported a 29% response rate to cisplatin in ovarian cancer patients who were resistant to alkylating agents. Cisplatin is now established as a cornerstone in the combination chemotherapy of ovarian cancer. Responsiveness of ovarian carcinoma to other classes of anticancer drugs has been disappointing. The relative inactivity of other agents in comparison to those of the alkylating class has been attributed to their employment as "second-line" therapy. Stanhope et al. (1977) reported a meager 6% response rate among 347 patients who received a second drug regimen, regardless of the response to initial chemotherapy.

In contrast to the alkylating agents, which attack the DNA molecule directly, another class of chemotherapeutic agents, the antimetabolites, exerts an antitumor effect by inhibiting the synthesis of DNA. Since these drugs act primarily during the phase of DNA synthesis in the mitotic cycle (S phase), they are maximally effective against small tumor populations in which the growth fraction is high. A consistently low activity of fluorouracil and methotrexate is not surprising since ovarian carcinomas considered evaluable in clinical trials have palpable and therefore bulky tumor masses with a presumably low growth fraction.

Antibiotic chemotherapeutic agents intercalate with the DNA molecule, but in contrast to alkylating agents, they interfere with DNA function rather than with its structure. Dactinomycin, which has not been used as a single agent in ovarian cancer, has been included in drug combinations, particularly those that have been effective against malignant germ cell tumors. Although doxorubicin (Adriamycin) has been promising, a meager 20% response rate was obtained in collected series. Vincristine, a vinca alkaloid that interferes with mitotic spindle formation, has shown no activity in the epithelial ovarian cancers but is an important component of the VAC regimen for germ cell tumors.

Although combination chemotherapy of ovarian cancer was initiated by Greenspan's use of thiotepa and methotrexate in the early 1960s, evidence of superiority over single alkylating agent therapy has emerged only in recent years (Table 9–11).

Young et al., in 1978, reported the first study that demonstrated improved survival in advanced ovarian cancer with a combination drug regimen in a prospective comparison with an alkylating agent. Eighty previously untreated patients were randomized to receive either melphalan in conventional doses, or a combination of hexamethylmelamine, cyclophosphamide, methotrexate, and fluorouracil (Hexa-CAF). Treatment with the combination regimen attained a significantly increased overall response rate (75%

TABLE 9–11.

Response Rates of Advanced Ovarian Carcinoma to Combination Chemotherapy

Investigators	Agents*	No. of Patients	% Responses
Young et al. (1978)	Hexa-CAF	40	75
Edmonson et al. (1979)	D-C	99	45
Delgado et al. (1979)	CHF	12	83
Parker et al. (1980)	D-C	41	83

*D-C = doxorubicin and cyclophosphamide; CHF = cyclophosphamide, hexamethylmelamine, and fluorouracil.

vs. 54%), more complete responses (33% vs. 16%), and longer median survival (29 vs. 17 months). The combination regimen was most effective in patients with minimal residual disease. Patients achieving complete remission documented by operative restaging had a long survival, and 60% of these women were free of disease for at least 4 years. Significant prolongation of survival depended on the attainment of a complete response.

At the Mayo Clinic (Edmonson et al., 1979), 111 patients with advanced ovarian cancer were randomized to receive either cyclophosphamide alone or cyclophosphamide and doxorubicin. In patients with bulky disease, the two regimens had comparable response rates and survival rates. However, in patients with minimal residual disease, the combination regimen achieved a significant increase in both response rate and duration of survival.

Parker et al. (1980) at the Brigham and Women's Hospital and Dana Farber Cancer Institute have also evaluated the role of combination chemotherapy (doxorubicin and cylophosphamide) in advanced ovarian cancer. Objective response was noted in 34 of 41 (83%) patients without prior cytotoxic chemotherapy but in only 2 of 12 patients (17%) who had failed a single alkylating agent or radiotherapy. This study emphasizes the marked reduction of activity in advanced ovarian cancer as well as the lack of success of initiating therapy with an alkylating agent and then later attempting to save patients suffering relapse with more aggressive combination drugs.

Several recent studies have therefore consistently indicated that combination chemotherapy induces a higher response rate with prolonged survival compared with single alkylating agents in the treatment of advanced ovarian cancer. However, the greater effectiveness of combination chemotherapy appears to be limited to patients with minimal residual disease at the onset of treatment.

Although survival with combination chemotherapy has been prolonged, it is still unclear if long-term cure is improved vs. single alkylating agents. Louie et al. (1986) reported that only 9 (15%) of 62 patients with advanced ovarian cancer who were treated with cisplatin-based combination chemotherapy were alive at 4 years.

Clinical examination and radiographic studies have limited capabilities to detect small foci of persistent intraperitoneal disease. An elevation in the CA-125 level strongly indicates persistent tumor. However, even if the CA-125 value is normal, about one half of the patients will be found to have tumor at second-look surgery (Berek et al., 1986).

Second-look exploratory laparotomy is the most accurate way of determining tumor status following primary therapy. Only about 40% of patients who are clinically free of disease have pathologically normal second-look surgeries (Ho et al., 1987). Furthermore, one half of the patients with normal second-look surgeries still develop recurrent ovarian tumor. In addition, no improvement in survival accrued to advanced-stage platinum-treated patients who underwent second-look surgery compared with similar patients who did not undergo the procedure (Chambers et al., 1988). The performance of second-look surgery has not yet been demonstrated to significantly affect long-term survival. Second-look operations may be best limited to experimental protocols where precise measurement of tumor size may be important.

Several second-line therapies are currently being evaluated in patients with persistent ovarian cancer. Howell et al. (1987) reported a median survival of more than 4 years in patients with refractory but small volume (less than 2 cm) ovarian cancer treated with intraperitoneal platinum. In addition, following whole abdominal irradiation, 70% of patients with small-volume persistent well- or moderately differentiated tumors were free of disease at 3 years (Schray et al., 1988). Furthermore, radiolabeled monoclonal antibodies have recently been employed in patients with persistent small-volume (less than 2 cm) tumors, and 9 (56%) of 16 patients had an objective response (Epenetos et al., 1987). The optimal second-line therapy has not been determined, but currently there are several encouraging options.

Supportive Treatment.—A major advance in the treatment of advanced ovarian carcinoma has been the development of safe and effective parenteral nutrition. Intravenous hyperalimentation has enabled these nutritionally depleted patients with disordered GI function to undergo the rigors of extensive operation and intensive chemotherapy. Short-term hyperalimentation may have a palliative effect in advanced cases, but it must be used judiciously to avoid prolongation of a hopeless and miserable existence.

The natural history of ovarian cancer often

results in a protracted terminal phase. The patient is beleaguered with frequent nausea and vomiting, discomfort from a distended abdomen, dyspnea due to pleural effusions, and intermittent bouts of partial bowel obstruction. Operation for presumed bowel obstruction should be avoided, since isolated points of obstruction are rare and the surgeon is faced with adherent bowel and mesentery laden with tumor masses. Intermittent gastric or intestinal intubation may afford temporary relief.

The physician's interaction with the patient and her family is of the greatest importance. Empathy must be tempered with hope and encouragement, but the patient's complete trust in her physician cannot be sacrificed by patent untruths, however well meaning.

REFERENCES

Afridi MA, Vongtama V, Tsukada Y, et al: Dysgerminoma of the ovary: Radiation therapy for recurrence and metastases. *Am J Obstet Gynceol* 1976; 126:190.

Arey LB: The origin and form of the Brenner tumor. *Am J Obstet Gynecol* 1961; 81:743.

Asadourian LA, Taylor HB: Dysgerminoma: An analysis of 105 cases. *Obstet Gynecol* 1969; 33:370.

Aure JC, Hoeg K, Kolstad P: Clinical and histologic studies of ovarian carcinoma. *Obstet Gynecol* 1971; 37:1.

Baker TG: Radiosensitivity of mammalian oocytes with particular reference to the human female. *Am J Obstet Gynecol* 1971; 110:746.

Barber HRK, Graber EA: The PMPO syndrome (postmenopausal palpable ovary syndrome). *Obstet Gynecol* 1971; 38:921.

Barbieri RL, Niloff JM, Bast RC Jr, et al: Elevated serum concentrations of serum CA125 in patients with advanced endometriosis. *Fertil Steril* 1986; 45:630.

Barbieri RL, Rein M, Hornstein MD, et al: Rat Leydig cell and granulosa cell 17-ketosteroid reductase activity: Subcellular localization and substrate specificity. *Am J Obstet Gynecol* 1988a; 159:1564.

Barbieri RL, Ryan KJ: Hyperandrogenism, insulin resistance, and acanthosis nigricans syndrome: A common endocrinopathy with unique pathophysiologic features. *Am J Obstet Gynecol* 1983; 147:90.

Barbieri RL, Smith S, Ryan KJ: The role of hyperinsulinemia in the pathogenesis of ovarian hyperandrogenism. *Fertil Steril* 1988b; 50:197.

Bast RC Jr, Feeney M, Lazarus H, et al: Reactivity of a monoclonal antibody with human ovarian carcinoma. *J Clin Invest* 1981; 68:1331.

Bennington JL, Ferguson BC, Haber SL: Incidence and relative frequency of benign and malignant ovarian neoplasms. *Obstet Gynecol* 1968; 32:627.

Berek JS, Knapp RC, Malkasian GD, et al: CA125 serum levels correlated with second-look operations among ovarian cancer patients. *Obstet Gynecol* 1986; 67:685.

Björkholm E, Silfverswärd C: Prognostic factors in granulosa-cell tumors. *Gynecol Oncol* 1981; 11:261.

Block E: Quantitative morphological investigations of the follicular system in woman. *Acta Anat* 1952; 14:108.

Cangir A, Smith J, Van Eys J: Improved prognosis in children with ovarian cancers following modified VAC (vincristine sulfate, dactinomycin and cyclophosphamide) chemotherapy. *Cancer* 1978; 42:1234.

Chambers SK, Chambers JT, Kohorn EI, et al: Evaluation of the role of second-look surgery in ovarian cancer. *Obstet Gynecol* 1988; 72:404.

Clark DGC, Hilaris B, Roussis C, et al: The role of radiation therapy (including isotopes) in the treatment of cancer of the ovary (results of 614 patients treated at Memorial Hospital, New York, N.Y.), in Ariel IM (ed): *Progress in Clinical Cancer*. New York, Grune & Stratton, vol 5, 1973.

Climie ARW, Health LP: Malignant degeneration of benign cystic teratomas of the ovary. *Cancer* 1968; 22:824.

Cramer DW, Cutler SJ: Incidence and histopathology of malignancies of the female genital organs in the United States. *Am J Obstet Gynecol* 1974; 118:443.

Cramer DW, Hutchison GB, Welch WR, et al: Factors affecting the association of oral contraceptives and ovarian cancer. *N Engl J Med* 1982a; 307:1047.

Cramer DW, Hutchison GB, Welch WR, et al: Determinants of ovarian cancer risk: I. Reproductive experiences and family history. *J Natl Cancer Inst* 1983; 71:711.

Cramer DW, Welch RW, Hutchinson GB, et al: Dietary animal fat in relation to ovarian cancer risk. *Obstet Gynecol* 1984; 63:833.

Cramer DW, Welch WR, Scully RE, et al: Ovarian cancer and talc—a case-control study. *Cancer* 1982b; 50:372.

Creasman WT, Fetter BF, Hammond CB, et al: Germ cell malignancies of the ovary. *Obstet Gynecol* 1979; 53:226.

Curry SL, Smith JP, Gallagher HS: Malignant

teratoma of the ovary: Prognostic factors and treatment. *Am J Obstet Gynecol* 1978; 131:845.

Cutler SJ, Myers MH, Green SB: Trends in survival rates of patients with cancer. *N Engl J Med* 1975; 293:122.

Cutler SJ, Myers MH, White PC: Who are we missing and why? *Cancer* 1976; 37:421.

Decker DG, Malkasian GD, Taylor WF: Prognostic importance of histologic grading in ovarian carcinoma. *Natl Cancer Inst Monogr* 1975; 42:9.

Decker DG, Webb MJ, Holbrook M: Radiogold treatment of epithelial cancer of the ovary: Late results. *Am J Obstet Gynecol* 1973; 115:751.

Delclos L, Smith JP: Tumors of the ovary, in Fletcher G (ed): *Textbook of Radiotherapy*. Philadelphia, Lea & Febiger, 1973.

Delgado G, Schein P, MacDonald J, et al: L-PAM vs cyclophosphamide, hexamethylmelamine, and 5-fluorouracil (CHF) for advanced ovarian cancer. *Proc Am Assoc Cancer Res* 1979; 20:434.

Dembo AJ: Abdominopelvic radiotherapy in ovarian cancer: A 10-year experience. *Cancer* 1985; 55:2285.

Dembo AJ, Bush RS, Beale FA, et al: Ovarian carcinoma: Improved survival following abdominopelvic irradiation in patients with a completed pelvic operation. *Am J Obstet Gynecol* 1979; 134:793.

Edmonson HJ, Fleming TR, Decker DG, et al: Different chemotherapeutic sensitivities and host factors affecting prognosis in advanced ovarian carcinomas versus minimal residual disease. *Cancer Treat Rep* 1979; 63:241.

Epenetos AA, Munro AJ, Stewart S, et al: Antibody-guided irradiation of advanced ovarian cancer with intraperitoneally administered radiolabeled monoclonal antibodies. *J Clin Oncol* 1987; 5:1890.

Faddy MJ, Gosden RG, Edwards RG: Ovarian follicle dynamics in mice: A comparative study of three inbred strains and an F1 hybrid. *J Endocrinol* 1983; 96:23.

Fathalla MF: Factors in the causation and incidence of ovarian cancer. *Obstet Gynecol Surv* 1972; 27:751.

Feuillan PP, Pescovitz OH, Cutler GB, et al: Precocious puberty: Mechanism, evaluation and management, in Barbieri RL, Schiff I (eds): *Reproductive Endocrine Therapeutics*. New York, Alan R Liss Publishers, 1988, pp 311–336.

Finkler NJ, Benacerraf B, Lavin PT, et al: Comparison of serum CA125, clinical impression and ultrasound in the preoperative evaluation of ovarian masses. *Obstet Gynecol* 1988; 72:659.

Fox H, Agrawal K, Langley FA: A clinicopathologic study of 92 cases of granulosa cell tumor of the ovary with special reference to the factors influencing prognosis. *Cancer* 1975; 35:231.

Gershenson DM: Menstrual and reproductive function after treatment with combination chemotherapy for malignant ovarian germ cell tumors. *J Clin Oncol* 1988; 6:270.

Gershenson DM, Del Junco G, Herson J, et al: Endodermal sinus tumor of the ovary: The M.D. Anderson experience. *Obstet Gynecol* 1983; 61:94.

Gershenson DM, Wharton JT, Kline RC, et al: Chemotherapeutic complete remission in patients with metastatic ovarian dysgerminoma. *Cancer* 1986; 58:2594.

Goodman AL, Hodgen GD: The ovarian triad of the primate menstrual cycle. *Recent Prog Horm Res* 1983; 39:1.

Gordon A, Lipton D, Woodruff JD: Dysgerminoma: A review of 158 cases from the Emil Novak Ovarian Tumor Registry. *Obstet Gynecol* 1981; 58:497.

Graham J, Graham R: Ovarian cancer and asbestos. *Environ Res* 1967; 1:115.

Graham JB, Graham RM, Schueller E: Preclinical detection of ovarian cancer. *Cancer* 1964; 17:1414.

Griffiths CT: Surgical resection of tumor bulk in the primary treatment of ovarian carcinoma. *Natl Cancer Inst Monogr* no 42, 1975, pp. 101–104.

Griffiths CT, Fuller AF Jr: Intensive surgical and chemotherapeutic management of advanced ovarian cancer. *Surg Clin North Am* 1978; 58:131.

Griffiths CT, Grogan RH, Hall TC: Advanced ovarian cancer: Primary treatment with surgery, radiotherapy and chemotherapy. *Cancer* 1972; 29:1.

Hacker NF, Berek JS, Lagasse L, et al: Primary cytoreductive surgery for epithelial ovarian cancer. *Obstet Gynecol* 1983; 61:413.

Hart WR, Norris HJ: Borderline and malignant mucinous tumors of the ovary. *Cancer* 1973; 31:1031.

Hertig AT, Gore HM: Tumors of the ovary and fallopian tube, in *Tumors of the Female Sex Organs:* part 3, section 9, fascicle 33, *Atlas of Tumor Pathology*. Washington, DC, Armed Forces Institute of Pathology, 1961.

Ho AG, Beller U, Speyer JL, et al: A reassessment of the role of second-look laparotomy in advanced ovarian cancer. *J Clin Oncol* 1987; 5:1316.

Holtz F, Hart WR: Krukenberg tumors of the ovary—a clinicopathologic analysis of 27 cases. *Cancer* 1982; 50:2438.

Howell SB, Zimm S, Markman M, et al: Long-term survival of advanced refractory ovarian carcinoma patients with small-volume disease treated with intraperitoneal chemotherapy. *J Clin Oncol* 1987; 5:1607.

Ireland K, Woodruff JD: Masculinizing ovarian tumors. *Obstet Gynecol Surv* 1976; 31:83.

Jacobs AJ, Deppe G, Cohen CJ: Combination chemotherapy of ovarian granulosa cell tumor with cis-platinum and doxorubicin. *Gynecol Oncol* 1982; 14:294.

Javaheri G, Lifchez A, Valle J: Pregnancy following removal of and long-term chemotherapy for ovarian malignant teratoma. *Obstet Gynecol* 1983; 61:8s.

Jones GES: Some newer aspects of the management of infertility. *JAMA* 1949; 141:1123.

Judd HL, Judd GE, Lucas WE, et al: Endocrine function of the postmenopausal ovary: Concentrations of androgens and estrogens in ovarian and peripheral vein blood. *J Clin Endocrinol Metab* 1974; 39:1020.

Kent SW, McKay DG: Primary cancer of the ovary. *Am J Obstet Gynecol* 1960; 80:430.

Killick S, Elstein M: Pharmacologic production of luteinized unruptured follicles by prostaglandin synthetase inhibitors. *Fertil Steril* 1987; 47:773.

Koninckx PR, Heyns WJ, Corvelyn PA, et al: Delayed onset of luteinization as a cause of infertility. *Fertil Steril* 1978; 29:266.

Knapp RC, Friedman EA: Aortic lymph node metastases in early ovarian cancer. *Am J Obstet Gynecol* 1974; 119:1013.

Knauf S, Urbach GI: A study of ovarian cancer patients using a radioimmunoassay for human ovarian tumor-associated antigen OCA. *Am J Obstet Gynecol* 1980; 138:1222.

Krepart G, Smith JP, Rutledge F, et al: The treatment for dysgerminoma of the ovary. *Cancer* 1978; 41:986.

Kurman RJ, Craig JM: Endometrioid and clear cell carcinoma of the ovary. *Cancer* 1972; 29:1653.

Kurman R, Norris HJ: Embryonal carcinoma of the ovary. *Cancer* 1976a; 38:2420.

Kurman R, Norris HJ: Endodermal sinus tumor of the ovary: A clinical and pathological analysis of 71 cases. *Cancer* 1976b; 38:2404.

Kurman R, Norris HJ: Malignant mixed germ cell tumors of the ovary. *Obstet Gynecol* 1976c; 48:579.

Lauchlan SC: The secondary müllerian system. *Obstet Gynecol Surv* 1972; 27:133.

Limber GK, King RE, Silverberg SG: Pseudomyxoma peritonaei: A report of ten cases. *Ann Surg* 1973; 178:587.

Linder D, McCain BK, Hecht F: Parthenogenic origin of benign ovarian teratomas. *N Engl J Med* 1975; 292:63.

Lobo R: Endocrine therapy of hyperandrogenism, in Barbieri RL, Shiff I (eds): *Reproductive Endocrine Therapeutics.* New York, Alan R Liss Publishers 1988, pp 101–126.

Louie KG, Ozols RF, Myers CE, et al: Long-term results of a cisplatin-containing combination chemotherapy regimen for the treatment of advanced ovarian carcinoma. *J Clin Oncol* 1986; 4:1579.

MacDonald PC, Grodin JM, Edman CD, et al: Origin of estrogen in a postmenopausal woman with a nonendocrine tumor of the ovary and endometrial hyperplasia. *Obstet Gynecol* 1976; 47:644.

Malkasian GD Jr, Knapp RC, Lavin PT, et al: Preoperative evaluation of serum CA125 levels in premenopausal and postmenopausal patients with pelvic masses: Discrimination of benign from malignant disease. *Am J Obstet Gynecol* 1988; 159:341.

Malkasian GD, Symmonds RE: Treatment of unilateral encapsulated ovarian dysgerminoma. *Am J Obstet Gynecol* 1964; 90:379.

Marik J, Hulka J: Luteinized unruptured follicle syndrome: A subtle cause of infertility. *Fertil Steril* 1978; 29:270.

McKay DG: The origins of ovarian tumors. *Clin Obstet Gynecol* 1962; 5:1181.

Miles PA, Norris HJ: Proliferative and malignant Brenner tumors of the ovary. *Cancer* 1972; 30:174.

Norris HJ, Chorlton I: Functioning tumors of the ovary. *Clin Obstet Gynecol* 1974; 17:189.

Norris HJ, Jenson RD: Relative frequency of ovarian neoplasms in children and adolescents. *Cancer* 1972; 30:713.

Norris HJ, Taylor HE: Prognosis of granulosatheca tumors of the ovary. *Cancer* 1968; 21:255.

Norris HJ, Zirkin HJ, Benson WL: Immature (malignant) teratoma of the ovary: A clinical and pathologic study of 58 cases. *Cancer* 1976; 37:2359.

Novak ER, Kutchmeshgi J, Mupas R, et al: Feminizing gonadal stromal tumors. *Obstet Gynecol* 1971; 38:701.

Page DC, de la Chapelle A: The paternal origin of X chromosomes in XX males determined using restriction fragment length polymorphisms. *Am J Hum Genet* 1984; 36:565.

Parker LM, Griffiths CT, Yankee RA, et al: Combination chemotherapy with Adriamycin-cyclophosphamide for advanced ovarian carcinoma. *Cancer* 1980; 46:669.

Perez CA, Walz BJ, Jacobson PL: Radiation therapy in the management of carcinoma of the ovary. *Natl Cancer Inst Monogr* 42:119, 1975.

Piver MS, Mettlin CJ, Tsukada Y, et al: Familial ovarian cancer registry. *Obstet Gynecol* 1984; 64:195.

Piver MS, Sinks L, Barlow JJ, et al: Five-year remissions of metastatic solid teratoma of the ovary. *Cancer* 1976; 38:987.

Robboy SJ, Scully RE: Ovarian teratoma with glial implants on the peritoneum. *Hum Pathol* 1970; 1:643.

Rogers LW, Julian CG, Woodruff JD: Mesonephroid carcinoma of the ovary: A study of 95 cases from the Emil Novak Tumor Registry. *Gynecol Oncol* 1972; 1:76.

Romero R, Schwartz PE: Alpha fetoprotein determinations in the management of endodermal sinus tumors and mixed germ cell tumors of the ovary. *Am J Obstet Gynecol* 1981; 141:126.

Santesson L, Kottmeier HL: General classification of ovarian tumors, in Gentil F, Junqueira AC (eds) *Ovarian Cancer*. UICC monograph series, vol 2. New York, Springer-Verlag, New York, 1968.

Schray M, Martinez A, Cox R, et al: Radiotherapy in epithelial ovarian cancer: Analysis of prognostic factors based on long-term experience. *Obstet Gynecol* 1983; 62:373.

Schray M, Martinez A, Howes AE, et al: Advanced epithelial ovarian cancer: Salvage whole abdominal irradiation for patients with recurrent or persistent disease after combination chemotherapy. *J Clin Oncol* 1988; 6:1433.

Scully RE: Gonadoblastoma: A review of 74 cases. *Cancer* 1970a; 25:1340.

Scully RE: Recent progress in ovarian cancer. *Hum Pathol* 1970b; 1:73.

Serov SF, Scully RE: *Histological Typing of Ovarian Tumors*. International Histological Typing of Tumors, no 9. Geneva, World Health Organization, 1973.

Smith JP, Rutledge F: Advances in chemotherapy for gynecologic cancer. *Cancer* 1975; 36:669.

Smith JP, Rutledge F, Wharton JT: Chemotherapy of ovarian cancer: New approaches to treatment. *Cancer* 1972; 30:1565.

Stanhope CR, Smith JP, Rutledge FN: Second-trial drugs in ovarian cancer. *Gynecol Oncol* 1977; 5:51.

Stenwig JT, Hazekamp JT, Beecham JB: Granulosa cell tumors of the ovary: A clinicopathological study of 118 cases with long-term follow-up. *Gynecol Oncol* 1979; 7:136.

Taylor MH, De Petrillo AD, Turner AR: Vinblastine, bleomycin and cisplatin in malignant germ cell tumors of the ovary. *Cancer* 1985; 56:1341.

Thomas GM, Dembo AJ, Hacker NF, et al: Current therapy for dysgerminoma of the ovary. *Obstet Gynecol* 1987; 70:268.

Tobachman JK, Tucker MA, Kane R, et al: Intraabdominal carcinomatosis after prophylactic oophorectomy in ovarian cancer-prone families. *Lancet* 1982; 2:795.

Waldstreicher J, Santoro NJ, Hall JE, et al: Hyperfunction of the hypothalamic-pituitary axis in women with polycystic ovarian disease. Indirect evidence for partial gonadotropin desensitization. *J Clin Endocrinol Metab* 1988; 66:165.

Webb MJ, Decker DG, Mussey E: Factors influencing survival in stage I ovarian cancer. *Am J Obstet Gynecol* 1973; 116:222.

Wiltshaw E, Kroner T: Phase II study of *cis*-dichlorodiammine platinum II in advanced adenocarcinoma of the ovary. *Cancer Chemother Rep* 1976; 60:55.

Woodruff JD, Telinde RW: The histology and histogenesis of ovarian neoplasia. *Cancer* 1976; 38:411.

Wynder EL, Dodo H, Barber HR: Epidemiology of cancer of the ovary. *Cancer* 1969; 23:352.

Young RC, Chabner BA, Hubbard SP, et al: Prospective trial of melphalan (L-PAM) versus combination chemotherapy (Hexa-CAF) in ovarian adenocarcinoma. *N Engl J Med* 1978; 199:1261.

Zurawski VR Jr, Knapp RC, Einhorn N, et al: An initial analysis of preoperative serum CA125 levels in patients with early stage ovarian carcinoma. *Obstet Gynecol* 1988; 30:7.

10   The Breast

Robert L. Shirley, M.D.

GENERAL CONSIDERATIONS

The characteristics that separate human beings from the lampreys, sharks, fishes, frogs, lizards, and birds are mammary glands. Officially, subphylum Vertebrata, class Mammalia includes those vertebrates that have breast and hair development.

The human breast is as central to the psychological core of *Homo sapiens* as any physical structure. The breast offered—breast received, nursing-suckling interrelationship is primal. The female human breast has become the center of literary and commercial emphasis because of exaggerated emphasis on sexual social behavior.

The breast is a challenge to the gynecologist in the continuous struggle to secure early cancer detection. Unfortunately, many gynecologists do not examine the breasts as part of a routine physical examination. This group of subspecialists may consider themselves "pelvicologists" instead of recognizing that the Greek root *gyne* refers to the whole woman.

DEVELOPMENT AND PHYSIOLOGIC ALTERATIONS

Growth and development of the embryonic skin lead to the formation of specialized skin appendages. Specific sweat glands develop a specialized function, such as lacrimal and scent, but the most elaborate pattern is exemplified in the mammary glands. These develop along the milk line extending obliquely from each axilla to the homolateral pubic mons. In the human, the mammary glands differentiate on the ventral surface of the chest centered in the fourth thoracic segment slightly lateral to the midclavicular line.

Approximately 15 sweat glands bud inward in the region of each nipple, with an early branching that forms the anlage of future growth. Surrounding these primary papillae is another group of sudoriferous glands surrounding the nipple. They, in turn, develop into mammary-like areolar glands (the follicles of Montgomery).

At thelarche, usually age 9 to 11 years, the breast ducts enter a second growth phase with further extension of the duct systems. This coincides with pubic and axillary hair growth, stimulated by the increased secretion of estrogens and growth hormone. Menarche follows 1 or 2 years later. The expanding growth center of the breast may form a temporary round firm mass, which resembles a fibroadenoma. This usually appears in the superolateral portion of the subareolar region. This temporary condensation disappears gradually in about 3 months.

The breast duct systems further elongate and branch during the pubertal phase and form the final adult breast. The cyclic menstrual changes in breast tissue are often quite marked during the third, fourth, and fifth decades. A concerted effect of estrogen, progesterone, and prolactin induces epithelial and stromal cell hypertrophy as well as intracellular edema. These changes occur during the luteal phase and often peak at ovulation and menstruation.

The changes of pregnancy represent the final chapter of breast growth and development. Acinar development at the distal end of each terminal duct occurs under the influence of increasing levels of progesterone, estriol, other estrogens, and prolactin. The production and release of milk are finally realized with the release of prolactin and oxytocin at the time of parturition.

During the postmenopausal years the breast epithelium becomes atrophic, and the previously dense stroma is replaced by fat. This fatty metamorphosis is a progressive process throughout old age.

ANATOMY

The paired hemispheres of breast tissue are attached on their planoconcave surface against the fascia of the ventral chest wall from the parasternal to the anterior axillary line covering the second through seventh ribs. Vascular supply is from the axillary vessels through the upper outer quadrants and through perforating internal mammary vessels via the parasternal and intercostal spaces.

The innervation of the breast enters the breast skin and the substance from the lateral segmental sensory nerves of the second through sixth thoracic segments. Hyperextension injuries of the neck will commonly irritate one or more of these nerves, causing a patient to complain of breast pain.

The functional unit of the mammary gland is the lactiferous lobe. The distal end of each lobe empties through the nipple, where it is firmly supported by dense connective tissue. Just below the nipple the lactiferous duct is wider for 1.5 to 2.0 cm. This preterminal dilatation is named the lactiferous sinus and represents a milk reservoir for the lactating breast. Associated with the distensibility of the subareolar duct system is a reduction in the supporting connective tissue. This makes the subareolar portion of the breast much softer than the more peripheral breast tissue. In many cases palpation of the subareolar area reveals a cuplike depression, which is surrounded by a ring of nodular peripheral breast tissue of a more dense nature. This can simulate the apex of a volcano mountain.

The distribution of lobes throughout the breast is quite asymmetric. Fewer than 20% of the ducts are formed in the medial half of the breast. Approximately 30% extend deep below the areolar region in the central portion of the breast. More than 50% of the ducts branch laterally, mostly upward in the tail of Spence toward the axilla extending over and under the pectoralis muscle group.

The supporting structures of the breast are fascial. The breast is contained in a fascial envelope, its superficial layer being subcutaneous and its deep layer adjacent to the fascia of the chest wall muscles. Fascial septa separate each lactifer-

ous lobe into a separate entity. These fascial partitions extend from the deep to the superficial fascial envelope. In the superior aspect of the breast, these fascial supports are thickest, presumably because of gravity traction, and are called Cooper's ligaments. This area presents a dense sensation to palpation in many larger breasts, called by some "Cooper's thickening."

The fat of the breast composes a significant proportion of the breast volume. It occurs as a 1 to 3 cm layer between the skin and the superficial fascia. With age, as atrophic changes affect the ductal and stromal elements, replacement by fatty metamorphosis characterizes the senile breast. The fatty tissue in the most dependent portion of the breast often becomes edematous and indurated as a function of gravity and dependency. This indurated area is know as the inframammary ridge. It is quite dense in some older women, and its medialmost portion can mimic a tumor.

The lymphatics of the breast drain mostly to the axilla and then medially along the axillary vein. Most of these lymphatics drain around and under the pectoral muscles, although some pathways do exist through and between the musculature (Rotter's nodes). The medial and centromedial areas of the breast contain lymphatics that course toward the sternum, perforate the intercostal spaces, and drain into the internal mammary chain inside the thorax. Lesser pathways of drainage include epigastric, supraclavicular, and anterior cervical lymphatics.

DISEASES OF THE BREAST

Inflammation

Inflammation in the breast most freqently occurs during the puerperium. Although maceration and traumatic dermatitis of the areolar skin occur with suckling, these are usually mild. Obstruction of the outflow of milk in the lactiferous duct occurs occasionally, usually in the nipple itself. With continued milk production behind the obstructed area, increased pressure develops within all branches of the obstructed lobe. This fullness and pain represent a "caked" segment of breast tissue. Proper treatment of this condition includes efforts to relieve the obstruction with manual expression of milk, suckling along with reduction in the luminal pressure of the lactiferous system by the local application of cold compresses or ice packs, or both. Cold application reduces the breast metabolism and thereby inhibits milk production. Conversely, application of heat to the engorged lactating breast will increase milk production and induce further intraluminal pressure increase.

Continuing congestion of a lactiferous unit will lead to segmental mastitis with increased pain and systemic manifestations. When fever appears with mastitis and there is no evidence of abscess formation, resolution will usually follow the addition of broad-spectrum antibiotics to the ice and drainage program.

After approximately 1 week of continued mastitis, abscess formation may occur. This requires drainage by large-needle aspiration or surgical incision. Radial incisions should be avoided because of resulting unsightly scars. Appropriate antibiotics should be instituted after specific bacteriologic sensitivity studies. Cultures of puerperal breast abscesses usually show staphylococci or streptococci.

Nonseptic inflammation can occur at any time following trauma or spontaneous rupture of macrocystic disease into the breast tissue. These inflammatory reactions are often prolonged in resolution. If continued improvement occurs and there are no signs of malignancy, conservative therapy is indicated. However, in many cases biopsies must be carried out to exclude inflammatory carcinoma. Aspiration for culture and cytologic examination can be very helpful in supporting a plan for either conservative or operative treatment.

Breast Discharges

After "priming" effects of more than 5 months of pregnancy, with elevated production of estrogens, progesterone, and prolactin, the onset of breast milk secretion is stimulated by the withdrawal of estrogen and progesterone and continued pituitary prolactin release. The breast acini and lobular epithelium respond by milk production in the presence of proper nutrition and cell energy levels. This requires caloric energy, rest, hydration, insulin, cortisol, and thyroxine support.

In addition to epithelial secretion, the breast duct systems require oxytocin stimulation of their musculature to effect the milk let-down or excretory phase of lactation. Oxytocin release as a reflex response follows stimulation of the cervix or chest wall structures.

Coincident with the onset of lactation, the supporting stroma of the breast undergoes an edematous phase. This engorgement can be delayed or suppressed by exogenous sex steroid administration at the time of delivery.

After experiencing lactation, the breast may maintain a low-grade secretory activity throughout life. Therefore, it is not unusual to find a pigmented nipple secretion from both breasts of a multiparous patient. The source of this pigment is not clear. Normal breast secretions do not contain blood. Tests for occult blood are therefore helpful in evaluating a green or brown discharge from the nipple.

Patients who present with spontaneous, nonpuerperal lactation should be evaluated by measurement of serum prolactin levels and by thyroid function tests. Elevations of prolactin should be further characterized by repeating the prolactin levels, obtaining computed tomography scans or magnetic resonance scans of the sella turcica, and obtaining measurements of visual fields to detect prolactinomas or parapituitary tumors. Treatment of hyperprolactinemia can usually be successful with oral bromocriptine. Patients failing to respond or maintain their response should be considered for pituitary surgery or irradiation. Psychotropic drugs, such as phenothiazines or haloperidol, can cause hyperprolactinemia and nonpuerperal lactation. Occasionally, chest wall trauma or surgery can cause galactorrhea.

Unilateral discharge that is clear and sticky or that contains blood requires further evaluation (Leis and Pilnik, 1970). Cytologic study of this fluid is of some value. The first fluid expressed is usually hypocellular and yields little cytologic information. Breast material prepared for cytologic examination must be placed on a slide with some special features for adherence. A thin coating of albumin or a totally frosted slide will suffice. Serial smears will demonstrate increased cytologic material since the fluid from the higher levels of the lactiferous system contains more cells. A persistent, bloody discharge is an indication for segmental resection of the involved lobe.

Technique of Nipple Flap Duct Resection

Careful inspection of the location of the duct within the nipple helps locate the lobe involved. Confirmatory evidence is obtained by milking the segment suspected and demonstrating further discharge. A periareolar incision is performed in the appropriate quadrant, and undermining of the skin centrally and peripherally permits sufficient retraction of the areolar skin to expose the lactiferous ducts. A meticulous dissection is necessary under the nipple to avoid disruption of the thin-walled lactiferous sinuses. Duct ectasia, if present, will be apparent grossly at this point in the dissection. Gentle occlusion of the suspected duct when identified should be followed by further milking action to confirm its positive identity. When the involved duct or ducts are identified, they are transected. With gentle traction on the transected ducts, segmental dissection and removal of the involved lobe can be completed. Extensive branching of the duct system is found early in the dissection, and the lactiferous lobe broadens quickly. A gradually tapering dissection will not include the entire lobe.

Indolent drainage or crusting may occur with any skin disease of the nipple. Nevertheless, because Paget's disease may appear as a benign, inflammatory process, the gynecologist should be suspicious of this disease whenever the nipple appears abnormal. Unfortunately, this malignant ulceration of the nipple has been treated frequently as eczema for weeks or months before diagnosis. If the biopsy results reveal Paget's disease and no masses are detectable in the breast, the cure rate by modified radical mastectomy approximates 90%. The glass slide contact smear for cytologic study will often expedite the diagnosis of Paget's disease.

Breast Pain

Pain in one or both breasts is a common complaint. Frequently this symptom does not represent breast disease but is referred to the breast from other regional disorders. Neck injuries are commonly followed by cervical and thoracic nerve root radiculitis. If the radicles involved include the upper thoracic segments, breast pain may be the only complaint. Similarly, pain arising from the rib and costal cartilages will often present as breast pain. Local palpation with rib compression will localize the pain to its musculoskeletal source. The diffuse anterior thoracic attachment of the pectoral muscles makes them a common source of breast-related pain. Active adduction of the arm by the patient will exacerbate this pain and clearly localize it to the muscle.

Painful engorgement and edema of the breast during the luteal phase of the menstrual cycle are a difficult problem. Dietary salt restriction may be helpful.

Suppression of the biphasic fluctuations of estrogen and progesterone associated with the normal menstrual cycle may reduce breast discomfort. This may be accomplished by the use of an oral contraceptive with low estrogen content. Similar suppression may be obtained by continuous administration of progestins such as medroxyprogesterone acetate in a dose of 20 mg daily. Methyltestosterone exerts an antiestrogenic effect on the breast and is usually given as a 10-mg sublingual tablet one or two times daily. If, however, the monthly dose exceeds 300 mg, some patients may note acne, hoarseness, or increased facial hair growth. Danazol and tamoxifen as potent antiestrogens, although quite expensive, have been successful in controlling difficult cases of mastodynia.

A host of other therapies that are less disturbing to the patient's metabolism have traditionally been offered to women suffering from pain associated with benign cyclic breast changes. Vitamin E therapy (400–600 units/day) has been associated with improved symptoms in many patients treated. Elimination of cigarettes, caffeine, and other methylxanthines and reduction of stress factors has been proposed by Minton et al. (1979) to quiet the overactive cyclic adenosine monophosphate–guanosine monophosphate associated with hyperplastic fibrocystic breasts. In our experience, this seems effective. Administration of vitamins A, B-complex, and C, as well as iodine and selenium, have also been recommended.

Inflammatory conditions in the breast usually produce pain. The comforting admonition that pain is not a sign of serious trouble is often relayed to patients complaining of breast pain. It must be remembered that approximately 20% of patients with breast cancer complain of pain in the area of their tumor. Of course, the vast majority of those with inflammatory breast cancer complain of pain. Immediate aspiration, cytologic examination, and bacteriologic cultures will help expedite the differential diagnosis and distinguish between inflammation and tumor.

LUMPS IN THE BREAST

Carcinoma

Carcinoma of the breast most often presents as a lump. Careful evaluation of breast lumps with maximum acuity is a significant contribution to patient care. Appropriate and rapid use of ancillary procedures assures maximum diagnostic evaluation.

Conditions that present as a dominant lump include carcinoma, fibrocystic disease, fibroadenomas, giant fibroadenomas or sarcomas, fat necrosis, and other uncommon breast lesions. These include galactoceles, sebaceous cysts, histiocytomas, leiomyomas, lipomas, adenolipomas, granular cell tumors, neurofibromas, sarcoidosis, and tuberculosis.

Carcinoma usually presents as a painless, firm, deep-seated mass. Local infiltration may cause fixation of the tumor to the chest wall. This is elicted by adduction of the arm to set the pectoral muscles and fascia. Fixation or edema of the skin are other signs of advancing malignancy. Altered vascularity and increased metabolism of the tumor produce increased heat as measured by thermography or skin erythema after alcohol applications. The characteristic palpable mass that exhibits density contrast on mammograms and the gritty sensation of the needle tip at the time of aspiration are due to the very dense reaction in the stroma adjacent to the tumor, the desmoplastic response. Cytologic findings of the needle aspirate are suspicious or positive for malignancy in 95% of cases. Needle, incisional, or excisional biopsy is necessary to confirm the diagnosis. Ulceration of the skin and satellite-tumor nodules in the same breast indicate advanced disease.

Mirror-image biopsy of the opposite breast or upper outer quadrant site is recommended at the time of definitive surgery. Screening for evidence of metastatic disease by radioactive bone scanning and by measurement of liver and bone enzymes should precede therapy. At the time of original diagnosis and workup, it is wise to register the status of tumor markers from the same blood sampling. These levels may be valuable in general prognosis and in assessment of further therapy. The carcinoembryonic antigen (CEA) is being used for this purpose. Table 10-1 shows primary tumor, regional node, and metastasies (TNM) staging.

Proper treatment for breast cancer is undergoing reevaluation at this time. Two characteristics of the disease make it difficult to plan therapeutic stratagems. First is the multifocal nature of the process. Careful examination of cancerous breasts by Gall and later by Gallagher has revealed multiple foci of cancer origin in up to 50% of cases. Results of random biopsies of the opposite breast show bilateral disease in up to 20% of cases both in Urban's (1969) experience and in our

TABLE 10-1.

Staging System for Cancer of the Breast

T	Primary tumor measurement, preoperative (rule or caliper, xeromammography)
T0	No tumor
TIS	Preinvasive carcinoma (CIS), noninfiltrating intraductal carcinoma or Paget's disease of nipple and no demonstrable tumor
T1	Tumor size 2 cm
T1a	No fixation to pectoral fascia and/or muscle
T1b	Fixation to pectoral fascia and/or muscle
T2	Tumor size 2-5 cm
T2a	No fixation to pectoral fascia and/or muscle
T2b	Fixation to pectoral fascia and/or muscle
T3	Tumor size more than 5 cm
T3a	No fixation to pectoral fascia and/or muscle
T3b	Fixation to pectoral fascia and/or muscle
T4	Tumor of any size with direct extension to chest wall or skin (not including skin dimpling or nipple retraction)
T4a	Fixation to chest wall
T4b	Edema, infiltration or ulceration of skin (including peau d'orange), or satellite nodules confined to the same breast
T4c	Both (T4a and T4b)
N	Regional lymph nodes
N0	No palpable homolateral axillary nodes
N1	Movable homolateral axillary nodes
N1a	Metastasis not suspected
N1b	Metastasis suspected
N2	Fixed homolateral axillary nodes
N3	Homolateral supraclavicular or infraclavicular nodes or edema of the arm
M	Distant metastases
M0	No evidence of distant metastases
M1	Distant metastases present, including skin involvement beyond the breast area

Stage-Grouping

TIS	Carcinoma in situ			
Invasive carcinoma				
Stage I	T1a	N0	or N1a	M0
	T1b	N0	or N1a	M0
Stage II	T0	N1b		
	T1a	N1b		
	T1b	N1b		
	T2a	N0	or N1a	M0
	T2b	N0	or N1a	
	T2a	N1b		
	T2b	N1b		
Stage III	Any T3	with any N		
	Any T4	with any N		M0
	Any T	with	N2	
	Any T	with	N3	
Stage IV	Any T		Any N	with M1

own. The second problem in breast cancer treatment lies in the fact that up to 70% of the patients have disseminated disease at the time of diagnosis. At this time, programs of castration, antiestrogenic treatment, and chemotherapy given as adjuvant therapy have not made impressive inroads on ultimate recurrence.

A dramatic clinic alert from the National Cancer Institute in 1988 pointed out that all patients with breast cancer, with or without regional lymph node metastases, apparently benefit from adjuvant therapy. This therapy includes chemotherapy for younger patients and hormonal therapy with tamoxifen for patients more than age 50 years, especially for those patients with estrogen or progesterone receptors in their tumors. It should be carefully noted that this benefit was measured in both disease-free survival and in long-term survival. Although these results are encouraging, both immediate and late detrimental side effects from chemotherapy can be expected. Late complications of tamoxifen, such as genital tract tumors, osteoporosis, or vascular disease, have not been ruled out (Early Breast Cancer Trialists' Collaborative Group, 1988). The possibil-

ity that adjuvant immunotherapy might make an important difference should be explored.

Either total mastectomy with axillary lymph node sampling or removal of the tumor followed by total breast tangential radiation with 5,000 to 6,000 rad and axillary node sampling seem interchangeably adequate for local control. Treatment of metastatic disease is diverse and depends on the estrogen and progesterone receptor assays of the tumor, as well as on the clinical setting within which the metastases arise. Probably the discovery of effective preventive measures and improvements in early detection are the only real hopes for improvement in breast cancer survival.

Breast Carcinoma in Situ

There are two breast carcinomas in situ (CIS). Both confer a 10-fold increased risk of subsequent invasive cancer relative to that of comparable women who have never undergone a breast biopsy.

The first, noninvasive intraductal carcinoma (IDC), occurs mostly in postmenopausal women, has trebled in frequency with the use of modern film screen mammography, and signifies an in-

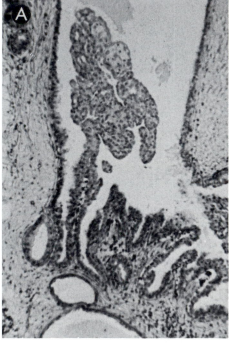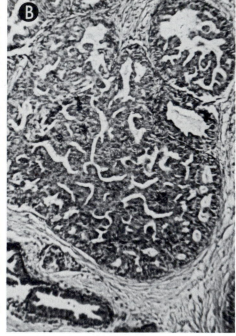

FIG 10–1.
Examples of breast epithelial hyperplasia. **A,** intraductal papilloma: benign overgrowth in the duct lumen. **B,** intraductal hyperplasia: benign overgrowth fills ducts. *(Continued.)*

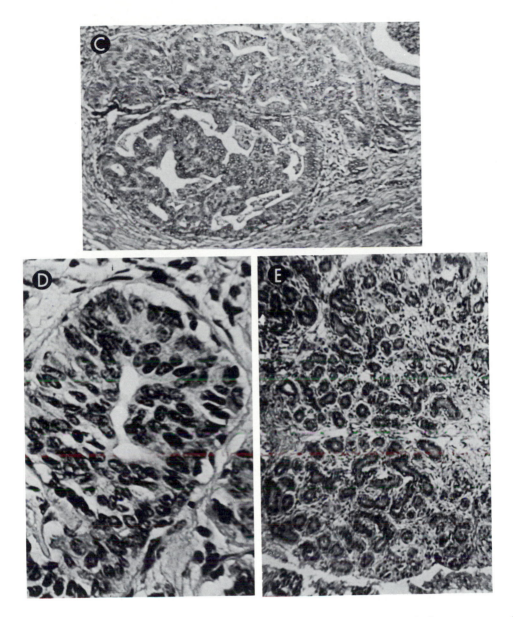

FIG 10—1 (cont.).

C, intraductal carcinoma: necrotic areas are evident. Cellular atypia may be mild. **D,** atypical blunt duct adenosis: benign acting but may appear wild. **E,** lobular hyperplasia: active lobule may precede CIS and carcinoma simplex.

creased cancer risk of the same segment of the same breast in which it arises (Fig 10—1).

The second form, lobular carcinoma in situ (LCIS), is seen mostly in premenopausal women, is always found coincidentally in about 2.5% of breast biopsy specimens for any reason, and signifies an increased risk of cancer for both breasts equally.

The fine clustered calcifications associated with IDC are surely responsible for its more frequent detection recently. There are no identifying characteristics of LCIS except the careful evaluation by pathologists of all material obtained at all breast resections.

Recommended preventive surgery for these lesions is simple mastectomy in the case of IDC and bilateral simple mastectomy in the case of LCIS. Growing interest in radiotherapy or simply close surveillance after wide excision of the lesions is being investigated. In practice, the commonest management of IDC is total mastectomy. The commonest course for the LCIS patient is close surveillance (Shirley, 1987).

Fibrocystic Disease

Dominant lumps due to fibrocystic disease are common. Large cysts, 1 to 10 cm in diameter, are easily evacuated by aspiration. Up to 80 ml of cyst fluid may be removed. This fluid may be spread on a slide for cytologic study or mixed with 50% alcohol for cell-block histologic study. If aspiration-evacuation of a cyst returns the breast to normal, follow-up examination in 3 or 4 weeks is suggested.

No longer should patients with a previous diagnosis of fibrocystic changes be denied health insurance. A consensus of 30 breast pathology experts was held in New York, Oct 3 to 5, 1985, to establish the relationship of fibrocystic disease to breast cancer. The following classification was established comparing the risk of subsequent invasive breast cancer associated with various fibrocystic diagnoses with the risk of comparable women who had never undergone a breast biopsy (Table 10–2).

It is reasonable to reassure a woman complaining of pain or lumpiness in her breasts that she does not have a serious problem. The time has come to recognize that women's breasts are often normally lumpy, painful, or tender. "Fibrocystic change" is not a disease. It is not helpful to initiate a lifelong career of worrying by telling a patient that she is "cystic" (Shirley, 1987).

Comparison of breast hyperplasia to atypical hyperplasia of the endometrium is tempting. Similar age groups and hormonal influences are shared by the two conditions. The progression from atypical hyperplasia to carcinoma, however, is better established in the endometrium.

Recurrent discomfort, cysts, and tumor formation are common in some women. Attempts at therapy similar to that for cyclic congestion symptoms are occasionally successful, but, unfortunately, a few patients in their fourth decade are plagued by relentless and progressive fibrocystic disease.

Fibroadenomas

Fibroadenomas usually present as characteristic firm, round, nontender mobile masses, which

TABLE 10–2.

Diagnosis and Risk Status*†

Diagnosis	Risk Status
Adenosis, sclerosing or florid	No increased risk
Apocrine metaplasia	No increased risk
Macrocysts, microcysts, or both	No increased risk
Duct ectasia	No increased risk
Fibroadenoma	No increased risk
Fibrosis	No increased risk
Hyperplasia, mild	No increased risk
Mastitis (inflammation)	No increased risk
Periductal mastitis	No increased risk
Squamous metaplasia	No increased risk
Hyperplasia, moderate or florid, solid or papillary	Slightly increased risk (1.5–2 times)
Papilloma with fibrovascular core	Slightly increased risk (1.5–2 times)
Atypical hyperplasia (borderline lesion), ductal or lobular	Moderately increased risk (5 times)

*From Winchester DP: The relationship of fibrocystic disease to breast cancer. *Am Coll Surg Bull* 1986; 71:29. Used by permission.
†Mild hyperplasia exists when the epithelium is greater than two, but not more than four, cells deep. Moderate and florid hyperplasia refer to more extensive degrees of epithelial proliferation. "Atypical hyperplasia" (ductal or lobular) as used here refers to lesions that have some features of CIS but not enough to make an unequivical diagnosis of CIS, the so-called borderline lesion.

commonly occur in young women. Their subcutaneous location has led to the term *poppability*, which describes their unusual mobility. During attempted aspiration, they "bite" the needle with a rubbery tenacity that makes smooth withdrawal difficult. The aspirate usually reveals scant cellular material with benign duct cells and fibroblasts on cytologic examination.

Although the diagnosis of fibroadenoma is usually obvious in most cases, removal is still recommended. A carcinoma does occasionally masquerade as a fibroadenoma, and mammography may not be helpful in detecting early malignancy. Furthermore, a few fibroadenomas posses unusual growth potential and may progress to the "giant" fibroadenoma or cystosarcoma phyllodes. Existing fibroadenomas grow dramatically under the influence of high levels of estrogen. This may occur during pregnancy, and the very rapid growth may suggest a malignant lesion. The mass should be excised under local anesthesia as soon as it is detected.

Fat Necrosis

Fat necrosis has been mentioned previously in the discussion of inflammatory processes. Unfortunately, this lesion may look and feel exactly the same as carcinoma. Therefore, it is important to use all of the adjunctive diagnostic procedures before proceeding to surgery. Aspiration is usually less gritty than with cancer, and the cytologic examination is characterized by inflammatory cells. Mammography is not always helpful in making a precise diagnosis.

Other Lumps

Adolescent breast buds, prominent subareolar lactiferous sinuses, thickenings of Cooper's ligament, prominent inframammary ridges, and the more prominent tail of Spence have been described. Both breasts should be examined and compared to determine the normality of lumplike findings. Fat lobules and hormonally stimulated breast lobules may seem to be dominant lumps if the patient is examined during the luteal phase. Reexamination on day 5, 6, or 7 of the next menstrual cycle will reveal the temporary and cyclic nature of these masses.

Techniques of Evaluating Breast Lumps

Friction-Free Examination

The breast skin can be rendered friction free by the use of powder, thin lubricating jelly, or warm soap and water, thus improving an appreciation of breast structures by palpation. Previous biopsy sites are better delineated as saucerized defects or linear suture line densities. Subareolar prominences can be distinguished as a circular ring of uniform structures. Improved delineation of questionable areas in the breast by this simple approach will reduce the incidence of unnecessary breast resections and, perhaps more important, will increase the incidence of patients having early malignancy detected.

The hot rinse after the soap and water examination serves two purposes. The soap is removed to avoid an itchy aftermath, and the hot compress effect tends to promote nipple discharge and will improve the yield of nipple discharge samples that can be tested for occult blood. Bloody or sticky yellow nipple secretions should be further evaluated. Guaiactivity in the nipple secretion also should be investigated (Chaudary et al., 1982).

Aspiration Cytology

Needle aspiration of the breast is a simple procedure. The mass or area of suspicion is held between two fingers of the left hand. Cutaneous spray with ethyl chloride until the skin is blanched provides adequate anesthesia for this puncture. A 20-gauge needle attached to a 10-ml syringe is quickly thrust into the center of the area. This syringe and needle are previously prepared by aspirating a small amount of Ringer's lactate into the dead space of the syringe and needle lumen. When the fluid is expressed, approximately 0.05 ml of fluid remains in the lumen of the needle and syringe tip. After insertion of the needle, vigorous suction is applied to the syringe while multiple small tracts are made in the breast tissue.

Aspirated cyst fluid is spread thinly on an albumin-coated or totally frosted slide and sprayed with cytologic fixative and submitted as a Papanicolaou smear. If no cyst fluid is obtained, the contents of the needle are expressed onto a similar slide, and it is rocked to and fro until the vehicular fluid is evaporated. It is then sprayed with the cytologic fixative (Abele et al., 1983; Bell et al., 1983; Fig 10–2).

Aspiration of "vagomas," or questionable areas of thickening or lumpiness for cytology, will help to reduce the error factor involved in evaluating these difficult areas often found during breast examination. The traditional use of mammography and follow-up examination for observation of changes has a built-in failure rate of approximately 20% of cases and a delay in many more cases. Use of aspiration cytology in this setting can improve our speed and accuracy of diagnosis.

Mammography

Mammography has become an important diagnostic procedure for the detection of breast cancer even in the presence of a normal physical examination. The procedure is of major assistance in screening high-risk and difficult to examine patients. This technique not only is accurate in predicting a diagnosis but also scans the remainder of the breast tissue for nonpalpable disease. Mammograms cannot, repeat *not,* be substituted for biopsy of a dominant mass in the breast. Densities and fine-speckled calcifications are suspicious findings that are due to the dense stromal reaction around a breast malignancy. Spiculation, or radiating lines, and the skin changes of thickening or retraction are suspicious findings presumably due

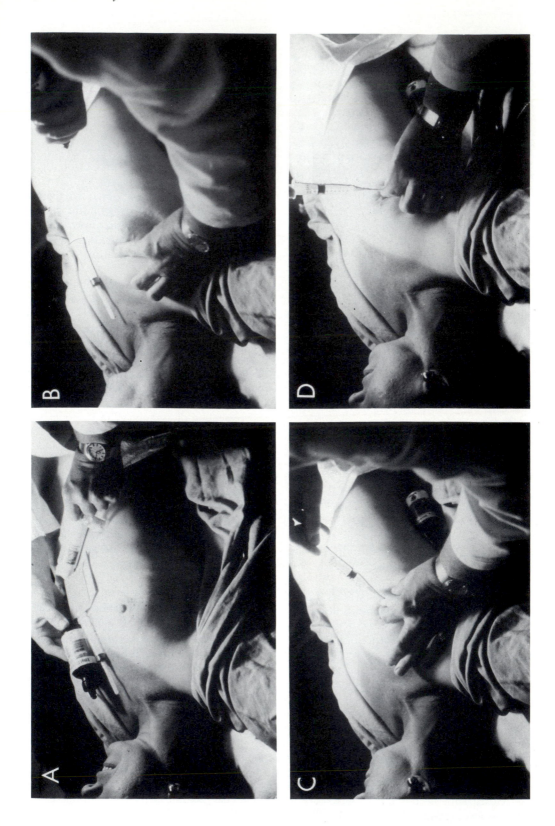

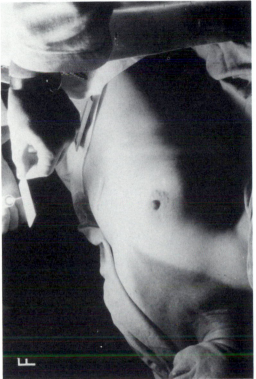

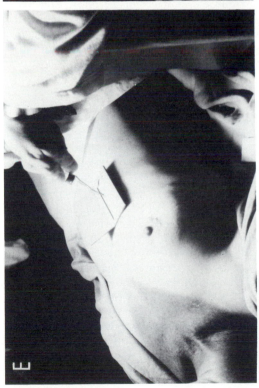

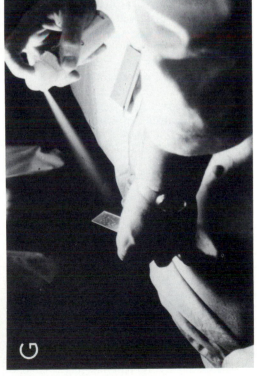

FIG 10–2.

Fine-needle aspiration of the breast for cytologic study. **A,** necessary equipment is shown: syringe (10 ml) and needle (20 gauge), ethyl chloride, cytology spray fixative, and totally frosted slide. **B,** appropriate area of breast is sprayed to an ice spot with ethyl chloride. **C,** puncture of area with syringe-needle combination premoistened with Ringers's lactate is followed by firm suction traction on the syringe. **D,** multiple-tract aspiration of the area is facilitated by pinching the skin up with the needle when backing up to start a new tract. **E,** the dead-space fluid and cellular material are sprayed on the totally frosted glass slide. **F,** the cellular material is gently and evenly spread out. **G,** the still-moist (slightly) smear is sprayed with cytology fixative.

to adjacent infiltration by carcinoma. Despite the excellent diagnostic aid provided by mammography, up to 25% of cancers do not show characteristics that permit an early diagnosis of malignancy. Obviously, then, biopsy must be performed when a persistent dominant mass is detected.

Another inadequacy of mammography is the impervious density of the breast tissue in young women. Mammography will detect an increasing number of breast cancers after the age of 40 years, since, as breast tissue is replaced by fat, radiation detectability improves.

A federally funded breast demonstration project showed significant pickups by mammography only after age 45 years (Eddy et al., 1988). However, the American Cancer Society has recommended *mammography between age 35 and 40 years. It should be repeated every 1 or 2 years from age 40 to 50 years and then yearly.* Tort risk management would suggest that we comply.

Dr. Daniel Kopans, director of mammography at the Massachusetts General Hospital, suggests a slight modification of the American Cancer Society guidelines. His plan is to perform annual mammograms from age 40 to 50 years and then to space them out progressively as women get older. This plan would focus on the age when CIS and other premalignant states can be found with a greater frequency as breast imaging technology continues to improve (Shirley, 1987).

Modern mammography can indeed detect ductal carcinoma at earlier stages (Fig 10–3). Clinicians should seek mammography for their patients with modern film-screen or xerogram equipment, with dedicated mammogram technicians, and with radiologists who are in the habit of using magnifying lenses to look for faint calcifications.

Thermography

Continued research may ultimately improve the techniques and interpretation of thermographic mammometry. The wide variety of heat distribution in various breast diseases markedly reduces the precision of thermographic diagnosis. Thermography is seldom employed at the Boston Hospital for Women division of the Brigham and Women's Hospital.

Ultrasound

Although diagnostic ultrasound seems totally safe, its applicability to breast imaging is limited.

Both contact and immersion ultrasonography are able to document that a dominant mass is fluid filled or solid. Of course, fine-needle aspiration can obtain this information more directly.

Breast Biopsy

A complete evaluation of any lump in the breast is possible only by excisional biopsy and histologic examination of the tissue. In women over the age of 50 years, any dominant breast lump is an indication for immediate excision. In younger patients, especially if menstruation is still occurring, reexamination should be scheduled after the next menstrual period and excision performed if the mass remains or becomes larger.

Technique of Breast Biopsy.—Three major considerations affect the choice of the incision for biopsy. First, a relatively central location is desirable so that the subsequent mastectomy incision will not be compromised. Second, the cosmetic appearance of the scar is usually excellent if the skin incision is areolar or periareolar. Langer's lines in the skin of the breast are generally circumferential around the breast globe. Last, radial incisions should *never* be made in the breast skin. Within the substance of the breast, however, radial or elliptical incisions should be used in young women to preserve potential lactational function. Extensive skin undermining is sometimes necessary to reach the tumor or to ensure adequate exposure for proper dissection and closure of the breast excision site.

Incision within the breast to achieve removal of the lesion with a margin of normal breast tissue and a properly elliptical biopsy defect can be confusing if the breast is distorted with traction by hooks, clamps, or forceps. A freehand scalpel incision is usually preferred. This scalpel blade should be small to avoid cutting the retracted skin edges.

Hemostasis is best achieved after the biopsy specimen has been removed. The wound is packed tightly with sponges, and then a search for significant "bleeders" will systematically reveal the vessels to be sutured, ligated, or coagulated. Compression suture-ligatures may be necessary if the vessel is detected in dense breast tissue. Minor oozing from the cut edge of the breast tissue can be controlled by compression approximation of the cut edges. The breast-closing sutures should all be held as an entire row of sutures to assure a smooth closure. Premature tying of one suture will make subsequent suture placement difficult

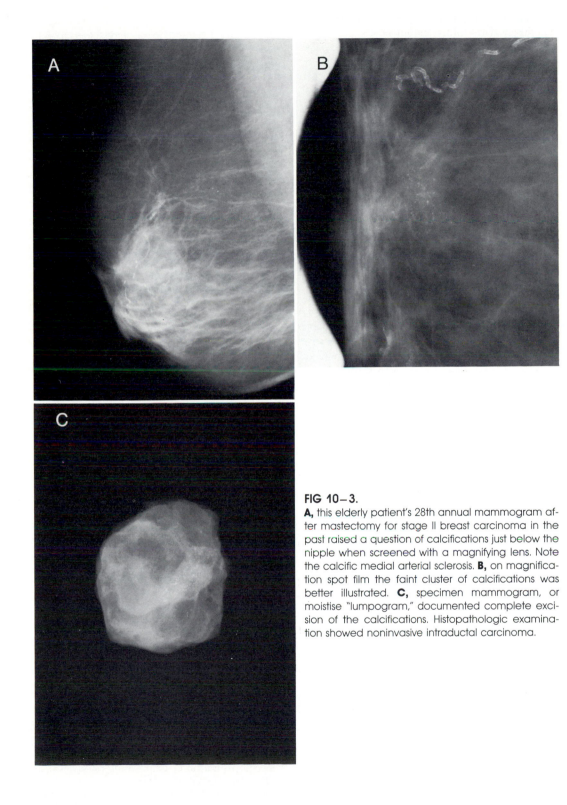

FIG 10–3.
A, this elderly patient's 28th annual mammogram after mastectomy for stage II breast carcinoma in the past raised a question of calcifications just below the nipple when screened with a magnifying lens. Note the calcific medial arterial sclerosis. **B,** on magnification spot film the faint cluster of calcifications was better illustrated. **C,** specimen mammogram, or moistise "lumpogram," documented complete excision of the calcifications. Histopathologic examination showed noninvasive intraductal carcinoma.

and lead to a distorted lumplike biopsy site that will falsely alarm future examiners.

Compression dressing for 6 hours can be changed to a light dressing before discharge of the patient on the night of biopsy. Firm support with few limitations in activity are the general rules of postoperative care. Subcutaneous cuticular closure of the skin with polyglycolic acid suture material allows for the most trouble-free recovery.

Biopsy to investigate mammographic abnormalities is a special problem. By careful measurements of the x-rays and the patient's breast, an accurate estimation of the location is possible. Calcific densities may be verified by radiographic study of the biopsy specimen. Partial slicing, or "bread-loafing," of the specimen before x-ray will help the pathologist find the calcific area.

Areas of density or radiating lines of spiculation cannot be verified by specimen radiology because their appearance depends on relative density within the breast tissue. Biopsy of a nonpalpable mammogram abnormality requires preoperative localization by placement of a Kopan's wire or other similar radiopaque marker in the vicinity of the designated area. Repeat mammography then pinpoints the area to be resected and allows a clear diagnostic evaluation with minimal breast tissue removal. This system has been quite helpful in avoiding the embarrassing nuisance of missing the target shadow.

Abnormal biopsy material should be submitted in ice for determination of estrogen and progesterone-binding protein of the tumor. A fresh portion of tumor, 1 by 1 by 1 cm, shipped in dry ice should be rushed to a laboratory equipped to perform these assays.

EARLY DETECTION OF BREAST CANCER

With judicious use of the aforementioned tools and biopsy of all dominant masses, the detection of breast cancer before the stage of regional or distant metastases should be relatively more common. The grouping of patients at especially high risk for the development of breast cancer allows the focus of special attention on them for early detection. Identifiable patients for inclusion in this type of diagnostic breast clinic include:

1. Patients with previous unilateral breast cancer.

TABLE 10–3.

Stage I Rates of Breast Cancer at the Brigham and Women's Hospital

Period	Stage I Rate (%0)
1905–1946	36
1947–1961	42
1964–1967	52
1971	54
1972	67
1973	64
1974	50
1975	81

2. Patients whose previous biopsies have revealed epithelial abnormalities with premalignant potential, such as intraductal hyperplasia, papillomatosis, lobular neoplasia, or carcinoma in situ (see Fig 10–1).
3. Patients with two epidemiologic risk factors from the following:
   a. Mother, sister, or daughter with breast cancer.
   b. Blood relatives with premenopausal breast cancer.
   c. Blood relatives with bilateral breast cancer.
   d. Nulliparous patients or patients whose first pregnancy was after the age of 30 years (Cole and MacMahon, 1973).

Another helpful adjuvant to encourage early diagnosis is to lower the threshold for biopsy. Patients who are not suspicious for malignancy may be biopsied as outpatients or day-service patients and discharged the same day. If the patient knows that no provisions for immediate mastectomy have been made, her breast sampling process will be much less of an ordeal.

Success in early breast cancer detection is manifested by a significant percentage of the patients having negative lymph nodes at the time of treatment. Improvement in the stage I rate of breast cancer cases at the Brigham and Women's Hospital is depicted in Table 10–3.

REFERENCES

Abele JS, Miller TR, Goodson WH, et al: Fine-needle aspiration of palpable breast masses. *Arch Surg* 1983; 118:859.

Bell DA, et al: Role of aspiration cytology in the

diagnosis and management of mammary lesions in office practice. *Cancer* 1983; 51:1182–1189.

Brooks PG, Gart S, Heldfond A, et al: Measuring the effect of caffeine restriction of fibrocystic disease. *J Reprod Med* 1981; 26:279.

Chaudary MA, et al: Nipple discharge: The diagnostic value of testing for occult blood. *Ann Surg* 1982; 196:651.

Cole P, MacMahon B: Epidemiology of breast cancer. *J Natl Cancer Inst* 1973; 51:21.

Early Breast Cancer Trialists' Collaborative Group: Effects of adjuvant tamoxifen and of cytotoxic therapy on mortality in early breast cancer: An overview of 61 randomized trials among 28,896 women. *N Engl J Med* 1988; 319:1681.

Eddy DM, Hasselblad V, McGivney W, et al: The value of mammography screening in women under age 50 years. *JAMA* 1988; 259:1512.

Haagensen CD: *Diseases of the Breast*. Philadelphia, WB Saunders Co, 1971.

Leis HP Jr, Pilnik S: Nipple discharge. *Hosp Med,* November 1970, p 29.

Minton JP, Foecking MK, Webster DJI, et al: Caffeine, cyclic nucleotides, and breast disease. *Surgery* 1979; 86:105.

Reid DE, Christian CD: *Controversy in Obstetrics and Gynecology,* ed 2. Philadelphia, WB Saunders Co, 1974.

Shirley RL: Breast diseases: Old axioms and new concepts. *Postgrad Obstet Gynecol* 1987, vol 7.

Urban JA: Biopsy of the "normal breast" in treating breast cancer. *Surg Clin North Am* 1969; 49:291–301.

Winchester DP: The relationship of fibrocystic disease to breast cancer. *Am Coll Surg Bull* 1986; 71:29.

11 _____ Endometriosis*

Robert L. Barbieri, M.D.

Mark D. Hornstein, M.D.

Although endometriosis was described in detail more than 100 years ago, it continues to be one of the unsolved, enigmatic diseases affecting women. The first known report was written by Rokitansky in 1860, but following this only a few scattered reports appeared until about 1900, when Cullen and Meyer published extensive descriptions of their findings. Yet in 1921, Cattell and Swinton were able to document fewer than 20 reports of endometriosis in the world literature. In the same year, Sampson (1921) published the first of his series of reports, recording for posterity his theory of retrograde menstruation and implantation as the causative factor in the disease. His articles awakened wide interest, even controversy, in the subject, and today his theory kindles as much heated debate among physicians as it did following publication of his first reports.

Definitions.—Endometriosis may be defined as the presence of functioning endometrial tissue outside of the uterus but is usually confined to the pelvis in the region of the ovaries, uterosacral ligaments, cul-de-sac, and uterovesical peritoneum. The development and extension of endometrial tissue into the myometrium is termed adenomyosis. This disease entity seems unrelated histogenetically and is characterized by a different clinical situation. It should be iterated that the term endometriosis implies proliferating growth and function (usually bleeding) in an extrauterine site. An endometrioma may be defined as an area of endometriosis, usually in the ovary, that has enlarged sufficiently to be classified as a tumor.

*From Barbieri RL: *Curr Probl Obstet Gynecol Fertil* 1989; 12:9–31. Used by permission.

When an endometrioma is filled with old blood, resembling tarry or chocolate-colored syrupy fluid, it is commonly known as a "chocolate cyst." It should be remembered, however, that a corpus luteum hematoma may have an identical gross appearance, so that all chocolate cysts should not be considered to be caused by endometriosis without pathologic confirmation. Even in bona fide endometriomas, the histologic picture may be confusing, since endometrial glands and stroma may become compressed by the pressure of the trapped blood, and the pathologist is unable to make a specific diagnosis. If the endometriosis is not completely burned out, close examination of the wall usually reveals numerous hemosiderin-laden macrophages, lymphocytes, and patches of condensed endometrial stroma without glands.

ETIOLOGY

The two most popular theories of histogenesis are the transport theory and the coelomic metaplasia theory.

The transport theory states that viable fragments of endometrium are carried to intraperitoneal sites by retrograde regurgitation through the oviducts or by transport via lymphatics or vascular channels. The vast majority of endometriotic implants are thought to arise from the regurgitation of small fragments of endometrium via the fallopian tubes. In support of the transport theory are the following observations: (1) during menstruation, retrograde regurgitation of desquamated endometrium has been observed at laparoscopy or laparotomy; (2) some desquamated menstrual endometrium is viable and can seed and grow in intraperitoneal locations; and (3) endometrial tissue can be found in pelvic lymphatic channels. The transport theory also provides a possible explanation for the presence of endometriosis in old laparotomy or laparoscopy sites and for the presence of endometriosis in such distant sites as the lung, pleura, arm, thigh, and pelvic lymph nodes.

The coelomic metaplasia theory states that the ovarian epithelium and pelvic peritoneal mesothelium are capable of differentiating into müllerian elements such as endometrium. The stimuli that cause the transformation of these epithelial elements into endometrium are poorly characterized. Inflammatory processes, however, such as the irritation of the pelvic peritoneum by regurgitated menstrual blood or acute infection, may be important stimuli for metaplasia.

The majority of authorities favor the retrograde transport theory over the coelomic metaplasia theory as the most likely explanation for the original source of endometriotic implants. There are, however, a number of findings yet to be explained by supporters of the retrograde transport theory, most important: Why don't all women with retrograde menstruation develop endometriosis? One possible answer to this question is that there is a dose response effect; only those women with retrograde menstruation of large amounts of endometrium develop endometriosis. Epidemiologic evidence that supports this concept will be presented later.

Another possibility is that immunologic surveillance varies among women and that women with deficiencies in certain immune functions fail to eradicate small implants of endometrium regurgitated into the peritoneal cavity.

A key concept in understanding the etiology of endometriosis is that hormonal factors are of central importance in the pathogenesis of this disease. The importance of hormonal factors is highlighted by the following clinical observations: (1) endometriosis is uncommon prior to the menarche and occurs infrequently after the menopause; (2) ovarian ablation usually results in complete and prompt regression of ectopically located endometrial glands and stroma (although scar tissue may persist); (3) endometriosis is rarely observed in amenorrheic women but is common in women with uninterrupted cyclic menstruation for more than 5 years; (4) endometriosis improves or stabilizes during episodes of physiologically induced (pregnancy) or artificially induced (hormonal)

amenorrhea; and (5) frequent pregnancies, if initiated early in reproductive life, appear to prevent the development of endometriosis.

Little experimental evidence concerning the hormonal requirements of the endometrial implants of endometriosis is available, but it is known that normal endometrium and the implants of endometriosis contain estrogen, androgen, and progesterone receptors. It is likely that the endometriotic implants retain patterns of hormonal responsiveness similar to those of normal endometrial cells. The following observations are true in normal endometrium: (1) estrogen in physiologic doses stimulates endometrial hyperplasia in a dose-dependent fashion if unopposed by progesterone, (2) androgens produce atrophy of the endometrium, (3) physiologic doses of progesterone support endometrial growth and secretory changes, and (4) pharmacologic doses of progestational agents produce a decidual reaction when adequate estrogen is present and atrophy when a hypoestrogenic environment exists (Table 11–1). To test the hypothesis that implants of endometriosis retain hormonal responses similar to those of normal endometrium, DiZerega et al. (1980) studied the effects of estrogen, progesterone, and placebo on the growth of peritoneal endometriotic implants in castrated monkeys. Estrogen alone was able to support the growth of the endometriotic tissue in the peritoneal cavity. In a hypoestrogenic, hypoprogestational environment, the endometriotic tissue atrophied. Progesterone alone was also able to support the growth of the endometriotic tissue. These hormonal responses of endometriotic tissue form the physiologic underpinning for effective hormonal therapy.

The pelvic peritoneum and ovary are the commonest anatomic sites involved by endometriosis, and both the peritoneal fluid and the ovaries contain very high concentrations of estradiol. In normal ovulatory women, the circulating estradiol

TABLE 11–1.

The Effects of Estrogens, Androgens, and Progestins on Endometrial Tissue

	Physiologic Doses	Pharmacologic Doses
Estrogens	Growth	Hyperplasia
Androgens	—	Atrophy
Progestins	Secretory changes	Decidual reaction

concentration usually does not exceed 0.4 ng/ml. However, the concentration of estradiol in cul-de-sac fluid is in the range of 1 ng/ml, and the concentration of estradiol in ovarian follicular fluid can be in the range of 1,000 ng/ml. The high local concentration of estradiol in peritoneal fluid and in the ovary probably plays an important role in supporting the growth of endometriotic implants.

PATHOLOGY

The four basic structures seen microscopically in endometriosis are endometrial epithelium, glands or glandlike structures, stroma, and hemorrhage (Fig 11–1). Continuing function in areas of endometriosis tends to destroy its microscopic characteristics; thus, Hertig's observation, "the more advanced the lesion clinically, the poorer the histologic detail," is the most descriptive. Early lesions, particularly those in the cul-de-sac, if excised in toto and properly oriented for the pathologist, usually demonstrate classic histology, whereas the large endometrial cysts of the ovary, obvious to the gynecologist at the operating table, may show only hemosiderin-laden macrophages with varying amounts of fibrous connective tissue and inflammatory cells. It is important, however, to remember that it is endometrial stroma that is responsible for bleeding in endometriosis, not the glands or epithelium. The presence of stroma alone is diagnostic of the disease, and the experienced gynecologic pathologist usually makes the diagnosis of endometriosis without difficulty. The presence of a decidual reaction or a typical "naked nuclei" cellular pattern surrounded by a delicate reticulum or spiral arterioles with adjacent predecidua, either with or without old or recent hemorrhage, is sufficient to permit the diagnosis to be made without glands.

The commonest site of endometriosis is the ovary, and in about 50% of patients both ovaries are involved. Other areas and organs affected (in order of incidence) are the posterior cul-de-sac, anterior uterovesicle peritoneum, posterior broad ligament, uterosacral ligaments, fallopian tube, uterus, rectovaginal septum, sigmoid colon, cervix, vulva, vagina, umbilicus, small intestine, laparotomy or episiotomy scars, ureter and bladder mucosa, arm, leg, pleura, and lung (Fig 11–2).

Endometriosis may have many visual manifestations. The classic visual appearance of endometriosis is the "powder burn" lesion, a small

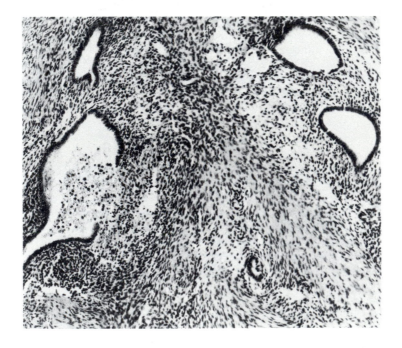

FIG 11–1.
Endometriosis of uterosacral ligament. Typical endometrial glands and stroma are evident in the fibrous connective tissue of the ligament.

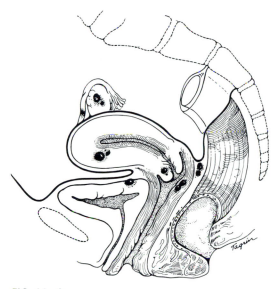

FIG 11–2.
Common sites of pelvic endometriosis.

punctate brown or purple discoloration of the peritoneum or ovarian surface. Endometriosis, however, may also appear as small blue, pink, or white lesions. Red flamelike lesions may appear on the peritoneum. Endometriotic lesions may also be invisible to the human eye. Published reports describe the occurrence of microscopic foci of endometriosis on the pelvic peritoneum that cannot be visually detected by the surgeon. The benign endometrial cyst of the ovary varies from microscopic size to a mass 8 to 10 cm in diameter. The cysts may be multiple in the early stages of the disease but subsequently coalesce into a single large cyst. During the early stage of development, endometriotic cysts are usually mobile and have smooth surfaces. As growth progresses, however, and surface bleeding occurs, the cyst becomes densely adherent to surrounding structures, particularly to the serosa of the sigmoid colon. The convex border (lateral aspect) of the ovary is more often involved and may become adherent to the ileum or lateral pelvic peritoneum. Frequently the ovary shows multiple areas resembling "powder burns" as a result of changes in blood pigments. Minute red or blue cystic areas (raspberry or blueberry spots) with adjacent puckering may be identified on the ovarian surface but are noted more often on the uterosacral ligaments or pelvic peritoneum. The lining of the endometrial cyst varies from red to dark brown, depending on the extent and duration of bleeding. The

cyst wall may be thin and smooth or thick and velvety, depending on the preponderance of fibrous tissue or functioning endometrium within it. If discrete papillary or polypoid lesions are found within the cyst cavity, the possibility of malignancy should be considered. The contents of the cyst are usually thick, resembling chocolate syrup or tar.

The uterosacral ligaments or rectovaginal peritoneum may be involved separately, or there may be a fused mass incorporating both structures (Fig 11–3). The discovery of bluish red or brown nodules with surrounding areas of puckering on the uterosacral ligaments, adjacent cul-de-sac, peritoneum, or serosa of the sigmoid is a characteristic finding, and if these reach adequate size, they may be palpated easily on rectovaginal examination. Eventually an intensive fibrous connective tissue reaction occurs, with fusion of the rectosigmoid to the back of the cervix and vagina. Masses of this type may become so firm that malignancy is suspected.

The lower genital tract may occasionally be the site of endometriosis; lesions of the cervix, vagina, and vulva have been reported. Usually there is a history of antecedent trauma, such as cervical cauterization or conization, vulvar surgery, or episiotomy. Surface endometriosis of this variety is almost certainly derived from implantation of viable endometrium and, in general, responds actively to estrogen and progesterone. When endometriosis involves the portio vaginalis of the cervix, the gross examination is usually pathognomonic, with blue-black, elevated nodules, either discrete or confluent, evident on speculum examination.

The round ligament is occasionally the site of endometriosis, and if the lesion exceeds 0.5 cm in diameter, it can usually be palpated by examination of the inguinal areas. Subjective complaints in the region of the internal inguinal ring or canal of Nuck are frequently cyclic and may be correlated with the menses.

Small bowel involvement is rare (about 0.1%–0.2%) but may lead to an erroneous preoperative diagnosis. With scarring there is often twisting or coiling about the lesion with resultant symptoms of nausea, diarrhea, and crampy midabdominal or periumbilical pain. When lesions invade the bowel mucosa, patients may present with rectal bleeding. Cyclic monthly hematochezia associated with the menses is highly suggestive of intestinal endometriosis. Grossly, the mucosal

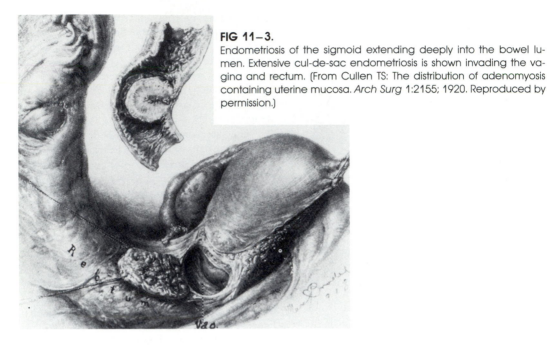

FIG 11–3.
Endometriosis of the sigmoid extending deeply into the bowel lumen. Extensive cul-de-sac endometriosis is shown invading the vagina and rectum. (From Cullen TS: The distribution of adenomyosis containing uterine mucosa. *Arch Surg* 1:2155; 1920. Reproduced by permission.)

surface is usually smooth with subjacent fibrosis and scarring. In extensive pelvic endometriosis, several loops of ileum may be involved by contiguity so that resection of the areas is necessary. Similarly, the serosa of the appendix is often involved.

Urinary tract endometriosis is not common but probably occurs more often than is reported in the literature. The involvement of the serosal surface of the bladder is seen rather frequently but is usually asymptomatic. By the time the muscularis or mucosa is involved, the patient usually has noted cyclic hematuria and pain. Cystoscopy may show typical bluish "mulberry" lesions, and endoscopic biopsy usually confirms the diagnosis. Ureteral involvement has been reported and probably explains some cases of idiopathic, unilateral hydronephrosis in women (Fig 11–4). Cyclic flank pain, fever, and pyuria may occur as a result of intermittent ureteral obstruction. The excretory urogram may show beginning ureteral dilatation if obtained at the optimum time in the cycle. A tentative diagnosis may be confirmed by noting cessation of symptoms and improvement in the urogram following prolonged periods of induced anovulation.

Several cases are now on record of biopsy-proved pleural and pulmonary endometriosis in which a hematogenous or lymphatic mode of dissemination must be postulated.

In summary, the pathologic process of endometriosis, although microscopically benign, produces extensive havoc in the pelvis as important structures are gradually involved. The process is unique in that it spreads in a cancer-like manner, which produces fibrosis and scarring. The end result may be ovarian destruction, oviduct deformity, bladder dysfunction, large bowel obstruction, and ureteral constriction.

Malignancy in endometriosis is rare. Criteria for the diagnosis of carcinoma arising in endometriosis were outlined by Sampson in 1925 and are still acceptable, namely: (1) the ovary must be the site of benign endometriosis, (2) there must be a genuine adenocarcinoma, and (3) a transition from benign to malignant areas must be demonstrated. Of interest is the observation that many cases of clear cell carcinoma of the ovary are associated with endometriosis (Scully et al., 1966).

EPIDEMIOLOGY

The epidemiology of endometriosis is poorly defined, and the incidence and risk factors for endometriosis are the subject of much controversy. The main problem hindering a clear exploration of the epidemiology of endometriosis is that this disease can be only definitively diagnosed by a surgical procedure (laparoscopy or laparotomy).

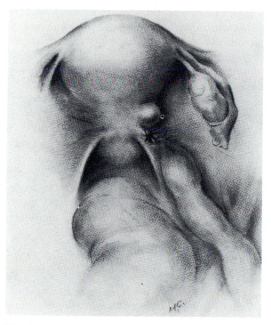

FIG 11–4.
Endometriosis invading the right uterosacral ligament, with fibrosis producing marked hydroureter. (Courtesy of Dr. Thomas Leavitt.)

Ethical considerations preclude random laparoscopy of large groups of women, so until a noninvasive method of diagnosing endometriosis is discovered, investigation of the epidemiology of endometriosis will be hampered by methodologic problems.

Endometriosis can occur in women between the ages of 10 and 60 years. The average age at first diagnosis is 27 years. Most women with endometriosis have had symptoms of the disease for 2 to 5 years prior to diagnosis.

Endometriosis is an exceedingly common gynecologic problem, but precise incidence and prevalence figures are not available. A study of discharge records from acute care, nonfederal hospitals in 1980 revealed that approximately 8% of all women with gynecologic admissions had endometriosis as a discharge diagnosis (Cramer, 1987). Of all women admitted to the hospital, 0.6% had a discharge diagnosis of endometriosis. Of all women between the ages of 15 and 44 years, 0.9% had a discharge diagnosis of endometriosis. These and similar studies suggest that in the general population of reproductive age women, the prevalence of endometriosis is at least 1%. In certain high-risk populations, the prevalence of endometriosis is much higher. For example, in female partners of infertile couples, the prevalence of endometriosis in the women is approximately 30% to 50%.

Genetic factors may play a role in endometriosis. Familial clustering of endometriosis is a common clinical observation. In families with endometriosis, the disease is often confined to the maternal line and is seven times commoner in first-degree relatives than in the general population. In future studies, evaluation of DNA polymorphism may allow the identification of specific genes involved in the development of endometriosis.

Menstrual factors appear to play an important role in the development of endometriosis. Women with the disease report menstrual cycles of less than 27 days with greater than 8 days of menstrual flow much more often than women without endometriosis (Table 11–2; Cramer et al., 1985). Women with müllerian anomalies in whom normal menstrual egress is blocked by cervical stenosis or vaginal septa often develop endometriosis. Of special interest, women with double uteri and only one blocked uterine outflow tract often develop endometriosis on the pelvic structures contralateral to the blocked outflow tract but not on the ipsilateral pelvic structures. These findings support the concept that increasing amounts of retrograde menstruation increase the risk of developing endometriosis.

TABLE 11–2.

Menstrual Characteristics in Relation to Relative Risk for Endometriosis*

	Relative Risk for Endometriosis
Cycle (days)	
≤ 27	2.1
28–34	1.0
≥ 35	0.6
Duration of flow	
≤ 7	1.0
≥ 8	2.4
Menstrual pain	
None	1.0
Mild	1.7
Moderate	3.4
Severe	6.7

*From Cramer DW: Epidemiology of endometriosis, in Wilson EA (ed): *Endometriosis.* New York, Alan R Liss, 1987, pp 5–22. Used by permission.

Other epidemiologic studies suggest that prolonged use of low-dose oral contraceptives and multiple pregnancies may decrease the risk of developing endometriosis. Both exposures probably decrease the cumulative amount of retrograde menstruation. Of special interest are recent studies that suggest that conditioning exercise may be associated with a decreased risk of developing endometriosis. For example, Cramer et al. (1985) observed that women who exercise regularly, who started exercising before age 15 years, and who exercise more than 7 hours/week are at a low risk of developing endometriosis. These findings have important public health implications.

CLINICAL FEATURES

Symptoms

The characteristic symptoms associated with endometriosis are (1) progressive, acquired, severe pain associated with or occurring just prior to menstruation; (2) dyspareunia; (3) painful defecation; (4) premenstrual staining and hypermenorrhea; (5) suprapubic pain, dysuria, and hematuria; and (6) infertility (Table 11–3). Some patients do not have "acquired" dysmenorrhea but state that they have always had painful periods. Most, however, will admit to a recent increase in the severity of their pain. In many patients the pain cannot be classified as dysmenorrhea but is actually premenstrual and varies from mild discomfort to severe pain that is characteristically in the lower abdomen, is usually bilateral, and is often associated with a sense of rectal pressure. A constant soreness in the lower abdomen or pelvis throughout the cycle that is aggravated just before the menses or during coitus may be the only complaint. The pain in endometriosis is of un-

known cause but is probably related to miniature menstruation and bleeding and to the release of prostaglandins. That the pain is due to intermittent stimulation and withdrawal of hormones is substantiated by the fact that dysmenorrhea is not evident if amenorrhea is induced.

Pain is not always associated with endometriosis even when the disease is extensive. Bilateral, large ovarian endometriomas frequently are not symptomatic unless rupture occurs. On the other hand, incapacitating pelvic discomfort may be associated with minimal amounts of active endometriosis. Often the surgeon can find only puckering and scarring of the posterior cul-de-sac with an adherent rectosigmoid to account for the multiplicity of symptoms.

Signs

Endometriosis cannot be definitively diagnosed by physical examination; however, many women with endometriosis have physical findings that suggest the presence of the disease (see Table 11–3). Women with endometriosis may have tender uterosacral ligaments, which on palpation may be thickened ("banjo strings") and nodular. Rectovaginal examination may demonstrate a thickened rectovaginal septum and an indurated cul-de-sac. In women with endometriomas, fixed adnexal masses may be noted.

DIAGNOSIS AND STAGING

Although the diagnosis of endometriosis may be suggested by history and physical examination, it can be made definitively only by laparoscopy or laparotomy.

In patients with mild to moderate endometriosis, laparoscopy reveals the classic "powder burn" lesions, which consist of small (less than 5 mm) purple, blue, or red spots visible on the pelvic peritoneum. Scarring and adhesions are commonly seen in association with cases of moderate to severe endometriosis. Evaluation of ovarian masses by laparoscopy is difficult, and the definitive diagnosis of ovarian endometriomas should not be made by laparoscopic evaluation. Aspiration of ovarian masses at the time of laparoscopy may increase the number of endometriomas accurately diagnosed during this procedure. Biopsy of small endometriotic lesions via the laparoscope can be helpful to confirm the diagnosis. However,

TABLE 11–3.

Symptoms and Signs of Endometriosis

Symptoms
Progressive dysmenorrhea
Dyspareunia
Infertility
Premenstrual staining
Painful defecation
Signs
Cul-de-sac induration
Uterosacral ligament nodularity
Fixed ovarian masses

it should be remembered that some endometriotic implants may contain only stroma with hemorrhage, thus making the diagnosis difficult for the pathologist.

Currently, intensive efforts are being made to develop noninvasive methods of diagnosing endometriosis. In women with endometriomas, ultrasound can help confirm the mass and provide a noninvasive method of following the size of the mass. Pelvic ultrasound, however, is of little value in screening for endometriosis because ultrasound cannot diagnose peritoneal implants or adhesions. Recent studies suggest that nuclear magnetic resonance imaging (MRI) may be the noninvasive procedure with the highest sensitivity and specificity for diagnosing endometriosis (Nishimura et al., 1987). Many endometriotic implants have relatively unique and intense relaxation signals, allowing their identification. Much more research is needed to clarify the role of MRI in the diagnosis of endometriosis. The high cost of MRI studies may preclude the widespread clinical application of this technique.

Recently, our laboratory has described the clinical utility of the measurement of serum CA-125 for the diagnosis of endometriosis. The history of this development will be reviewed. In the late 1970s, Drs. Robert C. Knapp and Robert C. Bast produced a panel of monoclonal antibodies to membrane antigens of human ovarian epithelial cancers. They accomplished this goal by immunizing Balb/C mice with tumor cells from a human serous papillary cystadenocarcinoma. Spleen cells from the immunized mice were fused with cells from the P3/NS-1 plasmacytoma cell line. The fused cells were then diluted so that only one cell was present in each culture well. As the cells grew, each culture well contained only one clonal colony of homogeneous daughter cells. Because each daughter cell was derived from the same parental cell, each culture well contained only one type of antibody, a monoclonal antibody. Evaluation of hundreds of clones revealed one antibody that was of particular interest. This monoclonal antibody was designated OC-125 (Bast et al., 1981). The antigenic determinant defined by OC-125 was designated CA-125. With the use of the monoclonal antibody OC-125 and the biotin-avidin immunoperoxidase technique, various tissues were screened for the antigenic determinant CA-125. In adult human tissues, CA-125 was detected in the endocervix, endometrium, fallopian tube, peritoneum, pleura, and pericardium. In human fetal tissues, CA-125 was detected in the müllerian epithelium, amnion, umbilical epithelium, peritoneum, pleura, and pericardium. The normal adult and fetal ovary were both negative for CA-125. The majority of human epithelial ovarian cancers were positive for CA-125. Endometriomas were also noted to stain with the antibody OC-125 (Fig 11–5). CA-125 has been partially purified and noted to be a complex membrane glycoprotein with a molecular weight of greater than 200 kilodaltons (kD). On

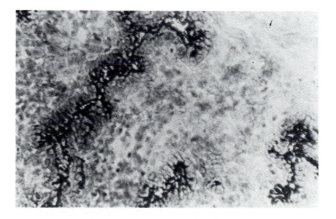

FIG 11–5.
Cryostat section of ovarian endometrioma stained with OC-125 antibody and the avidin-biotin immunoperoxidase technique and counterstained with hematoxylin. Normal ovarian tissue present in the upper right portion of the figure does not stain with OC-125 antibody. The endometrioma tissue stains with the OC-125 antibody. (From Barbieri RL: Elevated concentrations of CA-125 in patients with advanced endometriosis. *Fertil Steril* 1986; 45:630. Reproduced by permission.)

the basis of these observations, it was suggested that CA-125 was an "oncofetal" coelomic epithelial differentiation antigen. The precise function of CA-125 is still unknown.

Bast et al. (1983) hypothesized that CA-125 might be present in the peripheral circulation because of "shedding" of CA-125 from membrane surfaces. To test this hypothesis, they developed a sensitive immunoradiometric assay to detect CA-125 in the blood. Evaluation of the blood test for CA-125 revealed the following striking findings: (1) greater than 80% of patients with ovarian cancer had elevated blood levels of CA-125, and (2) less than 1% of apparently healthy controls had elevated blood levels of CA-125 (Bast et al., 1983). Modest elevations in blood CA-125 levels were also noted occasionally in four clinical situations other than ovarian carcinoma: (1) in pregnant women in the first trimester, (2) in women with acute pelvic inflammatory disease, (3) postoperatively in women undergoing gynecologic surgery, and (4) in some patients with endometriosis.

To further investigate the relationship between elevated blood CA-125 levels and endometriosis, Barbieri et al. (1986) prospectively measured serum CA-125 preoperatively in 147 consecutive patients undergoing diagnostic laparoscopy or laparotomy. They noted that patients with advanced endometriosis (stages III and IV) had elevated blood CA-125 levels compared with women with normal diagnostic laparoscopies (66.5 units/ml vs. 8.2 units/ml, $p < 0.001$) (Fig 11–6).

Patients with stage II endometriosis also had serum CA-125 levels greater than controls (17.3 units/ml vs. 8.2 units/ml, $p < 0.05$), but there was a considerable overlap in the CA-125 levels between these two groups. For the diagnosis of stages III and IV endometriosis, serum CA-125 measurements had a sensitivity of 0.54, a specificity of 0.96, a positive predictive value of 0.58, and a negative predictive value of 0.96 in a population with an incidence of stage III/IV endometriosis of 9% (Barbieri et al., 1986). These results have been confirmed by other investigators (Table 11–4).

Serum CA-125 measurements may also have value in monitoring disease activity. Our group and other investigators have observed that after effective surgical or medical therapy of endometriosis, serum CA-125 levels decrease. Recurrence of disease is often associated with an increase in the serum CA-125 level (Fig 11–7; Barbieri et al., 1986).

An important unanswered question is, Why is the CA-125 level elevated in the blood of women with advanced endometriosis? We believe that two mechanisms may be responsible for elevated blood levels of CA-125. First, endometriotic lesions appear to have a greater membrane concentration of CA-125 than normal endometrium. This observation suggests that even if endometriosis arises from retrograde transport, it must still undergo a "biochemical coelomic metaplasia" to express more of the CA-125 antigen. Second, the inflammation associated with endometriosis may increase the rate at which CA-125 is shed from the membranes of endometriotic lesions and increase the rate at which CA-125 enters the circulation (leaky capillary endothelium). This "inflammation mechanism" may also explain why some patients with acute pelvic inflammatory disease also have elevated blood levels of CA-125 (Barbieri, 1986)

The major problem with the clinical applica-

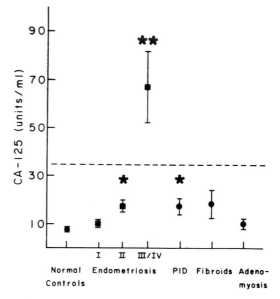

FIG 11–6.
CA-125 concentrations prior to diagnostic laparoscopy or laparotomy. Mean ± SEM. *$p < 0.05$, **$p < 0.001$ compared with controls. Normal controls were patients with visually normal pelvic organs at the time of diagnostic laparoscopy. (From Barbieri RL: Elevated concentrations of CA-125 in patients with advanced endometriosis. *Fertil Steril* 1986; 45:630. Reproduced by permission.)

TABLE 11–4.

Serum CA-125 Concentration in Women With Endometriosis

	Investigator			
	Barbieri et al. (1986)	Pittaway and Fayez (1986)	Malkasian et al. (1986)	Fedele et al. (1988)
Disease Status	Serum CA-125 (units/ml)			
Normal controls	8	8	—	16
Endometriosis				
Stage I	10	14	30	23
Stage II	17	23	28	24
Stage III/IV	67	33	53	33

tion of serum CA-125 measurements for diagnosis of endometriosis is that most patients with endometriosis have stage I or II disease, and serum CA-125 has very low sensitivity (0.17) for the diagnosis of stage I and II disease. However, it may be possible to develop a more sensitive and specific blood test for endometriosis. If endometriotic lesions contain membrane antigens that are specific for the disease, it may be possible to develop antibodies to these antigens. If these antigens appear frequently in the circulation of patients with endometriosis but not in patients without endometriosis, a useful blood test for endometriosis could be developed. A blood test for endometriosis would represent a significant advance in gynecology.

A critical concept is that endometriosis is a heterogeneous disease, ranging in severity from minimal to severe. Therefore, surgical pathological staging is of utmost importance for planning therapy, determining prognosis, communicating with other physicians, and standardizing research reporting. In the 1970s, Acosta and Kistner both proposed descriptive clinical staging systems. These systems have been generally replaced by the revised American Fertility Society (AFS) staging system (Fig 11–8; American Fertility Society, 1985).

In the AFS staging system, points are assigned for severity of endometriosis based on the size and depth of the implant and for the severity of adhesions. The points are summed and patients assigned to one of four stages: stage I—minimal disease, 1 to 5 points; stage II—mild disease, 6 to 15 points; stage III—moderate disease, 16 to 40 points; and stage IV—severe disease, more than 40 points. Although the point assignments in the AFS system are relatively arbitrary, it is an excellent system for clinical research in part because its components are easily entered into a computerized data base.

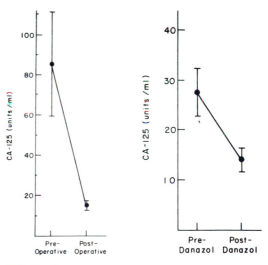

FIG 11–7.
A, preoperative and postoperative serum CA-125 concentrations in six patients with advanced endometriosis who had total abdominal hysterectomy–bilateral salpingo-oophorectomy (TAH-BSO). Postoperative serum CA-125 concentration was measured 3 months after surgery. **B,** serum CA-125 concentrations before and after danazol therapy in 10 patients with endometriosis. Patients underwent laparoscopy before and after danazol therapy to monitor disease activity. American Fertility Society endometriosis score before therapy was 26, and after therapy was 14.

Patient's Name _____   Date_____

Stage I   (Minimal) - 1-5
Stage II   (Mild)   - 6-15   Laparoscopy_____ Laparotomy_____ Photography_____
Stage III (Moderate) - 16-40   Recommended Treatment_____
Stage IV   (Severe)   - >40
Total_____   Prognosis_____

PERITONEUM	**ENDOMETRIOSIS**	<1cm	1-3cm	>3cm
	Superficial	1	2	4
	Deep	2	4	6
OVARY	R Superficial	1	2	4
	Deep	4	16	20
	L Superficial	1	2	4
	Deep	4	16	20

	POSTERIOR CULDESAC OBLITERATION	Partial		Complete
		4		40

	ADHESIONS	<1/3 Enclosure	1/3-2/3 Enclosure	>2/3 Enclosure
OVARY	R Filmy	1	2	4
	Dense	4	8	16
	L Filmy	1	2	4
	Dense	4	8	16
TUBE	R Filmy	1	2	4
	Dense	4*	8*	16
	L Filmy	1	2	4
	Dense	4*	8*	16

*If the fimbriated end of the fallopian tube is completely enclosed, change the point assignment to 16.

Additional Endometriosis: _____   Associated Pathology: _____

_____   _____

_____   _____

_____   _____

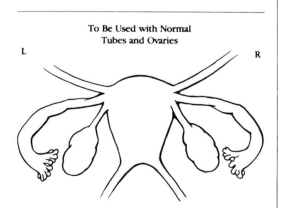

To Be Used with Normal
Tubes and Ovaries

L   R

To Be Used with Abnormal
Tubes and/or Ovaries

L   R

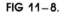

FIG 11–8.
Revised AFS classification for endometriosis. (Courtesy of the American Fertility Society.) (Continued.)

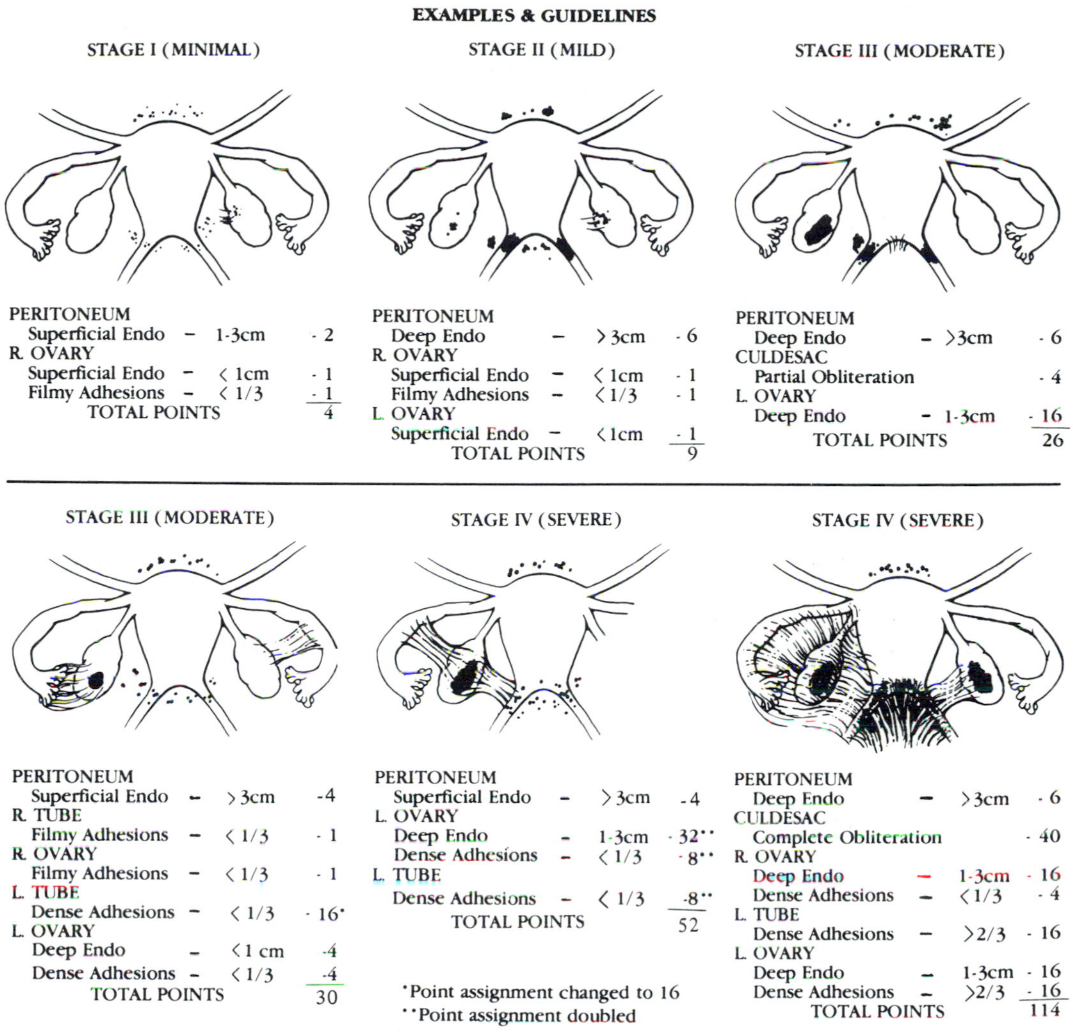

EXAMPLES & GUIDELINES

STAGE I (MINIMAL)

PERITONEUM
  Superficial Endo — 1-3cm · 2
R. OVARY
  Superficial Endo — < 1cm · 1
  Filmy Adhesions — < 1/3 · 1
      TOTAL POINTS 4

STAGE II (MILD)

PERITONEUM
  Deep Endo — > 3cm · 6
R. OVARY
  Superficial Endo — < 1cm · 1
  Filmy Adhesions — < 1/3 · 1
L. OVARY
  Superficial Endo — < 1cm · 1
      TOTAL POINTS 9

STAGE III (MODERATE)

PERITONEUM
  Deep Endo — > 3cm · 6
CULDESAC
  Partial Obliteration · 4
L. OVARY
  Deep Endo — 1-3cm · 16
      TOTAL POINTS 26

STAGE III (MODERATE)

PERITONEUM
  Superficial Endo — > 3cm · 4
R. TUBE
  Filmy Adhesions — < 1/3 · 1
R. OVARY
  Filmy Adhesions — < 1/3 · 1
L. TUBE
  Dense Adhesions — < 1/3 · 16*
L. OVARY
  Deep Endo — < 1 cm · 4
  Dense Adhesions — < 1/3 · 4
      TOTAL POINTS 30

STAGE IV (SEVERE)

PERITONEUM
  Superficial Endo — > 3cm · 4
L. OVARY
  Deep Endo — 1-3cm · 32**
  Dense Adhesions — < 1/3 · 8**
L. TUBE
  Dense Adhesions — < 1/3 · 8**
      TOTAL POINTS 52

*Point assignment changed to 16
**Point assignment doubled

STAGE IV (SEVERE)

PERITONEUM
  Deep Endo — > 3cm · 6
CULDESAC
  Complete Obliteration · 40
R. OVARY
  Deep Endo — 1-3cm · 16
  Dense Adhesions — < 1/3 · 4
L. TUBE
  Dense Adhesions — > 2/3 · 16
L. OVARY
  Deep Endo — 1-3cm · 16
  Dense Adhesions — > 2/3 · 16
      TOTAL POINTS 114

FIG 11–8 (cont.).
Revised AFS classification for endometriosis. (Courtesy of the American Fertility Society).

The importance of staging endometriosis is highlighted by recent reports that most patients with untreated stage I endometriosis have a fecundity potential no different from that of the general population (Seibel et al., 1982). This observation indicates that stage I endometriosis may have a prognosis quite different than stage II, III, or IV endometriosis.

CLINICAL PRESENTATION AND TREATMENT

Most patients with endometriosis present with pelvic pain, infertility, or a pelvic mass.

Therapeutic considerations differ for each presentation (Table 11–5). For most women with a persistent adnexal mass, surgical removal of the mass is the treatment of choice. Surgical removal of adnexal masses is simultaneously diagnostic and therapeutic. The surgical removal of an endometrioma should be followed by the development of a long-term treatment plan, because the majority of young women who have had an endometrioma surgically removed will have a recurrence of their endometriosis within 5 years. The sequential resection of multiple, recurrent endometriomas may often result in the development of premature menopause. For young patients, long-term hormonal therapy may be necessary to prevent the re-

TABLE 11–5.

Management Strategies in the Treatment of
Endometriosis Based on the Presenting Complaint

| | Pelvic Pain* | | |
Stages	Family Not Completed	Family Completed	Infertility
I and II	Hormonal therapy	Hormonal therapy	Expectant management, hormonal therapy, or laparoscopic surgery
III and IV	Hormonal therapy, surgery, or both	Hormonal therapy, surgery, or both (TAH/BSO considered)	Conservative surgery with preoperative or postoperative (or both) hormonal therapy; IVF

*Fertility not an immediate issue.

petitive recurrence of endometriomas. In many instances, this can be accomplished after the resection of an endometrioma by instituting a long-term course of combined estrogen-progestogen oral contraceptives used in a noncyclic manner.

Clinical evidence suggests that moderate and severe endometriosis can cause subfertility and infertility. The mechanisms responsible for this association include mechanical factors and a host of other poorly characterized processes. For example, it is clear that if both ovaries are completely covered by adhesions, there will be an inability for the egg and sperm to interact, resulting in infertility. Less clearly defined is the possibility that an ovarian endometrioma will disrupt egg maturation by intraovarian mechanisms.

Much effort has recently focused on defining abnormalities in the peritoneal environment of women with endometriosis. Pelvic endometriosis is often associated with diffuse pelvic inflammation and an increase in peritoneal fluid volume and the number of activated peritoneal macrophages. These activated peritoneal macrophages are capable of phagocytosis of sperm and secretion of esterases, peroxidases, proteolytic enzymes, cytokines, and lymphokines. These secretions may create an environment hostile to egg and sperm function and interaction (Haney, 1988).

In general, it is our clinical opinion that women who are subfertile or infertile, with stage III or IV endometriosis, should have surgery in an attempt to remove all endometriotic implants and adhesions. In addition, we advise all women with infertility and endometrioma(s) to have the endometrioma(s) removed, in the belief that removal improves follicular development and provides pathologic diagnosis of the ovarian cyst.

There is no strong scientific evidence to support the hypothesis that minimal (stage I) or mild (stage II) endometriosis causes infertility. Thus, it is not surprising that there are no controlled clinical studies demonstrating that the treatment of mild or moderate endometriosis cures infertility. In fact, the few randomized prospective studies that have been completed suggest that the treatment of women with minimal or mild endometriosis does not improve fecundability compared with women with endometriosis who were not treated (Seibel et al., 1982). The use of hormonal or surgical therapy for the treatment of infertility associated with mild or moderate endometriosis is a clinical decision to be made jointly by the physician and patient after all alternatives have been explored.

Approximately 40% of women with advanced endometriosis and infertility will be unable to conceive even after surgical and medical therapy. For these women, in vitro fertilization and embryo transfer (IVF-ET) or gamete intrafallopian transfer (GIFT) are viable treatment options. In most large series, the success of IVF-ET or GIFT for the treatment of endometriosis is similar to the success of these technologies for the treatment of tubal factor infertility. In general, the clinical pregnancy rate is in the range of 20% per oocyte retrieval (Jones et al., 1984); however, patients with stage I or II endometriosis have a higher clinical pregnancy rate than patients with stage III or IV disease.

One exception to this observation is that women with advanced endometriosis who have had multiple previous ovarian cystectomies for endometriomas often respond poorly to ovarian hyperstimulation and develop less than the expected number of mature ovarian follicles. In turn, the poor response to ovulation induction decreases the clinical pregnancy rate for this group of women. The mechanism or mechanisms responsible for this observation are unclear. However, multiple ovarian cystectomies for endometriomas may be associated with the resection of a significant proportion of the total oocyte population (Hornstein et al., 1989).

Sporadic reports have suggested that endometriosis may be associated with an increased incidence of spontaneous abortions and luteal phase defects. Recent studies suggest that the association between endometriosis and an increased risk of spontaneous abortion is spurious and probably was due to selection bias (Pittaway, 1988). It is also unlikely that there is an important association between endometriosis and luteal phase defects. In 100 consecutive patients with endometriosis who had an endometrial biopsy in the late luteal phase of the cycle, none had an out of phase endometrium. These data from our practice suggest that luteal phase deficiency is not especially common in women with endometriosis (Barbieri et al., 1982).

Pelvic pain is one of the commonest presentations of women with endometriosis. Women with pelvic pain that is not relieved by antiprostaglandins such as ibuprofen or that causes significant disability (absenteeism from work or school) should consider undergoing a diagnostic laparoscopy. If endometriosis is diagnosed, hormonal treatment of the disease will completely or partially relieve the pain in 90% of treated patients. In young women with endometriosis and severe pelvic pain, long-term hormonal therapy may be required. Surgery to remove endometriotic implants and scar tissue may provide temporary relief from pain, but without postoperative hormonal therapy, the endometriosis will usually recur postoperatively, resulting in the return of the pelvic pain. In general, women with severe endometriosis who are more than 40 years old and have completed their families are probably best treated by a definitive surgical procedure (hysterectomy and bilateral oophorectomy).

TREATMENT

Patients with endometriosis typically present with complaints of pelvic pain, a pelvic mass, or infertility. Therapeutic interventions should be designed to adequately address the patient's specific problem. Therapy will be discussed under five headings: (1) prophylaxis, (2) observation and analgesia, (3) hormonal therapy, (4) conservative operation, and (5) extirpative operation.

Prophylaxis

Manipulations that produce amenorrhea or cause endometrial atrophy are likely to decrease the chance of developing endometriosis. Early and frequent pregnancies appear to effectively decrease the frequency of endometriosis, but this therapeutic strategy is incompatible with the life plans of most patients. Exercise-induced amenorrhea may prove to be an effective prophylactic modality but may also be difficult to achieve for many women.

There is suggestive evidence that women who have been taking oral contraceptives for prolonged periods of time, especially those with a potent progestin and a minimal amount of estrogen, may have a diminished chance of subsequently developing endometriosis. This is based on the observation that these agents produce endometrial atrophy and lessen menstrual flow, thus preventing tubal reflux of menstrual debris into the peritoneal cavity.

Observation and Analgesia

For some women with endometriosis, expectant management is a viable therapeutic option. For instance, some women with pelvic pain and minimal endometriosis may prefer therapy with analgesics over hormonal therapy with danazol or gonadotropin-releasing hormone (GnRH) agonists. For some young women with infertility and minimal or mild endometriosis, the best way to improve the patient's fecundability may be to ensure that there are no other confounding infertility factors rather than treating the endometriosis.

Hormonal Therapy

During the past 40 years, the medical management of endometriosis has become significantly more sophisticated. In the early 1950s, the high-dose estrogen regimen of Karnaky was the only available hormonal treatment for endometriosis. In the 1960s and 1970s, Kistner's "pseudopregnancy" and "progestin-only" regimens dominated the medical management of endometriosis. During the 1980s, danazol has become the primary hormonal agent used in the treatment of endometriosis. It is likely that the 1990s will witness the ascendancy of the GnRH agonists for the treatment of endometriosis. These advances have significantly expanded the hormonal armamentarium of the gynecologist treating endometriosis. Proper use of these agents requires a thorough understanding of the hormonal responses of endometriotic tissues and an appreciation of the pharmacologic properties of the available agents.

The central dogma that guides the hormonal therapy of endometriosis is the belief that steroid hormones are the major regulators of growth and function of endometriotic tissue. The majority of endometriotic implants contain estrogen receptors, progesterone receptors, and androgen receptors. In general, estrogen stimulates the growth of these implants, and androgens induce their atrophy. The role of progesterone in the regulation of endometriotic tissue is controversial. Progesterone alone may actually support the growth of endometriotic tissue. However, the synthetic 19-nor progestogens, which are derivatives of testosterone and have androgenic properties, appear to inhibit the growth of endometriotic tissue.

The polarity of response of endometriotic tissue to androgens and estrogens is the yin and yang on which all current hormonal therapy of endometriosis is based. Three observations complicate this simplistic conceptualization. First, a small percentage of endometriotic implants (about 5%) do not contain significant concentrations of either estrogen or progesterone receptors.

These lesions may be relatively resistant to hormonal therapy. Second, microheterogeneity within endometriotic lesions may make the steroid receptor-positive cell populations more susceptible to hormonal manipulations than the steroid receptor-negative cell populations. Third, some endometriotic lesions that contain progesterone receptors do not demonstrate typical functional (increased 17β-hydroxysteroid dehydrogenase enzyme activity) or structural (secretory changes) responses to progesterone stimulation. This observation suggests that in some endometriotic implants the intranuclear steroid receptors are uncoupled from their site of action (DNA).

The polarity of response of endometriotic tissue to androgens and estrogens is the basis for the two hormonal strategies that are most often used to treat endometriosis. One basic strategy is to create an acyclic, low-estrogen hormonal environment. The low estrogen levels cause atrophy of the endometriotic tissues. The acyclic environment helps minimize the chance of miniature "menstruation" in the endometriotic implants and prevents reseeding of implants from the retrograde transport of normal endometrium during menstruation. An acyclic, low-estrogen environment is best produced by bilateral oophorectomy or with the use of GnRH agonists. The second basic strategy is to produce a hormonal environment high in androgens. Danazol therapy is the best example of this strategy. The high-androgen environment directly produces atrophy of endometriotic implants. The high-androgen strategy also results in low, acyclic estrogen levels by interfering with ovarian follicular development. Table 11–6 summarizes these different strategies.

TABLE 11–6.

Hormonal Strategies for Endometriosis Treatment

Hormone Strategy	Examples	Estradiol Concentration (pg/ml)	Unwanted Effects
I. Low estrogen, low androgen	GnRH agonists	20	Vasomotor symptoms, bone loss
	Bilateral oophorectomy	20	Irreversible sterility, vasomotor symptoms, bone loss, lipid changes
II. Low estrogen, high androgen	Danazol	40	Weight gain, acne, oily skin, hirsutism, voice changes

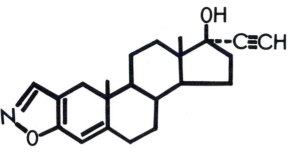

FIG 11–9.
Structure of danazol.

Danazol

Danazol is an isoxazole derivative of the synthetic steroid 17-ethinyltestosterone (Fig 11–9). The pharmacology of danazol is exceedingly complex and is best discussed in terms of the molecular pharmacology of the drug (Barbieri and Ryan, 1981). Current laboratory findings suggest that danazol interacts with only two major classes of proteins: (1) steroid hormone receptors and (2) enzymes of steroidogenesis. The entire pharmacologic profile of danazol (and danazol's metabolites) can be explained by danazol's interaction with these two classes of proteins.

Danazol and Steroid-Binding Proteins.— In the first systematic screening of the interaction of danazol with steroid-binding proteins, our laboratory reported that danazol binds to intracellular androgen, progesterone, and glucocorticoid receptors (Barbieri et al., 1979). Subsequently, numerous other investigators have confirmed our original findings (Table 11–7).

The interaction of a steroid with an intracellular steroid receptor system can result in three possible outcomes: (1) the steroid can produce the biological effects characteristic of that intracellular receptor system (agonist), (2) the steroid can block the biologic effects typically seen after stimulation of the receptor system (antagonist), and (3) the steroid can produce a mixed pattern of agonistic and antagonistic effects. For example, in androgen receptor bioassays (prostatic growth), danazol appears to be a potent androgen agonist. As previously noted, androgens induce atrophy in endometriotic implants. The androgenic effect of danazol is one of the main pharmacologic means by which this drug produces atrophy in endometriotic tissue.

Danazol has been reported to bind to intranuclear estrogen receptors. However, the affinity of the danazol-estrogen receptor interaction is so weak that this interaction is not believed to have clinical significance. Danazol interacts with glucocorticoid receptors, and preliminary evidence suggests that it is a weak glucocorticoid agonist. Danazol also binds to intranuclear progesterone

TABLE 11–7.

Interaction of Danazol With Intracellular Androgen, Progesterone, and Estrogen Receptors and With Circulating Steroid-Binding Proteins

	Affinity of Danazol for Receptor	Biologic Consequence
Intracellular receptor system		
Androgen	High affinity	Androgen agonist
Progestin	Moderate affinity	Mixed progestin agonist-antagonist
Estrogen	Low affinity	No estrogenic effects
Circulating steroid-binding proteins		
Sex hormone–binding globulin	Moderate affinity	Causes large increase in free testosterone
Corticosteroid-binding globulin	Moderate affinity	Causes small increase in free cortisol

receptors, but its effects in bioassays for progesterone are exceedingly complex. In some bioassays, danazol induces secretory changes in the endometrium, suggesting that danazol is a progesterone agonist. In other systems, however, danazol is able to block the effect of progesterone in the Clauberg assay (a test substance is given to estrogen-primed immature rabbits and endometrial histologic studies are performed to assess progestational changes). Thus, in this circumstance, danazol behaves as an antiprogesterone. Given these diverse bioassay findings, it may be best to classify danazol as a mixed agonist-antagonist with respect to the progesterone receptor system.

In addition to binding to intracellular steroid receptors, danazol also interacts with circulating steroid hormone–binding globulins. Danazol can displace testosterone from sex hormone–binding globulin (SHBG) and cortisol from corticosteroid-binding globulin. Of these two interactions, the danazol-induced increase in the percentage of "bioavailable testosterone" is clinically the more important. In normal women, 40% of testosterone is bioavailable (non-SHBG bound). In women taking danazol, 80% or more of the circulating testosterone is bioavailable (Table 11–8; Nilsson et al., 1982). Therefore, part of the androgenic properties of danazol in the human may be due to the dramatic increase in bioavailable androgens caused by danazol. In addition, the observation that danazol can bind to circulating steroid-binding proteins significantly complicates the interpretation of serum total steroid concentrations in patients receiving this drug.

In summary, danazol is an androgen and glucocorticoid agonist and a mixed agonist-antagonist with respect to the progesterone receptor system. Part of danazol's androgenic behavior

TABLE 11–8.

Percent of Testosterone Bound to Sex Hormone–Binding Globulin, Bound to Albumin, and Free in Women Receiving Danazol*

	Normal Women	Women Receiving Danazol
SHBG bound	60.1	18
Albumin bound	38.6	79.4
Free testosterone	1.3	2.6

*From Nilsson B: Danazol and gestogen displacement of testosterone and influence of sex hormone binding capacity. *Fertil Steril* 1983; 39:505. Used by permission.

may be due to its ability to displace testosterone from SHBG, resulting in an increase in bioavailable testosterone. Danazol's poor binding to estrogen receptors suggests that it has no significant effects in this receptor system. Steroid receptors regulate cell function in a large number of diverse tissues. The effects of danazol on cell function in a variety of steroid receptor-containing tissues will be reviewed briefly.

By acting as an androgen agonist, danazol decreases LH and FSH secretion in castrate animals. One of danazol's main metabolites, ethinyltestosterone, also suppresses LH and FSH secretion in castrate animals by acting as a progesterone agonist (Desaulles and Krahenbul, 1964). Although danazol suppresses LH and FSH in castrate animals, the effects of danazol on LH and FSH in animals with intact gonads are complex. The weight of evidence suggests that in women with ovaries, danazol administration does not produce a significant decrease in basal serum LH or FSH levels. This can be explained by the fact that danazol exerts a mild suppressive effect on pituitary secretion of LH and FSH but simultaneously causes a decrease in circulating estradiol levels (by direct actions on the ovary), which, in turn, stimulates a rise in LH and FSH levels. The overall effect is that danazol does not produce any significant change in basal serum LH or FSH levels in premenopausal women receiving this drug.

Danazol's androgenic properties directly suppress the growth of endometrial and endometriotic tissues. Danazol's lack of estrogenic effects facilitates the androgen-mediated inhibition of growth.

Danazol's androgenic properties probably contribute to the decreased high-density lipoprotein (HDL) cholesterol levels observed in women receiving danazol. The atherogenic risk caused by the decrease in HDL cholesterol levels remains to be fully quantitated, but patients with low HDL cholesterol levels may be at increased risk of developing atherosclerosis. Danazol's androgenic and mixed progestational effects probably contribute to the mild increase in insulin resistance observed in women receiving this drug.

Danazol's androgenic properties play a major role in altering the production rates of a large number of liver proteins. Danazol increases the production of the following liver proteins: prealbumin, Cl-esterase inhibitor, haptoglobin, transferrin, antithrombin III, prothrombin, and plasminogen. Danazol decreases the production of these liver proteins: SHBG, thyroxine-binding globulin, and pregnancy zone protein.

Substantial evidence is accumulating that steroid hormones play a major role in the regulation of the immune system. Glucocorticoid and progestogenic agonists appear to be the most important steroid regulators of the immune system. Danazol, a drug known to interact with both progesterone and glucocorticoid receptors, has been reported to be effective in the treatment of idiopathic thrombocytopenic purpura and systemic lupus erythematosis. Recent in vivo and in vitro studies have demonstrated that danazol can directly suppress leukocyte function (Hill et al., 1987).

Danazol and Enzymes of Steroidogenesis.—In 1977, our laboratory was the first to report that danazol inhibits multiple enzymes of steroidogenesis (Barbieri et al., 1977a, 1977b). We observed that concentrations of danazol similar to those in the circulation of women taking 800 mg/day of the drug (2 μmol/L) inhibit multiple enzymes involved in ovarian, testicular, and adrenal steroidogenesis. These enzymes include (1) 3β-hydroxysteroid dehydrogenase isomerase; (2) the 17-hydroxylase, 17-20-lyase complex; (3) 17β- hydroxysteroid dehydrogenase; (4) 11β-hydroxylase, and (5) 21-hydroxylase (Barbieri et al., 1980, 1981). Steingold and colleagues (1986) reported data that demonstrate that danazol inhibits steroidogenesis in vivo. They compared the estradiol rise caused by the administration of urinary LH and FSH in five normal women treated with danazol and five normal women not treated with danazol. Danazol treatment resulted in a 50% decrease in serum estradiol. This suggests that danazol inhibited the effects of exogenous gonadotropins by a direct action on the ovary. These investigators also provided evidence that danazol is an inhibitor of the ovarian 17-hydroxylase enzyme in vivo in a second experiment, in which all the experimental subjects were given dexamethasone. The purpose of this manipulation was to ensure that all serum C-21 and C-19 steroids were derived from the ovary. One half of the subjects were then treated with danazol. In the women treated with danazol, a significant increase in serum pregnenolone along with a concomitant decrease in serum 17-hydroxypregnenolone, androstenedione, and dehydroepiandrosterone was observed (Steingold et al., 1986). These studies suggest that danazol blocks ovarian estrogen production by inhibiting enzymes of steroidogenesis.

As previously noted, an acyclic, high-androgen, low-estrogen environment is extremely hostile to the growth of endometriotic tissue. Danazol produces a high-androgen environment because (1) danazol is inherently androgenic, and (2) danazol produces high levels of bioavailable testosterone by displacing testosterone from SHBG. A high-androgen environment directly inhibits the growth of endometriotic tissue. Danazol produces a low-estrogen environment by (1) inhibiting follicular growth by decreasing LH secretion (and FSH secretion) and (2) inhibiting follicular estrogen secretion via a direct action on follicular steroidogenesis. In addition, the acyclic endocrine environment produced by danazol minimizes the chance of menstruation, which prevents the "reseeding" of the peritoneum with new implants of the retrograde transported endometrium. The acyclic endocrine environment may also decrease pelvic pain by inhibiting bleeding in the endometriotic implants.

Guidelines concerning the use of danazol continue to evolve. The following discussion highlights the areas of consensus and the breadth of disagreement concerning the use of danazol.

Selection of Patients for Therapy.—Most clinicians agree that patients with a suspected diagnosis of endometriosis must have confirmation of the diagnosis by laparoscopy or laparotomy prior to initiation of therapy.

Initiation of Therapy.—Danazol should be initiated after the completion of a normal menses. It is important that danazol not be administered to a pregnant woman. Female pseudohermaphroditism is common in female offspring of mothers treated with danazol during the first and second trimesters (Duck and Katayama, 1981). Danazol is an effective contraceptive agent (less than 1% incidence of ovulation) at doses of 400 to 800 mg/day. However, patients with poor medication compliance can become pregnant on these doses of danazol because they are taking the drug in an intermittent fashion. Pregnancy testing and careful uterine examinations during danazol therapy will ensure the early detection of an unintended pregnancy. At doses of danazol less than 400 mg/day, the incidence of ovulation is substantial, thus barrier contraceptive should be used. In addition, women taking more than 400 mg/day of danazol should use a barrier contraceptive if their medication compliance is poor.

Dosage.—Danazol in doses of 200 mg/day or greater produces pain relief in the majority of patients with endometriosis. However, doses of at least 400 mg of danazol are required to reliably induce amenorrhea (Table 11–9; Biberoglu and Behrman, 1981). Given these considerations and a desire to minimize costs, we start most patients on 200 mg of danazol twice daily. For patients with severe endometriosis, consideration can be given to using danazol at a dose of 200 mg four times daily.

Cessation of menses and serum estradiol levels are good clinical and laboratory monitors of danazol therapy. Many experienced clinicians believe that the maximal therapeutic effect of danazol occurs if menses are completely suppressed. The greater the degree of estrogen suppression, the greater the likelihood that amenorrhea will occur. The interval between drug administration appears to play an important role in determining the degree of estrogen suppression. For example, in one study, the mean serum estradiol concentration was 40% lower in patients receiving 200 mg of danazol every 6 hours than in patients receiving 400 mg of danazol every 12 hours (Dickey et al., 1984).

Duration of Therapy.—Initial trials investigating the efficacy of danazol evaluated a 6-month therapy regimen. This therapy interval need not be followed rigidly. Individualization of care is important when danazol is used to treat endometriosis. For example, in the patient with advanced endometriosis who is scheduled for conservative

laparotomy, a 12-week preoperative course of danazol might be appropriate. For the patient with painful endometriosis who does not desire pregnancy and who is adamantly opposed to surgery, a 52- to 78-week course of danazol is not unreasonable if side effects and laboratory parameters are carefully monitored.

Side Effects.—In our experience, more than 75% of patients receiving danazol will complain of one or more side effects (Barbieri et al., 1982). The major side effects seen with danazol therapy (in decreasing order of frequency) are weight gain, edema, decreased breast size, acne, oily skin, hirsutism, deepening of the voice, headache, hot flashes, changes in libido, and muscle cramps. Significant weight gain (2–10 kg) is not uncommon.

Contraindications.—In nonpregnant, nonbreast-feeding patients with documented endometriosis, relatively few absolute contraindications to danazol therapy exist. Danazol is metabolized largely via hepatic mechanisms and has been reported to produce mild changes in liver function tests (elevated serum transaminase levels) in some patients. Therefore, in patients with hepatic dysfunction, danazol is relatively contraindicated. Since danazol can induce marked fluid retention, patients with severe hypertension, congestive heart failure, or borderline renal function may experience deterioration of their medical condition after danazol therapy is begun.

Timing of Attempts at Conception After Completion of Therapy.—Dmowski and Cohen (1978) have reported a high number of second-

TABLE 11–9.

Dose Response Characteristics of Danazol in the Treatment of Endometriosis After 6 Months of Treatment

Daily Dose of Danazol (mg)	Percentage of Women With		
	Amenorrhea	Symptomatic Improvement	Objective Improvement
100	29	54	67
200	38	86	79
400	86	74	66
600	88	96	91

*From Biberoglu K, Behrman SJ: Dosage aspects of danazol therapy in endometriosis: Short-term and long-term effectiveness. *Am J Obstet Gynecol* 1981; 139:645. Used by permission.

and third-trimester intrauterine fetal deaths in patients who conceived within the first three cycles after discontinuation of danazol. They suggest that this degree of fetal wastage may be secondary to implantation in an atrophic endometrium and that following a course of danazol, one full menstrual cycle with normal flow and duration be observed prior to any attempts to conceive. In contrast to these observations, Daniell and Christianson (1981) observed no increase in fetal wastage in patients conceiving within 3 months of completing a course of danazol. Barbieri, Evans, and Kistner (1982) confirmed that danazol therapy was not associated with increased fetal wastage. Further information is needed to resolve these discrepancies.

Use of Danazol With Surgery in the Treatment of the Infertility of Endometriosis.—In patients with infertility and advanced stages of endometriosis, surgery is usually necessary to repair anatomic abnormalities and to remove implants of endometriosis. Little experimental data concerning the value of danazol in the preoperative or postoperative management of endometriosis are available. Some experienced clinicians suggest that danazol has little value in the preoperative management of endometriosis, whereas others believe that danazol may improve the prognosis for infertile women with endometriosis by decreasing the number and size of endometriotic areas, thereby minimizing the extent of surgery. In addition, the preoperative use of danazol eliminates the chance of traumatizing a corpus luteum. Use of danazol in the postoperative management of the infertile patient with endometriosis is also controversial. Most conceptions following surgical therapy occur within the first 12 months after surgery. Therefore, by treating surgical patients with danazol for a prolonged period postoperatively, the time interval with the highest fertility potential may be passed over. It is our belief that danazol should be used in most patients preoperatively and that short courses of postoperative danazol therapy should be reserved for women with residual disease.

Use in the Treatment of Endometriosis in Patients Not Desiring Fertility.—For the patient older than 40 years with symptomatic endometriosis who has completed her family, definitive therapy consisting of TAH-BSO is usually recommended. However, some patients may want to postpone or avoid major surgery. For these patients a trial of danazol may be reasonable. For the young symptomatic patient with endometriosis who intends to delay pregnancy, danazol therapy is highly effective in relieving symptoms and physical findings.

Treatment of Endometriomas.—No systematic study assessing the effect of danazol on endometriomas has been reported. Clinical experience suggests that danazol can often reduce the size of small endometriomas but that it is unusual for danazol to cause complete regression of an endometrioma. In general, danazol is more effective in causing regression of peritoneal endometriotic implants of small diameter than in ablating cysts. Large ovarian masses generally require surgical exploration.

Use in Metastatic Endometriosis.—For the majority of patients with endometriosis involving organs outside the pelvis, TAH-BSO is necessary. Certain patients, however, will refuse surgery, and others are extremely poor operative risks. In these patients, danazol therapy is an alternative of last resort. Danazol has been successful in the treatment of pulmonary endometriosis, bowel obstruction, and ureteral obstruction caused by endometriosis. However, once hormone therapy is discontinued, the disease often recurs.

Recurrence Rates After Therapy for Endometriosis.—A major problem in the treatment of endometriosis is that the disease tends to recur unless definitive surgical therapy is performed. Following a course of danazol therapy, the recurrence of symptoms and physical findings is at least 20% per year and is generally higher in patients with endometriomas (Barbieri et al., 1982). A second course of danazol therapy is often successful in inducing a remission of disease symptoms and physical findings.

Danazol vs. Pseudopregnancy.—Very little data that directly compare the efficacy of danazol vs. a pseudopregnancy regimen in the treatment of endometriosis are available. The results of one small, prospective, randomized trial of danazol vs. a combination of mestranol and norethynodrel have been reported by Noble and Letchworth (1979). A total of 86% of the patients treated with danazol reported improvement in their symptoms. Only 30% of the pseudopregnancy group reported symptomatic improvement, and improvement in objective findings was demonstrated in 84% of patients treated with danazol compared with only 18% of patients on the pseudopregnancy regimen. Side effects were a major problem for patients receiving both therapeutic regimens. Only 4% of the danazol group but 41% of the pseudopregnancy group discontinued therapy because of side effects. In a retrospective study of 438 patients, Mettler and Semm (1984) found that patients with endometriosis treated medically had a higher fertility rate when treated with danazol (45%) than when treated with lynestrenol (32%). However, it is difficult to assess the validity of the results of either study because of several deficiencies in design. The clinical impression of those who have used danazol extensively is that it is more effective than pseudopregnancy in the treatment of endometriosis.

Gonadotropin-Releasing Hormone Agonist Therapy

Gonadotropin-releasing hormone is a hypothalamic decapeptide that controls LH and FSH secretion. In primates, pulses of GnRH in the range of one pulse per hour are associated with a normal pattern of LH and FSH secretion, normal follicular and corpus luteum development, and cyclic menses. Administration of GnRH at a high pulse rate (more than five pulses per hour) or in a continuous fashion produces an initial increase in LH and FSH secretion, followed by a drastic decrease in LH and FSH secretion with cessation of ovarian follicular activity, hypoestrogenism, and amenorrhea. This may be due to downregulation or desensitization of pituitary GnRH receptors by continuous infusion of GnRH (Knobil, 1980).

The natural decapeptide GnRH has a short half-life because of its degradation by tissue and circulating peptidases. Therefore, it is difficult to produce a constant circulating concentration using native GnRH. By the chemical alteration of amino acids 6 and 10 of GnRH, analogues can be synthesized that have two useful properties: high affinity for the pituitary GnRH receptor and a very long half-life due to the resistance to cleavage by endopeptidases. Initially, many investigators believed that these synthetic derivatives of GnRH would be superagonists and potent fertility-enhancing agents, hence the term GnRH agonists. Unexpectedly, however, GnRH agonists proved to be potent inhibitors of gonadal function. Their administration to men or women causes a transient 1- to 2-week increase in the production of LH and FSH by the pituitary gland and then a dramatic and sustained decrease in pituitary production of bioactive LH and FSH. The ability of the GnRH agonists to downregulate pituitary secretion of gonadotropins has not been fully explained. Numerous GnRH agonists, including nafarelin, leuprolide, buserelin, goserelin, histrelin, and tryptorelin, are currently being evaluated in clinical trials (Table 11–10). Currently, no GnRH agonist is effective when given orally. These agents, however, can be administered by monthly intramuscular depot injections or implants or by daily subcutaneous injections or nasal spray (Table 11–11).

Treatment with GnRH agonists results in the reversible suppression of gonadal steroid production in men and women. Consequently, many diseases that are modulated by the gonadal steroids testosterone and estradiol can be successfully treated with GnRH agonists.

For example, GnRH agonists have been reported to be successful in the treatment of endometriosis, leiomyomata uteri, polycystic ovarian disease, precocious puberty, and premenstrual syndrome and as an adjuvant for the induction of ovulation in women and in the treatment of prostatic cancer in men.

Henzl and associates (1988) have reported on the comparative efficacies of danazol and the

TABLE 11–10.

Structures of Gonadotropin-Releasing Hormone Agonists With Documented Efficacy in the Treatment of Endometriosis

Native GnRH	*p* Glu-His-Trp-Spr-Tyr-Gly-Leu-Arg-Pro-Gly-NH2		
		6	10
Leuprolide		D-Leu	-NHEt
Buserelin		D-Ser(*t*Bu)	-AzA-Gly
Nafarelin		D-NAL(2)	—

TABLE 11-11.

Doses of Gonadotropin-Releasing Hormone Agonists
Used in the Treatment of Endometriosis

Leuprolide acetate	0.5–1.0 mg subcutaneously daily
Leuprolide acetate–Depo formulation	3.75–7.5 mg intramuscularly monthly
Nafarelin	0.4–0.8 mg intranasally daily

GnRH agonist nafarelin in the treatment of endometriosis. In our opinion, this study was the best-designed and best-executed trial of drug therapy for endometriosis ever reported (Barbieri, 1988). The study was large, randomized, and double blind and included an objective assessment of the response to therapy by a comparison of laparoscopic examinations performed before and after treatment. The investigators tested two dosages of nasal nafarelin (400 and 800 μg/day) and one dosage of oral danazol (800 mg/day). Drug therapy was continued for 6 months. More than 80% of the patients treated with either nafarelin or danazol had symptomatic and objective improvement in their condition. Nafarelin and danazol were found to be quantitatively similar in efficacy (Fig 11–10). However, the side effects of the two drugs differed substantially. The women receiving danazol reported weight gain, edema, and myalgia and had increased circulating levels of serum aspartate aminotransferase and alanine aminotransferase and decreased levels of HDL cholesterol. In contrast, the principal side effects reported by women receiving nafarelin were hot flashes, decreased libido, and vaginal dryness.

The women treated with nafarelin did not have notable decreases in HDL cholesterol levels or increases in serum aspartate aminotransferase and alanine aminotransferase levels. Since estrogen is a major regulator of bone density in women, it should be expected that the hypoestrogenic state induced by GnRH agonists may produce a decrease in bone mass. Henzl and colleagues (1988) did not report on the effect of nafarelin on bone mass. In their discussion of nafarelin, however, they note that therapy with this drug is probably associated with an appreciable loss of spinal trabecular bone mass, although this loss may be partially reversible after therapy is discontinued.

For women who cannot tolerate danazol therapy, treatment with GnRH agonists represents an important therapeutic alternative (Barbieri, 1988).

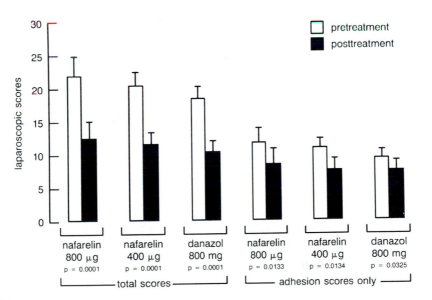

FIG 11-10.

Pretreatment and posttreatment American Fertility Society endometriosis scores in women receiving 6 months of nasal nafarelin or oral danazol therapy. (From Henzl M, Corson SL, Moghissi K, et al: Administration of nasal nafarelin as compared with oral danazol for endometriosis: A multicenter double-blind comparative clinical trial. *N Engl J Med* 1988; 318:485. Reproduced by permission.)

Guidelines for the use of leuprolide or na-farelin for the treatment of endometriosis are similar to those outlined for the use of danazol: (1) document the presence of endometriosis by laparoscopy or laparotomy, (2) ensure that the patient is not pregnant, (3) employ the drug at a dose that will induce amenorrhea, (4) consider a treatment interval of 6 months, and (5) monitor side effects carefully.

Pseudopregnancy Regimens

In response to chronic, noncyclic stimulation by both estrogen and progesterone, the endometrium becomes inactive and demonstrates decidualization. Figures 11–11 and 11–12 illustrate this phenomenon. This observation is the basis for the use of uninterrupted combined estrogen-progestogen agents in the treatment of endometriosis (Kistner, 1958, 1960). There is no evidence that any one preparation of estrogen-progestogen pill is uniquely effective in the treatment of endometriosis. Therefore, any combined estrogen-progestogen preparation may be employed; however, oral contraceptives utilizing an androgenic progestin have theoretical appeal. A standard regimen would employ 0.03 mg of ethinyl estradiol with 0.3 mg of norgestrel (Lo/Ovral) daily. The hormones are given every day for 3 to 4 months. For 1 week the medication is discontinued, and a light menstrual bleed may occur at this time. The medication is then reinstituted for another course. If clinically significant breakthrough bleeding occurs, the hormone dosage can be increased to 0.05 mg of ethinyl estradiol with 0.5 mg of norgestrel (Ovral) daily.

In our experience, a pseudopregnancy regimen is especially useful in the management of dysmenorrhea due to endometriosis in the young patient. For example, for a 17-year-old teenager with mild endometriosis with incapacitating dysmenorrhea, we will often prescribe a pseudopregnancy regimen as previously described. For the teenage patient, a pseudopregnancy regimen is less expensive and often better tolerated than danazol.

Progestin-Only Regimens

Numerous progestins (e.g., medroxyprogesterone acetate, norethindrone acetate, norgestrel acetate, and lynestrenol) have been used as single

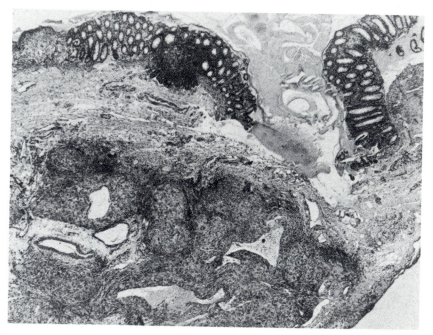

FIG 11–11.
Biopsy of a mass in the rectovaginal septum during the 14th week of pregnancy. Rectal mucosa is seen at the top of the section. Approximately two thirds of the rectal wall has been replaced by endometriotic tissue made up of inactive glands and decidua. The endometrial stroma (as decidua) is packed in whorl-like accumulations. (From Kistner RW: The use of steroidal substances in endometriosis. *Clin Pharmacol Ther* 1960; 1:525. Reproduced by permission.)

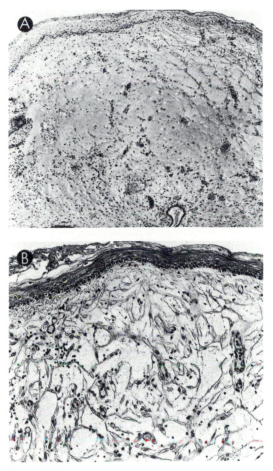

FIG 11–12.
Biopsy of an area of vaginal endometriosis after 12 weeks of continuous norethyndrel with ethinyl estradiol therapy. **A,** there is evidence of marked generalized edema throughout the endometriosis. Under the vaginal epithelium the decidua is well maintained, but most of it is undergoing necrosis. **B,** high-power view of **A.** An unusual pattern of decidual change is present. Most decidual cells remain as naked nuclei or as a cytoplasmic strand in an edematous stroma. A few lymphocytes and macrophages are present and suggest an absorptive process of the necrotic endometriosis. (From Kistner RW: The treatment of endometriosis by inducing pseudopregnancy with ovarian hormones. *Fertil Steril* 1959; 10:549. Reproduced by permission.)

agents for the treatment of endometriosis (Semm and Mettler, 1980). In general, these agents produce a hypoestrogenic-acyclic hormonal environment by suppressing ovarian follicular activity via inhibition of LH and FSH secretion. In addition, these agents may have direct effects on endo-

metriotic tissue androgen and progesterone receptors. As noted earlier, many synthetic progestins are weak androgen agonists.

A major problem with the use of progestins as single agents is that large doses must be given to produce an acyclic-hypoestrogenic environment. These high doses are often associated with side effects such as bloating, weight gain, depression, and irregular uterine bleeding. Parenteral administration of large doses of medroxyprogesterone acetate in depot form can be effective in the treatment of endometriosis (dose range 150 mg every 3 months to 150 mg every month). However, this drug is not recommended as a first-line agent because it can produce prolonged amenorrhea after termination of therapy, and the long-term safety of the agent is still controversial. Oral administration of 30 to 50 mg of medroxyprogesterone acetate daily can be effective in the treatment of endometriosis.

Surgical Treatment

In contemplating surgical treatment of endometriosis, one should always bear in mind that functioning ovarian tissue is necessary for the continued activity of the disease. Therefore, the successful treatment of endometriosis depends on a knowledge of when it is reasonably safe or desirable to maintain ovarian function and when it is necessary to eliminate it. It is quite obvious that ovarian function should be conserved in treating very early and, perhaps, symptomless lesions and eliminated when the pelvic organs are hopelessly invaded by endometriosis or when fertility is no longer a concern. Unfortunately, from the standpoint of definite surgical indications, the majority of cases will fall between these two extremes and may present problems in surgical judgment seldom encountered in any other pelvic disease. As our knowledge of the life history of endometriosis has increased, there has been a definite tendency to become more conservative, particularly in the treatment of early and borderline cases. In general, it is believed that one should err on the side of conservatism. This belief is based on the fact that endometriosis (1) usually progresses slowly over a period of years, (2) is not inherently and only very rarely becomes malignant, and (3) regresses at the menopause.

Current surgical options include laparoscopic surgery, conservative surgery via a laparotomy, and extirpative surgery.

Laparoscopic Surgery

The diagnosis of endometriosis requires laparoscopy or laparotomy, so there is an efficiency to the suggestion that at the time of a diagnostic laparoscopy, an attempt should be made to excise all endometriotic implants and adhesions. Laparoscopic surgery for advanced endometriosis requires 2 to 3 hours of operative time, advanced technical skills on the part of the surgeon, and specialized equipment. Minimal and mild endometriosis can often be surgically treated at the time of diagnostic laparoscopy without significantly prolonging operative time and with a minimum of special skills and equipment. Laparoscopic treatment of endometriosis utilizes a two- or three-puncture technique. Two lower abdominal incisions are often necessary to grasp specific pelvic organs and to allow the utilization of unipolar or bipolar electocautery or laser for lysis of adhesions and ablation of implants. Ablation of the uterosacral ligaments at laparoscopy may decrease pain in some patients. There have been no studies directly comparing the efficacy of electrocautery and laser in the treatment of endometriosis associated infertility. Laser surgery has the theoretical advantage, however, that the depth of tissue injury induced is often less than that produced by cautery. Advances in laparoscopic surgery are discussed in more detail in Chapter 22.

Conservative Surgery Technique

If childbearing function is to be preserved, operative procedures should be as conservative as possible. The approach can usually be through a suprapubic transverse incision. Thorough exploration of the pelvic and abdominal organs should be performed routinely and the decision reached whether conservative or definitive surgery should be performed. It is important to stress good infertility surgical technique. Gentle handling of tissues and meticulous hemostasis are important in minimizing subsequent adhesion formation. The uterus is frequently found to be adherent to the rectosigmoid. These adhesions are separated either by blunt or sharp dissection in the midline so that the uterus can be brought forward. Traction sutures of 1-0 Mersilene may be placed around the round ligaments to lift the corpus forward and out of the cul-de-sac (Fig 11–13). With the uterus held forward, further adhesions may then be separated under direct vision. As previously

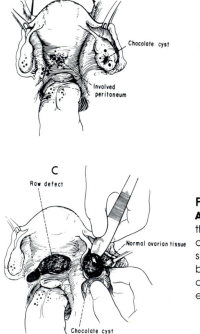

FIG 11–13.
A, the uterus is drawn forward using traction sutures placed around the round ligaments. Areas of endometriosis are shown on the ovaries, posterior aspect of the uterus, and anterior surface of the sigmoid colon. **B,** serosa of posterior aspect of the uterus involved by endometriosis is excised. Alternatively, endometriotic lesions in this area can be fulgurated. **C,** endometrioma of the right ovary is excised, preserving as much normal ovarian cortex as possible.

mentioned, the use of hormonal agents for 6 to 12 weeks preoperatively may make the surgery easier to perform. Endometrial implants on the uterosacral ligaments or in the cul-de-sac may be excised, fulgurated by electrocautery, or vaporized by laser. Because some pain transmitting nerve fibers from the uterus course through the uterosacral ligaments, some gynecologists cut or fulgurate them in the hope of reducing postoperative dysmenorrhea.

Endometrial cysts of the ovary should be excised. These cysts are usually adherent and do not separate as freely as corpus luteum or follicular cysts. After as much of the cyst as possible has been removed, the walls of the ovary are reapproximated with several mattress stitches of fine Vicryl suture, and the surface is closed with a running, locked stitch of 4-0 Vicryl suture. Occasionally all ovarian tissue is destroyed, and oophorectomy is necessary. Nevertheless, it is remarkable how frequently an ovarian cyst can be enucleated and a fairly thick capsule of functioning cortical tissue left in situ. We have had the experience of performing unilateral salpingo-oophorectomy (USO) and resection of 90% of the remaining ovary and of being rewarded by subsequent ovulation and pregnancy. This is not always the case, however, and some patients have premature menopause following such surgery.

Early implantations on the surface of the peritoneum, wherever they are located, may be excised or destroyed with cautery or the laser. Conservative operations may also be accompanied by correction of uterine displacement, relief of cervical stenosis, and removal of any other concomitant pelvic pathology to aid in the prevention of a recurrence of the condition. Presacral neurectomy, in which the superior hypogastric plexus is divided and ligated, may be performed at the same time to reduce pain associated with endometriosis in women who wish to preserve childbearing.

The use of intraoperative, intraperitoneal adjuvants to prevent adhesion formation has become widespread in gynecologic surgery without substantial experimental evidence to support its efficacy. Glucocorticoids, promethazine, high molecular weight dextran (Hyskon), and heparin all have been used in this effort. In addition, some gynecologists have advocated the postoperative use of nonsteroidal anti-inflammatory drugs such as ibuprofen to reduce adhesion formation associated with pelvic surgery.

In recent years, Hyskon (a water-soluble glucose polymer of 32% dextran 70 in 10% dextrose) has become popular among gynecologic surgeons. It is widely used as a distending medium for hysteroscopy and is frequently used to prevent adhesions as well (Rosenberg and Board, 1984). The mechanism of action in minimizing adhesions is unknown but probably occurs due to several of its properties. It is hyperosmolar, so it induces a temporary ascites separating serosal layers. It also may inhibit coagulation of fibrin on traumatized serosal surfaces. The solution is easily administered by pouring 50 to 100 ml over the pelvic viscera prior to closing the peritoneum.

Serious side effects, including anaphylaxis, vulvar edema, and pleural effusions, have been reported (Reisner, 1984; Tulandi, 1987). These complications can be prevented by the prophylactic intravenous use of low molecular weight dextran (Promit). Promit is a monovalent hapten that prevents the formation of immune complexes of dextran-reactive immunoglobulin (IgG) and thus impedes the occurrence of allergic phenomena. Promit should be given several minutes before the use of Hyskon.

Recent studies have also shown some reduction in postoperative adhesions when antiprostaglandins have been used postoperatively (Jarrett and Dawood, 1986). The use of Hyskon with an antiprostaglandin has provided greater adhesion reduction than when either agent was used alone (DeLeon et al., 1986).

Despite a number of studies showing benefits from the use of these adhesion prevention modalities, some investigators have found no benefit to their use. Simple use of Ringer's lactated solution may provide protection against adhesions equal to that achieved by other means and produces fewer side effects (Fayez and Schneider, 1987).

Since leiomyomas of the uterus are found in about 15% of patients with endometriosis, single or multiple myomectomy should be carried out as part of the conservative approach. A uterine suspension is sometimes performed. The uterosacral ligaments are plicated in the midline. This accomplishes forward fixation of the uterus, and the shortened uterosacral ligaments effect a backward pull on the cervix, producing a more normal anatomic position.

Hormonal therapy is generally given for approximately 3 months after surgery if all areas of endometriosis cannot be excised; then concerted efforts toward conception are made. About one half of women so treated will become pregnant if no other cause for infertility exists.

The incidence of pregnancy following conservative surgery varies widely and is dependent on such factors as extent of the disease, age of the patient, frequency of coitus, previous parity, and the presence of other pelvic pathologic lesions (leiomyomas, tubal disease, or adhesions) at the time of surgery. It seems reasonable to expect that approximately 40% to 70% of patients who are desirous of childbearing will become pregnant after conservative surgical treatment for endometriosis. Most pregnancies will occur within the first 12 months following conservative surgery.

Extirpative Surgery

As mentioned earlier, the treatment of choice for most women with advanced endometriosis who have completed their family is TAH-BSO. From a pathophysiologic viewpoint, it is the bilateral oophorectomy and the concomitant hypoestrogenism that provide relief from the disease process. Many authorities recommend TAH with unilateral salpingo-oophorectomy (USO) for the treatment of endometriosis. These authorities argue that leaving one ovary in situ will prevent the sequelae of an early surgical menopause. Although this is true, approximately 50% of women treated with TAH-USO will require reoperation because of persistent endometriosis. In our opinion the 50% failure rate associated with TAH-USO for advanced endometriosis makes this an unattractive option. However, in cases of mild to moderate endometriosis, TAH-USO may be a reasonable treatment choice.

When definitive surgery for advanced endometriosis is performed, it is important to remove all functioning ovarian tissue. We have seen many women with advanced endometriosis who allegedly have had TAH-BSO and present with persistent symptoms of disease activity. Uniformly, these women have serum estradiol and FSH concentrations in the premenopausal range. These laboratory studies demonstrate the presence of residual ovarian activity. The high frequency of this scenario has prompted us to make the following recommendations. First, during TAH-BSO for advanced endometriosis, the infundibulopelvic vessels should be ligated high on the pelvic side wall through an incision in the retroperitoneum. Second, every attempt should be made to remove the ovaries en bloc along with adherent peritoneal surfaces. Third, after TAH-BSO, serum FSH and estradiol levels should be monitored monthly until these hormones enter the menopausal range.

Large bilateral ovarian endometrial cysts with extensive peritoneal endometriosis and numerous pelvic adhesions or with marked invasion of the rectosigmoid and rectovaginal space constitute the most urgent indications for radical removal of all the pelvic organs, regardless of the age of the patient.

From the operative standpoint, early or moderately advanced endometriosis offers no unusual difficulties, but extensive endometriosis may present many technical problems. Endometriosis, in contrast to pelvic inflammatory disease, produces an extremely dense type of pelvic adhesions with almost complete absence of planes of cleavage. Therefore, much of the dissection must be done with sharp instruments, and the danger of damage to adherent structures is thereby increased. This hazard may be diminished by the use of preoperative danazol or GnRH agonists.

A hysterectomy and BSO can usually be done on patients with large ovarian endometrial cysts and extensive pelvic adhesions and even on those with marked invasion of the rectovaginal septum. This may be facilitated by incising the posterior peritoneum above the insertion of the uterosacral ligaments. The endopelvic fascia and rectosigmoid may then be reflected, and the danger of fistula formation is minimized. At times, it may be necessary to leave a considerable portion of the implants attached to the bowel or other pelvic structures, but these remnants will regress along with other müllerian tissue in the pelvis following removal of the ovaries, a fact of great importance in the treatment of this disease. A few cases where this atrophy did not occur have been reported; one may suspect, however, that not all ovarian tissue was completely removed in some of these cases.

As we have repeatedly emphasized, hypoestrogenism "cures" most cases of endometriosis. Paradoxically, most women who have undergone TAH-BSO for advanced endometriosis can use low-dose estrogen replacement therapy without reactivating the endometriosis. In our practice, if significant endometriosis is still present after TAH-BSO, we will wait 3 to 6 months prior to initiating estrogen replacement therapy. At that time we prescribe 0.625 mg of conjugated equine estrogens (CEEs) daily or its equivalent. With this regimen, fewer than 10% of patients should have reactivation of their disease. If the disease does recur, the hormone replacement can be discontinued. Some authorities believe that residual endometriotic implants can undergo malignant transformation when stimulated by continuous unopposed estrogen replacement. These authorities recommend adding a cyclic progestin to the CEE. No well-controlled scientific data to evaluate this practice are available.

REFERENCES

American Fertility Society: Revised American Fertility Society classification of endometriosis. *Fertil Steril* 1985; 43:351.

Barbieri RL: CA-125 in patients with endometriosis. *Fertil Steril* 1986; 45:767.

Barbieri RL: New therapy for endometriosis. *N Engl J Med* 1988; 318:512.

Barbieri RL, Canick JA, Makris A, et al: Danazol inhibits steroidogenesis. *Fertil Steril* 1977a; 28:809.

Barbieri RL, Canick JA, Ryan KJ: Danazol inhibits steroidogenesis in the rat testis in vitro. *Endocrinology* 1977b; 101:676.

Barbieri RL, Evans S, Kistner RW: Danazol in the treatment of endometriosis: Analysis of 100 cases with a 4 year follow-up. *Fertil Steril* 1982; 37:737.

Barbieri RL, Hornstein MD: Medical therapy for endometriosis, in Wilson EA (ed): *Endometriosis*. New York, Alan R Liss, 1987, pp 111–140.

Barbieri RL, Lee H, Ryan KJ: Danazol binding to rat androgen, glucocorticoid, progesterone and estrogen receptors: Correlation with biological activity. *Fertil Steril* 1979; 31:182.

Barbieri RL, Niloff JN, Bast RC, et al: Elevated serum concentrations of CA-125 in patients with advanced endometriosis. *Fertil Steril* 1986; 45:630.

Barbieri RL, Osathanondh R, Ryan KJ: Danazol inhibition of steroidogenesis in the human corpus luteum. *Obstet Gynecol* 1981; 57:722.

Barbieri RL, Osathanondh R, Stillman RJ, et al: Danazol inhibits human adrenal 21- and 11α-hydroxylation. *Steroids* 1980; 35:251.

Barbieri RL, Ryan KJ: Danazol: Endocrine pharmacology and therapeutic applications. *Am J Obstet Gynecol* 1981; 141:453.

Bast RC, Feeney M, Lazarus H, et al: Reactivity of a monoclonal antibody with human ovarian carcinoma. *J Clin Invest* 1981; 68:1331.

Bast RC, Klug TL, St John E, et al: A radioimmunoassay using a monoclonal antibody to monitor the course of epithelial ovarian cancer. *N Engl J Med* 1983; 309:883.

Biberoglu KO, Behrman SJ: Dosage aspects of danazol therapy in endometriosis: Short-term and long-term effectiveness. *Am J Obstet Gynecol* 1981; 139:645.

Cattel RB, Swinton NW: Endometriosis with particular reference to conservative treatment. *N Engl J Med* 1936; 241:341.

Cramer DW: Epidemiology of endometriosis, in Wilson EA (ed): *Endometriosis*. New York, Alan R Liss, 1987, pp 5–22.

Cramer DW, Wilson E, Stillman RJ, et al: The relation of endometriosis to menstrual characteristics, smoking and exercise. *JAMA* 1985; 225:1904.

Cullen TS: Adenomyoma of the round ligament. *Bull Johns Hopkins* 1896; 7:112.

Daniell JF, Christianson G: Combined laparoscopic surgery and danazol therapy for pelvic endometriosis. *Fertil Steril* 1981; 35:521.

DeLeon FD, Odan J, Hudkins P, et al: Orally and parenterally administered ibuprofen for postoperative adhesion prevention. *J Reprod Med* 1986; 31:1019.

Desaulles PA, Krahenbuhl C: Comparison of the anti-fertility and sex hormone activities of sex hormones and derivatives. *Acta Endocrinol* 1964; 47:444.

Dickey RP, Taylor SN, Curole DN: Serum estradiol and danazol: I. Endometriosis response, side effects, administration interval, concurrent spironolactone and dexamethasone. *Fertil Steril* 1984; 42:709.

DiZerega GS, Barber DL, Hodgen GD: Endometriosis: Role of ovarian steroids in initiation, maintenance and suppression. *Fertil Steril* 1980; 33:649.

Dmowski WP, Cohen MR: Antigonadotropin (danazol) in the treatment of endometriosis. *Am J Obstet Gynecol* 1978; 130:41.

Duck SC, Katayama KP: Danazol may cause pseudohermaphroditism. *Fertil Steril* 1981; 35:230.

Fayez JA, Schneider PJ: Prevention of adhesion formation by different modalities of treatment. *Am J Obstet Gynecol* 1987; 157:1184.

Fedele L, Vercellini P, Arcaini L, et al: CA 125 in serum, peritoneal fluid, active lesions, and endometrium of patients with endometriosis. *Am J Obstet Gynecol* 1988; 158:166.

Friedman AJ, Barbieri RL: Leuprolide acetate: Applications in gynecology. *Curr Probl Obstet Gynecol Fertil* 1988; 11:205.

Haney AF: Pelvic endometriosis: Etiology and pathology. *Semin Reprod Endocrinol* 1988; 6:287.

Henzl MR, Corson SL, Moghissi K, et al: Administration of nasal nafarelin as compared with oral danazol for endometriosis: A multicenter double-blind comparative clinical trial. *N Engl J Med* 1988; 318:485.

Hill JA, Barbieri RL, Anderson DJ: Immunosuppressive effects of danazol in vitro. *Fertil Steril* 1987; 48:414.

Hornstein MD, Barbieri RL, McShane PM: The

effects of previous ovarian surgery on the follicular response to ovulation induction in an in vitro fertilization program. *J Reprod Med* 1989; 34:277.

Jarrett JC, Dawood MY: Adhesion formation and uterine tube healing in the rabbit: A controlled study of the effects of ibuprofen. *Am J Obstet Gynecol* 1986; 155:1186.

Jones HW, Acosta AA, Andrews MC, et al: Three years of in vitro fertilization at Norfolk. *Fertil Steril* 1984; 42:826.

Kistner RW: The use of newer progestins in the treatment of endometriosis. *Am J Obstet Gynecol* 1958; 75:264.

Kistner RW: The use of steroidal substances in endometriosis. *Clin Pharmacol Ther* 1960; 1:525.

Knobil E: The neuroendocrine control of the menstrual cycle. *Recent Prog Horm Res* 1980; 36:53.

Malkasian GD Jr, Podratz KC, Stanhope CR, et al: CA 125 in gynecologic practice. *Am J Obstet Gynecol* 1986; 155:515.

Mettler L, Semm K: Three-step therapy of genital endometriosis in cases of human infertility with lynestrenol, danazol or gestrinone administration in the second step, in Raynaud JP (ed): *Medical Management of Endometriosis.* New York, Raven Press, 1984, pp 233–247.

Meyer R: Uber endometrium in der tube sowie uber die hierausentstehenden wirklichen und virmantlichen folgen. *Zentralbl Gynakol* 1927; 51:1482.

Nilsson B, Sodergard R, Damber MG, et al: Danazol and gestagen displacement of testosterone and influence of sex hormone binding capacity. *Fertil Steril* 1982; 38:48.

Nishimura K, Togashi K, Itoh K, et al: Endometrial cysts of the ovary: MR imaging. *Radiology* 1987; 162:315.

Noble AD, Letchworth AT: Medical treatment of endometriosis: A comparative trial. *Postgrad Med J* 1979; 55(suppl 5):37.

Pittaway DE: Endometriosis and spontaneous abortion. *Semin Reprod Endocrinol* 1988; 6:257.

Pittaway DE, Fayez JA: The use of CA-125 in the diagnosis and management of endometriosis. *Fertil Steril* 1986; 46:790.

Reisner LS: Anaphylaxis to intraperitoneal dextran. *Anesthesiology* 1984; 60:259.

Rosenberg SM, Board JA: High molecular weight dextran and human infertility surgery. *Am J Obstet Gynecol* 1984; 148:380.

Rokitansky C: Über uterusdrusen-neubilding im uterus und ovarialsarcomen. *ZKK Gesellch d Arzte zu Wein* 1860; 37:577.

Sampson JA: Perforating hemorrhagic (chocolate) cysts of the ovary. *Arch Surg* 1921; 3:245.

Sampson JA: Endometrial carcinoma of the ovary arising in endometrial tissue in that organ. *Arch Surg* 1925; 10:1.

Scully RE, Richardson GS, Barlow JF: The development of malignancy in endometriosis. *Clin Obstet Gynecol* 1966; 9:384.

Seibel MM, Berger MJ, Weinstein FG, et al: The effectiveness of danazol on subsequent fertility in minimal endometriosis. *Fertil Steril* 1982; 38:534.

Semm K, Mettler L: Technical progress in pelvic surgery via operative laparoscopy. *Am J Obstet Gynecol* 1980; 138:121.

Steingold KA, Lu JKH, Judd HL, et al: Danazol inhibits steroidogenesis by the human ovary in vivo. *Fertil Steril* 1986; 45:649.

Tulandi T: Transient edema after intraperitoneal instillation of 32% dextran 70: A report of five cases. *J Reprod Med* 1987; 32:472.

12   Evaluation of the Infertile Couple

Mitchell S. Rein, M.D.

Isaac Schiff, M.D.

The definition of infertility is 1 year of unprotected coitus without conception. The term *primary infertility* is applied to the couple who has never achieved a pregnancy; *secondary infertility* implies that at least one previous conception has taken place. The purpose of the present chapter is to review the investigation of the infertile couple. Because more and more infertile couples are seeking help in achieving a pregnancy, the importance of an efficient and systematic evaluation cannot be overstated. A thorough infertility investigation has four important purposes:

1. It attempts to offer an explanation for the infertility.
2. It furnishes a basis for therapy.
3. It provides a prognosis that enables couples to make realistic decisions regarding their treatment options.
4. It provides an emotional foundation for maintaining their psychological well-being.

EPIDEMIOLOGY

The epidemiology of infertility is best understood in the context of the probability of fertility. *Fecundability* is defined as the probability of conceiving during a monthly cycle and provides the basis for estimating fertility over time. The fecundability of "normal" couples using no contraception has been estimated to be about 20% to 25% per cycle (Cramer et al., 1979). Based on a fecundability of 20% to 25%, 50% of couples should conceive after 3 to 4 months and 95% after 12 months. This cumulative fertility is a simple function of fecundability. It provides a basis for the clinical rule that 12 months of unprotected intercourse may define a fertility problem. Using this definition, the National Survey of Family Growth estimates 10% to 15% of couples may be classified as infertile (Mosher, 1982, 1985).

Data from several sources suggest maternal age may affect fecundability. A multicenter French study evaluated cumulative fertility rates in 2,193 multiparous women with azoospermic husbands who underwent artificial donor insemination (Schwartz and Mayaux, 1982). The cumulative fertility after 12 cycles of insemination declined after age 30 years. The cumulative fertility after 12 cycles of insemination was 73% for women younger than 25 years, 74.1% for those 26 to 30 years of age, 61.5% for those 31 to 35 years of age, and only 53.6% for women more than 35 years of age. Data extrapolated from the 1976 National Survey of Family Growth similarly suggest a decline in fecundity with increasing maternal age (Table 12–1; Hendershot et al., 1982). A substantial decline in fertility after age 30 years has also been observed among Hutterite women (Tietze, 1957). In summary, fecundity in women is maximal around the age of 25 years, and the incidence of infertility increases after the age of 30 years.

It is important to categorize the nature of the fertility problem based on the pathophysiological source in the man or woman. The major categories of infertility are male factor, 35%; ovulatory factors, 20%; tubal factor, 20%; cervical factor, 5%; endometriosis, 10%; and unexplained, 10%. It has been estimated that 25% to 35% of all infertility problems are of multiple origin.

TABLE 12–1.

The Influence of Age on the Cumulative Pregnancy Rate*

Age Group (yr)	Conceiving in 12 mo. (%)
20–24	86
25–29	78
30–34	63
35–39	52

*Adapted from Hendershot GE, Mosher WD, Pratt WF: Infertility and age: An unresolved issue. *Fam Plan Perspect* 1982; 14:287.

Presumptive etiological factors have been identified for some categories of infertility. Iatrogenic factors (conization and cautery), sexually transmitted diseases (Horne et al., 1973), and smoking (Phipps et al., 1987) have been associated with cervical factor. Pelvic inflammatory disease (PID) has been strongly associated with tubal factor (Westrom, 1983). The increasing incidence of ectopic pregnancy and infertility is largely attributed to the increasing incidence of PID. Other risk factors for tubal factor include endometriosis, diethylstilbestrol (DES) exposure, intrauterine device (IUD) use, and smoking. Although oral contraceptive pills (OCPs) seem to protect against PID, they may not be beneficial for tubal factor due to the poorer protection against *Chlamydia* (Washington et al., 1985). Risk factors for endometriosis include menstrual irregularities, dysmenorrhea, and a family history of endometriosis (Cramer et al., 1986). Exercising and smoking appear to have a protective effect for endometriosis. The etiological factors associated with ovulatory dysfunction include smoking, exercise, body habitus, and genetic factors. Hereditary factors associated with premature ovarian failure (POF) include x chromosome deletions and errors of galactose metabolism. Multiple factors have been associated with male factor infertility; these will be discussed under the evaluation of male factor.

The prognosis for infertile couples appears to be strongly affected by their clinical diagnoses, as demonstrated in a group of almost 1,300 infertile couples (Collins et al., 1984). The cumulative conception rates are shown in Figure 12–1. Couples with ovulatory disorders seem to have the best prognosis (Collins et al., 1984; Dor et al.,

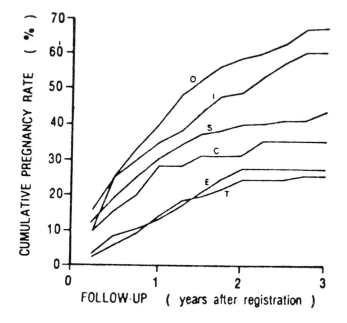

FIG 12–1.

Cumulative pregnancy rates and primary clinical diagnoses among infertile couples. *(O),* ovulatory disorders; *(I),* unexplained; *(S),* male factor; *(C),* cervical factor; *(E),* endometriosis; *(T),* tubal factor. (From Collins JA: A proportional hazards analysis of the clinical characteristics of infertile couples. *Am J Obstet Gynecol* 1984; 148:527. Used with permission.)

1977). The relatively poor prognosis observed with tubal factor and male factor may improve as a result of the advances of in vitro fertilization. The duration of infertility is also a predictor of subsequent pregnancies (Collins et al., 1984a; Weir and Cicchinelli, 1964). Couples with less than a 3-year history of infertility are more likely to conceive. A prior pregnancy with the same partner may be the most powerful predictor of subsequent pregnancy (Collins et al., 1984a; Dor et al., 1977).

In summary, pregnancy rates appear to correlate best with the age of the female, underlying diagnosis, duration of infertility, and pregnancy history. Based on the epidemiological data, any couple interested in having children who have not conceived after 1 to 2 years of unprotected intercourse with adequate coital exposure are reasonable candidates for an infertility evaluation. Earlier investigation may be recommended in women more than age 35 years or younger women with obvious risk factors such as oligomenorrhea or a history of PID.

THE INITIAL VISIT

A detailed interview is the critical first step in an infertility evaluation. A major goal during the initial visit is to obtain the necessary basic information while at the same time educating the couple so that they can adequately prepare for what is often an emotionally and physically demanding evaluation. Information regarding infertility, reproductive physiology, and the subsequent investigation is important. During the initial visit both partners should be present and interviewed together. On the premise that infertility is often a syndrome of multiple origin, an adequate investigation requires inquiring about all possible etiologies in both the husband and wife. Besides obtaining a complete medical, surgical, and gynecological history, the physician should elicit information regarding the psychological, emotional, and sexual behaviors of both partners. This should include questions regarding sexual habits, frequency of intercourse, sexual dysfunction, stability of the relationship, and the motivation to achieve a successful pregnancy. Certain couples may benefit from specific instructions regarding the timing and frequency of intercourse. A frequency of two to three times per week without the use of lubricants or douches is usually adequate. Coitus every 36 to 48 hours 3 to 4 days before and after the calculated day of ovulation is optimal. The disruption of spontaneous sexuality should be discouraged.

The important historical points in the evaluation of the male and female partners are outlined in Tables 12–2 and 12–3. Separate physical examinations should follow. During the physical examination of the woman, particular attention should be given to the height, weight, hair distribution, and presence of galactorrhea, as well as to the pelvic examination. Since a semen analysis should be obtained early in the investigation, examination of the man by a urologist is often recommended if there is a semen abnormality.

An explanation of the causes of infertility provides an ideal introduction to the nature of the subsequent evaluation. The schedule for the planned investigation should be flexible; however, in most cases, the majority of the investigation should be completed within 3 to 6 months. The

TABLE 12–2.

Important Historical Points in Men

Duration of infertility
Prior pregnancies, fertility in other relationships
Medical and surgical history (childhood illnesses, venereal diseases, trauma)
Medications
Alcohol, cigarette, marijuana use
Occupational exposures (excessive heat, chemical radiation)
Sexual dysfunction
Tight-fitting underwear, hot baths, saunas
Previous tests and therapy for infertility

TABLE 12–3.

Important Historical Points in Women

Duration of infertility
Detailed menstrual history
Prior pregnancies
Fertility in other relationships
Prior contraceptive use (OCPs, IUD)
Frequency of intercourse, sexual dysfunction
Gynecological history (PID, endometriosis, fibroids, cervical dysplasia)
DES exposure
Medical and surgical history
Medications
Previous tests and therapy for infertility

sequence in which specific infertility tests should be offered will depend on the etiological factors that are suggested by the history and physical examination. These specific tests will be discussed in the context of the multiple causes of infertility.

MALE FACTOR

Male factor is frequently cited as the commonest cause of infertility. However, this is somewhat misleading since the present tests available for the evaluation of the man do not easily separate normal fertile men from men with reduced fertility. The evaluation of the man is limited not only by a large overlap in the semen parameters among fertile and subfertile men but also by the wide fluctuations among sequential semen specimens from the same individual. Since it is relatively rare to identify a male partner with azoospermia (no sperm in the ejaculate), it is often difficult to implicate male factor as the principal cause for a couple's infertility. Despite its limitations, the semen analysis remains the primary screening test for male factor infertility. In our institution, if the semen analysis is persistently abnormal, the patient is referred to a urologist for examination and further evaluation. A number of different schemes to categorize the multiple causes of male infertility have been devised. The causes of male infertility are outlined in Table 12–4.

A karyotype, vasography, and testicular biopsy may be recommended for patients with azoospermia or severe oligozoospermia. Endocrine studies measuring serum testosterone, luteinizing hormone (LH), follicle-stimulating hormone (FSH), thyroid-stimulating hormone (TSH), and prolactin levels should be considered for patients with azoospermia, oligozoospermia, or oligoasthenospermia (poor motility). Immunological factors may be suggested by sperm agglutination, oligoasthenospermia, or poor cervical mucous penetrability. Immunological infertility will be further discussed in the section on cervical factor. Microbiological studies should be recommended if there is any suggestion of genital tract infections.

The interpretation and clinical value of the various tests available for the evaluation of seminal fluid, sperm cell properties, and sperm cell function will be presented after a brief review of male reproductive physiology.

TABLE 12–4.

The Causes of Male Infertility

Anatomical factors
  Varicocele
  Cryptorchidism
  Ductal obstruction (Young's syndrome)
  Congenital Anomalies (hypospadias, epispadias, cystic fibrosis, testicular hypoplasia or aplasia, and partial or total absence of the vas deferens)
Endocrine factors
  Gonadotropin deficiency
  Kallmann's syndrome
    Pituitary tumors (Cushing's disease, acromegaly)
    Dwarfism
    Hypothyroidism
  Fertile eunuch syndrome
  Enzymatic defects in testosterone synthesis
  Androgen receptor deficiency
  Congenital adrenal hyperplasia
Genetic factors
  Klinefelter's syndrome
  Down syndrome
  47 XYY
  Autosomal translocations
Inflammatory factors
  Orchitis
  Epididymitis
  Prostatitis
  Urethritis
Immunological factors
  Systemic
  Local
Sexual dysfunction and faulty coital technique
  Impotence
  Retrograde ejaculation
  Premature ejaculation
  Spermicidal lubricants
Exogenous factors
  Medication (antihypertensives, antipsychotics, antidepressants, cimetidine, chemotherapy)
  Radiation
  Alcohol
  Marijuana
  Trauma
  Excessive heat (hot tubs)
  Cigarettes

Male Reproductive Physiology

The testes contain two cell types (Fig 12–2). Sertoli cells containing spermatogonia line the seminiferous tubules. The interstitial tissue is composed of the androgen-producing Leydig cells. The epididymis is a reservoir for sperm storage and the site of sperm maturation. The vas defer-

SEMINIFEROUS TUBULE

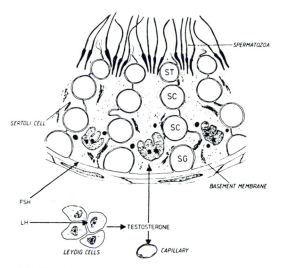

FIG 12–2.
Spermatogenesis. A schematic illustration of the cellular composition and structural relationship between different cell types in the testis. (Adapted from Hargreave TB: *Male Infertility.* New York, Springer-Verlag, p.89.)

ens connects the epididymis with the ejaculatory ducts. The prostate, seminal vesicles, and the bulbourethral (Cowper's) glands secrete the seminal fluid. The anatomy of the male reproductive tract is depicted in Figure 12–3.

Spermatogenesis is the process of formation and development of the spermatozoon. The transformation of spermatogonia into spermatids involves a series of mitotic and meiotic divisions. The differentiation of spermatids into mature spermatozoa is termed *spermiogenesis*. In man, spermatogenesis is a continuous process, and approximately 74 days are required for the conversion of spermatogonia into spermatozoa. When spermatozoa enter the epididymis, they are functionally inactive; however, after an average of 12 days of further maturation, they are capable of progressive motility.

The endocrinology of spermatogenesis involves pituitary secretion of LH and FSH and the testicular secretion of testosterone and inhibin. Whereas LH stimulates Leydig cell synthesis and secretion of testosterone, FSH stimulates Sertoli cell secretion of inhibin. High levels of intratesticular testosterone are required to support spermatogenesis.

During ejaculation, the contents of the distal vas deferens and prostatic fluid are initially released and followed soon after by the release of seminal vesicle secretions. Although semen coagulates during ejaculation to form a gel, liquefaction occurs within 20 to 30 minutes due to the proteolytic enzymes in prostatic fluid. Seminal spermatozoa are not capable of fertilization. The process by which sperm acquire the ability to fertilize ova is termed *capacitation*. This poorly defined series

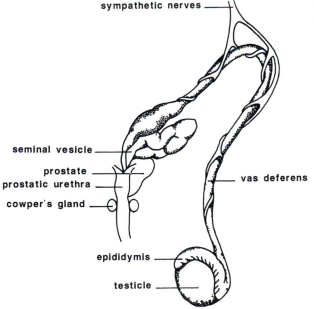

FIG 12–3.
Anatomy of the male reproductive tract.

of biochemical and biophysical changes in the sperm surface membrane gives sperm the capacity to undergo the acrosome reaction. Capacitation appears to take place in the cervical mucus. However, a period of time in the female reproductive tract is not required since sperm are capable of fertilization in vitro.

The acrosome reaction involves the breakdown and fusion of the sperm plasma membrane with the outer acrosomal membrane (Fig 12–4; Bedford, 1970). Several enzymes within the acrosome appear to be important for sperm penetration of the cumulus cell mass, corona radiata, and zona pellucida. Species-specific sperm receptors exist on the zona pellucida. During sperm penetration, the oocyte initiates the cortical reaction, the process by which further sperm are prevented from penetrating the oocyte. The cortical reaction involves the breakdown and dispersion of the secretory granules that lie just below the vitelline membrane (Barros and Yanagimachi, 1971).

Diagnostic Tests

Semen Analysis

Since no laboratory test that definitively predicts the potential for fertility has been developed, the semen analysis remains the primary diagnostic test for evaluating male factor. The basic semen analysis measures volume, pH, fructose, liquefaction, round cells, sperm density, motility, and morphology. Prior to obtaining the semen specimen, the patient is instructed to abstain from ejaculation for a minimum of 48 hours and no longer than 7 days. The optimal period of sexual abstinence has not been determined. Frequent ejaculation does not appear to affect sperm density. It may be associated with decreased semen volume and therefore decreased total motile sperm (Hargreave and Nillson, 1983). In contrast, infrequent ejaculation appears to be associated with decreased sperm motility and therefore should be discouraged. There is no scientific data to support the recommendation that having intercourse every other day is more likely to result in a conception than having intercourse every day. The method of choice for collection is masturbation with avoidance of potential spermicidal lubricants. These specimens should be collected in a clean container and brought to the laboratory within 1 to 2 hours. Several (two or three) samples should be analyzed over a period of 1 to 3 months due to individual fluctuations. The semen analysis may be evaluated by an experienced technician or semiautomated computers.

Normal semen volumes range from 2 to 6 ml. A very small or very large semen volume may be associated with abnormal semen parameters due to a disturbance in the ejaculatory ducts. The

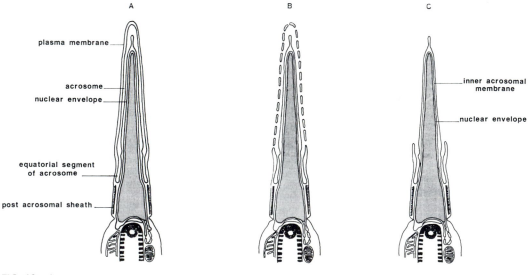

FIG 12–4.
Diagramatic representation of the acrosome reaction. *A,* intact unreacted spermatozoon; *B,* the acrosome reaction; *C,* acrosome-reacted spermatozoon.) (Adapted from Mortimer D: Male factor in infertility: II. Sperm function testing. *Curr Probl Obstet Gynecol,* 1985, vol 8, no. 8.)

patient with persistently increased semen volumes may benefit from collecting and examining the ejaculate in two parts (split ejaculate). The absence of fructose and an acidic pH may suggest seminal vesicle dysfunction or ejaculatory duct obstruction. The absence of liquefaction may result in relatively immobilized spermatozoa. Leukocytospermia may be suggested by an elevated pH and an abnormal number of round cells (greater than 1×10^6/ml). However, white blood cells (WBCs) are often difficult to distinguish from immature germ cells by conventional microscopy. An abnormal number of immature germ cells may be the result of a defect in spermatogenesis and therefore may warrant an endocrine evaluation. The development of improved techniques for detecting leukocytospermia is currently in progress. An immunoperoxidase staining technique specific for WBCs has recently been described (Wolf and Anderson, 1988).

The interpretation of sperm density, motility, and morphology may be difficult for several reasons. As previously mentioned, there are wide fluctuations in sequential semen analyses from the same individual, as well as significant overlap between fertile and subfertile men. Further difficulty correlating semen parameters with fertility potential occurs because fertility is a function of both partners and not the man alone. An additional drawback is that the semen analysis does not measure all of the functional properties of spermatozoa such as capacitation, cervical mucous interaction, penetrating ability, and fertilization. The predictive inadequacy of the seminal parameters is illustrated by the difficulty determining the lower limits of the fertile range. This is further exemplified by the relatively high pregnancy rates of vasovasotomized men with oligozoospermia, and by the normozoospermic men who fail to penetrate their partner's ova at the time of in vitro fertilization. Nevertheless, among all the tests and parameters available, sperm density, motility, and morphology have been most consistently correlated with fertility status.

Sperm density is a measure of the number of sperm in the ejaculate per milliliter. Based on studies of "fertile" men undergoing vasectomy (Derrick and Johnson, 1974; Nelson and Bunge, 1974) and follow-up studies of infertile groups (Smith et al., 1977; Bostofte et al., 1982), the lower limit of the fertile range appears to be 5 million sperm/ml. Studies comparing sperm density and in vitro fertilization rates seem to suggest

a slightly higher cutoff for the "normal" range between 10 and 20 million sperm/ml (Battin et al., 1984; Hirsch et al., 1986; Mahadevan and Trounson, 1984). Despite these recent studies, the most widely accepted lower limit of the "normal" range continues to be 20 million sperm/ml, based on the landmark studies of MacLeod and Gold (1951a). When a higher cutoff is applied, there is an increase in sensitivity at the expense of a decrease in specificity. In our institution, patients with persistent sperm density less than 20 million/ml are considered to have male factor infertility and are often referred for further urological evaluation. In contrast, the lower cutoff of 5 million sperm/ml is often used for therapeutic recommendations such as donor insemination. Because of the possible association between polyzoospermia and poor motility and penetrability, patients with persistent sperm densities greater than 250 million sperm/ml are also recommended for urological evaluation.

The assessment of sperm motility is as important as the determination of sperm density. Sperm motility should be evaluated within 2 hours after the specimen is produced. Sperm motility is most often expressed as the percentage of progressively motile sperm; however, similar to sperm density, estimating the percentage of progressively motile sperm does not accurately separate fertile men from subfertile men. The recommended lower limits of normal motility range between 20% and 60% (Bostofte et al., 1984; Chong et al., 1983; McLeod and Gold, 1951b; Amelar et al., 1980; Pryor, 1981). Data obtained from in vitro fertilization suggest that a cutoff of 50% motility has significant prognostic value (Mahadevan and Trounson, 1984). In our institution, sperm motility persistently less than 50% warrants further urological evaluation.

In an attempt to improve the predictive value of the semen analysis, the analysis of sperm movement has expanded to include the evaluation of linear velocity and the amplitude of lateral head displacement. Various computer technologies have been developed for the evaluation of sperm movement; however, the clinical usefulness of more complex motility data remains to be determined.

Sperm morphology is another semen parameter that appears to be loosely associated with fertility potential. All semen specimens contain a certain percentage of abnormal spermatozoa. Morphological abnormalities may involve the sperm head, midpiece, or tail. Abnormalities of the head are most frequently associated with infertility (Bostofte et al., 1985). Based on a number of clinical studies, the recommended cutoffs for normal sperm morphology range from 40% to 60% normal forms (Bostofte et al., 1985; Mahadevan and Trounson, 1984). In our institution, patients with persistently fewer than 50% morphologically normal spermatozoa are considered to have teratozoospermia and are referred for urological evaluation. Although abnormal morphology is often associated with reduced sperm density and motility, isolated abnormalities of sperm morphology are not uncommon (Rogers et al., 1983; Kruger et al., 1986). In fact, using strict criteria, recent studies suggest that sperm morphology may be a powerful predictor of successful in vitro fertilization (Kruger et al., 1986, 1988).

Although separate evaluation of each seminal variable is important, there may be some advantages of combining semen variables. Mathematical manipulations allow for the expression of the total number of motile sperm and the total number of morphologically "normal" motile sperm per ejaculate. The combination of seminal variables avoids the interpretation of several different "normal" standards. Although a total motile count less than 20 million has been associated with lower pregnancy rates (Small et al., 1987), the prognostic superiority of combining semen variables remains to be established.

Although the semen analysis remains the primary screening test for male factor infertility, additional diagnostic tests have been developed in an attempt to define more precisely the reproductive potential of sperm. The majority of these tests assess the functional properties of spermatozoa, and the sperm penetration assay (SPA) has been widely applied to clinical practice. Unfortunately, as in the case of the semen analysis, the SPA has significant limitations.

Sperm Penetration Assay

The SPA, also known as the zona-free hamster egg penetration test, was developed in an attempt to improve the evaluation of male factor infertility. This assay is believed to assess the ability of sperm to (1) undergo capacitation and the acrosome reaction, (2) fuse with and penetrate the egg membrane, and (3) undergo nuclear decondensation. Sperm are washed free of seminal plasma and incubated in a protein-enriched medium that promotes capacitation. After incubation, motile sperm are separated and used to inseminate hamster eggs that have previously been enzyme-treated so that the cumulus and zona pellucida have been removed. Therefore, the SPA does not test the ability of sperm to penetrate the zona pellucida. Sperm from a donor of proved fertility is always tested simultaneously as a positive control. Following several hours of insemination, the hamster eggs are examined for sperm penetration. Penetration rates less than 10% to 15% are considered abnormal. Although the initial studies suggested a high degree of sensitivity and specificity (Rogers et al., 1979; Karp et al., 1981), more recent studies have been unable to substantiate these excellent early results (Margalioth et al., 1983; Wickings et al., 1983). After reviewing the world's literature, Mao and Grimes (1988) concluded that the validity, reproducibility, and utility of the SPA have not been established. They recommend that the SPA not be used to evaluate infertile couples. However, interpreting the clinical value of the SPA is particularly difficult when comparing results from different laboratories. The potential utility of an adequately standardized SPA has recently been emphasized (Bronson and Rogers, 1988).

The utility of the SPA for predicting success during in vitro fertilization remains controversial. Although an abnormal SPA is not always associated with an inability to penetrate human eggs, there does appear to be a correlation between the SPA and in vitro fertilization rates. The SPA appears to be less predictive of fertilization success or failure for patients with abnormal semen parameters than for patients with unexplained or tubal factor infertility (Margalioth et al., 1986; Aitken, 1985). The long-term prognostic ability of the SPA is difficult to determine since prospective studies have yielded different results. Aitken and co-workers (1984) found that 0% was the only SPA value diagnostic of infertility. At the present time, whether additional information is gained from the SPA when compared to the traditional semen analysis remains uncertain. In our institution, the SPA is often recommended for couples with long-standing unexplained infertility. If one realizes its limitations, the SPA may also be offered to couples with persistently abnormal semen analyses. Whereas a markedly abnormal SPA may have prognostic and therapeutic implications, a normal test result should not be regarded as reassuring. Needless to say, further studies are required to better define the clinical utility of the SPA.

Future Diagnostic Studies

A variety of new methods have been described to evaluate sperm function. The hypo-osmotic swelling test measures the functional integrity of sperm membranes by placing specimens in hypo-osmotic fluids (Jeyendran et al., 1984). This assay has been correlated with successful in vitro fertilization (Van der Ven et al., 1986). Several monoclonal antibodies that can be used to detect the acrosome reaction of human sperm are available (Wolf et al., 1985). These immunofluorescence assays assess whether a sperm population has the capacity to undergo the acrosome reaction. The hemizona test assesses the ability of spermatozoa to bind to the zona pellucida (Burkman et al., 1988). The human zona pellucida is bisected with one half of the zona incubated with donor sperm and the other hemizona incubated with the sperm from an infertility patient. These tests are presently limited to research protocols, and further studies will be required to demonstrate their clinical utility.

CERVICAL FACTOR

The uterine cervix appears to have several important roles in reproduction and is often considered the gateway to the upper reproductive tract. During parturition, massive dilatation of the cervix is required for a normal vaginal delivery. In the nonpregnant state, its primary physiological function is the secretion of cervical mucus, which functions as a biological valve. During midcycle, cervical mucus facilitates the transport of spermatozoa. At other times during the menstrual cycle, cervical mucus functions as a barrier by preventing the passage of foreign material into the upper reproductive tract.

Cervical factor is best defined as the midcycle interaction of spermatozoa and cervical mucus. The postcoital test (PCT) remains the standard test for assessing the cervical factor and is recommended early in the evaluation of most infertile couples. The clinical value of the multiple in vitro studies such as the slide test (Miller and Kurzrok, 1932), the capillary tube test (Kremer, 1965), and the in vitro cervical mucus penetration test (Alexander, 1981) remains to be demonstrated. At the present time, the in vitro tests for cervical factor are rarely employed in clinical practice. In the next section, the physiology of cervical mucus will be reviewed and the evaluation of cervical factor in infertility will be discussed.

Cervical Mucus Physiology

Cervical mucus is a heterogeneous secretion produced primarily by the secretory cells of the endocervix. The cervical mucus pool may contain a small amount of endometrial, tubal, and follicular fluid, cellular debris from the uterus, cervix, and vagina, and leukocytes. Cervical mucus contains 92% to 98% water. The physical properties of cervical mucus are due to the major constituents, which are mucinous glycoproteins. Biochemical studies have demonstrated that cervical mucus is a fibrillar system, and the mucin fibrils originate in the endocervical canal (Gibbons and Mattner, 1971). Other constituents of cervical mucus include carbohydrates, lipids, proteins, proteolytic enzymes, and inorganic salts. During coitus, 200 to 500 million spermatozoa are delivered to the cervix and posterior vaginal fornix; however, less than 200 attain close proximity to the egg (Settlage et al., 1973). Moghissi (1985) has described several functional properties of the cervix and its secretions that are important for sperm migration: (1) the cervix appears to be the site of sperm capacitation, (2) the fibrillar structure of cervical mucus contributes to sperm transport, (3) the nutrients in cervical mucus provide a supplemental energy source for sperm, (4) cervical mucus protects sperm from the hostile acidic environment of the vagina, (5) cervical mucus has a filtering effect, and (6) the cervical crypts are responsible for the storage and gradual release of spermatozoa to the upper reproductive tract.

The physical properties and certain constituents of cervical mucus display cyclic variations. The secretion of cervical mucus by the endocervical glands is stimulated by estrogen and inhibited by progesterone. The estrogen effect may be assayed by gross inspection or by microscopic examination. Around the time of ovulation, the mucus forms a thin, continuous thread as it is pulled apart—a phenomenon called *Spinnbarkeit*. This physical characteristic is a function of increasing levels of estrogen and disappears after the appearance of progesterone. Microscopically, when preovulatory mucus is allowed to dry on a slide, it reveals a characteristic crystallization pattern called *ferning*. Preovulatory mucus also becomes more profuse, watery, alkaline, and acellular. Cyclic changes in the physical properties and chemical constituents of cervical mucus may influence sperm migration. Despite individual variation, sperm penetrability begins around the ninth day of the menstrual cycle and is optimal around the time of ovulation (Moghissi et al., 1964, 1972). Within 1 to 2 days after ovulation, sperm migration is usually inhibited (Moghissi, 1966). A scoring system to evaluate the quality of cervical mucus is illustrated in Table 12–5 (Belsey et al., 1980).

The Postcoital Test

The PCT, also known as the *Sims-Huhner test*, was first described in 1866 by Marion Sims (Sims, 1866); however, Huhner is credited for popularizing the test as an index of sperm–cervical mucus interaction. The PCT remains an integral part of the routine evaluation of the infertile couple. The clinical value of the PCT in predicting fertility remains controversial. The major problem with the PCT is that it lacks standardization, and as a result, there is considerable disagreement regarding the timing and interpretation.

The PCT should be performed as close to the time of ovulation as possible. The couple is in-

structed to abstain from intercourse for 2 days prior to having intercourse for the test. Douches or intravaginal medications should not be used during the 48 hours preceding the test. A nonlubricated speculum is inserted into the vagina and a sample of cervical mucus obtained. A number of techniques for collecting cervical mucus have been described. A long, narrow, dressing forceps with a small oval aperture at the tip is often used (Fig 12–5). Alternatively, if the cervical os is too small to admit a metal instrument, an angiocatheter and syringe may be used to aspirate a sample of cervical mucus. The cervical mucus should be placed on a glass slide, covered with a cover slip, and examined under the microscope. The number of spermatozoa per high-power field, percent motility, and the quality of forward progression should be noted. Whenever possible, the quality of the cervical mucus should be determined as previously described.

The controversy regarding the timing of the PCT in relation to coitus has been recently addressed (Taymor and Overstreet, 1988). Several authors have recommended performing the PCT between 2 and 3 hours after coitus since this is the time when sperm concentration is at a maximum (Treadway et al., 1975; Davajan, 1985). In contrast, many authors recommend delaying the PCT until at least 6 hours after coitus, emphasizing the role of the cervix as a reservoir for spermatozoa. Moghissi (1976b) recommends perform-

TABLE 12–5.
Evaluating the Quality of Cervical Mucus*

Amount_____	Viscosity_____
0 = 0	0 = thick, highly viscous
1 = 0.1 ml	1 = intermediate viscosity
2 = 0.2 ml	2 = mildly viscous
3 = 0.3 ml	3 = normal
Ferning_____	Cellularity_____
0 = no crystallization	0 = 11 cells/HPF†
1 = atypical pattern	1 = 6–10 cells/HPF
2 = primary and secondary stems	2 = 1–5 cells/HPF
3 = tertiary and quartenay stems	3 = 0 cells/HPF
Spinnbarkeit_____	Total score_____
0 = < 1 cm	> 10 = normal
1 = 1–4 cm	5–10 = unfavorable
2 = 5–8 cm	< 5 = hostile
3 = >9 cm	

*Adapted from Belsey MA, Eliasson R, Gallegos AJ, et al: *Laboratory Manual for Examination of Human Semen and Semen-Cervical Mucus Interaction.* Geneva, World Health Organization, 1980.
†HPF = high-power field.

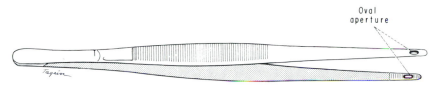

FIG 12–5.
Long dressing forceps adapted for collection of seminal fluid from the endocervical canal.

ing the PCT initially at 6 to 8 hours after coitus. Taymor and Overstreet (1988) also emphasize the importance of sperm longevity, as well as the impracticality of having intercourse several hours before going to the physician's office. They recommend having intercourse "at bedtime" and performing the PCT at 10 to 16 hours after coitus. In our unit, we also recommend performing the PCT at 10 to 16 hours after coitus, allowing for greater flexibility in the timing of intercourse. However, if the initial PCT is abnormal, earlier timing should be considered.

As previously mentioned, the clinical value of the PCT in predicting subsequent fertility is highly controversial. Well-designed prospective studies that demonstrate significant prognostic value for the PCT (Hall et al., 1982; Jette and Glass, 1972) are balanced by equally well-designed studies that demonstrate no predictive value (Collins et al., 1984b). The lack of predictive value is further supported by several laparoscopic studies in which peritoneal fluid was recovered around the time of ovulation and examined for spermatozoa (Asch, 1976; Stone, 1983). Stone (1983) observed numerous motile sperm in the peritoneal fluid in 56% of patients with poor to absent cervical mucus and repetitively poor PCT results (less than five sperm per HPF). In contrast, sperm was recovered from only 53% of control subjects with normal PCT results. Although the studies do not support abandoning the PCT, they do point out some of its limitations in the evaluation of sperm migration and sperm longevity.

Because of conflicting studies, there is also some debate about what constitutes a normal PCT result. Moghissi's (1976) criteria for a normal PCT result is 10 or more sperm with directional motility per HPF. Several other investigators contend that five or more actively motile sperm per HPF may be considered satisfactory (Davajan and Kunitake, 1969; Treadway et al., 1975). Jette and Glass (1972) have observed that a PCT result with greater than 20 motile sperm

per HPF is associated with an increased likelihood of pregnancy and a normal semen analysis. Although often quoted, these authors have emphasized that no specific number of motile spermatozoa in the PCT result should be judged as "normal."

Interpretation of the PCT result is further complicated by difficulty in determining the day of ovulation. "Abnormal" cervical mucus is often the result of inaccurate timing with respect to ovulation. Therefore, if the initial PCT result is abnormal and associated with unfavorable cervical mucus, it should be repeated with additional testing to determine the day of ovulation (see the discussion of ovulation prediction). If ovulation cannot be determined with a reasonable degree of accuracy, serial PCTs should be considered.

The multiple causes of an abnormal PCT result are listed in Table 12–6. Persistently abnormal PCT results suggest either oligoasthenospermia, abnormal cervical mucus, faulty coital technique, or abnormal cervical mucus–spermatozoa interaction. Male factor infertility is often suggested when multiple abnormal PCT results are

TABLE 12–6.
Causes of an Abnormal Postcoital Test

Male factors
  Oligospermia
  Oligoasthenospermia
  Sexual dysfunction
Abnormal cervical mucus
  Poor timing
  Hypoestrogenism
  Cervical stenosis
  Cervical varicosities
  Cauterization and cryotherapy
  Cervicitis
  Clomiphene citrate
  Cervical prolapse
Abnormal sperm-cervical mucus interaction
  Idiopathic
  Immunological

associated with a persistently abnormal semen analysis.

Abnormal cervical mucus may be due to hormonal, anatomical, or infectious etiologies. Any hypoestrogenic state may be associated with unfavorable cervical mucus. Subtle abnormalities in follicular maturation may lead to a relatively low level of preovulatory estradiol and abnormal cervical mucus. Clomiphene citrate has been clearly associated with poor PCT results (Graff, 1971; Maxson et al., 1984). The mechanism may be related to an antiestrogen effect at the level of the cervix. Anatomical defects that may contribute to abnormal cervical mucus include the hypoplastic cervix and cervical stenosis. Anatomical variations in the position of the cervix are unlikely to contribute to a poor PCT result. Varicosities of the hypoplastic endocervical canal have been associated with extreme friability and scant cervical mucus (Scott et al., 1977). Cervical stenosis may be associated with scant cervical mucus and is most commonly the result of a previous cervical conization. Extensive cauterization or cryotherapy of the endocervix, significant cervical prolapse, and acute and chronic cervicitis may also be associated with abnormal cervical mucus. The role of *Mycoplasma* and *Chlamydia* in infertility will be discussed toward the end of the chapter. Faulty coital technique may be suspected when the semen analyses and cervical mucus are relatively normal, and there are no spermatozoa seen on the PCT result. This may be the result of male or female sexual dysfunction (or both) such as impotence, premature or retrograde ejaculation, or vaginismus. In addition, the partners of extremely obese women may not be able to fully penetrate the vagina and deposit their semen in the posterior fornix.

Abnormal cervical mucus–sperm interaction is often suggested when the PCT result is poor and the cervical mucus and semen analysis are normal. In the majority of cases, no specific cause for abnormal cervical mucus–sperm interaction can be identified. However, an immunological cause should be suspected when all spermatozoa are immotile, shaking, or displaying poor forward progression.

The immunology of the male and female reproductive tract has recently been reviewed (Alexander and Anderson, 1987; Hill and Anderson, 1988). Both cellular and humoral immunity appear to contribute to reproductive failure. In vitro, the soluble products of macrophages and lymphocytes inhibit sperm motility (Hill et al., 1987) and penetrability (Hill et al., 1989). Clinically there appears to be a relationship between immunity to sperm and infertility (Bronson et al., 1984; Haas et al., 1980; Menge et al., 1982).

Antisperm antibodies have been isolated from semen, cervical mucus, and male and female serum. These antibodies may be secreted locally within the reproductive tract and occur independently from those in the serum, or they may be associated with circulating serum antibodies (Rumke, 1974; Uehling, 1971). The presence of sperm antibodies in semen and cervical mucus is more strongly associated with reproductive impairment when compared to serum. The precise mechanisms by which antisperm antibodies contribute to infertility remain to be elucidated, but they may interfere with sperm transport, gamete interaction, and macrophage phagocytosis (Bronson et al., 1981; London et al., 1984).

Bronson and co-workers (1984) have emphasized that immunity to sperm is not an all-or-nothing phenomenon. The extent to which antisperm antibodies are present in the reproductive tract appears to influence the degree of fertility impairment. For example, when less than 50% of sperm were antibody bound, the number of motile sperm in the PCT result was no different from that in antibody-negative couples (Bronson et al., 1984). In addition, spontaneous remission of immunity to sperm has been reported (Bronson et al., 1984). The etiology of antisperm antibodies appears to be multifactorial. An increased incidence has been associated with vasectomy (Shulman et al., 1972), genital tract infections (Witkin and Toth, 1983) and gastrointestinal exposure to sperm (Bronson et al., 1984).

A relationship between decreased fertility and antisperm antibodies has been more clearly established in men when compared to women. In a study of 254 infertile men, Rumke et al. (1974) demonstrated that the prognosis for future pregnancy was inversely correlated with antibody titers. More recently, Ayvaliotis et al. (1985) have shown that when more than 50% of the spermatozoa in the ejaculate are found to have surface-bound immunoglobulins, the pregnancy rate is 15%, compared with 67% when less than 50% of the sperm are antibody bound. The role of immunologic factors in the cervical mucus and upper reproductive tract remains unclear. Nevertheless, patients with persistent unexplained infertility have a significantly higher incidence of sperm antibodies in their cervical mucus (18.4%) when compared with patients with persistent, explained infertility (7.1%; Moghissi et al., 1980).

Several different assays for the detection of antisperm antibodies have been described. The incidence of abnormal test results varies according to the patient population, the individual test, and the titer that is considered abnormal. The Isojima immobilization test result is abnormal in 5% to 10% of women with unexplained infertility (Isojima et al., 1968). No single assay has proved to be superior. This is not surprising since immunity to sperm may lead to a number of different functional abnormalities. A brief description and the relative advantages and disadvantages of several of the tests for antisperm antibodies are outlined in Table 12–7.

We recommend obtaining an antisperm antibody profile in all couples with poor PCT results. However, there is a poor correlation between an abnormal PCT result and the presence of antisperm antibodies (Collins, 1988a; Ainmelk et al., 1982), since approximately one third of female patients with antisperm antibodies have a satisfactory PCT result (Moghissi, 1985). The PCT should not be used as the sole screening test for antisperm antibodies, and couples with long-standing unexplained infertility or a history of recurrent or chronic genital tract infections should be recommended an antisperm antibody profile. In our institution, the antisperm antibody profile may consist of male and female serum, cervical mucus, and semen. The direct immunobead test is used to detect antisperm antibodies in cervical mucus and semen. The Kibrick sperm agglutination, Isojima sperm immobilization, and the indirect Immunobead tests are used to detect antisperm antibodies in serum.

THE OVARIAN FACTOR

Ovulatory disorders include anovulation, oligo-ovulation, and luteal phase defects. Regular menstrual cycles occurring at intervals of 25 to 35 days, particularly when associated with molimina, suggest ovulation. In contrast, ovulatory disorders are often associated with irregular menstrual cycles, oligomenorrhea, or amenorrhea. A history of obesity, excessive weight loss, galactorrhea, hirsutism, or acne is often associated with ovulatory disorders. The major clinical entities associated with anovulation and infertility are the polycystic

TABLE 12–7.

Tests for Detecting Sperm Immunity*

Isojima's immobilization test (complement-dependent cytotoxy)
  Measures the ratio of motile sperm in control and test serum
  Tests for IgG, IgM (IgAs do not fix complement)
  Highly specific; lacks sensitivity (false negatives common)
Kibrick, Friberg-Trey agglutination test (sperm agglutination)
  Classical serum tests, measures agglutinating antibodies
  False positives result from nonspecific binding
Enzyme-linked immunosorbent assay (ELISA)
  Antiglobulin binds to human immunoglobulin on sperm surface
  False positives and false negatives result from fixation process and membrane damage (i.e. membrane extracts may not contain relevant antigens)
Fluorescein-conjugated antiglobulins
  False positives common
Radiolabeled antiglobulin assay
  High specificity and sensitivity when used with living sperm
  Does not determine regional specificity of binding
  Does not determine proportion of antibody-bound sperm
Mixed agglutination reaction
  Uses sensitized Rh-positive red blood cells and IgG antiglobulin
  Limitations similar to those of radiolabeled antiglobulin assay
Immunobead test
  Detects sperm coating immunoglobulins in seminal plasma and cervical mucus
  Subclass specific (IgM, IgG, IgA)
  Can determine regional specificity
  Can determine proportion of antibody-bound sperm

*Adapted from Bronson R, Cooper G, Rosenfeld D: Sperm antibodies: Their role in infertility. *Fertil Steril* 1984; 42:171.

ovary syndrome (PCOS), premature ovarian failure (POF), hyperprolactinemia, and hypothalamic amenorrhea. Certain disorders of the adrenal and thyroid gland may be associated with ovulatory dysfunction. Luteal phase defects appear to be a relatively uncommon cause of infertility. Following a discussion of these major clinical diagnoses, the techniques for documenting ovulation and an adequate luteal phase will be presented.

Polycystic Ovarian Disease

In 1935, Stein and Leventhal called attention to the syndrome PCOS. It has become increasingly clear that PCOS is a heterogeneous disease. As originally described, the hallmark features of this disorder are androgen excess and chronic anovulation. Clinically, the commonest symptoms associated with PCOS are hirsutism (90%), menstrual irregularities (90%), and infertility (75%). Obesity is found in approximately 50% of cases. In the past, the diagnosis was based on the anatomical findings of polycystic or sclerocystic ovaries. However, approximately one third of women with symptoms and hormonal parameters suggestive of PCOS may have normal-appearing ovaries. The ovaries are large, and the surface appears thickened, pale, and smooth. When the ovary is bisected, numerous cystic follicles may be identified beneath the capsule (Fig 12–6). Microscopically there is fibrosis of the cortical stroma with areas of hyalinization (Fig 12–7). Examination of the cystic follicles reveals an unusual activity of the theca interna cells with luteinization. Corpora albicans and corpora lutea are usually absent, but on occasion one or more may be identified. Although at one time this microscopic picture was thought to be pathognomonic of PCOS, present evidence suggests that it is merely representative of prolonged periods of anovulation from various causes. Polycystic ovaries may be observed in women with specific causes of hyperandrogenism, including Cushing's syndrome, congenital adrenal hyperplasia, ovarian and adrenal tumors, hyperprolactinemia, hypothyroidism, and acromegaly.

There is no universal agreement regarding the pathophysiology of PCOS. Recent reviews have suggested a multifactorial etiology (Barbieri et al., 1988). At least five major systems may contribute to the development of PCOS: (1) hypothalamus and pituitary, (2) ovary, (3) skin, (4) adrenal, and (5) pancreas. The characteristic biochemical abnormalities include ovarian hyperandrogenism, adrenal hyperandrogenism, inappropriate gonadotropin secretion, peripheral hyperestrogenism, and hyperinsulinemia. It has been suggested that these hormonal abnormalities represent a vicious cycle of events that perpetuate PCOS.

The inappropriate gonadotropin secretion involves an elevated level of LH and a normal or low level of FSH (Lobo et al., 1983b). The mechanisms that are responsible for the inappropriate gonadotropin secretion remain to be fully elucidated. Centrally, a relative deficiency of dopamine (Yen, 1980) and a relative excess of norepinephrine (Lobo et al., 1983a) may contribute to the elevated secretion of LH. Peripherally, relatively constant levels of estrogen result from the extraglandular conversion of androstenedione to estrone. Since estrogen may enhance LH secretion, the chronic secretion of estrogen in PCOS may contribute to the persistently elevated levels of LH. The suppression of FSH and the resultant anovulation may be partially due to the chronically elevated levels of estrogen, an increased secretion of inhibin, or both (Tanabe et al., 1983). Several investigators have suggested that the primary defect in the PCOS lies in the hypothalamus. It is possible that an increase in endogenous gonadotropin-releasing hormone (GnRH) may contribute to the increased LH level. Several studies have demonstrated an increased LH pulse frequency and amplitude in PCOS, suggesting a

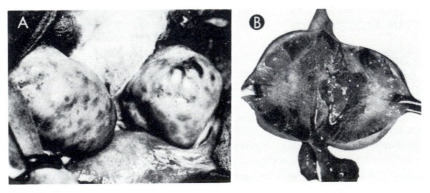

FIG 12–6.
Polycystic ovaries. **A,** gross appearance. **B,** on bisection.

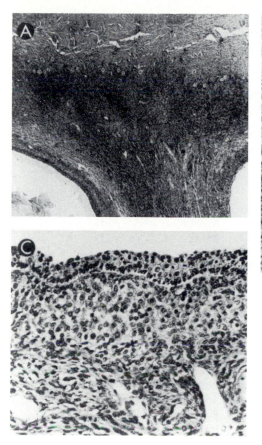
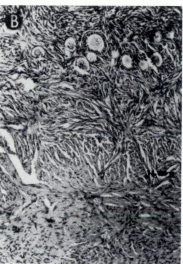

FIG 12–7.
Microscopic appearance of polycystic ovaries. **A,** low-power view. Note cystic follicles and collagenous character of the cortex. **B,** higher-power view. Numerous primordial follicles are seen in the zone between the normal cortex and the hyperplastic fibrotic cortex. **C,** high-power view showing the wall of a cystic follicle with a narrow layer of granulosa cells toward the lumen of the cyst and a wide layer of luteinized theca cells.

lowered threshold for pituitary LH release. In combination, the relatively constant levels of estrogen may contribute to the increased sensitivity of the pituitary to GnRH stimulation of LH release and decreased pituitary sensitivity to GnRH stimulation of FSH release.

Several lines of evidence suggest that the adrenal gland may be important in the pathogenesis of PCOS. Approximately 50% of patients with PCOS have elevated levels of dehydroepiandrosterone sulfate (DHEAS; Hoffman and Lobo, 1983; Lobo, 1984). The mechanism of excess adrenal androgen production in PCOS is unknown. However, patients with PCOS and elevated levels of DHEAS appear to have adrenals that are extremely sensitive to adrenocorticotropin (ACTH) stimulation (Chang et al., 1982).

The association of hyperinsulinemia with PCOS has been manifested clinically by acanthosis nigricans and termed the HAIR-AN syndrome (Barbieri, 1983). The severity of the insulin resistance is strongly correlated with the degree of hyperinsulinemia, which, in turn, is highly correlated with the severity of the hyperandrogenism. The hyperinsulinemic state appears to cause the hyperandrogenism and not vice versa. This is supported by the observation that the insulin resistance and acanthosis nigricans are not affected by lowering ovarian androgen production (Barbieri et al., 1988).

Because PCOS is a heterogeneous syndrome, there has been considerable debate regarding the diagnostic criteria. The criteria of Lobo (1986) are listed in Table 12–8. However, some patients

TABLE 12–8.

Diagnostic Criteria for Polycystic Ovary Syndrome*

Perimenarcheal onset of menstrual irregularity
Androgen excess
Chronic anovulation
Inappropriate gonadotropin secretion (LH:FSH >3)
Obesity
Euprolactinemia

*Adapted from Lobo RA: Polycystic ovary syndrome, in Mishell DR, Davajan V (eds): *Infertility, Contraception and Reproductive Endocrinology.* Oradell, NJ, Medical Economic Books, 1986.

considered to have PCOS may not meet these strict criteria. The most consistent finding in PCOS appears to be a mildly elevated serum testosterone level, usually in the range of 70 to 120 ng/dl. In patients with a serum testosterone level greater than 150 ng/dl, the diagnosis of ovarian stromal hyperthecosis is more likely, and the possibility of an androgen-secreting tumor must be excluded. The presence of mild hyperandrogenism does not differentiate between PCOS, congenital adrenal hyperplasia (CAH), and Cushing's syndrome. Distinguishing differential diagnoses of PCOS, CAH, and Cushing's syndrome may be accomplished with an ACTH stimulation test and dexamethasone suppression test, respectively.

Premature Ovarian Failure

Premature ovarian failure is defined as a failure of ovarian estrogen production in the setting of hypergonadotropism before age 35 years. The etiology of POF appears to be multifactorial. Most cases are idiopathic. Recent evidence supports the hypothesis that a specific genetic defect may cause POF (Krauss et al., 1987). It may be the result of a reduced number of primordial follicles or an increased rate of atresia. Infectious and iatrogenic destruction of primordial follicles may occur as a result of mumps oophoritis, irradiation, or chemotherapy. Documentation of antiovarian antibodies and the association of POF with other immunologic endocrine disorders supports the hypothesis that POF may be an autoimmune disease (Alper and Garner, 1985). An increased incidence of POF has also been associated with abnormal galactose metabolism (Kaufman et al., 1979).

The clinical presentation of POF is quite variable. Patients may present at varying ages with amenorrhea, infertility, or both. Symptoms suggestive of the menopause, including hot flashes, vaginal dryness, sleep disturbances, and mood disturbances, may be present. Ovarian failure may be temporary, with spontaneous return of menstrual function. Associated autoimmune disorders include Addison's disease, thyroiditis, hypoparathyroidism, diabetes, pernicious anemia, myasthenia gravis, and vitiligo. Because of the associated polyendocrine autoimmune syndromes, patients should be screened for diabetes, anemia, and thyroid, adrenal, and parathyroid insufficiency. The diagnosis is confirmed by elevated gonadotropin levels, particularly FSH. All patients less than 30 years of age with POF should have a chromosomal analysis to identify any patients with a Y chromosome who are at risk for the development of a gonadal tumor.

Hyperprolactinemia

The association of ovulatory dysfunction and hyperprolactinemia is well documented (Jacobs, 1976). The primary mechanism appears to be inhibition of pulsatile GnRH secretion, resulting in a hypoestrogenic state (Monroe et al., 1981). Elevated prolactin levels may also cause direct inhibition of steroidogenesis at the level of the ovary (McNatty et al., 1973). A number of clinical conditions may cause elevated circulating prolactin levels. These include pituitary tumors, various medications, chest wall trauma, chronic renal insufficiency, hypothyroidism, the empty sella syndrome, pituitary stalk transection, and, rarely, nonpituitary tumors. Medications that commonly cause hyperprolactinemia include phenothiazines, tricyclic antidepressants, estrogen-containing medications, including oral contraceptive agents, butyrophenones, metoclopramide, reserpine, amphetamines, and methyldopa (Aldomet). Transient elevations of prolactin have also been associated with beer and protein ingestion, herpes zoster, nipple stimulation, stress, sexual intercourse, and hypoglycemia. Although associated galactorrhea is common, not all women with hyperprolactinemia have this symptom. Even though pituitary adenomas tend to be associated with high levels of prolactin, they may be associated with any degree of hyperprolactinemia. Therefore, we recommend radiographic evaluation with either computed tomography or magnetic resonance imaging for all patients with persistent hyperprolactinemia regardless of the absolute level.

Hypothalamic Amenorrhea

Hypothalamic amenorrhea is a diagnosis of exclusion. Despite multiple etiologic factors, the primary mechanism appears to be an alteration in GnRH secretion. This results in decreased gonadotropin secretion, a failure in the stimulation of follicular development, and a diminution in gonadal steroidogenesis. Therefore, any process resulting in a disturbance of GnRH production may lead to hypothalamic amenorrhea. In contrast to PCOS, hypothalamic amenorrhea is associated with a hypoestrogenic state. Hypothalamic amenorrhea must be distinguished from other forms of hypoestrogenic amenorrhea such as hyperprolactinemia, POF, and Asherman's syndrome (see the discussion of the uterine factor). The diagnosis is confirmed by normal or low gonadotropin levels and a normal progestin challenge. The commonest causes of hypothalamic amenorrhea include exercise, weight loss, and stress. Rare causes include anorexia nervosa, Kallmann's syndrome, and nonfunctional hypothalamic pituitary tumors. In a large percentage of cases, there may be no obvious underlying cause. The commonest clinical problem associated with hypothalamic amenorrhea is infertility. In contrast to patients with POF, symptoms of estrogen deficiency are relatively rare.

Luteal Phase Defect

A luteal phase defect refers to a relative deficiency in the secretion of progesterone by the corpus luteum. Progesterone is important for the implantation of the embryo and the maintenance of early human pregnancy. The progesterone deficiency may be in the amount or duration (or both) of secretion. The short luteal phase refers to a shortening of the interval between ovulation and the onset of menses to 10 days or less. The short luteal phase may be associated with a normal peak value of progesterone. The inadequate luteal phase refers to a luteal phase of normal length with lower than normal progesterone secretion. The incidence of luteal phase defect as a pathological condition is difficult to determine. This is partially related to the probable high incidence among the normal female population. The incidence of luteal phase defect as a cause for in-

fertility in an unselected, infertile population has been estimated to be between 2% and 4% (Jones and Pourmand, 1962). However, the frequency of luteal phase defects appears to be much higher in certain clinical situations. For example, patients with recurrent miscarriages appear to have an incidence as high as 35% (Phung et al., 1979). Luteal phase defects also appear to be commoner in patients with hyperprolactinemia. Other conditions that contribute to ovulatory disorders, such as strenuous exercise, significant weight loss, and hyperandrogenism, may be associated with an increased incidence of luteal phase defect. Luteal phase defects also appear to be commoner at the extremes of reproductive life. The anovulatory patient requiring ovulation induction may demonstrate a residual luteal phase defect. This appears to be particularly common among women treated with clomiphene citrate for anovulation (Garcia et al., 1977).

A lack of uniform diagnostic criteria also makes it difficult to determine the incidence of luteal phase defects. The endometrial biopsy appears to be the gold standard for diagnosing luteal phase defects. The most widely accepted criterion for diagnosing a luteal phase defect is endometrial dating, which lags behind the time in the cycle by more than 2 days when derived retrospectively in two separate cycles. Attempts have been made to utilize a midluteal serum progesterone level for the diagnosis of luteal phase defect. A midluteal serum progesterone level of greater than 10 ng/ml has been associated with adequate luteal function (Hull et al., 1982). The basal body temperature chart is notoriously inaccurate for detecting luteal phase defects. However, evidence of a luteal phase of less than 11 days on basal body temperature charts does appear to correlate with the presence of a short luteal phase (Downs and Gibson, 1983). Although the importance of luteal phase defect as a primary cause of infertility remains to be proved, a small percentage of infertility patients appear to have reproducible evidence of luteal phase defects.

Thyroid Disease

Both hyperthyroidism and hypothyroidism may be associated with menstrual irregularities and ovulatory dysfunction. The underlying mechanism appears to be related to alterations in the metabolism of androgens and estrogens. Thyroid disease may also be associated with abnormalities in gonadotropin secretion. Although many studies suggest a clear association between clinical hypothyroidism and ovulatory disorders, studies demonstrating an association between hyperthyroidism and ovulatory disorders are lacking. Hypothyroidism and hyperthyroidism appear to be associated with decreased libido, and this may be another mechanism of thyroid-related infertility.

Although rare reported cases of pregnancy in patients with hypothyroidism and myxedema exist, myxedematous women appear to be anovulatory (Hodges et al., 1952; Montoro et al., 1984). Hypothyroidism is associated with alterations in the metabolism of testosterone and estradiol. There is a decrease in sex hormone–binding globulin levels, an increase in the metabolic clearance rate of testosterone, an increase in the conversion of androstenedione to testosterone, and an increase in the conversion of testosterone to estradiol (Gordon et al., 1969). In hypothyroidism, the chronic anovulation appears to be the result of alterations in the metabolism of estradiol and inappropriate estrogen feedback. There is a shift in the normal 2-hydroxylation with an increase in 16-hydroxylation, resulting in an increase in the estriol level (Fishman et al., 1962). Yen (1986) has postulated that this increase in the level of the less potent estriol results in inappropriate feedback, abnormal gonadotropin secretion, and chronic anovulation. Hypothyroidism may also be associated with hyperprolactinemia, offering an additional mechanism for the abnormal gonadotropin secretion associated with hypothyroidism.

Despite its popularity, the efficacy of thyroid hormone therapy for euthyroid women remains unsubstantiated. Several well-controlled clinical studies have demonstrated no benefit from the use of thyroid hormone in euthyroid, infertile women (Yen, 1986; Buxton and Herrman, 1954). The role of thyroid hormone therapy for patients with subclinical hypothyroidism (i.e., elevated TSH level and normal thyroxine and triiodothyronine levels) remains unclear and warrants further investigation. In comparison, patients with clinical hypothyroidism may benefit from thyroid hormone replacement with a resumption of normal ovulatory function. In patients with panhypopituitarism, it is imperative that the adrenal insufficiency be corrected before thyroid hormone replacement is initiated since this may result in fatal adrenal insufficiency.

Hyperthyroidism may also be associated with menstrual irregularities due to alterations in testosterone and estradiol metabolism. There is an increase in the level of plasma sex hormone–binding globulin, a decrease in the metabolic clearance rate of androgens and estrogens, an increase in the level of plasma testosterone, an increase in the conversion of testosterone to androstenedione, and an increase in the concentration of estrone (Gordon et al., 1969; Ruder et al., 1971; Chopra and Tulchinsky, 1974). Hyperthyroidism is also associated with an increase in 2-hydroxylation (Fishman et al., 1965). The menstrual irregularities associated with hyperthyroidism appear to be related to inappropriate feedback with elevated LH secretion and normal FSH secretion (Southern et al., 1974). This is similar to the inappropriate gonadotropin secretion associated with PCOS. However, despite a clear pathophysiological basis, an association between hyperthyroidism and infertility remains to be demonstrated.

Adrenal Disease

Certain disorders of the adrenal may be associated with ovulatory disorders. Autoimmune adrenal insufficiency (Addison's disease) may be associated with POF as part of a number of syndromes of polyglandular failure (Neufeld et al., 1981). Cushing's syndrome, characterized by an overproduction of glucocorticoids, may mimic PCOS by producing obesity, hirsutism, menstrual irregularities, and enlarged polycystic ovaries. Cushing's syndrome may result from an overproduction of ACTH or the autonomous production of glucocorticoids. Cushing's disease is the result of pituitary ACTH hypersecretion and hypercortisolism. The clinical manifestations of Cushing's syndrome are listed in Table 12–9. The mechanisms by which Cushing's syndrome lead to ovulatory dysfunction are not clear. Similar to PCOS, there appears to be an increase in the peripheral production of estrogen, which results in inappropriate acyclic feedback. In addition, there appears to be an abnormality in the pulsatile secretion of GnRH (Yen, 1986). As previously mentioned, patients with Cushing's syndrome may be distinguished from PCOS with a dexamethasone suppression test. Dexamethasone (1 mg) is given at bedtime, and a fasting cortisol level is measured the following morning. If the plasma cortisol level is less than 5 μg/100 ml, the diagnosis of Cushing's syndrome is excluded.

TABLE 12–9.

Clinical Manifestations of Cushing's Syndrome

Symptom	%
Obesity	95
Moon face	95
Hypertension	85
Glucose intolerance	80
Menstrual irregularities	75
Androgen excess	72
Striae	67
Proximal muscle weakness	65
Easy bruisability	55
Osteoporosis	55
Depression	50

Though an abnormal value of greater than 5 µg/ 100 ml is not diagnostic, it does warrant further evaluation.

The adult-onset form of CAH may also mimic PCOS. The subject of CAH has been recently reviewed (White et al., 1987). Relative deficiencies of 21-hydroxylase and 11-hydroxylase may be associated with hirsutism, menstrual irregularities, and ovulatory dysfunction. Because of these enzymatic defects, the normal biosynthetic pathways are interrupted, and an accumulation of adrenal androgens results. Since there appears to be a strong genetic predisposition, a family history of hirsutism, menstrual disorders, and infertility may be suggestive of CAH. In our institution, a fasting, morning 17-hydroxyprogesterone level is often obtained in the *follicular* phase as a screening test. A morning, follicular-phase 17-hydroxyprogesterone concentration greater than 4 ng/ml strongly suggests the diagnosis of late-onset CAH. A morning, follicular-phase 17-hydroxyprogesterone less than 2 ng/ml suggests that CAH is not present. The diagnosis of CAH may be confirmed with a cosyntropin (Cortrosyn) stimulation test, which demonstrates markedly elevated levels of 17-hydroxyprogesterone (New et al., 1983).

TECHNIQUES FOR PREDICTING AND DETECTING OVULATION

Besides pregnancy, recovering an ovum from the female genital tract is the only direct evidence of ovulation. This is impractical for clinical practice. Therefore, a variety of diagnostic tests that indirectly predict and detect ovulation are commonly employed. The diagnostic tests commonly used to confirm ovulation include the basal body temperature (BBT) chart, midluteal serum progesterone level, and the endometrial biopsy. The diagnostic tests that predict the time of ovulation include the BBT chart and the serial assessment of plasma or urinary LH levels.

Basal Body Temperature Chart

All infertility patients should be instructed to take their temperature with a basal thermometer. The BBT chart not only can provide indirect evidence of ovulation but may also aid in the timing of intercourse, inseminations, and other diagnostic procedures such as the postcoital test. The reading is taken each morning and recorded on a chart, with day 1 corresponding to the first day of menses (Fig 12–8). Basal body temperature thermometers show a range of only a few degrees and are easier to read. The reading is most accurate when taken immediately on awakening, before any activity. During the follicular phase, the temperature will usually range between 97° F and 98° F. During the luteal phase, the temperature is generally greater than 98° F. The mechanism for the elevation in temperature appears to be related to the thermogenic properties of progesterone on the central nervous system. It is often difficult to pinpoint the exact day of ovulation. A significant rise in temperature is not noted until 2 days after the LH peak and coincides with a rise in the serum progesterone level to greater than 4 ng/ml (Moghissi et al., 1972). Ovulation probably occurs on the day prior to the first temperature elevation and may be marked by a dip in the temperature to the lowest level of the cycle. This is supported by the observation that the most likely time for conception based on a single artificial insemination is the day before the temperature rise (Newill and Katz, 1982). The absence of a biphasic temperature pattern is suggestive but not diagnostic of anovulation. In approximately 75% of monophasic cycles, hormonal evidence of ovulation has been documented (Bauman, 1981; Moghissi, 1976). A slow rise in a biphasic chart is not necessarily an indication of an ovulatory disorder. However, a temperature elevation of less than 10 days' duration is suggestive of a luteal phase defect. In summary, the BBT chart is very helpful when it is clearly biphasic. When the chart is monophasic or difficult to interpret, another diagnostic method should be pursued.

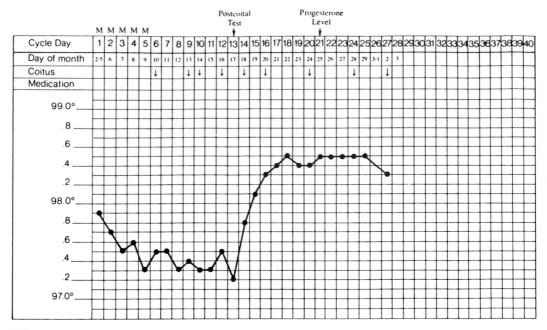

FIG 12—8.
Basal body temperature chart. This example of a BBT chart indicates a biphasic pattern with notations for the days of menstruation *(M)*, and the timing of coitus (solid circle).

Midluteal Serum Progesterone

A single, midluteal serum progesterone level greater than 3 ng/ml is indirect evidence of ovulation. However, there is a poor correlation between the serum progesterone level and endometrial biopsy in the evaluation of luteal phase defects (Shangold et al., 1983). Nevertheless, a midluteal phase progesterone level of greater than 10 ng/ml has been associated with adequate luteal function (March, 1987), since this level has been found in the midluteal phase of cycles during which conception has occurred (Hull et al., 1982; Hammond and Talbert, 1982). These discrepancies may be partially due to the pulsatile nature of progesterone secretion. Although extremely accurate for confirming ovulation, a single midluteal serum progesterone level is much less reliable for evaluating the adequacy of the luteal phase.

Endometrial Biopsy

The finding of secretory endometrium on an endometrial biopsy is additional indirect evidence of ovulation. Although relatively safe and rarely significantly uncomfortable, the endometrial biopsy should not be performed routinely for con-

firmation of ovulation due to the availability of accurate noninvasive studies. The role of the endometrial biopsy in the infertility investigation is for the diagnosis of luteal phase defects. The biopsy should be performed 2 to 3 days prior to the expected menses. A sensitive serum pregnancy test should be offered to the patient in an attempt to prevent the interruption of an early pregnancy. A pelvic examination should precede the biopsy so that the position and size of the uterus can be determined. The cervix is exposed with a speculum and cleansed with an antiseptic reagent. Premedication with a nonsteroidal anti-inflammatory agent and a paracervical block with 1% to 2% chloroprocaine (Nesacaine) may minimize patient discomfort. A tenaculum is attached to the anterior cervix. The specimen is obtained by placing a Duncan, Novak, or Pipelle curet high in the anterior uterine fundus and using a firm stroke from the fundus to the cervix (Fig 12—9). The tissue is immediately fixed in Bouin's solution. The interpretation of the endometrial biopsy is based on the dating criteria of Noyes (Noyes et al., 1950). Proliferative endometrium is diagnostic of anovulation. Dated secretory endometrium should be compared with the retrospectively derived cycle day. The first day of bleeding is considered cycle

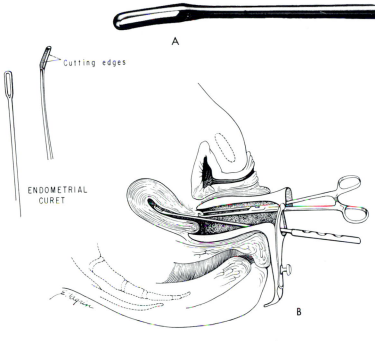

FIG 12–9.
A, cutting edge of Duncan curet. This instrument can be introduced easily through an undilated nullipa- rous cervical os. *B,* proper technique of endometrial biopsy with the Duncan curet.

day 28. A luteal phase defect is suggested by a lag in the dating by more than 2 days. Because of the relative frequency of a luteal phase defect in a single cycle, most investigators advocate two abnormal biopsy results before diagnosing a luteal phase defect.

Ultrasound Monitoring

Serial ultrasound examinations can demonstrate the growth of a follicle. The disappearance of a dominant follicle combined with the presence of free fluid in the cul-de-sac suggests follicular rupture and is presumptive evidence of ovulation. Ultrasound may also be helpful in assessing corpus luteum formation. Because of the wide range of the preovulatory follicle's diameter (17–26 mm), ultrasound examination appears to be an inaccurate predictor of ovulation. Ultrasound monitoring is also rarely used as a primary diagnostic aid for confirming ovulation.

Ultrasound examination may be useful in the diagnosis of the luteinized, unruptured follicle syndrome (LUFS). The LUFS is characterized by a normal pattern of gonadotropin secretion, regular menses, and no evidence of follicular rupture (Mareck and Hulka, 1978). The absence of follicular rupture is associated with entrapment of the oocyte and subsequent luteinization. The LUFS has been associated with unexplained infertility, endometriosis, and pelvic adhesions. Ultrasound criteria include the persistence of an echo-free dominant follicle beyond 36 hours after the LH peak (Richie, 1985). The absence of stigmata of ovulation at laparoscopy has also been suggestive of LUFS. There is no general agreement regarding the incidence of LUFS among the fertile or infertile patient population. At the present time, a causal relationship between LUFS and infertility remains to be established since the LUFS does not appear to be recurrent. Therefore, routine ultrasound evaluation of infertile couples for LUFS is not recommended (Katz, 1988). The major usefulness of ultrasound monitoring appears to be limited to the timing of human chorionic gonadotropin (hCG) administration during ovulation induction protocols and perhaps in the evaluation of unexplained infertility.

Luteinizing Hormone Monitoring

The measurement of daily preovulatory serum LH levels appears to be the gold standard for predicting ovulation. Ovulation occurs approximately 34 to 36 hours after the onset of the LH surge (Hoff et al., 1983). A twofold rise above the baseline serum LH level is suggestive of the onset of the LH surge. The accuracy of monitoring the serum LH level must be weighed against the relative inconvenience and significant cost of daily blood testing. More recently, simple inexpensive urinary LH ovulation detection kits have become readily available. The accuracy of these kits compared to serum LH and BBT charts for timing intercourse and inseminations remains controversial. Several studies have demonstrated that certain home urinary LH assays are quite accurate (Elkind-Hirsch et al., 1986; Vermesh et al., 1987). Several new techniques are currently being investigated for their accuracy of predicting ovulation. These include salivary detection kits for LH and progesterone and the determination of salivary or vaginal electrical resistance (Fernando et al., 1987).

TUBAL AND PERITONEAL FACTORS

The etiological factors for tubal disease, pelvic adhesions, and endometriosis have been previously described. Interestingly, there are no identifiable risk factors in approximately 50% of patients with subsequently documented tubal or peritoneal factors (Rosenfeld et al., 1983). Therefore, the routine infertility evaluation commonly includes a test for tubal patency. Alternatively, some clinicians recommend postponing an evaluation of tubal patency in certain situations such as the anovulatory patient undergoing ovulation induction with clomiphene citrate or the infertile couple with moderate to severe male factor.

Hysterosalpingography

In the past, uterotubal insufflation (Rubin's test) was used as a screening procedure to determine tubal patency. Hysterosalpingography (HSG) has replaced uterotubal insufflation as the most commonly employed screening method due to the increased accuracy and additional information gained from HSGs. In addition to assessing tubal patency, the HSG may provide useful information about the uterine cavity (see the discussion of uterine factors). The HSG is a nonoperative, outpatient procedure that is often performed in conjunction with the department of radiology. The procedure is scheduled before ovulation, usually between cycle day 5 and 11, to prevent the possible irradiation of a fertilized ovum. The patient is placed in the dorsolithotomy position. After the position of the uterine fundus is determined, a single-tooth tenaculum is placed on the anterior cervix and a cannula snugly inserted into the cervical canal. A sterile, radiopaque contrast medium is slowly injected through the cannula. The injection phase of the procedure is best visualized under fluoroscopy. When a fluoroscopic screen is not available, radiographs should be taken after the sequential injection of 3 to 5 ml of dye. Depending on the size of the uterus, 8 to 10 ml of contrast material may be required.

A film should be taken when the uterine cavity is filled. The HSG often provides evidence suggesting proximal tubal obstruction. Several studies have demonstrated that among infertile women with abnormal HSGs, the site of tubal obstruction appears to be cornual approximately 50% of the time (Rice et al., 1986; Gabos, 1976; Hutchins, 1977). Salpingitis isthmica nodosa (SIN) was first described in 1887 (Chiari, 1887) and is a rare cause of proximal tubal obstruction. Salpingitis isthmica nodosa is characterized by numerous small diverticuli involving the interstitial segment or isthmus (or both) of the fallopian tube. Although the etiology remains unknown, SIN is often found in association with chronic inflammation. A second radiograph is taken as the ampullae fill. The presence of mucosal rugae appears to be a favorable prognostic factor for subsequent pregnancy, and the absence of rugae suggests damaged tubal epithelium. Young and co-workers (1970) demonstrated a 60.7% pregnancy rate in cases with rugal folds compared with a 7.3% pregnancy rate when rugal folds were absent. A distal tubal occlusion is suggested when there is partial filling of the fallopian tube with dye but no peritoneal spillage. This may occur in the isthmic, ampullary, or fimbrial portion of the fallopian tube and is often associated with radiographic evidence of hydrosalpinges. An irregular distribution of loculated dye around the fimbriated end of the tube suggests periadnexal adhesions. Whenever possible, a final radiograph demonstrating free intraperitoneal contrast material should be taken to document tubal patency. Figure 12–10 shows the normal findings obtained by HSG and the findings seen in chronic PID. The accuracy of HSG will be discussed in the following section on laparoscopy.

The optimal contrast medium for HSGs remains controversial (Soules and Spadoni, 1982). Currently we are using a water-soluble contrast medium, meglumine diatrizoate (Renografin-60), and obtain excellent quality radiographs. The disadvantages of water-contrast medium include increased abdominal cramping and poorer resolution. The use of water-soluble rather than oil contrast medium avoids the potential complications of lipid granulomas and lipid embolization. Lipid embolization is the result of the injection of dye into the myometrium with subsequent intravasation into the venous or lymphatic system. Siegler (1974) has reported nine deaths attributable to

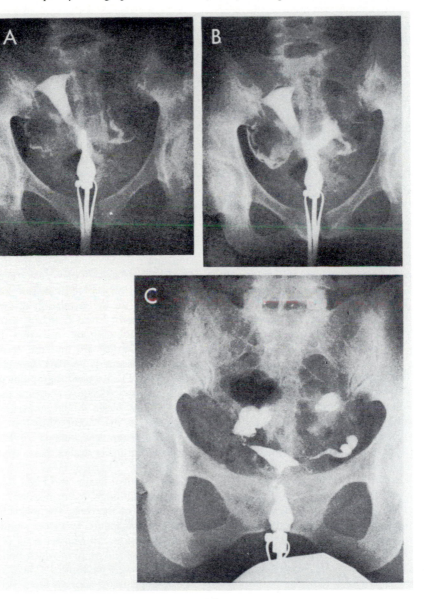

FIG 12–10.
Hysterosalpingograms. **A,** visualization of uterus and both oviducts in a normal patient. **B,** second film showing free passage of the dye from the oviduct into the peritoneal cavity. **C,** patient with chronic PID and bilateral hydrosalpinges.

the intravasation of dye. Bateman et al. (1980) have reported 13 cases of dye intravasation in a series of 533 HSGs performed with oil contrast medium. However, only six of these patients had embolization of dye, and there was no associated morbidity or mortality. These authors state that the use of fluoroscopy allows for early detection of intravasation and minimizes complications. Whenever there is evidence of intravasation, injection should be discontinued immediately, regardless of the contrast media employed. The appearance of intravasation includes a network of streak-like opacities adjacent to the uterine cavity extending toward the pelvic side walls and subsequently migrating in a cephalad direction.

The use of fluoroscopy combined with the use of the less viscous contrast dye ethiodized oil (Ethiodol) may minimize the risk of a fatal oil embolus. The popularity of ethiodized oil in certain centers is due to its possible value as a therapeutic agent. Despite numerous anecdotal cases, the therapeutic benefit of an HSG remains controversial. Although several studies have demonstrated no increase in the pregnancy rate following an HSG (Alper et al., 1986), several studies do seem to suggest an increased pregnancy rate (Palmer, 1960). Moreover, several studies suggest an increased pregnancy rate with oil contrast compared to water-soluble contrast medium (Gillespie, 1965; DeCherney et al., 1980). De-Cherney et al. (1980) studied 339 patients over a 4-month period and demonstrated a 29% pregnancy rate with oil medium compared to 13% with water-soluble medium. The mechanisms by which an HSG may enhance fertility include (1) a mechanical lavage of a partially obstructed tube, (2) stimulation of the tubal cilia, and (3) perturbation of a hostile peritoneal environment in that ethiodized oil has been shown to inhibit macrophage phagocytosis of spermatozoa in vitro (Surrey and Meldrum, 1987).

The absolute contraindications for performing an HSG include a possible pregnancy and a history of PID. Relative contraindications include a history suggestive of PID, recent uterine instrumentation, and iodine allergy. The risk of PID following HSG has been estimated between 1% and 3% (Rice et al., 1986; Stumpf and March, 1980). A sedimentation rate may be helpful for screening patients at risk for an acute flare of PID. Although routine antibiotic prophylaxis has not been demonstrated to be efficacious (Stumpf and March, 1980), patients at risk for an acute flare of PID may benefit from antibiotic therapy

(Pitaway et al., 1983). In our unit, all patients are recommended antibiotic prophylaxis with doxycycline for 3 to 5 days. For patients at significant risk for an acute flare of PID, laparoscopy with tubal lavage is recommended in lieu of HSG for the evaluation of tubal patency.

Laparoscopy

Laparoscopy with tubal lavage is considered the gold standard for evaluating tubal patency and other peritoneal factors. Laparoscopy offers the advantage of directly visualizing the pelvic anatomy. During laparoscopy, in addition to assessing tubal patency with the instillation of blue dye, the appearance of the fimbria, the anatomical relationship between the fimbria and the ovary, and the presence of periadnexal adhesions and endometriosis can be determined. The technique of laparoscopy is thoroughly reviewed by Wheeless and Katayama (1985). Laparoscopy is usually performed under general anesthesia as a day surgical procedure. However, the procedure may be performed under sedation with local anesthesia or regional anesthesia. The patient is placed in the lithotomy position, and a cannula is placed through the cervical canal for the injection of indigo carmen dye. A thin Verres needle is placed through an infraumbilical incision into the peritoneal cavity for the instillation of carbon dioxide. Approximately 2 to 3 L of CO_2 provides an adequate pneumoperitoneum so that the larger trochar may be inserted into the peritoneal cavity. The laparoscope is inserted through this trochar (Fig 12–11). A second suprapubic puncture may be necessary to adequately expose the pelvic anatomy. Tubal lavage should be performed with indigo carmen dye to assess tubal patency.

The diagnostic accuracy of HSG has been evaluated in many studies that compare HSG and laparoscopy. Although HSG is not a perfect predictor of tubal factor, the HSG is in agreement with the findings at laparoscopy approximately two thirds of the time. The major inadequacy of HSG is the failure to detect significant periadnexal adhesions. El Minawi et al. (1978) studied 352 cases of infertility in which both laparoscopy and HSG were performed. There was complete agreement in 56.7% of the cases. Pelvic adhesions were suggested by HSG in 76 cases compared with 151 cases documented by laparoscopy. Moreover, laparoscopy was able to document pelvic adhesions or endometriosis in 57% of patients with previously unexplained infertility (El Minawi

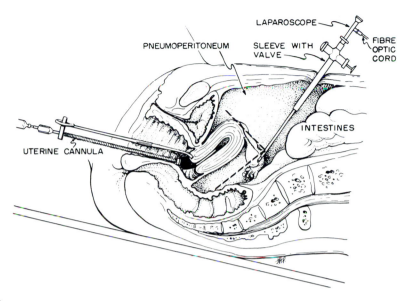

FIG 12–11.
Schematic diagram of pelvis at laparoscopy. (From Cohn MR: *Laparoscopy, Culdoscopy, and Gynecog-* *raphy.* Philadelphia, WB Saunders Co, 1970. Reproduced by permission.)

et al., 1978). Collins et al. (1988b) have estimated the aggregate sensitivity and specificity of HSG to be 76% and 83%, respectively. Therefore, laparoscopy will be required among women with a normal HSG to identify a certain percentage of patients with tubal and peritoneal factors. The decision when to proceed with laparoscopy when the HSG is normal should be individualized based on the history, physical examination, and the remainder of the initial infertility evaluation.

In contrast, whenever the HSG suggests a tubal factor, laparoscopic confirmation is essential due to the relatively high incidence of false positives. The commonest cause of a false positive HSG is cornual spasm. In an attempt to eliminate the complication of cornual spasm, Hutchins (1977) studied 62 patients under general anesthesia. This study revealed that 45 of 62 patients (73%) with proximal tubal occlusion on HSG had laparoscopic evidence of normal oviducts with evidence of tubal patency by methylene blue insufflation. Because of the high incidence of false cornual obstruction, a minimum of three separate tubal studies should be performed before the diagnosis of proximal tubal obstruction is confirmed.

The commonest laparoscopic finding is postinfective tubal disease (Collins et al., 1988b). This may include pelvic adhesions, phimotic fimbria, hydrosalpinges, or tubal obstruction. Significant pelvic adhesions may also be the result of previous abdominal surgery. Myomectomy, ruptured appendicitis, or any other cause of peritonitis may lead to pelvic adhesion formation. Endometriosis is the second commonest laparoscopic finding. The prevalence of endometriosis among women undergoing diagnostic laparoscopy for infertility has been reported between 5% and 25%. Laparoscopic visualization, biopsy, or both are required for the diagnosis of endometriosis since there are no specific screening tests or clinical findings. The subject of endometriosis is extensively reviewed in Chapter 11.

The American Fertility Society's classifications of adnexal adhesions, distal tubal occlusion, and endometriosis is based on laparoscopic findings and provides a rational foundation for therapy (American Fertility Society, 1988; Buttram, 1985). Recent advances in operative laparoscopy and laser technology have allowed for lysis of adhesions, fulguration of endometriosis, and tubal reconstruction at the time of diagnostic laparoscopy. The techniques of diagnostic and operative laparoscopy are further discussed in Chapter 22.

Future Diagnostic Procedures

Although HSG is an adequate screening procedure for assessing tubal patency, and laparoscopy can accurately confirm tubal patency and detect peritoneal factors, there is presently no procedure available to evaluate the functional integrity of the fallopian tube. Tubal patency does not confirm ovum pickup or gamete or embryo transport. Although fallopian tube physiology remains poorly understood (see Chapter 8), the ciliated tubal epithelial cells are thought to be important for ovum and embryo transport. Salpingoscopy allows for the endoscopic evaluation of the endosalpinx and may help identify an abnormal mucosal pattern, intratubal adhesions, or both. The technique of salpingoscopy may allow for a better understanding of tubal physiology, including the mechanisms of bidirectional tubal motility. Salpingoscopy may be performed at the time of laparoscopy or laparotomy. Shapiro and co-workers (1988) recently reported 17 patients who underwent salpingoscopy at the time of laparoscopy or laparotomy and found a 23.5% discordance rate between the fimbrial appearance at surgery and the salpingoscopic findings. They suggest that salpingoscopy may aid in the often difficult therapeutic decision between reconstructive tubal surgery and in vitro fertilization.

UTERINE FACTORS

Although uterine abnormalities are often associated with recurrent pregnancy loss, they are not generally considered a cause of infertility. The association between uterine factors and infertility remains unclear since the hormonal and immunological prerequisites for normal implantation and early embryo development remain poorly understood. A large number of progesterone-dependent endometrial and decidual proteins have been characterized and may be important for the implantation of the embryo (Bell et al., 1986).

The association of DES exposure and infertility may be partially the result of uterine factors. Uterine leiomyomas or fibroids are often implicated as a cause for infertility, even though well-controlled epidemiological and clinical studies are lacking. A review of the literature suggests that fibroids alone are an infrequent cause of infertility (Buttram and Reiter, 1981). The mechanisms by which fibroids may cause infertility include mechanical obstruction of sperm transport and suboptimal implantation. Although the majority of the uterine proteins described have been produced from the endometrium and decidua, the myometrium appears to be hormonally active as well. Recently, the myometrium and uterine fibroids have been shown to secrete prolactin (Wal-

ters et al., 1983; Daly et al., 1984). The clinical significance of uterine and fibroid prolactin remains to be elucidated. Before myomectomy is considered as a primary procedure, the other potential causes of infertility should be evaluated and treated. In patients undergoing myomectomy, the preoperative gestational size and location of the leiomyomas are important prognostic factors with regard to subsequent fertility (Buttram and Reiter, 1981).

Congenital uterine anomalies such as uterine didelphys and uterine septa are also much more commonly associated with midtrimester loss and early fetal wastage when compared with infertility (Fig 12–12). Asherman's syndrome (intrauterine synechiae) is commonly associated with amenorrhea, menstrual irregularities, habitual abortion, and poor obstetric outcome. It is rarely associated with infertility. Nevertheless, patients with severe intrauterine adhesions may have mechanical obstruction of sperm migration as well as an unfavorable endometrial environment for implantation (Schenker and Margalioth, 1982).

Although the significance of uterine factors may be difficult to determine, women at high risk for intrauterine pathology are those with a history of DES exposure, fibroids, previous curettage, and previous spontaneous abortion. Hysterosalpingography often suggests possible asymptomatic uterine factors. The diagnostic accuracy of HSG for the evaluation of uterine factors has been evaluated in many studies that compare HSG and hysteroscopy (Taylor, 1977; Valle, 1980; Fayez et al., 1987). Hysterosalpingography is considered an excellent screening test for uterine factors since it is associated with a high sensitivity (i.e., false negative diagnoses are uncommon). However, because of its increased accuracy, hysteroscopy remains the gold standard for the evaluation of uterine factors and is required to confirm any suspected diagnoses as well as determine the extent of the disease. The techniques of diagnostic and operative hysteroscopy are extensively discussed in Chapter 22.

UNEXPLAINED INFERTILITY

Perhaps the most frustrated patients, and the most frustrating to take care of, are the couples with unexplained infertility. Moghissi and Wallach (1983) have defined unexplained infertility as "any couple who has failed to establish a

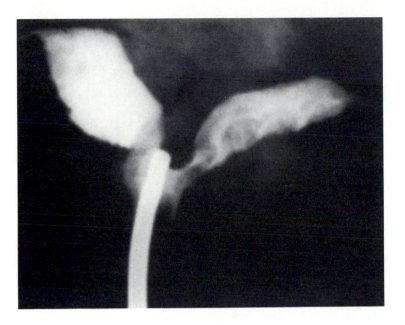

FIG 12–12.
Hysterosalpingogram demonstrating a congenital uterine anomaly. This may represent a bicornuate uterus or a uterine septum. Laparoscopic and hyst- eroscopic visualization of the external and internal uterine surface are required to distinguish these two entities.

pregnancy despite an evaluation that uncovers no obvious reason for infertility or after correction of the factor(s) identified as responsible for the infertility." The incidence of unexplained infertility appears to be decreasing, most likely as a result of improvements in the diagnostic evaluation. In recent reviews, the incidence of unexplained infertility has been estimated to be approximately 15% (Templeton and Penny, 1982). Although unexplained infertility may represent the inability of the present diagnostic tests to identify a potential cause, it may alternatively represent a lack of understanding of some aspect of the reproductive process.

Coulam and co-workers (1988) have suggested that additional testing may reduce the incidence of unexplained infertility. Therefore, if the initial evaluation of BBT, semen analysis, PCT, HSG, and laparoscopy are all normal, additional testing should be considered. In our institution, this may include an endometrial biopsy for luteal phase defects, antisperm antibodies for immunologic infertility, a sperm penetration assay to evaluate sperm function, *Mycoplasma* cultures, and serial ultrasound monitoring for luteinized, unruptured follicle syndrome. If this additional evaluation fails to identify a particular etiology, empiric therapy should be considered.

MYCOPLASMA AND CHLAMYDIA

Despite a large body of literature, the role of subclinical genital tract infections in infertility remains enigmatic. In particular, the role of *Mycoplasma* in infertility remains rather controversial. Although *Chlamydia* appears to be clearly associated with tubal factor and male factor infertility, its role in cervical factor infertility remains unclear.

Isolation rates of *Mycoplasma* (*Ureaplasma urealyticum, Mycoplasma hominis*) vary depending on a number of socioeconomic factors as well as the number of sexual partners. Whether there is a significant difference between fertile and infertile patient populations remains controversial since clinical studies have provided conflicting results (Gnarpe and Friberg, 1972; DeLouvois et al., 1974; Matthews et al., 1975). Several studies suggest that there may be an increased incidence of *Ureaplasma urealyticum* in certain etiological categories of infertility. For example, couples with male factor and unexplained infertility appear to have an increased incidence of *Ureaplasma urealyticum* (Cassell et al., 1983; Idriss et al., 1978). In the male, subclinical genital tract infections, including *Mycoplasma*, have been found to be associated with decreased sperm motility (Fowlkes et al., 1975), and adequate therapy appears to be associated with an improvement (Swenson et al., 1979). Unfortunately, well-controlled, prospective studies of the subsequent pregnancy rates have yielded conflicting results (Toth et al., 1983; Hinton et al., 1979; Harrison et al., 1975). Several other mechanisms of *Mycoplasma*-related male infertility that have been proposed include the association of antisperm antibodies (Witkin and Toth, 1983) and abnormal egg penetration (Busolo and Zanchetta, 1985). In comparison, there is insufficient evidence to support a primary role for *Mycoplasma* in tubal factor or cervical factor infertility. Several studies have demonstrated that *Ureaplasma urealyticum* does not alter the physiological characteristics of cervical mucus or sperm penetration and viability (Rehewi et al., 1978; Idriss et al., 1978). In summary, critical analysis of epidemiological studies fails to provide significant evidence that *Mycoplasma* is causally related to infertility. In our institution, patients with male factor and unexplained infertility are offered cultures for *Mycoplasma,* since these couples may benefit from antibiotic therapy. Although a follow-up culture may have prognostic value (Toth et al., 1983), repetitive courses of antibiotics should be discouraged. There is no role for routine *Mycoplasma* cultures or empiric treatment with doxycycline.

Unlike *Mycoplasma, Chlamydia trachomatis* has clearly been identified as an etiologic agent for infertility. *Chlamydia* has been shown to be a major pathogen in acute salpingitis and therefore has been associated with tubal factor infertility. Several studies have demonstrated that at least 20% of cases of acute salpingitis have been associated with chlamydial infection. However, whether patients previously exposed to *Chlamydia* are at risk for tubal factor infertility remains controversial. Several studies suggest that serological evidence of previous chlamydial infection is associated with an increased risk of asymptomatic tubal disease (Moore et al., 1982; Jones et al., 1982).

Although leukocytospermia and acute chlamydial urethritis are associated with abnormal semen parameters, the importance of subclinical chlamydial infection in male factor infertility remains controversial (Hellstrom et al., 1987). Similarly, there is presently no evidence to suggest that previous or asymptomatic chlamydial infection is associated with cervical factor infertility. However, these studies are not available since asymptomatic *Chlamydia* cervicitis is rather uncommon in the infertility patient population. In our institution, only patients with evidence of leukocytospermia, active cervicitis, or acute PID are recommended cultures for *Chlamydia* and, if positive, antibiotic therapy.

SUMMARY

The investigation of the infertile couple requires a thorough and systematic approach. The initial evaluation should be explained to the couple in the context of the multiple causes of infertility. The basic evaluation should include a semen analysis, PCT, documentation of ovulation, and assessment of tubal patency. If the initial evaluation is normal, diagnostic laparoscopy should be considered to exclude the possibility of pelvic adhesions and endometriosis. The results of the basic workup should be reviewed with the couple. In the majority of cases, the probable cause or causes for the infertility can be determined. This provides a basis for rational therapy. If the initial evaluation does not reveal an explanation for the infertility, additional testing should be recommended. Regular review sessions are essential to provide the couple with additional treatment options, emotional support, and a realistic prognosis for future fertility. The treatment of infertility will be discussed in the next chapter.

REFERENCES

Ainmelk Y, Nemirovsky M, Belisle S, et al: Primary infertility. Correlation between sperm migration test and humoral immunity. *Int J Fertil* 1982; 27:52.

Aitken RJ: Diagnostic value of the zona-free hamster oocyte penetration test and sperm movement characteristics in oligospermia. *Int J Androl* 1985; 8:348.

Aitken RJ, Best FSM, Warner P, et al: A prospective study of the relationship between semen quality and fertility in cases of unexplained infertility. *J Androl* 1984; 5:297.

Alexander JA: Evaluation of male infertility with an in-vitro cervical mucus penetration test. *Fertil Steril* 1981; 36:201.

Alexander NT, Anderson DJ: Immunology of semen. *Fertil Steril* 1987; 47:192.

Alper MM, Garner PR: Premature ovarian failure: Its relationship to autoimmune disease. *Obstet Gynecol* 1985; 66:27.

Alper MA, Garner PR, Spence JH, et al: Pregnancy rates after hysterosalpingography with oil- and water-soluble contrast media. *Obstet Gynecol* 1986; 68:6.

Amelar RD, Dubin L, Schoenfeld C: Sperm motility. *Fertil Steril* 1980; 34:197.

American Fertility Society: The American Fertility Society classifications of adnexal adhesions, distal tubal occlusion, tubal occlusion secondary to tubal ligation, tubal pregnancies, mullerian anomalies and intrauterine adhesions. *Fertil Steril* 1988; 49:944.

Asch RH: Laparoscopic recovery of sperm from peritoneal fluid in patients with negative or poor Sims-Huhner test. *Fertil Steril* 1976; 27:1111.

Ayvaliotis B, Bronson R, Rosenfeld D, et al: Conception rates in couples where autoimmunity to sperm is detected. *Fertil Steril* 1985; 43:739.

Barbieri RL, Ryan KJ: Hyperandrogenism, insulin resistance, acanthosis nigricans. A common endocrinopathy with distinct pathophysiological features. *Am J Obstet Gynecol* 1983; 147:90.

Barbieri RL, Smith S, Ryan KJ: The role of hyperinsulinemia in the pathogenesis of ovarian hyperandrogenism. *Fertil Steril* 1988; 50:197.

Barros C, Yanagimachi R: Induction of zona reaction in golden hamster eggs by cortical granule material. *Nature* 1971; 233:2368.

Bateman BG, Nunley WC Jr, Kitchin JD: Intravasation during hysterosalpingography using oil-base contrast media. *Fertil Steril* 1980; 34:439.

Battin DA, Vargyas JM, Fumihiko S, et al: In vitro fertilization rates of male factor patients. *Fertil Steril* 1984; 41:42S.

Bauman JE: Basal body temperature: Unreliable method of ovulation detection. *Fertil Steril* 1981; 36:729.

Bedford JM: Sperm capacitation and fertilization in mammals. *Biol Reprod* 1970; 2(suppl):128.

Bell SC, Patel SR, Kirwan PH, et al: Protein synthesis and secretion by the human endometrium during the menstrual cycle and the effect of progesterone in vitro. *J Reprod Fertil* 1986; 77:221.

Belsey MA, Eliasson R, Gallegos AJ, et al: *Laboratory Manual for Examination of Human Semen and Semen-Cervical Mucus Interaction*. Geneva, World Health Organization, 1980.

Bostofte E, Serup J, Rebbe H: Relation between sperm count and semen volume, and pregnancies obtained during a 20-year follow-up period. *Int J Androl* 1982; 5:267.

Bostofte E, Serup J, Rebbe H: Relation between number of immobile spermatozoa in pregnancies obtained during a 20-year follow-up period. *Andrologia* 1984; 16:136.

Bostofte E, Serup J, Rebbe H: The clinical value of morphological rating of human spermatozoa. *Int J Fertil* 1985; 30:31.

Bronson R, Cooper G, Rosenfeld D: Ability of antibody-bound human sperm to penetrate zona-free hamster ova in vitro. *Fertil Steril* 1981; 36:778.

Bronson R, Cooper G, Rosenfeld D: Sperm antibodies: Their role in infertility. *Fertil Steril* 1984; 42:171.

Bronson RA, Rogers BJ: Pitfalls of the zona-free hamster egg penetration test: Protein source as a major variable. *Fertil Steril* 1988; 50:851.

Burkman LJ, Coddington CC, Franken DR, et al: The hemizona assay (HZA): Development of a diagnostic test for the binding of human spermatozoa to the hemizona pellucida to predict fertilization potential. *Fertil Steril* 1988; 49:688.

Busolo F, Zanchetta R: The effect of *Mycoplasma hominis* and *Ureaplasma urealyticum* on hamster egg in vitro penetration by human spermatozoa. *Fertil Steril* 1985; 43:110.

Buttram BC, Reiter RC: Uterine leiomyomata: Etiology, symptomatology, and management. *Fertil Steril* 1981; 36:433.

Buttram VC: Evolution of the revised American Fertility Society's classification of endometriosis. *Fertil Steril* 1985; 43:347.

Buxton CL, Herrman WL: Effect of thyroid hormone on menstrual disorders and sterility. *JAMA* 1954; 155:1035.

Cassell GH, Younger BJ, Brown MB, et al: Microbiologic study of infertile women at the time of diagnostic laparoscopy. *N Engl J Med* 1983; 308:502.

Chang RJ, Mandel FP, Wolfsen AR, et al: Circulating levels of plasma adrenocorticotropin in polycystic ovary disease. *J Clin Endocrinol Metab* 1982; 54:1265.

Chiari H: zur Pathologischen Anatomie des Eileitercatarrhs. *Z Heilkunde* 1887; 8:457.

Chong AP, Walters CA, Weinrieb SA: The neglected laboratory test. *J Androl* 1983; 4:280.

Chopra IJ, Tulchinsky D: Status of estrogen-androgen balance in hyperthyroid men with Grave's disease. *J Clin Endocrinol Metab* 1974; 38:269.

Collins JA: Diagnostic assessment of the infertile female partner. *Curr Probl Obstet Gynecol Fertil* 1988a; 2:27.

Collins JA: Diagnostic assessment of the infertile female partner. *Curr Probl Obstet Gynecol Fertil* 1988b; 11:27.

Collins JA, Garner JB, Wilson EH, et al: A proportional hazards analysis of the clinical characteristics of infertile couples. *Am J Obstet Gynecol* 1984a; 148:527.

Collins JA, So Y, Wilson EH, et al: The postcoital test as a predictor of pregnancy among 355 infertile couples. *Fertil Steril* 1984b; 41:703.

Coulam CB, Moore SB, O'Fallon W: Investigating unexplained infertility. *Am J Obstet Gynecol* 1988; 158:1374.

Cramer DW, Walker AN, Schiff I: Statistical methods in evaluating the outcome of infertility therapy. *Fertil Steril* 1979; 32:80.

Cramer DW, Wilson E, Stillman RJ, et al: The relation of endometriosis to menstrual characteristics, smoking and exercise. *JAMA* 1986; 255:1904.

Daly DC, Walters CA, Pryor JC, et al: Prolactin production from proliferative phase leiomyoma. *Am J Obstet Gynecol* 1984; 148:1059.

Davajan V: Postcoital testing, in Mishell DR, Davajan V (eds): *Infertility, Contraception, and Reproductive Endocrinology*. Oradell, NJ, Medical Economics Co, 1985.

Davajan V, Kunitake GM: Fractional in-vivo and in-vitro examination of postcoital cervical mucus in the human. *Fertil Steril* 1969; 20:197.

DeCherney AH, Kort H, Barner JB, et al: Increased pregnancy rate with oil soluble hysterosalpingography dye. *Fertil Steril* 1980; 33:407.

DeLouvois J, Blades M, Harrison RF, et al: Frequency of mycoplasma in fertile and infertile couples. *Lancet* 1974; 1:1073.

Derrick FC, Johnson J: Reexamination of "normal" sperm count. *Urologie* 1974; 3:99.

Dor J, Homburg R, Rabau E: An evaluation of etiologic factors and therapy in 665 infertile couples. *Fertil Steril* 1977; 28:718.

Downs KA, Gibson M: Basal body temperature graph and the luteal phase defect. *Fertil Steril* 1983; 40:466.

Elkind-Hirsch K, Goldzieher JW, Gibbons WE, et al: Evaluation of the Ovu-Stick urinary luteinizing hormone kit in normal and stimulated menstrual cycles. *Obstet Gynecol* 1986; 67:450.

El Minawi MF, et al: Comparative evaluation of laparoscopy and hysterosalpingography in infertile patients. *Obstet Gynecol* 1978; 51:29.

Fayez JA, Mutie G, Schneider PJ: The diagnostic value of hysterosalpingography and hysteroscopy in infertility investigation. *Am J Obstet Gynecol* 1987; 156:558.

Fernando RS, Regas J, Betz G: Prediction of ovulation with the use of oral and vaginal electrical measurements during treatment with clomiphene citrate. *Fertil Steril* 1987; 47:409.

Fishman J, Hellman L, Zumoff B: Influence of thyroid hormone on estrogen metabolism in man. *J Clin Endocrinol Metab* 1962; 22:389.

Fishman J, Hellman L, Zumoff B, et al: Effect of thyroid on hydroxylation of estrogen in man. *J Clin Endocrinol Metab* 1965; 25:365.

Fowlkes DM, Dooher GB, O'Leary WM: Evidence by scanning electron microscopy for an association between spermatozoa and t-mycoplasmas in men of infertile marriage. *Fertil Steril* 1975; 26:1203.

Gabos P: A comparison of hysterosalpingography and endoscopy: An evaluation of tubal function in infertile women. *Fertil Steril* 1976; 27:238.

Garcia J, Jones GS, Wentz AC: The use of clomiphene citrate. *Fertil Steril* 1977; 28:707.

Gibbons RA, Mattner P: The chemical and physical characteristics of the cervical secretion and its role in reproductive physiology, in Sherman AI (ed): *Pathways to Conception*. Springfield, Ill, Charles C Thomas, Publisher, 1971.

Gillespie HW: The therapeutic aspect of hysterosalpingography. *Br J Radiol* 1965; 38:301.

Gnarpe H, Friberg J: *Mycoplasma* in human reproductive failure. *Am J Obstet Gynecol* 1972; 114:727.

Gordon GG, Southern AL, Rochimoto S, et al: Effect of hyperthyroidism and hypothyroidism on the metabolism of testosterone and androstenedione in man. *J Clin Endocrinol Metab* 1969; 29:164.

Graff G: Suppresion of cervical mucus during clomiphene therapy. *Fertil Steril* 1971; 22:209.

Haas GG, Cines DB, Schreiber AD: Immunologic infertility: Identification of patients with antisperm antibody. *N Engl J Med* 1980; 180:303.

Hall MG, Savage PE, Bromham DR: Prognostic value of the postcoital test: Prospective study based on time-specific conception rates. *Br J Obstet Gynaecol* 1982; 89:299.

Hammond MG, Talbert LM: Clomiphene citrate therapy of infertile women with low luteal phase progesterone levels. *Obstet Gynecol* 1982; 59:275.

Hargreave TB, Nillson S: Seminology, in Hargreave TB (ed): *Male Infertility*. New York, Springer-Verlag New York, 1983.

Harrison RF, Blades M, Delouvois J, et al: Doxycycline treatment in human infertility. *Lancet* 1975; 1:605.

Hellstrom WJG, Schachter J, Sweet RL, et al: Is there a role for *Chlamydia trachomatis* in genital *Mycoplasma* in male infertility? *Fertil Steril* 1987; 48:337.

Hendershot GE, Mosher WD, Pratt WF: Infertility and age: An unresolved issue. *Fam Plan Perspect* 1982; 14:287.

Hill JA, Anderson DJ: Immunological Mechanisms of Female Infertility, in Johnson PM (ed): *Bailliere's Clinical Immunology and Allergy: Immunologic Disease in Pregnancy.* London, Balliere Tindall, 1988, p 551.

Hill JA, Cohen J, Anderson DJ: The effects of lymphokines and monokines on human sperm fertilizing ability in the hamster egg penetration test. *Am J Obstet Gynecol* 1989; 160:1154.

Hill JA, Haimovici F, Anderson DJ: Effects of soluble products of activated lymphocytes and macrophages (lymphokines and monokines) on human sperm motion parameters. *Fertil Steril* 1987; 47:460.

Hinton RA, Egdell LM, Andrews BE, et al: A double blind crossover study of the effect of doxycycline on *Mycoplasma* infection and infertility. *Br J Obstet Gynaecol* 1979; 86:379.

Hirsch I, Gibbons WE, Lipshultz LI, et al: In vitro fertilization in couples with male factor infertility. *Fertil Steril* 1986; 45:659.

Hodges RE, Hamilton AG, Keetel WC: Pregnancy in myxedema. *Arch Intern Med* 1952; 90:863.

Hoff JD, Quigley ME, Yen SS: Hormonal dynamics at mid-cycle: A re-evaluation. *J Clin Endocrinol Metab* 1983; 57:792.

Hoffman D, Lobo RA: The prevalence and significance of elevated DHEA-S levels in anovulatory women. *Fertil Steril* 1983; 39:404.

Horne HW, Hertig AT, Kundsin RB, et al: Subclinical endometrial inflammations and T-mycoplasma. *Int J Fertil* 1973; 18:226.

Hull MGR, Savage PE, Bromham DR, et al: The value of a single serum progesterone measurement in the mid-luteal phase as a criterion of a potentially fertile cycle ("ovulation") derived from treated and untreated conception cycles. *Fertil Steril* 1982; 37:355.

Hutchins CJ: Laparoscopy and hysterosalpingography in the assessment of tubal patency. *Obstet Gynecol* 1977; 49:325.

Idriss WM, Patton WC, Taymor ML: On the etiologic role of *Ureaplasma urealyticum* (t-mycoplasma) infection in infertility. *Fertil Steril* 1978; 30:293.

Isojima S, Li T, Ashitaka Y: Immunologic analysis of sperm-immobilizing factor found in sera of women with unexplained sterility. *Am J Obstet Gynecol* 1968; 101:677.

Jacobs HS: Prolactin and amenorrhea. *N Engl J Med* 1976; 295:954.

Jette NT, Glass RH: Prognostic value of the postcoital test. *Fertil Steril* 1972; 23:29.

Jeyendran RS, Van der Ven HH, Perez-Pelaez M, et al: Development of an assay to assess the functional integrity of the human sperm membrane and its relationship to other semen characteristics. *J Reprod Fertil* 1984; 70:219.

Jones GES, Pourmand K: An evaluation of etiologic factors and therapy in 555 private patients with primary infertility. *Fertil Steril* 1962; 13:389.

Jones RB, Ardery BR, Huy SL, et al: Correlation between serum antichlamydial antibodies and tubal factor as a cause of infertility. *Fertil Steril* 1982; 38:553.

Karp LE, Williamson RA, Moore DE, et al: Sperm penetration assay: Useful test in evaluation of male fertility. *Obstet Gynecol* 1981; 57:620.

Katz E: The luteinized unruptured follicle and other ovulatory disorders. *Fertil Steril* 1988; 50:839.

Kaufman F, Kogut MD, Donnell GN, et al: Ovarian failure in galactosemia. *Lancet* 1979; 2:737.

Krauss CM, Turksoy NR, Atkins L, et al: Familial premature ovarian failure due to an interstitial deletion of the long arm of the X chromosome. *N Engl J Med* 1987; 317:125.

Kremer J: A simple sperm penetration test. *Int J Fertil* 1965; 10:209.

Kruger TF, Acosta AA, Simmons KF, et al: Predictive value of abnormal sperm morphology in in vitro fertilization. *Fertil Steril* 1988; 49:112.

Kruger TF, Menkveld R, Stander FSH, et al: Sperm morphologic features as a prognostic factor in in vitro fertilization. *Fertil Steril* 1986; 46:1118.

Lobo RA: The role of the adrenal in polycystic ovary syndrome. *Semin Reprod Endocrinol* 1984; 2:251.

Lobo RA: Polycystic ovary syndrome, in Mishell DR, Davajan V (eds): *Infertility, Contraception and Reproductive Endocrinology.* Oradell, NJ, Medical Economic Books, 1986.

Lobo RA, Granger LR, Paul WL, et al: Psychological stress and increases in urinary norepinephrine metabolites, platelet serotonin and adrenal androgens in women with polycystic ovary syndrome. *Am J Obstet Gynecol* 1983a; 145:496.

Lobo RA, Kletsky OA, Campeau JD, et al: Elevated bioactive luteinizing hormone in women with the polycystic ovary syndrome. *Fertil Steril* 1983b; 39:674.

London SN, Haney AF, Weinberg JB: Diverse humoral and cell-mediated effects of antisperm antibodies on reproduction. *Fertil Steril* 1984; 41:907.

MacLeod J, Gold RZ: The male factor in fertility and infertility: II. Spermatozoan counts in 1000 men of known fertility and in 1000 cases of infertile marriages. *J Urol* 1951a; 66:436.

MacLeod J, Gold RZ: The male factor in fertility and infertility: III. Analysis of motile activity. *Fertil Steril* 1951b; 2:187.

Mahadevan MM, Trounson AO: The influence of seminal characteristics on the success rate of human in vitro fertilization. *Fertil Steril* 1984; 42:400.

Mao C, Grimes DA: The sperm penetration assay: Can it discriminate between fertile and infertile men? *Am J Obstet Gynecol* 1988; 159:279.

March CM: Update: Luteal phase defects. *Endocr Fert Forum* 1987; 10(4):3.

Mareck J, Hulka JF: Luteinized unruptured follicle syndrome: A subtle cause of infertility. *Fertil Steril* 1978; 29:270.

Margalioth EJ, Laufer N, Navot D, et al: Reduced fertilization ability of zona-free hamster ova by spermatozoa from male partners of normal infertile couples. *Arch Androl* 1983; 10:67.

Margalioth EJ, Navot D, Laufer N, et al: Correlation between the zona-free hamster egg sperm penetration assay and human in vitro fertilization. *Fertil Steril* 1986; 45:665.

Matthews CD, Elmslie RG, Clapp KH, et al: The frequency of genital mycoplasma infection in human fertility. *Fertil Steril* 1975; 26:988.

Maxson WS, Pittaway DE, Herbert CM, et al: Antiestrogenic effect of clomiphene citrate: Correlation with serum estradiol concentrations. *Fertil Steril* 1984; 42:356.

McNatty KP, Sawers RS, McNeilly AS: A possible role for prolactin in control of steroid secretion by the human graafian follicle. *Nature* 1973; 250:653.

Menge AC, Medley NE, Mangione CM, et al: The incidence and influence of antisperm antibodies in infertile human couples on sperm-cervical mucus interactions and subsequent fertility. *Fertil Steril* 1982; 38:439.

Miller EG Jr, Kurzrok R: Biochemical studies of human semen. *Am J Obstet Gynecol* 1932; 24:19.

Moghissi KS: Cyclic changes of cervical mucus in normal and progestin-treated women. *Fertil Steril* 1966; 17:663.

Moghissi KS: Accuracy of basal body temperature for ovulation detection. *Fertil Steril* 1976a; 27:1415.

Moghissi KS: Postcoital test: Physiologic basis, technique, and interpretation. *Fertil Steril* 1976b; 27:117.

Moghissi KS: The cervix in infertility, in Hammond MG, Talbert LM (eds): *Infertility: A Practical Guide for the Physician.* Oradell, NJ, Medical Economics Co, 1985.

Moghissi KS, Dabich D, Levine J, et al: Mecha-

nism of sperm migration. *Fertil Steril* 1964; 15:15.

Moghissi KS, Sacco AJ, Borin K: Immunologic infertility: I. Cervical mucus antibodies and postcoital tests. *Am J Obstet Gynecol* 1980; 136:941.

Moghissi KS, Syner FN, Evans TN: A composite picture of the menstrual cycle. *Am J Obstet Gynecol* 1972; 114:405.

Moghissi KS, Wallach EE: Unexplained infertility. *Fertil Steril* 1983; 39:5.

Monroe SE, Levine L, Chany RJ, et al: Prolactin-secreting pituitary adenomas: V. Increased gonadotropin responsivity in hyperprolactinemic women with pituitary adenomas. *J Clin Endocrinol Metab* 1981; 52:1171.

Montoro MN, Collea JA, Frasier SN, et al: Successful outcome of pregnancy in women with hypothyroidism. *Ann Intern Med* 1984; 94:31.

Moore DF, Foy HM, Daling JR: Increased frequency of serum antibodies to *Chlamydia trachomatis* in infertility due to distal tubal disease. *Lancet* 1982; 2:574.

Mosher WD: Infertility trends among U.S. couples: 1965–1976. *Fam Plan Perspect* 1982; 14:22.

Mosher WD: Reproductive impairments in the United States, 1965–1982. *Demography* 1985; 22:415.

Nelson CMK, Bunge RG: Semen analysis: Evidence for changing parameters of male fertility potential. *Fertil Steril* 1974; 25:503.

Neufeld M, MacLaren NK, Blizzard RM: Two types of autoimmune Addison's disease associated with different polyglandular autoimmune (PGA) syndromes. *Medicine* (Baltimore) 1981; 60:355.

New MI, Lorenzen F, Lerner AJ, et al: Genotyping steroid 21-hydroxylase deficiency: Hormonal reference data. *J Clin Endocrinol Metab* 1983; 57:320.

Newill RG, Katz M: The basal body temperature chart in artificial insemination by donor pregnancy cycles. *Fertil Steril* 1982; 38:431.

Noyes RW, Hertig A, Rock J: Dating the endometrial biopsy. *Fertil Steril* 1950; 1:3.

Palmer A: Ethiodol hysterosalpingography for the treatment of infertility. *Fertil Steril* 1960; 11:311.

Phipps WR, Cramer DW, Schiff I, et al: The association between smoking and female infertility as influenced by cause of the infertility. *Fertil Steril* 1987; 48:377.

Phung TT, Byrd JR, McDonough PG: Etiologies and subsequent reproductive performance of 100 couples with recurrent abortion. *Fertil Steril* 1979; 132:389.

Pitaway DE, Wynfield AC, Maxin W, et al: Prevention of acute pelvic inflammatory disease after hysterosalpingography: Efficacy of doxycycline prophylaxis. *Am J Obstet Gynecol* 1983; 47:623.

Pryor JB: Seminal analysis. *Clin Obstet Gynecol* 1981; 8:571.

Rehewi MSE, Thomas AJ, Haveze SE, et al: *Ureaplasma urealyticum* (t-mycoplasma) and seminal plasma in spermatozoa from infertile and fertile volunteers. *Eur J Obstet Gynecol Reprod Biol* 1978; 8:247.

Rice JB, London SN, Olive DL: Re-evaluation of hysterosalpingography in infertility investigation. *Obstet Gynecol* 1986; 67:718.

Richie WG: Ultrasound in the evaluation of normal and induced ovulation. *Fertil Steril* 1985; 43:167.

Rosenfeld DL, Seidman SM, Bronson RA, et al: Unsuspected chronic pelvic inflammatory disease in the infertile female. *Fertil Steril* 1983; 39:44.

Rogers BJ, Bentwood BJ, van Campen H, et al: Sperm morphology assessment as an indicator of human fertilizing capacity. *J Androl* 1983; 4:119.

Rogers BJ, van Campen H, Ueno M, et al: Analysis of human spermatozoal fertilizing ability using zona-free ova. *Fertil Steril* 1979; 32:664.

Ruder H, Corvol P, Mahoudeau JA, et al: Effects of induced hyperthyroidism on steroid metabolism in man. *J Clin Endocrinol Metab* 1971; 33:382.

Rumke P: The origin of immunoglobulins in semen. *Clin Exp Immunol* 1974; 12:287.

Rumke P, Van Amstell N, Messer EN, et al: Prognosis of fertility of men with sperm agglutinins in the serum. *Fertil Steril* 1974; 25:393.

Schenker JG, Margalioth EJ: Intrauterine adhesions: An updated appraisal. 1982; 37:593.

Schwartz D, Mayaux MJ: Female fecundity as a function of age: Results of artificial insemination in 2193 nulliparous women with azoospermic husbands. Fed Des Sentres d'Etude et de Conservation du Sperme Humain. *N Engl J Med* 1982; 306:404.

Scott JZ, Nakamura RM, Mutch J, et al: The cervical factor in infertility: Diagnosis and treatment. *Fertil Steril* 1977; 28:1289.

Settlage, DSF, Motoshima M, Treadway DR: Sperm transport from the external cervical os to the fallopian tubes in women: A time and quantitation study. *Fertil Steril* 1973; 24:655.

Shangold M, Berkley A, Gray J: Both midluteal serum progesterone levels and late luteal endometrial histology should be assessed in all infertile women. *Fertil Steril* 1983; 40:627.

Shapiro BS, Diamond MP, DeCherney AH: Salpingoscopy: An adjunctive technique for evaluation of the fallopian tube. *Fertil Steril* 1988; 49:1076.

Shulman S, Zappi E, Ahmed U, et al: Immunologic consequences of vasectomy. *Contraception* 1972; 5:269.

Siegler AM: *Hysterosalpinography*. New York, Medcon Press, 1974.

Sims JM: *Uterine Surgery*. New York, William Woods Co, 1866.

Small DRJ, Collins JA, Wilson EH, et al: The interpretation of semen analysis among infertile couples. *Can Med Assoc J* 1987; 136:829.

Smith KD, Rodriguez-Rigau LJ, Steinberger E: Relation between indices of semen analysis and pregnancy rate in infertile couples. *Fertil Steril* 1977; 28:1314.

Soules MR, Spadoni LR: Oil vs. aqueous media for hysterosalpingography: A continuing debate based on many opinions and few facts. *Fertil Steril* 1982; 38:1.

Southern AL, Olivo J, Gordon G, et al: The conversion of androgens to estrogens in hyperthyroidism. *J Clin Endocrinol Metab* 1974; 38:207.

Stone SC: Peritoneal recovery of sperm in patients with infertility associated with inadequate cervical mucus. *Fertil Steril* 1983; 40:802.

Stumpf PG, March CM: Febrile morbidity following hysterosalpingography: Identification of risk factors and recommendations for prophylaxis. *Fertil Steril* 1980; 33:487.

Surrey E, Meldrum DR: Pregnancy rates after hysterosalpingography with oil-and-water-soluble contrast media. *Obstet Gynecol* 1987; 69:830.

Swenson CE, Toth A, O'Leary WM: *Ureaplasma urealyticum* in human infertility: The effect of antibiotic therapy on semen quality. *Fertil Steril* 1979; 31:660.

Tanabe K, Gagliano P, Channing CP, et al: Levels of inhibin-F activity and steroids in human follicular fluid from normal women and women with polycystic ovarian disease. *J Clin Endocrinol Metab* 1983; 57:24.

Taylor PJ: Correlations in infertility, symptomatology, hysterosalpingography, laparoscopy, and hysteroscopy. *J Reprod Med* 1977; 8:339.

Taymor ML, Overstreet JW: Some thoughts on the postcoital test. *Fertil Steril* 1988; 50:702.

Templeton AA, Penny GC: The incidence, characteristics, and prognosis of patients whose infertility is unexplained. *Fertil Steril* 1982; 37:175.

Tietze C: Reproductive span and rate of reproduction among Hutterite women. *Fertil Steril* 1957; 8:89.

Toth A, Lesser M, Brooks C, et al: Subsequent pregnancies among 161 couples treated for t-mycoplasma genital tract infection. *N Engl J Med* 1983; 308:505.

Treadway DT, Settlage DF, Nakamura RM, et al: Significance of timing of postcoital evaluation of cervical mucus. *Am J Obstet Gynecol* 1975; 121:387.

Uehling DT: Secretory IgA in seminal fluid. *Fertil Steril* 1971; 22:769.

Valle RF: Hysteroscopy and the evaluation of female infertility. *Am J Obstet Gynecol* 1980; 137:425.

Van der Ven HH, Jeyendran RS, Al-Hasani S, et al: Correlation between human sperm swelling in hypoosmotic medium (hypoosmotic swelling test) and in vitro fertilization. *J Androl* 1986; 7:140.

Vermesh M, Kletzky OA, Davajan V, et al: Monitoring techniques to predict and detect ovulation. *Fertil Steril* 1987; 47:259.

Walters CA, Daly DC, Chapitis J, et al: Human myometrium: A new potential source of prolactin. *Am J Obstet Gynecol* 1983; 147:639.

Washington AE, Gove S, Schachter J: Oral contraceptives, *Chlamydia trachomatis* infection, and pelvic inflammatory disease. *JAMA* 1985; 253:2246.

Weir W, Cicchinelli AL: Prognosis for the infertile couple. *Fertil Steril* 1964; 15:625.

Westrom L: Effect of acute pelvic inflammatory disease on fertility. *Am J Obstet Gynecol* 1983; 146:153.

Wheeless CR, Katayama KP: Laparoscopy and tubal sterilization, in Mattingly RF, Thompson JD (eds): *Operative Gynecology,* ed 6. Philadelphia, JB Lippincott Co, 1985.

White PC, New MI, Dupont B: Congenital adrenal hyperplasia. *N Engl J Med* 1987; 316:1519.

Wickings EJ, Freischem CW, Langer K, et al: Heterologous ovum penetration test and seminal parameters in fertile and infertile men. *J Androl* 1983; 4:261.

Witkin SS, Toth A: Relationship between genital tract infections, sperm antibodies in seminal fluid, and infertility. *Fertil Steril* 1983; 40:805.

Wolf D, Boldt J, Byrd W, et al: Acrosomal status evaluation in normal ejaculated sperm with monoclonal antibodies. *Biol Reprod* 1985; 32:1157.

Wolf H, Anderson DJ: Immunohistologic characterization and quantitation of leukocyte subpopulations in human semen. *Fertil Steril* 1988; 49:497.

Yen SSC: The polycystic ovary syndrome. *Clin Endocrinol* 1980; 12:177.

Yen SSC: Chronic anovulation caused by peripheral endocrine disorders, in Yen SSC, Jaffe RB (eds): *Reproductive Endocrinology.* Philadelphia, WB Saunders Co, 1986.

Young PE, Egan JE, Barlow JJ, et al: Reconstructive surgery for infertility at the Boston Hospital for Women. *Am J Obstet Gynecol* 1970; 108:1092.

13   Infertility Treatment

Robert M. Wah, M.D.

Veronica Ravnikar, M.D.

Today's physician working with infertile couples has a broad and successful therapeutic armamentarium to offer. As medical science gains a deeper understanding of the reproductive process, more specific therapies are developed. There is reason for relative optimism in the treatment of infertility today.

For some indications, physicians are very successful in treating infertile couples. However, along with the development of new reproductive technologies has come many ethical questions. Due to our ability to manipulate the reproductive process, issues such as donor gametes, donor embryos, surrogate motherhood, host uteri, and the rights of a pre-embryo have become ethical dilemmas for today's society (American Fertility Society, 1986a). These are examples of where our technological abilities have progressed faster than our ability to develop ethical guidelines regarding these new technologies.

The goal of this chapter is to familiarize the reader with current techniques used in the treatment of infertility. Some of these techniques may not be available to every practitioner due to the technical complexities involved. Utilization of some of these therapies may require referral of patients to centers that offer these treatment modalities. In addition to outlining currently available reproductive technologies, we will also attempt to provide a glimpse of future techniques and directions currently being pursued in the treatment of infertility. Although advances in the treatment of infertility have been made on many fronts, this chapter will focus on artificial insemination, ovulation induction, and assisted reproductive technologies. Other issues such as immunological infertility treatment, infectious disease-related infertility, and microsurgery are dealt with in detail elsewhere.

ARTIFICIAL INSEMINATION

One of the oldest treatments of infertility still in current use is artificial insemination (Table 13–1). It was first described in 1790 when a cloth merchant with severe hypospadias was told to collect his semen in a warm syringe and inject it into his wife's vagina. The man's wife did become pregnant, and thus began a long history of anecdotal and uncontrolled studies claiming increased success rates with artificial insemination, husband (AIH). Despite its long history of use, AIH has never been proved to be more effective than normal intercourse except when significant abnormalities preventing deposition of sperm in close proximity to the uterus and cervix are documented. In many studies, the treatment independent pregnancy rate is nearly 20% (Nachtigall et al., 1979). Artificial insemination rarely improves on this rate of success except in those cases where there is severe hypospadias, retrograde ejaculation, impotence, or significant uterine malposition. One benefit of AIH may be that more attention is placed on timing of insemination than with natural intercourse. In some couples, this may increase chances for pregnancy. The reason this technique has persisted in being used is that practitioners believe that there is some potential benefit, there is very little risk involved with the procedure, and there is minimal cost or inconvenience involved.

A variation of artificial insemination is the treatment called artificial insemination, donor

TABLE 13–1.

Indications for Artificial Insemination Techniques

Technique	Indications
Artificial insemination, husband (AIH)	Abnormalities preventing deposition of sperm close to cervix Impotence Hypospadias Retrograde ejaculation Uterine malposition
Artificial insemination, donor (AID)	Azoospermia Severe oligospermia/asthenospermia High risk of paternally inherited disease
Intrauterine insemination (IUI)	Cervical factor infertility Male factor infertility Unexplained infertility

Miscellaneous procedures
    IUI with menotropins (Pergonal) superovulation
    Sperm processing to influence gender selection
	Unexplained infertility
	Male factor infertility
	Prevention of sex-linked diseases

(AID). Donor semen is used in place of husband's semen for artificial insemination. The indications for the use of donor insemination are azoospermia, severe sperm morphology or motility defects, and high genetic risk of paternally inherited disorders. Artificial insemination, donor was originally described in 1884 when it was used for the treatment of a couple with azoospermia and the woman became pregnant (Hard, 1909). The use of AID has progressed today to where it is commonly used in many infertility clinics. It has been estimated that there are 30,000 AID births per year in the United States (Office of Technology Assessment, 1988).

The success rates with AID appear to be dependent on the male diagnosis requiring donor insemination. In those couples where there is azoospermia, the pregnancy rates are higher with AID than in those couples with oligospermia. Azoospermic couples have approximately a 60% to 80% pregnancy rate, whereas the oligospermic couples have approximately a 50% pregnancy rate. In a review of AID at Boston Hospital for Women, Albrect and associates (1982) reported cumulative rates of conception of 68% for oligospermic couples and 92% for azoospermic couples. These rates differ slightly from those normally reported because the life table method was used to correct for variable periods of and losses to follow-up (Cramer et al., 1979). The reason

for the discrepancy between oligospermic and azoospermic couples is believed to be that women married to oligospermic men who seek infertility treatment represent a selected population with decreased fertility unable to compensate for the oligospermia. These women are more likely to have a concomitant female factor involved with the infertility, such as an ovulatory dysfunction or peritoneal factors. The average number cycles required for pregnancy is approximately three cycles in multiple studies of AID (Batzer and Corson, 1987). Using frozen semen, some programs have equivalent success rates to using fresh (Bordson et al., 1986; Hammond et al., 1986). Other investigators (Richter et al., 1984) have demonstrated a higher success rate using fresh semen vs. frozen for AID. In this study, patients used both fresh and frozen sperm in alternating cycles. The cycle fecundity was 19% using fresh sperm and 5% using frozen. The use of frozen semen has many advantages over fresh semen with regard to transmission of infectious diseases. At the current time, the use of fresh semen in donor programs is not advised (American Fertility Society, 1988).

The technique of artificial insemination is either to place the semen in the external os and in the posterior vaginal fornix with the woman in the dorsal lithotomy position or to place the semen into a cervical cup against the cervix and have the patient remove the cup at home several hours later (American Fertility Society, 1986b). There appears to be no difference in the success rates between these two techniques.

Success rates may be more related to the timing of the artificial insemination. Until recently, the timing was based on prior menstrual cycles by monitoring basal body temperature charts; however, this method is only mildly successful in predicting ovulation. A recent development is the ability for patients to test their urine at home for luteinizing hormone (LH; Corson, 1986). By monitoring their urine, patients can check for the LH surge that precedes ovulation, thus giving advance notice of impending ovulation. The start of the LH surge begins about 32 hours before ovulation, and the peak of the LH surge precedes ovulation by approximately 12 to 24 hours (World Health Organization Task Force, 1980). The urine LH surge lags 4 to 6 hours behind serum levels. Most authors recommend insemination the day after the urine LH surge is detected. Two urine LH detection kits that use a double monoclonal antibody enzyme-linked technique were compared by Vermesh and others (1987). Ovustick (Monoclonal Antibodies, Inc.) uses one antibody against the alpha subunit and the other against the beta subunit of LH and predicted ovulation on day 1 after the surge in 88% of patients. First Response (Tambrands, Inc.) uses both antibodies against the beta subunit of LH and predicted ovulation on the day of the surge in 54% of patients.

Other methods of predicting ovulation include serum LH measurement (less than 40 mIU/ml) and ultrasound monitoring of follicle growth (Queenan et al., 1980). These techniques are much more involved than the simple determination of urine LH. They should be reserved for those patients in whom the urine LH kits are not predictive of ovulation. In discussing insemination timing, one must remember that sperm survives in the female reproductive tract for 2 days or longer and that the oocyte is viable for about 24 hours after ovulation. Theoretically, insemination does not have to be done precisely at the moment of ovulation.

Donor insemination raises many moral and ethical questions. There are very few laws governing donor insemination procedures. Some states have enacted laws concerning the legal status of a child born from donor insemination. In 29 states that have enacted laws concerning artificial donor insemination, the husband of the mother of a child born by artificial donor insemination is the legal father of that child (Baylson, 1987). Most donor insemination programs are set up to protect the confidentiality of the donor as well as the offspring of the donor.

Concerning infectious disease, donor programs regularly screen their donor applicants for high-risk behavior that may expose them to sexually transmitted diseases. Periodic cultures for gonorrhea and *Chlamydia* are taken, along with serum titers for hepatitis B. Donors are also screened for any family history of inherited diseases. These precautions have come under new scrutiny in light of the problem of acquired immune deficiency syndrome (AIDS). There currently is no method of directly determining the presence of the human immunodeficiency virus (HIV) in bodily fluids. Current methods of detection are limited to the determination of antibodies raised against HIV. These antibodies can take 60 days or longer to form after initial infection with the virus. In other words, a donor may be infectious but have a normal antibody titer during this time. Because of these detection limitations as well as the lack of a cure for AIDS, programs should discontinue the use of fresh semen in donor insemination programs.

The current method for using frozen semen involves quarantining the semen for a specific amount of time, 60 to 180 days, until a second follow-up HIV antibody titer is determined to be normal. The current recommendations from the Food and Drug Administration (FDA), Centers for Disease Control (CDC), and the American Fertility Society (1988) is that fresh semen no longer be used in donor insemination programs and that frozen semen be quarantined for a minimum of 180 days with a follow-up normal HIV antibody titer being determined before the quarantined semen is released for donor insemination. If methods become available to treat or cure the AIDS disease or the ability to detect the virus directly in bodily fluids without waiting for a host antibody response becomes available (McDonough, 1988), this long expensive quarantine period may be avoided. Until that time, the safety of the donor semen recipient must take precedence over cost of such a quarantine or any perceived lower success rate with frozen semen.

A more recent variation on the concept of artificial insemination is IUI of washed sperm. The direct intrauterine placement of semen is precluded by the irritating nature of seminal components such as prostaglandins. If the seminal elements are washed away and only the sperm is isolated, IUI can take place safely. The theory behind IUI is to place an increased number of sperm higher in the reproductive tract closer to the oocyte. This is accomplished by bypassing the cervix and directly placing the sperm into the uterine cavity.

There are three main indications for IUI: (1) male factor, (2) cervical factor, and (3) unexplained infertility. Male factor problems amenable to IUI are oligospermia, asthenospermia, and abnormal semen volume or consistency. Cervical factors are abnormal cervical mucus, distorted cervical architecture, and poor postcoital tests. Immunological infertility may be treated with IUI if antibodies are present in cervical mucus but not serum (Huszar and DeCherney, 1987). The timing of IUI appears to be the same as in other methods of insemination, that is, the day after the urine LH surge is detected.

Different methods of sperm isolation have been explored in various studies as well. In most centers, semen is centrifuged to collect the sperm as a pellet. From this pellet, sperm are allowed to swim free, and those sperm that swim away from the pellet are collected in a "swim up" procedure (Lopata et al., 1976). During this procedure, sperm may undergo capacitation. This appears to select the motile sperm from the semen sample. This process increases the percentage of motile sperm deposited in uterus. Berger and associates (1985) compared albumin gradients, silica (Percoll) gradients, swim up, and centrifugation with simple washing. They measured progressive motility, recovery percentage, and hamster ova penetration rates after sperm isolation. The silica gradient technique yielded the best results in their analysis. The swim up technique is simplest to perform and has been successful for many centers (Huszar and DeCherney, 1987), including ours.

At the Brigham and Women's Fertility Unit, the washed sperm for IUI is concentrated to a volume of 0.3 ml of human tubal fluid (Irvine Scientific). A small volume is desirable to avoid uterine distention and spasm. The sample is loaded into a 16-gauge, 12-in. Teflon catheter (Intercath, Deseret Medical, Inc.). The catheter is then inserted through the cervical os into the uterine cavity. The sperm are injected with a small air bolus behind to clear the catheter. The process is done with as little manipulation as possible. For some patients with a sharply angled cervical canal, placement of a cervical tenaculum may be needed for traction. This increases the likelihood of uterine cramping. The patient remains in the modified dorsal lithomy position for 10 minutes. The vast majority of our patients find that the procedure causes little or no discomfort. The IUI procedure not only has minimal discomfort but also presents minimal risk to patients. Two theoretical risks are infection and induction of antisperm antibodies by exposure to high quantities of sperm. In actual practice, these risks rarely become realities (Makler, 1987).

Evaluating the literature for success rates of IUI is problematic. There are wide variations in patient selection, sperm preparation, technique, timing of ovulation, and methods of data analysis. There is also a consistent lack of control groups in these studies. Table 13−2 summarizes recent published studies on IUI. Results from a single center with a large number of patients represent success rates when the above variables are held constant may be more illustrative. Makler (1987) reported on 438 patients. They had male factor (292), cervical factor (110), and unexplained factor (36) infertility. The success rates were 29% for male factor, 40% for cervical factor, and 22% for unexplained infertility. The overall pregnancy rate was 31% with successful cervical and male factor patients requiring an average 2.4 cycles and 3.0 cycles for the unexplained group. In 1,492 treatment cycles, there were no cases of pelvic inflammatory disease resulting from IUI.

Current investigation to improve IUI success rate involves examining different media and addition of compounds such as relaxin (Lessing et al., 1985), caffeine (Harrison, 1978), and other constituents (Fakih et al., 1986) to improve the quality of sperm function. Sperm parameters have been improved in vitro, but proved increases in vivo have not been demonstrated.

In addition to modifying sperm function in the sperm wash process, other investigators have tried to separate sperm carrying the X or Y chromosome to influence gender selection. Two techniques that show promise are a gradient technique to isolate Y sperm (Ericsson et al., 1973) and a chromatographic technique to isolate X sperm (Steeno et al., 1975; Quinlivan et al., 1982). Beernink and Ericsson (1982) reported 79% male deliveries in 84 patients at various centers. To date, the cumulative multicenter results show 75% boys born in 343 patients (Corson and Batzer, 1987). The chromatographic method has had a 75% success in obtaining girls in 52 deliveries (Corson and Batzer, 1987). Studies of this

TABLE 13—2.

Summary of Intrauterine Insemination Success Rates

Author (yr)	No. of Patients	No. of Pregnancies	%	Comments
Cervical factor				
Confino et al. (1986)	37	19	51	
DiMarzo and Rakoft (1986)	14	6	43	Other female factors present
Byrd et al. (1987)	29	10	35	
Huszar and DeCherney (1987)	93	18	19	Includes idiopathic patients
Makler (1987)	110	44	40	
Sunde et al. (1988)	5	0	0	
Lalich et al. (1988)	65	15	23	Includes secondary factors and female immune
TOTAL	353	112	31	
Male factor				
Confino et al. (1986)	27	0	0	
DiMarzo and Rakoff (1986)	9	2	22	
Byrd et al. (1987)	21	9	43	
Huszar and DeCherney (1987)	77	22	29	
Makler (1987)	292	84	29	
Sunde et al. (1988)	40	8	20	
Lalich et al. (1988)	63	10	16	Includes secondary factors and male immune factors
TOTAL	529	135	26	
Unexplained factor				
Byrd et al. (1987)	18	7	39	
Makler (1987)	36	8	22	
Sunde et al. (1988)	11	1	9	
Lalich et al. (1988)	10	4	40	Includes secondary factors
TOTAL	75	20	27	
TOTAL (all diagnoses)	957	267	28	

type need to have a larger study sample to be statistically significant (Moore and Gledhill, 1988). Medical reasons for controlling gender selection are related to the prevention of sex-linked diseases. The American Fertility Society (1986a) does not advocate gender selection for nonmedical reasons.

A variation on the theme of IUI is coupling IUI with human menopausal gonadotropin (hMG) hyperstimulation of the woman. The theory is that by hyperstimulating the woman, there will be not only an increased number of sperm in the reproductive tract but also an increased number of oocytes. Although in theory this technique appears to be promising, there have not been many controlled studies to examine the issue.

Many different adjuncts have been tried to improve IUI success rates. Cruz and associates (1986) compared IUI and intracervical insemination (ICI) in couples with all women undergoing simultaneous superovulation with hMGs. They reported a 14% pregnancy rate with IUI couples vs. 2% in the ICI group. The total group was 49 undergoing 182 cycles. Dodson and others (1987b) reviewed 148 cycles in 85 patients using hMG/IUI and reported an overall cycle fecundity rate of 0.16 ranging from 0 to 0.40 depending on the infertility diagnosis in each woman. This cycle fecundity approaches that found with in vitro fertilization (IVF). The authors admitted this was an uncontrolled retrospective study and did not advocate the empirical use of hMG/IUI until conclusive studies can be done. A recent report by Serhal and associates (1988) describes their study of three groups of patients. Group 1 underwent IUI, group 2 had hMG with natural intercourse, and group 3 had hMG and IUI. Group 3 had a pregnancy rate of 41%, which was significantly higher then group 2 (12%) or group 1 (7%). All 62 patients had primary unexplained infertility of 6 to 11 years' duration. They also advocated the use of hMG/IUI prior to IVF or gamete intrafallopian transfer (GIFT) procedures. As noted with IUI studies, large controlled studies from a single institution will be helpful in assessing efficacy of this procedure.

OVULATION INDUCTION

The induction of ovulation represented a new and radical departure from prior treatments of infertility. For the first time physicians were able to medically treat an infertility disorder as opposed to using surgical or mechanical methods. The therapy of ovulation induction grew in synchrony with basic science knowledge of the intricate workings of the hypothalamic-pituitary-ovarian axis. Treatment of women with pure ovulatory dysfunction is both successful and highly satisfying for physicians. The three modalities that we will discuss for induction of ovulation are the use of clomiphene citrate (CC), hMGs, and gonadotropin-releasing hormones (GnRHs).

Clomiphene Citrate

Clomiphene citrate is a synthetic nonsteroidal molecule found to initiate ovulation. The initial studies were performed by Kistner and Smith

(1960) using a predecessor of CC called MER-25 (Figure 13–1). Clomiphene citrate was synthesized in 1956. Clinical trials were begun on MRL-41, code name for CC, in 1960 by Greenblatt et al. (1961) and Kistner (1965). The Merrell Drug Company obtained FDA approval for the use of CC in humans in 1967, under the trade name Clomid. Clomiphene citrate is also available from Serono Labs as Serophene. Clomiphene citrate has proved to be a highly effective agent in initiating ovulation in anovulatory women. It has gained widespread use with minimal side effects or complications.

Clomiphene citrate is a triphenylethylene derivative. Other medications derived from triphenylethylene are chlorotrianisene (TACE, Merrell Dow) and tamoxifen (Fig 13–2). Clomiphene citrate used commercially is a racemic mixture of the cis and trans stereoisomers. Currently, controversy exists as to which of the two stereoisomers are responsible for CC's ovulation initiating effect. It may be that both isomers are necessary for the effect to exist.

Clomiphene citrate is rapidly absorbed in the gastrointestinal tract. It is metabolized in the liver and excreted in the feces. There is enterohepatic circulation whereby metabolites of CC are altered by enteric bacteria resulting in reabsorption of the CC molecule. When CC is labeled with carbon 14, an average of 51% of an orally administered dose was excreted by 5 days (Adashi, 1986).

Despite widespread clinical use of CC for more than 20 years, the precise mechanism of action of this medication is still unclear (Adashi, 1984). Clomiphene citrate like other triphenylethylene derivatives appears to bind with estrogen receptors. The most widely proposed mechanism for the action of CC is that it binds with estrogen receptors in the hypothalamus without exerting estrogenic effects. By blocking native estrogen's negative feedback effects on the hypothalamus, CC leads to increased GnRH pulse frequency by

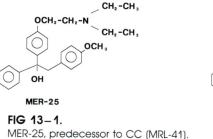

MER-25

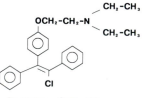

Clomiphene (MRL-41)

FIG 13–1.
MER-25, predecessor to CC (MRL-41).

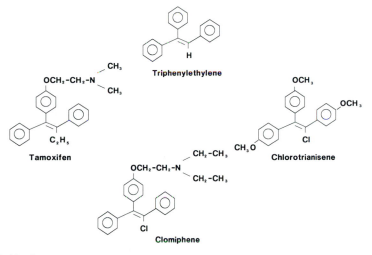

FIG 13–2.
Triphenylethylene and its derivatives tamoxifen, clomiphene, and chlorotrianisene.

the hypothalamus. This leads to increased pituitary gonadotropin secretion, which then stimulates the ovary. To be effective, CC requires an intact hypothalamic-pituitary-ovarian axis. Pituitary or ovarian lesions such as Sheehan's syndrome or premature ovarian failure will usually not respond to CC therapy. Clomiphene citrate is very effective in polycystic ovarian disease where the hypothalamic-pituitary-ovarian axis is intact but not properly coordinated to effect successful ovulation. The clinical use of CC involves establishment of the diagnosis of anovulation. A male factor as well as other endocrinological abnormalities such as thyroid dysfunction or hyperprolactinemia should be ruled out.

Although CC's primary effect appears to be centered on the hypothalamus, it also may affect the pituitary, ovary, cervix, and vagina in its binding to estrogen receptors. The effects of CC on the pituitary and ovary remain controversial, with some investigators claiming an estrogen antagonist effect and others demonstrating an agonist effect. Clinically, the antagonistic effect of CC on the reproductive tract may be seen in women who develop poor cervical mucus. Another side effect of CC is development of a luteal phase defect, which may represent altered ovarian function, endometrial function, or both (Jones et al., 1970). The various effects of CC in these tissues were well summarized by Adashi (1984). Obviously, much more work is needed before the complex properties of this intriguing molecule are fully understood.

The method of administration is straightforward. An oral dose of 50 mg of CC is given daily on days 5 to 9 of the menstrual cycle. If ovulation does not result after this regimen, the dosage is increased by 50 mg increments daily each cycle up to a maximum of 250 mg/day. Gysler and associates (1982) found in their 10-year experience that 86% of their patients ovulated on a regimen of 150 mg CC/day or less, with more than 50% ovulating at the 50 mg/day dose. A positive correlation between CC dosage and the patient's weight was reported by Shepard and associates (1979). Patients with higher ponderal indices required higher dosages of clomiphene citrate. Nevertheless, use of CC at dosages higher than 150 mg/day is of limited success and may be necessary only in selected obese patients.

There are various methods for monitoring ovulation on CC therapy. The least expensive and least invasive method is monitoring of the basal body temperature. Intercourse should be timed between 4 and 5 days after the last pill is taken. More extensive methods for monitoring CC therapy are to measure the serum estradiol level approximately days 12 to 14 of the cycle and to measure the progesterone level in the midluteal phase, approximately day 21 (Adashi, 1986). If there are any questions regarding the luteal phase, an endometrial biopsy for precise dating of the endometrium should be performed. Another method of following follicular development is using abdominal or vaginal ultrasound studies.

There are several modifications of these regimens for those patients who do not respond with ovulation. One method proposed is to increase the length of dosage from 5 to 8 days per cycle (Lobo et al., 1982). In those patients with elevated adrenal androgen levels (dehydroepiandrosterone sulfate [DHEAS] level greater than 2 µg/ml), Daly and associates (1984) recommend suppressing the adrenal androgen levels with 0.5 mg of dexamethasone in the follicular phase of the cycle. For those patients who develop poor cervical mucus, estrogen therapy may be added using 1.25 mg of conjugated estrogens or its equivalent on day 10 of the CC cycle and continuing until day 14 (Hammond, 1984). Nevertheless, high doses of estrogen should be avoided, because they may inhibit ovulation. In those patients receiving CC who have follicular growth but do not ovulate, O'Herlihy and co-workers (1982) were successful using ultrasound to follow follicular growth and administering 5,000 IU of human chorionic gonadotropin (hCG) when the follicle was 18 mm or larger. With this regimen, 92% of their patients ovulated, with 76% of them conceiving.

Once ovulatory cycles are achieved with CC, the regimen should be continued for four to six cycles. If no pregnancy occurs, the following treatment plan for these "CC failures" is advised (Table 13–3). A well-timed postcoital test should be done to rule out CC effects on cervical mucus. An endometrial biopsy should be done since luteal phase defects have been reported in up to 50% of patients on CC therapy (Jones et al., 1970). Tubal status should be evaluated by hysterosalpingogram. Any male factor or endocrinological testing not done prior to CC use should be completed. Finally, if the evaluation remains normal, laparoscopy should be performed.

In examining the efficacy rates of CC therapy, one finds approximately an 80% ovulation rate. Approximately 75% of patients will ovulate at either the 50 or 100 mg/day dose (Gysler et al.,

1982). These rates of ovulation have not changed substantially since the early clinical trials in the 1960s. Pregnancy rates unfortunately do not match ovulation rates, with only approximately one half of those women with successful ovulation achieving pregnancy. This discrepancy most likely represents other infertility factors present in the couple in addition to ovulatory dysfunction. Clomiphene citrate may also cause a luteal phase defect, poor cervical mucus, or poor follicular development, leading to a decreased pregnancy rate. Another explanation may be that the data analysis contributes to the discrepancy. Hammond and associates (1983) demonstrated a fecundity rate of 0.22 in women on CC therapy with no other infertility factors compared to a fecundity of 0.247 in women discontinuing diaphragm use.

The complications and contraindications of CC are few (Table 13–4; Asch and Greenblatt, 1976). Ovarian enlargement occurs in approximately 13.6% of patients treated. Another significant side effect is vasomotor flushing, occurring in approximately 11% of patients. In the menopausal woman, hot flashes are believed to be due to hypothalamic deprivation of estrogen because of the diminished production by the postmenopausal ovary. In patients treated with CC, this hypothalamic deprivation is thought to represent estrogen receptor blockade in the hypothalamus.

Visual symptoms in patients on CC therapy have been estimated to occur in approximately 1.5% of patients. These symptoms have been described as blurring, spots, or flashing. There appears to be an increase in symptoms with an in-

TABLE 13–3.

Evaluation for Clomiphene Citrate Failures

Postcoital test
Endometrial biopsy
Hysterosalpingogram
Male factor testing
Other endocrinological testing
Diagnostic laparoscopy

TABLE 13–4.

Complications and Contraindications to Clomiphene Citrate Use

	%
Complications (Asch and Greenblatt, 1976)	
Ovarian enlargement	13.6
Vasomotor symptoms	11.0
Multiple gestations	7.9
Visual symptoms	1.5
Contraindications	
Pregnancy	
Ovarian cysts	
Hepatic disease	
Visual symptoms	
Premature ovarian failure	
(Anecdotal reports of pregnancy have been made.)	

crease in total dosage. The visual symptoms are totally reversible on discontinuation of therapy.

Multiple gestations occur in approximately 7.9% of patients on CC therapy. Of these patients, 6.9% are twins, and 0.5% are triplets. This is to be compared with the approximately 1% incidence of twinning in normal population. Clomiphene citrate therapy can cause multiple gestations because it initiates an increased GnRH pulse frequency and subsequent increases in pituitary follicle-stimulating hormone (FSH) and LH secretion. This leads to stimulation and development of several ovarian follicles. There does not appear to be an increased incidence of congenital anomalies in those pregnancies resulting from CC initiation of ovulation (Lunenfeld et al., 1986).

There are several contraindications to the use of CC. Since the primary indication is anovulation, which is often accompanied by amenorrhea, pregnancy must be carefully ruled out prior to initiation of therapy. Preexisting ovarian cysts present a relative contraindication to further ovarian stimulation prompted by CC use. Patients with liver disease should not be treated with CC due to hepatic metabolism of the drug. In patients who develop visual symptoms while taking the medication, discontinuation would be prudent. To be successful, CC requires an intact hypothalamus, pituitary, and ovary. In those patients with lesions in these organs, CC should not be used. There have been, however, some anecdotal reports of pregnancy recorded with CC in ovarian failure patients (Davis and Ravnikar, 1989).

The use of CC in normal ovulating women is controversial. Vandenberg and Yen (1973) demonstrated that use in normal ovulating women will raise serum estradiol levels to 1,200 pg/ml. This suggests multiple follicles developing, which may increase chances for pregnancy. The risks of CC use in these women are disruption of normal ovulation, inducement of a luteal phase defect, or poor cervical mucus. Although CC is a therapy with many unexplained effects and uses, it has no role as a nonspecific therapy for unexplained infertility. It should not be thought of as an all-purpose "fertility" pill.

HUMAN GONADOTROPINS

Pituitary extracts of FSH were used by Gemzell and associates in 1958 to induce ovulation. Unfortunately, pituitary extracts yielded very small amounts of material with which to work. It was not until hMGs were isolated and purified from the urine of postmenopausal women that widespread use of gonadotropins for induction of ovulation was possible. In 1962, Lunenfeld and associates used hMG to induce ovulation in two women. Both of these women conceived. The use of hMG for ovulation induction quickly became part of the infertility treatment armamentarium. With more widespread use and increased application of hMG, worldwide demand has increased dramatically in recent years. To meet this demand, researchers are turning to molecular recombinant technology to commercially produce LH, FSH, and hCG.

The use of human gonadotropins for ovulation induction is complex and varied. A standard protocol for their use does not exist. Many variations are being used by practitioners tailored to the needs of individual patients. Extensive monitoring of serum estradiol levels and follicle growth by ultrasound methods have decreased the complication rate of gonadotropin use (Smith et al., 1980). These techniques often require substantial laboratory and radiology support. Because this level of support is not available to all practitioners, it may often be necessary to refer infertility patients to centers that have this capability for the use of human gonadotropins. This section will attempt to review the pharmacology and mechanism of action for human gonadotropins. The clinical use and indications as well as the complications and success rates of this ovulation-inducing therapy will also be described.

The use of human gonadotropins directly induces ovulation, unlike CC use, which initiates ovulation. The gonadotropins directly stimulate the ovary, bypassing the pituitary and the hypothalamus. Luteinizing hormone, FSH, and hCG are glycoproteins consisting of an alpha subunit and a beta subunit. The alpha subunit is the same in the three glycoproteins, with the molecular specificity being conferred by the beta subunit. Luteinizing hormone is approximately 28 kilodaltons (kD) in molecular weight, with FSH being 33 kD and hCG being 38 kD. Luteinizing hormone and hCG have a high degree of structural similarity. Human chorionic gonadotropin is used to simulate the midcycle LH surge. Premenopausal women produce between 500 and 1,000 IU of LH/day. In contrast, postmenopausal women produce approximately 3,000 to 4,000

IU daily (Catt and Pierce, 1986). Gonadotropins in the postmenopausal woman are excreted in the urine, where they can be isolated for use in ovulation induction. Human chorionic gonadotropin is produced in the placenta in increasing amounts with progressing gestational age. Commercial preparations of human gonadotropins are currently all manufactured by Serono Laboratory. Pergonal comes as a lyophilized powder containing 75 IU of FSH and 75 IU of LH. Metrodin is purified FSH with 75 IU contained in each ampule. Profasi HP consists of 10,000 USP units of hCG/ampule in a lyophilized powder. All of these preparations require addition of sterile diluent and intramuscular administration. These agents are well absorbed parenterally; the plasma half-life of LH is 30 minutes, and that of FSH is twice as long at 60 minutes. The half-life of hCG is approximately 8 hours in the plasma. These agents are cleared in the liver and kidneys, with approximately 10% to 20% of gonadotropins being excreted in the urine (Catt and Pierce, 1986).

Human gonadotropins are currently being used for a wide variety of indications (Table 13–5). The primary indication for use is anovulation secondary to hypothalamic pituitary failure or hypothalamic amenorrhea. Pergonal is also used in those patients who fail to ovulate on maximum dosages of CC or who fail to conceive after six ovulatory cycles on CC therapy. Patients with PCO disease usually do better with CC ovulation initiation than with Pergonal induction (Jones et al., 1987). However, those patients who fail CC use will occasionally benefit from Pergonal use. Menotropins has also been used to treat those patients who have failed all other modalities of treatment for a luteal phase defect. In those patients who have no identified source of their infer-

tility, Pergonal is occasionally a treatment of last resort (Wang and Gemzell, 1979). Human menopausal gonadotropins have also been used in patients with premature ovarian failure. Such use remains controversial. In the small series where ovarian failure patients are treated with Pergonal, they are first primed with oral estrogens to suppress their endogenous gonadotropins (Check and Chase, 1984). The most recent new indication for use of hMGs is for ovulation induction of multiple follicles for assisted reproductive technologies (IVF and GIFT).

Metrodin is purified FSH, which is obtained by running hMGs through a system that adsorbs the LH molecule onto gel columns. This results in a highly purified FSH product. Each ampule of Metrodin contains less than 1 IU of LH. The primary indication for Metrodin is polycystic ovarian disease, in which the CH/FSH ratio is elevated. Success rates are expected to be higher with a pure FSH formulation. Many protocols have been investigated to treat patients with polycystic ovarian disease, including low and intermediate dose FSH without hCG and FSH with hCG. Despite the theoretical advantage of using FSH to reestablish the LH/FSH ratio in these patients, success rates with Metrodin appear to be no greater than that which can be obtained with Pergonal (Claman and Seibel, 1986).

The exact details of ovulation induction techniques with hMGs varies from practitioner to practitioner (Diamond and Wentz, 1986). Although most physicians use an individualized protocol of increasing the hMG dose as indicated, Abbasi et al. (1987) reported on an increased ovulation rate using a "step down" regimen vs. a "step up" regimen in monkeys. The primary goals of all of these different methods, however, is to obtain one or more mature follicles that measure 15 to 20 mm by ultrasound coupled with a serum estradiol level between 500 and 1,000 pg/ml. When this occurs, hCG (5,000–10,000 USP units) is given intramuscularly to stimulate ovulation by mimicking the LH surge. If the estradiol level is more than 2,000 pg/ml, the risks of hyperstimulation are high, and consideration for withholding hCG should be made.

The following protocol is used at the Fertility and Endocrine Unit of the Brigham and Women's Hospital for administration of human gonadotropins for ovulation induction. All patients are completely evaluated prior to use of hMG, with tubal, uterine, and male factors being

TABLE 13–5.

Indications for Human Menopausal Gonadotropin Ovulation Induction

Hypothalamic amenorrhea
CC failures
Polycystic ovarian disease
Luteal phase defects unresponsive to other
  treatments
Unexplained infertility
Premature ovarian failure
Assisted reproductive technologies (in vitro
  fertilization)

corrected prior to treatment. The patients and their partners are given a class taught by a fertility nurse practitioner that covers the use, benefits, side effects, and techniques of hMG ovulation induction. Informed consent is obtained at this time. During this class, the patients and their partners are taught the proper techniques to self-administer the gonadotropins. The ovulation induction is monitored with both serum estradiol levels and ultrasound scanning of ovarian follicles. Nearly all of our patients undergo vaginal ultrasound scanning at this time. A cycle starts at the time of menses when a baseline ultrasound scan is obtained. A starting dose of 150 IU of Pergonal (two ampules) is given on the fourth day of the menstrual cycle. This dosage is continued without monitoring until cycle day 9 when the patient has blood drawn and an ultrasound performed. Our laboratory uses an iodine 125 estradiol double antibody assay kit (Pantex) for daily estradiol determinations. This allows rapid and accurate determinations of estradiol values, which provides the physicians with the estradiol levels by 3 P.M. each day. Treatment is individualized, based on the estradiol level and the ultrasound follicular measurements. On day 9, if the estradiol level is less than 150 pg/ml, the Pergonal dosage is increased. If the level is between 150 and 300 pg/ml, the dosage remains the same. The patient calls in for her dosage instructions for that evening, which she administers at 8 P.M. Estradiol levels should increase at an exponential rate (Wilson et al., 1982) with no more than a doubling of the value every 24 hours. When the estradiol value is between 500 and 1,000 pg/ml, and the dominant follicle reaches a maximum diameter between 15 and 20 mm, the patient is instructed to use 5,000 USP units of hCG. Intercourse or artificial insemination is then advised at 24 and 48 hours after hCG administration. Patients are counseled to seek care if symptoms of hyperstimulation occur. A serum level of β-hCG is obtained if abnormal menses or amenorrhea occurs. Metrodin therapy is carried out in a similar fashion; however, the usual starting dosage is one ampule (75 IU).

Adjuvants are used with Pergonal in selected clinical situations. In those patients with polycystic ovarian disease who fail to achieve pregnancy on hMG/hCG therapy alone, 0.5 mg of dexamethasone daily is used for adrenal suppression prior to and concomitant with hMG use (Evron et al., 1983). In patients with polycystic ovarian disease or premature surges of LH, the use of GnRH agonist has been employed to downregulate endogenous pituitary release of gonadotropins. Once these endogenous gonadotropins are suppressed, Pergonal treatment is then initiated for ovulation induction (Dodson et al., 1987a). In patients treated with GnRH agonists, the Pergonal requirement is increased.

Human menopausal gonadotropins have also been combined with CC in various ovulation induction protocols. Kistner (1976) and March et al. (1976) found that such a combination reduced the amount of Pergonal necessary for successful ovulation induction. However, in a review of the literature by Kemmann and Jones (1983), no improvement in pregnancy rates with this combined regimen was found. The newest area of research is to combine hMG with growth hormone, which increases the granulosa cell responsiveness. This leads to a decrease in the amount of Pergonal used and a possible increase in the quality of the follicular response (Owen et al., 1988).

Ever since its introduction into clinical use in 1962, Pergonal use has been associated with two major complications (Table 13–6): multiple gestations and ovarian hyperstimulation. Because Pergonal therapy bypasses endogenous hypothalamic-pituitary feedback monitoring systems, it becomes incumbent on the physician to carefully monitor patients on such therapy to decrease the risk of hyperstimulation and multiple gestations. Prior to the availability of rapid serum estradiol measurements and ultrasound measurements of follicular size, physicians could monitor their patients only by clinical methods such as examination of cervical mucus for ferning and spinnbarkheit and cervical dilatation (Insler et al., 1972). With the advent of more precise monitoring, complications of ovulation induction with human gonadotropins should be minimized while maximizing ovulation and pregnancy rates. In a recent review, Yeh and Ravnikar (1988) summarized published studies of hMG therapy since

TABLE 13–6.

Complications of Human Menopausal Gonadotropin Use

Ovarian hyperstimulation
Multiple gestations
Spontaneous abortion
Ectopic pregnancy
No increase in congenital or chromosomal abnormalities

1980. These studies represent current monitoring techniques and induction protocols used today. In their summary, there was a total of 2,504 patients in 10 studies. All studies used urinary or serum estrogen levels for monitoring except one, which strictly used ultrasound measurements of ovarian follicle growth. There were 7,952 cycles, 86% of which were ovulatory, with 44% of the patients becoming pregnant. The pregnancy rate per ovulatory cycle was 19%. The rate of ovarian hyperstimulation was 6.3%, ranging from less than 1% to 13%. Multiple birth comprised 24% of those patients achieving pregnancy, with a range of 12% to 30%. The spontaneous abortion rate was 20%, ranging from 8% to 28%.

In the discussion of the complications of Pergonal therapy, prevention of complications by close monitoring was described. However, despite meticulous monitoring, a certain number of patients undergoing ovulation induction with human gonadotropins will suffer ovarian hyperstimulation, multiple gestations, and other complications. Ovarian hyperstimulation is massive luteinization of follicles, which can become symptomatic 5 to 7 days after hCG is administered. Hyperstimulation ranges from mild to severe in degree (Rabau et al., 1967). Patients with excessive weight gain, painful abdominal distention, nausea, or shortness of breath after hCG administration should be evaluated for hyperstimulation. If hCG is not given, hyperstimulation will not occur. In most cases, if the ovaries are larger than 10 cm or a rapid weight gain greater than 4.5 kg occurs, patients require hospitalization for careful monitoring. Hospital therapy consists of intravenous (IV) fluids, careful monitoring of hematocrit values, blood chemistries, and vital signs. Pelvic and abdominal examinations should be kept to a minimum to prevent ovarian rupture. Major complications of severe hyperstimulation include respiratory embarrassment, pleural effusions, hyperviscosity with thromboembolism, hypovolemia, and shock. Rarely, ultrasonographically guided paracentesis is required to remove excessive fluid. When conception does not occur, the ovarian cysts subside in 20 to 40 days (Schenker and Weinstein, 1978).

Multiple gestations that occur as a result of Pergonal therapy carry many increased risks, including spontaneous abortion, premature delivery, and increased perinatal morbidity and mortality (Schenker et al., 1981). With careful monitoring, the majority of multiple gestations will be

twins. In those patients with higher numbers of gestational sacs, some practitioners have begun experimentation with ultrasonically guided reduction of gestational sacs (Birnholz et al., 1987). The possibility of this becoming a future therapy for Pergonal-induced multiple gestations carries many moral and ethical dilemmas.

The increased spontaneous abortion rate with Pergonal therapy, approximately 29%, is believed to be due to poor luteal development, hyperestrogenemia causing an increase in tubal motility, and the multiple pregnancy rate (Ben-Rafael et al., 1983). Ectopic and heterotopic pregnancies are also more likely with hMG use (Falk and Lackritz, 1977; Eckshtein et al., 1978). There is no indication that pregnancies resulting from Pergonal treatment have any increased incidence of congenital abnormalities (Lunenfeld et al., 1986).

At the Fertility and Endocrine Unit of Brigham and Women's Hospital, the average cost of Pergonal therapy per patient per cycle is approximately $2,000. In addition to these direct costs, there is the cost of lost time from work that the patient has to bear. The majority of costs of each Pergonal cycle involve the careful monitoring process. This meticulous monitoring is a prophylaxis against the significant complications of ovarian hyperstimulation and multiple gestations. Attempts to economize therapy by reducing these preventive measures will increase the risk to the patient as well as increase long-term costs, should hospitalization be required for ovarian hyperstimulation or complications of multiple gestations.

GONADOTROPIN-RELEASING HORMONE

Ovulation induction has also been accomplished using GnRH (Santoro, 1988). Gonadotropin-releasing hormone is a decapeptide secreted by the hypothalamus, which stimulates the pituitary to release gonadotropins. Its structure was determined in 1971. It is available commercially as Factrel (Ayerst Laboratories). To be effective, GnRH is given exogenously in a pulsatile fashion to mimic normal hypothalamic secretion (Reid et al., 1981). It requires parenteral administration through IV (Santoro et al., 1986; Jansen et al., 1987) or subcutaneous (Hurley et al., 1984) indwelling catheter. Small portable pumps that administer 1-minute pulses every 60 to 90 minutes are available. Usual dosages range from 5 to 20 µg/pulse. Lower doses are possible using the IV route. Therapy is begun day 1 to 5 of the cycle and continues until menses or pregnancy results.

Gonadotropin-releasing hormone therapy is effective in Kallmann's syndrome (Crowley and McArthur, 1980) and hypothalamic amenorrhea (Hammond et al., 1979). Ovulation occurs in 85% to 100% of treatment cycles. Luteal phase defects and poor cervical mucus have also been treated with GnRH therapy (Loucopoulos and Ferin, 1987). Patients with polycystic ovarian disease have a lower success rate with GnRH therapy. This may reflect a pituitary response abnormality or an inability to override an abnormal endogenous hypothalamic release of GnRH. Adjuncts that have been tried include GnRH with CC (Eshel et al., 1988) or GnRH agonist pretreatment for pituitary suppression followed by Factrel administration (Filicori et al., 1988). Increased success rates have been noted in small groups of patients. Complications are mild hyperstimulation of the ovary, multiple births, as well as hematomas and phlebitis secondary to the indwelling catheters used with the portable pumps. To be effective, this therapy relies on an adequately responsive pituitary and ovaries. With further study and refinement, this form of therapy may become more widespread for ovulation induction.

ASSISTED REPRODUCTIVE TECHNOLOGIES

In vitro fertilization and embryo transfer (ET) are the best known examples of assisted reproductive technology (ART). Assisted reproductive technology consists of assisting the reproductive process by bringing together female and male gametes, manipulating the resultant embryo, or both. Historically, ET was first described in the 1890s when a rabbit embryo was flushed free from one animal and transferred into the uterus of another animal and a mixed litter resulted, providing evidence of successful embryo transfer (Heape, 1891). Human IVF was reported by Rock and Menkin at the Free Hospital for Women in Boston in 1944. Oocytes were obtained at the time of laparotomy, and no ET was attempted. Chang was the first to describe successful pregnancy and delivery after fertilization outside the body by mixing rabbit gametes together in 1959. This work was followed by many researchers in various laboratories using both animal and human models. Finally, in 1978, Louise Brown was born, a product of the first successful IVF and ET in the world as described by Steptoe and Edwards (1978). Since that first success in human IVF, there has been a virtual explosion of development in the field of assisted reproductive technology (Table 13–7).

TABLE 13–7.

The History of Assisted Reproductive Technology

Yr	Investigators	Results
1891	Heape	Rabbit embryo transferred from one animal to another.
1944	Rock and Menkin	Human IVF, no ET.
1959	Chang	Pregnancy and delivery from rabbit IVF and ET. Embryo transfer.
1978	Steptoe and Edwards	Pregnancy and delivery from human IVF and ET.
1986	Society of Assisted Reproductive Technology (SART)	311 infants born from 485 pregnancies resulting from 2,864 ETs in the United States.
1987	SART	1,858 infants born from 1,964 pregnancies resulting from 9,919 ETs, GIFT procedures, or frozen ETs in the United States.

Assisted reproductive technology is conceptually a simple process (Fig 13–3). Oocytes are harvested from the female in either natural or stimulated cycles. These are mixed with sperm and incubated until embryos are formed. These resultant embryos are then transferred back into the uterine cavity for implantation. Despite the rapid advancement of knowledge in the various components in this process, many mysteries still remain unsolved. This section will review ARTs by its components: patient selection, ovulation induction, oocyte retrieval, sperm preparation, fertilization, embryo transfer, and finally, success rates with complications and costs. Other modalities and new horizons in ART will be outlined as well.

As the success rates of IVF have increased, its use has been considered for more and more indications (Jones, 1986). Initially it was used for tubal or mechanical factor infertility to bring together gametes that could not previously meet due to tubal or peritoneal blockage. Male factor infertility could also be treated with IVF because it brought gametes closer together than normal intercourse or artificial insemination. This procedure has met with limited success in many centers. In male factor couples, the rate of failed fertilization is higher than other patient groups. The use of IVF for unexplained infertility has also been employed. By dissection of the reproductive process into its component parts, unexplained infertility patients may succeed despite a previously normal evaluation. Patients suffering from infertility due to immunological causes may also ben-

efit from these new ARTs with removal of immunological barriers to fertility by bringing gametes together outside the body. Reproductive failure may still occur in these patients in the form of early and recurrent miscarriages.

In the selection of patients appropriate for IVF, age is also an important factor. Live-born birth rates with IVF in women after the age of 39 years are very low. In a study of 118 patients more than 39 years old, Fishel and associates (1985) had only 7 live births (6%). They noted a high percentage of spontaneous abortions (56% of clinical pregnancies) in this age group. In addition to the high abortion rate, this age group also has a higher cancellation rate due to poor ovulation induction. At the current time the IVF program at Brigham and Women's Hospital accepts female patients up to 39.5 years of age. It is believed that this is to protect the patients from going through a very strenuous process with dismal expectations of success.

Ovulation induction for IVF programs uses the same agents as described in the section on ovulation induction, namely, CC, hMGs, pure FSH, and GnRH agonists. The goals of ovulation induction for IVF, however, are different. The goal is to stimulate multiple follicles for oocyte retrieval. In the first IVF pregnancy described by Steptoe and Edwards (1978), the woman's natural ovulatory cycle was used. However, since that time it has become obvious that success rates and efficient use of the IVF team are higher with ovulation induction.

The protocol for ovulation induction in the

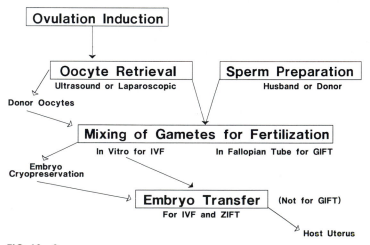

FIG 13–3.
Sequence of events in ART.

Brigham and Women's Hospital IVF program is patterned after the work of Meldrum and associates (1987). It begins on day 2 of the patient's menstrual cycle with three ampules (75 IU/ampule) of Pergonal daily from day 2 to 5. On the morning of day 6, an ultrasound and serum estradiol level are obtained. All patients are then placed on a split Pergonal 2/2 dose from day 6 onward. Patients who weigh greater than 68 kg are started on this split dose regimen from day 2 on. Therapy is then individualized based on oocyte measurements by ultrasound and serum estradiol levels. When an estradiol level greater then 500 pg/ml and at least two follicles with an maximum diameter of 16 mm are obtained, hCG (10,000 USP units) is given. Oocyte retrieval is scheduled for 36 hours after hCG administration. A serum estradiol level is drawn the morning after hCG administration, and an ultrasound is performed prior to oocyte retrieval.

In those patients with elevated adrenal androgen levels (DHEAS level greater than 2 μg/ml), 0.5 mg of dexamethasone (Daly et al., 1984) is given daily until pregnancy is detected. In those patients with premature luteinization as evidenced by a plateau in estradiol values, a fall in estradiol level of greater than 30% after hCG administration, or poor egg or embryo quality, progesterone and LH values are obtained from serum in the late follicular phase to confirm the diagnosis. If the diagnosis is confirmed, GnRH agonist is used for ovarian suppression prior to ovulation induction with Metrodin or Pergonal. The protocol with GnRH agonist is based on studies by Serafini et al. (1988), where they had a 93% oocyte retrieval rate in patients on GnRH agonist therapy vs. 18% in those without. The patients on GnRH agonist therapy had a 45% pregnancy rate per transfer, and patients without such therapy had an 8% rate.

Research in the field of ovulation induction continues to progress with nearly as many different protocols for ovulation induction being available today as there are IVF programs. The main goal and concern for any ovulation induction protocol is to obtain oocytes of high quality and number.

Until very recently, the retrieval phase of IVF involved a laparoscopy with oocyte retrieval under direct visualization. This technique has now been replaced in most centers by ultrasound directed aspiration of ovarian follicles (Schulman et al., 1987). The ultrasound may be directed transabdominally or transvaginally, with the retrieval needle being directed transvesically, transurethrally, or transvaginally. We currently use transvaginal ultrasound with a transvaginal needle for retrieval (Fig 13–4). The advantages of the ultrasound retrieval method are decreased cost to the patient and decreased discomfort and risk sec-

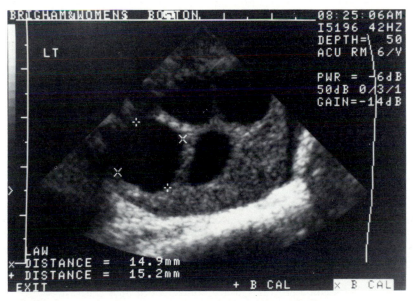

FIG 13–4.
Image of ovary with multiple follicles as seen with vaginal ultrasound.

ondary to the avoidance of general anesthesia and laparoscopy. There appears to be no difference in the oocyte quality or success of IVF in those programs using ultrasound retrieval (Lewin et al., 1986). Theoretically, there may be an advantage of using ultrasound oocyte retrieval in that there is no oocyte exposure to the gases used for pneumoperitoneum and laparoscopy or general anesthetic agents.

In a man who has a history or suspicion of male factor, a pre-IVF sperm preparation is done to anticipate potential problems. In addition, the couple is counseled about the availability of donor insemination at the time of IVF. Sperm is washed twice in medium with gentle centrifugation. After the final centrifugation, the swim up technique is used to isolate sperm of good motility. This procedure accomplishes sperm capacitation. As mentioned earlier, other separation techniques such as albumin gradients, silica gradients, or centrifugation with washing were evaluated by Berger et al. (1985). In those patients with sperm antibodies in the semen, the semen sample is collected by ejaculation directly into the media to dilute out the antibodies. Research is currently underway to determine what the ideal medium is for sperm preparation and gamete incubation (Han and Kiessling, 1988). The various media that have been tried include Hams F10, Tyrodes, Earles, Follicular Fluid, and various combinations of these with added human and bovine sera for protein. In those patients without a male factor problem, we use approximately 50,000 sperm/oocyte/ml. This concentration is increased in those patients with male factor up to 500,000 sperm per oocyte. When the GIFT procedure is performed, approximately 50,000 sperm per side are used.

The fertilization phase of IVF is entered after the addition of sperm to oocytes. Insemination is delayed 6 to 8 hours after oocyte collection. There are many variables involved with the fertilization step. First, gamete quality must be considered. Oocytes are graded, after isolation, from germinal vesicles to postmature, depending on the status of the cumulus cells (Marrs et al., 1984). Sperm is graded after isolation through a swim up technique. The maintenance of high-quality control in the laboratory is essential for maximizing fertilization rates. The incubation medium, gas environment, and incubators all have a major impact on the fertilization process. Quality control is usually measured with mouse embryo development in these three crucial elements of the

laboratory. The absence of embryotoxic elements is assumed if two-cell mouse embryos can progress. The results of fertilization can be an embryo with just pronuclei present or with two cells, four cells, or eight cells .(Fig 13–5). Immature oocytes are occasionally incubated for an additional 12 to 24 hours prior to insemination for a higher fertilization rate (Marrs et al., 1984). In most programs, fertilization occurs 60% to 80% of the time in those patients without significant male factor infertility.

The IVF process is most strenuous on patients up to and including the fertilization step. The woman goes through the most difficult part by undergoing the ovulation induction and oocyte retrieval step. The couple next endures the waiting process to hear the news about fertilization outcome.

The technique of ET is relatively simple. Most centers use a side port catheter to prevent clogging of the catheter as it is advanced through the cervix. The embryos are loaded into the catheter in a minimal volume, usually less than 25 μl, and the small catheter is passed into the uterine cavity with or without an introducer. Minimal manipulation of the cervix is employed to decrease the risk of intrauterine irritation and contraction. The ET catheter is placed in the fundal portion of the uterine cavity. The embryos are then injected with minimal pressure, and the catheter is held in place for 1 minute. The catheter is removed slowly and gently so as not to disrupt the intrauterine environment. The catheter is then examined microscopically to rule out retention of embryos on the catheter tip. The timing of ET is approximately 48 to 72 hours after oocyte retrieval. In vivo, it is believed that gametes spend 3 or more days in the fallopian tube and that the embryo arrives into the endometrium cavity some 3 to 5 days after ovulation (Diaz et al., 1980). Concern that the current transfer timing in IVF may be placing the embryos into the endometrium cavity 1 to 2 days ahead when arrival occurs in vivo has been raised.

The number of embryos transferred is correlated with success rates in IVF. When one embryo is transferred, the success rate is 10% to 15%. When two embryos are transferred, approximately 20% to 26% success rate is achieved, and when three embryos are transferred, the success increases to 33% (Fishel et al., 1985). There appears to be no increase in success rates when the number of embryos transferred is greater than

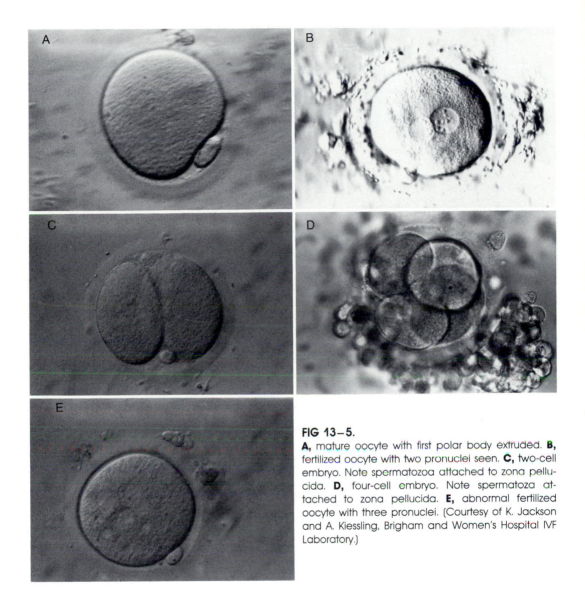

FIG 13–5.
A, mature oocyte with first polar body extruded. **B,** fertilized oocyte with two pronuclei seen. **C,** two-cell embryo. Note spermatozoa attached to zona pellucida. **D,** four-cell embryo. Note spermatoza attached to zona pellucida. **E,** abnormal fertilized oocyte with three pronuclei. (Courtesy of K. Jackson and A. Kiessling, Brigham and Women's Hospital IVF Laboratory.)

three (Wood et al., 1985). However, multiple gestation rates do increase with the number of embryos transferred. Our current protocol calls for the transfer of between three and four embryos, if available.

After embryo transfer, patients are observed at bed rest for 2 to 3 hours. They are then sent home to minimal activity for 24 to 48 hours. Vaginal activity is restricted for 1 week following ET. Normal ovarian physiology is most likely disrupted at the time of aspiration of multiple follicles for oocyte retrieval in IVF. Vargyas et al. (1986) noted a decrease in progesterone level after ovarian aspiration, although the level was

higher than in unstimulated patients. Most programs support the luteal phase with progesterone either via intramuscular or suppository route. Progesterone support is used until 14 days after transfer when a serum β-hCG is used to determine pregnancy. If results of the pregnancy test are negative, the progesterone is discontinued.

Success rates in ARTs are defined as number of pregnancies ongoing at 6 weeks per ET procedure. To evaluate success rates in the United States, the AFS has established the subgroup SART (Table 13–8). It maintains a registry of programs across the United States that report their ART experience in a uniform manner. Cur-

TABLE 13—8.

Outcome of in Vitro Fertilization Treatment per Embryo Transfer Procedure at Society of Assisted Reproductive Technology Programs*

Yr	No. of Clinics	Total No. Transfers	Clinical Pregnancies†		Abortions‡		Ectopic Pregnancies‡		All Deliveries†		Multiple Deliveries†	
			No.	%	No.	%	No.	%	No.	%	No.	%
1985	41	2,389	337	14	140	42	20	6	257	11	N/A	
1986	41	2,864	485	17	151	31	22	5	311	11	N/A	
1987	96	7,561	1,367	18	344	25	103	7	991	13	235	3.1

*Data from Medical Research International: In vitro fertilization/embryo transfer in the United States: 1985 and 1986 results from the National IVF/ET Registry. *Fertil Steril* 1988; 49:212; Medical Research International: In vitro fertilization/embryo transfer in the United States; 1987 results from the National IVF-ET Registry. *Fertil Steril* 1989; 51:13.
†Rate as percentage of transfers.
‡Rate as percentage of clinical pregnancies.

rently 120 programs report their data to SART. In the report covering 1985 and 1986, 41 clinics reported their data (Medical Research International, 1988), and in the report covering 1987, 96 clinics reported (Medical Research International, 1989). In 1985, data were available on 2,389 IVF cycles with embryos transferred. The overall pregnancy rate per transfer was 14.1%. In 1986, there were 2,864 cycles with ET, with a pregnancy rate per transfer of 16.9%. In 1987, the pregnancy rate per transfer was 18% in 7,561 transfers. Experience with ARTs appears to be important; those reporting in 1986 with less than 16 transfers had one half the clinical pregnancy rate of those clinics with more experience, 8.5% vs. 16.9%. At the Brigham and Women's Hospital IVF Program from April 1987 to June 1988, 134 patients were treated with IVF. The clinical pregnancy rate per transfer was 29%.

Complications from the IVF procedure are rare. The major risk of ovulation induction is ovarian hyperstimulation. This is decreased by fastidious oocyte retrieval, which prevents retention of a large number of ovarian follicles. The risks of oocyte retrieval is infection and bleeding, as well as damage to adjacent structures (Howe et al., 1988). The major complication of the IVF procedure is spontaneous abortion. In 1987 from the IVF registry, 25% of the clinical pregnancies resulted in a miscarriage. This is a decline from 42% in 1985. Multiple gestations are another potential complication from ART, with approximately 20% of pregnancies involving multiple gestations. Another pregnancy complication from ART is heterotopic pregnancy, where an intrauterine gestation is accompanied by a tubal gestation. Although this complication is rarely encoun-

tered in coitally related pregnancies, it must be kept in mind as a potential complication of ART (Rein et al., 1989). Chromosomal abnormalities from ovulation induction and ART have been a concern. A recent paper found no increase in chromosomal abnormalities in embryos or oocytes derived from ovulation induction or IVF (Whambsy et al., 1987).

The stress involved with going through any program of ART should not be overlooked. Psychological support through peer groups and trained social workers is advised for all programs. At Brigham and Women's IVF program, all patients are seen by a trained social worker as part of the orientation to the IVF program.

There are other modalities and exciting new horizons in the field of ART. The GIFT procedure involves the same steps as IVF up until oocyte retrieval (Asch et al., 1987). At this point, as opposed to IVF with fertilization occurring in the IVF laboratory, oocytes and sperm are transferred immediately back into the fallopian tube, where their mixture provides for fertilization. The advantages of the GIFT procedure are a decreased need for embryology laboratory support. For some patients with moral or religious reservations to IVF, the GIFT procedure allows fertilization to occur in the body of the woman. The GIFT procedure does require a laparoscopy for transfer of the gametes to the fallopian tube, and in most cases the same laparoscopy is used for oocyte retrieval. In the 1987 IVF National Registry, 71 clinics reported a 25% clinical pregnancy rate in 1968 GIFT procedures (Medical Research International, 1989). A variation of the GIFT procedure is the zygote intrafallopian transfer procedure (Hamori et al., 1988). It involves the transfer of a fertilized oocyte into a fallopian tube. Proponents of this procedure believe that there is some nurturing quality to time spent by the embryo in the fallopian tube prior to implantation in the uterus.

Another major development in ART is the cryopreservation of embryos and oocytes (Trounson, 1986). Although cryopreservation of sperm has been available for a long time, only recently have successful pregnancies resulted from cryopreserved embryos. The technology for cryopreservation of oocytes is much more complex and less successful. In 1985, the National IVF Registry had 26 cycles reported with using frozen embryos. This increased to 112 cycles with 7 clinical pregnancies in 1986. In 1987, 39 clinics performed 490 frozen ETs, which resulted in 50 pregnancies.

The ability to manipulate male and female gametes outside the body has also opened up new opportunities for donor combinations. It is now possible to have donor sperm, donor oocytes, or donor embryos to be used for various indications (Navot et al., 1986). In those women without a uterus but intact ovaries, some centers have tried to provide a surrogate or host uterus where a couple's gametes are placed together, yielding an embryo that is then transferred into the surrogate or host uterus.

To increase embryo fertilization rates, oocyte manipulation has also been attempted. The zona pellucida presents the major barrier to sperm. Researchers have attempted to bypass this barrier by various methods, including zona-dissolving biochemical treatment, (Kiessling et al., 1988), zona drilling by micropipettes, (Gordon et al., 1988) zona cracking or fracturing and microinjection of sperm directly into ooplasm. These techniques are at the research stage; however, they do provide a glimpse of potential uses of ART.

Physicians are more successful in helping couples overcome infertility today than at any other time in history. To keep this in perspective, however, one must not lose sight of the development of infertility treatments. In a recent entertaining dissertation on the history of infertility, DeCherney and Harris (1986) outline the development of infertility diagnoses and treatment from Egyptian times to the 20th century. Although our past knowledge of reproduction may seem rudimentary and the treatments crude, one must remember that previous practitioners during their own time had the same conviction in their

treatment abilities that we have today. Many of the things that we hold as absolute truth today may be regarded as folly in the future.

REFERENCES

Abbasi R, Kenigsberg D, Danforth D, et al: Cumulative ovulation rate in human menopausal/human chorionic gonadotropin-treated monkeys: "Step-up" versus "step-down" dose regimens. *Fertil Steril* 1987; 47:1019.

Adashi EY: Clomiphene citrate: Mechanism(s) and site(s) of action—a hypothesis revisited. *Fertil Steril* 1984; 42:331.

Adashi EY: Clomiphene citrate initiated ovulation: A clinical update. *Semin Reprod Endocrinol* 1986; 4:255.

Albrecht BH, Cramer D, Schiff I: Factors influencing the success of artificial insemination. *Fertil Steril* 1982; 37:792.

American Fertility Society: Ethical considerations of the new reproductive technologies. *Fertil Steril* 1986a; 46(suppl 1):1s.

American Fertility Society: New guidelines for the use of semen donor insemination. *Fertil Steril* 1986b; 46(suppl 2):95s.

American Fertility Society: Revised new guidelines for the use of semen donor insemination. *Fertil Steril* 1988; 49:211.

Asch RH, Balmadeda JP, Ellsworth LR, et al: Preliminary experiences with gamete intra fallopian transfer (GIFT). *Fertil Steril* 1987; 45:366.

Asch RH, Greenblatt RB: Update on the safety and efficacy of clomiphene citrate as a therapeutic agent. *J Reprod Med* 1976; 17:175.

Batzer R, Corson SL: Indications, techniques, success rates and pregnancy outcome: New directions with donor insemination. *Semin Reprod Endocrinol* 1987; 5:45.

Baylson MM: A medical advancement in the search of legal theory—artificial insemination by donor and the law. *Semin Reprod Endocrinol* 1987; 5:69.

Beernink FJ, Ericsson RJ: Male sex preselection through sperm isolation. *Fertil Steril* 1982; 38:493.

Ben-Rafael Z, Dor J, Mashiacch S, et al: Abortion rate in pregnancies following ovulation induced by human menopausal gonadotropin/human chorionic gonadotropin. *Fertil Steril* 1983; 39:157.

Berger T, Marrs RP, Moyer DL: Comparison of techniques for selection of motile spermatozoa. *Fertil Steril* 1985; 43:268.

Birnholz JC, Dmowski WP, Binor Z, et al: Selective continuation of gonadotropin induced multiple pregnancy. *Fertil Steril* 1987; 48:873.

Bordson BL, Ricci E, Dickey RP, et al: Comparison of fecundability with fresh and frozen semen in a therapeutic donor insemination. *Fertil Steril* 1986; 46:446.

Byrd W, Ackerman GE, Carr BR, et al: Treatment of refractory infertility by transcervical intrauterine insemination of washed spermatozoa. *Fertil Steril* 1987; 48:921.

Catt KJ, Pierce JG: Gonadotropic hormones in the adenhypophysis, in Yen SSC, Jaffe RB (eds): *Reproductive Endocrinology,* ed 2. Philadelphia, WB Saunders Co, 1986, p 75.

Chang MC: Fertilization of rabbit ova in vitro. *Nature* 1959; 184:406.

Check JH, Chase JS: Ovulation induction in hypergonadotropic amenorrhea with estrogen and human menopausal gonadotropin therapy. *Fertil Steril* 1984; 42:919.

Claman P, Seibel MM: Purified human follicles stimulating hormone for ovulation induction: A critical review. *Semin Reprod Endocrinol* 1986; 4:277.

Confino E, Friberg J, Dudkiewicz AB, et al: Intrauterine inseminations with washed human spermatozoa. *Fertil Steril* 1986; 46:55.

Corson SL, Batzer FR: Human gender selection. *Semin Reprod Endocrinol* 1987; 5:81.

Corson SL: Self prediction of ovulation using a urinary LH test. *J Reprod Med* 1986; 31(suppl):760.

Cramer DW, Walker AM, Schiff I: Statistical methods in evaluating the outcome of infertility therapy. *Fertil Steril* 1979; 32:80.

Crowley WF Jr, McArthur JW: Stimulation of the normal menstrual cycle in Kallman's syndrome by pulsatile administration of luteinizing hormone releasing hormone (LHRH). *J Clin Endocrinol Metab* 1980; 51:173.

Cruz RI, Kemmann E, Brandeis VT, et al: A prospective study of intrauterine insemination of processed sperm from men with oligoasthenospermia in superovulated women. *Fertil Steril* 1986; 46:673.

Daly DC, Walters CA, Soto-Albors CE: A randomized study of dexamethasone in ovulation induction with clomiphene citrate. *Fertil Steril* 1984; 41:844.

Davis OK, Ravnikar VA: Ovulation induction with clomiphene citrate in a patient with ovarian failure: A case report. *J Reprod Med* 1989; 33:559.

DeCherney AH, Harris TC: The barren woman throughout history, in DeCherney AH (ed): *Reproductive Failure.* New York, Churchill Livingstone, 1986.

Diamond MP, Wentz AC: Ovulation induction with human menopausal gonadotropins. *Obstet Gynecol Surv* 1986; 41:480.

Diaz S, Ortez ME, Croxatto HB: Studies on the duration of ovum transport by the human oviduct. *Am J Obstet Gynecol* 1980; 137:116.

DiMarzo SJ, Rakoff JS: Intrauterine insemination with husband's washed sperm. *Fertil Steril* 1986; 46:470.

Dodson WC, Hughes CL, Whitesides DB, et al: The effect of leuprolide acetate on ovulation induction with human menopausal gonadotropins in polycystic ovary syndrome. *J Clin Endocrinol Metab* 1987a; 65:95.

Dodson WC, Whiteside DB, Hughes CL, et al: Superovulation with intrauterine insemination in the treatment of infertility: A possible alternative to gamete intra fallopian transfer and in vitro fertilization. *Fertil Steril* 1987b; 48:441.

Eckshtein N, Ismajowich B, Yedwab G, et al: Combined tubal and multiple intrauterine pregnancies following ovulation induction. *Fertil Steril* 1978; 30;707.

Ericsson RJ, Langevin CN, Mishino M: Isolation of fractions rich in human Y sperm. *Nature* 1973; 246:421.

Eshel A, Abdulwahid NA, Armar NA, et al: Pulsatile luteinizing hormone releasing hormone therapy in women with polycystic ovary syndrome. *Fertil Steril* 1988; 49:956.

Evron S, Navot D, Laufer N, et al: Induction of ovulation with combined human menopausal gonadotropins and dexamethasone in women with polycystic ovarian disease. *Fertil Steril* 1983; 40:183.

Fakih H, MacLusky N, DeCherney A, et al: Enhancement of human sperm motility and velocity in vitro: Effects of calcium and creatinine phosphate. *Fertil Steril* 1986; 46:938.

Falk RJ, Lackritz RM: Bilateral simultaneous dual pregnancies after ovulation induction with clomiphene menotropin combination. *Fertil Steril* 1977; 28:32.

Filicori M, Campaniello E, Michelacci L, et al: Gonadotropin-releasing hormone (GnRH) analog suppression renders polycystic ovarian disease patients more susceptible to ovulation induction with pulsatile GnRH. *J Clin Endocrinol Metab* 1988; 66:327.

Fishel SB, Edwards RG, Purdy JM, et al: Implantation, abortion, and birth after in vitro fertilization using the natural menstrual cycle or follicular stimulation with clomiphene citrate and human menopausal gonadotropin. *J In Vitro Fertil Embryo Transfer* 1985; 2:123.

Gemzell CA, Diczfalusy E, Tillinger KG: Clinical effect of human pituitary follicle stimulating hormone. *J Clin Endocrinol Metab* 1958; 18:1333.

Gordon JW, Grunfeld L, Garrisi GJ, et al: Fertilization of human oocytes by sperm from infertile males after zona pellucida drilling. *Fertil Steril* 1988; 50:68.

Greenblatt RB, Barfield WE, Jungck EC, et al: Induction of ovulation with MRL-41. Preliminary report. *JAMA* 1961; 178:101.

Gysler M, March CM, Mishell DR, et al: A decade's experience with an individualized clomiphene treatment regimen, including its effect on the post-coital test. *Fertil Steril* 1982; 37:161.

Hammond CB, Weibe RH, Haney AF, et al: Ovulation induction with luteinizing hormone releasing hormone in amenorrheic infertile women. *Am J Obstet Gynecol* 1979; 135:924.

Hammond MG: Monitoring techniques for improved pregnancy rates during clomiphene ovulation induction. *Fertil Steril* 1984; 42:499.

Hammond MG, Halme JK, Talbert LM: Factors affecting the pregnancy rate in clomiphene citrate induction of ovulation. *Obstet Gynecol* 1983; 62:196.

Hammond MG, Jordan S, Sloan CS: Factors in affecting pregnancy rates in a donor insemination program using frozen semen. *Am J Obstet Gynecol* 1986; 155:480.

Hamori M, Stuckensen JA, Rumpf D, et al: Zygote intrafallopian transfer (ZIFT): Evaluation of 42 cases. *Fertil Steril* 1988; 50:519.

Han HD, Kiessling AA: In vivo development of transferred mouse embryos conceived in vitro in simple and complex media. *Fertil Steril* 1988; 50:159.

Hard AD: Artificial impregnation. *Med World* 1909; 27:163.

Harrison RF: Insemination of husband's semen with and without the addition of caffeine. *Fertil Steril* 1978; 29:532.

Heape W: Preliminary note on the transplantation and growth of ova within a uterine foster-mother. *Proc R Soc Lond (Biol)* 1891; 48:547.

Howe RS, Wheeler C, Mastroianni L, et al: Pelvic infection after transvaginal ultrasound guided ovum retrieval. *Fertil Steril* 1988; 49:726.

Hurley DM, Bryan R, Outch K, et al: Induction of ovulation and fertility in amenorrhea of women by pulsatile low dose gonadotropin releasing hormone. *N Engl J Med* 1984; 310:1069.

Huszar G, DeCherney A: The role of intrauterine insemination in the treatment of infertile couples: The Yale experience. *Semin Reprod Endocrinol* 1987; 5:11.

Insler B, Melmed H, Eichenbrenner I, et al: The cervical score: A simple semiquantitative method for monitoring of the menstrual cycle. *Int J Gynecol Obstet* 1972; 10:223.

Jansen RPS, Handelsman DJ, Boylan LM, et al:

Pulsatile intravenous gonadotropin releasing hormone for ovulation induction in infertile women. Safety and effectiveness with outpatient therapy. *Fertil Steril* 1987; 48:33.

Jones HW Jr: Indications for in vitro fertilization, in HW Jones, GS Jones, GD Hodgen, et al (eds): *In Vitro Fertilization.* Baltimore, Williams & Wilkins, Co, 1986.

Jones GS, Maffezzoli RD, Strott CA, et al: Pathophysiology of reproductive failure after clomiphene induced ovulation. *Am J Obstet Gynecol* 1970; 108:87.

Jones KP, Ravnikar VA, Schiff I: Results of human menopausal gonadotropin therapy at the Boston Hospital for Women 1979–1981. *Int J Fertil* 1987; 32:131.

Kemmann E, Jones JR: Sequential clomiphene citrate–menotropin therapy for induction or enhancement of ovulation. *Fertil Steril* 1983; 39:772.

Kiessling AA, Loutradis D, McShane PM, et al: Fertilization in trypsin treated oocytes. *Ann NY Acad Sci* 1988; 541:614–620.

Kistner RW: Induction of ovulation with clomiphene citrate. *Obstet Gynecol Surv* 1965; 20:873.

Kistner RW: Sequential use of clomiphene citrate and human menopausal gonadotropin in ovulation induction. *Fertil Steril* 1976; 27:72.

Kistner RW, Smith OW: Observations on the use of nonsteroidal estrogen antagonist: MER-25. *Surg Forum* 1960; 10:725.

Lalich RA, Marut EL, Prins GS, et al: Life table analysis of intrauterine insemination pregnancy rates. *Am J Obstet Gynecol* 1988; 158:980–984.

Lessing JB, Brenner SH, Schoenfeld C, et al: The effect of relaxin on the motility of sperm in freshly thawed human semen. *Fertil Steril* 1985; 44:406.

Lewin A, Laufer N, Rabinowitz A, et al: Ultrasonically guided oocyte collection under local anesthesia: The first choice method for in vitro fertilization—a comparative study with laparoscopy. *Fertil Steril* 1986; 46:257.

Lobo RA, Granger LR, Davajan V, et al: An extended regimen of clomiphene in women unresponsive to the standard therapy. *Fertil Steril* 1982; 37:762.

Loucopoulos A, Ferin N: The treatment of luteal phase defects with pulsatile infusion of gonadotropin releasing hormone. *Fertil Steril* 1987; 48:933.

Lunenfeld B, Blankstein J, Kotev-Emeth S, et al: Drugs used in ovulation induction: safety of patient and offspring. *Hum Reprod* 1986; 1:435.

Lunenfeld B, Sulimovici S, Rabau E, et al: L'induction de l'ovulation dans les amenorrhees hypophysaires par un traitement combine de gonadotrophines urinaires menopausiques et de gonadotrophines chorioniques. *CR Soc Fr Gynecol* 1962; 32:346.

Makler A: Washed and treated insemination in the treatment of idiopathic infertility. *Semin Reprod Endocrinol* 1987; 5:35.

March CM, Tredway DR, Mishell DR: Effect of clomiphene citrate upon amount and duration of human menopausal gonadotropin therapy. *Am J Obstet Gynecol* 1976; 125:699.

Marrs RP, Saito H, Yee B: Effect of variation of in vitro culture techniques upon oocyte fertilization-embryo development in human in vitro procedures *Fertil Steril* 1984; 41;519.

McDonough PG: Editor's comments. *Fertil Steril* 1988; 50:831.

Medical Research International: In vitro fertilization/embryo transfer in the United States: 1987 results from the National IVF-ET Registry. *Fertil Steril* 1989; 51:13.

Medical Research International: In vitro fertilization/embryo transfer in the United States: 1985 and 1986 results from the National IVF-ET Registry. *Fertil Steril* 1988; 49:212.

Meldrum DR, Chetkowski R, Steingold KA, et al: Evolution of a highly successful in vitro fertilization–embryo transfer program. *Fertil Steril* 1987; 48:86.

Moore DH, Gledhill BL: How large should my study be so that I can detect an altered sex ratio? *Fertil Steril* 1988; 50:21.

Nachtigall RD, Faure N, Glass RH: Artificial insemination of husband's sperm. *Fertil Steril* 1979; 32:141.

Navot D, Laufer N, Kapolovic J, et al: Artificially induced endometrial cycles and establishment of pregnancies in the absence of ovaries. *N Engl J Med* 1986; 314:806.

Office of Technology Assessment: *Artificial Insemination Practice in the United States*. No. 052-003-011-298. Washington, DC, US Government Printing Office, August 1988.

O'Herlihy C, Pepperell RJ, Robinson HP: Ultrasound timing of human chorionic gonadotropin administration in clomiphene stimulated cycles. *Obstet Gynecol* 1982; 59:40.

Owen E, Homburg R, Eshel A, et al: Combined growth hormone and gonadotropin treatment for ovulation induction. Paper presented at the American Fertility Society Meeting, Atlanta, October 1988.

Queenan JT, Obrien GD, Bains LM, et al: Ultrasound scanning of ovaries to detect ovulation in women. *Fertil Steril* 1980; 34:99.

Quinlivan WLG, Preciado K, Long GL, et al: Separation of human X and Y spermatozoa by albumin gradient and cephadex chromatography. *Fertil Steril* 1982; 37:104.

Rabau E, Siresee RDM, David A, et al: Human menopausal gonadotropins for anovulation and sterility. *Am J Obstet Gynecol* 1967; 96:92.

Rein MS, DiSalvo D, Friedman AF: Heterotopic pregnancy associated with in vitro fertilization and embryo transfer: A possible role for routine vaginal ultrasound. *Fertil Steril* 1989; 51:1057–1058.

Richter MA, Haning RV, Shapiro S: Artificial donor insemination: Fresh versus frozen semen; the patient as her own control. *Fertil Steril* 1984; 41:277.

Rock J, Menkin MF: In vitro fertilization and cleavage of human ovarian eggs. *Science* 1944; 100:105.

Santoro N, Wierman ME, Filicori M, et al: Intravenous administration of pulsatile gonadotropin releasing hormone in hypothalamic amenorrhea: Effects of dosage. *J Clin Endocrinol Metab* 1986; 62:109.

Schenker JG, Weinstein D: Ovarian hyperstimulation syndrome: A current survey. *Fertil Steril* 1978; 30:255.

Schenker JG, Yarkoni S, Granat M: Multiple pregnancies following induction of ovulation. *Fertil Steril* 1981; 35:105.

Schulman JD, Dorfmann AD, Jones SL, et al: Outpatient in vitro fertilization using transvaginal ultrasound guided oocyte retrieval. *Obstet Gynecol* 1987; 69:665.

Serafini P, Stone B, Kerin J, et al: An alternative approach to control ovarian hyper stimulation in "poor responders" pretreatment with a gonadotropin analog. *Fertil Steril* 1988; 49:90.

Serhal PF, Katz M, Little V, et al: Unexplained infertility—the value of Pergonal superovulation combined with intrauterine insemination. *Fertil Steril* 1988; 49:602.

Shepard MK, Balmaceda JP, Leija CG: Relationship of weight to successful reduction of ovulation with clomiphene citrate. *Fertil Steril* 1979; 32:641.

Smith DJ, Picker RH, Sinosisch M, et al: Assessment of ovulation by ultrasound and estradiol levels during spontaneous and induced cycles. *Fertil Steril* 1980; 33:387.

Steeno O, Adimoelja A, Steeno J: Separation of X and Y bearing human spermatozoa with a Cephadex gel filtration method. *Andrologia* 1975; 7:95.

Steptoe PC, Edwards RG: Birth after reimplantation of a human embryo. *Lancet* 1978; 2:366.

Sunde A, Kahn J, Molne K: Intrauterine insemination. *Hum Reprod* 1988; 3:97.

Trounson A: Preservation of human eggs and embryos. *Fertil Steril* 1986; 46:1.

Vandenberg G, Yen SSC: Effect of antiestrogenic action of clomiphene during the menstrual cycle: Evidence for a change in feedback sensitivity. *J Clin Endocrinol Metab* 1973; 37:356.

Vargyas J, Kletzky O, Marrs RP: The effect of laparoscopic follicular aspiration on ovarian steroidogenesis during the early preimplantation period. *Fertil Steril* 1986; 45:221.

Vermesh M, Kletzky OA, Davajan V, et al: Monitoring techniques to predict and detect ovulation. *Fertil Steril* 1987; 47:259.

Wang CF, Gemzell C: Pregnancy following treatment with human gonadotropins in primary unexplained infertility. *Acta Obstet Gynecol Scand* 1979; 58:141.

Wilson EA, Jawad MJ, Hayden TL: Rates of exponential increase of serum estradiol concentrations in normal and human menopausal gonadotropin-induced cycles. *Fertil Steril* 1982; 37:46.

Wood C, McMaster R, Rennie G: Factors influencing pregnancy rates following in vitro fertilization and transfer. *Fertil Steril* 1985; 43:245.

World Health Organization Task Force on Methods for the Determination of the Fertile Period: Temporal relationships between ovulation and defined changes in the concentration of plasma estradiol-17 beta, luteinizing hormone, follicle stimulating hormone and progesterone. *Am J Obstet Gynecol* 1980; 138:383.

Whamsby H, Fredga K, Liedholm P: Chromosome analysis of human oocytes recovered from preovulatory follicle and stimulated cycle. *N Engl J Med* 1987; 316:121.

Yeh J, Ravnikar VA: Induction of ovulation with human LH-FSH and human FSH, in Barbieri RL, Schiff I (eds): *Reproductive Endocrine Therapeutics*. New York, Alan R Liss, 1988, p 25.

14 _____ Recurrent Abortion

Joseph A. Hill, M.D.

Veronica A. Ravnikar, M.D.

Recurrent abortion is generally defined as the occurrence of three or more clinically detectable pregnancy losses prior to the 20th week of gestation. To encompass all of the studies that attempt to define the etiologies for habitual miscarriage in this chapter, we will broaden this definition to include women with preclinical pregnancy loss and women who have had term births, especially stillbirths or anomalous live infants, or two consecutive miscarriages. Evaluation of recurrent spontaneous abortion should be initiated on the couple's request after the second fetal loss if there are no previous term births (Harger et al., 1983).

Many potential etiologies for recurrent abortion have been proposed (Table 14–1). In this chapter, attention will first be given to causes of abortion intrinsic to the developing fetus itself, that is, genetic abnormalities that result in abortion. In fact, it must be emphasized that chromosomal aberrations, either in the couples or the abortus, remain the only proved cause for spontaneous fetal loss. A description of factors exogenous to the fetus will also be given. For example, anatomical, infectious, environmental, and immunological factors that have been associated with abortion will be discussed. Since many of these factors have not themselves been tested in a double-blind, randomized fashion to prove a causative relationship to abortions, we must be careful in the interpretation of some of these associations. Nevertheless, associations should not be entirely dismissed as being unimportant.

Chromosomal abnormalities, hormonal defects, and immunological mechanisms are responsible in most cases for first trimester losses. Structural abnormalities are associated with miscarriages in the second trimester, although first trimester losses may also occur.

GENERAL INCIDENCE

Preclinical Losses

The classic study performed at the Parkway Hospital in Boston was the first to describe morphological abnormalities in the preimplantation embryo (Hertig et al., 1959). Thirty-four fertilized human ova were recovered during the first 17 days of development from 210 fertile women considered optimal for the probability of early conception. On histological analysis, only 24 of the 34 eggs were considered normal. The remaining 10 showed growth disorganization. An analysis of the data according to the time postovulation (deduced by basal body temperature charts and coital times) revealed that the greatest ovular loss occurred prior to day 20 of the menstrual cycle, the preimplantation stage.

Currently available biochemical tests may potentially detect these preclinical losses. Nevertheless, determining beta-subunit human chorionic gonadotropin (β-hCG) levels can detect only post implantation, preclinical pregnancy losses (occurring 10 days after conception onward; Batzer, 1980). Secretory trophoblast is necessary for the production of hCG. Measuring β-hCG assays in cycles of normal women or a population of infertile women has demonstrated a high incidence of subclinical abortions. Approximately 61.9% of conceptions detected by β-hCG assays in 207 cycles were lost prior to 12 weeks, and the majority of these losses occurred without the mother's

TABLE 14–1.

Potential Etiologies for Recurrent Abortion

I. Genetic
   A. Multifactorial
   B. Chromosomal
      1. Pure history
      2. Mixed history
II. Anatomical
   A. Congenital
      1. Incomplete müllerian
         fusion or septum
         reabsorption
      2. Diethylstilbestrol (DES)
         exposure
      3. Uterine artery anomalies
   B. Acquired
      1. Uterine synechine
      2. Leiomyomas
      3. Endometriosis
      4. Cervical incompetence
III. Endocrine
   A. Luteal phase insufficiency
   B. Androgen overproduction
   C. Prolactin excess
   D. Hypothyroidism
   E. Diabetes mellitus
IV. Immunological
V. Miscellaneous
   A. Environmental
   B. Drugs
   C. Radiation
   D. Placentation abnormalities
   E. Infections
   F. Medical illness

knowledge (Chartier et al., 1979). When sensitive serial measurements of blood β-hCG are used, the risk of pregnancy in exposed ovulatory cycles is 59.6% (Edmonds et al., 1982). A more recent study using a more specific immunoradiometric assay of urinary hCG followed 221 healthy fertile women through a total of 707 menstrual cycles. In this study, 198 pregnancies were identified, but of these, 22% ended before the pregnancy was clinically detected. The incidence of pregnancy loss after implantation, including clinically recognized spontaneous abortions, was 31% (Wilcox et al., 1988).

Clinical Pregnancy Loss

A spontaneous miscarriage will present with the following physical signs: severe pelvic cramp-ing, bleeding, and the passage of clots, fetal tissue, or both. On physical examination of such individuals, note should be made of vital signs, uterine size on bimanual examination (along with the presence or absence of any adnexal masses), and dilatation of the cervix with or without the presence of tissue at the os. A hematocrit reading and blood typing for ABO and Rh subgroups are required. The bleeding from the miscarriage may be profound, requiring transfusion. RhoGAM ($Rh_o(D)$ immune human globulin) should be administered in the Rh-negative mother. On further evaluation, note should be made of the passage of fetal tissue spontaneously, the presence of villi on the curetted specimen, or both. An ectopic pregnancy can at times mask itself as a spontaneous miscarriage.

A spontaneous abortion may be further classified as complete or incomplete. In the latter case, a dilatation and evacuation may be needed to remove the remaining tissue. A missed abortion is a pregnancy loss detected by the failure of appropriate uterine growth or fetal growth (by scan), an empty gestational sac (by scan), or the lack of fetal heart tones (by Doppler ultrasound or scan when appropriate).

A threatened abortion is one that presents with bleeding and cramping in the first half of pregnancy. Approximately one half of these will abort. An inevitable abortion is one in which the membranes have ruptured and cervical dilatation has occurred. An incomplete abortion is one in which only part of the membranes or fetal tissue has passed. The cervix may be dilated, and the patient may have profuse bleeding necessitating curettage.

To do chromosomal karyotyping on the conceptus, it is important that the specimen is handled in a sterile fashion and placed in saline by the patient (if passed at home) or by the physician (after dilation and curettage of the uterus). Ironically, it is usually the abnormal concepti that are macerated (especially after a missed abortion) and grow poorly in tissue culture. The advent of chorionic villi biopsy may be helpful in detecting abnormal concepti. Once an abnormal pregnancy is identified or once a pregnancy is identified in a high-risk habitual aborter, a quick karyotypic analysis can be made (Cadkin and Sabbagha, 1980).

The routine biophysical and biochemical profile used to monitor pregnancies today is that of real-time ultrasonic imaging of the fetal crown-rump length, the gestational sac, the fetal heart beat, and β-hCG measurements on serial assays. The gestational sac can be visualized by 5 to 6 weeks' gestation (menstrual dates), and by 8 weeks fetal echoes can be determined within the sac. The absence of fetal echoes by 8 weeks' gestational age is consistent with a blighted ovum. For an ultrasonic demonstration of a normal intrauterine fetus and a blighted ovum, see Figures 14–1 and 14–2.

The majority of miscarriages prior to 12 weeks' gestation are chromosomally abnormal. In a recent study, the overall rate of chromosomal anomalies in 1,356 karyotyped specimens was 39.8%. The vast majority (94%) occurred in embryos less than 30 mm (Byrne et al., 1985). The most frequent abnormalities are autosomal trisomy, followed by sex chromosome monosomy, and then triploidy. Maternal age is the prevailing factor for fetal autosomal trisomy; one fourth of such abnormalities occur in young mothers, and three fourths of such abnormalities occur in women more than 35 years of age (Creasy, 1988). In 9 studies of more than 1,200 couples with habitual abortion, 7.2% had a chromosomal structural abnormality in 1 parent. Therefore, the workup of a couple with habitual abortion (three

or more) should include their chromosomal analyses (Creasy, 1988).

Morphologically, the tissue recovered will appear as either a macerated fetus, an intact empty sac, or an empty sac with or without a cord stump. On ultrasonographic evaluation, they appear as empty gestational sacs or fetuses with crown-rump lengths that lag behind the norm for the developmental stage (usually less than 5 mm). In defining the phenotypic expressions of triploidy in 40 spontaneous abortions, Harris et al. (1981) found that the following characteristics predominated on gross specimen analysis: cystic placental villi (short of molar degeneration), limb and facial developmental defects, and anachronistic development of retinal pigment. Therefore, it is advisable to detail the phenotype of such pregnancies via morphological analysis and ultrasonography, since it may be difficult to determine the genotype of such specimens by conventional chromosomal analysis.

Serial trends in the patient's hormonal profiles can be evaluated. There is a predictable rise in the level of hCG in the first trimester of pregnancy (Lagrew et al., 1983). With knowledge of menstrual dating, serial low levels of hCG prior to the first 60 days of pregnancy may predict poor fetal outcome. The exponential linear rise in pe-

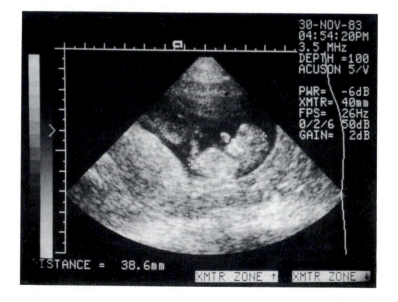

FIG 14–1.
Ultrasound scan showing a 10-week, 5-day-old intrauterine fetal gestation (crown-rump length 38.6 mm; Acuson 128 imaging; 3-MHz transducer). (Courtesy of Dr. Beryl Benacerraf.)

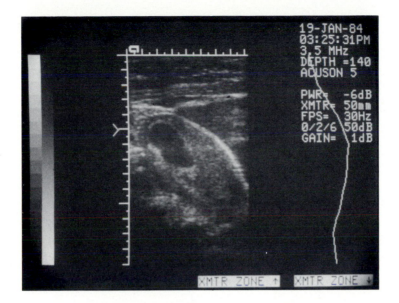

FIG 14–2.
Ultrasound scan showing blighted ovum with empty sac and no fetal heartbeat (Acuson 128 imaging; 3-MHz transducer). (Courtesy of Dr. Beryl Benacerraf.)

ripheral β-hCG titers detected by radioimmunoassay is depicted in Figure 14–3). A doubling time of hCG plasma concentration compatible with normal, early gestational growth has been reported as 1.4 to 2.0 days.

Finally, after a miscarriage there is slow clearance of hCG from the peripheral circulation. After an induced abortion in the first trimester, the mean time for clearance of hCG to a level of 2 mIU/ml was 37.5 ± 6.4 days. Second trimester abortions have a mean clearance time of 27.4 ± 4.8 days. Despite hCG levels as high as 35 mIU/ml, luteinizing hormone (LH) and follicle-stimulating hormone (FSH) peaks resume within 2 weeks. Contraception in individuals should be suggested immediately after a fetal loss due to this early time of ovulatory recovery (Marrs et al., 1979).

INCIDENCE OF SPONTANEOUS ABORTION

The incidence of spontaneous abortion and its recurrence risks have been analyzed both retrospectively and prospectively in large population studies. Knowledge of these statistics is important since the more pessimistic the figures, the more optimistic any mode of therapy for spontaneous losses will appear.

The classical studies by Malpas in 1938, reviewed in Warburton and Fraser (1961), initially formed the basis for evaluation of couples with habitual abortion until they were critiqued by Warburton and Fraser in 1961. Malpas devised a mathematical model (later revised by Eastman) to estimate the risk of abortion recurrence after prior pregnancy loss. According to Malpas the risk of abortion with the first pregnancy was estimated as 18%; according to the mathematical model, the risk increased to 84% after three consecutive abortions. The risk of miscarriage for a recurring cause was set at 1%, which is misleading since different etiologies for miscarriage have different rates of recurrence.

Subsequently, Warburton and Fraser (1964) retrospectively studied 2,134 families in which every woman interviewed had at least 1 living child. The abortion rate as a whole was 14.7 ± 0.4%. The subsequent rates were as follows: 12.3% with no history of previous miscarriage, 23.7% with one previous abortion, 26.2% with two previous losses, 32.2% with three, and 35.9% with four prior losses. In conclusion, a woman with one previous abortion has a 25% to 30% chance of aborting in each successive pregnancy providing

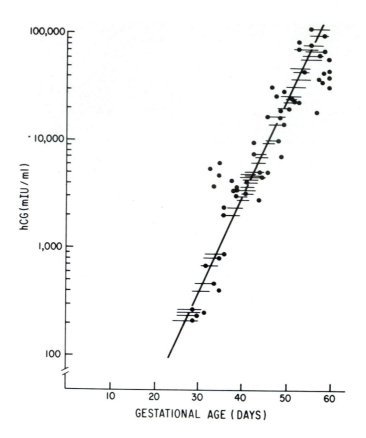

FIG 14–3.

Exponential increase in maternal serum hCG concentrations during the first 60 days' gestation. Regression equation: Day of test = 5.073 Ln (hCG concentrations) − 0.1322, r^2 = 0.8263, F = 275.9, $p<0.0001$. After 60 days' gestation, there is a wide individual variation in hCG values. (From Lagrew D, et al: Determination of gestational age by serum concentrations of human chorionic gonadotropin. *Obstet Gynecol* 1983; 62:37–40. Reproduced by permission.)

she has had one living child. These data may, therefore, not apply to women who have never had a living child.

Poland et al., (1977) in a prospective analysis of 472 patients and 638 pregnancies determined a higher overall rate of 22.1% if there were no live children. After one spontaneous abortion, there was a 19% chance of recurrence; the rate increased to 47% after three spontaneous abortions. This work justifies an investigation for the cause of repetitive abortion after the second miscarriage if there is no living child.

The use of newer gynecologic technologies to monitor pregnancies has provided further detail in regard to timing of most miscarriages. The incidence of miscarriage after ultrasound diagnosis of a viable pregnancy at 8 to 12 weeks' gestation is 3.2% (Simpson, 1987), implying that most chromosomally abnormal abortuses occur prior to 8 weeks' gestation. Therefore, the 15% to 20% incidence figure of fetal loss referred to previously applies to the "window" of time before 8 weeks when the majority of pregnancy losses occur. One of the most important applications of the study is that we can compare the loss rate that occurs with newer genetic screening technologies such as chorionic villus sampling against this natural loss rate. A recent seven-center study reports the loss rate with this procedure at 7.2% (including termination of abnormal pregnancies and spontaneous miscarriages; Rhodes et al., 1989). Against the background rate of 15% to 20%, this rate becomes acceptable.

There is an epidemiological relationship between increased maternal age and trisomic abortuses. However, a woman who has an abortus with monosomy X is younger on the average than a woman who has a live birth or a woman who has an abortion without an anomaly (Stein, 1983). This suggests an environmental determinant predisposing to monosomy. The effect of maternal age on the incidence of abortion shows an increased risk of 23% at ages 30 to 34 years, increasing to 48% at ages 35 to 39 years. Paternal age does not appear to be a major factor in the risk of miscarriage with chromosomally abnormal abortuses. However, it has been implicated in inducing new dominant mutations (Freedman, 1981).

Autosomal recessive inheritance, X-linked disorders, and neural tube defects are multifactorial genetic disorders associated with recurrent abortion. Anencephaly is the predominant feature in neural tube disorders, and most of these infants are girls. Abortion risk is not otherwise increased in mothers who have live-born infants with a wide variety of defects of a multifactorial nature (Warburton and Fraser, 1964).

A statistically significant association between ectopic pregnancies and prior spontaneous abortion has been implicated. However, a higher rate of chromosomal anomalies in the ectopic pregnancies beyond that expected for gestational age has not been demonstrated to date (Elias et al., 1981).

Previous induced abortions were once thought to statistically increase the chance of subsequent pregnancy failure (Madore et al., 1981). These data, however, have been challenged by several large series. A review of 5,003 records of consecutive deliveries at the Brigham and Women's Hospital (Schoenbaum, 1980) between 1975 and 1976 reported no increased risk for poor pregnancy outcome in women with a single prior induced abortion. However, offspring of secundigravidas with a proximate spontaneous abortion had an increased frequency of short gestations, low birth weights, low Apgar scores, and congenital malformations.

Jansen (1982) comprehensively analyzed the published series on pregnancies after infertility treatment. Ovulation induction with bromocriptine in hyperprolactinemic anovulation, artificial insemination with donor semen for azoospermia, and operation for endometriosis had an abortion incidence that approached the norm for the general population. Abortion incidences accompanying other modes of therapy were found to be higher. Induction of ovulation with clomiphene

citrate (Clomid) and the human menopausal gonadotropin Pergonal is associated with a higher rate of miscarriage (19.3% and 22.7%, respectively). Artificial insemination with husband's semen and salpingostomy for distal tube occlusion were also associated with higher than normal abortion rates (24.3% and 26.7%, respectively). The reasons suggested by Jansen (1982) for such may be postovulatory aging of the secondary oocyte, polyspermy, sperm selection at a normal tubal isthmus, sperm aging after ejaculation, and delayed or accelerated embryo transport due to pharmacologically induced steroid hormone levels that are in excess of the norm.

In conclusion, it is important to consider all of these factors in a patient's history when one is evaluating a couple for recurrent abortion (see Table 14–1). A knowledge of these studies offers the appropriate incidence figures in counseling patients.

ETIOLOGICAL FACTORS

Abortions tend to occur at the same developmental state in consecutive pregnancies (Poland et al., 1977). A conceptus in an early pregnancy loss is more likely to have a cytogenetic abnormality, whereas a late abortion is generally due to maternal or environmental factors.

Cytogenetic Etiology

Karyotypic analysis of 1,498 abortuses of less than 12 weeks' gestation revealed 38.52% to be normal and 61.48% to be abnormal. The most frequent aneuploid karyotype found was autosomal trisomy (52%), followed by sex chromosome monosomy (15.3%) (Boue et al., 1973). More specific staining techniques highlighting certain areas of the chromosomes (Q banding) can delineate deletions of chromosomal complements that can later be traced to a parental source for the structural rearrangement. A cytogenetic study of 27 spontaneous abortions analyzed by this technique revealed 59% with chromosomal anomalies (McConnell and Carr, 1975). Trisomy was found in 9 of 16; the chromosomes involved were no. 2, 8, 14, 16, and 22. The frequency of these different trisomic forms among abortuses is different from those at birth. Trisomy 16 compromises nearly one third of all anomalies seen in early losses, yet this malformation rarely proceeds to the stage of a recognizable embryo (Stein, 1981).

Presumably, sporadic problems during gametogenesis, namely, anaphase lag and nondisjunction during meiosis, are causative for the development of these abnormal embryos. However, a small percentage of these will be due to a parental carrier state of a cytogenetic abnormality. In fact, the incidence of significant chromosomal rearrangements is higher in persons with histories of repetitive miscarriage.

Khudr (1974), in his review of the cytogenetics of habitual abortion, found that 6.2% of the couples with recurrent miscarriage had a balanced translocation, whereas the incidence in the general population was less than 1%.

Structural chromosomal variations of the reciprocal (between metacentric or submetacentric chromosomes) or robertsonian (between acrocentric chromosomes) variety are found more frequently in women with a history of repetitive fetal wastage. In 24 of 41 women with translocations, 16 of the 24 were of the D/D variety. This has been corroborated by succeeding authors; 31.2% of 16 couples with habitual abortion had balanced translocations in the female partner (Heritage et al., 1978). Some studies show lower or higher incidence figures for parental chromosomal translocations depending on their referral base. Two-hundred couples with two or more spontaneous miscarriages and a mixed obstetric history were found to have a 3.7% incidence of balanced translocation in either parent. Forty eight of these had two or more abortions with an 8.4% incidence of balanced translocations. With four miscarriages, the risk increased to 10% (Michels et al., 1982). Studies from other centers, however, may dispute these high figures. One recent report described significant chromosomal anomalies in only 1.8% of couples with a history of prior miscarriage (Fitzsimmons et al., 1983). With two or more spontaneous abortions, the incidence went up to 2.3%.

When the pedigree of a couple with fetal loss is analyzed, it is important to clarify all previous obstetrical outcomes. The risk of parental translocation is higher if there is a history of abortions only and no term live births. The yield on chromosomal analysis of parents is also higher if abortion histories are interspersed with stillbirths and live-born infants with congenital anomalies.

After a history of two or more abortions, especially in the absence of a live birth, it is therefore reasonable to obtain parental chromosomal analysis, looking specifically for structural rearrangements, deletions, X chromosome mosaicism, and inversions of chromosomes. If a chromosomal abnormality is detected in the couple, no therapy is currently available. Donor embryo transfer may be applicable in the future for chromosomal aberrations in the woman. If the man is the carrier, artificial donor insemination may be offered. If an affected couple succeeds in carrying a pregnancy beyond 12 weeks, a second trimester amniocentesis should be offered.

There is a controversial subgroup of patients who are karyotypically normal but who still suffer repeated pregnancy wastage with recurrent aneuploidy in fetal specimens (Boue et al., 1973). In studying a subgroup of women (30 of 473) who had karyotyped abortuses, there was an increased incidence of an abnormal abortus if the previous one was abnormal despite normal parental chromosomal analyses. If the previous abortus was normal, however, there was a greater likelihood that the second would be normal also. Furthermore, in an analysis of 1,384 abortal specimens, the mothers who delivered a chromosomally normal abortus more often had a history of repeated abortion. Those in whom a chromosomally abnormal abortus was miscarried tended to have fewer repeated abortions but had an increased incidence of premature births of children with Down's syndrome. It is hypothesized that the group of women who had multiple miscarriages but who themselves had normal chromosomal complements underwent repeated nondisjunctional events in their gametes. Therefore, it has been suggested that women with repeat trisomic abortuses and repeated multiple nonkaryotyped miscarriages should undergo second trimester amniocentesis if a subsequent pregnancy proceeds past 12 weeks' gestation to exclude the possibility of trisomy.

Anatomical Factors

Anatomical causes for spontaneous abortion are either congenital or acquired. Generally, but not exclusively, these causative factors induce a miscarriage in the second trimester and manifest themselves with cramping and bleeding. If the symptoms occur in the latter part of the second trimester when fetal viability is assumed, the presentation is that of premature labor, and tocolysis may be instituted. These anatomical defects may be described using hysterosalpingography and hysteroscopy (combined, when appropriate, with laparoscopy; Kistner and Patton, 1975a).

Müllerian Anomalies

Failure of fusion of the müllerian ducts or incomplete septum reabsorption in the female embryo can result in many distinct abnormalities of uterine development (Fig 14–4; Kistner and Patton, 1975). These abnormalities of fusion have been classically divided into two groups (Semmens classification). Group 1 consists of uteri of single müllerian origin: the didelphic uterus, the unicornuate uterus, and the bicornuate uterus with one rudimentary horn. Group 2 consists of uteri of dual müllerian origin: the bicornuate uterus, septate uterus, and the arcuate uterus. Buttram (1983) proposed a broader grouping:

Class 1. Müllerian agenesis
Class 2. Unicornuate uterus
Class 3. Uterine didelphys
Class 4. Uterus bicornuis
  A. Complete
  B. Partial
  C. Arcuate
Class 5. Septate uterus
  A. Complete
  B. Partial
Class 6. Diethystilbestrol anomalies

Patients with a hemiuterus (Semmens group 1 and Buttram classes 2 and 3) have better reproductive function than those with a double uterus (Semmens group 2 and Buttram classes 4, 5, and 6), the overall rates of late abortion being 17.3%

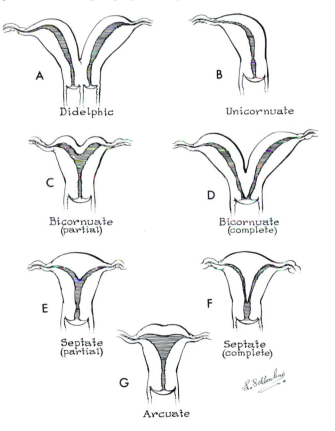

FIG 14–4.
Nonobstructive maldevelopment of the uterus. **A,** uterus didelphys. **B,** unicornuate uterus. **C,** a partial bicornuate uterus as evidenced by the external configuration. **D,** a complete bicornuate uterus as evidenced by the external configuration and a double cervix. **E** and **F,** septate uterus, partial and complete, as evidenced by a normal external configuration of the uterus and the septum, which can be diagnosed only by radiographic means. **G,** arcuate uterus, which is the mildest form of malformation and seldom associated with reproductive difficulties. (From Jones HW, Jones GS: *Am J Obstet Gynecol* 1953; 65:325. Reproduced by permission.)

and 34.7%, respectively. Nevertheless, both anomalies are manifested by repetitive pregnancy loss, usually in the second trimester or with premature delivery.

Depending on clinical suspicion of a uterine defect, the incidence has been variously reported as 0.06% to 0.48% in the general population (Green and Harris, 1976). Since some of these are found initially at delivery, it is mandated that a complete workup to exclude other causes of abortion be performed prior to surgical correction of the defect for the purpose of alleviating habitual abortion. The etiology of müllerian defects is unknown; familial aggregates have been reported. The mode of inheritance may be polygenic or multifactorial, although an autosomal recessive pattern has been implicated (Verp et al., 1983). It is important to exclude renal abnormalities (by intravenous pyelogram or ultrasound) in patients with uterine anomalies (Marshall and Beisel, 1978).

The classical surgical corrective procedures used are the Jones technique (the excision of a wedge of fundal uterus), the Strassman technique (first performed on, and still mainly applicable to, bicornuate uteri), and the Tompkins technique for unification of a subseptate uterus (Jones, 1981; Barnes et al., 1980).

Rock and Jones (1977), reporting from an updated series in their institution from 1964 through 1975, found that only one in five patients with uterine malformations (mainly the septate variety) had reproductive difficulties. The actual cause for reproductive loss in septate or bicornuate uteri has been postulated to be due to vascular insufficiency and inadequate endometrial development, which result in an abnormal placentation. Once the diagnosis is made by laparoscopy and hysteroscopy, surgical correction can be achieved. In a series reported from the Brigham and Women's Hospital using the Tompkin's technique for uterine septum, 17 of 20 patients had successful term pregnancies, with 86% conceiving in 11 months (McShane et al., 1983). This is not unlike the 77% success rate reported with the wedge technique (Rock and Jones, 1977). The Tompkin's technique is being replaced by hysteroscopic resection (Daly et al., 1983). This obviates the necessity of a cesarean section, which is usually required after a traditional metroplasty. Both cervical incompetence and uterine synechiae are potential complications of metroplasty.

Ironically, women who took the nonsteroidal estrogen DES due to their own poor reproductive performance produced daughters with anatomical abnormalities that may lead to increased pregnancy wastage. There is interest in the variety of ways that DES can cause reproductive difficulties, since the majority of these women are now in the childbearing age group. Many studies have concentrated on the reproductive performance of DES daughters and show different incidences of spontaneous abortion. The majority of these correlate with a higher incidence of the latter if severe uterine or cervical (or both) structural changes were produced by the DES. Kaufman et al. (1980) reported on 267 DES-exposed offspring, of whom 69% demonstrated a uterine abnormality that was associated with poor pregnancy outcome. The spontaneous abortion rate in their series (both first and second trimester) was 32%. The commonest roentgenographic finding in this series was a T-shaped uterus with a cavity less than 2.5 cm long (measured by planimetry). Thirty-nine percent of women with an abnormal tubogram had a spontaneous abortion. Of 119 pregnancies in 93 women, only 45% resulted in a term delivery (Kaufman et al., 1981). Nevertheless, no suitable surgical procedure for correcting a typical T-shaped DES uterus exists (Fig 14–5). Herbst and associates (1981) noted that the presence of cervicovaginal ridges increased the incidence of abortion; in their series, this included a 27% abortion rate compared with 16% in controls. Finally, Schmidt et al. (1980) at the University of North Carolina reported on 276 female offspring of women who had taken DES during pregnancy. Of 106 female offspring who attempted pregnancy, there were 129 conceptions and 58 live births. The fetal wastage was 43% for the first pregnancy and 37% for all pregnancies;

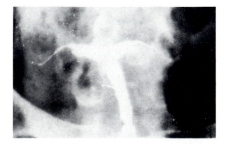

FIG 14–5.
Tubogram of patient exposed to DES in utero during mother's first trimester of pregnancy. Note T-shaped uterus.

25% were due to spontaneous abortions. Barnes et al. (1980), in the series from the National Cooperative Diethylstilbestrol Adenosis Project, disagreed with these findings. They reported an increased risk ratio of any unfavorable outcome of pregnancy among DES-exposed daughters as 1.69 ($p < 0.01$), and the risk ratio of abortion was 1.61. Ironically, 26 women with structural uterine defects had a 16.7% miscarriage rate, whereas the 184 who did not have a noted structural defect had a rate of 27.7%. In the studies that have reported an increased incidence of miscarriage, cervical incompetence is implicated.

A recent prospective study from the University of Pennsylvania suggests aggressive management of all DES-exposed patients with prophylactic cerclage, regardless of cervical findings in tubogram (Ludmir et al., 1987). This is a very controversial view. In individuals with typical DES changes (cervicovaginal ridges) and history of previous miscarriage, a cerclage certainly would not be inappropriate. Individual patient decisions must be made balancing the morbidity of a cerclage procedure against the potential of future loss.

Anomalies of the uterine artery have also been proposed as a predisposing factor for habitual abortion. Compromised uterine blood supply may predispose to miscarriages due to placental insufficiency.

Uterine Synechiae

Intrauterine adhesions (Asherman's syndrome) are generally caused by iatrogenic means—traumatic curettage after a delivery and especially a missed abortion. A metroplasty and extensive excision or cautery of submucous myomas can also cause such adhesions as can postabortal or postpartum endometritis. Another infrequent cause is genital tuberculosis. Clinically, the diagnosis is suspected in an individual with postcurettage or postsurgical amenorrhea who has biphasic basal body temperatures and luteal serum progesterones levels yet does not respond to estrogen-progesterone administration with withdrawal menstrual flow. Suspicion is heightened if filling defects are demonstrated on a hysterosalpingogram, but the diagnosis is made more accurately by hysteroscopy. The latter is both a diagnostic and therapeutic modality, since these adhesions can be graded and cut during hysteroscopy (Siegler and Vallee, 1988). The degree of intrauterine scarring is most closely correlated with the menstrual pattern, that is, the more severe cases have complete amenorrhea. In a combined series (Schenker and Margalioth, 1982), 40% of women with untreated Asherman's syndrome suffered habitual or missed abortions. When such persons are treated with hysteroscopic lysis of adhesions and oral conjugated estrogen (treatment length and doses vary) for 1 month, the abortion rate decreased to 25%. March and Israel (1981) were able to show that in 84 pregnancies in women with intrauterine adhesions, only 16.7% resulted in the delivery of a viable infant. Following treatment, 39 pregnancies resulted in a term gestation in 87.2%.

The ability to diagnose and treat intrauterine synechial with hysteroscopy has aided our therapy in this syndrome. No standardized regimen of hormonal or antibiotic therapy exists. Nevertheless, most series report beneficial results with combined use of an intrauterine device (or Foley catheter) and hormonal therapy (2.5 mg of Premarin/day for 1 month) to regenerate the endometrial lining.

Uterine Leiomyomas

Submucous leiomyomas (fibroids) may disturb endometrial function or encroach on the cavity of the uterus to such a degree that normal implantation is compromised. Large intramural leiomyomas may produce hyperirritability or dysfunction of the endometrium, resulting in abortion. The location of the fibroid appears to be more important than its overall size. Fibroids grow to larger dimensions during pregnancy due to the increases in estrogen and progesterone secretion. In this way, they can create a greater problem during pregnancy than that which would be predicted by the size prior to pregnancy. Surgical correction via myomectomy is indicated in patients who have experienced repetitive miscarriage when no other cause for abortion is found. If the uterine cavity is entered during myomectomy, a cesarean section is indicated at delivery of a subsequent term birth.

Excision of uterine leiomyomas under hysteroscopic control has been described (Siegler and Vallee, 1988). With hysteroscopic and laparoscopic control, morcellation of submucous leiomyomas can be performed using diathermic cautery or laser. The pedunculated myomas with a distinct stalk are most conducive to removal by such a procedure. There are no large series to date to compare overall morbidity figures. However, such hysteroscopic resection, even if limited only to the pedunculated type of myomas, decreases morbidity since it negates the need for a laparotomy for myomectomy and a subsequent cesarean section for delivery. These procedures, however, should be performed only by surgeons skilled in hysteroscopy. The patient must be prepared for laparotomy in the event of uncontrollable bleeding.

Pelvic Endometriosis

Although controversial, the frequency of miscarriage appears to be inversely related to the severity of documented endometriosis in an affected individual. A recent survey tabulated 34% of 226 pregnancies ending in a first trimester spontaneous abortion prior to conservative surgical treatment of the disease. This was compared with an incidence of 13% of pregnancies in control, primary infertility patients ($n = 128$). Mild endometriosis was associated with a greater incidence of miscarriage (49% in 87 patients) compared with 24% in severely afflicted patients ($n = 107$). Rock et al. (1981) found a 49% abortion risk in women with endometriosis; the figure was reduced to 20% if conservative surgery was chosen. Dmowski and Cohen (1978) also indicated an increased incidence of second and third trimester intrauterine fetal deaths in conceptions occurring within three cycles of discontinuation of danazol (Danocrine) pseudopregnancy therapy for endometriosis. This was not found in a 4-year study performed in Kistner's practice in which, after danazol therapy for endometriosis, there was no increase in the miscarriage rate (Barbieri et al., 1982). These individuals, however, were advised not to conceive immediately after stopping danazol therapy.

What exactly causes miscarriages associated with endometriosis is speculative at this time. It may be related to the increased levels of peritoneal fluid prostaglandin-like compounds (thromboxane B_2 and 6-ketoprostaglandin $F_{1\alpha}$; Drake et al., 1981), or it may be related to poor luteal function. Immunological factors have also been proposed (reviewed by Hill and Anderson, 1988a).

Cervical Incompetence

Classically, the diagnosis of an incompetent cervix (Fig 14–6) is made by history: painless dilatation between the 16th and 28th week of pregnancy with symptoms of pelvic pressure and increased mucoid discharge.

If a no. 18 cervical dilator can be inserted into the cervix in the nonpregnant state and a typical obstetrical history is elicited, a diagnosis of incompetence is made. A hysterosalpingogram can also aid the diagnosis. Quite typically, in the absence of obstructed tubes, there is backflow of the dye through the cervix; the cervical isthmus is also widened to greater than 1 cm. Ultrasound criteria for diagnosing cervical incompetence during pregnancy have been developed (Michaels et al., 1989). Patients who developed cervical incompetence during the pregnancy necessitating a

FIG 14–6.
Incompetent cervical os seen during the 32nd week of gestation. The cervix is widely patulous and the membranes clearly visible. (From Easterday CL, Reid DE: *N Engl J Med* 1959; 260:687. Reproduced by permission.)

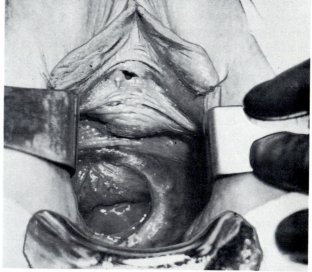

cerclage had a combination of the following depicted by weekly ultrasound examinations: membrane protrusion through the cervix, progressive herniation, cervical dilatation, and cervical shortening.

The causes of cervical incompetence are either traumatic (i.e., multiple dilatation and curettage procedures and wide conization of the cervix) or anatomical (congenital; i.e., a history of DES exposure in utero or collagen matrix abnormalities). The frequency of pregnancy wastage ascribed to an incompetent cervix varies greatly. However, it is generally believed to be ascribed as the causative factor in about one of five midtrimester losses. A preconceptual (Lash) procedure or a postconceptual suture (Shirodkar or MacDonald) around the incompetent cervix can be used.

In the presence of cervicitis, vaginal infection, or rupture of membranes, the operation is contraindicated. The best results with postconceptual suture are achieved if minimal cervical dilatation is achieved. The prognosis for success is much poorer if membranes are bulging through a dilated cervix.

Harger's (1980) series from Magee Women's Hospital, Pittsburgh (1971–1978), drew from a retrospective analysis of 251 cerclage procedures (Shirodkar or MacDonald) in 105 selected women. Fetal survival was markedly improved from 20% to 80% in elective cases and reached an average of 60% if the procedure was performed in a nonemergent situation. Morbidity attributed to the cerclage procedure consisted of chorioamnionitis in 1.2% of the individuals; the remainder was due to cervical lacerations. Cervical scarring and elective cesarean section rates were significantly increased (16%–25%). It has, therefore, been suggested that cervical cerclage be performed as soon as the diagnosis of cervical incompetence is made. The risk of chorioamnionitis is increased 2.6-fold, and premature rupture of the membranes prior to the 32nd week may occur if the procedure is delayed or done under emergent conditions (Charles and Edwards, 1981).

Endocrine Factors

Luteal phase defects are broadly defined as abnormalities in the functioning of the corpus luteum, which create problems in progesterone production. These deficiencies in luteal progesterone secretion are believed to be a cause of early first trimester reproductive failure. Such defects were found to occur spontaneously in 3.5% of patients with primary infertility but in 25.0% of patients with repeated miscarriages. Recent reports estimate the incidence to be higher among the population of infertile patients, with Rosenberg et al. (1980) reporting an incidence of 8.1%, Wentz (1980) reporting 19%, and Seeger-Jones et al. (1970) reporting 29.5% (the latter figure also includes the incidence in women receiving clomiphene citrate therapy).

Luteal phase insufficiency is characterized by insufficient progesterone secretion by the corpus luteum. Menses usually occurs 6 to 9 days after ovulation. Reduced estradiol-17β and FSH secretion occur during the follicular phase, an aberrant thermal response per basal body temperature recording, and a midluteal progesterone level of less than 10 ng/ml may also be demonstrated. If these are suggestive of a defect, the diagnosis is made by two consecutive-month, well-timed endometrial biopsies in the late luteal phase with the expected secretory pattern defined by Noyes et al. (1950). The specific criteria for diagnosis are still very controversial, as is the exact treatment modality. A 29.5% incidence of luteal phase insufficiency per the Noyes et al. (1950) criteria in 144 infertile patients on initial biopsy has been reported but declined to 19% after two biopsies. Furthermore, 29.5% of 44 patients on clomiphene citrate therapy have been noted to have an inadequate luteal phase by biopsy (Wentz, 1980). Downs et al. (1983) reported that conception rates with luteal phase defects of greater than 5 days were significantly improved with clomiphene citrate therapy (79% conception rate), whereas those with a delay of less than 5 days were not. Therefore, two or more endometrial biopsy specimens that are out of phase and a defect that is not equivocal are the criteria for luteal phase inadequacy.

It is suggested that luteal phase defects may be due to central defects in LH pulse mechanics in the luteal phase, to an ovarian defect in progesterone production, or both. DiZerega and Hodgen (1981) have described luteal phase dysfunction "as a sequence of aberrant folliculogenesis." Their work in the primate model demonstrated aberrations in FSH secretion and, hence, a central defect caused defective corpus luteum progesterone production, which could be overcome by treatment with menotropins. These defects in follicular development can be pharmacologically induced (e.g., with clomiphene citrate or Pergonal treatment) or associated with hyperprolactinemia (St. Michael and DiZerega, 1983). An ovarian defect causing poor progesterone output can be due to deficiencies of low-density lipoprotein synthesis (i.e., individuals with abetalipoproteinemia) or low-density lipoprotein delivery to the corpus luteum (possibly due to defective vascularization of the corpus luteum; Carr et al., 1982). A very rare defect creating absence of stromal cytosol receptors for progesterone, which is clinically demonstrated by absence of secretory endometrial changes, has also been documented (Keller et al., 1979).

Much more work in deciphering the actual causes of poor luteal functioning is needed. In the past, this entity has been treated empirically with exogenous progesterone. This is still a subject of great controversy; two separate double-blind placebo-controlled studies have found conflicting results (Goldzieher, 1964; Daya, 1988).

The successful use of supplemental progesterone, either intramuscular (12.5 mg of progesterone in oil) or by vaginal suppositories (25 mg twice daily), has been proposed by some investigators, although these studies have not been performed in a double-blind fashion (Rosenberg et al., 1980; Soules et al., 1981). The use of progesterone supplementation in pregnancy has not been acknowledged as efficacious by the Food and Drug Administration. In fact, their use has been loosely implicated with an increase in the incidence of congenital heart defects (Heinonen et al., 1977), although this is a subject of continuing debate (Chez, 1978). More recent studies (Katz et al., 1985) have been unable to document progestogen teratogenicity in the first trimester. In patients who may have a poorly vascularized corpus luteum, exogenous progesterone supplementation may be the treatment of choice. Currently, many in vitro fertilization programs are employing the use of progesterone supplementation after follicle aspiration for ovum recovery with no apparent adverse sequelae.

The ovulatory-induction agent clomiphene citrate has been favored as a treatment modality for inadequate luteal phase progesterone production, even though clomiphene itself has been associated with luteal phase insufficiency (Quagliarello and Weiss, 1979; Soules et al., 1981; Hammond and Talbert, 1982). It is important to try to identify the cause for poor luteal progesterone production. When hyperprolactinemia is identified as

a probable contributing factor to poor luteal progesterone production, bromocriptine (Parlodel) can successfully reverse the defect. Androgen overproduction may also contribute to luteal phase insufficiency, resulting in spontaneous abortion.

Abnormal maternal thyroid function has not been conclusively demonstrated to increase the incidence of miscarriage. An indirect association with the presence of thyroid antibodies and Down's syndrome in younger mothers has been implicated; this may indirectly relate to the slight increase in spontaneous losses seen in hypothyroidism (Fralkow, 1967).

Maternal diabetes has not been causally related to the incidence of first trimester abortions (Crane and Wahl, 1981). However, when compared with a control population correlating abnormally high levels of glycosylated hemoglobin levels (Hb A_{1c}); a higher rate of spontaneous miscarriage was demonstrated (Wright et al., 1983). The implication is that with poorer diabetic control, the possible incidence of miscarriage is greater, reinforcing the need for strict diabetic control even prior to a contemplated pregnancy.

Infectious Etiology

Many infections have been proposed as causative factors for habitual abortion; however, the two most commonly associated infections are *Mycoplasma* and *Ureaplasma*. *Mycoplasma hominis* and *Ureaplasma urealyticum* (T-mycoplasma, or T-strains) can be isolated frequently from the female genital tract. The T-strains have been associated with early fetal wastage. In fact, T-mycoplasma was first identified and described in abortal specimens from a spontaneous miscarriage (Horne et al., 1974). The issue of whether or not the infection is caused by the abortal process itself has been raised. The mechanism whereby an infectious agent may cause poor embryonic development requires elucidation.

There have been many studies detailing improved pregnancy outcome in women treated for T-mycoplasma, although these studies have not demonstrated a direct causal relationship and have been disputed by others. Although T-mycoplasma may be an opportunistic infection in an individual who has had multiple miscarriages, it still may be prudent to culture and treat such individuals. T-mycoplasma is very sensitive to tetracyclines. It is important not to treat habitual aborters empirically with tetracyclines but, rather, to obtain cultures and antibiotic susceptibility testing prior to prescribing therapy. The usual course of therapy is for both partners to take 100 mg of doxycycline twice daily for 10 days. If tetracycline is prescribed to the woman, therapy should be given in the follicular phase.

Part of the difficulties in obtaining reliable results may be in the collection of specimens for T-mycoplasma. Urine should be cultured simultaneously to increase the detection rate of the organism. In men, semen is a better source of culture than urine or urethral swabbings.

Uterine toxoplasmosis infections in developing countries have also been implicated as causative factors in habitual miscarriage (Stray-Pederson and Lorentzyn-Styr, 1977). However, these organisms were found only in the endometrium of postabortal women and did not appear in the serological screening of patients. Colonization by this organism may be a result of ascending infection rather than the cause of the miscarriage. Further studies are needed before other microbiological factors can be causally associated with repeated fetal wastage.

Immunological Factors

The immune system is a complex, integrated system that has evolved to protect the individual from non-self tissue, yet the maternal immune system does not normally react adversely to the conceptus. The embryo, fetus, and trophoblast are natural immunological targets due to their paternally inherited gene products and tissue-specific differentiation antigens (Hill and Anderson, 1988b). An immunological etiology for habitual abortion has been proposed for many couples with an otherwise unexplained etiology for their reproductive failure. The principal mechanisms that have been proposed to explain immune rejection of the engrafted conceptus are listed in Table 14–2.

Lack of Suppressor Cells and Suppressor Factors

A deficiency of immune suppressor cells in the endometrium and decidua have been proposed to cause spontaneous abortion. Support for this theory comes from a study where endometrial curettings were performed on failing chemical pregnancies in humans after in vitro fertilization and embryo transfer (Nebel, 1984). A mononu-

TABLE 14–2.

Immunological Mechanisms Implicated in Spontaneous Abortion

Lack of suppressor cells and suppressor factors
Induction of major histocompatibility antigen (MHC) expression
Lack of blocking factors
Antibodies to phospholipids
Soluble products of activated immune cells

clear cell infiltrate deficient in suppressor cells was seen in the curettings. Suppressor cells have also been reported to be decreased in the decidua of women with a missed abortion (Daya et al., 1985). Significantly increased helper/suppressor lymphocyte ratios have been found in endometrial biopsy specimens from nonpregnant women with a history of recurrent abortion compared with fertile controls (Xu et al. 1988). Macrophage activation and function, normally suppressed in pregnancy, have been observed to be enhanced in the decidua from women with spontaneous abortion (Hill, 1989). Further studies are needed before causal relationships can be ascribed, because these results may represent the effect of abortion rather than cause.

Induction of Major Histocompatibility Antigen Expression

The major histocompatibility complex is the complex of genes on chromosome 6 that is responsible for production of human leukocyte antigens (HLA), some complement components, and immune response genes. Human leukocyte antigen comprises the MHC in humans. Human leukocyte antigens are antigens that determine immunological compatibility of tissues and organs. Immunological recognition of these antigens can lead to graft rejection. Class I MHC antigens encoded by the HLA region A, B, and C are important mediators of rejection responses by cytotoxic T lymphocytes. Class II antigens, encoded by HLA-D, present antigens to helper T lymphocytes and initiate immune responses.

The lack of class I MHC antigens on syncytotrophoblast, together with the atypical nature of HLA antigen expression on cytotrophoblast and the complete absence of Class II MHC determinants on any form of trophoblast, precludes trophoblast involvement as either a classical immunogen for maternal sensitization or a target for MHC-directed cytotoxic T cells (Billington,

1988). Class I MHC antigen expression, however, may be induced in trophoblast by the T-helper lymphocyte product interferon-γ, or IFN-γ (Anderson and Berkowitz, 1985). T-helper cells predominate in the endometrium of some women with recurrent abortion, and on activation, these cells can secrete IFN-γ (Steeg et al., 1982). This could then induce class I MHC antigen expression, providing a mechanism for cytotoxic T-cell attack, ending in abortion.

Lack of Blocking Factors

A presumed role for blocking of potentially deleterious maternal immune rejection responses by maternal antibodies produced against fetal-trophoblast antigens has been proposed by many investigators to explain the success of normal pregnancy. The first hypothesis concerned HLA within the MHC. This hypothesis was based on the observation that animal reproductive performance was enhanced when there were mating pair differences in MHC antigens (Beer and Billingham, 1977). These animal studies prompted investigation into possible parental HLA sharing and potential fetal HLA homozygosity as a cause of recurrent miscarriage in humans. Initial reports based on limited sample sizes suggested that this association was valid. These observations, together with the report of an uncharacterized pregnancy serum factor–inhibiting lymphocyte proliferation in mixed lymphocyte culture (MLC; Rocklin et al., 1976), led to the concept that HLA heterozygosity is necessary for the production of blocking factors (presumably antibodies), which must be developed for successful pregnancy, and that a lack of blocking factors are associated with habitual abortion (Rocklin et al., 1976; Beer et al., 1981; Unander and Olding, 1983; McIntyre et al., 1983; Mowbray et al., 1983). However, more recent HLA typing studies from larger study groups indicate no clear association between sharing of specific HLA alleles and recurrent miscarriage (reviewed by Risk and Johnson, 1989). Furthermore, HLA data from a closed community of Hutterites also indicate that MHC heterozygosity is not an essential requirement for successful gestation (Ober et al., 1983). Similarly, many inbred animal strains have been successfully bred for generations.

Another potential HLA-linked antigen system has been proposed to explain habitual abortion. This antigen system has been termed the *trophoblast-lymphocyte cross-reactivity* (TLX) *antigen system*. These antigens were originally derived from polyclonal rabbit antisera that cross-reacted with polymorphic antigens on peripheral blood lymphocytes and trophoblast (Faulk et al., 1978). It has been proposed that HLA antigen sharing is a marker for TLX antigen homozygosity and that such a situation inhibits the generation of blocking factors as determined by MLC, which are believed necessary for successful pregnancy. The importance of the TLX antigen system remains undefined and theoretical. In fact, the clinical relevance of TLX in reproductive failure may have been overestimated, as recent evidence indicates that TLX is simply the complement receptor (Purcell et al., 1989). Moreover, serum factors that inhibit MLC responses are an inconsistent phenomena because blocking activity is not always detected in the serum of women with normal pregnancy (Rocklin et al., 1982). The role for any blocking immunoglobulin effector in pregnancy is also seriously challenged by the fact that normal pregnancy can occur in both B cell–deficient agammaglobulinemic mice and women (Rodger, 1985). Therefore, current evidence indicates that neither HLA heterozygosity nor the production of blocking antibodies are necessary for successful pregnancy. Most investigators who have reported that the lack of blocking antibody is a cause of habitual abortion have compared groups of women with multiple miscarriages to those with multiple live births. This comparison could represent differences that are the result of multiple live births rather than the cause of habitual abortion (Sargent et al., 1988).

Antiphospholipid Antibodies

Antiphospholipid antibodies are autoantibodies detected by standard tests for syphilis, lupus anticoagulant test (activated partial thromboplastin time, Russell's viper venom), or an enzyme-linked immunoabsorbent assay for anticardiolipin antibody. These autoantibodies have been associated with both venous and arterial thrombosis, thrombocytopenia, and poor obstetrical outcome, including abortion. Thrombosis occurs in 25% to 33% of people with the lupus anticoagulant (Gastineau et al., 1985) and in more than 75% of patients with high levels of IgG anticardiolipin antibodies (Harris et al., 1986).

The mechanism of fetal loss in women with these autoantibodies is unclear, although placental vessel thrombosis resulting in infarction and placental insufficiency have been proposed. The suggested mechanism is that antiphospholipid antibodies cause increased platelet aggregation secondary to decreased prostacyclin production and increased thromboxane by vascular endothelium (Carreras et al., 1981). However, fetal vessel thrombosis and placental infarction are inconsistently found in the placenta of an aborted fetus from women with antiphospholipid antibodies (Rustin et al., 1987).

Retrospective studies associate the lupus anticoagulant and anticardiolipin antibodies with recurrent fetal loss (Lockshin et al., 1985, 1987; Lubbe et al., 1983; Branch et al., 1985). Affected women usually have high titers of antibodies over an extended period of time (Lockshin et al., 1987). Therefore, the diagnosis of antiphospholipid-related fetal loss should be based on high-titer antibodies determined on more than one occasion several weeks apart (Harris, 1988). Prospective collaborative studies are needed to determine the antibody levels and isotopes associated with fetal loss, as well as the overall importance of antiphospholipid antibodies in recurrent reproductive failure.

Soluble Products of Activated Immune Cells

Advances in immunology have enabled studies on the effects of soluble mediators of immuno-logical responses, collectively termed *cytokines,* on reproductive cells and their functions (Anderson and Hill, 1988). Cytokines are divided into products of activated macrophage-monocyte populations called *monokines* and those of activated lymphocytes called *lymphokines.* Many of these cytokines have been shown to interfere with reproductive processes in vitro, including embryo development (Hill et al., 1987) and trophoblast proliferation (Berkowitz et al., 1988), and have been proposed to be a potential mechanism for immunological infertility and recurrent spontaneous abortion (Hill and Anderson, 1988c). The proposed model is illustrated in Figure 14–7. These factors may achieve cytotoxic effects directly and indirectly in a nonpaternal/fetal-MHC restricted manner, since macrophages do not require MHC antigens for activation, and T-helper lymphocytes can become activated without target cell MHC antigens being involved if they are programmed by activated macrophages. Therefore, maternal macrophages residing in the decidua of susceptible women may become activated by trophoblast antigens, sperm antigens, or both, expressed on either the embryo or early trophoblast (Hill and Anderson, 1988b) or stimulated by microbial or viral antigens (Hill and Anderson, 1988c). On macrophage activation, monokines, such as interleukin-1 Il-1 and tumor-necrosing factor, and other soluble factors, such as free oxy-

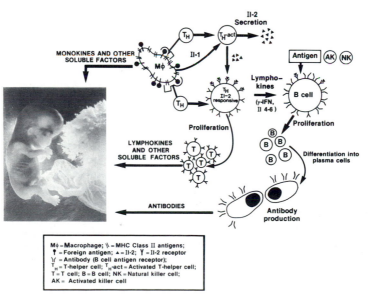

FIG 14–7.
Cellular immunity for abortion.

gen radicals, hormones (e.g., prostaglandins), chemicals (e.g., hydrogen peroxide), and enzymes, that could have detrimental effects on early pregnancy may also be released (Anderson and Hill, 1988).

Such monokines as Il-1 play a pivotal role in initiating an immune response by stimulating the release of interleukin-2, a lymphokine secreted by Il-1-activated T lymphocytes. Interleukin-2, in turn, can stimulate the proliferation and differentiation of other lymphocytes causing the secretion of other cytokines. Some of these cytokines either directly or indirectly through activation of other cytocidal mediators (natural killer cells, cytotoxic cells, and antibodies) may have toxic effects on the developing conceptus. Preliminary studies suggest that trophoblast and sperm antigens may stimulate macrophages and lymphocytes from some women with habitual abortion to secrete soluble factors that are toxic to either embryos, trophoblast, or both (Hill et al., 1989). Further studies are needed before the clinical relevance of these factors are verified. Not all cytokines are necessarily detrimental to reproductive efficiency. Many cytokines are potential growth factors and may be involved in facilitating immune regulation at the maternal-fetal interface effecting the continual maintenance and ultimate success of pregnancy.

Immunotherapy for Recurrent Abortion

Two forms of immunotherapy have been devised for recurrent abortion: immunostimulation and immunosuppression. The rationale for immunotherapy involving immunostimulation was originally based on the concept that immunological recurrent abortion was due to maternal immunological recognition abnormalities in response to pregnancy. The foundation supporting the use of this form of immunotherapy is based on three suppositions: (1) that there is an antifetal maternal cell-mediated immune response that develops in all pregnancies that must be blocked; (2) blocking antibodies develop in all successful pregnancies; and (3) in the absence of blocking antibodies, maternal rejection (i.e., abortion) of the fetus occurs (Sargent et al., 1988). As previously described, the validity of these assertions are as yet unproved. Many immunization regimens, consisting of paternal (Beer et al., 1985) or third-party unmatched leukocytes (Taylor and Faulk, 1981), trophoblast vesicle fluid (Johnson et al., 1988), or donor seminal plasma (Coulam, 1988)

have been devised and implemented in uncontrolled clinical trials, with purported success being attributed to induction of maternal antibodies blocking fetal rejection. This experimental effect has not been conclusively demonstrated to be attributable to an antibody. Only one controlled trial has been reported to date, indicating 78% success in recurrent aborting women immunized with paternal leukocytes compared with 37% in recurrent aborting women receiving their own leukocytes (Mowbray et al., 1985). The validity of the placebo effect in this study, however, remains obscure since those women receiving their own leukocytes did not develop any inflammation at the injection site, unlike those receiving paternal leukocytes. This is potentially very important, because supportive psychotherapy alone has claimed similarly high success rates (Stray-Pederson and Stray-Pederson, 1988). Studies to date have not eliminated the possibility that the potential benefit of this form of therapy may be due not to the generation of antibodies but to a phenomena known as *antigenic competition*. This is the situation in which one T lymphocyte–dependent antigen can block the response to another (Roit, 1980). Thus, the maternal host may not be able to mount an immune response that is detrimental to the conceptus due to down regulation caused by the previous antigenic challenge (i.e., antigenic leukocytes).

Immunostimulation procedures are not necessarily innocuous. Anaphylaxis and serum sickness may be produced by multiple administrations of foreign antigens. Another potential hazard is the transmission of non-A, non-B hepatitis, human immunodeficiency virus, or other viruses. ABO and other blood group incompatibilities are also potential concerns. Graft-vs.-host reactions in immunized women are other possibilities. Physicians should also be aware of the potential for severe fetal growth retardation in offspring of immunized women (Menge and Beer, 1985).

The rationale for immunotherapy involving immunosuppression is based on the concept that an adverse maternal immune response, either humoral (involving autoantibodies) or cellular (involving cytokines), contributes to reproductive failure. Immunosuppressive therapy has been recommended for women with recurrent abortion attributable to antiphospholipid antibodies. Treatment with corticosteroids to abrogate adverse autoantibody production and low-dose aspirin to inhibit thromboxane may theoretically enhance pregnancy outcome. Patient selection criteria for treatment, optimal timing, and dosage regimens remain to be determined. As yet, there have been no appropriately controlled trials reported for evaluating therapy. Other immunosuppressive agents are needed because corticosteroids may have serious adverse side effects not only for the woman receiving such medication but for her developing conceptus as well.

Treatment modalities are needed for habitual abortion. The cure, however, must be scientifically well founded and more innocuous than the disease. A thorough understanding of the potential immunological mechanisms of reproductive failure are prerequisite before successful strategies of prevention can be formulated. Until these mechanisms are firmly elucidated and the safety and efficacy of immunotherapy (either stimulation or suppression) are clearly and scientifically established by concomitant multicenter randomized double-blind placebo and unrelated antigen-controlled trials and birth registries to follow possible adverse sequelae, the routine use of immunotherapy is inadvisable.

Miscellaneous Factors

Chronic medical illnesses, especially those involving compromised blood flow such as cardiac and renal disease, have been associated with abortion. Cause and effect mechanisms are difficult to affirm, although any condition compromising placental blood flow could lead to pregnancy failure.

Environmental pollutants have been implicated in reproductive failure. Heavy metal toxicity, carbon tetrachloride, trichoroethylene, and benzene are all associated with spontaneous abortion. Drugs such as folic acid antagonists, inhalation anesthetics, ethanol, and nicotine are also factors for miscarriage.

Excess alcohol consumption is an especially vibrant issue in today's society, with many recent studies showing direct susceptibility of the early embryo to the effects of alcohol. The most prominent study showing a statistical increase in miscarriage rates was noted in a large series where twice the rate of abortions occurred in women who had more than two drinks per week (overall minimum of 1 oz per week; Kline et al., 1980). It was assumed by the authors that alcohol may be a chronic fetal poison inducing miscarriage. The threshold level for producing such an effect was

low and may be debatable. Ernhart et al. (1987) showed that the critical period for alcohol teratogenicity was the time of conception, but the threshold to produce such an effect was much higher than the Kline study: 3 or more oz of absolute alcohol daily (six drinks per day).

Smoking has also been found to increase the risk of spontaneous abortions. Women who smoke 10 cigarettes daily have a tendency to have more abortions (Hemminki et al., 1983). However, assignment of adverse fetal effects to the use of one drug or behavioral characteristic is difficult. Patients who drink two or more alcoholic drink per day tend to be heavy smokers of cigarettes and marijuana. The effects of these various chemical teratogens on reproductive failure are diverse (Kurzel and Cetrullo, 1985).

Ionizing radiation has been associated with spontaneous abortion, although the critical dose necessary for this effect is not well elucidated. There is no scientific evidence substantiating the claim that video display terminals or microwave ovens cause spontaneous abortion.

Abnormalities of placentation have been associated with second trimester pregnancy loss. These rare abnormalities are most commonly due to circumvallate placenta and placenta marginata.

DIAGNOSTIC ASSESSMENT

Evaluation of the couple with recurrent abortion may be initiated after the second miscarriage and certainly after the third spontaneous loss. Couples should be advised to delay conception for at least two menstrual cycles after experiencing a miscarriage. During this interim, preconception assessment of potential etiologies for pregnancy loss can be initiated. A general history including past medical, surgical, genetic, and psychological histories should be obtained. Description and sequence of all prior pregnancies including reports on the histological assessment of prior abortuses is important. A history of uterine instrumentation, pelvic infection, or in utero exposure to DES, drugs, radiation, and environmental pollutants is important. Family history of reproductive difficulties may also be important.

A general physical examination should be performed looking for signs of metabolic illness. Particular attention should be given to the pelvic examination. The cervix should be evaluated for anatomical abnormalities associated with DES exposure, lacerations, and infections. Uterine enlargement or irregularity should also be noted.

Laboratory studies are warranted, depending on the history and physical findings. A complete blood cell count and erythrocyte sedimentation rate may be indicated, as well as blood chemistries including glucose level and a urinalysis. Thyroid function studies should be obtained. The woman's blood type and Rh factor should also be determined. TORCH (toxoplasmosis, rubella, cytomegalovirus, and herpes simplex) titers may be indicated. A peripheral blood karotype should be obtained on both partners. A timed luteal phase endometrial biopsy should be obtained, and if endometrial asychrony is found and confirmed on a subsequent biopsy, serum prolactin level and androgen profile (testosterone, dehydroepiandrosterone sulfate) are warranted. Endocervical and urine cultures for mycoplasma may be in order. Repeat cultures following therapy should be performed to ensure eradication. Immunological assessment includes antiphospholipid antibody determination (anticardiolipid antibody and activated partial thromboplastin time or Russell's viper venom) and maternal serum and midcycle cervical mucous collection for antisperm antibodies. The latter is warranted since sperm antigens are expressed on the developing embryo and early trophoblast. Embryotoxic and trophoblastoxic factor determinations are experimental and therefore are neither substantially nor currently available. Assessment of potential HLA sharing or MLC results are unnecessary as previously discussed. Hysterosalpingography may be indicated, followed by hysteroscopy and laparoscopy should an anatomical defect be suspected.

Once a pregnancy is established, close monitoring is prudent. Serial progesterone determinations in the luteal phase of a conception cycle and early gestation have been recommended, but their usefulness is controversial. Serial quantitive β-hCG determinations followed by ultrasound monitoring for fetal viability are reassuring measures. Later in pregnancy, fetal assessment includes maternal serum α-fetoprotein determination. Chorionic villi biopsy or amniocentesis may also be warranted. Should another miscarriage occur, phenotypic, cytogenetic, and histological analyses of the abortus are necessary. Above all, a caring and supporting attitude on the part of the physician toward the couple experiencing habitual abortion is essential in helping them through the trying process of evaluation and either the success or failure of a subsequent pregnancy.

PROGNOSIS

The prognosis for a couple with recurrent abortion subsequently delivering a normal child depends on the etiology of their miscarriages. Two studies have determined the prognosis for a normal child when the etiology of recurrent abortion was presumed to be due to genetic, müllerian, endocrine, or unknown factors. These studies do not delineate the potential increase in prognostic rates for potential immune causes of recurrent abortion. Tho et al. (1982) studied 110 couples from 1968 through 1977 and selected those with poor reproductive performance on the basis of (1) two or more histologically documented abortions and (2) one or more abortions associated with a phenotypically abnormal child. Harger et al. (1983) studied 155 couples from 1977 through 1981 who had had at least two or more consecutive pregnancy losses, with at least three occurring in 106 women.

In the Tho et al. (1982) study, a genetic etiology was found in 25% of the cases, and this had the poorest prognosis. Müllerian anomalies were found in 15%, with an overall success rate of term pregnancy following surgical correction of 60%. The best prognosis was in the "endocrine" group found to have retarded endometrial development; this group represented 23%, with an overall success rate of 91% following hormonal supplementation.

In the Harger et al. (1983) study, 15.4% of the couples demonstrated chromosomal anomalies, and in 27% there was a uterine morphological abnormality. The incidence of an abnormal finding did not increase with repetitive abortions following the second abortion arguing in favor of starting an evaluation after the second miscarriage (Table 14–3). There was a high rate of abnormal antinuclear antibody titers in asymptomatic women in this study, however, antiphospholipid antibodies (anticardiopin antibodies lupus anticoagulant) were not ascertained. Also, a high rate of colonization with T-mycoplasma is reported, although a significant number of these patients who remained culture positive after treatment had suc-

TABLE 14–3.

Abnormal Laboratory Test Results Associated With Recurrent Pregnancy Losses*†

| | No. of Pregnancy Losses | | | | | | | |
| | ≥ 4 | | 3 | | 2 | | Total | |
Test	No.	%	No.	%	No.	%	No.	%
Karyotype	5/88	5.7	12/112	10.7	4/72	5.6	21/272	7.7
Hysterosalpingogram	8/30	27	11/45	24	11/37	30	30/112	27
Thyroid function	0/30		2/52	3.9	0/37		2/119	1.7
Antinuclear antibody	1/32	3.1	5/51	10	3/37	8.1	9/120	7.5
Cervical culture								
M. hominis	7/40	18	8/61	13	7/46	15	22/147	15
U. urealyticum	22/40	55	27/61	44	22/46	48	71/147	48

*Adapted from Harger JH, Archer DF, Marchese SG, et al: Etiology of recurrent pregnancy losses and outcome of subsequent pregnancies. *Obstet Gynecol* 1983; 62:574–581.
†Abnormal test result/total number of tests performed. The chance that a given diagnostic test will be abnormal does not increase linearly with an increasing number of pregnancy losses.

TABLE 14–4.

Relationship Between Apparent Cause of Pregnancy Losses and Prognosis of Subsequent Pregnancies*

| | Next Pregnancies | | Abortions | | Stillbirths | | Live Births | |
Abnormality	No.	%	No.	%	No.	%	No.	%
Cytogenetic (total)	18	100	4	25		0	14	78
Balanced translocation		8		2		0		6
X-chromosome mixoploidy		5		1		0		6
Pericentric inversion		3		1		0		2
Uterine (total)	15	100	3	20	2	13	10	67
Intrauterine synechiae		5		1		1		3
Subseptate or bicornuate		4		1		0		3
Other		6		1		1		4
Abnormal antinuclear antibody level	7	100	3	43		—	4	57
Cervical culture positive for U. urealyticum	4	100	11	27		0	29	73
Successful therapy		19		6		0		13
Unsuccessful therapy		7		1		0		6
Not treated		14		4		0		10

*Adapted from Harger JH, Archer DF, Marchese SG, et al: Etiology of recurrent pregnancy losses and outcome of subsequent pregnancies. *Obstet Gynecol* 1983; 62:574–581.

cessful pregnancies. The overall prognosis for subsequent live births was good if the diagnostic evaluation was normal (77%) or abnormal (71%; Table 14–4). A factor contributing to recurrent pregnancy loss was found in 68% of women with three or more losses, and diagnostic studies that gave the highest yield were hysterosalpingogram, peripheral lymphocyte karyotypes, and cervical cultures for T-mycoplasma.

With the exception of inborn genetic errors in one or both partners of the recurrent aborting couple, the probability of a subsequent normal pregnancy and delivery may be as high as 60% to 90%. This is both clinically important and relevant to the practicing physician evaluating such couples, especially since many of the presumed etiologies and treatment modalities for pregnancy failure remain controversial.

REFERENCES

Alberman E, Elliott M, Creasy M, et al: Previous reproductive history in mothers presenting with spontaneous abortion. *Br J Obstet Gynecol* 1975; 82:366–373.

Anderson DJ, Berkowitz RS: Gamma-IFN enhance expression of Class I MHC antigens in the weakly HLA (+) human choriocarcinoma cell line BeWo, but does not induce MHC expression in the HLA-negative choriocarcinoma cell line jar. *J Immunol* 1985; 138: 2498.

Anderson DJ, Hill JA: Criteria for the use of lymphokines and monokines in reproductive test systems. *Fertil Steril* 1987; 48:894.

Anderson DJ, Hill JA: Cell-mediated immunity in infertility. *Am J Reprod Immunol Microbiol* 1988; 17:22–30.

Barbieri RL, Evans S, Kistner R: Danazol in the treatment of endometriosis: Analysis of 100 cases with a four year followup. *Fertil Steril* 1982; 37:737–746.

Barnes AB, Colton T, Gunderson J, et al: Fertility and outcome of pregnancy in women exposed *in utero* to diethylstilbestrol. *N Engl J Med* 1980; 302:609–613.

Batzer FR: Hormonal evaluation of early pregnancy. *Fertil Steril* 1980; 34:1–13.

Beer AE, Billingham RE: Histocompatibility gene polymorphisms and maternal-fetal interaction. *Transplant Proc* 1977; 9:1393–1401.

Beer AE, Quebbeman JF, Ayers JWI, et al: Major histocompatibility complex antigens, maternal and paternal immune responses and chronic habitual abortions in humans. *Am J Obstet Gynecol* 1981; 141:987.

Beer AE, Semprini AE, Zhu X, et al: Pregnancy outcome in human couples with recurrent spontaneous abortions: 1) HLA antigen profiles; 2) HLA antigen sharing; 3) Female serum MLR blocking factors; and 4) Paternal leukocyte immunization. *Exp Clin Immunogenet* 1985; 2:137.

Berkowitz RS, Hill JA, Kurtz CB, et al: Effects of products of activated leukocytes (lymphokines and monokines) on the growth of malignant trophoblast cells *in vitro*. *Am J Obstet Gynecol* 1988; 158:199–203.

Billington WD: Maternal-fetal interaction in normal human pregnancy, in Johnson PM (ed): *Clinical Immunology and Allergy*. London, Bailliere Tindall, 1988, pp 527–549.

Boue J, Boue A: Chromosomal analysis of two consecutive abortions in each of 43 females. *Hum Genet* 1973; 19:275–280.

Boue J, Boue A, Lazar P: Retrospective and prospective epidemiologic studies of 1,500 karyo-typed spontaneous human abortions. *Teratology* 1975; 11–12:11–26.

Boue JG, Boue A, Lazar P, et al: Outcome of pregnancies following a spontaneous abortion with chromosomal anomalies. *Am J Obstet Gynecol* 1973; 116:806–812.

Branch DW, Scott JR, Kochenour NK, et al: Obstetric complications associated with the lupus anticoagulant. *N Engl J Med* 1985; 313:1322–1326.

Buttram VS: Mullerian anomalies and their management. *Fertil Steril* 1983; 40:159–163.

Byrne J, Warburton D, Kline J, et al: Morphology of early fetal deaths and their chromosomal characteristics. *Teratology* 1985; 32:297–315.

Cadkin AV, Sabbagha RE: Abnormal pregnancy, in *Diagnostic Ultrasound Applied to Obstetrics and Gynecology*. New York, Harper & Row, Publishers, 1980, pp 149–164.

Carr BR, MacDonald PC, Simpson ER: The role of lipoproteins in the regulation of progesterone secretion by the human corpus luteum. *Fertil Steril* 1982; 38:303–311.

Carreras LO, Defreyn G, Machin SJ, et al: Arterial thrombosis, intrauterine death and the "lupus" anticoagulant: Detection of immunoglobulin interfering with prostacycline formation. *Lancet* 1981; 1:244–246.

Charles D, Edwards WE: Infectious complications of cervical cerclage. *Am J Obstet Gynecol* 1981; 141:1065–1071.

Chartier M, Roger M, Barrat J, et al: Measurement of plasma human chorionic gonadotropin (hCG) and B hCG activities in the late luteal phase: Evidence for the occurrence of spontaneous menstrual abortions in infertile women. *Fertil Steril* 1979; 31:134–135.

Chez R: Proceedings of the symposium, progesterone, progestins and fetal development. *Fertil Steril* 1978; 30:21–26.

Coulam CB: Treatment of recurrent spontaneous abortion. *Am J Reprod Immunol Microbiol* 1988; 17:149.

Crane JP, Wahl N: The role of maternal diabetes in repetitive spontaneous abortion. *Fertil Steril* 1981; 36:477–479.

Creasy R: The cytogenetics of spontaneous abortion in humans, in Beard RW, Sharp F (eds): *Early Pregnancy Loss*. New York, Springer-Verlag New York, 1988, pp 293–304.

Daly DC, Jaban N, Walters C, et al: Hysteroscopic resection of the uterine septum in the presence of a septate cervix. *Fertil Steril* 1983; 39:560–563.

Daya S, Burrows E: Progesterone profiles in luteal phase defect cycles and outcome of progesterone treatment in patients with recurrent abortion. *Am J Obstet Gynecol* 1988; 158:225–232.

Daya S, Clark DA, Devlin MC, et al: Preliminary characterization of two types of suppressor cells in the human uterus. *Fertil Steril* 1985; 44:778–785.

DiZerega GS, Hodgen GD: Luteal phase dysfunction infertility: A sequel to aberrant folliculogenesis. *Fertil Steril* 1981; 35:489.

Dmowski WP, Cohen MR: Antigonadotropin (danazol) in treatment of endometriosis. *Am J Obstet Gynecol* 1978; 130:41.

Downs KA, Gibson M: Clomiphene citrate for luteal phase defects. *Fertil Steril* 1983; 40:466–468.

Drake TS, O'Brien WF, Ramwell PW, et al: Peritoneal fluid thromboxane B2 and 6-keto prostaglandin F$_{1-alpha}$ in endometriosis. *Am J Obstet Gynecol* 1981; 140:401–404.

Edmonds DK, Lindsay KI, Miller JF, et al: Early embryonic mortality in women. *Fertil Steril* 1982; 38:447–453.

Elias S, LeBeau M, Simpson JL, et al: Chromosome analysis of ectopic human conceptuses. *Am J Obstet Gynecol* 1981; 141:698–703.

Elles RG, Williamson R, Neazi M, et al: Absence of maternal contamination of chrionic villi used for fetal-gene analyses. *N Engl J Med* 1983; 308:1433–1435.

Ernhart CB, Sokol RJ, Martier S, et al: Alcohol teratogenicity in the human: A detailed assessment of specificity, critical period, and threshold. *Am J Obstet Gynecol* 1987; 156:33–39.

Faulk WP, Temple A, Louins RE, et al: Antigens of human trophoblast: A working hypothesis for their role in normal and abnormal pregnancies. *Proc Natl Acad Sci USA* 1978; 75:1947–1951.

Fitzsimmons J, Wapner R, Jackson L: Repeated pregnancy loss. *Am J Med Genet* 1983; 16:7–13.

Fralkow PJ: Thyroid antibodies, Down's syndrome and maternal age. *Nature* 1967; 214:1253–1254.

Freedman JM: Genetic disease in the offspring of older fathers. *Obstet Gynecol* 1981; 57:745–749.

Gastineau DA, Kazimer FS, Nichols WL, et al: Lupus anticoagulant: An analysis of the clinical and laboratory feature of 219 cases. *Am J Hematol* 1985; 19:265–275.

Goldzeiher JW: Double-blind trial of a progestinin habitual abortion. *JAMA* 1964; 188:651–654.

Green LK, Harris RE: Uterine anomalies: Frequency of diagnosis and obstetric complications. *Obstet Gynecol* 1976; 47:427–429.

Hammond MG, Talbert LM: Clomiphene citrate therapy of the infertile woman with low luteal phase progesterone levels. *Obstet Gynecol* 1982; 59:275–279.

Harger JH: Comparison of success and morbidity in cervical cerclage procedures. *Obstet Gynecol* 1980; 56:543–548.

Harger JH, Archer DF, Marchese SG, et al: Etiology of recurrent pregnancy losses and outcome of subsequent pregnancies. *Obstet Gynecol* 1983; 62:574–581.

Harris EN: Clinical and immunological significance of antiphospholipid antibodies, in Beard RW, Sharp F (eds): *Early Pregnancy Loss: Mechanisms and Treatment*. New York, Springer-Verlag New York, 1988; pp 43–65.

Harris EN, Chan JKH, Asherson RA: Thrombosis, recurrent fetal loss and thrombocytopenia: Predictive valve of the anticardiolipin antibody test. *Arch Intern Med* 1986; 146:2153–2159.

Harris MJ, Poland BJ, Dill FJ: Triploidy in 40 human spontaneous abortuses: Assessment of phenotype in embryos. *Obstet Gynecol* 1981; 57:600–606.

Heinonen OP, Slone D, Monson RR, et al: Cardiovascular birth defects and antenatal exposure to female sex hormones. *N Engl J Med* 1977; 196:67–70.

Hemminki K, Mutanen P, Saloniemi I: Smoking and the occurrence of congenital malformations and spontaneous abortions: Multivariate analysis. *Am J Obstet Gynecol* 1983; 145:61.

Herbst AL, Hubby MM, Azizi F, et al: Reproductive and gynecologic surgical experience in diethystilbestrol-exposed daughters. *Fertil Steril* 1981; 141:1019–1028.

Heritage DW, English SC, Young RB, et al: Cytogenetics of recurrent abortions. *Fertil Steril* 1978; 29:414–417.

Hertig AT, Rock J, Adams EC, et al: Thirty-four fertilized human ova, good, bad and indifferent, recovered from 210 women of known fertility. *Pediatrics* 1959; 23:202–211.

Hill JA: Macrophage phagocytic function in normal pregnancy and spontaneous abortion [abstract]. Presented at the Society for Gynecologic Investigation, San Diego, March 1989.

Hill JA, Anderson DJ: The embryo as an immunologic target in infertility and recurrent abortion, in Mather S, Fredericks CW (eds): *Perspectives in Immunoreproduction: Conception and Contraception*. New York, Hemisphere Publishing Corp, 1988a, pp 261–267.

Hill JA, Anderson DJ: Immunological mechanisms of female infertility, in Johnson PM (ed): *Clinical Immunology and Allergy*. Bailliere Tindall, London, 1988b, pp 551–575.

Hill JA, Anderson DJ: Cell-mediated immune mechanisms in recurrent spontaneous abortion, in Talwar GP (ed): *Contraceptive Research for Today and the Nineties,* New York, Springer-Verlag New York, 1988c, p 171.

Hill JA, Haimovici FR, Anderson DJ: Products of activated lymphocytes and macrophages inhibit mouse embryo development *in vitro. J Immunol* 1987; 139:2250–2254.

Hill JA, Haimovici F, Schiff I, et al: Reproductive antigens (sperm and trophoblast) stimulate the production of embryo and trophoblast toxic factors in women with recurrent spontaneous abortion [abstract]. Soc Gynecol Invest. San Diego, March 1989.

Horne HW, Kundsin RB, Kosasa TS: The role of *Mycoplasma* infection in human reproductive failure. *Fertil Steril* 1974; 25:380–388.

Jansen RPS: Spontaneous abortion incidence in the treatment of infertility. *Am J Obstet Gynecol* 1982; 143:452–473.

Johnson PM, Chia KV, Hart CA, et al: Trophoblast membrane transfusion for unexplained recurrent miscarriage. *Br J Obstet Gynecol* 1988; 95:342–347.

Jones HW: Reproductive impairment and the malformed uterus. *Fertil Steril* 1981; 26:137–148.

Katz Z, Lancet M, Skornik J, et al: Teratogenicity of Progestogens given during the first trimester of pregnancy. *Obstet Gynecol* 1985; 65:775.

Kaufman RH, Adam E, Bender G, et al: Upper genital tract changes and pregnancy outcome in offspring exposed *in utero* to diethystilbestrol. *Am J Obstet Gynecol* 1980; 137:299–308.

Keller DW, Wiest WH, Askin FB, et al: Pseudocorpus luteum insufficiency: A local defect of progesteronee action on endometrial stroma. *Fertil Steril* 1979; 48:127–132.

Khudr G: Cytogenetics of habitual abortion: A review. *Obstet Gynecol Surg* 1974; 29:299–310.

Kim HJ, Ksu LYF, Paduc S, et al: Cytogenetics of fetal wastage. *N Engl J Med* 1975; 293:844–847.

Kistner RW, Patton GW: Endoscopy, in Kistner RW, Patton GW (eds): *Atlas of Infertility Surgery.* Boston, Little, Brown & Co, 1975a, pp 21–44.

Kistner RW, Patton GW: Surgery of the uterus, in Kistner RW, Patton GW (eds): *Atlas of Infertility Surgery.* Little, Brown & Co, Boston, 1975b, pp 65–93.

Kline J, Stein ZA, Shrout P, et al: Drinking during pregnancy and spontaneous abortion. *Lancet* 1980; 2:176.

Kurzel RB, Cetrullo CL: Chemical teratogenesis and reproductive failure. *Obstet Gynecol Surv* 1985; 40:397.

Lagrew D, Wilson EA, Jawad J: Determination of gestational age by serum concentrations of human chorionic gonadotropin. *Obstet Gynecol* 1983; 62:37–40.

Lockshin MD, Druzin MC, Goei S, et al: Antibody to cardiolipin as a predictor of fetal distress or death in pregnant patients with systemic lupus erythematosus. *N Engl J Med* 1985; 313:1322–1326.

Lockshin MD, Quamar T, Druzin MC, et al: Antibody to cardiolipin, lupus anticoagulant and fetal death. *J Rheumatol* 1987; 14:259–262.

Lubbe WF, Butler WS, Palmer SJ, et al: Fetal survival after prednisolone suppression of natal lupus anticoagulant. *Lancet* 1983; 1:1361–1363.

Ludmir J, Landon MB, Gabbe SG, et al: Management of the Diethylstilbestrol-exposed pregnant patient: A prospective study. *Am J Obstet Gynecol* 1987; 157:665–669.

Madore C, Hawes WE, Many F, et al: A study of the effects of induced abortion on subsequent pregnancy outcome. *Am J Obstet Gynecol* 1981; 139:516–521.

March CM, Israel R: Gestational outcome following hysteroscopic lysis of adhesions. *Fertil Steril* 1981; 36:455–459.

Marrs RP, Kletzky OA, Howard WF, et al: Disappearance of human chorionic gonadotropin and resumption of ovulation following abortion. *Am J Obstet Gynecol* 1979; 135:6, 731–736.

Marshall FF, Beisel DS: The association of uterine and renal anomalies. *Obstet Gynecol* 1978; 51:559–562.

McConnell HD, Carr DH: Recent advances in the cytogenetic study of human spontaneous abortions. *Obstet Gynecol* 1975; 45:547–552.

McIntyre JA, Faulk WP, Verhulst SJ, et al: Human trophoblast-lymphocyte cross-reactive (TLX) antigens define on alloantigen system. *Science* 1983; 222:1135–1137.

McShane P, Reilly RJ, Schiff I: Pregnancy outcomes following Tompkins metroplasty. *Fertil Steril* 1983; 40:190–194.

Menge A, Beer AE: The significance of human leukocyte antigen profiles in human infertility, recurrent abortion, and pregnancy disorders. *Fertil Steril* 1985; 43:693.

Michaels W, Thompson HO, Schreiber FR, et al: Ultrasound surveillance of the cervix during pregnancy in diethylstilbestrol-exposed offspring. *Obstet Gynecol* 1989; 73:230.

Michels VV, Medrano C, Venne VL, et al: Chromosome translocations in couples with multiple spontaneous abortions. *Am J Hum Genet* 1982, 34:507–513.

Mowbray JF, Gibbings C, Liddell H, et al: Controlled trial of treatment of recurrent spontaneous abortion by immunization with paternal cells. *Lancet* 1985; 1:941–943.

Mowbray JF, Gibbings CR, Sidgewick AS, et al: Effects of transfusion in women with recurrent spontaneous abortion. *Transplant Proc* 1983; 15:869–899.

Nebel C: Malimplantation: A cause of failure after IVF and ET. *Am J Reprod Immunol* 1984; 6:56.

Noyes RW, Hertig A, Rock J: Dating the endometrial biopsy. *Fertil Steril* 1950; 1:3.

Ober C, Martin AO, Simpson JL: Shared HLA antigens and reproductive performances among Hutterites. *Am J Hum Genet* 1983; 35:994–1004.

Poland BJ, Miller JR, Jones DC, et al: Reproductive counseling in patients who have had a spontaneous abortion. *Am J Obstet Gynecol* 1977, 127:685–691.

Purcell DFJ, Brown MA, Russell SM, et al: The cDNA cloning of human CD46, an antigen system incorporating TLX and MCP (abstract). Presented at the 4th International Congress of Reproductive Immunology, Kiel, FRG, July 1989.

Quagliarello J, Weiss G: Clomiphene citrate in the management of infertility associated with shortened luteal phases. *Fertil Steril* 1979; 31:373–377.

Rhodes GG, et al: The safety and efficacy of chorionic villus sampling for early prenatal diagnosis of cytogenetic abnormalities. *N Engl J Med* 1989; 320:609–617.

Risk JM, Johnson PM: Genetic studies of the MHC regimen in human recurrent spontaneous abortion, in Gill T, Wegman T (eds): *The Molecular and Cellular Immunobiology of the Maternal-Fetal Interface.* New York, Oxford University Press, 1989.

Rock JA, Guzeck DS, Sengos C, et al: The conservative surgical treatment of endometriosis: Evaluation of pregnancy success with respect to the extent of the disease as characterized using contemporary classification systems. *Fertil Steril* 1981; 35:131.

Rock JA, Jones HA: The clinical management of the double uterus. *Fertil Steril* 1977; 28:793–806.

Rocklin RE, Kitzmiller JL, Carpenter CB, et al: Maternal-fetal relation: Absence of an immunologic blocking factor from the serum of women with chronic abortions. *N Engl J Med* 1976; 295:1209–1213.

Rocklin RE, Kitzmiller JL, Garvoy MR: Maternal-fetal relation II: Further characterization of an immunologic blocking factor that develops during pregnancy. *Clin Immunol Immunopathol* 1982; 22:305.

Rodger JC: Lack of a requirement for a maternal humoral immune response to establish or maintain successful allogenic pregnancy. *Transplantation* 1985; 40:372–375.

Roit IM: *Essential Immunology.* Boston, Blackwell Scientific Publications, 1980, p 102.

Rosenberg SA, Luciano AA, Riddick DH: The luteal phase defect: The relative frequency of, and encouraging response to, treatment with vaginal progesterone. *Fertil Steril* 1980; 34:17–20.

Rustin MHA, Bull HA, Dowel DA: Presence of the lupus anticoagulant in patients with systemic lupus erythematosus does not cause inhibition of prostacycline production. *Thromb Haemost* 1987; 58:390.

St Michel P, DiZerega GS: Hyperprolactinemia and luteal phase dysfunction infertility. *Obstet Gynecol Surv* 1983; 38:248–254.

Sargent IL, Wilkins T, Redman CWG: Maternal immune responses to the fetus in early pregnancy and recurrent miscarriage. *Lancet* 1988; 2:1099–1104.

Schenker JS, Margalioth EJ: Intrauterine adhesions: An updated appraisal. *Fertil Steril* 1982; 37:593–610.

Schmidt G, Fowler WC, Talbert L, et al: Reproductive history of women exposed to diethylstilbestrol *in utero. Fertil Steril* 1980; 33:21–24.

Schoenbaum S, Monson RR, Stubblefield PG, et al: Outcome of delivery followed an induced or spontaneous abortion. *Am J Obstet Gynecol* 1980; 136:19–24.

Scott JR: Immunologic aspects of recurrent spontaneous abortion. *Fertil Steril* 1982; 38:301–302.

Seegar-Jones G, Maffezzoli RD, Strott CA, et al: Pathophysiology of reproductive failure after clomiphene-induced ovulation. *Am J Obstet Gynecol* 1970; 108:847–867.

Semmens JP: Congenital anomalies of the female genital tract. *Obstet Gynecol* 1962; 19:328–350.

Siegler AM, Vallee RF: Therapeutic hysteroscopic procedures. *Fertil Steril* 1988; 50:685–701.

Simpson JL, Mills JL, Holmes LB, et al: Low fetal loss rates after ultrasound proved viability in early pregnancy. *JAMA* 1987; 258:2555–2557.

Soules MR, Hughes CL, Askel S, et al: The function of the corpus luteum of pregnancy and ovulatory dysfunction and luteal phase deficiency. *Fertil Steril* 1981; 36:31–40.

Steeg P, Moore RN, Johnson HM, et al: Regulation of murine macrophage in antigen expression by a lymphokine with immune interferon activity. *J Exp Med* 1982; 156:1780.

Stein Z: Early fetal loss. *Birth Defects* 1981; 17:95–111.

Stetten G, Rock JA: A paracentric chromosomal inversion associated with repeat pregnancy wastage. *Fertil Steril* 1983; 40:124–126.

Stray-Pedersen B, Lorentzen-Styr A-M: Uterine *Toxoplasma* infections and repeated abortions. *Am J Obstet Gynecol* 1977; 128:716–721.

Stray-Pedersen B, Stray-Pedersen S: Recurrent abortion: The role of psychotherapy, in Beard RW, Ship F (eds): *Early Pregnancy Loss: Mechanisms and Treatment*. New York, Springer-Verlag New York, 1988, pp 433–440.

Taylor C, Faulk WP: Prevention of recurrent abortion with keukocyte transfusions. *Lancet* 1981; 2:68–70.

Tho SPJ, Byrd JR, McDonough PG: Chromosome polymorphism in 110 couples with reproductive failure and subsequent pregnancy outcome. *Fertil Steril* 1982; 38:688–693.

Unander M, Olding LB: Habitual abortion: parental sharing of HLA antigen, absence of maternal blocking antibody and suppressing of maternal lymphocytes. *Am J Reprod Immunol* 1983; 4:171–178.

Verp MS, Simpson JL, Elias S, et al: Heritable aspects of uterine anomalies: I. Three familial aggregates with mullerian fusion anomalies. *Fertil Steril* 1983; 40:80–90.

Warburton D, Fraser FC: On the probability that a woman who has had a spontaneous abortion will abort in subsequent pregnancies. *Br J Obstet Gynaecol* 1961; 68:784–787.

Warburton D, Fraser FC: Spontaneous abortion risks in man: Data from reproductive histories collected in a medical genetics unit. *Hum Genet* 1964; 16:1–25.

Wentz AC: Endometrial biopsy in the evaluation of infertility. *Fertil Steril* 1980; 33:121–124.

Wilcox AJ, Weinberg CR, O'Connor JF, et al: Incidence of early loss of pregnancy. *N Engl J Med* 1988; 319:189–194.

Wright AW, Pollack A, Nicholson H, et al: Spontaneous abortion and diabetes mellitus. *Postgrad Med J* 1983; 59:295–298.

Xu C, Hill JA, Anderson DJ: Identification of T-lymphocyte subpopulations in normal and abnormal endometrial biopsies. Presented at the Society for Gynecologic Investigation, Atlanta, March 1987.

15

Gestational Trophoblastic Diseases

Ross S. Berkowitz, M.D.

Donald P. Goldstein, M.D.

Gestational trophoblastic diseases (GTDs) encompass a group of interrelated diseases including molar pregnancy, invasive mole, placental site trophoblastic tumor, and choriocarcinoma that have varying propensities for invasion and spread. Gestational trophoblastic tumors (GTTs) are one of the rare human malignancies that are highly curable even with widespread metastases (Goldstein and Berkowitz, 1982; Bagshawe, 1976). Although GTTs most commonly follow a molar pregnancy, they may ensue after any gestation. Important advances have been made in the diagnosis, treatment, and follow-up of patients with molar pregnancy and GTT. This chapter will review these advances and discuss basic principles in management based on the clinical experience accumulated at the New England Trophoblastic Disease Center (NETDC).

EPIDEMIOLOGY

The reported incidence of gestational trophoblastic disease varies dramatically in different regions of the world. The frequency of molar pregnancy in Asian countries is 7 to 10 times greater than the reported incidence in North America or Europe (Bracken, 1984). Although hydatidiform mole occurs in Taiwan in 1 per 125 pregnancies, the incidence of molar gestation in the United States is about 1 per 1,500 live births. Variations in the incidence rates of molar pregnancy result partly from differences between reporting hospital-based vs. population-based data.

The high incidence of molar pregnancy in some populations has been attributed to socioeconomic and nutritional factors. We have observed in a case-control study that the risk for complete molar pregnancy progressively increases with decreasing levels of consumption of dietary carotene (vitamin A precursor) and animal fat (Berkowitz et al., 1985). Parazzini et al. (1988) also reported from Italy that low carotene consumption was associated with GTD. Regions with a high incidence of vitamin A deficiency correspond to areas with a high frequency of molar pregnancy. Dietary factors such as carotene may therefore explain the regional variations in the incidence of molar pregnancy.

The risk of having a molar pregnancy also increases with advanced maternal age (Bracken, 1987). Women older than age 40 years have a 5- to 10-fold greater risk of having a molar gestation. Ova from older women may be more susceptible to abnormal fertilizations.

MOLAR PREGNANCY

Complete vs. Partial Molar Pregnancy

Pathologic and Chromosomal Features

Hydatidiform mole may be categorized as either complete or partial based on gross morphology, histopathology, and karyotype (Table 15–1).

Complete moles have no identifiable embryonic or fetal tissues. The chorionic villi have generalized swelling and diffuse trophoblastic hyperplasia (Fig 15–1). Complete moles usually have a 46,XX karyotype, and the molar chromosomes are derived entirely from paternal origin (Kajii and Ohama, 1977). Complete moles appear to arise from a defective ovum that has been fertilized by a haploid sperm, which then duplicates its own

TABLE 15–1.

Histopathologic and Chromosomal Features of Complete Versus Partial Molar Pregnancy

	Complete Mole	Partial Mole
Fetal or embryonic tissue	Absent	Present
Hydatidiform swelling of chorionic villi	Diffuse	Focal
Trophoblastic hyperplasia	Diffuse	Focal
Scalloping of chorionic villi	Absent	Present
Trophoblastic stromal inclusions	Absent	Present
Karyotype	46,XX (mainly); 46,XY	Triploid (mainly); diploid

chromosomes (Yamashita et al., 1979). Although most complete moles have a 46,XX chromosomal pattern, about 10% of complete moles have a 46,XY karyotype (Pattillo et al., 1981). The molar chromosomes in the 46,XY complete mole are also derived entirely from paternal origin.

Partial hydatidiform moles are characterized by the following pathologic features: (1) varying-sized chorionic villi with focal swelling and focal trophoblastic hyperplasia (Fig 15–2), (2) marked villous scalloping and prominent stromal trophoblastic inclusions, and (3) identifiable fetal or embryonic tissues (Szulman and Surti, 1978a). Partial moles generally have a triploid karyotype that

results from the fertilization of an apparently normal ovum by two sperm (Szulman and Surti, 1978b). When fetuses are identified with partial moles, they generally have stigmata of triploidy, including growth retardation and multiple congenital anomalies. However, infrequently, partial moles may have a diploid chromosomal pattern.

Complete Molar Pregnancy

Presenting Signs and Symptoms

Vaginal Bleeding.—Vaginal bleeding is the commonest presenting symptom in patients with complete mole, occurring in 97% of our patients

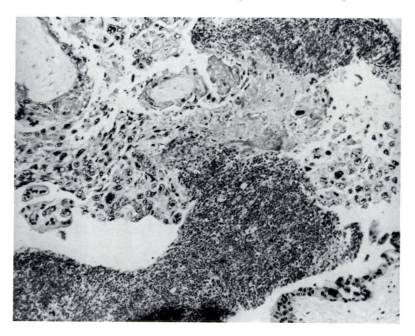

FIG 15–1.

Hydatidiform mole showing hyperplasia and anaplasia of epithelial elements. Note syncytial border of villus at lower right and "tissue culture" growth of pure trophoblast in center.

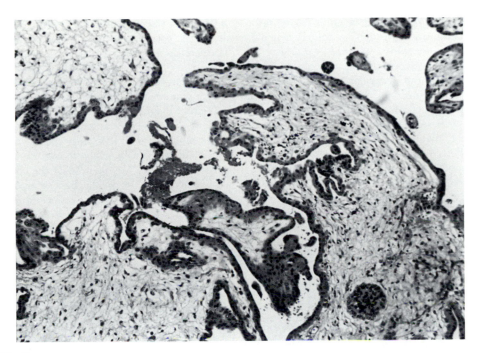

FIG 15—2.
Photomicrograph of partial mole demonstrating varying-sized chorionic villi with focal trophoblastic hyperplasia and villous scalloping and stromal trophoblastic inclusions.

(Berkowitz and Goldstein, 1981). The endometrial cavity may be expanded by large volumes of retained blood. When the intrauterine clots undergo oxidation and liquefaction, prune juice–like fluid may leak into the vagina.

Excessive Uterine Size.—The uterus is larger than expected for gestational age in one half of our patients with complete mole. The endometrial cavity may be expanded by both chorionic tissue and retained clot. Excessive uterine size is generally associated with markedly elevated human chorionic gonadotropin (hCG) levels because the uterus is expanded by chorionic tissues with hyperplastic trophoblast. Although excessive uterine size is one of the classic signs of complete molar pregnancy, one half of the patients with complete mole lack this clinical finding.

Preeclampsia.—Preeclamptic toxemia is diagnosed in 27% of our patients with complete mole. Although preeclampsia is often associated with hypertension and hyperreflexia, eclamptic convulsions rarely occur. Toxemia develops almost exclusively in patients with markedly elevated hCG values and excessive uterine enlarge-ment. Curry et al. (1975) also reported that 81% of their patients with molar pregnancy and toxemia had excessive uterine size. The diagnosis of hydatidiform mole should be considered in any patient who develops toxemia early in pregnancy.

Hyperemesis Gravidarum.—Hyperemesis requiring antiemetic or intravenous (IV) therapy (or both) occurred in 26% of our patients with complete mole. Infrequently, patients may develop severe electrolyte disturbances and require parenteral fluids. Hyperemesis develops primarily in patients with excessive uterine size and markedly elevated hCG levels. Although the etiology of hyperemesis is still debated, Masson et al. (1985) reported high serum hCG levels in the first trimester in women with nausea and vomiting.

Hyperthyroidism.—Hyperthyroidism was diagnosed in 7% of our patients with complete mole. These patients may present with tachycardia, warm skin, and tremor. The diagnosis of hyperthyroidism is confirmed by detecting elevated serum levels of free thyroxine (T_4) and triiodothyronine (T_3). If hyperthyroidism is suspected, β-adrenergic blockers should be administered prior to evacuation since anesthesia or surgery may precipitate thyroid storm. Thyroid storm may be manifested by hyperthermia, convulsion, atrial fibrillation, or cardiovascular collapse. β-Adrenergic blockers may prevent or rapidly reverse many of the metabolic and cardiovascular complications of thyroid storm.

Some investigators have suggested that hCG is the thyroid stimulator in patients with molar pregnancy (Nisula and Taliadouros, 1980). Positive correlations between serum hCG and serum total T_4 or total T_3 concentrations have been observed in some but not all studies. However, we measured thyroid function tests in 47 patients with complete mole and observed no significant correlation between serum hCG levels and free T_4

or T_3 index values (Amir et al., 1984). The identity of the thyrotropic factor in molar pregnancy has therefore not been clearly delineated.

Trophoblastic Embolization.—Two percent of patients with complete mole develop acute respiratory distress presumably due to trophoblastic embolization to the pulmonary vasculature (Kohorn, 1987). Patients may experience tachypnea and tachycardia in the recovery room after molar evacuation. Auscultation of the chest usually reveals diffuse rales, and chest roentgenogram may demonstrate bilateral pulmonary infiltrates (Fig 15–3). The signs and symptoms of respiratory distress generally resolve within 72 hours with cardiovascular and respiratory support.

Respiratory distress usually develops in pa-

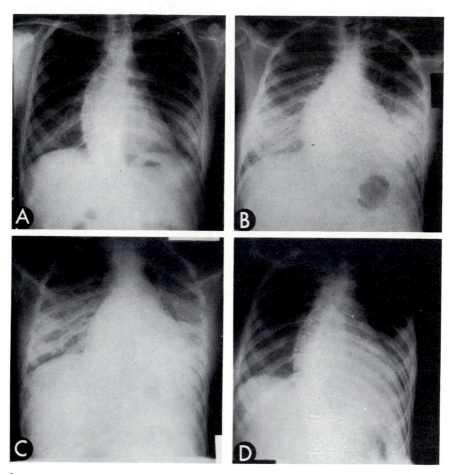

FIG 15–3.
A–D, chest roentgenograms of patient in whom trophoblastic embolization developed immediately following suction evacuation of molar pregnancy. The condition generally runs its course in 72 to 96 hours, as shown by complete clearing of both lung fields **(D).**

tients with markedly enlarged uteri. Twiggs et al. (1979) reported that 12 (27%) of 44 patients with a molar pregnancy of at least 16 weeks' size developed pulmonary complications.

Interestingly, Hankins et al. (1987) detected only minimal trophoblastic cells in the pulmonary arterial blood of six women undergoing evacuation of large molar pregnancies. None of these women developed significant pulmonary compromise or hemodynamic instability. Hankins et al. (1987) speculated that pulmonary compromise in patients with mole may be due at least in part to the cardiopulmonary changes induced by preeclampsia, anemia, hyperthyroidism, and vigorous transfusion therapy.

Theca Lutein Ovarian Cysts.—Prominent theca lutein ovarian cysts (more than 6 cm in diameter) develop in about one half of our patients with complete mole (Berkowitz and Goldstein, 1981). The cysts contain amber-colored or serosanguineous fluid and are usually bilateral and multilocular. Ovarian enlargement occurs almost exclusively in patients with markedly elevated hCG levels. The formation of theca lutein cysts may also be related to increased serum levels of prolactin (Osathanondh et al., 1986). Although theca lutein cysts are usually noted at presentation, they may also develop shortly after uterine evacuation. The mean time for spontaneous regression of theca lutein cysts is 8 weeks (Montz et al., 1987). Montz et al. (1987) reported that only 3 of 99 patients with theca lutein cysts developed acute surgical complications (torsion or rupture). If patients have marked symptoms of pelvic pressure, theca lutein cysts may be aspirated percutaneously under ultrasound control or during laparoscopy.

Partial Molar Pregnancy

Presenting Signs and Symptoms

Patients with partial molar pregnancy usually do not present with the clinical features that are characteristic of complete mole. These patients generally present with the signs and symptoms of missed or incomplete abortion. Eighty-one patients were followed with partial mole at the NETDC between January 1979 and August 1984 (Berkowitz et al., 1986a). Excessive uterine size and preeclampsia were noted in only three and two patients, respectively. Szulman and Surti (1982) also reported that only 9 (11%) of 81 pa-

tients with partial mole had excessive uterine enlargement. None of our patients had prominent theca lutein ovarian cysts, hyperthyroidism, or hyperemesis. Preevacuation hCG values were measured in 30 patients and exceeded 100,000 mIU/ml in only 2 (7%). The diagnosis of partial mole may be considered only after histologic review of curettage specimens.

Ultrasonography and Diagnosis of Hydatidiform Mole

Ultrasonography is sensitive and reliable in detecting a complete molar pregnancy. Because of marked swelling of the chorionic villi, complete mole produces a characteristic vesicular sonographic pattern. If a normal pregnancy is present, the gestational sac should be visualized from the 6th to the 10th week of gestation, and the fetal head should be identified after the 14th week of gestation. However, it may be difficult to distinguish an early mole from degenerating chorionic tissues. Molar chorionic villi in the first trimester may be too small to visualize on ultrasound. Human chorionic gonadotropin measurement at the time of sonography may help in differentiating a complete mole from a missed abortion.

Ultrasonography may also contribute to the diagnosis of partial molar pregnancy. Sixty-one of our patients with partial mole, who were clinically thought to have an incomplete or missed abortion, underwent a preevacuation pelvic ultrasound. Pelvic ultrasound suggested molar disease in 16 (26.2%) of these patients due to the presence of multiple cystic spaces in the placenta.

Natural History

Complete hydatidiform moles are well recognized to have a potential for developing uterine invasion or distant spread. Following molar evacuation, uterine invasion and metastasis occur in 15% and 4% of the patients, respectively (Berkowitz and Goldstein, 1986).

We reviewed 858 patients with complete mole to identify factors that predispose to postmolar tumor. At the time of presentation, 41% of the patients had the following signs of marked trophoblastic proliferation: hCG level more than 100,000 mIU/ml, uterine size more than gestational age, and theca lutein cysts more than 6 cm in diameter. After evacuation, 31% of these patients developed uterine invasion, and 8.8% developed metastases. The risk for persistent tumor is considerably less for patients who do not present with signs of marked trophoblastic growth. Following molar evacuation, only 3.4% of these patients developed invasion, and 0.6% developed metastases. Therefore, patients with complete moles and markedly elevated hCG levels and excessive uterine size are at increased risk of developing postmolar tumor and are categorized as high risk.

An increased risk of postmolar GTT has also been observed in women older than 40 years. Tow (1966) reported that 37% of women older than 40 years with molar pregnancy developed persistent tumor. Complete moles in older women are more frequently aneuploid, and this may be related to their increased potential for local invasion and metastasis.

Eight (9.9%) of our 81 patients with partial mole developed nonmetastatic persistent GTT (Berkowitz et al., 1985). These eight patients were all thought to have missed abortion before evacuation. None of the eight patients had theca lutein cysts, markedly elevated hCG levels, or excessive uterine size. Patients with partial mole who developed persistent tumor did not have clinical characteristics that distinguished them from other patients with partial mole.

The risk of developing persistent GTT after partial mole has been reported from zero to 11% (Table 15–2) (Berkowitz et al., 1988). Patients with persistent tumor after partial mole generally have nonmetastatic disease. However, both Wong et al. (1986) and Stone et al. (1976) have reported two patients with metastatic tumor following partial molar pregnancy.

TABLE 15–2.

Persistent Tumor After Partial Molar Pregnancy

Series	Patients (no.)	Persistent Tumor (no.)
Stone and Bagshawe (1976)	194	5*
Vassilakos et al. (1977)	56	0
Czernobilsky et al. (1982)	25	1
Lawler et al. (1982)	15	0
Szulman and Surti (1982)	49	2
Wong and Ma (1984)	35	4*
Berkowitz et al. (1985)	81	8
Ohama et al. (1986)	56	0
TOTAL	511	20(3.9%)

*Two patients had metastases.

Treatment

After a molar pregnancy is diagnosed, the patient is carefully evaluated for possible medical complications, including preeclampsia, electrolyte imbalance, hyperthyroidism, and anemia. The patient is first stabilized, and then a decision must be made concerning the most appropriate method of evacuation.

If the patient no longer desires to preserve fertility, hysterectomy may be performed, and prominent theca lutein ovarian cysts may be aspirated at the time of surgery. Although hysterectomy eliminates the risks of local invasion, it does not prevent metastasis.

Suction curettage is the preferred method of evacuation regardless of uterine size in patients who desire to preserve fertility (Berkowitz et al., 1987b). As the cervix is being dilated, the surgeon may encounter brisk uterine bleeding due to the passage of retained blood. Shortly after suction evacuation is commenced, uterine bleeding is generally controlled, and the uterus rapidly regresses in size. If the uterus is larger than 14 weeks' size, one hand should be placed on top of the fundus and the uterus massaged to stimulate uterine contraction. When suction evacuation is thought to be complete, a sharp curettage should be performed to remove any residual molar tissue. The curettings from suction and sharp curettage are separately submitted for pathologic review.

Prophylactic Chemotherapy

The use of prophylactic chemotherapy at the time of molar evacuation remains controversial (Goldstein, 1974). However, several investigators have reported that chemoprophylaxis reduces the risk of postmolar tumor.

Between July 1965 and June 1979 at the NETDC, 247 patients with complete mole received actinomycin D prophylactically at the time of evacuation. Uterine invasion subsequently developed in only 10 (4%) patients, and no patient developed metastases. Furthermore, all 10 patients who developed local invasion later achieved remission after only one additional course of chemotherapy.

Kim et al. (1986) performed an important randomized, prospective trial of chemoprophylaxis in patients with complete mole. Chemoprophylaxis reduced the incidence of postmolar tumor from 47% to 14% in patients with high-risk mole. However, chemoprophylaxis did not significantly influence the occurrence of persistent tumor in patients with low-risk mole.

We have recently reviewed our experience with prophylactic actinomycin D in patients with high-risk complete mole (Berkowitz et al., 1987b). Only 10 (11%) of 93 patients with high-risk complete mole developed postmolar tumor after prophylactic actinomycin D. Chemoprophylaxis failure more commonly occurred in patients with markedly elevated hCG values. Prophylactic chemotherapy may be of benefit in patients with high-risk complete moles, particularly when hormonal follow-up is unavailable or unreliable.

Hormonal Follow-up

After molar evacuation, all patients must be followed with hCG measurements to assure remission. Patients are followed with weekly hCG values until they are normal for 3 weeks and then monthly values until they are normal for 6 months.

Patients are encouraged to use effective contraception during the entire interval of follow-up. Intrauterine devices should not be inserted until the patient achieves normal hCG levels because of the risk of uterine perforation. If the patient does not desire surgical sterilization, she is then confronted with the choice of using either oral contraceptives or barrier methods.

The incidence of postmolar tumor has been reported to be increased in patients who used oral contraceptives (Stone et al., 1976). However, data from the University of Southern California and the NETDC indicate that oral contraceptives do not increase the risk of postmolar trophoblastic disease (Morrow et al., 1985; Berkowitz et al., 1981b). The contraceptive method also did not influence the mean hCG regression time. We therefore believe that oral contraceptives may be safely prescribed after molar evacuation.

GESTATIONAL TROPHOBLASTIC TUMORS

After a molar pregnancy, persistent GTT may have the histologic pattern of either molar tissue or choriocarcinoma. However, following a nonmolar gestation, persistent GTT may have only the histologic features of choriocarcinoma. Gestational choriocarcinoma does not contain chorionic villous structures but is composed of sheets of both cytotrophoblast and syncytiotrophoblast (Fig 15–4).

Placental site trophoblastic tumor (PSTT) is an uncommon variant of choriocarcinoma (Finkler et al., 1988). It is composed almost entirely of cytotrophoblast and does not contain chorionic

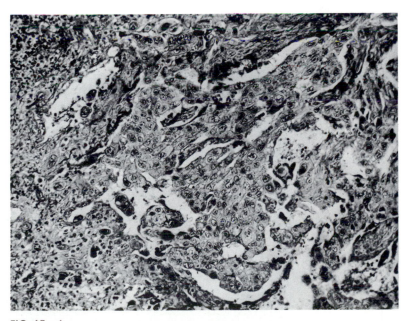

FIG 15–4.
Typical plexiform arrangement of trophoblastic cells in choriocarcinoma.

villi. It secretes very limited amounts of hCG, and therefore a large tumor burden may be present before hCG levels are detectable.

Natural History

Nonmetastatic Disease

Locally invasive GTT develops in 15% of patients following molar evacuation and infrequently after other gestations (Berkowitz and Goldstein, 1981). Trophoblastic tumor may perforate through the myometrium, producing intraperitoneal bleeding, or may erode into uterine vessels, causing vaginal hemorrhage. Bulky necrotic tumor may serve as a nidus for uterine infection (Fig 15–5).

Metastatic Disease

Metastatic GTT occurs in 4% of patients after molar evacuation and infrequently following other pregnancies. Metastatic GTT is often associated with choriocarcinoma. Choriocarcinoma has a propensity for early vascular invasion with widespread dissemination. The commonest metastatic sites are the lung (80%), vagina (30%), brain (10%), and liver (10%). Because trophoblastic tumors are perfused by fragile vessels, metastases are often hemorrhagic. Patients may present with signs and symptoms of bleeding from metastases such as hemoptysis or acute neurologic deficits. Cerebral and hepatic metastases are uncommon unless there is concurrent involvement of the lungs, vagina, or both.

Staging System

The Federation of International Gynecology and Obstetrics has begun to report data on GTT using an anatomic staging system (Table 15–3). Stage I includes all patients with persistently elevated hCG levels and tumor confined to the uterine corpus. Stage II comprises all patients with tumor outside of the uterus but localized to the vagina, pelvis, or both. Stage III includes all patients with pulmonary metastases with or without uterine, vaginal, or pelvic involvement. Stage IV patients have far-advanced disease with involvement of the brain, liver, kidneys, or gastrointestinal (GI) tract. Patients with stage IV disease are in the highest risk category because they are most likely to be resistant to chemotherapy. Stage IV tumors generally have the histologic pattern of choriocarcinoma and commonly follow a nonmolar pregnancy.

It is also helpful to employ prognostic variables to predict the likelihood of drug resistance and to assist in selecting appropriate chemotherapy. The World Health Organization has published a prognostic scoring system based on one developed by Bagshawe that reliably predicts the potential for chemotherapy resistance (Table 15–4). When the prognostic score is 8 or greater, the patient is considered high risk and requires intensive combination chemotherapy to achieve remission. In general, patients with stage I disease have a low-risk score, and patients with stage IV disease have a high-risk score. Therefore, the dis-

FIG 15–5.
Uterine choriocarcinoma with massive destruction of uterine wall.

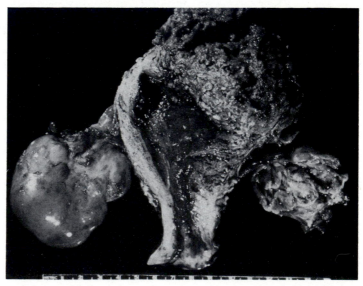

TABLE 15–3.

Staging of Gestational Trophoblastic Tumors

Stage
I Confined to uterine corpus
II Metastases to pelvis and vagina
III Metastases to lung
IV Distant metastases

tinction between low and high risk applies primarily to stage II and III GTT.

Diagnostic Evaluation

The optimal management of GTT requires a thorough evaluation of the extent of the disease prior to treatment. All patients with persistent tumor should undergo a thorough assessment, including a complete history and physical examination, hCG levels, and hepatic, thyroid, and renal function tests. The metastatic workup should include a chest roentgenogram, ultrasonography of the abdomen and pelvis, head computed tomography (CT) scan, and, in some cases, selective angiography of abdominal and pelvic structures.

Head CT scan has facilitated the early detection of asymptomatic cerebral lesions (Fig 15–6; Athanassiou et al.). Human chorionic gonadotropin levels are measured in the cerebrospinal fluid (CSF) in patients with choriocarcinoma or metastases (or both) to detect cerebral tumor. Bagshawe and Harland (1976) have reported that a plasma/CSF hCG ratio less than 60 strongly suggests CNS involvement by GTT.

Management of Stage I Gestational Trophoblastic Tumor

Tables 15–5 and 15–6 review the NETDC protocol for the management of stage I disease and the results of therapy. The selection of treatment is based mainly on the patient's desire to preserve fertility.

If the patient no longer wishes to retain fertility, hysterectomy with adjuvant single-agent chemotherapy may be performed as primary treatment. Adjuvant chemotherapy is administered for three reasons: (1) to reduce the likelihood of disseminating viable tumor cells at surgery, (2) to maintain a cytotoxic level of chemotherapy in the bloodstream and tissues in case viable tumor cells are disseminated at surgery, and (3) to treat any occult metastases that may be already present at the time of surgery. Occult pulmonary metastases may be detected by CT scan in about 40% of patients with presumed nonmetastatic disease (Mutch et al., 1986). Chemotherapy may be safely administered at the time of hysterectomy without increasing operative complications.

TABLE 15–4.

Scoring System Based on Prognostic Factors

Prognostic Factors	Score*			
	0	1	2	4
Age (yr)	$\leq$39	>39		
Antecedent pregnancy	Hydatidiform mole	Abortion	Term	
Interval[†]	4	4–6	7–12	>12
hCG (IU/L)	10^3	10^3–10^4	10^4–10^5	>10^5
ABO groups (F × M)		O × A A × O	B AB	
Largest tumor, including uterine tumor		3–5 cm	>5 cm	
Site of metastases		Spleen Kidney	GI tract Liver	Brain
Metastases identified (no.)		1–4	4–8	>8
Prior chemotherapy			Single drug	$\geq$2 drugs

*The total score for a patient is obtained by adding the individual scores for each prognostic factor. Total score: $\leq$4, low risk; 5–7, middle risk; $\geq$8, high risk.
†Interval: time (mo.) between end of antecedent pregnancy and start of chemotherapy.

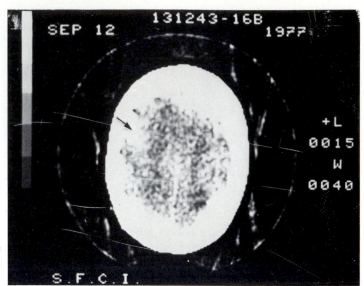

FIG 15–6.
Computed tomographic scan of large intracranial metastasis of choriocarcinoma showing filling defect.

Twenty-three patients were treated by primary hysterectomy and adjuvant chemotherapy at the NETDC, and all achieved complete remission with no additional therapy.

Nonmetastatic PSTT patients should be treated with hysterectomy because of their poor response to chemotherapy. Because PSTT is generally resistant to chemotherapy, there are few, if any, long-term survivors with metastases despite intensive multimodal therapy.

Single-agent chemotherapy is the preferred treatment in patients with stage I disease who de-

sire to retain fertility. Primary single-agent chemotherapy induced complete remission in 283 (94.6%) of 299 patients with stage I GTT. The remaining 16 resistant patients subsequently attained remission with either combination chemotherapy or surgical intervention. If the patient is resistant to chemotherapy and wants to preserve fertility, local uterine resection may be considered. When local resection is planned, ultrasound, arteriogram, or both may identify the site of resistant tumor.

TABLE 15–5.

Treatment Protocol at the New England Trophoblastic Disease Center for Stage I Gestational Trophoblastic Tumor

Initial
  Single-agent chemotherapy or hysterectomy with
    adjunctive chemotherapy
Resistant
  Combination chemotherapy
  Hysterectomy with adjunctive chemotherapy
  Local resection
  Pelvic infusion
Follow-up
  hCG
    Weekly until normal × 3
    Monthly until normal × 12
Contraception
  12 consecutive mo. of normal hCG levels

Management of Stage II and III Gestational Trophoblastic Disease

The NETDC protocol for the management of stage II and III disease and the results of treatment are outlined in Tables 15–7 to 15–9. Although low-risk patients are treated with primary single-agent chemotherapy, high-risk patients are managed with primary combination chemotherapy.

Between July 1965 and December 1986, 25 patients with stage II disease were treated at the NETDC, and all achieved remission. Single-agent chemotherapy induced complete remission in 15 (88.2%) of 17 low-risk patients. In contrast, only two of eight high-risk patients achieved remission with single-agent treatment.

Vaginal metastases may bleed profusely because they may be highly vascular and friable (Fig

TABLE 15—6.

Results of Stage I, Confined to Uterine Corpus, at the New England Trophoblastic Disease Center, July 1965—December 1986*

Remission Therapy	Patients, no. (%)	Remissions, no. (%)
Initial	308 (95.1)	
Sequential MTX/act D		283 (91.9)
Hysterectomy		23 (7.5)
MAC		2 (0.6)
Resistant	16 (4.9)	
MAC		10 (62.5)
EMA		1 (6.2)
Hysterectomy		2 (12.5)
Local uterine resection		2 (12.5)
Pelvic infusion		1 (6.2)
TOTAL	324	324 (100)

*MTX = methotrexate; act D = actinomycin D; MAC = methotrexate, actinomycin D, and cyclophosphamide; EMA = etoposide, methotrexate, and actinomycin D.

15–7). Bleeding may be controlled by packing the hemorrhagic lesion or performing wide local excision. The administration of one or two courses of chemotherapy may result in avascular planes around the vaginal tumor. Infrequently, angiographic embolization of the hypogastric arteries may be required to control hemorrhage from vaginal metastases.

Between July 1965 and December 1986, 103 patients with stage III tumors were managed at the NETDC, and 102 (99%) attained complete remission. Single-agent chemotherapy induced complete remission in 63 (87%) of 72 patients with low-risk disease and in 13 (42%) of 31 patients with high-risk disease. All patients who were resistant to single-agent treatment later achieved remission with combination chemotherapy.

Thoracotomy has a limited role in the management of stage III GTT. Thoracotomy should be performed if the diagnosis is seriously in question. Furthermore, if a patient has a persistent viable pulmonary nodule despite intensive chemotherapy, pulmonary resection may be performed. However, an extensive metastatic survey should be obtained to exclude other sites of persistent tumor. It is important to emphasize that fibrotic nodules may persist indefinitely on chest roentgenogram after complete gonadotropin remission is achieved.

Hysterectomy may be required in patients with metastatic GTT to control uterine hemorrhage or sepsis. Furthermore, in patients with bulky uterine tumor, hysterectomy may reduce the tumor burden and thereby limit the need for chemotherapy.

TABLE 15—7.

Treatment Protocol at the New England Trophoblastic Disease Center for Stage II and III Gestational Trophoblastic Tumor

Low risk*	
Initial	Single-agent chemotherapy
Resistant	Combination chemotherapy
High risk*	
Initial	Combination chemotherapy
Resistant	Second-line combination chemotherapy
Follow-up	
hCG	Weekly until normal × 3 Monthly until normal × 12
Contraception	12 consecutive mo. of normal hCG levels

*Local resection optional.

Management of Stage IV Gestational Trophoblastic Tumor

Tables 15–10 and 15–11 outline the NETDC protocol for the management of stage IV disease and the results of treatment. These pa-

TABLE 15–8.

Results of Stage II, Metastases to Pelvis and Vagina, at the New England Trophoblastic Disease Center, July 1965–December 1986*

Remission Therapy	Patients, no. (%)	Remissions, no. (%)
Low risk	17 (68.0)	
Initial		
Sequential MTX/act-D		15 (88.2)
Resistant		2 (11.8)
MAC		
High risk	8 (32.0)	
Initial		
Sequential MTX/act D		2 (25.0)
MAC		4 (50.0)
Resistant		
MAC		1 (12.5)
CHAMOCA		1 (12.5)
TOTAL	25	25 (100)

*MTX = methotrexate; act D = actinomycin D; MAC = methotrexate, actinomycin D, and cyclophosphamide; CHAMOCA = Bagshawe multiagent regimen.

TABLE 15–9.

Results of Stage III, Metastases to Lung, at the New England Trophoblastic Disease Center, July 1965–December 1986*

Remission Therapy	Patients, no. (%)	Remissions, no. (%)
Low risk	72 (69.9)	
Initial		
Sequential MTX/act D		63 (87.5)
Resistant		
MAC		9 (12.5)
High risk	31 (30.1)	
Initial		
Sequential MTX/act D		13 (41.9)
MAC		12 (38.7)
Resistant		
MAC		2 (6.4)
CHAMOCA		1 (3.2)
5-FU-adria		1 (3.2)
VPB		1 (3.2)
TOTAL	103	102 (99.0)

*MTX = methotrexate; act-D = actinomycin D; MAC = methotrexate, actinomycin D, and cyclophosphamide; CHAMOCA = Bagshawe multiagent regimen; 5-FU-adria = 5-fluorouracil and Adriamycin; VPB = vinblastine, cis-platinum, and bleomycin.

tients are at high risk for developing rapidly progressive disease despite intensive therapy.

All patients with stage IV disease should be treated with intensive combination chemotherapy and the selective use of radiation therapy and surgery (Surwit and Hammond, 1980). Before 1975, only 6 (30%) of 20 patients with stage IV disease attained complete remission. However, af-

ter 1975, 12 (75%) of 16 patients with stage IV tumors achieved remission. This dramatic improvement in survival resulted from intensive multimodal therapy.

The management of hepatic metastases is particularly difficult and challenging. If a patient is resistant to systemic chemotherapy, hepatic arterial infusion of chemotherapy may induce com-

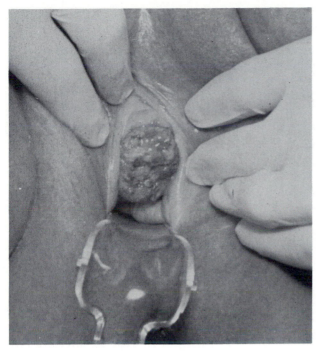

FIG 15–7.
Fungating suburethral metastasis of choriocarcinoma with necrosis and infection.

plete remission in selected cases. Hepatic resection may also be required to control bleeding or to excise resistant tumor (Fig 15–8).

If cerebral metastases are detected, whole brain irradiation is promptly instituted at our center. The risk of spontaneous cerebral hemorrhage

TABLE 15–10.
Treatment Protocol at the New England Trophoblastic Disease Center for Stage IV Gestational Trophoblastic Tumor

Initial
  Combination chemotherapy
    Brain
      Whole head irradiation (3,000 rad)
      Craniotomy to manage complications
    Liver
      Resection to manage complications
Resistant*
  Second-line combination chemotherapy
Follow-up
  hCG
    Weekly until normal × 3
    Monthly until normal × 24
Contraception
  24 consecutive mo. of normal hCG levels

*Local resection optional.

may be reduced by the concurrent use of chemotherapy and brain irradiation (Weed and Hammond, 1980). Brain irradiation may be both hemostatic and tumoricidal. Yordan et al. (1987) recently reported that deaths due to CNS involvement occurred in 11 (44%) of 25 patients treated with chemotherapy alone but in none of 18 patients treated with brain irradiation and chemotherapy.

However, Athanassiou et al. (1983) have reported excellent remission rates in patients with cerebral metastases who were treated with chemotherapy alone. Eighty percent of their patients with cerebral lesions achieved sustained remission with intensive combination chemotherapy, including high-dose IV and intrathecal methotrexate. Excellent cure rates can, therefore, be attained in patients with cerebral metastases with intensive chemotherapy alone.

Craniotomy should be performed to manage life-threatening complications and thereby provide the opportunity for chemotherapy to induce complete remission. Craniotomy may be necessary to provide acute decompression or to control bleeding (Fig 15–9). Infrequently, cerebral metastases that are resistant to chemotherapy may be amenable to resection. Fortunately, patients with

TABLE 15—11.

Results of Stage IV, Distant Metastases, at the New England Trophoblastic Disease Center, July 1965—December 1986*

Remission Therapy†	Remissions no. (%)	
Before 1975		
Initial		
Sequential MTX/act D	5	
Resistant		
MAC	1	6/20 (30)
After 1975		
Initial		
Sequential MTX/act D	2	
MAC	2	
Resistant		
High-dose MTX/act D	4	12/16 (75)
MAC	1	
CHAMOCA	1	
VPB	1	
EMA	1	

*MTX = Methotrexate; act D = actinomycin D; MAC = methotrexate, actinomycin D, and cyclophosphamide; CHAMOCA = Bagshawe multiagent regimen; VPB = vinblastine, cis-platinum, and bleomycin; EMA = etoposide, methotrexate, and actinomycin D.
†Radiotherapy and surgery used when indicated.

cerebral metastases who achieve remission generally have no residual neurologic deficits.

Follow-up

All patients with stage I, II, and III GTT are followed with weekly hCG values until they are normal for 3 weeks and then monthly values until they are normal for 12 months. Patients are encouraged to use contraception during the entire interval of follow-up.

Patients with stage IV disease are followed with weekly hCG values until they are normal for 3 weeks and then monthly values until they are

FIG 15—8.
Liver showing diffuse involvement with choriocarcinoma.

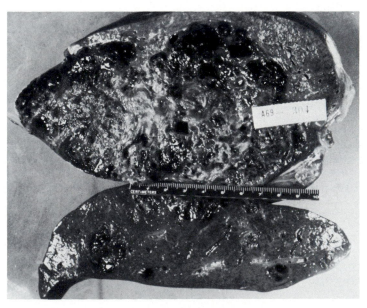

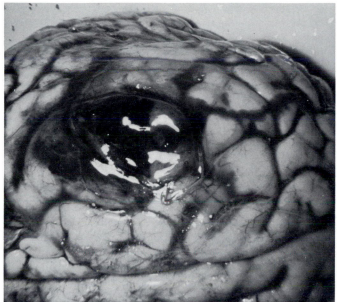

FIG 15–9.
Cerebral metastasis of choriocarcinoma with recent hemorrhage.

normal for 24 months. These patients require prolonged follow-up because they have an increased risk of late recurrence.

Chemotherapy

Single-Agent Chemotherapy

Selection of Single-Agent Chemotherapy.— Single-agent chemotherapy with either actinomycin D or methotrexate has induced comparable and excellent remission rates in both nonmetastatic and metastatic GTT (Osathanondh et al., 1975). An optimal regimen should maximize the cure rate while minimizing the toxicity.

Methotrexate and folinic acid has been the preferred single-agent regimen in the treatment of GTT at the NETDC since 1974 (Berkowitz et al., 1986b). Between September 1974 and September 1984, 185 patients with GTT were treated with primary methotrexate–folinic acid at the NETDC. Complete remission was induced with methotrexate–folinic acid in 162 (87.6%) patients, and 132 (81.5%) of these patients required only one course of methotrexate–folinic acid to achieve remission. Methotrexate–folinic acid induced remission in 147 (90.2%) of 163 patients with stage I GTT and in 15 (68.2%) of 22 patients with low-risk stage II and III GTT. Resistance to methotrexate–folinic acid was commoner in patients with choriocarcinoma, me-

tastases, and pretreatment hCG levels greater than 50,000 mIU/ml. Following methotrexate–folinic acid, thrombocytopenia, granulocytopenia, and hepatotoxicity occurred in only 11 (5.9%), 3 (1.6%), and 26 (14.1%) patients, respectively. No patient required platelet transfusions or developed sepsis due to myelosuppression. Methotrexate–folinic acid not only induces an excellent remission rate with minimal toxicity but also effectively limits chemotherapy exposure (Berkowitz et al., 1981a).

Administration of Single-Agent Chemotherapy.—The hCG level is measured weekly after each course of chemotherapy, and the hCG regression curve serves as the primary basis for determining the need for further treatment. After the first treatment, further chemotherapy is withheld as long as the hCG level is falling progressively. Additional single-agent chemotherapy is not administered at any predetermined or fixed time interval. A second course of chemotherapy is administered under the following conditions: (1) the hCG level plateaus for more than 3 consecutive weeks or reelevates, and (2) the hCG level does not decline by one log within 18 days after completing the first treatment.

If a second course of methotrexate–folinic acid is required, the dosage of methotrexate is unchanged if the patient's response to the first treatment was adequate. An adequate response is defined as a fall in the hCG level by one log following a course of chemotherapy. When the response to the first treatment is inadequate, the dosage of Mtx is increased 2 mg/kg in four divided doses. If the response to two courses of methotrexate–folinic acid is inadequate, the patient is considered to be resistant to methotrexate and actinomycin D is promptly substituted.

Combination Chemotherapy

Modified triple therapy with methotrexate–folinic acid, actinomycin D, and cyclophosphamide had been the preferred combination drug regimen at the NETDC (Berkowitz et al., 1984). Ten (71.4%) of 14 patients with high-risk metastatic GTT achieved complete remission with modified triple therapy. However, triple therapy is inadequate as an initial treatment in metastatic patients with a high-risk score (score greater than 8) (DuBeshter et al., 1987). Triple therapy induced remission in only 5 (45%) of 11 patients with a high-risk score.

Etoposide (VP16) has been demonstrated to be a new effective antitumor agent in GTT. Primary oral etoposide induced complete sustained remission in 56 (93.3%) of 60 patients with nonmetastatic or low-risk metastatic GTT (Wong et al., 1986). Bagshawe (1984) has reported an 83% remission rate in patients with a high-risk score using a new combination regimen that includes etoposide. This new regimen includes etoposide, methotrexate, actinomycin D, cyclophosphamide, and vincristine and may currently be the preferred treatment for patients with a high-risk score. The optimal combination drug regimen will most likely include methotrexate, actinomycin D, and etoposide and perhaps other agents administered in the most dose-intensive manner (Surwit, 1987).

Patients who require combination chemotherapy must be treated intensively to attain remission. We administer combination chemotherapy as frequently as toxicity permits until the patient attains three consecutive normal hCG levels. After the patient achieves normal hCG levels, additional chemotherapy is administered to reduce the risk of relapse.

SUBSEQUENT PREGNANCIES

Pregnancies After Hydatidiform Mole

Patients with complete molar pregnancies can anticipate normal reproduction in the future (Berkowitz et al., 1987a). Patients with complete moles who were treated at the NETDC had 1,048 later pregnancies between June 1965 and December 1986. These pregnancies resulted in 723 (69.0%) full-term live births, 81 (7.7%) premature deliveries, 7 (0.6%) ectopics, and six (0.6%) stillbirths (Table 15–12). First-trimester spontaneous abortion occurred in 174 (16.6%) pregnancies, and major and minor congenital malformations were detected in only 34 (4.2%) infants. Primary cesarean section was performed in only 29 (14.1%) of 205 subsequent full-term and premature births between January 1979 and December 1986.

Limited information is available regarding the later pregnancy experience in patients with partial mole (Berkowitz et al., 1987a). Between June 1965 and December 1986, patients with partial mole at the NETDC had 50 subsequent gestations that resulted in 37 (74%) full-term live births, 1 (2%) stillbirth, 1 (2%) partial mole, and no premature deliveries. First-trimester spontaneous abortion occurred in seven (14%) pregnancies, and major or minor congenital anomalies were detected in only one (2.6%) infant. The preliminary data concerning subsequent conceptions after partial mole are therefore reassuring.

When a patient has had a molar pregnancy, she is at increased risk of developing molar disease in later conceptions. Nine (1 : 150) of our patients have had at least two consecutive molar gestations. Patients may have an initial complete or partial mole and then in a later pregnancy develop

TABLE 15–12.

Subsequent Pregnancies in Patients With Complete Mole at the New England Trophoblastic Disease Center, June 1965–December 1986

Outcome	No. (%)
Term delivery	723 (69.0)
Stillbirth	6 (0.6)
Premature delivery	81 (7.7)
Spontaneous abortion	
First trimester	174 (16.6)
Second trimester	17 (1.6)
Therapeutic abortion	26 (2.6)
Ectopic	7 (0.6)
Repeat mole	14 (1.3)
Total no. of pregnancies	1,048
No. deliveries (%)	
Congenital malformations	34/810 (4.2)
Primary cesarean section	29/205 (14.1)*

*January 1979–December 1986.

the other type of molar disease. Most important, three of our patients have had a normal subsequent term pregnancy after two prior molar gestations.

It therefore seems prudent to obtain an ultrasound in the first trimester of any subsequent pregnancy to confirm normal gestational development. Furthermore, the placenta or products of conception from later pregnancies should undergo pathologic review. An hCG measurement should also be obtained 6 weeks after the completion of any future pregnancy to exclude occult trophoblastic mischief.

Pregnancies After Gestational Trophoblastic Tumor

Patients with GTT who are successfully treated with chemotherapy can also expect normal reproduction in the future (Walden and Bagshawe, 1976; Berkowitz et al., 1987a). Patients with GTT who were treated with chemotherapy at the NETDC had 324 pregnancies between June 1965 and December 1986. These later pregnancies resulted in 227 (70.0%) full-term live births, 14 (4.3%) premature deliveries, three (0.9%) ectopic pregnancies, and 6 (1.8%) stillbirths (Table 15–13). First-trimester spontaneous abortion occurred in 51 (15.8%) pregnancies, and major and minor congenital anomalies were detected in only 5 (2.0%) infants. It is particularly reassuring that the frequency of congenital

malformations is not increased, because chemotherapy may be teratogenic and mutagenic. Primary cesarean section was performed in only 20 (14.3%) of 141 subsequent full-term and premature deliveries between January 1979 and December 1986. Later pregnancies have no increased risk for obstetrical complications either prenatally or intrapartum.

Song et al. (1988) performed cytogenetic studies on the peripheral lymphocytes from 94 children from subsequent pregnancies and reported no increase in chromosomal aberrations. The growth and development of these children were also evaluated and proved to be normal.

TABLE 15–13.

Subsequent Pregnancies in Patients With Gestational Trophoblastic Tumors at the New England Trophoblastic Disease Center, June 1965–December 1986

Outcome	No. (%)
Term delivery	227 (70.0)
Stillbirth	6 (1.8)
Premature delivery	14 (4.3)
Spontaneous abortion	
First trimester	51 (15.8)
Second trimester	7 (2.2)
Therapeutic abortion	15 (4.7)
Ectopic pregnancy	3 (0.9)
Repeat molar pregnancy	1 (0.3)
Total no. of pregnancies	324
No./deliveries (%)	
Congenital malformations	5/247 (2.0)
Primary cesarean section	20/141 (14.3)*

*January 1979–December 1986.

REFERENCES

Amir SM, Osathanondh R, Berkowitz RS, et al: Human chorionic gonadotropin and thyroid function in patients with hydatidiform mole. *Am J Obstet Gynecol* 1984; 150:723–728.

Athanassiou A, Begent RHJ, Newlands ES, et al: Central nervous system metastasis of choriocarcinoma: 23 years experience at the Charing Cross Hospital. *Cancer* 1983; 52:1728–1735.

Bagshawe KD: Risks and prognostic factors in trophoblastic neoplasia. *Cancer* 1976; 38:1373–1385.

Bagshawe KD: Treatment of high-risk choriocarcinoma. *J Reprod Med* 1984; 29:813–820.

Bagshawe KD, Harland S: Immunodiagnosis and monitoring of gonadotropin-producing metastases in the central nervous system. *Cancer* 1976; 38:112–118.

Berkowitz RS, Goldstein DP: Pathogenesis of gestational trophoblastic neoplasms. *Pathobiol Ann* 1981; 11:391–411.

Berkowitz RS, Goldstein DP: Management of molar pregnancy and gestational trophoblastic tumors, in Knapp RC, Berkowitz RS (eds): *Gynecologic Oncology.* New York, Macmillan Publishing Co, 1986, pp 425–443.

Berkowitz RS, Goldstein DP, Bernstein MR: Modified triple chemotherapy in the management of high-risk metastatic gestational trophoblastic tumors. *Gynecol Oncol* 1984; 19:173–181.

Berkowitz RS, Goldstein DP, Bernstein MR: Natural history of partial molar pregnancy. *Obstet Gynecol* 1986a; 66:677–681.

Berkowitz RS, Goldstein DP, Bernstein MR: Ten years experience with methotrexate and folinic acid as primary therapy for gestational trophoblastic disease. *Gynecol Oncol* 1986b; 23:111–118.

Berkowitz RS, Goldstein DP, Bernstein MR:

Partial molar pregnancy: A separate entity. *Contemp Obstet Gynecol* 1988; 31:99–102.

Berkowitz RS, Goldstein DP, Bernstein MR, et al: Subsequent pregnancy outcome in patients with molar pregnancy and gestational trophoblastic tumors. *J Reprod Med* 1987a; 32:680–684.

Berkowitz RS, Goldstein DP, DuBeshter B, et al: Management of complete molar pregnancy. *J Reprod Med* 1987b; 32:634–639.

Berkowitz RS, Goldstein DP, Jones MA, et al: Methotrexate with citrovorum factor rescue—reduced chemotherapy toxicity in the management of gestational trophoblastic neoplasms. *Cancer* 1981a; 45:423–426.

Berkowitz RS, Goldstein DP, Marean AR, et al: Oral contraceptives and postmolar trophoblastic disease. *Obstet Gynecol* 1981b; 58:474–478.

Bracken MB, Brinton LA; Hayashi K: Epidemiology of hyatidiform mole and choriocarcinoma. *Epidemiol Rev* 1984; 6:52–75.

Curry SL, Hammond CB, Tyrey L, et al: Hyatidiform mole—diagnosis, management and long-term follow-up of 347 patients. *Am J Obstet Gynecol* 1975; 45:1–8.

Czernobilsky B, Barash A, Lancet M: Partial moles: A clinicopathologic study of 25 cases. *Obstet Gynecol* 1982; 59:75–77.

DuBeshter B, Berkowitz RS, Goldstein DP, et al: Metastatic gestational trophoblastic disease: Experience at the New England Trophoblastic Disease Center, 1965–1985. *Obstet Gynecol* 1987; 69:390–395.

Finkler NJ, Berkowitz RS, Driscoll SG, et al: Clinical experience with placental site trophoblastic tumors at the New England Trophoblastic Disease Center. *Obstet Gynecol* 1988; 71:854–857.

Goldstein DP: Prevention of gestational trophoblastic disease by use of actinomycin-D in molar pregnancies. *Obstet Gynecol* 1974; 43:475–479.

Goldstein DP, Berkowitz RS: *Gestational Trophoblastic Neoplasms—Clinical Principles of Diagnosis and Management.* Philadelphia, WB Saunders Co, 1982, pp 1–301.

Hankins G, Wendel GD, Snyder RR, et al: Trophoblastic embolization during molar evacuation—central hemodynamic observations. *Obstet Gynecol* 1987; 69:368–372.

Kajii T, Ohama K: Androgenetic origin of hyatidiform mole. *Nature* 1977; 268:633–634.

Kim DS, Moon H, Kim KT, et al: Effects of prophylactic chemotherapy for persistent trophoblastic disease in patients with complete hydatidiform mole. *Obstet Gynecol* 1986; 67:690–694.

Kohorn EI: Clinical management and the neoplastic sequelae of trophoblastic embolization associated with hydatidiform mole. *Obstet Gynecol Surv* 1987; 42:484–488.

Lawler S, Fisher RA, Pickthall V, et al: Genetic studies on hyatidiform moles: I. The origin of patial moles. *Cancer Genet Cytogenet* 1982; 5:309–320.

Masson GM, Anthony F, Chau E: Serum chorionic gonadotrophin (hCG), schwangersschaftsprotein 1 (SP1), progesterone and oestradiol levels in patients with nausea and vomiting in early pregnancy. *Br J Obstet Gynecol* 1985; 92:211–215.

Montz FJ, Schlaeth JB, Morrow CP: Natural history of theca lutein cysts. *Gynecol Oncol* 1987; 26:414.

Morrow P, Nakamura R, Schlaerth J, et al: The influence of oral contraceptives on the postmolar human chorionic regression curve. *Am J Obstet Gynecol* 1985; 151:906–914.

Mutch DG, Soper JT, Baker ME, et al: Role of computed axial tomography of the chest in staging patients with nonmetastatic gestational trophoblastic disease. *Obstet Gynecol* 1986; 68:348–352.

Nisula BC, Taliadouros GS: Thyroid function in gestational trophoblastic neoplasia—evidence that the thyrotropic activity of chorionic gonadotropin mediates the thyrotoxicosis of choriocarcinoma. *Am J Obstet Gynecol* 1980; 138: 77–85.

Ohama K, Ueda K, Okamoto E, et al: Cytogenetic and clinicopathologic studies of hyatidiform moles. *Obstet Gynecol* 1986; 68:259—262.

Osathanondh R, Berkowitz RS, deCholnoky C, et al: Hormonal measurements in patients with theca lutein cysts and gestational trophoblastic disease. *J Reprod Med* 1986; 31:179–182.

Osathanondh R, Goldstein DP, Pastorfide GB: Actinomycin D as the primary agent for gestational trophoblastic disease. *Cancer* 1975; 36:863–866.

Parazzini T, LaVecchia C, Mangili G, et al: Dietary factors and risk of trophoblastic disease. *Am J Obstet Gynecol* 1988; 158:93–100.

Pattillo RA, Sasaki S, Katayama KP, et al: Genesis of 46, XY hydatidiform mole. *Am J Obstet Gynecol* 1981; 141:104–105.

Song H-Z, Wu P-C, Wang Y, et al: Pregnancy outcomes after successful chemotherapy for choriocarcinoma and invasive mole: Long-term follow-up. *Am J Obstet Gynecol* 1988; 158:538–545.

Stone M, Dent J, Kardana A, et al: Relationship of oral contraception to development of tro-

phoblastic tumour after evacuation of a hydatidiform mole. *Br J Obstet Gynaecol* 1976;
83:913–916.

Surwit EA: Management of high-risk gestational
trophoblastic disease. *J Reprod Med* 1987;
32:657–662.

Surwit EA, Hammond CB: Treatment of metastatic trophoblastic disease with poor prognosis. *Obstet Gynecol* 1980; 55:565–570.

Szulman AE, Surti U: The syndromes of hydatidiform mole: I. Cytogenetic and morphologic correlations. *Am J Obstet Gynecol* 1978a;
131:665–771.

Szulman AE, Surti U: The syndromes of hydatidiform mole: II. Morphologic evolution of
the complete and partial mole. *Am J Obstet
Gynecol* 1978b; 132:20–27.

Szulman AE, Surti U: The clinicopathologic profile of the partial hydatidiform mole. *Obstet
Gynecol* 1982; 59:597–602.

Tow WSH: The influence of the primary treatment of hydatidiform mole on its subsequent
course. *J Obstet Gynaecol Br Commonw* 1966;
73:545–552.

Twiggs LB, Morrow CP, Schlaerth JB: Acute
pulmonary complications of molar pregnancy.
Am J Obstet Gynecol 1979; 135:189–194.

Vassilakos P, Riotton G, Kajii T: Hyatidiform
mole: Two entities. *Am J Obstet Gynecol* 1977;
127:167–170.

Walden PAM, Bagshawe KD: Reproductive performance of women successfully treated for
gestational trophoblastic tumors. *Am J Obstet
Gynecol* 1976; 125:1108–1114.

Weed JC Jr, Hammond CB: Cerebral metastatic
choriocarcinoma: Intensive therapy and prognosis. *Obstet Gynecol* 1980; 55:89–94.

Wong LC, Choo YC, Ma HK: Primary oral
etoposide therapy in gestational trophoblastic
disease, an update. *Cancer* 1986; 58:14–17.

Wong LC, Ma HK: The syndrome of partial
mole. *Arch Gynecol* 1984; 234:161–164.

Yamashita K, Wake N, Araki T, et al: Human
lymphocyte antigen expression in hydatidiform
mole: Androgenesis following fertilization by a
haploid sperm. *Am J Obstet Gynecol* 1979;
135:597–600.

Yordan EL Jr, Schlaerth J, Gaddis O, et al: Radiation therapy in the management of gestational choriocarcinoma metastatic to the central nervous system. *Obstet Gynecol* 1987;
69:627–630.

16 _____ Menopause

Brian W. Walsh, M.D.

Isaac Schiff, M.D.

Menopause denotes the permanent cessation of menses. This is but one aspect of the climacteric, during which time women undergo endocrine, somatic, and psychological changes. These changes are related both to aging and to estrogen depletion; it is not possible to quantify the respective effects of each. This chapter will address the consequences of declining estrogen production in postmenopausal women as well as the possible beneficial value of replacement therapy.

AGING OF THE OVARY

The mean age of women at the menopause is 51 years (McKinlay et al., 1972), with approximately 4% of women undergoing a natural menopause prior to age 40 years (Fig 16–1). The age at menopause is not influenced by prolonged periods of hypothalamic amenorrhea, number of pregnancies, or oral contraceptive use. Since the average age at menopause has not changed since antiquity (Amundsen and Diers, 1970), increases in life expectancy mean that American women today will spend one third of their lifetime after ovarian failure.

The aging process of the ovary appears to begin during fetal development. Although 7 million oogonia are present at 20 weeks' gestation, only 700,000 remain at birth (Schiff and Wilson, 1978). Following birth, the number of oocytes continues to decline even before the onset of puberty (Fig 16–2).

For several years prior to menopause, estradiol and progesterone production decline, despite the occurrence of ovulatory cycles (Sherman et al., 1976). This waning of ovarian follicular activity will reduce the negative feedback inhibition of estradiol on the hypothalamic-pituitary system, resulting in a gradual rise in follicle-stimulating hormone (FSH). The remaining ovarian follicles are increasingly less responsive to FSH; menopause occurs when the residual follicles are refractory to elevated concentrations of FSH.

Estrogen production by the postmenopausal ovary is minimal (Fig 16–3). The major source of postmenopausal estrogens is adrenal androgens, particularly androstenedione, which undergoes aromatization by peripheral tissues to estrone. Typically 2.8% of androstenedione is converted to estrone, but higher rates are seen in obese women, who have more adipose tissue to aromatize androgens (Grodin et al., 1973). This explains in part why obese women have fewer menopausal symptoms than do thin women (Erlik et al., 1982). The mean postmenopausal concentration of estrone is 35 pg/ml, which exceeds the mean concentration of estradiol, 13 pg/ml (Vermeulen, 1976). The estradiol is produced by conversion from estrone.

The postmenopausal ovary continues to produce testosterone and androstenedione, primarily from stromal and hilar cells (Fig 16–4). The mean concentration of testosterone in postmenopausal women (approximately 250 pg/ml) is minimally lower than that in premenopausal women. In contrast, the mean postmenopausal concentration of androstenedione, 850 pg/ml, is less than that of premenopausal women, 1,500 pg/ml (Vermeulen, 1976). Since these postmenopausal androgens are no longer opposed by estrogens, they may lead to increased hair growth on the upper lip and chin.

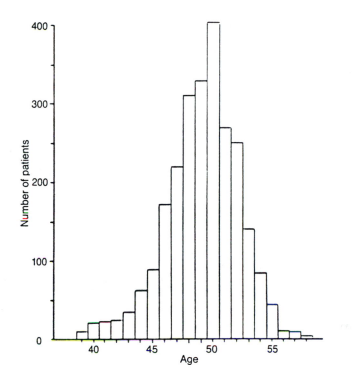

FIG 16–1.
Age of menopause in 2,000 women during a natural menopause. (From Gambrell RD Jr: The menopause: benefits and risks of estrogen-progesterone replace-ment therapy. *Fertil Steril* 1982; 37:457. Reproduced by permission.)

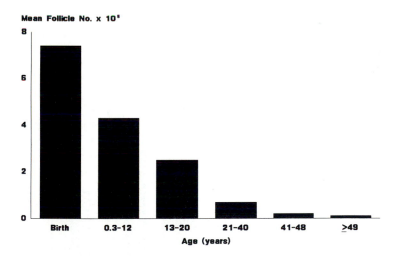

FIG 16–2.
Number of primordial oocytes in women throughout the life cycle. (From Nicosia SV: Morphological changes of the human ovary throughout life, in Serra GB (ed): *The Ovary*. Raven Press, New York, 1983, pp 57–81. Reproduced by permission.)

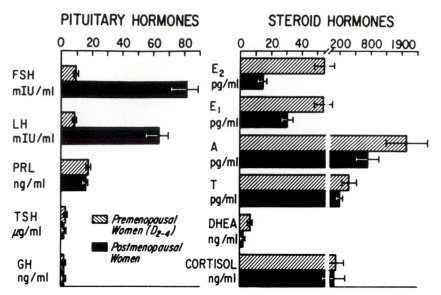

FIG 16–3.
Circulating concentrations of pituitary and steroid hormones in premenopausal (menstrual cycle day 2–4) and postmenopausal women. (From Yen SSC: The biology of menopause. *J Reprod Med* 1977; 18:28. Reproduced by permission.)

VASOMOTOR FLUSHES

One of the most frequent and troublesome symptoms for women at the climacteric is vasomotor flushes; approximately 60% of women will note hot flashes within 3 months of a natural or a surgical menopause. Of those women, 85% will have them for more than 1 year and 25% to 50% for up to 5 years (Thompson et al., 1973). Hot flashes will lessen in frequency and intensity with advancing age, unlike other sequelae of the menopause that progress with time.

Definitions and Pathophysiology

A *hot flash* is the subjective sensation of intense warmth of the upper body, which typically lasts for 4 minutes, but may range from 30 seconds to 5 minutes (Chang and Judd, 1979). This may follow a prodrome of palpitations or a sensa-

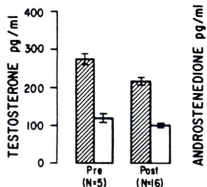
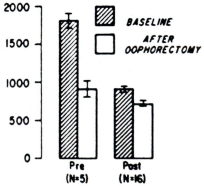

FIG 16–4.
Serum testosterone and androstenedione levels before and 6 to 8 weeks after bilateral oophorectomy. Five premenopausal *(Pre)* and 16 postmenopausal *(Post)* women were studied. (From Judd HL, Lucas WE, Yen SSC: Effect of oophorectomy on testosterone and androstenedione levels. *Am J Obstet Gynecol* 1974; 118:793. Reproduced by permission.)

tion of pressure within the head and is frequently accompanied by weakness, faintness, or vertigo. This episode usually ends in profuse sweating and a cold sensation.

Hot flashes typically occur more frequently at night, thereby awakening patients from sleep. Evidence that nocturnal flashes awaken patients was provided by Erlik et al. (1981b), who simultaneously recorded finger temperature and skin resistance as objective indices of vasomotor flushes while monitoring the stages of sleep using a sleep polygraph (electroencephalogram, electromyelogram, and electro-oculogram) (Fig 16–5). The waking episodes were indeed highly correlated with the occurrence of hot flashes. This reduced quality of sleep results in fatigue, which may then lead to such symptoms as irritability, poor concentration, and impaired memory.

A *vasomotor flush* is the objective component of this phenomenon, characterized by a visible ascending flush of the thorax, neck, and face. An increase in peripheral blood flow, particularly of the fingers, is the first observable event, occurring 1.5 minutes before the subjective sensation and 6 minutes before the peak increase in peripheral skin temperature (Fig 16–6). This increase in blood flow appears to be limited to the cutaneous vasculature and does not involve blood flow to

muscle; for this reason, blood pressure remains stable during a flush. Coincident with the rise in digital temperature and blood flow, core temperature falls (Mashchak et al., 1985). Thus, it appears that vasomotor flushes may be a physiologic consequence of a sudden lowering of the hypothalamic thermoregulatory set point; core temperature is reduced by activating cutaneous vasodilatation, causing increased distal blood flow and, consequently, heat loss. A rise in plasma luteinizing hormone (LH) level is the final event, reaching its peak 12 minutes after the onset of increased digital perfusion.

Etiology

Hot flashes are a consequence of the withdrawal of estrogens rather than of hypoestrogenism per se. They are therefore associated with the menopause, whether it be natural, surgical, or "medical" (i.e., hypoestrogenism induced by the use of long-acting gonadotropin-releasing hormone [GnRH] agonists or by danazol). The discontinuation of exogenous estrogens may also precipitate flushes; women with Turner's syndrome, who are hypoestrogenic, do not have hot flashes unless exogenous estrogens have been prescribed and are later withdrawn (Yen, 1977).

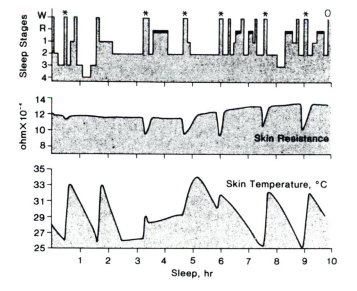

FIG 16–5.
Sleepgram and recordings of skin resistance and temperature in a postmenopausal subject with severe hot flashes. Asterisks denote objectively measured hot flashes. (From Erlik Y, Tataryn IV, Meldrum DR, et al: Association of waking episodes with menopausal hot flushes. *JAMA* 1981; 245:1741. Reproduced by permission.)

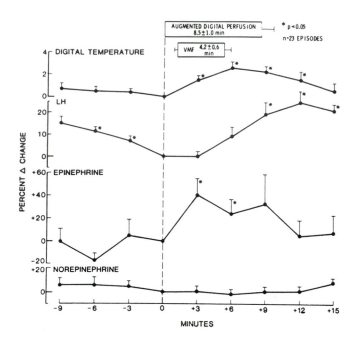

FIG 16–6.

Composite graph of objective parameters obtained in five symptomatic postmenopausal women. Data are normalized to the beginning of augmented digital perfusion (0 time). (From Mashchak CA, Kletsky OA, Artal R, et al: The relation of physiological changes to subjective symptoms in postmenopausal women with and without hot flushes. *Maturitas* 1985; 6:301. Reproduced by permission.)

Men also may have hot flashes, but as a consequence of testosterone withdrawal. In fact, 73% of men following orchiectomy for prostatic cancer will have flashes (Frodin et al., 1985). Treatment with estrogens will provide relief, but they may return if estrogen treatment is discontinued (Huggins et al., 1941). Androgens per se, independent of conversion to estrogen, suppress hot flashes, since the use of a nonaromatizable androgen, fluoxymesterone, was as active as methyltestosterone in relieving flashes in a man with testosterone insufficiency (DeFazio et al., 1984).

Obese women tend to be less troubled by hot flashes: Erlik et al. (1982) found asymptomatic women to weigh considerably more than severely symptomatic ones, even when matched for age, ovarian status, and years since menopause. Obese women are relatively "protected" from hot flashes because they are functionally less hypoestrogenic, for two reasons: (1) their increased adiposity allows for greater peripheral conversion of adrenal androgens into estrogen and estradiol (Grodin et al., 1973); and (2) they typically have lower sex hormone–binding globulins (Davidson et al., 1981), and so a greater proportion of their estrogens are unbound and can act on target tissues (Fig 16–7).

At one time LH was thought to play a role in the initiation of vasomotor flushes. This hypothesis was discarded when the use of exogenous LH (as in human menopausal gonadotropins) was not found to cause flashes. Careful analysis of the chronology of hot flashes subsequently identified the LH peak to be a late component (see earlier discussion). Moreover, vasomotor flushes do not require an intact pituitary; a total hypophysectomy will not prevent their occurrence (Larson, 1977). Vasomotor flushes therefore appear to be caused by an acute lowering of the hypothalamic thermoregulatory set point, precipitated by estrogen withdrawal. Stimulation of adjacent hypothalamic centers controlling LH release produces the associated peaks of LH.

Estrogen's effect on the hypothalamic thermoregulatory center may be mediated by neurotransmitters, such as norepinephrine (NE). As shown in Figure 16–8 (Berkow, 1987), the intraneuronal level of NE is regulated by the balance between the enzymes tyrosine hydroxylase (the rate-limiting step of NE synthesis from ty-

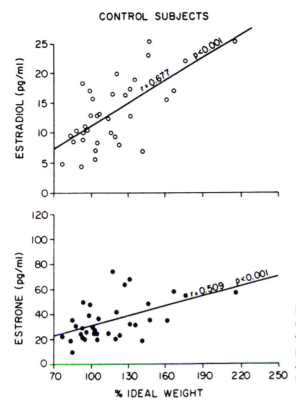

CONTROL SUBJECTS

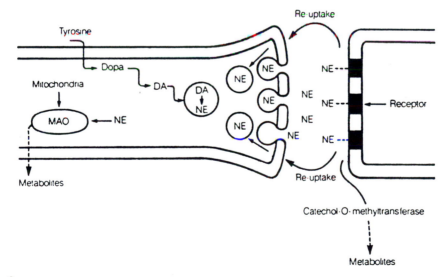

FIG 16–7.
Correlation of plasma estradiol and estrone levels with percentage of ideal weight in postmenopausal women. (From Judd HL, Davidson BJ, Frumar AM, et al: Serum androgens and estrogens in postmenopausal women. *Am J Obstet Gynecol* 1980; 136:859. Reproduced by permission.)

FIG 16–8.
Schematic representation of an adrenergic junction. Tyrosine is converted by the enzyme tyrosine hydroxylase to 3,4-dihydroxyphenylalanine *(Dopa)*, decarboxylated to dopamine *(DA)*, hydroxylated to form norepinephrine *(NE)*, and stored in vesicles. On release, NE interacts with adrenergic receptors. This action is terminated by reuptake of NE back into the prejunctional neurons. Norepinephrine is degraded into inactive metabolites by monoamine oxidase *(MAO)* and catechol-O-methyltransferase. (From Berkow R (ed): *The Merck Manual of Diagnosis and Therapy.* Rahway, NJ, Merck & Co, 1987, p 2472. Reproduced by permission.)

rosine) and monoamine oxidase (which irreversibly degrades NE to inactive metabolites). After synthesis, NE is stored in prejunctional vesicles. When released into the synaptic cleft, NE binds to postjunctional receptors to propagate a response, either excitatory or inhibitory. This action is terminated by the rapid reuptake of NE back into the prejunctional neuron.

In animals, estrogen has been found to have multiple effects on NE neurons. Estrogen stimulates tyrosine hydroxylase activity (Beattie et al., 1972), thereby increasing NE synthesis. In addition, estrogen reduces monoamine oxidase activity (Luine and McEwen, 1977) and so retards NE degradation. Both of these actions will increase the intraneuronal level of NE. Estrogen has also been shown to augment NE release (Paul et al., 1979) and inhibit NE reuptake (Nixon et al., 1974), thereby potentiating its effect on postjunctional receptors. Finally, estrogen also appears to increase the number of hypothalamic α_2-postsynaptic receptors (Johnson et al., 1985). All of these actions serve to enhance α_2-adrenergic activity. Since this work has been performed in animals, it is not definitively known if estrogen has the same effects in humans. Nevertheless, these findings do suggest that estrogens enhance α_2-adrenergic activity, and that estrogen withdrawal may lead to vasomotor flushes due to reduced α_2-adrenergic activity.

This hypothesis is consistent with the finding that α_2-agonists such as clonidine (Clayden et al., 1974), methyldopa (Aldomet; after conversion to its active form, methylnorepinephrine; Hammond et al., 1984), and lofexidine (Jones et al., 1985), have all been shown to reduce hot flashes (see later discussion). This is consistent with the fact that estrogen replacement does not produce immediate relief of flashes (see later discussion) but requires 2 to 4 weeks to exert its maximal effects (Haas et al., 1988); altering central NE metabolism would not be expected to be an instantaneous process. This alteration of NE metabolism would be expected to persist for a short time after estrogen withdrawal, explaining why hot flash relief continues after estrogens are discontinued. As well, endorphins may play a role in the etiology of hot flashes.

Diagnosis

A careful history and physical examination should be sufficient to make the diagnosis and exclude other conditions such as thyrotoxicosis, carcinoid tumor, pheochromocytoma, anxiety, diabetic insulin reaction, alcohol withdrawal, and diencephalic epilepsy. Menopause may be confirmed, if necessary, by demonstrating an elevated serum FSH level. However, the finding of a low serum estradiol level is not diagnostic, since premenopausal women frequently have low levels during menses.

Treatment

Estrogens

Since hot flashes are a consequence of estrogen withdrawal, the most effective form of therapy is estrogen replacement, having greater than 95% efficacy (Utian, 1975). By relieving hot flashes, particularly those occurring at night, estrogen replacement will improve sleep quality; estrogen treatment has been shown to reduce sleep latency and to increase rapid eye movement sleep (Schiff et al., 1979). In a double-blind, placebo-controlled study, estrogen use was found to decrease insomnia, irritability, and anxiety while improving memory (Campbell and Whitehead, 1977). Thus, those symptoms that appear to result from a chronic sleep disturbance are significantly improved by estrogen replacement.

A dose-response relationship between estrogen dose and hot flash frequency was demonstrated for transdermal estrogens (Steingold et al., 1985). After 3 weeks of treatment, flashes were reduced by 40% with a 0.025-mg dose, by 53% with a 0.05-mg dose, by 83% with a 0.10-mg dose, and by 91% with a 0.20-mg dose. Treatment with placebo had no effect.

Treatment with estrogen does not produce immediate relief of hot flashes; 2 to 4 weeks appears to be necessary. Haas (1988) studied 19 women who kept daily records of their flashes after starting treatment with transdermal estrogens (Fig 16–9). Hot flash frequency was not reduced until after 2 weeks of treatment, and maximal relief did not occur until 4 weeks. Thus, the adequacy of a particular dose in relieving flushes cannot be known until after 4 weeks' time; doses should not be adjusted more frequently than this. Haas also showed that hot flashes are significantly suppressed for more than 2 weeks after treatment is discontinued. It should be recognized that estrogen replacement is not a permanent cure for hot flashes; they will return when treatment is discontinued. For that reason, estrogens should

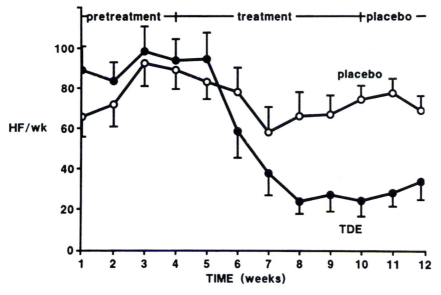

FIG 16–9.

Change in subjective hot flashes *(HF)* recorded by postmenopausal women treated with transdermal estrogen *(TDE)* and placebo. (From Haas S, Walsh B, Evans S, et al: The effect of transdermal estradiol on hormone and metabolic dynamics over a six-week period. *Obstet Gynecol* 1988; 71:671. Reproduced by permission.)

not be abruptly discontinued but should be slowly tapered over a number of weeks to months to avoid the return of hot flashes. The patient should be advised of this when terminating estrogen therapy.

Progestins

Women with endometrial cancer undergoing treatment with depomedroxyprogesterone acetate (Depo-Provera, or depo-MPA) were incidentally noted to have relief of their hot flashes. A double-blind randomized study of 47 patients evaluated the effects of 50, 100, and 150 mg of intramuscular depo-MPA on hot flashes. Hot flash frequency fell within 2 weeks after injection, became maximal at 4 weeks, and remained suppressed for the remainder of the 12 weeks of observation. A dose-response effect was also demonstrated, with 50 mg reducing flashes by 60%, 100 mg by 75%, and 150 mg by 85%. Placebo had no appreciable effect (Morrison et al., 1980). This temporal relationship in hot flash relief, as well as dose responsiveness, resembles that seen with transdermal estrogens (see earlier discussion). Unfortunately, the use of depo-MPA is associated with a high incidence of irregular vaginal bleeding, as well as a prolonged but unpredictable duration of action.

Oral MPA, with a considerably shorter and more predictable half-life, was evaluated in a randomized, double-blind, placebo-controlled study of 27 patients (Schiff et al., 1980). Twenty milligrams of MPA daily was found to reduce vasomotor flushes by 70% after 1 month's time; in comparison, placebo reduced flushes by 15%. A later study found 10 mg of MPA daily to reduce flush frequency by 87% compared with placebo after 4 weeks of treatment. Placebo reduced hot flashes by 25% (Albrecht et al., 1981).

The mechanism of action of progestins is unknown. It has been hypothesized that they too may act via central neurotransmitters, since they raise the hypothalamic thermoregulatory set point during the luteal phase of ovulatory women. Progestins are useful in patients for whom estrogen is contraindicated, but they may cause irregular vaginal bleeding, as well as abdominal bloating, breast tenderness, and mood changes.

Clonidine

Clonidine, an α-adrenergic agonist, significantly lowers hot flash frequency by 30% to 40% when used at doses of 0.1 and 0.2 mg twice daily. At these doses, patients frequently complain of dizziness and dry mouth (Laufer et al., 1982).

For that reason, the appropriate initial dose should be 0.05 mg twice daily, increasing to 0.1 mg twice daily if hot flashes persist and if there are no side effects. Clonidine tends to be tolerated best by hypertensive patients, who may be the best candidates for this nonhormonal treatment. Clonidine has been hypothesized to act as a central α-adrenergic agonist on the hypothalamus to "stabilize" the thermoregulatory center (see earlier discussion). The possibility also exists that it may act directly on the peripheral vasculature, to block the vasodilation that characterizes vasomotor flushes.

Other α-Adrenergic Agonists

Hypertensive women taking methyldopa were incidentally noted to have few hot flashes. Hammond et al. (1984) studied 10 women, randomizing them to either 250 mg of methyldopa three times daily or to placebo and then crossed over to the other treatment. Methyldopa was found to reduce flashes by 20% compared with placebo according to subjective patient report. Similarly, another adrenergic agonist, lofexidine, was evaluated in five women, also using a randomized, double-blind, crossover design (Jones et al., 1985). The initial dose of lofexidine was 0.1 mg twice daily, increasing by increments of 0.1 mg every 2 weeks until flashes were abolished, until side effects (dry mouth, fatigue, and headache) were intolerable, or until a maximum dose of 0.6 mg twice daily was reached. At the maximum tolerated dose, patients had 66% fewer hot flashes compared with placebo by subjective report. Thus, both of these α-adrenergic agonists, methyldopa and lofexidine, significantly reduce flashes, but side effects such as dry mouth, fatigue, and headache limit their use.

Bellergal

Bellergal, a preparation of ergotamine tartrate, belladonna alkaloids, and 40 mg of phenobarbital, has been shown to be 50% effective (Lebherz and French, 1969). It is unknown which of its components is responsible for its effectiveness. The usual dose is one tablet twice daily. Due to its addictive potential and the fact that safer alternative treatments are available, this medicine should rarely be necessary.

Other agents, such as tricyclic antidepressants and oxazepam, have been proposed for the treatment of hot flashes. Because they have not been compared with placebo, their therapeutic efficacy

remains unproved. Comparison with placebo is important, since many investigators have shown placebo to significantly reduce hot flashes.

OSTEOPOROSIS

Definition and Etiology

Osteoporosis is the progressive reduction in bone mass without qualitative abnormalities. It affects trabecular bone earlier than cortical bone, and its major consequence is fracture. The most frequent sites of fracture are the vertebral bodies, distal radius, and femoral neck.

Primary osteoporosis results from estrogen deficiency and constitutes 95% of all cases. Recent work suggests that estrogen receptors are present in bone, and so estrogen may act on bone directly (Komm et al., 1988). Alternatively, estrogen has been theorized to act by one of the following mechanisms:

1. Decreasing the sensitivity of bone to parathyroid hormone (PTH) without changing the amount of circulatory PTH.
2. Increasing calcitonin. This is consistent with the facts that (a) high estrogen states such as oral contraceptives and pregnancy are associated with elevated calcitonin levels (Lindsay and Sweeney, 1976); (b) men, who have greater bone mass than women, have higher calcitonin levels as well (Hillyard et al., 1978); and (c) calcitonin levels decline with age (Deftos et al., 1980) and menopause and rise with estrogen replacement (Stevenson et al., 1981).
3. Directly increasing intestinal calcium absorption.

Secondary osteoporosis is a consequence of any of the following disorders: glucocorticoid or heparin use, renal failure, hyperthyroidism, primary hyperparathyroidism, hyperadrenalism, dietary calcium deficiency, or upper gastrointestinal surgery.

Incidence

Peak bone mass is achieved at age 30 years, with men at all ages having a greater mass than women. Bone is then progressively lost with aging, at a rate of approximately 1% to 2% per year after age 40 to 50 years (Heanly, 1976). This loss is accelerated at the time of menopause, averaging 3.9% per year for 6 years (Fig 16–10; Horsman et al., 1977).

Individuals with a lower peak bone mass are more likely to develop significant osteoporosis, so that women are at a higher risk than men, whites and Asians more than blacks (Smith et al., 1973), and thin women more than obese ones (Dalen et al., 1975). This greater bone mass of obese women may be due to their increased weight, placing additional mechanical stress on their axial skeleton. An alternative explanation is that these women have greater endogenous estrogens due to (1) increased peripheral aromatization of androstenedione to estrone (Grodin et al., 1973) and (2) lower sex hormone–binding globulin with greater free estradiol levels (Davidson et al., 1981).

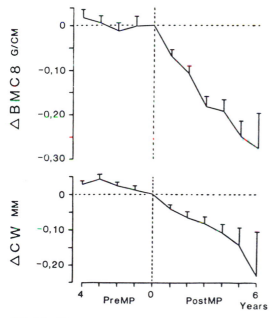

FIG 16–10.

Mean (± SEM) changes in bone mass, measured as bone mineral content (grams per centimeter) of the proximal *(BMC8)* forearm and mean cortical width *(CW)* (millimeters) of metacarpals 2, 3, and 4 of both hands. δ, changes from the last premenopausal *(PreMP)* year. Broken horizontal line gives values for the last premenopausal year (0), and the broken vertical line indicates the last premenopausal year. (From Falch JA, Oftebro H, Haug E: Early postmenopausal bone loss not associated with decrease in vitamin D. *J Clin Endocrinol Metab* 1987; 64:836. Reproduced by permission.)

The rate of bone loss varies greatly among individuals: women who smoke, drink alcohol, are sedentary, or consume low-calcium or high-protein or high-phosphate diets will lose bone mass more quickly (Daniell, 1976; Aloia et al., 1978; Matkovic et al., 1979; Licata et al., 1981). Family history is also a significant risk factor.

Twenty-five percent of women beyond age 60 years will show vertebral fractures on x-ray film, as will 50% of women beyond age 75 years (Alffam, 1964; Iskrant, 1968). Twenty-five percent of women beyond the age of 80 years will have a hip fracture (Gordon and Vaughan, 1976), with the annual incidence being 1.3% per year after age 65 years and 3.3% per year after age 85 years (Lindsay et al., 1984a). One of six women with hip fractures will succumb within three months (Gallagher and Nordin, 1973). The annual health care cost in the United States for these fractures is estimated to be $4 billion.

Diagnosis

Once osteoporosis has occurred, it may be difficult to reverse. For that reason, a number of radiological modalities have been developed to attempt to detect a loss of bone mass before fractures occur. Since osteoporosis affects trabecular bone earlier than cortical bone, those modalities that measure trabecular bone preferentially will be the most informative; however, this usually requires greater expense and radiation exposure.

Single-photon absorptiometry of the distal radius is inexpensive, easy to perform, and requires only 5 mrem of radiation. However, it measures 75% cortical bone and 25% trabecular bone, which is its primary limitation. In skilled hands, it has an accuracy within 5% and a precision of 2% to 4% (Dequeker and Johnston, 1981).

Dual-photon absorptiometry of the second to fourth vertebral body offers an advantage because it measures 60% cortical bone and 40% trabecular bone. It is more expensive, requires 5 to 15 mrem, and has an accuracy within 5% to 7% with a precision of 2% to 5% (Dequeker and Johnston, 1981).

Computed tomography of the vertebral body measures 5% cortical bone and 95% trabecular bone and so may detect changes over an interval as short as 6 months (Cann et al., 1980). It has the greatest radiation exposure (200 mrem) and expense and has a precision of 1% to 3%.

The most recent modality to be developed, quantitative digital radiography (QDR), provides high-resolution images with a high degree of precision (1%–2%) but a much lower radiation exposure (1–3 mrem; Kelly et al., 1988). Quantitative digital radiography requires less than 8 minutes per study, which is considerably faster than the time needed for dualphoton absorptiometry (20–45 minutes).

A nonradiological method has been proposed to identify those women who will be "fast bone losers" (i.e., greater than 3.1% loss per year of forearm bone mineral content) and would therefore benefit most by estrogen replacement. A single measurement of a fasting urinary calcium/creatinine ratio greater than 270 mmoles/mole, fasting urinary hydroxyproline/creatinine ratio greater than 11.2 mmoles/mole, serum alkaline phosphatase level greater than 120 µg/L, and a fat mass index less than 0.222 (calculated from height and weight) correctly identified 79% of the "fast losers" and 78% of the "slow losers." The discriminatory power of this method is less than ideal; the predictive value of an abnormal test result was only 53% (Christiansen et al., 1987).

Patients found to have osteoporosis or osteoporosis-related fractures should undergo careful history and physical examination to exclude an underlying etiology (see earlier discussion). Measurement of serum calcium, phosphate, and alkaline phosphatase levels, sedimentation rate, or serum protein electrophoresis may assist in identifying any of those disorders, but they will all be normal in patients with primary osteoporosis.

Prevention

As previously stated, established osteoporosis may not be significantly reversed; for this reason, the emphasis of medical management should be on prophylaxis rather than on treatment. Stopping smoking, reducing dietary phosphates, and, particularly, exercising regularly, will all act to preserve bone mass.

Estrogens have been clearly shown to prevent osteoporosis, causing decreased bone resorption (Fig 16–11; Christiansen et al., 1981), increased intestinal calcium absorption, and reduced renal calcium excretion (Lobo et al., 1983). Conjugated equine estrogens CCEEs, 0.625 mg, have been proved to be as effective as 1.25 mg in preventing bone loss as well as reducing the incidence of fractures (Fig 16–12; Weiss et al., 1980). Ethinyl estradiol (EE) and mestranol, 20 µg, have also been found to be effective (Lindsay et al., 1976); but this dose has a much greater effect on the liver than does 0.625 mg of CEEs (Mandel et al 1982b). Thus, nonsynthetic estrogens are preferable to synthetic ones. To be maximally effective, estrogens should be initiated

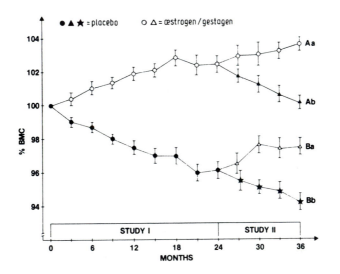

FIG 16–11.
Bone mineral content *(BMC)* as a function of time and treatment in 94 *(study I)* and 77 (study II) women soon after menopause. (From Christiansen C, Christiansen MS, Transbol I: Bone mass in postmenopausal women after withdrawal of estrogen/gestagen replacement therapy. *Lancet* 1981; 1:459. Reproduced by permission.)

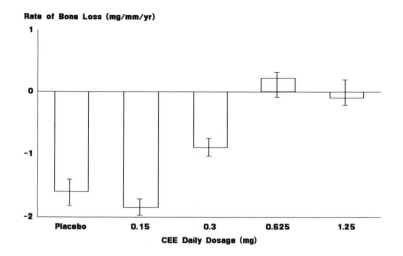

FIG 16–12.

Mean annual change (± SEM) in bone mass in women treated daily with placebo, 0.15, 0.3, 0.625, and 1.25 mg of oral CEEs. Bone mineral content measured by single-photon absorptiometry at the midpoint of the third right metacarpal. (Adapted from Lindsay R, Hart DM, Clark DM: The minimum effective dose of estrogen for prevention of postmenopausal bone loss. *Obstet Gynecol* 1984; 63:759.)

shortly after the menopause to prevent the rapid bone loss that occurs at that time. Treatment should continue for at least 6 years to substantially reduce the lifetime risk of fracture (Fig 16–13). Because there is no ideal method to identify which patients will develop osteoporosis, all postmenopausal women should discuss this therapy with their physicians. Measurement of baseline bone density may be helpful for patients when the decision to initiate estrogen replacement is difficult.

Progestins used alone have also been shown to restore urinary calcium/creatinine ratios, but preservation of bone mass has not yet been demonstrated (Lindsay et al., 1978). Appropriate doses are of 10 mg MPA daily (Mandel et al.,

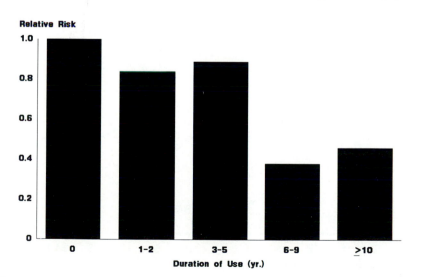

FIG 16–13.

Relative risk for hip or forearm fracture according to duration of postmenopausal estrogen use. (Adapted from Weiss NS, Ure CL, Ballard JH, et al: Decreased risk of fractures of the hip and lower forearm with postmenopausal use of estrogen. *N Engl J Med* 1980; 303:1195.)

1982), or 150 mg of depo-MPA intramuscularly every 3 months (Lobo et al., 1984a). Combined with estrogen, progestins may act synergistically to increase bone mass. A proposed mechanism is that progesterone may block glucocorticoid receptors located in bone (Manolagas and Anderson, 1978), preventing endogenous glucocorticoids from exerting their inhibitory effects on bone metabolism.

Calcium supplementation has been found to modestly reduce the rate of bone loss (Recker et al., 1977) but is not a substitute for estrogen therapy in preventing osteoporosis (Fig 16–14). However, it may serve as a useful adjunct to estrogen treatment, allowing a lower dose of estrogen to be used (Ettinger et al., 1984). Since the dietary intake of calcium necessary to maintain positive balance, 1,500 mg daily, exceeds that found in most diets, oral supplements are usually necessary to achieve this amount. Although increasing dietary calcium does not change the percent of calcium absorbed, it does increase the total amount. Caution should be used in patients with a history of renal stones.

Fluoride has been proposed for the treatment of osteoporosis. Its use has been complicated by a high incidence of side effects, including hematemesis, anemia, joint pain, and neurological symptoms. Moreover, the bone formed has been thought to be weak and brittle. More recently, a slow-release oral preparation of sodium fluoride, 25 mg twice daily, has been found to significantly increase lumbar bone mass as measured by dual-photon absorptiometry, with a low incidence of side effects. Cyclic treatment has been recommended to prevent osteoblasts from becoming re-fractory to fluoride-induced stimulation; 3 months of fluoride therapy are followed by a 2-month rest period. Calcium and vitamin D supplementation is added to this regimen (Pak et al., 1989).

GENITAL ATROPHY

Pathogenesis

The tissues of the lower portion of the vagina, labia, urethra, and trigone are of common embryonic origin, derived from the urogenital sinus, and are all estrogen dependent (Iosif et al., 1981). Following the loss of estrogen at menopause, the vaginal walls become pale, due to diminished vascularity, as well as thin, perhaps only three or four cells thick. The vaginal epithelial cells contain less glycogen, which prior to menopause has been metabolized by lactobacilli to create an acidic pH, thereby protecting the vagina from bacterial overgrowth. Loss of this protective mechanism leaves the thin, friable tissue vulnerable to infection and ulceration. The vagina also loses its rugae and becomes shorter and inelastic.

Patients may complain of symptoms secondary to vaginal dryness, such as dyspareunia and vaginismus, which may lead to diminished libido. They may also have symptoms secondary to vaginal ulceration and infection, such as vaginal discharge, burning, itching, or bleeding.

The urethra and urinary trigone undergo atrophic changes similar to those of the vagina. Dysuria, urgency, frequency, and suprapubic pain may occur in the absence of infection. A proposed mechanism is that the markedly thin urethral mu-

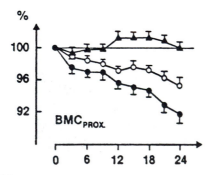
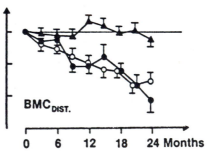

FIG 16–14.
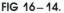
Bone mineral content of the proximal (BMC$_{PROX}$) and distal (BMC$_{DIST}$) radius of postmenopausal women treated with percutaneous estrogens *(solid triangle)*, calcium *(open circle)* and placebo *(solid circle)*.

(From Riis B, Thomsen K, Christiansen C: Does calcium supplementation prevent postmenopausal bone loss? *N Engl J Med* 1987; 316:173. Reproduced by permission.)

cosa may allow urine to come in close contact with sensory nerves. In addition, the menopausal loss of the resistance to urinary flow by thick, well-vascularized urethral mucosa has been hypothesized to contribute to urinary incontinence (Zinner et al., 1980)

Diagnosis

Atrophic vaginitis may be diagnosed by its typical appearance, but a biopsy specimen of all atypical lesions should be taken. If a discharge is present, it should be evaluated for pathogens such as *Candida, Neisseria gonorrhoeae, Chlamydia, Trichomonas,* and *Gardnerella*. If *Candida* is found, the patient should be screened for diabetes, since the low glycogen content of unestrogenized vaginal epithelial cells will not ordinarily support its growth. The presence of atrophy may be confirmed, if necessary, by a vaginal cell maturation index, obtained by scraping the lateral vaginal wall at the level of the cervix. The exfoliated cells may then be classified by degree of maturation,

with a small proportion of superficial cells indicating a high degree of vaginal atrophy.

Atrophic urethritis or trigonitis is diagnosed by ruling out the presence of infection. Urethroscopy will reveal a pale, atrophic urethra.

Treatment

Estrogen is the only effective therapy, with the dose required generally being less than that needed for hot flashes or osteoporosis. Thus, treatment for those conditions will also be adequate for genital atrophy. If this is the only indication for estrogen treatment, daily use for a minimum of 2 to 12 weeks is required to reverse the atrophic changes, followed by intermittent therapy, two to three times weekly. Usual daily oral doses are 0.3 or 0.625 mg of CEEs; 0.3, 0.625, or 1.25 mg of estrone; or 1 or 2 mg of micronized β-estradiol (Carr and MacDonald, 1983). Transdermal estradiol, 50 μg twice weekly, is also effective. Estrogens may also be administered vaginally, such as 0.3 mg of CEEs (Fig 16–15)

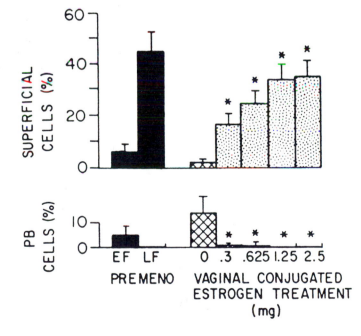

FIG 16–15.
Mean (± SEM) percent superficial and parabasal *(PB)* cells from vaginal exfoliative cytology. Premenopausal controls in the early follicular *(EF)* and late follicular *(LF)* phases of their cycles are compared with postmenopausal women before and after vaginal administration of various doses of conjugated estrogen. *Asterisk indicates significant difference (*p* < 0.05) from the untreated postmenopausal value. (From Mandel FP, Geola FL, Meldrum DR, et al: Biologic effects of various doses of vaginally administered conjugated equine estrogens in postmenopausal women. *J Clin Endocrinol Metab* 1983; 57:133. Reproduced by permission.)

(Mandel et al., 1983) or 0.2 mg of micronized β-estradiol (Gordon et al., 1979). Although they exert a local effect, they are rapidly absorbed systemically (Schiff et al., 1977). Thus, the addition of a progestational agent is advised for patients with an intact uterus.

If estrogens are contraindicated, water-soluble lubricants may relieve dyspareunia. Improvement of vaginal stenosis has been accomplished by the careful use of graduated vaginal dilators.

ATHEROSCLEROSIS

Estrogens have been hypothesized to protect against atherosclerosis, since American women at all ages have lower rates of cardiovascular disease (CVD) than do men of the same age. However, prior to menopause, women have approximately one fifth the CVD mortality of men, but after the menopause their mortality rapidly rises to become one half that of men (Fig 16–16; Lerner and Kannel, 1986). One explanation is that a premenopausal woman's estrogen confers protection, which is lost at menopause. This is supported by the observation that women who undergo a premature surgical menopause (i.e., bilateral oophorectomy) and do not use postmenopausal estrogens have significantly more CVD than do age-matched premenopausal controls. If they use postmenopausal estrogens, however, their incidence of CVD is the same as premenopausal women of the same age. Premature natural menopause, in contrast, was not found to increase CVD risk when controlled for age, smoking, and estrogen use (Coldnitz et al., 1987).

Epidemiologic studies have compared the incidence of CVD among postmenopausal estrogen users and nonusers. Retrospective case-control studies (Pfeffer et al., 1978; Ross et al., 1981; Bain et al., 1981) provided inconsistent results, although most found estrogen use to be associated with less CVD. Prospective cohort studies, which have fewer sources of bias, generally showed estrogen use to reduce CVD (Hammond et al., 1979; Bush et al., 1983; Burch et al., 1974; Petitti et al., 1979). One notable exception is the Framingham Study, which demonstrated an adverse effect (Wilson et al., 1985) or no effect (Eaker and Castelli, 1987) of estrogen treatment, depending on the inclusion criteria for CVD and the multiple regression model employed. In contrast, the Nurses' Health Study (Stampfer et al., 1985), the largest cohort study following 32,317 postmenopausal women for 2 to 4 years, identified 90 cases of nonfatal myocardial infarction (MI) or fatal coronary heart disease. The relative risk of coronary heart disease with estrogen use was significantly reduced to 0.5 (95% confidence

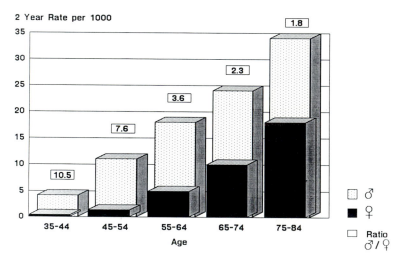

FIG 16–16.
Incidence of myocardial infarctions (MI) by age and sex (female, *solid bar*; male, *stippled bar*): 26 years of follow-up, Framingham study. Ratio of male to female MIs for each age group is noted at top of graph. (Adapted from Lerner DJ, Kannel WB: Patterns of coronary disease morbidity and mortality: A 26-year follow-up of the Framingham population. *Am Heart J* 1986; 111:383.)

interval [CI]: 0.3–0.8) for "ever" use and 0.3 (CI: 0.2–0.7) for current use. Adjustment for a number of cardiovascular risk factors did not alter these findings, arguing against any major physician bias to prescribe estrogens to healthier women. Therefore, the weight of evidence suggests that postmenopausal estrogen replacement protects against CVD.

The only attempts to reduce CVD by estrogen treatment have all been performed in men. Early trials, enrolling men after an MI, showed estrogen treatment to reduce serum cholesterol levels but not the incidence of a second event (Stamler et al., 1980; Oliver and Boyd, 1961). The Coronary Drug Project, consisting of 1,101 MI survivors, was terminated when excess thrombotic events were seen in the estrogen-treated group; CVD incidence was not reduced (Coronary Drug Project Research Group, 1973). This experience is similar to that seen in men with prostatic cancer treated with an estrogen, diethylstilbestrol, which appears to increase CVD, possibly by causing excessive fluid accumulation, leading to congestive heart failure, or by increasing thromboembolism (DeVogt et al., 1986). This adverse action of estrogen in men may have been the consequence of high estrogenic potency of the doses used and may not reflect the physiologic action of estrogens.

Since men and women have an equal incidence of CVD when matched for lipoprotein concentrations (Gordon et al., 1977), the sex difference in CVD may be a consequence of the characteristic sex differences in serum lipoprotein concentrations. Thus, premenopausal women appear to be protected against CVD by their typically lower low-density lipoprotein (LDL) levels and higher high-density lipoprotein (HDL) levels compared with men of the same age (Fig 16–17). However, coincident with the loss of estrogen, female LDL levels rise at the time of the menopause to exceed those of men (Kannel, 1987). It has been suggested that the loss of estrogen at the menopause causes this increase in LDL levels, since postmenopausal estrogen replacement has been found to lower LDL levels in a dose-dependent fashion by 4% to 11% (Notelovitz et al., 1983; Robinson and Lebeau, 1965). In contrast, HDL levels in women are unaffected by menarche (Orchard and Rodgers, 1980), menopause, and aging (Kannel, 1987). Thus, the HDL-raising effect of oral estrogens appears to

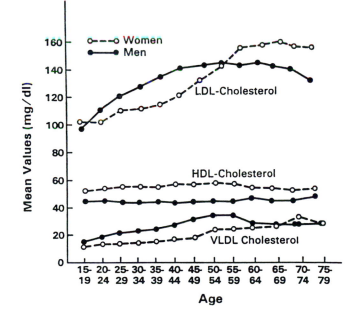

FIG 16–17.
Age and sex trends in lipoprotein cholesterol fractions, Framingham study. (From Kannel WB: Risk factors for coronary disease in women. Perspective from the Framingham study. *Am Heart J* 1987; 114:413. Reproduced by permission.)

be a pharmacological action of the high portal estrogen concentrations presented to the liver following intestinal absorption. Therefore, if endogenous estrogens protect against CVD, an effect on the level of LDL, rather than HDL, is the likely mechanism.

An alternative explanation has been proposed for the sex difference in CVD, since a semilogarithmic plot of female cardiovascular deaths against age shows that the rate of increase in the rate of CVD is constant throughout a woman's lifetime and is not accelerated after the menopause. In contrast, a similar analysis of male CVD shows a decline in the rate of increase after the onset of the "male climacteric," when testosterone levels wane (Fig 16–18; Heller and Jacobs,

1978). This decline in androgens may therefore be the major factor responsible for the lower female/male CVD ratio seen with increasing age. Androgens are known to adversely affect serum lipoprotein levels; both exogenous use (e.g., testosterone enanthate and methyltestosterone) and endogenous increases in androgen levels (occurring during puberty) have been found to lower HDL levels and raise LDL levels (Kirkland et al., 1987; Oliver and Boyd, 1956; Orchard and Rodgers, 1980).

Since there are no long-term randomized studies of postmenopausal estrogen replacement to address this issue, the beneficial effect of estrogen replacement on CVD remains unproved.

ESTROGENS

Pharmacology

Synthetic estrogens are chemical derivatives of estradiol. Ethinyl estradiol (EE) results from the addition of a 17 α-ethinyl group, which impedes catabolism by the liver, leading to its long half-life of 48 hours. The other commonly used synthetic estrogen, mestranol, must undergo demethylation by the liver to become EE, its active form. Because this demethylation is only 50% complete, mestranol has only one half of the potency of EE (Delforge and Ferrin, 1970; Briggs and Briggs, 1973; Schwartz and Hammerstein, 1973). These synthetic estrogens, when given orally, are more than 100 times as potent on a per weight basis as natural estrogens in stimulating the production of hepatic proteins (Mashchak et al., 1982). Since the minimum dose for therapeutic effect (10 µg), exceeds the lowest dose that markedly elevates hepatic globulin levels (5 µg) (Mandel et al., 1982b), these synthetic estrogens are not routinely recommended for postmenopausal use.

Nonsynthetic "natural" estrogens may be administered orally, vaginally, transdermally, or subcutaneously. Orally administered estradiol is rapidly converted in the intestinal mucosa to estrone, which is then presented to the liver, where 30% of an initial dose is conjugated with glucuronide on the first pass (Siddle and Whitehead, 1983). These conjugates undergo rapid renal and biliary excretion. The biliary conjugates are hydrolyzed by intestinal flora, allowing for 80% to be reabsorbed and returned to the liver. They may then be reconjugated and excreted or may enter the systemic circulation. This enterohepatic circula-

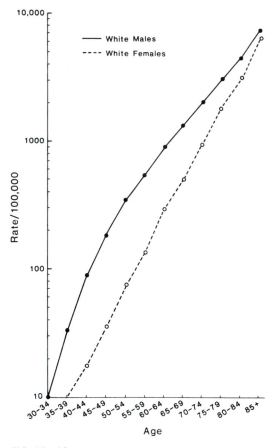

FIG 16–18.
Age-specific mortality rates for ischemic heart disease by sex (whites only, United States, 1977). (From Ross RK, Paganini-Hill A: Estrogen replacement therapy and coronary heart disease. *Semin Reprod Endocrinol* 1983; 1:19. Reproduced by permission.)

tion contributes to the prolonged effect of orally administered estrogens. Thus, patients with altered gut flora (e.g., antibiotic therapy) may not sufficiently hydrolyze these conjugates, thereby preventing reabsorption. They may thus require higher doses for a therapeutic effect. Also, patients chronically maintained on phenytoin therapy have enhanced glucuronidation and will more rapidly excrete estrogens (Englund and Johansson, 1978). They too may require higher doses.

The commonest nonsynthetic estrogens used orally are CEEs (0.625 mg), piperazine estrone sulfate (1.25 mg), and micronized estradiol-17β (1 mg). At these doses, the mean peak serum estradiol level will range from 30 to 40 pg/ml, similar to that of the premenopausal early follicular phase; the estrone level will range from 150 to 250 pg/ml (Lobo et al., 1984b). These doses are generally effective in relieving menopausal symptoms such as hot flashes as well as normalizing urinary calcium/creatinine ratios while having a minimal effect on the liver. In general, CEEs are twice as potent as estrone preparations (Mashchak et al., 1982); they contain up to 50% of the potent equine estrogens, including equilin and 17 α-dihydroequilin sulfates, with the remainder being estrone sulfate. These equine estrogens have a prolonged action, due in part to storage and slow release from adipose tissue, and have been detected in the blood as long as 13 weeks after administration (Whittaker et al., 1980).

Since the concentration of estrogen in the portal circulation after oral ingestion is four to five times that in the general circulation, there is more estrogen presented to hepatocytes than to cells of other organs. Thus, estrogens given orally will have a more profound effect on the liver than those given parenterally. Although many of these actions on the liver may potentially be deleterious, such as stimulating renin-substrate and coagulation factors, some effects may be beneficial, such as increasing HDL levels and decreasing LDL levels. Both of these effects on lipoprotein levels may reduce cardiovascular risk (Fig 16–19). In any case, appropriate doses of parenteral estradiol, given vaginally or transdermally, can result in therapeutic serum estradiol levels with relief of hot flashes and restoration of urinary calcium/creatinine ratios while having a minimal effect on the liver. In addition, estradiol will enter the systemic circulation directly without significant conversion to estrone, so that the serum estradiol level will exceed that of estrone, as is seen prior to menopause.

Parenteral estrogens may be given by the vaginal, transdermal, or subcutaneous route. Vaginal estrogens are absorbed and enter the systemic circulation, achieving one fourth of the circulatory level of an equal dose given orally (Deutsch et al., 1981). However, they exert a potent local effect; 0.3 mg of CEEs given vaginally produces the same degree of epithelial maturation as 1.25 mg

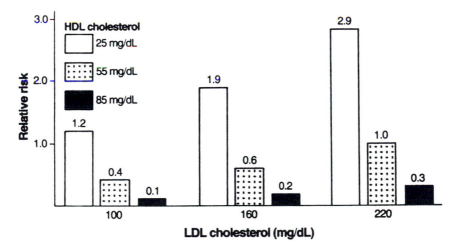

FIG 16–19.
Relative risk of coronary heart disease by HDL and LDL cholesterol levels. Framingham study of normotensive men aged 50 to 70 years, with 4 years' follow-up. (From Kannel WB: Lipids, diabetes, and coronary heart disease: Insights from the Framingham study. *Am Heart J* 1985; 110:1100. Reproduced by permission.)

given orally (Mandel et al., 1983; Geola et al., 1980). The continued use of estrogen vaginally will lead to increased circulatory levels due to enhanced transfer across a healthier, more vascularized epithelium (Siddle and Whitehead, 1983).

Subdermal estradiol pellets (25 mg) have been found to be effective but have variable life spans of 3 to 6 months and are difficult to remove. Transdermal skin patches, applied twice weekly, will provide constant serum estrogen levels: the 50 μg patch yields a mean serum estradiol level of 70 pg/ml and an estrone level of 50 pg/ml, which are usually adequate to significantly reduce hot flashes (Haas et al., 1988).

A comparison of the biological potencies of various estrogens on different organ systems is presented in Table 16–1.

Possible Side Effects

Estrogens may cause nausea, mastalgia, headache, and mood changes. A discussion of more serious risks follows.

Endometrial Neoplasia

Unopposed estrogen use (i.e., without the addition of a progestin) may induce endometrial hyperplasia and, ultimately, adenocarcinoma. These carcinomas associated with estrogen use are generally of early stage and low grade and are less apt to have invaded myometrium (Chu et al., 1982). The adjusted 5-year survival is 94% compared with 81% for estrogen nonusers (Elwood and Boyes, 1980), possibly due to one or more of the following: (1) women prescribed estrogens

TABLE 16–1.

Comparison of the Biological Potencies of Different Estrogen Preparations*

| | Dose Producing 50% Maximal Effect (mg) | | | | Dose Producing Premenopausal Status (mg) | | | |
| | Suppression | Induction | | | | | | |
	FSH	Angioten-sinogen	SHBG†	CBG‡	Vaginal Cytology	Urinary Ca/Cr§	Bone Density	Level Suppressing Ovulation (mg)
Oral								
Estrone	1.7	1.7	4.4	8.4			2.5	
Estradiol-17β	1.3	2.4	4.4	4.4			1.0	5.0
Conjugated equine estrogen	1.2	0.49	1.4	3.4	>1.25	0.625	0.625	3.75
Diethylstilbestrol	0.45	0.13	0.16	0.12				5.0
Ethinyl estradiol	0.01	0.004	0.007	0.001	0.005	0.01	0.02	0.05
Mestranol					0.020		0.024	0.08
Parenteral								
Transdermal estradiol-17β patch	0.100	—‖	—‖	—‖	0.10	0.05		
Transdermal estradiol-17β gel							3.0	
Vaginal estradiol	>2.5	—‖	—‖	—‖	0.3	1.25		
Vaginal conjugated estrogen	>2				0.2			

*Data from Mashchak, 1982; 144:511; Martinez-Menayton, 1969; Lagrelius, 1981; Christiansen, 1982 Geola, 1980; Lindsay, 1984; Horsman, 1983; Henzl, 1973; and Chetkowski, 1986.
†SHBG=sex hormone–binding globulin.
‡CBG=corticosteroid-binding globulin.
§Ca/Cr=calcium/creatinine.
‖No apparent effect at standard doses.

are generally in better health than nonusers; (2) they are followed more closely, allowing for earlier diagnosis; or (3) only well-differentiated endometrial neoplasms retain estrogen receptors, by which exogenous estrogens can provide a stimulus.

Retrospective case-control studies have found unopposed estrogen use to increase the risk of endometrial cancer twofold to fourfold, from 1 per 1,000 women (age 50–74 years) per year to 4 per 1,000 women per year, which is related to both the dose and duration (minimum 1–2 years) of estrogen use (Fig 16–20; Weiss et al., 1979). Reducing the dose, or treating cyclically, will not provide adequate protection (Schiff et al., 1982); progestins are mandatory in a patient with an intact uterus.

Progestins can both prevent and reverse hyperplasia. Studd et al. (1980), following 855 women with annual endometrial biopsies for up to 5 years, found a 15% incidence of hyperplasia among women taking 1.25 mg of unopposed Premarin. The addition of 7 days/month of a progestin reduced this incidence to 3%. Extending the duration of the progestin to 10 days further lowered the incidence to 2%; 13 days of treatment reduced this to essentially zero (Fig 16–21). Gambrell (1982a) found the combined use of progestin with estrogen to lower the incidence of endometrial cancer (71 per 100,000 women) to below that of untreated women (242 per 100,000) and of estrogen-only users (434 per

100,000), differences that were statistically significant. Gambrell et al., (1980) were also successful in completely reversing established endometrial hyperplasia in 94% of 258 women treated with progestins.

Whitehead et al. (1981) provided biochemical and histological evidence for the antihyperplastic effect of progestins on the endometrium. They found numerous progestins reverse the induction of estradiol and progesterone receptors produced by estrogen. Progestins, in addition, increase the activity of estradiol and isocitric dehydrogenases of the endometrium. The magnitude of these effects was more dependent on the duration of progestin therapy than on the dose. Specifically, 1 mg of norethindrone appeared to be as effective as 10 mg, and 150 µg of norgestrel was as effective as 500 µg.

Ovarian Neoplasia

Estrogen replacement may possibly increase the risk of endometrioid cancer of the ovary, which comprises 10% to 20% of all ovarian malignancies, but this has not been conclusively established (Weiss et al., 1982). It is not known if progestin use will reduce this risk, if it, indeed, exists.

Breast Neoplasia

There has been a suspicion, based on theoretical grounds, that estrogen use increases the risk of breast cancer, since (1) breast cancer can be an

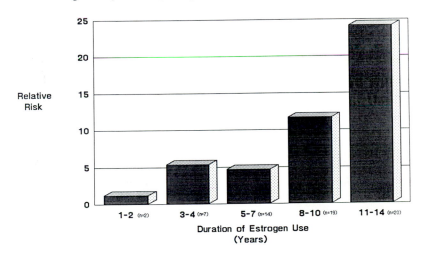

FIG 16–20.
Relative risk of endometrial cancer according to duration of postmenopausal estrogen use. (Adapted from Weiss NS, Szekely DR, English DR, et al: Endometrial cancer in relation to patterns of menopausal estrogen use. *JAMA* 1979; 242:261.)

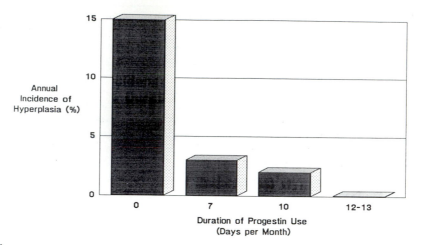

FIG 16–21.
Annual incidence of endometrial hyperplasia according to duration of progestin use per month. (Adapted from Studd JWW, Thorn MH, Patterson MEL, et al: The prevention and treatment of endometrial pathology, in Pasetto N, Paoletti R, Ambrus JL (eds): *The Menopause and Postmenopause.* MTP Press, Lancaster, England, 1980, p 127.)

estrogen-sensitive tumor, (2) estrogens can induce mammary tumors in rodents, and (3) women with prolonged endogenous estrogen exposure (e.g., early menarche, late menopause, nulliparity) are at increased risk of breast malignancies. However, postmenopausal estrogen replacement does not appear to substantially increase the risk of developing breast cancer. The largest epidemiological study to date investigating this issue is that by Brinton et al. (1986). This series consisted of 1,960 cases of breast cancer with 2,258 matched controls, identified through a breast screening program with 280,000 participants. The relative risk (RR) of breast cancer for all postmenopausal estrogen users was not increased at 1.03. When participants were analyzed for duration of estrogen use, exposures of 10 to 14 years had an RR of 1.28; for greater than 20 years, the RR was 1.47. Although the RR was not statistically significant for each stratum analyzed individually, a "trend test" did indicate an overall statistically significant increase in breast cancer with increasing duration of estrogen use. This increase is of a very small magnitude, however, with an approximate RR of 1.02 per year of estrogen use.

The possibility that the addition of a progestin may protect the breast, as it does the endometrium, has been suggested. Gambrell (1986) analyzed 69 cases of breast cancer and found 11 to be among combined estrogen and progestin users (incidence 66.8 per 100,000 women years) and 28 among estrogen-only users (incidence 142 per 100,000 women years). Although possibly suggesting a trend, this finding was not statistically significant ($p < 0.08$). Thus, the benefit of progestins in preventing breast cancer remains unproved. Moreover, this hypothesis is contrary to the fact that the mitotic activity of the breast increases during the luteal phase (peak endometrial mitosis is during the follicular phase; Anderson et al., 1982) and that progesterone induces mammary ductal growth in rodents (Dulbecco et al., 1982). A recent study of 208 women with breast cancer found no evidence of any protective effect of progestins against breast malignancy. In fact, the progestin users had a greater expected incidence of breast cancer, but this difference was not statistically significant (Bergkvist et al.). Because there is no good evidence that progestins will reduce the risk of breast cancer but may adversely affect lipoproteins and thus increase cardiovascular mortality, the use of progestins in women without a uterus is unnecessary and possibly detrimental.

Gallbladder Disease

On theoretical grounds, estrogen replacement is expected to increase cholelithiasis. Indeed, estrogens, both endogenous and exogenous, have been found to reduce the amount of chenodeoxycholic acid in bile (Bennion, 1977; Heuman et al., 1979). This is potentially significant, since chenodeoxycholic acid keeps cholesterol in aqueous solution and so inhibits cholesterol precipitation and stone formation.

The Boston Collaborative Drug Surveillance Program (1974) found the relative risk of gallbladder disease among estrogen users to be 2.5 (95% CI: 1.5–4.2). This may be an overestimate, since their control group consisted of hospital inpatients, nearly 30% of whom were admitted for treatment of fractures. Thus, their control group may be overrepresented by estrogen nonusers, which will lead to overestimation of the risk of gallbladder disease among estrogen users.

A more recent study (Kakar et al., 1988) found the relative risk of gallbladder disease in estrogen users to be only 1.2 (95% CI: 0.7–2.1). This lower relative risk, compared with that found by the Boston study, may be due to (1) the use of a more appropriate control group or (2) the fact that clinicians now generally use lower doses of estrogen for hormonal replacement (Ross et al., 1988).

Thromboembolic Disease

Oral contraceptives, particularly those with the highest estrogen content, are associated with thromboembolic disease (Inman, 1983). This appears to be a dose-response relationship; controlled epidemiological studies of physiological postmenopausal estrogen replacement have found no increase in thrombosis (Pfeffer and Van den Noort, 1976). Moreover, a consistent biochemical effect of estrogen replacement on the coagulation and fibrinolytic systems has not been identified.

Hypertension

Estrogen replacement, in general, may modestly lower blood pressure in many women (Mashchak and Lobo, 1985) but on occasion may induce or exacerbate hypertension in others (Crane et al., 1971). This idiosyncratic reaction to oral estrogens may be mediated by an increase in the hepatic production of renin substrate or by the production of an aberrant form (Shionoiri et al., 1983). In any case, this elevation in blood pressure is usually reversible on discontinuation of estrogen.

Glucose Tolerance

Although oral contraceptives are associated with impaired carbohydrate metabolism (Spel-

lacy, 1976), the lower doses used for estrogen replacement have not been linked to impaired glucose tolerance (Spellacy et al., 1978). Postmenopausal women with diabetes showed no change or an improvement of their disease with estrogen use, evidenced by lower glucose levels or reduced insulin requirements (Cantilo, 1941). This is consistent with the observation that estrogen appears to increase the binding of insulin to its receptor (Ballejo et al., 1983). Moreover, animal models have shown estrogen to improve experimentally induced hyperglycemia (Paik et al., 1982).

Contraindications

Absolute contraindications to postmenopausal estrogen replacement are:

1. Known or suspected endometrial or breast cancer.
2. Undiagnosed genital bleeding.
3. Active liver disease.
4. Active thromboembolic disease or a history of estrogen-related thromboembolic disease.

Relative contraindications are:

1. Chronic liver dysfunction. The liver's ability to metabolize estrogen is impaired, leading to excessive levels of estrogen. This may be compensated by using smaller and less frequent doses.
2. Preexisting uterine leiomyomas or active endometriosis. Estrogen use may prevent the involution of these conditions, which would be expected following the menopause.
3. Poorly controlled hypertension.
4. History of thromboembolic disease.
5. Acute intermittent porphyria. Estrogens are known to precipitate attacks.

PROGESTOGENS

Progestins are used primarily to reduce the risk of endometrial hyperstimulation caused by estrogen replacement. They may also be used to relieve hot flashes in patients who are not candidates for estrogen replacement.

Available Preparations

Progesterone and its derivatives are absorbed by the vaginal, rectal, and intramuscular routes. The oral route, although convenient and commonly used, provides a highly variable degree of absorption, with as much as a threefold difference between patients (Whitehead et al., 1980). For this reason, variable clinical effects may be seen among patients given the same oral dose. Following absorption, oral progestins are presented to the liver in high concentration, where they may greatly affect the hepatic metabolism of serum lipoproteins. These progestins are then rapidly and significantly metabolized by the liver to deoxycorticosterone (Ottoson et al., 1984).

Medroxyprogesterone acetate, 10 mg, is the most commonly used progestin in the United States and is effective against hyperplasia with minor effects on serum lipids. For those patients unable to tolerate this dose, 5 mg may be used. The 5-mg dose in most cases will offer similar protection against hyperplasia (Gibbons et al, 1986), except for the individual who poorly absorbs oral MPA. Medroxyprogesterone acetate given intramuscularly as its depot form is well absorbed but has a highly variable duration of effectiveness and is commonly associated with irregular vaginal bleeding. The usual dose is 50 to 150 mg intramuscularly every 1 to 3 months. The 50-mg dose is usually adequate to relieve hot flashes (Morrison et al., 1980), whereas the 150-mg dose is as effective as 0.625 mg of CEE in reducing urinary calcium/creatinine ratio to premenopausal levels (Lobo et al., 1984a).

Megestrol acetate is also effective in suppressing hot flashes and restoring calcium/creatinine ratios to premenopausal levels. Doses of 40 to 80 mg are generally required to exert these effects (Erlik et al., 1981a). Micronized progesterone, 200 to 300 mg, is also active against hyperplasia (Whitehead et al., 1987) without significantly altering serum lipid levels.

19-Nortestosterone derivatives are the progestins used in oral contraceptives and have partial androgenic properties with an adverse action on serum lipid levels (see the discussion that follows). Norethindrone (norethisterone, NET) was initially used in doses of 2.5 to 5 mg, but 1 mg (as is used in low-dose oral contraceptives) is equally effective against hyperplasia but has a much smaller impact on lipids. D,L-norgestrel, known for its more potent androgenic properties,

was similarly used in 0.5-mg doses, but it appears that 0.15 mg is equally effective (Whitehead et al., 1981). Of note is that only the L-isomer is biologically active, so that 0.15 mg of D,L-norgestrel is equivalent to 0.075 mg of levonorgestrel.

Adverse Effects

Progestins may produce abdominal bloating, mastalgia, headaches, mood changes, and acne. More important, all progestins, particularly the 19-nortestosterone derivatives (e.g., norgestrel and norethindrone) negatively affect serum lipid levels, especially HDL. A dose of 10 mg of MPA was found by two studies (Silfverstolpe et al., 1982; Tikkanen et al., 1981) to reduce HDL levels by 9% and 16%, differences that could not be shown to be statistically significant given the small number of patients studied (8 and 11, respectively). A dose of 500 μg of norgestrel (equivalent to 250 μg of levonorgestrel) decreases HDL levels by 12% to 22% (Hirvonen et al., 1981; Tikkanen et al., 1982) and 10 mg of norethindrone lowers HDL by 20% to 30% (Silfverstolpe et al., 1982; Hirvonen et al., 1981). These particular doses of norgestrel and norethindrone may be higher than necessary; in a small series, Whitehead et al. (1981) have shown that doses of 150 μg and 1 mg, respectively, are equally effective against hyperplasia. The effect of these lower doses on lipids awaits definitive study.

Of course, the net effect of a hormonal regimen on lipids depends on the particular estrogen and progestin used, as well as their dose, route, and frequency of administration. In general, progestins may negate, in whole or in part, the beneficial effect of estrogen on HDL and LDL levels. This may compromise the possible reduction in CVD observed with estrogen replacement. Moreover, the protective effect of progestins against breast cancer is unproved. Therefore, the use of progestins may be justified only for those women with an intact uterus for whom prevention of endometrial cancer is required.

TREATMENT REGIMENS

Prior to initiation of hormonal therapy, the patient should be evaluated by a careful history and physical examination, including blood pressure, breast and pelvic examination, stool guaiac, and Papanicolaou smear. Mammography should be performed to prevent prescribing estrogens to a patient with preexisting subclinical cancer of the breast and should be repeated yearly. Blood pressure should be monitored in 3 to 6 months and then yearly. Serum cholesterol level should be measured at least every 5 years, provided it remains less than 200 mg/dl. If the serum cholesterol level exceeds 200 mg/dl, follow-up should be arranged, as outlined in Tables 16–2 and 16–3. An endometrial biopsy should be performed prior to treatment if there is a history of abnormal vaginal bleeding or if the patient is at increased risk of having a preexisting endometrial hyperplasia. The endometrium should be sampled if a patient bleeds at any time other than during the drug-free interval or if the bleeding is heavy. This may be accomplished by Vabra aspiration or, if adequate tissue cannot be obtained, by fractional dilatation and curettage. Patients receiving unopposed estrogens for an extended time should have a biopsy performed before therapy is insti-

TABLE 16–2.

Recommended Follow-up Based on Initial Classification and Total Cholesterol Level*†

Recommended follow-up	
Total cholesterol level, <200 mg/dl	Repeat within 5 yr
Total cholesterol level, 200–239 mg/dl	
Without definite CHD or two other CHD risk factors‡	Dietary information and recheck annually
With definite CHD or two other CHD risk factors	Lipoprotein analysis; further action based on LDL-cholesterol level
Total cholesterol level, ≥240 mg/dl	Lipoprotein analysis; further action based on LDL-cholesterol level

*Adapted from the Expert Panel: Report of the National Cholesterol Education Program Expert Panel on detection, evaluation, and treatment of high blood pressure in adults. *Arch Intern Med* 1988; 148:36.
†Classification: <200 mg/dl = desirable blood cholesterol level; 200–239 mg/dl = borderline high blood cholesterol level; ≥240 mg/dl = high blood cholesterol level.
‡Risk factors are male gender, family history of premature coronary disease, cigarette use, hypertension, diabetes mellitus, low HDL-cholesterol level, definite vascular disease, and marked obesity.

TABLE 16–3.

Treatment Decisions Based on Low Density Lipoprotein–Cholesterol Levels and Classification*†

	Initiation Level (mg/dl)	Minimal Goal (mg/dl)
Dietary treatment		
Without CHD or two other risk factors	≥160	<160
With CHD or two other risk factors	≥130	<130
Drug treatment		
Without CHD or two other risk factors	≥190	<160
With CHD or two other risk factors	≥160	<130

*Adapted from the Expert Panel: Report of the National Cholesterol Education Program Expert Panel on detection, evaluation, and treatment of high blood pressure in adults. *Arch Intern Med* 1988; 148:36.
†Classification:<130 mg/dl = desirable LDL-cholesterol level; 130–159 mg/dl = borderline–High Risk LDL-cholesterol level; ≥160 mg/dl = high-risk LDL-cholesterol level.

tuted and yearly thereafter, regardless of bleeding, because the annual incidence of hyperplasia is 30% (Schiff et al., 1982).

As mentioned earlier, the most commonly used schedule of hormone replacement in the United States for women with intact uteri is cyclic, with 0.625 mg of CEE given days 1 through 25 each month and 10 mg of MPA given days 13 through 25. No hormones are given the remainder of the month. On this regimen, many patients will demonstrate withdrawal bleeding typically during the drug-free interval. For those patients who have previously undergone hysterectomy, the estrogen may be given continuously, and no progestin is needed (see earlier discussion).

This schedule may be modified by substituting another estrogen for CEE or another progestin for MPA. Equivalent starting doses of other oral estrogens would be 1 mg of micronized estradiol-17β and 1.25 mg of piperazine estrone sulfate. Parenteral estrogens, such as transdermal estradiol, may be particularly useful for those women whom one wishes to bypass the hepatic effects of oral estrogens (see earlier pharmacology discussion), such as those with a prior history of hepatic dysfunction, thrombosis, or hypertension. The typical starting dose of transdermal estradiol is 50 µg applied twice weekly. After 1 month's time, many patients will not demonstrate an adequate clinical response to this dose and will need to be increased to 100 µg; rarely is it necessary to use a dose higher than 100 µg.

To avoid withdrawal bleeding, Magos et al. (1985) proposed continuous rather than cyclic treatment. A dose of 0.625 or 1.25 mg of CEEs as needed to control symptoms is given continuously with 0.35 mg of NET. The dose of NET is serially increased by 0.35 mg until all bleeding is abolished, up to a limit of 2.1 mg. Most patients will initially have irregular vaginal bleeding, but by 1 year 95% will be amenorrheic. Higher doses of NET are required with 1.25 mg of CEEs. These higher doses are associated with abdominal bloating and mastalgia, which may cause the patient to discontinue therapy. The effect of this regimen on serum lipid levels is unknown. Norethindrone, 0.35 mg, is available in the United States only as Micronor, a progestin-only oral contraceptive. The use of 2.5 to 10 mg of MPA has been suggested as a substitute for NET in this schedule.

At present, there are insufficient data to indicate that all postmenopausal women must be treated with estrogen replacement. For that reason, the benefits and risks as they pertain to each individual patient should be reviewed with her in detail. She must ultimately decide whether to initiate therapy and give her informed consent.

REFERENCES

Albrecht BH, Schiff I, Tulchinsky D, et al: Objective evidence that placebo and oral medroxyprogesterone acetate therapy diminish menopausal vasomotor flushes. *Am J Obstet Gynecol* 1981; 139:631.

Alffam PH: An epidemiologic study of cervical and intertrochanteric fractures of the femur in suburban population. *Acta Orthop Scand* 1964; 65:1.

Aloia JF, Cohn SH, Ostuni JA, et al: Prevention of involutional bone loss by exercise. *Ann Intern Med* 1978; 89:356.

Amundsen DW, Diers CJ: The age of menopause in classical Greece and Rome. *Hum Biol* 1970; 42:79.

Anderson JJ, Ferguson DJP, Raab GM: Cell turnover in the "resting" human breast: Influence of parity, contraceptive pill, age, and laterality. *Br J Cancer* 1982; 46:376.

Bain C, Willett WC, Hennekins CH, et al: Use of postmenopausal hormones and risk of myocardial infarction. *Circulation* 1981; 64:42.

Ballejo G, Saleem TH, Khan-Dawood FS, et al: The effect of sex steroids on insulin-binding by target tissues in the rat. *Contraception* 1983; 28:413.

Beattie CW, Rodgers CH, Soyka LF: Influence of ovariectomy and ovarian steroids on hypothalamic tyrosine hydroxylase activity in the rat. *Endocrinology* 1972; 91:276.

Bennion LJ: Changes in bile lipids accompanying oophorectomy in premenopausal women. *N Engl J Med* 1977; 297:709.

Bergkvist LB, Adami HO, Persson I, et al: Risk of breast cancer after estrogen and estrogen-progestin replacement. *N Engl J Med* 1989; 321:293.

Berkow R (ed): *The Merck Manual of Diagnosis and Therapy.* Rahway, NJ, Merck & Co, 1987, p 2472.

Boston Collaborative Drug Surveillance Program: Surgically confirmed gallbladder disease, venous thromboembolism, and breast tumors in relation to postmenopausal estrogen therapy. *N Engl J Med* 1974; 290:15.

Briggs M, Briggs M: Effect of some contraceptive steroids on serum proteins in women. *Biochem Pharmacol* 1973; 22:2277.

Brinton LA, Hoover R, Fraymeni JF: Menopausal oestrogens and breast cancer risk: An expanded case-control study. *Br J Cancer* 1986; 54:825.

Burch JC, Byrd BF, Vaughn WK: The effects of long-term estrogen on hysterectomized women. *Am J Obstet Gynecol* 1974; 118:778.

Bush TL, Cavan LD, Barrett-Connor E: Estrogen use and all-cause mortality. *JAMA* 1983; 249:903.

Campbell S, Whitehead M: Estrogen therapy and the postmenopausal syndrome. *Clin Obstet Gynecol* 1977; 4:31.

Cann CE, Genant HK, Ettinger B: Spinal mineral loss in oophorectomized women. Determination by quantitative computer tomography. *JAMA* 1980; 244:2056.

Cantilo E: Successful responses in diabetes mellitus of the menopause provided by the antagonistic action of sex hormones on pituitary activity. *Endocrinology* 1941; 28:20.

Carr BR, MacDonald PC: Estrogen treatment of postmenopausal women. *Adv Intern Med* 1983; 28:491.

Chang RJ, Judd HL: Elevation of skin temperature of the finger as an objective index of postmenopausal hot flushes: Standardization of the techniques. *Am J Obstet Gynecol* 1979; 135:713.

Chetkowski RJ, Meldrum DR, Steingold KA, et al: Biologic effects of transdermal estradiol. *N Engl J Med* 1986; 314:1615.

Christiansen C, Christiansen MS, Transbol I: Bone mass in postmenopausal women after withdrawal of estrogen/gestagen replacement therapy. *Lancet* 1981; 1:459.

Christiansen C, Riis BJ, Rodbro P: Prediction of rapid bone loss in postmenopausal women. *Lancet* 1987; 1:1105.

Christensen MS, Hagen C, Christiansen L, et al: Dose-response evaluation of cyclic estrogen/gestagen in postmenopausal women: Placebo-controlled trial of its gynecologic and metabolic actions. *Am J Obstet Gynecol* 1982; 144:873.

Chu J, Schweid AI, Weiss NS: Survival among women with endometrial cancer: A comparison of estrogen users and nonusers. Am J Obstet Gynecol 1982; 143:569.

Clayden JR, Bell JW, Pollard P: Menopausal flushing: Double-blind trial of a nonhormonal medication. *Br Med J (Clin Res)* 1974; 1:409.

Coldnitz GA, Willett WC, Stampfer MJ, et al: Menopause and the risk of coronary heart disease in women. *N Engl J Med* 1987; 316:1105.

The Coronary Drug Project Research Group: Findings leading to discontinuation of the 2.5

mg/day estrogen group. *JAMA* 1973; 226:652.

Crane MG, Harris JJ, Windsor W: Hypertension, oral contraceptive agents, and conjugated estrogens. *Ann Intern Med* 1971; 74:13.

Dalen N, Hallberg D, Lamke B: Bone mass in obese subjects. *Acta Med Scand* 1975; 197:353.

Daniell HW: Osteoporosis and the slender smoker. *Arch Intern Med* 1976; 136:298.

Davidson BJ, Gambone JC, Lagasse LD: Free estradiol in postmenopausal women with and without endometrial cancer. *J Clin Endocrinol Metab* 1981; 52:404.

DeFazio J, Meldrum DR, Winer JH, et al: Direct action of androgen on hot flashes in the human male. *Maturitas* 1984; 6:8.

Deftos LJ, Weisman MH, William G, et al: Influence of age and sex on plasma calcitonin in human beings. *N Engl J Med* 1980; 302:1351.

Delforge JD, Ferrin J: A histometric study of two estrogens: Ethinyl estradiol and mestranol. *Contraception* 1970; 1:57.

Dequeker JV, Johnston CC (eds): *Noninvasive Bone Measurements.* Herndon, Va, IRL Press, 1981.

Deutsch S, Ossowski B, Benjamin I: Comparison between degree of systemic description of vaginally and orally administered estrogens at different dose levels in postmenopausal women. *Am J Obstet Gynecol* 1981; 139:967.

DeVogt HJ, Smith PH, Davone-Macaluso M, et al: Cardiovascular side effects of diethylstilbestrol, cyproterone acetate, and medroxyprogesterone acetate used for treatment of prostatic cancer. *J Urol* 1986; 135:303.

Dulbecco R, Henahan M, Armstrong B: Cell types and morphogenesis in the mammary gland. *Proc Natl Acad Sci USA* 1982; 79:7346.

Eaker ED, Castelli WP: Coronary heart disease and its risk factors among women in the Framingham study, in *Coronary Heart Disease in Women.* New York, Haymarket Doyma, 1987.

Elwood JM, Boyes DA: Clinical and pathologic features and survival of endometrial cancer patients in relation to prior use of estrogens. *Gynecol Oncol* 1980; 10:173.

Englund DE, Johansson EDB: Plasma levels of oestrone, oestradiol, and gonadotropins in postmenopausal women after oral and vaginal administration of conjugated equine estrogens. *Br J Obstet Gynaecol* 1978; 85:957.

Erlik Y, Meldrum DR, Judd HL: Estrogen levels in postmenopausal women with hot flushes. *Obstet Gynecol* 1982; 59:403.

Erlik Y, Meldrum DR, Lagasse LD, et al: Effect of megestrol acetate on flushing and bone metabolism in postmenopausal women. *Maturitas* 1981a; 3:167.

Erlik Y, Tataryn IV, Meldrum DR, et al: Association of waking episodes with menopausal hot flushes. *JAMA* 1981b; 245:1741.

Ettinger B, Cann L, Genant K: Menopausal bone loss: Effects of conjugated estrogen and/or high calcium diet. *Maturitas* 1984; 6:108.

The Expert Panel: Report of the National Cholesterol Education Program Expert Panel on detection, evaluation, and treatment of high blood pressure in adults. *Arch Intern Med* 1988; 148:36.

Falch JA, Oftebro H, Haug E: Early postmenopausal bone loss not associated with decrease in vitamin D. *J Clin Endocrinol Metab* 1987; 64:836.

Frodin T, Alund G, Varenhurst E: Measurement of skin blood-flow to assess hot flushes after orchiectomy. *Prostate* 1985; 7:203.

Gallagher JC, Nordin BEC: Oestrogens and calcium metabolism. *Front Horm Res* 1973; 2:98.

Gambrell RD: Clinical use of progestins in the menopausal patient. *J Reprod Med* 1982a; 27:531.

Gambrell RD: The menopause: Benefits and risks of estrogen-progestin replacement. *Fertil Steril* 1982b; 37:457.

Gambrell RD: Role of progestins in the prevention of breast cancer. *Maturitas* 1986; 8:1569.

Gambrell RD, Massey FW, Castaneda TA: The use of the progestagen challenge test to reduce the risk of endometrial cancer. *Obstet Gynecol* 1980; 55:732.

Geola FL, Fumar AM, Tataryn IV, et al: Biological effects of various doses of conjugated equine estrogens in postmenopausal women. *J Clin Endocrinol Metab* 1980; 51:620.

Gibbons WE, Lobo RA, Moyer DU, et al: A comparison of biochemical and morphological events mediated by estrogen and progestin on the endometrium of postmenopausal women. *Am J Obstet Gynecol* 1986; 154:456.

Gordon G, Vaughan C: *Clinical Management of the Osteoporoses.* Acton, Mass, Publishing Sciences Group, 1976.

Gordon T, Castelli WP, Hjortland MC, et al: High density lipoprotein as a protective factor against coronary heart disease. *Am J Med* 1977; 62:707.

Gordon WE, Hermann HW, Hunter DC: Safety and efficiency of micronized estradiol vaginal cream. *South Med J* 1979; 72:1252.

Grodin JM, Siiteri PK, MacDonald PC: Source of estrogen production in postmenopausal women. *J Clin Endocrinol Metab* 1973; 36:207.

Haas S, Walsh B, Evans S, et al: The effect of transdermal estradiol on hormone and metabolic dynamics over a six-week period. *Obstet Gynecol* 1988; 71:671.

Hammond CB, Jelousek FR, Leck L, et al: Effects of long term estrogen replacement therapy. *Am J Obstet Gynecol* 1979; 133:525.

Hammond MG, Hatley L, Talbert LM: A double-blind study to evaluate the effect of methyldopa on menopausal vasomotor flushes. *J Clin Endocrinol Metab* 1984; 58:1158.

Heanly RP: Estrogens and postmenopausal osteoporosis. *Clin Obstet Gynecol* 1976; 19:791.

Heller RF, Jacobs HS: Coronary heart disease in relation to age, sex, and the menopause. *Br Med J* 1978; 1:472.

Henzl MR, Moyer DL, Townsend D: Quantitation of the estrogenic effects of mestranol in human endometrium and vaginal mucosa. *Am J Obstet Gynecol* 1973; 115:401.

Heuman R, Larsson-Cohn U, Hammar M, et al: Effects of postmenopausal ethinyl estradiol treatment on gallbladder bile. *Maturitas* 1979; 2:69.

Hillyard CJ, Stevenson JC, MacIntyre I: Relative deficiency of plasma calcitonin in normal women. *Lancet* 1978; 1:961.

Hirvonen E, Malkonen M, Manninen V: Effects of different progestins. *N Engl J Med* 1981; 304:560.

Horsman A, Jones M, Francis R, et al: The effect of estrogen dose on menopausal bone loss. *N Engl J Med* 1983; 309:1405.

Horsman A, Simpson M, Kirby PA: Nonlinear bone loss in oophorectomized women. *Br J Radiol* 1977; 50:504.

Huggins C, Stevens RE, Hodges CU: Studies of prostatic cancer: II. The effects of castration in advanced carcinoma of the prostate. *Arch Surg* 1941; 43:209.

Inman WH: Adverse reactions to new drugs [letter]. *Br Med J (Clin Res)* 1983; 286:719.

Iosif CS, Batra S, Ek A, et al: Estrogen receptors in the human female lower urinary tract. *Am J Obstet Gynecol* 1981; 141:817.

Iskrant AP: The etiology of fractured hips in females. *Am J Public Health* 1968; 58:485.

Johnson AE, Nock B, McEwen B, et al: Estradiol modulation of noradrenergic receptors in the guinea pig brain assessed by tritium-sensitive film autoradiography. *Brain Res* 1985; 336:153.

Jones KP, Ravnikar VA, Schiff I: Effect of lofexidine on vasomotor flushes. *Maturitas* 1985; 7:135.

Judd HL, Davidson BJ, Frumar AM, et al: Serum androgens and estrogens in postmenopausal women. *Am J Obstet Gynecol* 1980; 136:859.

Judd HL, Lucas WE, Yen SSC: Effect of oophorectomy on testosterone and androstenedione levels. *Am J Obstet Gynecol* 1974; 118:793.

Kakar F, Weiss NS, Strite SA: Noncontraceptive estrogen use and risk of gallstone disease in women. *Am J Public Health* 1988; 78:564.

Kannel WB: Lipids, diabetes, and coronary heart disease: Insights from the Framingham study. *Am Heart J* 1985; 110:1100.

Kannel WB: Risk factors for coronary disease in women. Perspective from the Framingham study. *Am Heart J* 1987; 114:413.

Kelly TL, Slovik DM, Schoenfeld DA, et al: Quantitative digital radiography vs. dual photon absorptiometry of the lumbar spine. *J Clin Endocrinol Metab* 1988; 67:839.

Kirkland RT, Keenan BS, Probstfield JL, et al: Decrease in plasma high-density lipoprotein cholesterol levels at puberty in boys with delayed adolescence: Correlation with plasma testosterone levels. *JAMA* 1987; 257:502.

Komm BS, Terpening CM, Benz DJ, et al: Estrogen binding, receptor mRNA, and biologic response in osteoblast-like osteosarcoma cells. *Science* 1988; 241:81.

Lagrelius A: Treatment with oral estrone sulfate in the female climacteric: III. Effects on bone density and on certain biochemical parameters. *Acta Obstet Gynecol Scand* 1981; 60:481.

Larson IF: Hot flushes after hypophysectomy. *Br J Med (Clin Res)* 1977; 2:1356.

Laufer LK, Erlik Y, Meldrum DR, et al: Effect of clonidine on hot flashes in postmenopausal women. *Obstet Gynecol* 1982; 60:483.

Lebherz TB, French LT: Nonhormonal treatment of the menopausal syndrome. A double-blind evaluation of an autonomic system stabilizer. *Obstet Gynecol* 1969; 33:795.

Lerner DJ, Kannel WB: Patterns of coronary disease morbidity and mortality: A 26-year follow-up of the Framingham population. *Am Heart J* 1986; 111:383.

Licata AA, Bou E, Bartter FC, et al: Acute effects of dietary protein on calcium metabolism in patients with osteoporosis. *J Gerontol* 1981; 36:14.

Lindsay R, Dempster DW, Clemens T, et al: Incidence, cost and risk factors of fracture of the proximal femur in the USA, in Christiansen C, et al (eds): *Osteoporosis*. Denmark, Aalborg Stoftsbogturkkeri, 1984a, pp 311–315.

Lindsay R, Hart DM, Aitken JM, et al: Long-term prevention of postmenopausal osteoporosis by estrogens. *Lancet* 1976; 1:1038.

Lindsay R, Hart DM, Clark DM: The minimum effective dose of estrogen for prevention of postmenopausal bone loss. *Obstet Gynecol* 1984b; 63:759.

Lindsay R, Hart DM, Purdie D, et al: Comparative effects of oestrogen and a progestagen on bone loss in postmenopausal women. *Clin Sci* 1978; 54:193.

Lindsay R, Sweeney A: Urinary cyclic AMP in osteoporosis. *Scott Med J* 1976; 21:231.

Lobo RA, Brenner PF, Mishell DR: Metabolic parameters and steroid levels in postmenopausal women receiving lower doses of natural estrogen replacement. *Obstet Gynecol* 1983; 62:94.

Lobo RA, McCormack W, Singer F, et al: Depo-medroxyprogesterone acetate compared with conjugated estrogens for the treatment of postmenopausal women. *Obstet Gynecol* 1984a; 63:1.

Lobo RA, Mishell DR, Budoff PW, et al: Estrogen replacement therapy, in *Symposium Proceedings*. San Francisco, Abbott Pharmaceuticals, May 9–10, 1984b, p 9.

Luine VN, McEwen BS: Effect of estradiol on turnover of type A monamine oxidase in brain. *J Neurochem* 1977; 28:1221.

Magos AL, Brincat M, Studd JWW, et al: Amenorrhea and endometrial atrophy with continuous oral estrogen and progestin therapy in postmenopausal women. *Obstet Gynecol* 1985; 65:496.

Mandel FP, Davidson BJ, Erlik Y, et al: Effect of progestins on bone metabolism in postmenopausal women. *J Reprod Med* 1982a; 27(suppl 8):511.

Mandel FP, Geola FL, La JK, et al: Biologic effects of various doses of ethinyl estradiol in postmenopausal women. *Obstet Gynecol* 1982b; 59:673.

Mandel FP, Geola FL, Meldrum DR, et al: Biologic effects of various doses of vaginally administered conjugated equine estrogens in postmenopausal women. *J Clin Endocrinol Metab* 1983; 57:133.

Manolagas SC, Anderson DG: Detection of high-affinity glucocorticoid binding in rat bone. *J Endocrinol* 1978; 76:379.

Martinez-Menayton J, Rudel HW: Antiovulatory activity of several synthetic and natural estrogens, in Greenblatt RB (ed): *Ovulation*. Philadelphia, JB Lippincott Co, 1969, p 243.

Mashchak CA, Kletsky OA, Artal R, et al: The relation of physiological changes to subjective symptoms in postmenopausal women with and without hot flushes. *Maturitas* 1985; 6:301.

Mashchak CA, Lobo RA: Estrogen replacement therapy and hypertension. *J Reprod Med* 1985; 30(suppl):805.

Mashchak CA, Lobo RA, Dozono-Takano R, et

al: Comparison of pharmacodynamic properties of various estrogen formulations. *Am J Obstet Gynecol* 1982; 144:511.

Matkovic V, Kostial K, Simonovic I, et al: Bone status and fracture rates in two regions of Yugoslavia. *Am J Clin Nutr* 1979; 32:540.

McKinlay S, Jeffreys M, Thompson B: An investigation of the age of menopause. *J Biosoc Sci* 1972; 4:161.

Morrison JC, Martin DC, Blair RA, et al: The use of medroxyprogesterone acetate for the relief of climacteric symptoms. *Am J Obstet Gynecol* 1980; 138:99.

Nicosia SV: Morphological changes of the human ovary throughout life, in Serra GB (ed): *The Ovary.* New York, Raven Press, 1983, pp 57–81.

Nixon RL, Jamowsky DS, David JM: Effects of progesterone, estradiol, and testosterone on the uptake and metabolism of ^{3}H-norepinephrine, ^{3}H-dopamine, and ^{3}H-serotonin in rat synaptosomes. *Res Commun Chem Pathol Pharmacol* 1974; 7:233.

Notelovitz M, Gudat JC, Ware MD, et al: Lipids and lipoproteins in women after oophorectomy and the response to estrogen therapy. *Br J Obstet Gynaecol* 1983; 90:171.

Oliver MF, Boyd GS: Endocrine aspects of coronary sclerosis. *Lancet* 1956; 2:1273.

Oliver MF, Boyd GS: Influence of reduction of serum lipids on prognosis of coronary heart disease: A five year study using estrogen. *Lancet* 1961; 2:499.

Orchard TJ, Rodgers M: Changes in blood lipids and blood pressure during adolescence. *Br Med J* 1980; 280:1563.

Ottoson U-B, Carlstrom K, Dambes J-E, et al: Conversion of oral progesterone into deoxycorticosterone during postmenopausal replacement therapy. *Acta Obstet Gynecol Scand* 1984; 63:577.

Paik SG, Michelis MA, Kim YT, et al: Induction of insulin-dependent diabetes by streptozotocin: Inhibition by estrogens, potentiation by androgens. *Diabetes* 1982; 31:724.

Pak CY, Sakhaee K, Zerwekh JE, et al: Treatment of osteoporosis with intermittent slow release sodium fluoride: Augmentation of vertebral bone mass. *J Clin Endocrinol Metab* 1989; 68:150.

Paul SM, Axelrod J, Saadvedra JM, et al: Estrogen-induced efflux of endogenous catecholamines from the hypothalamus in vitro. *Brain Res* 1979; 178:499.

Petitti DB, Wingerd J, Pellegrin F, et al: Risk of vascular disease in women: Smoking, oral contraceptives, noncontraceptive estrogens and other factors. *JAMA* 1979; 242:1150.

Pfeffer RI, Van den Noort S: Estrogen use and stroke risk in postmenopausal women. *Am J Epidemiol* 1976; 103:445.

Pfeffer RI, Whipple GH, Kurosaki TT, et al: Coronary risk and estrogen use in postmenopausal women. *Epidemiology* 1978; 107:479.

Recker PR, Saville PD, Heany RP: Effect of estrogen and calcium carbonate on bone loss in postmenopausal women. *Ann Intern Med* 1977; 87:649.

Riis B, Thomsen K, Christiansen C: Does calcium supplementation prevent postmenopausal bone loss? *N Engl J Med* 1987; 316:173.

Robinson RW, Lebeau RJ: Effect of conjugated equine estrogens on serum lipids and the clotting mechanism. *J Atheroscler Res* 1965; 5:120.

Ross RK, Paganini-Hill A: Estrogen replacement therapy and coronary heart disease. *Semin Reprod Endocrinol* 1983; 1:19.

Ross RK, Paganini-Hill A, Mack TM, et al: Menopausal estrogen therapy and protection from death from ischemic heart disease. *Lancet* 1981; 1:858.

Ross RK, Paganini-Hill A, Roy S, et al: Past and present prescribing practices of hormone replacement. *Am J Public Health* 1988; 78:516.

Schiff I, Regestein Q, Tulchinsky D, et al: Effects of estrogens on sleep and psychological state of hypogonadal women. *JAMA* 1979; 242:2405.

Schiff I, Sela HK, Cramer D, et al: Endometrial hyperplasia in women on cyclic or continuous estrogen regimens. *Fertil Steril* 1982; 37:79.

Schiff I, Tulchinsky D, Cramer D, et al: Oral medroxyprogesterone acetate in the treatment of postmenopausal symptoms. *JAMA* 1980; 244:1443.

Schiff I, Tulchinsky D, Ryan KJ: Vaginal absorption of estrone and 17 β-estradiol. *Fertil Steril* 1977; 28:1963.

Schiff I, Wilson E: Clinical aspects of aging of the female reproductive system, in Schneider EL (ed): *The Aging Reproductive System.* New York, Raven Press, 1978, pp 9–28.

Schwartz U, Hammerstein J: The estrogenic potency of ethinyl estradiol and mestranol—a comparative study. *J Acta Endocrinol* 1973; 72:118.

Sherman BW, West JH, Korenman SG: The menopausal transition: Analysis of LH, FSH, estradiol, and progesterone concentrations during menstrual cycles of older women. *J Clin Endocrinol Metab* 1976; 42:629.

Shionoiri H, Eggena P, Barrett JD, et al: An increase in high-molecular weight renin substrate associated with estrogenic hypertension. *Biochem Med* 1983; 29:14.

Siddle N, Whitehead M: Flexible prescribing of estrogens. *Contemp Obstet Gynecol* 1983; 22:137.

Silfverstolpe G, Gustafson A, Samsoie G, et al: Lipid metabolic studies in oophorectomized women: Effect on serum lipids and lipoproteins of three synthetic progestagens. *Maturitas* 1982; 4:103.

Smith DM, Nance WE, Kang KW: Genetic factors in determining bone mass. *J Clin Invest* 1973; 52:2800.

Spellacy WN: Carbohydrate metabolism in male infertility and female fertility-control patients. *Fertil Steril* 1976; 27:1132.

Spellacy WN, Butri WC, Birk SA: Effect of estrogen treatment for one year on carbohydrate and lipid metabolism in women with normal and abnormal glucose tolerance test results. *Am J Obstet Gynecol* 1978; 131:87.

Stamler J, Katz LN, Pick R, et al: Effects of long-term estrogen therapy on serum cholesterol-lipid-lipoprotein levels and mortality in middle aged men with previous myocardial infarction. *Circulation* 1980; 22:658.

Stampfer MJ, Willett WC, Coldnitz GA, et al: A prospective study of postmenopausal estrogen therapy in coronary heart disease. *N Engl J Med* 1985; 313:1044.

Steingold KA, Laufer L, Chetkowski RJ, et al: Treatment of hot flashes with transdermal estradiol. *J Clin Endocrinol Metab* 1985; 61:627.

Stevenson JC, Abeyasekera G, Hillyard CJ, et al: Calcitonin and the calcium-regulating hormones in postmenopausal women: Effect of estrogens. *Lancet* 1981; 1:693.

Studd JWW, Thorn MH, Patterson MEL, et al: The prevention and treatment of endometrial pathology, in Pasetto N, Paoletti R, Ambrus JL (eds): *The Menopause and Postmenopause*. Lancaster, England, MTP Press, 1980, p 127.

Thompson B, Hart SA, Durno D: Menopausal age and symptomatology in general practice. *J Biol Sci* 1973; 5:71–82.

Tikkanen MJ, Nikkila EA, Kuusi T, et al: Different effects of two progestins on HDL. *Atherosclerosis* 1981; 40:365.

Tikkanen MJ, Nikkila EA, Kuusi T, et al: HDL

and lipatic lipase. *J Clin Endocrinol Metab* 1982; 54:1113.

Utian WH: Definitive symptoms of postmenopause incorporating use of vaginal parabasal cell index. *Front Horm Res* 1975; 3:74.

Vermeulen A: The hormonal activity of the postmenopausal ovary. *J Clin Endocrinol Metab* 1976; 42:247.

Weiss NS, Lyon JL, Krishnamurthy S, et al: Noncontraceptive estrogen use and the occurrence of ovarian cancer. *J Natl Cancer Inst* 1982; 68:95.

Weiss NS, Szekely DR, English DR, et al: Endometrial cancer in relation to patterns of menopausal estrogen use. *JAMA* 1979; 242:261.

Weiss NS, Ure CL, Ballard JH, et al: Decreased risk of fractures of the hip and lower forearm with postmenopausal use of estrogen. *N Engl J Med* 1980; 303:1195.

Whitehead MI, Siddle N, Lane G, et al: The pharmacology of progestogens, in Mishell DR (ed): *Menopause, Physiology and Pharmacology*. Chicago, Year Book Medical Publishers, 1987, p 326.

Whitehead MI, Townsend PT, Gill DK, et al: Absorption and metabolism of oral progesterone. *Br Med J (Clin Res)* 1980; 280:825.

Whitehead MI, Townsend PT, Pryse-Davies J, et al: Effects of estrogens and progestins on the biochemistry and morphology of the postmenopausal endometrium. *N Engl J Med* 1981; 305:1599.

Whittaker PG, Morgan MR, Dean PD: Serum equilin, estrone, and estradiol levels in postmenopausal women receiving conjugated equine estrogens. *Lancet* 1980; 1:14.

Wilson PWF, Garrison RJ, Castelli WP: Postmenopausal estrogen use, cigarette smoking, and cardiovascular morbidity in women over 50. *N Engl J Med* 1985; 313:1038.

Yen SSC: The biology of menopause. *J Reprod Med* 1977; 18:28.

Zinner NN, Sterling AM, Ritter RC: Role of urethral softness in urinary incontinence. *Urology* 1980; 16:115.

17 _____ Conception Control

Rapin Osathanondh, M.D.

OVERVIEW

The practice of birth control can be traced back to ancient societies of different racial and religious origins (Noonan, 1986). At present time, voluntary prevention of pregnancy (contraception) as well as termination of unwanted pregnancy (therapeutic induced abortion) are widely accepted for medical (parental or fetal indications) and socioeconomic reasons. In spite of the rapid advancement in reproductive biology, there still exist four general problems regarding birth control that may or may not be resolved in our time:

1. *There is no ideal contraceptive method.* All contraceptive methods available in the United States are safer than no contraception. However, it is impossible to make a contraceptive that is 100% effective (Vessey et al., 1982), is easy to use, is reversible, and has no side effects. For each woman, any method of contraception has advantages and disadvantages, as well as relative and absolute contraindications. A suitable method means that its benefits far outweigh the risks. For example, statistical calculations by Tietze and Lewit (1979) in the past decade suggest that the safest contraceptive practice for women at any age in the United States is the diaphragm or condom backed by early, legal abortion should the method fail (Ory, 1983; Tietze, 1977). Unfortunately, induced abortion may be costly or inaccessible in many localities. To guard against pregnancy and sexually transmitted diseases (STDs), a combination of the low-dose oral contraceptive pill and use of latex condom by the male partner may represent the safest choice for women less than 40 years of age who do not smoke cigarettes.

2. *Women who use contraceptives should see a gynecologist at least once each year.* Contraceptive-related problems may occur as direct or indirect results of contraceptive use. Increased coital activity or increased number of sexual partners may necessitate switching from one method of contraception to another. For example, studies before and after birth control pill use showed an increased incidence of bacteriuria in some women with a tendency for repeated bladder infection.

3. *Efficacies of most contraceptives have been shown to be dependent on the user's motivation.* The often quoted "actual use effectiveness" may not be applicable in many circumstances. For some women, an intrauterine device (IUD) may be more effective than the pill because of poor dosing compliance. For many women, the "natural family planning" method such as abstinence or the rhythm method is, in fact, unnatural and often results in high failure rates.

4. *There is an epidemic of unintended teenage pregnancies in the United States.* There has been a trend toward earlier and more frequent, unprotected intercourse among teenagers. An annual occurrence of more than 1 million unintended teenage pregnancies in the U.S. population is considered high when compared with that in other industrialized nations. Epidemiological data reveal that teenage marriage generally leads to eventual separation or divorce, less education, and low paying or no job. Recent national statistics has revealed an average of one out-of-wedlock child for every five live births. Moreover, approximately 3 million women aged 15 to 44 years who do not want to conceive currently do not practice contraception. This is a serious public health problem and a great concern for society.

ORAL CONTRACEPTIVE

Birth control pills (or "the pill") represent the most studied class of medications since 1960.

Oral contraceptives (OCs) are taken daily by more than 50 million women, most of whom are not at risk of developing serious side effects. It is very effective in preventing unwanted conception, with a crude contraceptive efficacy *(Pearl index)* of less than 2 pregnancies per 100 women years. Its effects are reversible, and there are many noncontraceptive health benefits (Table 17–1), some of which will last for years after use.*

Most OCs contain ethinyl estradiol, a synthetic estrogen, and a progestin (progesterone-like substance), and these are called *combined,* or *combination, OCs.* In the United States, since October 1988, each combined OC tablet contains between 20 and 50 μg of ethinyl estradiol or a pharmacologically similar steroid mestranol (Fig 17–1) plus one of the four progestins: norgestrel, norethindrone, norethindrone acetate, or ethynodiol diacetate. A much less popular type of OC contains a small dose of progestin without any estrogen and is known as a *minipill.* Unless the word "minipill" is specifically mentioned in this text, OC is generally understood as the combined pill.

Administration and Types

The first tablet is usually taken on the fifth day of menses, followed by one tablet daily for 21 days. For simplicity or better protection, some brands are begun either on the first day of bleeding or the first Sunday of the menstrual cycle. Withdrawal (anovulatory) bleeding generally occurs within 3 to 5 days after the 21-day regimen, and the routine is begun again on the fifth day of the new cycle. Thus, there is a 1-week "off" period with every 3-week "on." Most pharmaceutical manufacturers also provide a nonstop 28-day OC package in which the last seven tablets are hormonally inert placebo. The latter packaging system eliminates the need to remember the on or

off interval. Since each of the 21 hormonally active tablets contain the same amount of estrogen and progestin, this conventional OC is known as *monophasic.*

Because of recent publicity regarding the metabolic side effects of progestins, the *biphasic* and *triphasic pills* were produced to lower the total amount of progestin while mimicking the hormonal peak and trough levels within the physiological menstrual cycle (Ellis, 1987). Of the four types of *multiphasic pills* (Table 17–2), only one formulation contains slightly varying amounts of estrogen, whereas three others put 35 μg of estrogen in each hormonally active tablet. To date there has been no well-controlled studies with solid evidence for overall superiority of the multiphasic over the common monophasic low-dose pills. Theoretically, these multiphasic formulations may represent the safest choice for potential pill users.

Mechanisms of Action

Low daily dosage of two synergistic steroids in the pill prevents ovulation by centrally inhibiting the midcycle pituitary gonadotropins surge (Goldzieher, 1984; Orme et al., 1983; Rock et al., 1956; Sturgis and Albright, 1940). The pituitary gland may be unable to respond to the hypothalamic gonadotropin-releasing hormone while the woman is taking the OC (Dericks-Tan et al., 1983). This central effect consequently obliterates the endogenous (ovarian) estrogen and progesterone production and commonly leads to a diminished endometrial proliferation. In the OCs with lesser amounts of estrogen, occasional small surges of gonadotropins may appear. However, such levels are usually insufficient to stimulate ovarian follicles. A recent report of anecdotal cases of ovarian retention cysts in users of low-dose pills may challenge this general rule (Caillouette and Koehler, 1987).

Peripherally, OCs also exert antinidation effects involving decreased oviductal function, endometrial glycogen content, and cervical mucus (Goldzieher, 1984; Liskin, 1983a; Liskin and Blackburn, 1987; Rock et al., 1956; Umapathysivam and Jones, 1980). These peripheral effects are probably responsible for the major contraceptive effect of the minipill. The scant and dry cervical mucus renders the cervix impermeable to penetration by the sperm. Furthermore, atrophic out of phase endometrium with resultant amenorrhea

*Berkowitz et al., 1984; Brenner, 1988; Cancer and Steroid Hormone Study of the Centers for Disease Control and the National Institute of Child Health and Human Development, 1987a, 1987b; Centers for Disease Control Cancer and Steroid Hormone Study, 1983b, 1983c; Connell, 1984; Cramer et al., 1982; del Junco et al., 1985; Franceschi et al., 1984; Goldzieher, 1984; Hseih et al., 1984; Hulka et al., 1982; Kaufman et al., 1980; Linos et al., 1983; Newton, 1984; Ostensen and Husby, 1983; Pastides et al., 1983; Potts and Diggory, 1983; Rosenberg et al., 1982; Sturgis and Albright, 1940; Trapido, 1983; Vandenbroucke et al., 1982, 1986; Weiss and Sayvetz, 1980; Willett et al., 1981.

TABLE 17–1.

Patient Consent Form for Obtaining Birth Control Pills

Birth control pills, or oral contraceptives, are being used every day by more than 50 million women around the world for the prevention of unwanted pregnancy. There are many health benefits of taking birth control pills besides the prevention of pregnancy (noncontraceptive benefits). There are also risks associated with taking the pills. However, these risks (for stroke, blood clots, heart attack) are seen mostly among women more than 35 years old and especially among women 35 years or older who smoke. The risk for younger women is very small. According to the U.S. Food and Drug Administration, increased risk of breast cancer has not been demonstrated among pill users, but there may be a slight increase in the risk for cancer of the cervix. All women must have Papanicoloau tests at least once every year. Also, be sure to read the package insert that comes with your birth control pills.

Noncontraceptive benefits
1. The pills usually reduce menstrual cramps.
2. The pills generally protect women against having breast problems that are not cancer, cysts in the ovary, endometriosis (a disease that may cause severe menstrual cramps and infertility), and cancer of the ovary and the womb (uterus).
3. The pills decrease bleeding from the uterus and also reduce the risk of iron deficiency anemia in some women who bleed a lot with periods and in those who bleed irregularly.
4. The pills may protect women against rheumatoid arthritis.

Side effects

Minor side effects

If they do occur, stay on the pills through the third package cycle, and they will usually go away by then. If not, consult a physician or a nurse. A different brand of the pills may agree with you better.
1. Bleeding or spotting between periods.
2. Nausea (try taking the pill at bedtime to avoid feeling sick).
3. Weight gain from fluid retention.
4. Weight gain or loss due to change in appetite (should not be more than 2.3 kg [5lb]).
5. Breast tenderness, mild headache, tiredness, or mood changes.
6. Increased blood pressure.
7. Enlargement of "fibroid" tumors in some women.
8. Scant flow (less and less monthly bleeding) or missed periods.
9. Decreased sex drive. However, most pill users report increased sex drive.
10. Acne (pimple). However, most pill users see a decrease in acne problems. In addition, some women who use the pills may develop redness or darkening of the skin over their cheeks.
11. Eye irritation may occur in some pill users who wear contact lenses.

More serious side effects

These are rare. Notify a physician immediately if they do occur.
1. Severe abdominal pain or discomfort (due to a gallbladder problem, a rare tumor in the liver, or blood clots in the bowel).
2. Severe chest pain or shortness of breath (due to blood clots in the heart or lungs).
3. Severe leg pain (due to blood clots in the leg).
4. Severe headache (due to stroke or other problems in the brain).
5. Eye problems such as blurred vision (due to blood clots or inflamed nerve in the eye).

Patient's statement

I have read the above and understand that there are both benefits and risks associated with the use of birth control pills. I choose to take the pills because I believe that the benefits for me are greater than the risks.

_____   _____

Patient's Signature   Date

_____

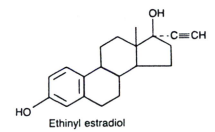

Ethinyl estradiol

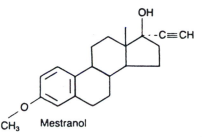

Mestranol

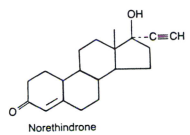

Norethindrone

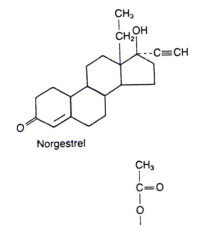

Norgestrel

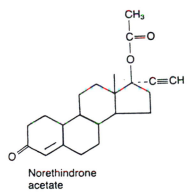

Norethindrone acetate

Ethynodiol diacetate

FIG 17—1.
Synthetic steroids used in oral contraceptives sold in the United States today. Estrogens: ethinyl estradiol and mestranol. Progestins: norethindrone, norethin- drone acetate, norgestrel, and ethynodiol diacetate. (Courtesy of P.G. Stubblefield, M.D.)

is not an uncommon finding. The minipill regimen does not totally abolish surges of luteinizing hormone (LH) or ovarian estrogens. However, it may partially block the central positive feedback response to endogenous estrogens, resulting in inadequate amplitudes of pituitary LH surges (Goldzieher, 1984; Liskin, 1983a; Litvak et al., 1970). Nevertheless, the reported pregnancy rate between 2 and 7 per 100 women years with this nonstop microdose progestin regimen is considerably higher than that observed with the combination OC. Irregular vaginal bleeding and increased

ectopic pregnancy rates among failure cases further reduce the minipill's popularity. At present, the minipill may be appropriate for a few women with cardiovascular disease who cannot tolerate any estrogenic stimulation of their renin-angiotensin-aldosterone axis and those with known hypersensitivity to synthetic estrogens.

Advantages

Oral contraceptives provide noncontraceptive benefits to the appropriate user and her society.

TABLE 17–2.

Oral Contraceptives Available in the United States*

	Estrogen (μg)	Progestin (mg)
Monophasic combination OC		
Loestrin 1/20	EE, 20	Norethindrone acetate, 1
Loestrin 1.5/30	EE, 30	Norethindrone acetate, 1.5
Ovcon 35	EE, 35	Norethindrone, 0.4
Brevicon, Modicon, Nelova 0.5/35	EE, 35	Norethindrone, 0.5
Genora 1/35, Gynex 1/35, Nelova 1/35, Norinyl 1+35, Ortho-Novum 1/35	EE, 35	Norethindrone, 1
Levlen, Nordette	EE, 30	D-Norgestrel, 0.15
Lo/Ovral	EE, 30	DL-Norgestrel, 0.3
Ovral	EE, 50	DL-Norgestrel, 0.5
Norlestrin 1/50	EE, 50	Norethindrone acetate, 1
Norlestrin 2.5/50	EE, 50	Norethindrone acetate, 2.5
Demulen	EE, 50	Ethynodiol diacetate, 1
Ovcon 50	EE, 50	Norethindrone, 1
Genora 1/50, Norinyl 1+50, Ortho-Novum 1/50	M, 50	Norethindrone, 1
Biphasic combination OC		
Ortho-Novum 10/11	EE, 35	Norethindrone, 0.5 (day 1–10), 1 (day 11–21)
Triphasic combination OC		
Tri-Norinyl	EE, 35	Norethindrone, 0.5 (day 1–7), 1 (day 8–16), 0.5 (day 17–21)
Ortho-Novum 7/7/7	EE, 35	Norethindrone, 0.5 (day 1–7), 0.75 (day 8–14), 1 (day 15–21)
Tri-Levlen, Triphasil	EE, 30–40–30	D-Norgestrel, 0.5 (day 1–6), 0.75 (day 7–11), 0.125 (day 12–21)
Progestin only (minipill)		
Micronor, Nor-QD		Norethindrone, 0.35
Ovrette		DL-Norgestrel, 0.075

*EE = ethinyl estradiol; M = mestranol, a methyl ester of EE converted by the liver into EE.

The pill protects the individual user from life-threatening ectopic pregnancy, reduces primary dysmenorrhea, and reduces the risks of benign and malignant gynecological problems as listed in the simplified consent form in Table 17–1. Society also benefits from the annual reduction of more than 50,000 hospitalizations and office visits, according to British and U.S. studies (Brenner, 1988; Connell, 1984; Rubin et al., 1982). After only 1 year of use, pill users may be protected from developing endometrial and ovarian cancer for 10 years (Brenner, 1988; Cancer and Steroid Hormone Study of the Centers for Dis-ease Control and the National Institute of Child Health and Human Development, 1987a, 1987b). The progestin in OCs reduces the number of estrogen and progesterone receptors in the endometrium. Furthermore, since ovulation does not occur, mitotic activity in the ovary, which is repeatedly high at the time of ovulation, is inhibited. There may be a delay in the return of ovulation following cessation of OC use with an initial prolongation of the follicular phase or a shortened luteal phase (Rice-Wray et al., 1967). In most cases, menses resume within 3 months, and fertility returns to the preexisting rate by the end of 2 years. If regular menstruation does not return within 6 months after cessation of OCs, hormonal evaluation is indicated. These particular users may have preexisting, slow-growing, pituitary microadenomas that can be treated successfully. The pill itself does not cause pituitary tumors (Pituitary Adenoma Study Group, 1983; Shy et al., 1983). Weight change, stress, or undiagnosed pregnancy may explain the postpill amenorrhea in other cases.

Disadvantages, Side Effects, and Contraindications

The pill must be taken daily and is considered a mild teratogen (Katz et al., 1985; Lammer and Cordero, 1986; Linn et al., 1983b). The user must devise her own system to ensure daily compliance. The pill should be taken at the same time every day. In addition, a backup method such as condoms or contraceptive sponges should be used concomittently in the first cycle of use when low-estrogen OCs may not provide a full protection. Lowering the content of ethinyl estradiol in each tablet from 50 to 30 μg significantly increased the pregnancy rate in users (Lawson et al., 1979). Simply put, the lower the hormonal content, the less danger from unwanted effects, but the higher the failure rate. Most gynecologists advise the user to take her previous day's pill if she forgets one and to take two pills each day for 2 days if she forgets two. If she forgets 3 days in a row, the pill may not be an appropriate contraceptive method for her.

Another disturbing side effect that can occur with or without missing the dose is intermittent or irregular *breakthrough uterine bleeding* (BTB). Breakthrough uterine bleeding during the first few months may resolve without treatment. Nonetheless, irregular bleeding could be a warning symptom that the OC's efficacy may be compromised in a particular user. Careful history should be obtained to rule out pregnancy, infection, or neoplastic bleeding. In many instances, watchful expectation may be preferred to conventional double dosing or adding more estrogen. Serious estrogen-related thromboembolic disorders appear to be dose dependent. If BTB exists or if it first occurs several months after pill initiation, switching to a more progestogenic pill usually solves the problem. Use of norgestrel-containing OCs may lessen the problem with irregular bleeding (Ravenholt et al., 1987). The al-

ternative of adding a low dose of estrogen or switching to a more estrogenic pill should be tried only after other approaches fail (Wessler et al., 1976).

Other estrogen-induced side effects, which are listed in the consent form's section on the minor side effects of OCs in Table 17–1 (Goldzieher et al., 1971), include nausea, vascular headaches, elevated blood pressure, weight gain due to fluid retention, tender breasts (mastalgia), increased mucoid vaginal discharge, cervical erosion (ectropion), or polyposis. A mild increase in blood pressure may occur due to activation of the renin-angiotensin-aldosterone system, hypervolemia, and decreased prostacyclin levels (Petitti and Klatsky, 1983). If the diastolic blood pressure is elevated (more than 90 mm Hg) in response to OC use, discontinuation should be considered. Synthetic estrogens in the pill induce increased hepatic protein levels (renin substrate, binding globulins, and most blood clotting factors) and decreased antithrombin III and plasminogen activators levels* (Table 17–3); Hypercoagulability will occur in pill users with a familial deficiency of antithrombin III. An undisputed pill-induced human tumor is hepatic adenoma, which is related to the use of synthetic estrogens (3.4 per 100,000 women per year); (Porter and Jick, 1981; Scott et al., 1984; Shar and Kew, 1982). Epidemiological studies have also disclosed twofold to fourfold increases in the diagnoses of cholelithiasis, postoperative deep vein thrombosis, pulmonary embolism (1 in 30,000 women per year), and cerebral thrombosis (1 in 30,000 women per year) among users of OCs with greater than 50 μg of synthetic estrogen when compared with nonusers.† The overall annual risk of venous thromboembolism may be one to two cases per 1,000 current users depending on the estrogen content in the pill, blood type, and perhaps race and lifestyle. This risk is lower in women with blood type O (Jick et al., 1969). The risk disappears after cessation of the pill and is not related to length of use. The effects of estrogen in reducing the activity of antithrombin III and plas-

---

*Beaumont et al., 1983; Gaspard, 1987; Lewis et al., 1983; Mammen, 1982; Seligsohn et al., 1984; von Kaulla et al., 1971.

†Beaumont et al., 1983; Brenner, 1984; Goldzieher, 1984; Newton, 1984; Petitti et al., 1979; Porter et al., 1985; Ramcharan et al., 1980; Royal College of General Practitioners' Oral Contraception Study, 1982; Stadel, 1981; Vessey et al., 1977; Vessey and Lawless, 1984.

TABLE 17–3.

Some Laboratory Values That Are Influenced by the Use of Combination Oral Contraceptive Pills

Values that may be increased
  Hematological
    Clotting factors (I, II, VII, VIII, IX, X, and XII)
    Antiplasmins and antiactivators of fibrinolysis
    Erythrocyte sedimentation rate
    Red and white blood cells and platelets
    Iron and iron-binding capacity
  Hepatic proteins and related tests
    α_1-globulins, α_2-globulins, and various binding globulins
    Renin, angiotensin, angiotensinogen, and aldosterone
    Bromosulfophthalein, bilirubin, and alkaline phosphatase
    Transaminases and transpeptidase
    Coproporphyrin and porphobilinogen
  Hormonal
    Growth hormone and insulin (and blood glucose)
    Urinary total estrogens
  Sterol and lipid
    Vitamin A
    Triglycerides and phospholipids
    Low density lipoprotein–cholesterol
  Others
    α_1-antitrypsin, C-reactive protein, serum copper, and ceruloplasmin
    Urinary xanthuric acid
    Positive results for antinuclear antibody and lupus erythematosus preparation
Values that may be decreased
  Hematological
    Folate and vitamin B_{12}
    Antithrombin III and fibrinolytic activity
  Hormonal
    Luteinizing and follicle-stimulating hormones
    Urinary pregnanediol and 17-ketosteroids
    Tri-iodothyronine resin uptake
  Others
    Glucose tolerance, zinc, magnesium, and ascorbic acid
    High density lipoprotein–cholesterol (HDL-C)
    Haptoglobulin and cholinesterase

change, as well as hypertension may also be related to progestins. Depression in some pill users may be due to pyridoxine deficiency with a resultant increase in the level of xanthurenic acid. Some medications, including certain antibiotics, anticonvulsants, and some sedatives, make OCs less effective‡ The most notorious is the antituberculous drug rifampin. Increased hepatic microsomal activity results in increased OC metabolism and decreased contraceptive effectiveness. In addition, disturbed intestinal function (enterohepatic circulation) or colonic bacterial milieu may lower the pill's efficacy. Commonly prescribed drugs that may decrease contraceptive effect of the pill include barbiturates, primidone, phenytoin, ampicillin, tetracycline, and griseofulvin. Backup contraceptive methods and the use of the 50 μg-estrogen pill may be required. Note also that the pill may delay elimination of theophylline drugs, and it may decrease the efficacy of oral anticoagulant preparations.

Long-term metabolic effects of progestins have recently been a subject for arguments with regard to the lowering of serum HDL-C and its consequence.§ One study revealed an increased mortality rate among pill users aged 25 to 34, 35 to 44, and more than 45 years due to circulatory diseases. Others have shown increased risk of coronary thrombosis and nonfatal myocardial infarction among pill users more than 30 years of age. However, close scrutiny later revealed that the risk was limited to those with hypertension, diabetes, and hyperlipidemia. As mentioned in Table 17–1, the greatest risk, estimated to be 1 in 5,000 women per year, was actually found among pill users more than 35 years of age who were smokers. Interestingly, the risk of coronary heart disease is not increased in former pill users and not correlated with the duration of OC use (Stampfer et al., 1988). The latter finding perhaps suggests that the pill-induced coronary vascular changes, if any, may be thrombotic and not

minogen activators are probably dose related (Mammen, 1982; von Kaulla et al., 1971; Wessler et al., 1976).

Untoward events related to progestins are decreased menses, reduced vaginal secretion, weight gain due to increased appetite, acne, leg cramps, fatigue, and sleepiness. Breakthrough uterine bleeding, chloasma, depression or mood

‡Brenner, 1988; Anonymous, 1980; Mattson et al., 1986; Newton, 1984; Orme et al., 1983; Potts and Diggory, 1983; Szoka and Edgren, 1988.

§Arntzenius et al., 1978; Bradley et al., 1978; Burkman, 1988; Connell, 1984; Engel et al., 1983; Gaspard, 1987; Gordon et al., 1977; Kay, 1982; Lincoln, 1984; Mann and Inman, 1975; Meade et al., 1980; Mishell, 1988b; Newton, 1984; Petitti and Klatsky, 1983; Petitti et al., 1979; Porter et al., 1985; Ramcharan et al., 1980; Royal College of General Practitioners' Oral Contraception Study, 1983; Stadel, 1981; Vessey and Lawless, 1984.

atherogenic in origin (Brenner, 1988). Progestins in the pills have been associated with an increased risk of atherosclerosis since they tend to lower the levels of serum HDL-C, especially the HDL_2 fraction.¶ In contrast, exogenous estrogens in the pill tend to raise HDL levels. Thus, the effects of a combination OC on users' lipid profile may depend on variable interactions between the relative estrogenicity of the estrogen vs. the antiestrogenicity and androgenicity of the progestin and the dose of the two hormones. Note, however, that the often quoted potency of a progestin in terms of delayed menses, withdrawal bleeding, or endometrial glycogen vacuoles may not be applicable in different women (Connell, 1984; Goldzieher, 1984; Lawson et al., 1979; Orme et al., 1983). Furthermore, some progestins have inherent estrogenic activity as they are converted in the body to estradiol. In fact, norethynodrel, which was the first progestin used in OCs, was highly estrogenic. All progestins in OCs are synthetic derivatives of 19-nortestosterone (meaning no carbon 19). Addition of an ethinyl group to carbon 17 results in an orally active steroid norethindrone as well as other *estrane* progestins, which include norethynodrel, norethindrone acetate, ethynodiol diacetate, lynestrenol, norgestrienone, norgesterone, and quingestanol acetate. More potent progestins (the *gonanes*) contain an ethyl group at C 13 (e.g., norgestrel and desogestrel). The active form of norgestrel is D-norgestrel (levonorgestrel). This 19-norsteroid stays in the body longer than other progestins. Unlike other progestins, levonorgestrel is unique in that its oral administration does not bring about any effects of "first-pass" hepatic metabolism. The third group of progestins (the *pregnanes*) are derivatives of 17-hydroxyprogesterone such as chlormadinone acetate, medroxyprogesterone acetate, megestrol acetate, and cyproterone acetate. Actually, there are at present 13 progestins used in more than 300 brand names of steroid contraceptives in various countries. Several progestins such as desogestrel, gestodene, and norgestimate (Fig 17–2) are popular in Europe and Asia, but they have not been approved for use in the United States (Eyong et al., 1988; Hahn et al., 1977). Oral contraceptives containing desogestrel (Org 2969) may be most beneficial for women with idiopathic hirsutism

¶Arntzenius et al., 1978; Bradley et al., 1978; Brenner, 1984; Burkman, 1988; Engel et al., 1983; Gaspard, 1987; Mishell, 1988b.

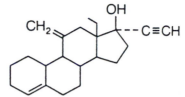

Desogestrel

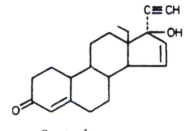

Gestodene

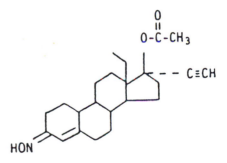

Norgestimate

FIG 17–2.
New progestins not yet available in the United States.

and selected patients with polycystic ovary syndrome (Mall-Haefeli et al., 1982; Rojanasakul et al., 1987; Samsioe, 1982; Sieberg et al., 1984). Desogestrel lacks intrinsic androgenicity (Mall-Haefeli et al., 1982; Samsioe, 1982). It does not interfere with the estrogen's capacity to induce an increase in sex hormone–binding globulin (Bergink et al., 1981). Consequently, combination OCs containing desogestrel increase the binding capacity for androgens, leading to a substantial decrease in free testosterone and free 5α-dihydrotestosterone (Rojanasakul et al., 1987). Active metabolites of desogestrel and norgestimate are 3-ketodesogestrel and norgestrel-related compounds, respectively.

Although the use of OCs reduces the incidence of benign breast disease, limited epidemiological and laboratory data have emerged almost every year suggesting an increased risk of breast cancer in pill users.[*] Specifically, worrisome findings with regard to breast cancer in pill users came out after the 1984 exoneration of the pill by Food and Drug Administration's (FDA's) panel of experts.[†] Because OCs have been available since 1960 and because the peak incidence of female breast cancer occurs between 55 and 74 years of age, any long-term latency effects of early pill use may not show up in this decade. Data implicating OC use with increased risks of cervical cancer[‡] and malignant melanoma have also appeared (Stevens et al., 1980). Epithelial abnormalities of the uterine cervix in many OC users are a matter of concern among epidemiologists with regard to transmission of the papilloma and human immunodeficiency viruses as well as *Chlamydia trachomatis* (Louv et al., 1989; Piot et al., 1988; Washington et al., 1985; World Health Organization, 1987b). Definite conclusions on the risks of breast and cervical cancer and malignant melanoma among pill users cannot be drawn based on presently available data because study designs have precluded the presence and influence of important confounding factors (Swann and

Petitti, 1982). An accepted fact is, however, that breast and some other gynecological tumors as well as certain adenocarcinomas and adenomas may be stimulated by sex steroids. Therefore, women with present or past history of such tumors should not use the pill.

The American College of Obstetricians and Gynecologists lists the following as absolute contraindications to the pill: thromboembolism or thrombotic disease, active or chronic (or both) liver disease, undiagnosed uterine bleeding, pregnancy, breast cancer, and estrogen-dependent neoplasia. Other strong contraindications should include history of coronary heart disease, stroke, hypertension, hyperlipidemia (especially type II hyperlipoproteinemia), smokers more than 40 years of age, cyanotic heart disease, sickle cell disease, severe headaches, active gallbladder disease, and conditions requiring total immobilization.[§]

Relative contraindications include smokers more than 35 years of age, moderate or severe cervical intraepithelial neoplasia (CIN), migraines, and certain types of diabetes mellitus. Diabetic women with elevated blood pressure, nephropathy, or retinopathy must be discouraged from using the pill. Many women with well-controlled diabetes or migraines have tolerated OC use and are happy with it. Use of low-dose OCs does not appear to alter the users' tolerance to 75-gm oral glucose load (Kasdorf and Kalkhoff, 1988). Impaired carbohydrate metabolism occurs with high-dose formulation containing norgestrel (Diamond et al., 1988). Oral contraceptive–induced insulin resistance is manifested by reduced peripheral tissue insulin sensitivity and may ameliorate with time (Kasdorf and Kalkhoff, 1988).

BARRIER METHOD AND SPERMICIDES

Condoms (Prophylactics)

The condom is without doubt the most popular but underreported mechanical contraceptive method for various justifiable reasons. It is disposable, is convenient to use, is inexpensively sold over the counter (OTC), and may help prevent

---

[*]Kalache et al., 1983; Longman and Buehring, 1987; McPherson et al., 1984, 1987; Meirik et al., 1986; Pike et al., 1983b; 1984; Secreto et al., 1983; Sturtevant, 1983; Swyer, 1983.

[†]Black et al., 1983; Brooks, 1984; Cancer and Steroid Hormone Study of the Centers for Disease Control and the National Institute of Child Health and Human Development, 1986; Centers for Disease Control Cancer and Steroid Hormone Study, 1983a; Hennekens et al., 1984; Janerick et al., 1983; Leads from the MMWR, 1984; Lincoln, 1984; Lipnick et al., 1986; Osborne et al., 1983; Paul et al., 1986; Rosenberg et al., 1984; Schlesselman et al., 1987, 1988; Stadel et al., 1985; Thomas, 1984; U.S. Health and Human Services, 1984; Vessey et al., 1983a; Vessey, 1984.

[‡]Clarke et al., 1985; Irwin et al., 1988; Lincoln, 1984; Royal College of General Practitioners' Oral Contraception Study, 198 ;Vessey et al., 1983b; Vessey and Lawless, 1984; World Health Organization, 1985.

[§]Arntzenius et al., 1978; Brenner, 1988; Connell, 1984; Engel et al., 1983; Freie, 1983; Gaspard, 1987; Gordon et al., 1977; Kay, 1982; Mann and Inman, 1975; Meade et al., 1980; Mishell, 1988b; Newton, 1984; Petitti and Klatsky, 1983; Porter et al., 1985; Stadel, 1981; Vessey and Lawless, 1984.

the spread of STDs. It should be used by pregnant women who have or are at risk for STD (Goldsmith, 1989). Its use may be indicated even though the couple is sterile. Regarding the feared viral transmission, condoms made of latex appear superior to other materials. However, the perfect barrier material has not yet been invented. Allergic reaction to latex is uncommon but has been reported. The chance of failure may be further reduced with the recently marketed condom prelubricated with a spermicide. The failure rate was theoretically estimated to be 3 per 1,000. Condoms cover the penis during coitus and serve as a reservoir to prevent the deposition of semen in the vagina. The prototype of a condom, made of animal products prior to the vulcanization of rubber, has been in use for centuries. Failures are related to the material itself or the manufacturing process and to the users' technical or mental difficulties (e.g., wearing the condom after some semen has been released into the vagina or sperm escaping out as a result of failure to withdraw before detumescence).

Spermicidal Agents

Most vaginal spermicides contain nonoxynol-9, a surface-active, nontoxic detergent that immobilizes sperm. It is available as cream, jelly, aerosol foam, foaming tablet, and suppository. The latest formulation comes from England in the form of a semitransparent square of contraceptive film that dissolves at body temperature into gel. Each product comes in 1% or 100 mg, but some contain as high as 5% or 28% of nonoxynol-9. It is also convenient and inexpensive, with a failure rate of 5 pregnancies per 100 women years. No association has been established between the use of vaginal spermicides and birth defects (Harlap et al., 1985; Louik et al., 1987; Warburton et al., 1987). These agents may lower the risk of STD. Vaginal or penile irritation due to local hypersensitivity to nonoxynol-9 may occur in some users, but this adverse effect is not common.

Another type of spermicide in preliminary trials with promising results is propranolol (Zipper et al., 1983). This drug kills sperm on contact. Its spermicidal property was first discovered in hypertensive men who became azoospermic following propranolol therapy. Among many β-sympathomimetic antagonists tested, propranolol showed the strongest spermicidal effect. The mechanism for this effect may be related to the

drug's lipophilic activity (Hong and Turner, 1982; Peterson and Freund, 1973).

Intravaginal Devices

The *diaphragm* is a barrier between the lower portion of the vaginal canal and the cervical canal. It is a latex rubber patch that is held in shape (Fig 17–3) by a circular, collapsible, metal frame with memory like a spring. The user must compress this circular spring rim to flatten and elongate it so that it can slip into her vagina while in a squatting or one-thigh-up position. There are four types of rim: coil, flat, wide seal, or arcing. The latter may be the easiest to insert correctly for full coverage of the cervical os. It comes in nine sizes based on the diameter of the circular rim (50–90 mm at 5-mm increments). The three sizes in the middle range (65, 70, and 75 mm). will fit most women. The proper size is determined by vaginal examination and trial with fitting rings. The correct size should be adequately large but not interfere with urination. The device rests in place under the urethra, and women with frequent cystitis may not be good candidates for using a diaphragm (Fihn et al., 1985; Ramahi and Richardson, 1988). Anatomical changes such as marked weight gain or loss or development of vaginismus may require refitting for a proper size of diaphragm. If it is used correctly with high motivation and compliance, its failure rate is theoretically less than 3 pregnancies per 100 women years. Spermicidal jelly should be applied on each side of diaphragm before insertion and the device left in for at least 6 hours after intercourse. It is then removed, washed, dried and put away until the next use. It must not be dusted with talcum powder since talc may increase the risk of ovarian cancer. Diaphragm use may lower the risks of pelvic inflammatory disease (PID) (Cramer et al., 1987; Kelaghan et al., 1982) and CIN; (Tatum and Connell-Tatum, 1981). There is a controversy regarding any association of toxic shock syndrome (TSS) and diaphragm use.

The *cervical cap* is much smaller than the diaphragm (see Fig 17–3) and must fit tightly over the cervix. It has a soft, nonmetal rim with a range of external diameter from 22 to 35 mm. Its cuplike shape fits right on the body of the cervix, with its circular rim toward the fornix. The Prentiff cavity rim, which is manufactured in England, has been approved by the FDA. Koch (1982) in Boston, who has been an active investigator, ad-

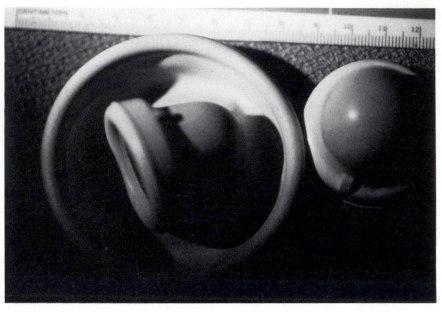

FIG 17–3.
Cervical caps (Prentiff Cavity Rim) compared with a diaphragm.

vises the use of a spermicidal jelly with high (3%–5%) concentration of nonoxynol-9 on the cervical side for contraceptive efficacy plus suction-cup effect. Such potent spermicides include Ramses (5%), Koromex (3%), or Shur-Seal (2%). It can be left in place for several days and must be removed if vaginal or menstrual bleeding occurs. To date, there has been no report of TSS in cap users. Initial users should have a Papanicolaou smear prior to the fitting and another 3 months thereafter. Increased risks of cervical erosion and CIN among cap users have been a concern. Other problems include widely different sizes and shapes of the cervix and difficulty in patient education toward correct placement of the cap relative to the diaphragm. Many women have great difficulty in finding their cervix. Others do not like to touch their own genitals, especially in certain cultures. On rare occasions when a user cannot remove her cap, a vaginal speculum is required. The cap will drop out of its place once the speculum is open inside the vagina. The cap's failure rate of 8 to 20 pregnancies per 100 women years is higher than that of the diaphragm. Several designs of custom-fit caps are under clinical trials. Such caps have a one-way valve to permit outflow of the uterine and cervical secretions while blocking sperm entrance.

The *vaginal contraceptive sponge* is a one-size-fits-all disposable barrier made of polyurethane containing 1 gm of nonoxynol-9 (enough for multiple acts of coitus). It is a convenient OTC product of modest price and will remain fully effective during 24 hours of use. Its failure rate is comparable to that of the diaphragm. Each sponge has a built-in loop for easy removal. The sponge is placed under tap water and immediately inserted into the vagina. Users are at a reduced risk of contracting STDs except candidiasis (Rosenberg et al., 1987). The risk of nonmenstrual TSS of 1 case per 2 million sponges is very low (Faich et al., 1986).

The *female condom* is another type of mechanical barrier that has been used off and on since the beginning of this century. Researchers in the United States, England, and Denmark are presently testing their devices. The type that has received FDA approval is a disposable seamless latex device fitting loosely inside the vagina and covering the perineum. It is aimed to prevent any contact with body secretions for the man and the woman. The rebirth of the female condom reflects the need for more protection against viral transmission. In fact, barrier contraceptives have gained immense popularity even though some users consider these barriers messy or inconvenient.

Such methods require manipulation of the genitalia at or near the time of coitus and thus require serious motivation for successful use.

INTRAUTERINE DEVICE

The IUD represents a highly effective means of birth control for a well-selected group of women (Liskin, 1982). It is a small plastic T-shaped rod or tiny circular ring made to fit easily inside the uterus. With an IUD in place, the uterus and oviducts become hostile to the sperm, oocyte, and the fertilized ovum (World Health Organization, 1987a). Consequently, 96% to 99% of all women wearing an IUD for 1 year will not conceive. Intrauterine device use is not associated with unwanted metabolic effects, and one device lasts a long time when compared to other reversible contraceptive methods. It is appropriate for women at low risk of STDs since its use is associated with an increased risk of PID and tubal infertility (Cramer et al., 1985; Daling et al., 1985). Since the IUD effectively prevents pregnancy, its use will not increase the overall incidence of tubal pregnancy. In fact, the incidence of ectopic pregnancies among 1,000 women using IUDs is significantly lower than would be the case among 1,000 women not using contraceptives. However, a high incidence of ectopic pregnancy has been observed among women who conceive while using an IUD, particularly the type that releases progesterone or D-norgestrel (Diaz et al., 1980). This may be analogous to the increased risk of ectopic pregnancy among minipill failure cases. Women who had an ectopic pregnancy or venereal disease such as gonorrhea or *Chlamydia* should not use an IUD.

Of all the FDA-approved IUDs, only two kinds are available in the United States: the Copper T-380A and the Progestasert. Both types are T shaped and radiopaque, but they differ in many aspects. The copper-containing IUD is superior to the noncopper device in contraceptive efficacy and perhaps lower relative risk of PID (Cramer et al., 1985; Sivin and Tatum, 1981; Zipper et al., 1969). Regarding the influence of type of device on the risk of PID, the worst record was observed with the Dalkon Shield and was attributed to poor design (Liskin, 1982). A significantly increased risk of PID in IUD wearers has been observed during the first few months after insertion (Burkman and the Women's Health Study, 1981). After that period, this risk may not be increased in copper-containing IUD wearers, especially those at low risk of contracting STDs. Salpingitis occurring more than a few months after insertion is likely due to STD and not the IUD (Lee et al., 1988). Women at high risk for developing PID include, in respective order of significance, those with a prior history of PID or STD, women with multiple sexual partners, nulliparous women less than 25 years of age, and single marital status (Cramer, 1989; Mishell, 1988a). They should be discouraged from using the IUD. Those at lowest risk of PID are parous women in a stable and mutually monogamous relationship. Because of its lack of metabolic effects, a copper-containing IUD may be ideal for an older parous woman who smokes cigarettes and does not want permanent sterilization.

Mechanism of Action

The IUD prevents fertilization and implantation by several postulated mechanisms, all of which are promptly reversible on removal of the device. It alters the intrauterine environment by inducing a local, sterile inflammatory response (foreign body reaction; Mishell et al., 1966). It is believed that leukocyte infiltration creates a hostile environment to the oocyte, sperm, and fertilized ovum. Two recent luteal phase studies of daily serum human chorionic gonadotropin (hCG) using highly sensitive assays led to the conclusion that implantation did not occur in IUD wearers (Segal et al., 1985; Sharpe et al., 1977; Wilcox et al., 1987). A controlled study of oocytes retrieved via tubal flushing strongly suggests that the IUD also inhibits fertilization process (World Health Organization, 1987a). Sperm may not reach the oocyte or are unable to penetrate the oocyte coverings. Alternatively, adverse tubal environment may damage the oocyte. Macrophage destruction of oocytes was shown in copper-containing IUD wearers. Copper may interfere with oocyte release or fimbria function, accelerate transport, or induce premature lysis of the ovum. In contrast to progesterone, copper inhibits the enzyme prostaglandin dehydrogenese in the local tissues (Kelly et al., 1983). The amount of copper absorbed into the systemic circulation is minute relative to the minimum daily dietary requirement. There have been rare cases of allergic skin lesions with pruritus due to intrauterine copper confirmed by standard skin tests (Romaguero and Grimalt, 1981).

Insertion Technique

The optimal time to insert an IUD is during menses when a woman is least likely to be pregnant. The user should have an opportunity to acquaint herself with any instructions and the informed consent form prior to the day of visit. Some women may require local anesthesia (paracervical block), especially when insertion is done on a day in the cycle between menses. Bimanual pelvic examination is performed to determine uterine size and position. The cervix is exposed with a speculum and cleansed with a local antiseptic, and its anterior lip is grasped with a tenaculum. Gentle traction to straighten the angle between the cervical canal and the uterine cavity is followed by probing the uterine cavity with a uterine sound to determine the internal direction and depth. The short-bladed (Moore-Graves) speculum may be required in case of acute anteflexion. The device is loaded into its inserter and gently slipped through the cervical canal. It is then freed within the uterine cavity by withdrawing the inserter tube over the plunger. This withdrawal technique reduces the risk of uterine perforation. Women wearing an IUD should report without delay any lower abdominal pain, fever and chill, unusual vaginal bleeding or spotting, pain during intercourse, or unpleasant vaginal discharge. A brief office visit should be offered 3 months after the insertion of the IUD and followed by annual checkup and cytological cervical smear.

Disadvantages, Adverse Effects, and Contraindications

Dysmenorrhea and *increased menstrual flow* are frequent IUD-related problems that may improve with short-term intermittent use of a nonsteroidal anti-inflammatory drug such as ibuprofen. This class of drugs (type I inhibitors) inhibits the biosynthesis of cyclic endoperoxides and prostaglandin E (PGE) and F (PGF) series. If these problems persist or worsen, the device should be removed, and the patient should be offered another choice of contraceptive. A new IUD (Ombrelle) has been designed so that its side arms will open

and close with uterine relaxation and contraction, respectively, with the hope of lowering the IUD-related dysmenorrhea incidence. Progestin-releasing IUDs were originally intended to alleviate both bleeding and dysmenorrhea problems. Unfortunately, such devices have been shown to increase the total number of days of bleeding and the incidence of midcycle spotting even though the volume of monthly blood loss is actually reduced. A report by World Health Organization (WHO) (1987a) Task Force on Psychological Research in Family Planning indicated that an increase in the number of days of bleeding may be less acceptable to women than an increase in the volume of bleeding. Another WHO study revealed no difference in dysmenorrhea complaints between the Progestasert and the Copper-7 users (Pizarro et al., 1979). Subsequently, those findings from WHO were confirmed by various independent investigators who reported similar removal rates between progestin-releasing IUDs and copper-containing or nonmedicated devices (Fylling and Fagerhol, 1979; Nilsson et al., 1981).

Another IUD-related problem that has received a careful review by Gupta and Woodruff (1982) concerns the unique organism *Actinomyces*. Reports have emerged since the past decade on the frequent *Actinomyces*-positive Papanicoloau smears among users of nonmedicated IUDs. There was also a high degree of association between true pelvic actinomycosis and the use of multifilamented tailed IUDs (which had since been discontinued). Although not common, true pelvic actinomycosis is a serious disease. A combination of PID and *Actinomyces*-positive Papanicoloau smear requires aggressive intravenous (IV) therapy with broad-spectrum antibiotics (Valicenti et al., 1982). Failure to obtain prompt clinical improvement would be strongly indicative of tubo-ovarian abscesses, which generally require surgical treatment. *Actinomyces*-positive Papanicoloau smears are less frequently found in conjunction with the use of copper-containing IUDs than with noncopper devices (Duguid et al., 1980). It has been postulated that copper may adversely affect the microbes as well as the gametes and the tubal mucosa.

The reported failure rate of the Copper T-380A is only 1 case annually per 100 users who are more than 25 years of age. However, one of every two current users who conceive will miscarry, and 1 of 20 IUD users who conceive will have *extrauterine pregnancy*. With an IUD in place, there is a high risk of sepsis among users who miscarry, particularly when the miscarriage occurs during the second trimester. Women who conceive while using an IUD should have the device removed or consider therapeutic-induced abortion since the risks and consequences are serious. An important risk is prematurity with or without sepsis (Toth et al., 1988). If an accidental pregnancy occurs after IUD use of more than 2 years, the risk of it being ectopic is high. Besides the IUD, contraceptive methods that predispose a user to ectopic pregnancy should the method fail include minipills, subdermal progestin implants, postcoital estrogen therapy, and most types of female sterilization.

Spontaneous expulsion of an IUD may occur in the first few months especially during menses. Disappearance of the IUD string may be the first sign of lost IUD that brings the patient back to her physician. Pregnancy must be ruled out, and when in doubt, a pelvic ultrasound is very helpful. High-resolution transabdominal and transvaginal ultrasound imaging by an experienced sonographer may reveal an abnormal position of IUD in the uterine wall or posterior wall of the cervix. In nonpregnant users with a question of lost IUD strings vs. a lost IUD, X-ray films of the abdomen and pelvis ultimately confirm its absence or presence, since most plastic devices have been impregnated with barium sulfate. Ultrasound guidance can facilitate the nontraumatic removal of an IUD with alligator forceps (Fig 17–4) when the string is not visible (Stubblefield et al., 1988). Failure of

this method of removal usually suggests that a part of the IUD has perforated the uterine wall, in which case laparoscopy is indicated. Partial expulsion of the stem of the T-shaped device may occur through the cervical canal. This may be associated with cramps, vaginal or cervical erosion with spotting, lacerations of the penis, and reduced contraceptive efficacy. The device must be removed and replaced.

In cases of *uterine perforation* with intraperitoneal protrusion of a copper-containing IUD, the device must be removed without delay because its tissue reactions will rapidly bring about severe adhesions and enclosure by the omentum. Downward displacement of the stem into the endocervix (mostly posteriorly) may require a slight upward dislocation before the whole device can be removed through the cervical canal.

Absolute contraindications to the use of IUD include a history of PID, STD, ectopic pregnancy, multiple male partners, purulent cervicitis, unresolved cervical neoplasia, undiagnosed genital bleeding, suspected pregnancy, Wilson's disease or known hypersensitivity to copper (for copper-containing IUD), valvular heart disease, genital actinomycosis, and any medical disorders predisposing to infection (Cramer, 1989). Relative contraindications include nulliparity, age less than 25 years, unmarried women who are not in a mutually monogamous relationship, recurrent vaginitis, anatomical derangement of the uterus (congenital anomalies, leiomyoma, cervical stenosis, etc.), painful heavy menses, anemia, rheumatic heart disease, or mitral valve prolapse (Cramer, 1989; World Health Organization, 1987a).

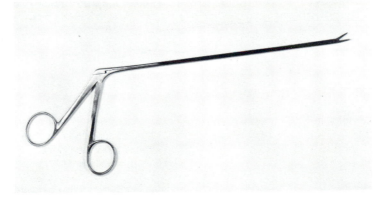

FIG 17–4.
Alligator forceps for IUD removal. (Courtesy of P.G. Stubblefield, M.D.)

POSTCOITAL TREATMENT AND MANAGEMENT OF SEXUAL ASSAULT VICTIMS

Treatment

The *morning-after pill* or *injection* represents the most practical step to terminate the natural development of a fertilized egg or eggs after an unprotected sexual intercourse. The original hormonal method to prevent fertilization or implantation of an already fertilized egg is by administration of high doses of a nonsteroidal estrogenic drug, diethylstilbestrol (DES), within 3 days of unprotected coitus (Table 17–4). Morris and van Wagenen (1966) were among the first to demonstrate the effectiveness of the so-called morning-after estrogenic pill for intercepting pregnancy in the rape victim. They reported 20 years ago that either DES or ethinyl estradiol tablets could be administered for this purpose (Morris and van Wagenen, 1966). Other estrogens that have been effectively used are conjugated estrogens, estradiol benzoate, and stilbestrol diphosphate (Cook et al., 1986; Dixon et al., 1980; Morris and van Wagenen, 1973). It should be mentioned that besides exogenous estrogens, a whole host of steroidal and nonsteroidal drugs such as antimetabolites, alkaloids, and prostaglandins can exert antifertility effects when administered postcoitally

(Shearman, 1973). These drugs will exert endocrine effects at local and possibly central levels, but the exact single mode of action for each type of morning-after pill, if any, has not been conclusively demonstrated.

Postcoital estrogen may prevent pregnancy by several postulated mechanisms, depending on the time of administration in the cycle. A fertilized egg normally reaches the uterine wall in 4 or 5 days, after which implantation of the blastocyst may or may not take place (Croxatto et al., 1972). One out of three midcycle exposures generally results in implantation of the blastocyst, which occurs on or after the sixth day from ovulation. Altered or asynchronic endometrial glandular and stromal development with resultant enzymatic and metabolic derangement such as reduced cellular carbonic anhydrase may render the secretory endometrium nonreceptive to implantation. Disturbances in the endogenous estrogen/progesterone ratio and decreased level of luteal progesterone may also be responsible for the drug's antifertility effects. A high dose of estrogen given during late follicular phase may suppress ovulation and often prevents the rise in basal body temperature (Gore et al., 1973; Johansson, 1973). Other hypotheses include interferences with sperm or tubal (or both) motility, sperm capacitation, fertilization, and viability of the zy-

TABLE 17–4.

Postcoital Antifertility Treatment From Selected Clinical Trials

Method	Regimen*
DES†	50 mg daily for 5 days
Ethinyl estradiol	5 mg daily for 5 days
Conjugated estrogens	30 mg daily for 5 days or 50 mg daily injection for 2 days
Ovral	Two tablets and two more 12 hr later
Danazol	400 mg and 400 mg 12 hr later
D-Norgestrel	0.4 mg within 3 hr of coitus
RU486	Midluteal 50 or 100 mg daily for 4 days regardless of time of coitus
Copper-T IUD	Insertion within 5 days of coitus

*Starting as soon as possible and within 2 or 3 days of coitus unless otherwise stated.
†Not recommended by manufacturer according to the package insert.

gote. However, once implantation has taken place, the pregnancy appears to be resistant to most steroids.

Continuation of an unrecognized pregnancy that has been exposed to the morning-after pill may theoretically result in certain birth defects. A controversy may exist as to whether such birth defects are directly related to sex steroid exposure during early pregnancy. Nevertheless, menstrual history should be carefully analyzed prior to any postcoital antifertility treatment. If a question of pregnancy arises, a rapid as well as a specific and sensitive pregnancy test should be performed and repeated at appropriate intervals. An informed consent form may be obtained before prescribing a specific postcoital antifertility therapy that includes its immediate and late untoward effects as well as recommendation of abortion in case of treatment failure. Failure rates for most methods are generally less than 2 per 100 isolated courses of treatment. The "actual" failure rates depend on the time of exposure in the cycle and other factors inherent to each method as well as type of subjects. Note, however, that a woman who requests postcoital antifertility therapy may choose to carry her unwanted pregnancy to term in the event of treatment failure. Interestingly, ectopic pregnancies were diagnosed in 10% of women whose postcoital estrogen therapy had failed (Morris and van Wagenen, 1967; Smythe and Underwood, 1975).

High doses of estrogen often produce uncomfortable bloated feeling, nausea, vomiting, as well as swelling of hands and feet. Estrogen treatment may likely induce spottings or menstrual disturbances for several cycles (i.e., shorter or longer than expected cycles). An antiemetic pill or rectal suppository (e.g., prochlorperazine) should be taken at least 30 minutes prior to therapy with high doses of estrogen. If vomiting occurs within 1 hour after a dose of estrogen is taken, that dose should be repeated. Morris and van Wagenen (1967) reported one serious complication from such high doses of estrogen. A woman with history of premenstrual fluid retention developed acute pulmonary edema from DES that resolved after supportive treatment and discontinuation of the drug. A history of venous thromboembolism, another possible complication of taking estrogen, certainly contraindicates the use of estrogenic morning-after pill.

The routine use of high doses of unopposed estrogen has been discouraged for the past decade not only due to its possible venous thromboembolic complications but also due to the recent awareness of its association with genital cancers. Consequently, the most popular morning-after pill to date is a combination of a potent progestin, DL--norgestrel, with 50 μg of ethinyl estradiol (Ovral). Postcoital antifertility treatment with this commonly available contraceptive pill (the *Yuzpe regimen*) consists of two tablets of Ovral, followed by two more tablets 12 hours later (Yuzpe et al., 1974, 1982). Like conventional high-dose estrogens, therapy must be initiated within 2 or 3 days after unprotected coitus and preferably with an antiemetic prophylaxis. About one half of women on this regimen may experience the frequent side effects of nausea and vomiting unless time-release antiemetic pills have been prescribed. This method is highly effective and has fewer side effects with a shorter duration of therapy than the conventional high-dose estrogen regimens (Rowlands, 1982).

A potent *progestin alone* such as D-norgestrel (levonorgestrel) can also be used as a morning-after pill (Kesseru et al., 1974). Other progestins that have been successfully tried for this purpose include clogestone, ethynodiol, norethindrone, norgestrienone, quingestanol acetate, and retroprogestagen. These progestins decidualize the endometrium, rendering it nonreceptive to implantation. In addition, they alter the cervical mucus, making it hostile to sperm penetration. Other possible antifertility effects are reduced sperm and tubal motility as well as reduced tubal secretions. Delayed ovulation and subsequent menstruation may occur with frequent isolated treatment (Craft et al., 1975). Increased intrauterine pH following postcoital administration of D-norgestrel appears to be associated with decreased number of motile sperm in intrauterine fluid (Kesseru et al., 1974). It should be mentioned among postcoital steroids that not only progestins but also *danazol* and *RU486* have been used for this clinical indication (Kubba et al., 1986; Lahteenmaki et al., 1988; Schaison et al., 1985).

In many areas of the world other than the United States, postcoital antifertility treatment of choice is insertion of a copper-containing IUD (preferably a small T-shaped device; Lippes et al., 1975). Definite advantages of insertion of the copper-containing IUD over steroidal drugs are in its longer, ongoing, protection up to several years if well tolerated and shorter duration of nausea or vagal reflex, usually less than 10 minutes. The latter can be blunted with premedication using doxylamine or diphenhydramine (or other antihistamines with inherent anticholinergic effects). Local anesthesia (paracervical block) may also be required for those with a tight internal cervical os. Inert (unmedicated) IUDs are not recommended because they require several days to achieve intended antifertility effects, whereas the released copper provides faster action after insertion. Women with a history of venous thromboembolism may be candidates for postcoital IUD, and a multiparous woman with mutually monogamous relationship represents an ideal candidate. Statistically, most pelvic infections that can be aggravated by the presence of an IUD will likely be diagnosed within 6 months of insertion, and a good number of such cases are evident shortly after insertion (Burkman and the Women's Health Study, 1981). The victim of unprotected coitus should receive an adequate dose of broad-spectrum parenteral antibiotic before IUD insertion. The antibiotic spectrum should cover both gonorrheal and chlamydial infections. Under trial is an IUD impregnated with chlorhexidine antiseptic, which is slowly released and may reduce insertion-related pelvic infections. Precautions, instructions, consent form, and follow-up for postcoital IUD are similar to postcoital steroid therapy. Progestin-releasing IUDs should not be used for postcoital contraception in view of the increased risk of ectopic pregnancy and prolonged spottings associated with progestin treatment (Diaz et al., 1980; Nilsson et al., 1981).

Management

Most sexual assault (rape) victims are females who range from pediatric-age to older-age groups. Rape is the most underreported violent crime. One third of all victims bear evidence of bodily harm besides genital trauma. A reported lifetime incidence of 1 victim for every 10 females is annually rising at an alarming rate, especially among victims in the older age groups. Rape is generally defined as any natural or unnatural act of sexual intimacy or intercourse forced on a person without consent, usually by force, threat of bodily injury, or the inability of the victim to give appropriate consent. This definition varies slightly from state to state.

Management of the victim reflects interplay between the medical and legal professions and in-

cludes (1) diagnosis and treatment of physical and mental trauma with objective documentation of assault as well as evidence collection and preservation, (2) prevention of pregnancy, and (3) prevention or treatment of STD. Beyond the acute management, follow-up and appropriate counseling are also important (Halbert and Darnell-Jones, 1978; Hicks, 1980).

The victim should be isolated from the mainstream of medical activity but should not be left alone for a long period of time. She should receive priority and compassionate care with full respect and concern. Most victims feel helpless and degraded, hence a nonjudgmental approach in obtaining a history and detail of events is crucial. In Massachusetts, the victim (or guardian) must consent to a full management protocol, which includes appropriate diagnostic methods, medical treatment, collection and release of evidence (specimens, clothing, photographs, etc.), before that particular sexual assault will be reported (i.e., the decision is the patient's). If possible, a brief description of the assault in the patient's own words should be recorded by only one clinician. Salient data include the date of last menstrual period, number of assailants, laceration on patient or assailant resulting in bleeding, orifice of penetration with or without ejaculation, use of any contraceptives, the victim's sexual activity within the last 5 days prior to the assault, and the victim's recent activities since the assault (e.g., wiping, washing, bathing or showering, douching, urinating, defecating, vomiting, teeth brushing, or clothes changing). Besides the physical findings on the victim's skin, hair, face, mouth, throat, breasts, abdomen, back, and extremities, general physical and emotional status should also be recorded. Complaints and findings, including foreign matter, should be recorded or collected in a standard rape kit with meticulous labelings. Pertinent materials to be collected are each fingernail scraping in separate test tube, foreign pubic hair from combing, about 10 of the victim's pubic hairs from cutting, and Polaroid photographs. Data related to the assault are kept in a chain of evidence pattern.

Pelvic examination must be performed with a nonlubricated, warm water-moistened, speculum. Examination of the vagina and cervix should be concentrated toward signs of pregnancy, parity, menstruation, trauma, infection, foreign material, and nature of fluid or discharge. The latter (from vaginal pool) are smeared and dried on glass slides and preserved for evidence. Motile sperms can be identified within 4 to 6 hours in saline preparation of vaginal fluid. However, acid phosphatase tablets are no longer used. Cellular antigens matching and modern DNA fingerprinting technique are highly reliable and specific even when applied years later on properly preserved specimens. Microbiological cultures are obtained from each orifice involved in the alleged assault. The risk of contracting STD is associated with the degree of sexual contact and the number of assailants. Sexually transmitted diseases associated with sexual assault (in respective order of frequencies) are gonorrheal (up to 13%), trichomonal, monilial, and *Gardnerella* (more than 6%), chlamydial (more than 4%), herpes (up to 4%), and treponemal (less than 1%) (Cates and Blackmore, 1984). Antibiotics of choice for prophylaxis are single-dose parenteral ceftriaxone and metronidazole (if trichomonads are present), followed by 1 week of oral doxycycline (Dattel et al., 1988; Washington et al., 1987). In cases of suspected pregnancy, a highly sensitive (qualitative) urinary pregnancy test using specific antibody against β-hCG can be expediently obtained prior to quantitative serum testing. Pregnancy interception and its small or unknown risk of potential damage in the event of retained embryo should be made clear to the patient. The victim's willingness or unwillingness to abort a pregnancy should be ascertained. Finally, the victim should receive appropriate instructions as to when and whom to contact for test results and whether to implement or cancel the postcoital antifertility hormone and antibiotic treatment.

The long-term consequences or prognosis may depend on the type and degree of assault (power rape, anger rape, or sadistic rape), the immediate and follow-up multilevel care provided, the support from her family and friends, and her preexistent adaptive behavior pattern (Amir, 1971; Nadelson et al., 1982).

LONG-ACTING PROGESTINS AND OTHER AGENTS

Progestin in certain forms with or without a synthetic estrogen can be injected intramuscularly or subdermally to provide a prolonged contraceptive effect for several months or even up to 3 years (Liskin, 1983a; Liskin and Blackburn, 1987). Two long-acting injectables widely used outside the United States are intramuscular de-

pomedroxyprogesterone acetate (depo-MPA) in microcrystalline suspension and subdermal D-norgestrel in Silastic carriers (Norplant-2) or biodegradable caprolactone carriers (capronor). These long-acting contraceptives have undergone extensive clinical trials. Other long-acting contraceptives contain norethindrone enanthate or combinations of dihydroxyprogesterone acetophenide and estradiol enanthate or medroxyprogesterone acetate (MPA) and estradiol cypionate.

The progestin depo-MPA was synthesized for contraceptive purpose almost 30 years ago. It was used in the "sequential" type of combination OC (brand name Provest), which had been discontinued along with other sequential pills. Nowadays, millions of women outside the United States have used and currently enjoy the protective effect of intramuscular depo-MPA (Rosenfield, 1974). The usual dose is 150 mg every 10 weeks. The failure rate is less than 0.5 pregnancy per 100 women years. Part of the reason that it is so effective is that its effect may last slightly longer than 10 weeks. Thus, users who delay receiving the next scheduled injection for a few weeks are still protected against accidental pregnancy. Its mechanisms of action are theoretically similar to those of the minipill. However, depo-MPA is much more reliable in consistently inhibiting ovulation. Estradiol levels during depo-MPA treatment are about those in the early follicular phase of normal (untreated) cycle. The problem is that after several years of treatment, resumption of ovulation and fertility may not occur for 1 year or even longer in some cases. Chronic intermenstrual spotting (from atrophic endometrium) may occur, and treatment is costly (Toppozada, 1977). In addition, a mild glucocorticoid effect in terms of weight gain is observed in most users. Thus, intramuscular depo-MPA may be appropriate only for thin multiparous women.

Norplant-2, originally made and approved for use in Finland, will release up to 80 μg of D-norgestrel daily during the first year of use and more than 30 μg/day in the third year. Such implants provide a blood level of D-norgestrel like that in a minipill user or one half to one fourth of a combination OC. The failure rate is about 1 pregnancy per 100 women years and even lower during the first year of use. Insertion technique (inner surface of the upper extremity) is fairly simple with the two Silastic rods in V-shaped arrangement under the skin (Fig 17–5) for easy removal. In one U.S. study, discontinuation was re-

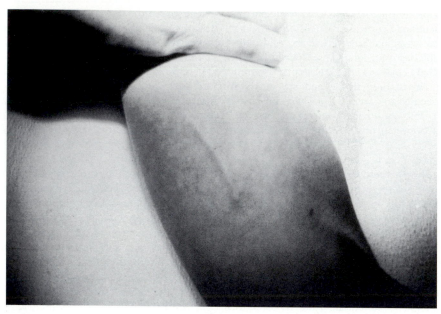

FIG 17—5.
Norplant-2 in situ (inner surface of the patient's upper arm). (Courtesy of PD Darney, MD)

quested by less than 10% of users due to unresolved weight gain or loss, headache, and menstrual abnormalities (Darney, 1988).

Other long-acting contraceptives under clinical trials include microcapsules, progestin or combined progestin-estrogen vaginal ring, once-per-month pill, and skin patch (Ginsburg and Moghissi, 1988). The vaginal Silastic ring is somewhat interesting since a user can insert and remove it by herself (Roy and Mishell, 1983). One ring lasts 3 months. It releases at a slow and relatively constant rate, the contraceptive steroid or steroids, which are easily absorbed by the vaginal mucosa into systemic circulation. It will not work if it is inserted just before coitus. However, once in use after one cycle, occasional removal of the vaginal ring for several hours will not decrease contraceptive protection. In a way, the vaginal ring is opposite to the barrier method in that users can remove this device in anticipation of sexual intercourse and then reinsert the vaginal ring after coitus. A 3-week on, 1-week off, schedule with the progestin-estrogen ring will bring about monthly withdrawal bleeding similar to the combination OC.

A safe and practical contraceptive pill for men has not been invented. Suppression of spermatogenesis has been demonstrated following treatment with exogenous testosterone or a combination of estrogen and testosterone. Unfortunately, long-term use of testosterone leads to hepatic dysfunction. Chinese physicians have utilized the cotton-plant pigment gossypol as an injectable or implantable contraceptive for men (Wu et al., 1986). Hypokalemia, hepatorenal dysfunction, and irreversible azoospermia have been observed in some subjects. Toxicological data from human trials may prevent approval for use in other countries (Anonymous, 1984).

REVERSIBLE METHODS WITH HIGH FAILURE RATES

Coitus interruptus (withdrawal of the penis before ejaculation) is perhaps the oldest contraceptive practice according to Catholic theologians and canonists (Noonan, 1986). Besides the demand for extreme self-control by the male partner, the method is not effective in real practice due to the escape of seminal fluid before orgasm and, in many instances, the unavoidable deposition of semen near the vaginal orifice. In other instances, when the woman has not achieved orgasm before penile withdrawal, she may require artificial stimulation for further gratification.

Lovemaking modifications for contraceptive purpose include orogenital and anal intercourse. The latter is commonly practiced in certain parts of the world, but most cultures have long condemned anal intercourse as unhealthy.

Postcoital douche is also an ancient contraceptive method intended to flush the semen out of the vagina. Water, vinegar solution, and various OTC products have been used. Certain douching solutions may possess a spermicidal effect. An example of folk method is to douche with diet Coca-Cola. This well-known carbonated drink actually has an in vitro spermicidal effect (Umpierre et al., 1985). Nevertheless, the effectiveness of postcoital douche is probably low since sperm can find their way into the cervical mucus almost instantly following ejaculation, and minutes later they can be found in the oviducts (Settlage et al., 1973). Thus, postcoital douche is considered an unreliable contraceptive method.

The *rhythm method (periodic abstinence),* considered unnatural by many couples, is another ineffective way to prevent unwanted conception. A woman's fertile period within each cycle may be crudely estimated from the calendar or basal body temperature or cervical mucus. Three factors that limit the method's effectiveness appear to be intraindividual variations in cycle length, variations in the length of survival of sperm, and actual use compliance. There have also been worrisome epidemiological data implying that an old sperm or an old egg may lead to an imperfect conceptus. However, such fears were not borne out in the Walnut Creek Study (Harlap et al., 1985).

Prolonged nursing is an unreliable contraceptive method and may turn out to be an unnatural way to nourish a well-grown child (McCann et al., 1981). Resumption of ovulation may occur before the first menstrual bleeding, and antiovulatory effect of lactation varies from woman to woman. Breast-feeding mothers should always use a reliable contraceptive such as a condom, diaphragm, sponge, or IUD.

STERILIZATION

Sterilization generally refers to a surgical procedure that is aimed to permanently block or remove male or female genital tracts so that fertilization will not occur. Permanency of sterilization should be the main consideration for any user who contemplates undergoing this surgical method of contraception. Reversal of sterilization requires major surgery and is not always successful (Henry et al., 1980).

Among effective methods for birth control, sterilization is the most frequently chosen by fertile men and multiparous women more than 30 years of age. In fact, the best contraception for an older multiparous woman in a stable and mutually monogamous relationship is male sterilization (vasectomy).

Vasectomy is an outpatient surgical procedure to excise a portion of the vas deferens. It requires local anesthesia and usually takes 15 minutes with experienced hands in a well-equipped facility. Complications, if they occur, are not serious and include hematoma or sperm leakage leading to granulomatous reactions (sperm granulomas). Semen analysis is required 1 and 2 months postoperatively since two sperm-free ejaculations will be considered a proof of sterility. Following vasectomy, it may take up to 20 ejaculations before the patient is azoospermic. Long-term deleterious effects of vasectomy have never been established. The fear of decreased virility or atherosclerosis is unfounded (Campbell, 1988; Goldacre et al., 1983; Liskin, 1983b; Massey et al., 1984).

Like vasectomy, most *female sterilization* methods are outpatient or day surgery procedures. Nevertheless, female sterilization is not as simple and convenient as vasectomy since the female genital tracts are located relatively deep in the pelvis. Risks of death (4 in 100,000) are less than that of one pregnancy and attributed primarily to anesthetic complications (Liskin and Rinehart, 1985; Peterson et al., 1983). There is also an increased risk of extrauterine pregnancy should the female sterilization fail. Attempts at blocking the oviducts via transcervical (transvaginal) extraperitoneal procedures have been recorded for 100 years, but none is acceptable thus far. Hysteroscopic methods for blocking the oviducts with silicone or caustic chemicals have been offered at some facilities. Such methods have never gained popularity because of high failure rates with an unacceptable risk of tubal pregnancy.

Female sterilization is commonly achieved by ligation or coagulation, with or without segmental removal of both oviducts. This tubal sterilization can be performed through two main intraperitoneal routes: the abdominal approach via laparoscopy or minilaparotomy and the vaginal approach via colpotomy or culdoscopy.

Laparoscopic tubal sterilization with bipolar cautery has been the popular choice for interval sterilization in the United States. This method requires elaborate equipment, but the procedural time is relatively short. *Minilaparotomy* has been an excellent choice for sterilization in the postpartum period when the oviducts are located high in the abdomen. It has also been used for interval sterilization under local anesthesia with the help of a uterine elevator device (Osathanondh, 1974). The latter technique is suitable in developing countries where most multiparous women are thin. With a thin abdominal wall, the required amount of local anesthetic drug will not exceed an allowable limit. The *vaginal tubal sterilization* is not commonly done because the method requires considerable technical expertise since intraperitoneal visualization is limited when compared with other interval sterilization methods. There is also an increased risk of ascending infection from the vagina when compared with abdominal incisions. Thus, broad-spectrum IV antibiotics should be given for prophylaxis in women who are undergoing vaginal tubal ligation.

Careful selection of the candidates with a discussion and a simplified consent form for tubal sterilization (Table 17–5) may obviate later regrets for the patient and for her physician as well. Ideal candidates are multiparous women more than 25 years of age. Nulliparous women and those younger than 25 years of age may, with a legitimate medical indication, benefit from sterilization provided that they have been counseled by another appropriate authority besides the operating gynecologist (Harrison and Cook, 1988).

Laparoscopic Tubal Sterilization*

Bipolar electrocoagulation is the method of choice using the two-puncture technique under general endotracheal anesthesia. It is much safer than the unipolar coagulation in avoiding accidental thermal injury to the bowel or neighboring structures, because the electric current will heat and coagulate only the oviductal tissues within the jaws of the electrocoagulation probe. Several contiguous fulgurations are preferred to the transection or segmental removal. The two-puncture technique offers better visualization and ease

*See also Chapter 22.

of manipulation of intra-abdominal organs. Immediate complications include anesthesia-related problems, damage to internal organs, and hemorrhage. Other problems that may occur following discharge are infection, hematoma, adhesions, unrecognized bowel injury, luteal phase pregnancy, and recanalization resulting in intrauterine or ectopic pregnancy (Neil et al., 1975; Schiff and Naftolin, 1974). Suboptimal anesthesia technique such as mask inhalation may result in fatal aspiration pneumonitis since pneumoperineum tends to induce regurgitation and aspiration of gastric contents. Local bleeding may occur if the tissue coagulation is inadequate. A major, life-threatening hemorrhage is rare; if it occurs, it requires immediate laparotomy to repair lacerations of blood vessels, and blood transfusion may be required. Unrecognized bowel burns may subsequently lead to symptoms analogous to ruptured appendicitis (Wheeless and Katayama, 1985). Bowel burns are rare with the use of regularly inspected and well-maintained bipolar instruments. Luteal phase pregnancy may be avoided if sterilization is performed during the first half of the cycle. Failure rate of most female sterilization methods is generally quoted as 2 per 1,000 operations performed. Most failures result from recanalization of the oviduct. However, if the procedure is hastily done without identifying the entire length of the oviduct to its fimbriated end, a round ligament could be mistaken for an oviduct. A high incidence of ectopic pregnancy has been reported with failures of electrocoagulation, especially after the obsolete unipolar method (51%; Liskin and Rinehart, 1985). Nevertheless, the general safety of laparoscopic sterilization and the absence of sequele in terms of menstrual or psychosocial problems have been amply documented (DeStefano et al., 1983; Liskin and Rinehart, 1985).

Beside electrocoagulation, mechanical constriction and obliteration of the oviduct can be accomplished with a Silastic Yoon band (Falope ring), a spring-loaded Hulka clip, and various other radiopaque, nonelectrical devices. Such devices may not be suitable for use on swollen oviducts (e.g., in the puerperium) or in the presence of some pelvic adhesions. The Falope ring is suitable for the single-puncture technique, which is employed primarily in outpatient laparoscopic sterilization under local anesthesia and monitored IV (conscious) sedation. However, several days of unique postoperative pain (more than that from electrocoagulation) may be expected after Falope

TABLE 17–5.

Patient Consent Form for Tubal Sterilization

Tubal sterilization is a surgical procedure to block your fallopian tubes so that fertilization will not occur. This procedure is more effective than any other birth control method but should be chosen only if you are sure that you want no more children because your tubes will become permanently blocked. Occasionally, women who have had tubal sterilization change their minds and want more children. Major surgery to reconstruct the tubes or in vitro fertilization is then necessary but not always successful.

Tubal sterilization can be performed by a laparoscopic procedure that requires small punctures of the abdomen or by a minilaparotomy procedure requiring a small surgical opening of the abdomen. Types of tubal sterilization include excision and ligation, methods involving surgical relocation of the tubes, constriction of each tube within a tight band, or by the passing of an electric current through the tubes. In general, complications of tubal sterilization may involve infection, bleeding, injuries to internal organs, or anesthetic complications. Damage to the bowel or blood vessels requiring major surgery and blood transfusion could happen, but these life-threatening complications are rare.

Your physician will discuss the choice of the procedure most suitable for you based on its advantages and disadvantages, balancing the possible risk of spontaneous healing that allows the tubes to open again against the complexity and complications of the various procedures. Spontaneous opening of the blocked tubes occurs in about 2 cases per 1,000 operations performed and may occur less often after surgical relocation of the tubes performed following childbirth or at the time of cesarean section. If your tubes heal in a way that leaves an opening, pregnancy may occur months or even years later. Such pregnancies can develop outside the womb (ectopic pregnancies) and cause severe bleeding. It is difficult to predict which women may develop these complications; therefore, you should report any irregularities of your period or pregnancy symptoms to your physician after tubal sterilization.

It is also possible that women may be pregnant at the time of tubal sterilization, especially those whose periods have not been normal or those having the operation in the last 2 weeks of their menstrual cycle. Your physician may perform a blood pregnancy test around the time of the operation if needed, but again, you should report any irregular periods or pregnancy symptoms to your physician after the tubal sterilization procedure.

Planned procedure:

Comments:

Patient's statement

I have read this consent form and understand that there are failure rates and risks associated with tubal sterilization. My physician has discussed the advantages and disadvantages of tubal sterilization. I consent to the planned procedure.

_____   _____

Patient's signature   Witness' signature

Date _____

rings application. The Hulka clip is probably the least traumatic to local tissues, but its failure rate is slightly higher than other methods. Major trauma to internal organs can be avoided or substantially reduced with the open laparoscopy technique. This technique is also practical if the procedure has to be performed under local anesthesia. The peritoneum is identified and entered through a small infraumbilical incision using the blunt, funnel-shaped, Hasson cannula (Hasson, 1982). Blind stabbings of the abdominal wall with Verres carbon dioxide needle and sharp trocar in conventional laparoscopy are avoided in this "open laparoscopy" method.

Minilaparotomy

Ligation and transection or resection of a portion of the oviduct may be electively performed during the puerperium and in the nonpregnant interval as well. Electrocoagulation can also be used in the minilaparotomy method of tubal sterilization. The simple "tie and cut" technique is usually a modification of the Pomeroy method.

There are techniques to relocate and bury the proximal portion of the transected oviduct to minimize failure. Uchida of Japan buries the ligated proximal stump of the tube retroperitoneally under the leaves of the broad ligament. The ligated distal stump remains intraperitoneal. The modified Irving method probably has the lowest failure rate, generally quoted as less than 0.1%. It is the sterilization method of choice immediately following cesarean delivery. The ligated proximal stump of the tube is buried into the uterine wall near the cornu. The original Irving's practice of burying the distal stump under the leaves of the broad ligament is not really necessary.

Safe timing for postpartum sterilization should be jointly determined by the obstetrician and anesthesiologist as well as the patient herself. In many circumstances, deferral until the patient is in optimal condition may be the best policy (American College of Obstetricians and Gynecologists Committee on Obstetrics, 1987). The parturient and pregnant women in second or third trimester are at an increased risk of regurgitation and aspiration of gastric contents. Following natural childbirth, many anesthesiologists prefer a routine waiting period of 6 hours to immediate postpartum sterilization. Any medical, obstetrical, neonatal survivability, or infectious problems

should override the original plan for immediate or puerperal sterilization (American College of Obstetricians and Gynecologists Committee on Obstetrics, 1987). With the advent of 24-hour broad-spectrum IV antibiotics for prophylaxis, there is no need for the patient to wait until 6 weeks postpartum before undergoing tubal ligation. In the absence of intrapartum of puerperal infection, minilaparotomy can be performed safely with prophylactic IV antibiotics before the complete involution of the uterus. Advantages are the easy access to the oviducts through a small abdominal incision and the patient's convenience in scheduling her surgery during allowable maternity leave.

Minilaparotomy can be performed under local anesthesia for interval sterilization or in conjunction with first trimester induced abortion. A device such as the Hulka tenaculum or a uterine elevator designed by Osathanondh (1974) will allow easy access to the oviduct via a small suprapubic incision. Women who have successfully undergone natural childbirth or a surgery under local anesthesia are good candidates. However, the patient should be of average body weight for her height and weigh less than 68 kg. Hypertension, hyperthyroidism, cardiac arrhythmia, and hypersensitivity to local anesthetics or epinephrine are contraindications. Local anesthetic solution containing a minimal amount of epinephrine is injected into the abdominal wall and the oviducts before ligation or electrocoagulation. Paracervical block anesthesia should be given before applying the uterine elevator or Hulka tenaculum. Intravenous drugs that are helpful include a parasympatholytic agent such as glycopyrrolate, a sedative (e.g., midazolam or droperidol), or an antihistamine (e.g., diphenhydramine), and the short-acting opioid fentanyl citrate. Dosage of these combined medications may be clinically adjusted and should not exceed the maximum allowable limits.

A sterilized woman may undergo a major surgery to unblock her Fallopian tubes. Success rates of the tubal reanastomosis depends on the method of sterilization. Those having had the clips, the Silastic bands, or the modified Pomeroy method, in respective order, are easier to reverse than the Irving, Uchida, or electrocoagulation method of sterilization. The most difficult to reverse is the blockade after unipolar cautery due to extensive tissue damage and frequent postoperative adhesions. Besides complications inherent to laparotomy and anesthesia, tubal pregnancy occurs at very high rates, especially after reversal of unipolar electrocoagulation (Henry et al., 1980; Wheeless and Katayama, 1985).

Patients with major uterine or pelvic pathology who request sterilization may benefit from hysterectomy. However, hysterectomy must not be viewed as a simple method of sterilization because it carries a higher complication rate than tubal sterilization.

PREGNANCY TERMINATION (THERAPEUTIC INDUCED ABORTION)

Pharmacotherapeutic Methods

Agents Disrupting Chorionic Villi

Progesterone Receptor Blockers.—Progesterone receptor blockers represent a new and important alternative in antifertility therapy. Such antiprogesterones are derivatives of norethindrone and are therefore within the class of 19-norsteroids.

A prototype of antiprogesterone, code named RU38.486, has been synthesized by Roussel-Uclaf Pharmaceutical Company in Romainville, France. Specifically, the addition of a functional group dimethylaminophenyl ring into the norethindrone molecule at the 11β-carbon position has resulted in this potent compound RU486, which can displace progesterone from its receptors (Baulieu and Segal, 1984). This receptor blocker appears to have no direct effect on ovarian production of progesterone. It has been approved for use in France and the People's Republic of China.

RU486, or mifepristone, has been used as an abortifacient in the first quarter of pregnancy, a morning-after pill, and in the treatment of Cushing's syndrome. In addition, the drug is being tried in the treatment of endometriosis. Its contraceptive efficacy as a once-per-month pill has so far been unreliable (Schaison, 1988).

RU486 effectively antagonizes progesterone actions on the gestational endometrium leading to eventual detachment of the chorionic villi and consequent decline in the peripheral blood levels of progesterone and hCG. When administered during midluteal phase, it blocks the effects of progesterone by displacing the natural steroid from its receptors on the secretory endometrium, with resultant induction of menses (Schaison et al., 1985). With this method of administration,

multiple sites of its action on the hypothalamic-hypophyseal-ovarian-endometrial axis have recently been proposed based on dynamic hormonal studies (Garzo et al., 1988). In the absence of progesterone, RU486 will exert mild progesterone-like effects (in estrogen-treated postmenopausal women leading to a further decrease in serum gonadotropin levels; Gravanis et al., 1985).

Besides its action within the female reproductive tract, RU486 also binds to the glucocorticoid receptors and thus antagonizes the actions of cortisol. In high doses, this drug may be beneficial in the treatment of Cushing's syndrome. Small and transient compensatory rises in plasma ACTH and cortisol levels have been shown following daily administration of 200 mg of RU486 for 4 days. This course of treatment is required for early pregnancy termination. Alternatively, a single oral dose of 600 mg has been employed with slightly less effectiveness (Grimes et al., 1988). A continued search by German scientists for an ideal antiprogesterone that lacks antiglucocorticoid effects has recently produced two other related compounds, ZK98.734 and ZK98.299 (Fig 17–6). The latter appear to have no antiglucocorticoid activity at all while being more effective abortifacients than RU486 in preliminary animal studies (Elger et al., 1987).

Oral or, more effectively, parenteral administration of RU486 has been shown to induce moderate uterine bleeding with significant decrease in hematocrit value, followed by complete expulsion of early (first-quarter) gestational products in 80% of the cases. The remaining 20% of the cases required dilatation and curettage (D&C). Bleeding in many cases occurred before the decrease in serum progesterone levels. Successful therapy is associated with an increase in plasma levels of $PGF_{2\alpha}$, myometrial contraction, favorable changes in the uterine cervix, and, in some patients, hormonal evidence of luteolysis. However, the most effective pharmacotherapy to terminate early gestation (and somewhat later gestation with fetal demise; Cabrol et al., 1985) is the administration of RU486 in combination with an otherwise subtherapeutic dose of a uterotonic prostaglandin (Table 17–6; Cameron and Baird, 1988). These two different classes of drugs are quite synergistic. A single, low dose of a prostaglandin drug administered toward the end of the course of RU486 treatment will ensure complete abortion without incurring systemic side effect of that prostaglandin. Note that RU486 has

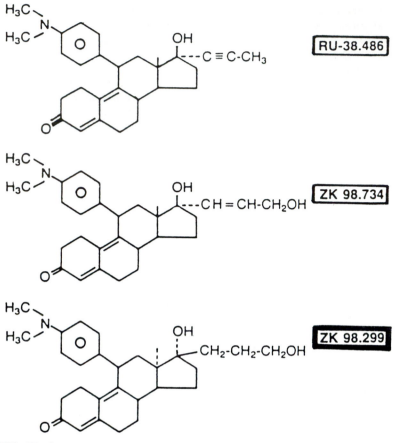

FIG 17–6.
Progesterone receptor blockers.

not been beneficial for terminating ectopic tubal pregnancy in limited, unpublished, clinical trials. Significant concentrations of this drug have been demonstrated in the umbilical plasma during second trimester therapeutic abortion, indicating that it is effectively transferred across the placental barrier (Frydmann et al., 1985). However, among the drug failure cases whose intrauterine pregnancy was not successfully terminated, there has been no fetal abnormality reported to date.

TABLE 17–6.

Therapeutic Abortion at 56 or Less Days of Amenorrhea*

Method	Completion Rate
RU486 150 mg/day orally for 4 days	60% (12/20)
PGE$_1$ analogue 1 mg vaginal pessary every 3 hr up to five doses	97% (29/30)
Vacuum aspiration	96% (27/28)
RU486 as above protocol plus only one dose of PGE$_1$ on day 3	95% (18/19)

*From Cameron IT, Baird DT: Early pregnancy termination: A comparison between vacuum aspiration and medical abortion using prostaglandin (16, 16 dimethyl-trans-δ$_2$-PGE$_1$ methyl ester) or the antiprogestogen RU486. *Br J Obstet Gynaecol* 1988; 95:271–276. Used by permission.

The plasma elimination half-life of RU486 is between 10 and 25 hours. Data on long-term untoward effects from repeated administration of RU486 are not available. A disadvantage of drug-induced abortion (vs. surgical evacuation) may be the unavailability of pathology specimens, especially in Asian countries where trophoblastic disease is prevalent.

Inhibitors of Progesterone Biosynthesis.— Inhibitors of progesterone biosynthesis such as aminoglutethimide (Salhanick, 1982), epostane (Crooij et al., 1988), or trilostane (van der Spuy et al., 1983) have been tried as moderately effective abortifacients up to 50 days of pregnancy (from last menstrual period [LMP]). However, unwanted effects at therapeutic antifertility doses include adrenocortical suppression and, in many cases, significant uterine bleeding due to incomplete miscarriage.

Aminoglutethimide is a bicyclic chemical compound with two optically active isomers. It inhibits major steroidogenic enzyme systems (cholesterol side-chain cleavage and aromatase) by blocking the terminal cytochrome P-450s. Besides its adrenal suppressive effects, which can be used for medical adrenalectomy, this drug may potentially depress the central nervous system and activate hepatic microsomal enzymes. Trilostane and epostane (Winthrop 24540 and 32729) are 4,5-epoxy steroids structurally related to testosterone and methyltestosterone, respectively. Each epoxy steroid blocks the biosynthesis of progesterone by inhibiting the enzyme 3β-hydroxysteroid dehydrogenase, with epostane being less suppressive to the adrenals than trilostane. Nevertheless, high doses of epostane (800 mg/day for 1 week) are usually required for early pregnancy termination. Although therapies with this class of drugs have not led to subsequent menstrual or ovulational disorder, this group of antifertility agents does not appear as promising as the progesterone receptor blockers.

Inhibitors of Folate Reductase.—Folate Reductase inhibitors have been used as abortifacients. However, these antimetabolites cannot be recommended as first-line drugs for terminating normal intrauterine pregnancy. The required duration of therapy appeared rather lengthy. The prototype oral agent 4-aminopteroylglutamic acid was originally tried for this purpose more than 30 years ago (Thiersch, 1952). All patients in that small series required either D&C or hysterotomy between 5 and 47 days after initiation of therapy. Interestingly, one such case of "medically indicated" therapeutic abortion with maternal tuberculosis resulted in a live fetus.

In the past 20 years, a common parenteral antimetabolite, methotrexate, has been successfully employed in the conservative treatment of placenta accreta. Blood transfusions, uterine packing, and antibiotics have also been required in such cases. Stormy, intensive, and protracted hospitalization typically followed before the patient recuperated with her uterus remaining intact. The availability of sensitive and specific serum hCG measurement together with high-resolution diagnostic ultrasound have led investigators in Asia, followed by a score of gynecologists in the United States, to use methotrexate in the pharmacotherapy of a small tubal or cervical pregnancy (Farabow et al., 1983; Ory, 1986; Oyer et al., 1988). It appears that methotrexate works well in destroying abnormal or ectopic trophoblastic cells but is not very effective against a large bulk of normal trophoblastic tissue. This is opposite to RU486, which works better on the normal intrauterine trophoblastic cells than on the ectopic ones. The benefit of methotrexate for tubal pregnancy should be weighed against the yet unknown long-term sequele of elevated serum hepatic transaminase levels. Such increased liver enzyme levels appear reversible on cessation of therapy. A fatal idiosyncratic reaction may occur when methotrexate is administered in conjunction with nonsteroidal anti-inflammatory drugs (Stockley, 1987).

It must be mentioned, however, that some patients with a small tubal pregnancy do not require any treatment except careful monitoring until tubal abortion or resorption occurs. Such patients later conceive with normal liveborn offsprings (Carp et al., 1986). Therefore, it could be reasoned that some patients reported in those methotrexate for ectopic series might have done all right without any treatment at all. Opponents of the methotrexate for ectopic treatment modality may label it a "radical" pharmacotherapy considering potential risks from this chemical agent when compared with their "conservative" treatment via minilaparotomy (salpingostomy) or pelviscopic surgery. Advocates, on the other hand, believe that any toxic sequele such as liver damage should be negligible based on long-term health of the majority of trophoblastic disease patients following oncolytic chemotherapy with methotrexate.

Uterotonic Agents

Prostaglandins.—Prostaglandins are long-chain 20-carbon derivatives of arachidonic acid produced in human tissues from phospholipids. They bear a common chemical structure of the C-20 prostanoic acid, which contains a cyclopentane ring between C-8 and C-12. Biosynthesis of such compounds in the uterine tissues requires the lysosomal enzyme phospholipase A_2 and a group of microsomal enzymes called *prostaglandin synthetase* (cyclo-oxygenase, isomerase, and reductase). Some prostaglandin drugs that will induce contractions of the gravid uterus include PGE_1, PGE_2, and its synthetic derivatives such as meteneprost potassium and sulprostone, $PGF_{2\alpha}$, and its 15-methyl analogue. They are extremely thermolabile in soluble forms and must be kept below $4°$ C until use.

Prostaglandin E_2 (dinoprostone) is available in a suppository (wax) or gel base (Rakhshani and Grimes, 1988). The vaginal suppository form of PGE_2 has been approved by the FDA for labor induction in case of fetal death up to 28 weeks of pregnancy. It is readily absorbed through the vaginal mucosa into the systemic circulation with resultant pharmacological effects as summarized in Table 17–7. The recommended dosage is 5 to 20 mg clinically adjusted (titrated) at safe intervals (usually every 3 or 4 hours) based on optimal uterotonic response vs. its undesirable systemic effects. The drug will stimulate the smooth muscles of the gravid uterus and gastrointestinal (GI) tract and will disturb the body's thermoregulatory center. Therefore, its common side effects include nausea, vomiting, diarrhea, and fever, respectively. Gastrointestinal side effects can be reduced by pretreatment medications with oral diphenoxylate with atropine (Lomotil) and an intramuscular

TABLE 17–7.

Systemic Effects of Prostaglandins

Contraction of pregnant uterus
Fever
Nausea and vomiting
Diarrhea
Increased intraocular pressure
Increased histamine level
Increased platelet aggregation
Decreased noradrenaline level

antinauseant such as prochlorperazine or phenoxyzine hydrochloride. Fever can be reduced with rectal acetaminophen and wet body sponge. Unlike $PGF_{2\alpha}$, PGE_2 will dilate the bronchial and most vascular smooth muscles (Table 17–8), resulting in moderate peripheral vasodilation and lowered diastolic blood pressure when large doses are used (Thaysson et al., 1981). Patients with active asthma or compromised cardiopulmonary hemodynamics will tolerate systemic PGE_2 much better than $PGF_{2\alpha}$.

Prior to labor induction with uterotonic prostaglandin, the degree of cervical effacement must be assessed. If the cervix is not well effaced, laminaria pretreatment is indicated regardless of cervical dilatation. The induction to delivery period is much shorter with adequate laminaria pretreatment of the cervix. After the products of conception have been expelled, routine inspection and gentle exploration of the uterine cavity with a large curette is strongly advised before discharging the patient. This can be accomplished under minimal sedation with or without local anesthesia. Since 1981, we have routinely used multiple laminaria tents plus one Lamicel in overnight preparation of the cervix before PG induction. With this special pretreatment, we have not had any cervical lacerations or uterine ruptures in more than 4,000 consecutive prostaglandin-induced midtrimester abortions. Use of a midtrimester dose of PGE_2 for pregnant women in the third trimester could lead to uterine rupture (Patterson et al., 1979; Valenzuela et al., 1980). Uterine rupture has also been reported after intra-amnionic injection of $PGF_{2\alpha}$ or 15-methyl $PGF_{2\alpha}$ (carboprost tromethamine) as well (Cederqvist and Birnbaum, 1980; Vergote et al., 1982). This complication tends to occur when a PG drug is administered in combination with oxytocin treatment. The uterine muscle near term pregnancy may be more sensitive to PG because of increased number of oxytocin receptors. Prostaglandin and oxytocin are strongly synergistic, and prostaglandin itself may induce an increase in oxytocin receptors. Thus, oxytocin should not be administered within 2 hours of the last prostaglandin dose.

Following an overnight laminaria preparation of the cervix, PGE_2 suppository can be inserted through the dilated cervical canal as the initial labor-inducing dose. This is done by compressing the PGE_2 wax onto the porous surface of the Lamicel at its distal pointed end. To keep the

TABLE 17–8.

Differences Between Prostaglandin $F_{2\alpha}$ and Prostaglandin $E_{2\alpha}$

	$PGF_{2\alpha}$	PGE_2
Uterine muscle		
Pregnant	Contract	Contract
Nonpregnant	Contract	Inhibit
Bronchial smooth muscle	Constrict	Dilate
Arterial perfusion		
Coronary	Decreased	Increased
Regional	Decreased	Increased
Aterial pressure		
Systemic	Increased	Decreased
Pulmonary	Increased	Increased
Central venous pressure	Increased	Decreased
Cardiac output and heart rate	Increased	Increased

drug in, one must snugly insert a large number of laminaria tents in the cervical canal immediately following this intrauterine, extra-amniotic, Lamicel-PGE_2 combination. This initial intrauterine dose may produce less systemic side effects than the vaginal application. The technique can also be used after rupture of membranes provided that all amniotic fluid has been manually expressed out of the uterus with suprapubic pressure.

15(S)-15-Methyl $PGF_{2\alpha}$ (carboprost tromethamine) has been used in combination with 64 ml of hypertonic (23.4%) saline for intra-amnionic abortion on our ambulatory service. Actually, this particular prostaglandin analogue has been approved for intramuscular use in case of postpartum hemorrhage due to atonic uterus (Bruce et al., 1982; Hankins et al., 1988). However, parenteral administration may produce, in some patients, severe untoward events, including cardiac arrhythmia, bronchoconstriction, pulmonary hypertension, increased intrapulmonary shunting, and arterial oxygen desaturation (Hankins et al., 1988). Unlike PGE_2, $PGF_{2\alpha}$ and its synthetic derivatives will stimulate the uterine contraction even in the nongravid state. Its efficacy following intra-amnionic injection for labor induction was described more than 10 years ago (Dingfelder et al., 1976; Karim and Sivasamboo, 1975). When our strict protocol of active management is used, the intra-amnionic injection to abortion time intervals for midtrimester abortion average 8 hours. Ninety-five percent of our patients who had prostaglandin abortions are discharged from our ambulatory unit within the same day. Free backflow of clear amniotic fluid must be seen at amniocentesis before the drug is injected into the amnionic sac. This caution is imperative because an accidental leakage of 15-methyl $PGF_{2\alpha}$ into the systemic circulation will result in cardiopulmonary side effects that may not abate as quickly as those caused by $PGF_{2\alpha}$. Dose-response study has revealed that 2 mg of 15-methyl $PGF_{2\alpha}$ and 64 ml of 23.4% saline (4 mEq/ml solution) are optimal for midtrimester intra-amnionic labor induction protocol. This protocol produces minimal or no systemic side effects when compared with the use of PGE_2 suppositories.

Misoprostol, a methyl analogue of PGE_1, has recently been approved by the FDA for use in the treatment of peptic ulcer disease. This oral agent has antisecretory activity up to 5 hours at the usual recommended dose (Monk and Clissold, 1987). However, it will exert a significant uterotonic effect in the first trimester of pregnancy at doses greater than 400 µg (Rabe et al., 1987).

Oxytocin.—Oxytocin, a neurohypophyseal octapeptide hormone, has been synthesized for clinical use in the induction of labor beyond the second trimester of pregnancy. Unlike prostaglandin, oxytocin is uterotonic only in the presence of adequate number of oxytocin receptors. It appears more potent than prostaglandin in causing contraction of the myoepithelial cells of the mammary gland, resulting in milk ejection. Thus, oxytocin nasal spray is available for stimulating initial milk letdown. Suckling is the only well-defined physiological stimulus for oxytocin release. Cervical dilatation is believed to be another stimulus for its release. Because of its similarity with vasopressin in amino acid sequence, oxytocin has $1/200$ the antidiuretic potency of vasopressin. If a concentrated oxytocin solution is to be infused for a prolonged period of time, a limited volume of electrolytes solution should be used instead of plain dextrose in water to avoid water intoxication with resultant hyponatremia and its consequences.

In midtrimester abortion, high-dose IV oxytocin is effective only when the patient's cervix is near or at full effacement (i.e., 90%–100%). Oxytocin will exert its uterotonic effect after the uterus has been adequately stimulated by an exogenous prostaglandin or other factors leading to local endogenous prostaglandin production. For midtrimester labor induction with a nonviable fetus, our IV oxytocin augmentation protocol requires 60 units in 500 ml of electrolyte solution at the initial rate of 10 ml/hour (equivalent to 20 mU/minute) using an infusion pump. The rate is increased at intervals and in increments of 10 ml/hour up to the limit of 60 ml/hour (120 mU/minute).

Two uterotonic agents that have fallen into disuse at our institution are buccal oxytocin citrate and the oxytocic alkaloid sparteine sulfate for intramuscular injection. The latter is very potent, but its uterotonic effect is difficult to titrate. In fact, many ergot alkaloids are potent uterotonics. They have been used in illegal abortions along with quinine tablets (Potts and Diggory, 1983).

Hypertonic and Locally Toxic Solutions.—
Hypertonic and locally toxic solutions have been used for intra-amnionic abortions long before the availability of prostaglandin drugs. They include 20% saline solution, 30% or 40% hyperosmolar urea, and the antiseptic acridine orange (acrinol) (Burkman et al., 1975; Kafrissen et al., 1984). Originally, hypertonic dextrose solution was also used, but its use was associated with high infection rate. Intra-amnionic injection of hypertonic or hyperosmolar solutions will induce a cascade of intrauterine events leading to prostaglandin release in the local tissues. Effective uterine contractions occur within several hours. Electrolyte and osmolar dynamics in these types of induced abortion have been described by many investigators (Anderson, 1968; Burkman et al., 1975; Frigoletto and Pokoly, 1971; Goodlin and Kresch, 1968). Too concentrated or too high a volume of saline solution may result in life-threatening disseminated intravascular coagulation or hypernatremia if accidentally injected into the uterine circulation.

Agents for Softening the Cervix

Hygroscopic devices (laminaria, Lamicel, and Dilapan) are considered an integral part of therapeutic abortion beyond the 12th week of pregnancy. They are placed in the cervical canal to achieve gentle and nontraumatic dilatation of the cervix. After adequate preparation of the cervix, the uterine evacuation procedure can be expediently accomplished by a trained physician with minimal risk of instrumental trauma and hemorrhage (Blumenthal, 1988).

Laminaria tent (Figure 17–7) is a dried stem

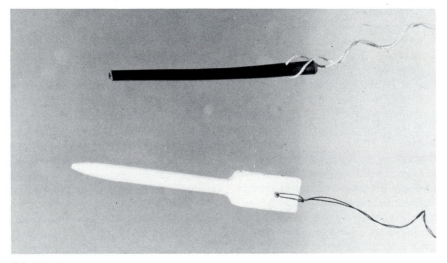

FIG 17–7.
A laminaria tent *(dark)* shown in comparison with a Lamicel *(white).*

of seaweed that feels like a wooden stick or a huge toothpick. It is 6 cm long and available in different widths based on the cross-section diameters at its tip, from 2 to 6 mm. At our institution, only the small-diameter (2- or 3-mm) laminaria tents are used (in large numbers per patient) because of the ease of insertion and greater surface area of exposure than small numbers of large tents. Two small laminarias work better than one large one. They are left in the cervical canal for at least 4 hours but preferably overnight before the uterine evacuation procedure. Insertion technique is described in Table 17–9.

Laminaria was actually used in Europe before World War II but was quickly abandoned because of sepsis (since it cannot be boiled). Its rebirth in modern-day obstetrics and gynecology came after the availability of gas sterilization with ethylene oxide and broad-spectrum antibiotics (Eaton et al., 1972; Hale and Pion, 1972; Newton, 1972). The device swells up three to four times its original diameter (Fig 17–8) and slowly

TABLE 17–9.

Laminaria Insertion Technique

1. Make sure the patient understands that laminaria insertion is the beginning and the most important part of the pregnancy termination procedure. If the patient is 18 weeks or more pregnant, an ultrasound imaging should be done to confirm the gestational age.
2. Do a pelvic examination to record the uterine size and axis, and then change gloves to put on sterile ones and insert speculum.
3. Prep the vagina and cervix with povidone-iodine (Betadine). Use diluted chlorhexidine gluconate (Hibiclens) if the patient is allergic to povidone-iodine.
4. Dip a small, long-stem, Q-tip swab in povidone-iodine, and gently sound the endocervix with it. Do not go in far beyond the internal os. The brownish staining of the Q-tip stem indicates the length of cervical canal.
5. If necessary, grasp the cervix with a long Allis clamp or straight ring forceps, taking care to grasp only a small fold of mucosa to minimize the patient's discomfort. A local (paracervical block) anesthesia may be required in case of cervical stenosis.
6. Grasp the laminaria at the string end with ring forceps and gently insert it until the laminaria tip with the string is flush with the external os. Always use the laminaria with the smallest diameter. For patients who are up to 12 weeks pregnant, insert two laminarias. For patients 13 to 17 weeks pregnant, insert three to five laminarias. For patients 18 weeks or more pregnant, insert three to five laminarias with one Lamicel as tolerated by the patient.
7. Dip folded 4 by 4 gauze in a small amount of povidone-iodine, lay it over the cervix, and tuck it gently into fornices. Lay a second (dry) 4 by 4 in. gauze over the first to pack the laminaria in place. Gently remove the speculum while holding the gauze sponges in place with ring forceps.
8. Have the patient remain lying in left lateral position for a few minutes to avoid syncope. Note in the chart the time of insertion and the number of laminarias and sponges inserted.
9. Be certain that the patient understands that she must return for laminaria removal the next day. Severe infection may result if one set of laminaria is left in situ for more than 48 hours. Inform the patient that the cramping with insertion will subside in a few minutes. Tell her to come back to the hospital at once if the membranes rupture, if bleeding occurs, or if she develops a fever. *Forbid coitus.* (Some patients had attempted coitus with laminarias in place; hence, give clear instructions against it.) The patient may take one or two acetaminophen tablets as needed for cramping, but *aspirin or other prostaglandin synthesis inhibitors should not be used.* Give the patient an instruction card that contains the above advice and precautions to read and keep with her in case she forgets the verbal information.

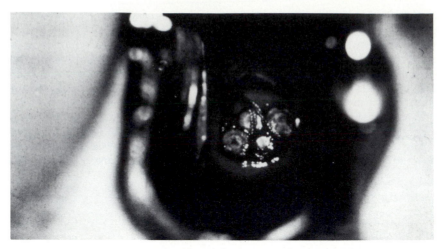

FIG 17–8.
Four laminaria tents that have been in the cervix overnight. (Courtesy of A.M. Altman, M.D.)

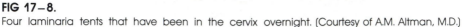

dilates the cervix. Following intracervical placement, the sonographical appearance of laminaria varies with time due to its hygroscopic nature (Hirsh and Levy, 1988). While exerting its effect, laminaria may produce moderate but tolerable crampy pain. Besides its hygroscopic (mechanical) action, use of laminaria is associated with significantly increased blood levels of prostaglandin metabolites (Ye et al., 1982). Following overnight placement, each laminaria tent becomes soft, as large as a cigarette, and easily removable. We prefer *Laminaria japonica* to the ones from Europe because of its uniform consistency and minimal hourglass (dumbbelling) effect. Whenever this phenomenon occurs, removal of such laminarias may be difficult and requires paracervical block anesthesia. Each laminaria should be grasped with ring forceps and the forceps then rotated 360 degrees before the incarcerated device can be pulled out.

Lamicel is a dried polyvinyl alcohol sponge stick impregnated with magnesium sulfate (see Fig 17–7). This hard and sharp stick will become softened and swells up with its spongy consistency immediately with its placement in the cervical canal. Each stick contains between 0.2 and 0.5 gm of magnesium sulfate, depending on its diameter. Minimal systemic absorption of magnesium sulfate may occur through the uterine tissue, but blood magnesium levels have not exceeded 4 mg/dl in our testing series. Through some poorly defined histochemical effects, Lamicel softens the cervix within 2 hours, making it pliable to gradual

dilatation with conventional instruments or with multiple *Laminaria japonica* tents. An overnight preparation of the cervix with one Lamicel plus three to five 4-mm laminarias on the day preceding labor induction has significantly shortened the prostaglandin induction to delivery interval and has thus far eliminated the risk of cervical rupture or cervicovaginal fistula (fistula cervicovaginalis laqueatica) (Ingvardsen and Eriksen, 1979). Paradoxical to its tocolytic effect, overnight preparation of the cervix with this magnesium sulfate device may enhance the effectiveness of prostaglandin-induced labor. Other investigators have effectively used Lamicel prior to suction evacuation of the uterus.

Dilapan, another hygroscopic cervical dilator, is a synthetic polymer similar to soft contact lens. It is recommended by its manufacturer for use within 4 hours of the abortion procedure on patients at or prior to 16 weeks of pregnancy. When compared with other hygroscopic dilators, this rather gluey and sticky device expands rapidly in and around the cervix. Thus, it may be difficult to remove the device within 2 hours of insertion.

Besides hygroscopic devices, intracervical or vaginal PGE_2 and other prostaglandin derivatives have been successfully used for softening the unfavorable (unripe) cervix (Fruzzetti et al., 1988). Meteneprost potassium, an analogue of PGE_2 in suppository form (10 mg), can induce adequate cervical softening within several hours of vaginal administration prior to first trimester induced abortion (Darney and Dorward, 1987; Osathanondh et al., 1985; Shapiro et al., 1982). Preparing the cervix with a low dose of PGE_2 or one of its synthetic derivatives will reduce the need for forceful, instrumental dilatation of the cervix prior to uterine evacuation. Minimal but well-tolerated prostaglandin-induced side effects should be expected.

Conventional Methods

More than 1 million therapeutic abortions have been reported in the United States each year, and there are probably as many unreported menstrual extraction or menstrual regulation procedures routinely performed in the physician's offices. In 1985, approximately one legal abortion was performed for every three live births in the United States (Leads from the MMWR, 1988). Most therapeutic abortions (95%) employ the *vacuum aspiration technique* and are safely accomplished in an outpatient facility (Wu, 1958). It is not a good contraceptive choice and should be used as the last resort. On the other hand, induced abortion is the best therapy to save the mother in case of severe cardiac, renal, metabolic, hepatic, hematological, or cerebrovascular disease (Bower et al., 1988). With rare and unusual indications, abortion in the third trimester may be justified strictly to save the mother's life. Appropriate fetal indications range from defects that are incompatible with extrauterine life, such as anencephaly, holoprosencephaly, and hypoplasia or agenesis of vital organs, to problems of chromosomal, metabolic, teratogenic, or infectious origin. Unique problems that combine the maternal and fetal indications for terminating the pregnancy are maternal neoplastic disease requiring radiation or chemotherapy, fetal death, and chorioamnionitis. With the latter diagnosis, the gravid uterus must be evacuated not only to save the mother but also to preserve her reproductive capability. Safe termination of pregnancy beyond 24 weeks from the LMP is justified in cases of fetal death or lethal malformation such as anencephaly (Chervenak et al., 1984; Osathanondh et al., 1980). Hysterotomy or gravid hysterectomy is rarely indicated when skilled physicians and modern techniques for uterine evacuation are readily available.

In general, complication rates from induced abortion increase with every advancing week of gestation (Grimes and Schulz, 1985; Ory, 1983; Tietze, 1977). Major complications as defined by the Centers for Disease Control Joint Program for the Study of Abortion (JPSA) include cardiac arrest, convulsions, death, endotoxic shock, fever for 3 days or more, hemorrhage necessitating transfusion, hypernatremia, injury to bladder, ureter, or intestine, pelvic infection with 2 or more days of fever and a peak of at least 40°C or with hospitalization for 11 days or more, pulmonary embolism or infarction, thrombophlebitis, major surgical treatment of complications, and wound disruption after hysterotomy or hysterectomy. Other complications not listed by the JPSA include retained pregnancy products or continuation of pregnancy, hematometra, and coagulopathy (Osathanondh et al., 1981; White et al., 1983). In addition, two or more induced abortions may increase the risk of subsequent first and second trimester loss (Hogue et al., 1982; Levin et al., 1980; Linn et al., 1983a; Stubblefield et al., 1984).

Menstrual extraction (miniabortion, minisuction, or menstrual regulation) is usually performed in a physician's office with a soft and flexible plastic cannula (sometimes referred to as *Karman cannula*). The cannula is attached to a special self-locking syringe or a small suction pump operated electrically or hydrostatically (Vabra aspirator). An experienced operator can perform this miniabortion up to 6 or 7 weeks from the patient's LMP without anesthesia. Most of the time, a 4-mm cannula or a recently available 3-mm cannula can be inserted into the gravid uterus without instrumental dilatation of the cervix. The patient may receive preoperative medications consisting of oral ibuprofen and diazepam (or sublingual lorazepam). An office pregnancy test using a rapid, specific, and sensitive assay is strongly advised before the minisuction to avoid unnecessary instrumentation of the uterine cavity. The minisuction evacuation can be accomplished within 5 minutes with in and out movement of the cannula while rotating it 360 degrees around its long axis. After the procedure is completed, the aspirated products of conception must be carefully inspected for the presence of trophoblastic villous tissue (chorionic villi; Fig 17–9). If only the decidual (hypertrophic gestational endometrial) tissue is obtained and the villous structure cannot be identified, ectopic pregnancy must be ruled out using an appropriate evaluation and treatment protocol. Bleeding (ruptured) tubal pregnancy with signs of peritoneal irritation may be observed shortly after minisuction of the uterine

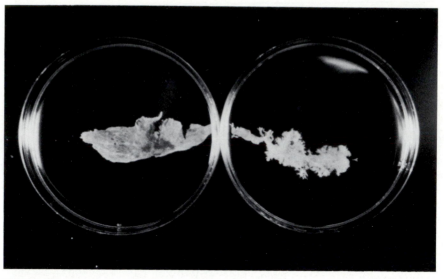

FIG 17–9.
Early pregnancy decidua *(left)* and trophoblastic villi *(right)*.

cavity of patients with unrecognized extrauterine gestation (Rubin et al., 1980). In spite of the obvious presence of villi, all patients should be reexamined several weeks thereafter due to the notoriously high incidence of retained POC or unrecognized continuation of intrauterine pregnancy. Many authorities advise routine pregnancy testing at the postoperative follow-up visit if the soft plastic catheter has been used for miniabortion.

Dilatation and suction evacuation (D&E) is the most frequently used procedure for terminating pregnancy up to 21 or 22 weeks from the LMP (Bowers et al., 1988; Grimes et al., 1977). Dilatation and suction evacuation beyond 15 weeks of pregnancy should be done only by qualified operators who possess a high degree of "touch and feel" aptitude. Another important consideration is the frequency of exposures to late midtrimester D&E that may be unaesthetic and may cause undesirable stress among dedicated staff. The latter problem may be avoided if a labor induction method is routinely available as an alternative.

Almost all of the D&E procedures at our institution (99%) are performed under local anesthesia with the use of chloroprocaine hydrochloride instead of lidocaine. Chloroprocaine hydrochloride has a wider safety margin and longer duration of action than lidocaine when injected into highly vascular tissues. Ideally, all D&Es should be done under local anesthesia if possible because

the procedural blood loss and the incidence of uterine perforation are much less than under general anesthesia. Procedural discomfort is blunted with appropriate IV medications and verbal distraction by a special nurse who has been trained to coach the patient before and during the procedure. This same nurse simultaneously monitors the patient's vital signs and respiration. We use midazolam, a short-acting anxiolytic benzodiazepine drug, not exceeding 2 mg plus fentanyl citrate not exceeding 100 µg for the monitored IV anesthesia, or conscious sedation. In addition, 25 mg of diphenhydramine hydrochloride may be required for its mild anticholinergic effects. Vasoactive agents such as atropine, epinephrine, or other pressor drugs such as vasopressin (Pitressin) are avoided. We believe that the cardiogenic risks of such vasoactive substances outweigh their claimed benefits of reducing blood loss or vagal reaction. In fact, many deaths from legal abortion in the United States are reportedly drug related (Cates and Jordaan, 1979; Centers for Disease Control Epidemiologic Notes and Reports, 1986). Proper training of the operator under direct hands on supervision and gentle manipulation with adequate dexterity will contribute to the uneventful completion of the procedure with minimal blood loss. The patient must fast for at least 7 hours due to delayed GI transit, especially during the late midtrimester. She should not go home by herself after the procedure. Abortion after 12 weeks from the

LMP should be preceded by adequate laminaria pretreatment of the cervix.

Blood typing (ABO and Rh), serum antibody screening, hematocrit value, and platelet count are routinely obtained at our institution before laminaria insertion. In addition, cervical cytology and screening for STD may be indicated in some patients.

At the time of the procedure, an IV line is inserted and secured in place for monitored IV medications. We use the no-touch technique in which only the portion of the instrument that will be in the uterus is kept sterile throughout the procedure. The operator should wear protective eye goggles or eyeglasses and a mask. Bimanual palpation of the uterine cervix and fundus should be performed to ascertain the direction of uterine axis. At this time, the sponges and laminaria tents may be digitally removed. The short-bladed (Moore-Graves) speculum is required for minimizing the angle between the cervical canal and the uterine axis (Fig 17–10). The anterior lip of the cervix is cleansed with an antiseptic solution and then injected with 3 ml of 1% chloroprocaine hydrochloride at the 12 o'clock position using a 22-gauge spinal needle. A single-toothed tenaculum is applied vertically with the inner jaw inside the cervical canal to include the whole thickness of the anterior lip of cervix within the bite. It is important to take a deep enough bite so that the tenaculum will not be inadvertently pulled out and tear through the cervix during the procedure. The rest of the cervix and vaginal fornices are cleansed, and the paracervical tissue is injected with 3 ml of the same anesthetic at 8, 4, 10, and 2 o'clock. The needle tip should reach the depth of only several millimeters within the submucosal (paracervical) tissue at or near the cervicovaginal junction. Preinjection aspiration is advised to avoid inadvertent leakage of the drug into a cervical branch of the uterine vein. The uterine sound should not be inserted into any gravid uterus before the D&E procedure since the risk of perforating the thin and soft uterine wall outweighs any information to be gained. The depth and axis of the uterine cavity change rapidly during the suction evacuation, and they should be gently assessed with a large curet but not with the uterine sound. The direction of the already dilated cervical canal can be assessed with a large cotton swab (a scopette). Should there be a need to forcefully dilate the cervix after removal of laminarias, we prefer dilators with tapered ends such as the Pratt dilator. The optimal diameter of the cannula for uterine evacuation (see Fig 17–10) generally correlates with the gestational age. For example, a

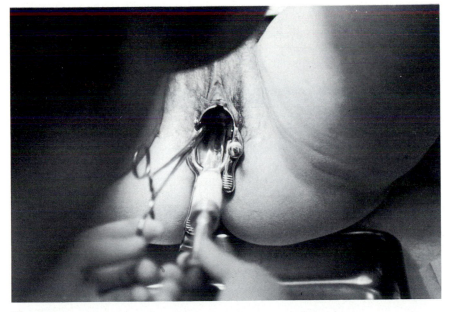

FIG 17–10.
A 16-mm rigid plastic cannula inserted through the cervical canal prior to suction evacuation of midtrimester uterus.

14-mm cannula is required for a complete evacuation of 13 to 15 weeks of pregnancy from the LMP. Five different sizes of rigid, clear plastic cannula with internal diameters of 8, 10, 12, 14, and 16 mm are frequently used in our institution. The ability to insert a large-bore cannula through the laminaria-pretreated cervix greatly facilitates a safe and expedient D&E beyond the first trimester of pregnancy. However, when the uterine size is greater than 16 weeks, most solid products of conception must be extracted with the Sopher forceps (Fig 17–11) because the parts are too large to be aspirated through the cannula. The large-bore cannula is required for the initial aspiration of amniotic fluid and for bringing the products of conception down to the lower uterine segment where the fetal parts can be safely extracted with Sopher forceps. Ideally, the hinge of the Sopher forceps should be at the level of the cervical canal. Note that the cannula must be connected to the hose and vacuum jar through a specially designed handle. This special handle is the key to the D&E technique since it allows the cannula to be rotated 360 degrees around its long axis while the hose remains immobile. The cannula is initially inserted just beyond the internal cervical os and rotated around the same cervicouterine axis while using a vacuum aspirating pressure between 50 and 60 cm Hg. Once the intrauterine volume has been reduced following the complete drainage of amniotic fluid, this cervicouterine axis may change, for example, from midposition to anteflexed or retroflexed. In most instances, the uterine cavity will eventually deviate toward the patient's right-hand side and remain in its resting dextrorotational axis. Whenever in doubt, a gentle exploration of the uterine cavity with a large curet will be required before advancing the cannula slightly deeper (to bring down the parts) and before the use of Sopher forceps. Only the large curet should be used for this exploration. At times, the operator's left hand may be placed on the abdomen to feel the fundus and to apply a suprapubic pressure. If the fetal calvarium cannot be easily brought down to a safe reach of the Sopher forceps, the patient should be given IV oxytocin using our high-dose protocol and the procedure temporarily halted. She can be brought back to the procedure room in 1 or 2 hours when the fetal calvarium is seen or digitally felt at or above the internal cervical os. This second-stage uterine evacuation can be easily and rapidly accomplished without pain or discomfort to the patient. In general, however, we do not administer any uterotonic agent during the D&E until after the fetal calvarium has been obtained for fear of trapping it up high or compressing it into the myometrium (Altman et al., 1985). The D&E procedure is considered complete after important fetal parts are identified and accounted for. Such fetal parts are the calvarium, spine, and tips of extremities. We routinely record the fetal footlength to corroborate the gestational age based on Streeter's data as modified by Moore (1973). The latter correlates well in our patient population. The fetal foot lengths at 10, 12, 14, 16, 18, 20, and 22 weeks from the LMP are 6, 9, 14, 20, 27, 33, and 39 mm, respectively. Induced abortions per-

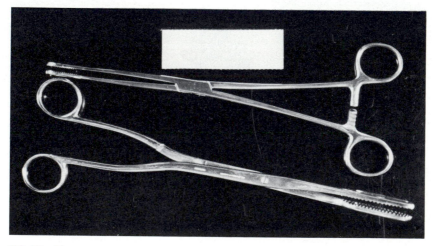

FIG 17–11.
Sopher forceps (with long jaws) compared with ordinary ring forceps.

formed between 8 and 10 weeks from the LMP should also yield a recognizable fetal part. Adding 6.5 to the crown-rump length in centimeters will provide an estimation of the gestational age in weeks during the first trimester.

It should be stressed that no descriptive text or "cookbook" manual on the D&E technique can replace the proper training with hands-on instruction by a skillful physician. At our institution, the resident physicians receive a minimum of 6 weeks of daily D&E training by a small number of experienced attending faculty members (Altman et al., 1985). This adequate training plus our well-defined protocol and dedicated nursing staff have enabled us to incorporate the D&E procedure within our emergency room management of patients with incomplete miscarriage (Brennan and Caldwell, 1987). Such patients safely and expediently undergo D&E under local anesthesia in our specially equipped emergency rooms.

Dilatation and labor induction is our abortion method of choice when the fetal biparietal diameters (BPDs) are between 50 and 55 mm. (The fetal BPD increases at an average of 0.43 mm/day or 3 mm/week.) This technique is also indicated whenever a completely well-preserved and intact fetus is to be obtained at the patient's request, usually for personal or genetic counseling reasons. On the other hand, several hours of effective labor in a patient whose cervix is not satisfactorily well prepared by laminarias may lead to favorable changes in the cervix and lower uterine segment to allow for a safe and easy D&E procedure. Because of our strict and active labor induction protocol, our complication rate is much less than that reported by the Centers for Disease Control (Grimes and Schulz, 1985; Kafrissen et al., 1984). The good record of our labor induction protocol is in contradistinction to the national statistics that showed higher serious complication rates with intra-amniotic prostaglandin. Our complication rate of less than 2% (based on the JPSA criteria) is not higher than that of our "late D&E" and may be attributed to the protocol, which is different from others'. First, the patient must undergo laminaria pretreatment of her cervix 20 hours before receiving any prostaglandin drug. Second, ultrasound imaging (Hornstein et al., 1986) and immediate coagulation screening tests as well as blood products are available on site (Osathanondh et al., 1981). Third, a full-time director of the unit (or his or her designate) will in-

stantly evaluate and, if necessary, perform the late D&E in case of excessive bleeding or prolonged labor. No patient is allowed to labor longer than 24 hours. Fourth, membranes are artificially ruptured after 4 hours of prostaglandin-induced labor. At this time, all amniotic fluid is expressed out with suprapubic pressure, and the cervical effacement is reassessed. If the cervix is still thick and long, intracervical PGE_2 at an appropriate dose will be administered with multiple Lamicel and laminaria tents, to be followed at 3-hour intervals with PGE_2 vaginal suppository treatment. Finally, all of our patients undergo uterine exploration and sharp curettage following delivery of the placenta. Otherwise, the placenta must be removed under local anesthesia within 2 hours of the fetal delivery.

We prefer intra-amnionic instillation of 2 mg of 15-methyl $PGF_{2\alpha}$, followed immediately by 64 ml of 23.4% saline (4 mEq/ml solution) using a three-way connecting tube. This procedure is similar to any diagnostic amniocentesis without the use of preoperative medications. However, a local anesthetic is used for infiltrating the abdominal wall because we use a long (9-cm) and large-bore (18-gauge) needle to demonstrate without doubt a free backflow of clear amniotic fluid before injecting the drugs. Actually, the prostaglandins are inactivated by the normal amniotic fluid. However, our carefully selected pharmacological dose is in excess and will set off an irreversible chain of intrauterine events leading to myometrial contractions within 1 hour of administration. The intra-amnionic injection produces less side effects than the extra-amnionic route. Following artificial rupture of the membranes, pretreatment medications are given at least 30 minutes before the first dose of PGE_2 is administered as described earlier. If the cervical effacement reaches 90%, the high-dose IV oxytocin infusion will be initiated so long as it is not within 2 hours of the last dose of prostaglandin. We do not routinely provide prophylactic antibiotics. However, we use broad-spectrum IV antibiotics liberally such as in undelivered patients after 10 hours of the artificial or spontaneous rupture of the membranes. Antibiotics are also prescribed following excessive procedural blood loss or if a degree of myometrial injury is strongly suspected and when a D&E procedure takes longer than 20 minutes to complete. Some well-controlled trials favor the routine use of a prophylactic antibiotic, but their small study populations limit any conclusive interpretation

(Darj et al., 1988; Park et al., 1985; Sonne-Holmes et al., 1981; Spence et al., 1982). We have arbitrarily defined our high-risk patients who may benefit from a course of antibiotic treatment from the time of laminaria insertion on the day before the D&E or labor induction. Such patients are those with fetal death, placenta previa, habitual abortions, Asherman's syndrome, an IUD, an orthopedic or cardiac prosthesis, trichomonads or koilocytosis on cervical cytology, a history of PID or STD or tubal pregnancy, sickle cell trait or disease, chronic hepatitis, IV drug abuse, tattoo, multiple male partners, and women from a correctional institute. We provide a preoperative prophylaxis against bacterial endocarditis not only for indicated cardiac patients but also for IV drug abusers. In addition, women with a dilated internal os due to incomplete, inevitable, or missed abortion with vaginal bleeding should receive antibiotics for prophylaxis. The spectrum of prescribed antibiotics should cover *Chlamydia trachomatis*. Twelve percent of women who requested legal abortion at our institution in 1986 had this organism, and the significance of this finding is being investigated.

Complications

Complications of induced abortion are reportedly dependent on two main factors: the gestational age (too early or too advanced) and the operator's experience (or inexperience). The recent U.S. National Statistics repeatedly showed that induced abortions performed between 7 and 12 weeks from the LMP were associated with less complications than those performed before or after this gestational age range, regardless of whether the complication rate or severity was looked at (Leads from MMWR, 1988; Ory, 1983). Increased risks of uterine trauma and hemorrhage occur in the D&E procedures performed by the resident when compared with those done by the experienced attending physician (Grimes and Schulz, 1985). Other risk factors include the use of general anesthesia, failure to adequately prepare the cervix with laminarias, parity, history of previous abortion, and the woman's age (Grimes et al., 1979; Ory, 1983; Schulz et al., 1983). With regard to the D&E, the risk of a cervical injury or related trauma is reduced with a history of a prior abortion, the use of laminaria, local anesthesia, and performance by an attending physician (Grimes and Schulz, 1985; Schulz et al., 1983). This risk is increased with age of 17

years or less, the use of general anesthesia, and performance by a physician in training. The risk factors for uterine perforation are similar to those for cervical injury except that multiparous women have three times the risk of nulliparous women (Cates et al., 1983).

Fortunately, two thirds of uterine perforations occur in the fundal region and are not associated with acute or uncontrollable hemorrhage. Obese patients and those with repeated cesarean scars may be at an increased risk of uterine perforation. Prompt recognition of this complication is the key to minimizing the damage. Undetected uterine perforation may lead to devastating generalized peritonitis from bowel injury and fatality. Acute problems associated with uterine perforation include lacerations of the uterine vessels leading to severe hypovolemia or expanding hematoma and injuries to intraperitoneal structures. Such problems dictate prompt laparotomy. A three-way indwelling catheter should be inserted into the urinary bladder prior to the laparotomy. Thus, methylene blue or indigo carmine can be readily injected intravesically should a question of bladder injury arise during this life-saving operation. Bleeding vessels can usually be ligated, in which case the uterine trauma is repaired and hysterectomy is not required. If forceps or suction has been applied intraperitoneally, the entire length of bowel should be inspected for any severe contusion or disruption of its blood supply. In the latter situation, an abdominal surgeon may decide to resect and reanastomose the damaged bowel. Most of the time, however, complete bowel rest with the help of intermittent nasogastric suction and broad-spectrum IV antibiotics will suffice. If the uterine perforation is promptly diagnosed before any intraperitoneal structure is damaged, the D&E procedure may be continued and readily accomplished under laparoscopic visualization. A delayed diagnosis of slowly expanding broad ligament hematoma in a hemodynamically stable patient may require only IV antibiotics and ultrasound imaging at follow-up intervals. A liquefied infected hematoma can be successfully drained under competent ultrasound guidance to abolish the stormy, febrile course and shorten the patient's incapacitation period. We have successfully used selective embolization of a damaged uterine vessel in patients with broad ligament hematoma as well as in patients with pathology-proved focal placenta accreta after adequate uterine packing and IV antibiotic treatment. Such conservative therapies are best preserved for nulliparous patients who fully understand the inherent procedural risks and sign the individualized informed consent form in the chart.

Another type of hemorrhagic complication of induced abortion is coagulopathy. It is not an infrequent problem after a fetal death of long duration with a large uterine size (beyond 13 weeks' gestation) and also after an intra-amnionic injection of a high volume of hypertonic saline. Coagulopathy may also occur in rare cases of otherwise routine D&E beyond 13 weeks since the LMP (Osathanondh et al., 1981; White et al., 1983). We therefore advise that midtrimester abortions be performed near or within a facility where blood products are readily available. Prolonged bleeding from the well-contracting, intact, empty uterus and from the tenaculum site should provoke a high index of suspicion. A tube of blood should be obtained to record the patient's clotting time, which may be prolonged, and any abnormal clot retraction or lysis. At the same time, a profile of blood coagulation tests should be immediately obtained. A severe depletion of platelets and fibrinogen that is disproportionate to the minor decrease in hematocrit value may promptly confirm this diagnosis. In general, coagulopathy in obstetrical hemorrhage is associated with a severe depletion of circulating fibrinogen before the decline of other clotting factors. A significant leakage of the thromboplastic fetal or trophoblastic tissue into the maternal circulation may be responsible for this postulated "consumptive" coagulopathy. It is frequently associated with violent uterine contractions or prolonged intrauterine manipulation in case of D&E for fetal death. Treatment requires infusion of cryoprecipitate and fresh plasma.

Another enigmatic complication of D&E that may occur within hours or several days postoperatively is hematometra. Some authorities call this complication the *postabortal syndrome* or the *redo syndrome* (Sands et al., 1974). It was first reported in 1974 as a unique type of uterine atony with an incidence of one in several hundred D&E cases. This syndrome is characterized by a painful and acutely tender enlargement of the uterus, which is full of dark liquid and clotted blood. The patient usually shows facial signs of general distress with sweating and tachycardia, but vaginal bleeding is not excessive. A repeat suction evacuation of the uterine cavity will promptly abolish

this puzzling phenomenon. Although the cause of this problem is unknown at this time, we prescribe an ergot and antibiotic drug in such cases for prophylaxis.

An acute drug reaction is a possible complication before or during a D&E procedure. If a toxic dose of the local anesthetic is inadvertently injected into the maternal circulation, convulsions, cardiac arrhythmias, and cardiovascular collapse may follow. The treatment consists of establishment and maintenance of an airway by endotracheal intubation with adequate ventilation of the patient. Adequate blood pressure is maintained with IV fluids and an appropriate sympathomimetic agent if necessary. However, this particular complication is preventable. Preinjection aspiration as described earlier must be practiced as a routine habit during the induction of paracervical anesthesia. The D&E should not be commenced within 3 minutes of paracervical anesthetic injections. Use of chloroprocaine hydrochloride and avoidance of epinephrine (or other pressor substances) in the highly vascular gravid tissues are also observed in our protocol. Premedication with 2 mg of IV midazolam may prevent a rare syndrome of chest wall stiffness caused by IV injection of an opioid such as fentanyl citrate. High doses of the latter drug may lead to a dose-related respiratory depression. An effective antidote is 0.4 mg of naloxone hydrochloride given intravenously.

A rare and unique respiratory embarrassment may occur during midtrimester D&E, especially with fetal death of long duration. It is characterized by signs of respiratory hypersecretion, coughing, and if not promptly corrected, bronchospasm. This syndrome is not related to an amniotic fluid embolism because it is self-limited and often occurs in cases of severe oligohydramnios or in "dry" fetal death. It is unlike a vasovagal reaction because of the presence of tachycardia and borderline elevation of blood pressure. It has been observed in association with violent uterine contractions, producing features analogous to inadvertent IV infusion of $PGF_{2\alpha}$. A similar problem has been described by Kohorn in collaboration with our group at the New England Trophoblastic Disease Center in 1978 as "trophoblastic embolization syndrome" following molar evacuation. The D&E procedure should be temporarily halted and the patient should be turned to her side. Intravenous diphenhydramine (25 mg) is slowly administered to reduce the secretion. Epinephrine should not be used for this type of bronchospasm because the patient's blood pressure may become too highly elevated (Silva et al., 1987), and epinephrine may produce an adverse cardiac effect in this situation. Bronchospasm in such cases is better relieved with an IV glucocorticoid such as 4 mg of dexamethasone than with the use of aminophylline, which is slow acting and produces tachycardia. With assurance and improved ventilation and respiration, the D&E procedure can proceed and be safely accomplished. On the other hand, amniotic fluid embolism can also occur during midtrimester abortion in rare cases following instrumental disruption of the placenta with a large volume of amniotic fluid in the uterine cavity or following abruptio placentae in cases of labor induction. It is usually associated with obvious signs of cardiopulmonary collapse and disseminated intravascular coagulation. Prompt arterial blood gas measurement, electrocardiogram, and ventilation-perfusion radionuclide scan will confirm the diagnosis. Effective resuscitation and successful management will require around the clock cardiopulmonary and hematological care by a team of a competent internist, gynecologist, anesthesiologist, hematologist or blood bank specialist, nurses, and laboratory personnel in a well-equipped intensive care facility. The uterus must be emptied as soon as the patient's cardiovascular status has been reasonably stabilized.

Delayed complications of induced abortion include different degrees of postabortal infection (Burkman et al., 1977) from endoparametritis to pelvic septic thrombophlebitis and thromboembolic events. Infection is usually associated with retained products of conception. Common symptoms are crampy pain with prolonged vaginal bleeding and low-grade fever. The uterus is tender, slightly enlarged, and "boggy." High-resolution ultrasound imaging with full bladder may confirm or exclude the diagnosis of retained products of conception. Treatment consists of IV antibiotics, an ergot alkaloid, and repeated uterine evacuation if indicated. Patients with a retained pregnancy or retained pregnancy products not infrequently have an unrecognized positional, anatomical, or congenital uterine anomaly. Such patients should undergo D&E under ultrasound guidance (Hornstein et al., 1986). The latter technique has also been useful in midtrimester D&E with known anatomical derangements and in patients with cervical stenosis.

Controversies exist as to the possibility of late sequelae of repetitive induced abortions with regard to premature delivery and low birth weight (Hogue et al., 1982). Most statistics have been derived from patients who have undergone primitive abortion techniques. Increasing experience and opportunities for proper training of physicians in the modern techniques of induced abortion may curtail those problems. One late sequele that is theoretically possible is Rh isoimmune disease (Litvak et al., 1970). A fail-safe mechanism can be devised in the quality assurance program using the nurse, physician, and patient education to ensure that Rh-negative patients will automatically receive adequate doses of Rh immune globulin for prophylaxis within 72 hours of induced abortion or miscarriage.

Selective Reduction of Multifetal Pregnancy

Successful in vitro fertilization, gamete intrafallopian transfer, and aggressive pharmacotherapy of infertility have led to an increase in a gestation with three or more fetuses. With a large number of fetuses in one gestation, each fetus is at a significantly increased risk of premature birth and its serious sequelae. The procedures to reduce multiple fetuses to only two (twins) have been performed with increasing experience and efficacy using ultrasound guidance. Early methods involved transcervical selective evacuation, transabdominal injection of air or hypertonic saline, needle disruption of a selected conceptus, and selective fetal exsanguination (Farquharson et al., 1987). Currently, the most popular method is an ultrasound-guided transabdominal injection of potassium chloride 2 or 3 mmole/embryo and in some cases 7 mmole/embryo at the end of the first trimester. Selective reduction procedures have also been performed in the second trimester for termination of a defective twin. The patient must be informed of known and unknown risks of losing some or all fetuses. Such risks have been described with and without undergoing the selective reduction procedure. The risks vary at different gestational ages and increase with an advanced maternal age. These risks include the syndrome of vanishing twins, trapped twins, twin-to-twin transfusion, and fetal disseminated intravascular coagulation. Dr. Richard L. Berkowitz, a respected investigator whose department probably holds the largest careful experience in this endeavor, has described possible, procedure-related, complications in a two-page informed consent form. Such complications include bleeding, infection, leakage of amniotic fluid, the need for repeating the procedure, risk of having to undergo D&E, or hysterectomy. Any infertile woman who has taken the risks of infertility treatment may be willing to take any known or unknown risks from the selective reduction of her multifetal pregnancy. With triplets, however, the risk/benefit ratio of undergoing a selective reduction procedure is unclear, especially at tertiary care maternity centers where triplets appear to do as well medically (physically) as twins do after birth. In this situation, the individual couple may take into account the quality of the offspring's life and perhaps the cost of upbringing. Thus, complex ethical and legal ramifications of the selective reduction procedure remain for further debates.

REFERENCES

Altman AM, Stubblefield PG, Schlam J, et al: Midtrimester abortion by laminaria and vacuum evacuation on a teaching service. *J Reprod Med* 1985; 30:601–606.

American College of Obstetricians and Gynecologists Committee on Obstetrics: Postpartum tubal sterilization: *Appropriate Timing of Surgery After Vaginal Delivery.* Committee Opinion no 50, 1987. Chicago, ACOG.

Amir M: *Patterns in Forcible Rape.* Chicago, University of Chicago Press, 1971.

Anderson ABM, Turnbull AC: Changes in amniotic fluid, serum and urine following the intra-amniotic injection of hypertonic saline. *Acta Obstet Gynecol Scand* 1968; 47:1–21.

Anonymous: Drug interaction with oral contraceptive steroids [editorial]. *Br Med J (Clin Res)* 1980; 281:93–94.

Anonymous: Gossypol prospects [editorial]. *Lancet* 1984; 1:1108–1109.

Arntzenius AC, van Gent CM, van der Voort H, et al: Reduced high-density lipoprotein in women aged 40–41 using oral contraceptives. *Lancet* 1978; 1:1221–1223.

Baulieu EE, Segal SJ (eds): *The Antiprogestin Steroid RU 486 and Human Fertility Control.* New York, Plenum, 1985.

Beaumont V, Lemort N, Beaumont JL: Evaluation of risk factors associated with vascular thrombosis in women on oral contraceptives. Possible role of anti-sex steroid hormone antibodies. *Artery* 1983; 11:331–344.

Bergink EW, Hamburger AD, de Jager E, et al: Binding of a contraceptive progestogen Org

2969 and its metabolites to receptor proteins and human sex hormone binding globulin. *J Steroid Biochem* 1981; 14:175–183.

Berkowitz GS, Kelsey JL, LiVolsi VA, et al: Oral contraceptive use and fibrocystic breast disease among pre- and postmenopausal women. *Am J Epidemiol* 1984; 120:87–96.

Black MM, Barclay THG, Polednak A, et al: Family history, oral contraceptive usage, and breast cancer. *Cancer* 1983; 51:2147–2151.

Blumenthal PD: Prospective comparison of dilapan and laminaria for pretreatment of the cervix in second-trimester induction abortion. *Obstet Gynecol* 1988; 72:243–246.

Bowers C, Devine PA, Chervenak FA: Dilation and evacuation during the second trimester of pregnancy in a woman with primary pulmonary hypertension. *J Reprod Med* 1988; 33:787–788.

Bradley DD, Wingerd J, Petitti DB, et al: Serum high density lipoprotein cholesterol in women using oral contraceptives, estrogens, and progestins. *N Engl J Med* 1978; 199:17–20.

Brennan DM, Caldwell M: Dilatation and evacuation performed in the emergency department for miscarriage. *J Emerg Nurs* 1987; 13:144–148.

Brenner PF: Oral combination contraceptives, in Bardin CW (ed): *Current Therapy in Endocrinology and Metabolism,* ed 3. Toronto, BC Decker, 1988, pp 195–198.

Brooks PG: The relationship of estrogen and progesterone to breast disease. *J Reprod Med* 1984; 29:530–538.

Bruce SL, Paul RH, Van Dorsten JP: Control of postpartum uterine atony by intramyometrial prostaglandin. *Obstet Gynecol* 1982; 59:47s–50s.

Burkman RT: Lipid and lipoprotein changes in relation to oral contraception and hormonal replacement therapy. *Fertil Steril* 1988; 49:(suppl):39S–50S.

Burkman RT, Atienza MF, King TM: Culture and treatment results in endometritis following elective abortion. *Am J Obstet Gynecol* 1977; 128:556–559.

Burkman RT, Atienza M, King TM, et al: Intra-amniotic urea as a midtrimester abortifacient: Clinical results and serum and urinary changes. *Am J Obstet Gynecol* 1975; 121:7–16.

Burkman RT and the Women's Health Study: Association between intrauterine device and pelvic inflammatory disease. *Obstet Gynecol* 1981; 57:269–276.

Cabrol D, D'Yvoire MB, Mermet E, et al: Induction of labor with mifespristone after intrauterine fetal death. *Lancet* 1985; 2:1019.

Caillouette JC, Koehler AL: Phasic contraceptive

pills and functional ovarian cysts. *Am J Obstet Gynecol* 1987; 156:1538–1542.

Cameron IT, Baird DT: Early pregnancy termination: A comparison between vacuum aspiration and medical abortion using prostaglandin (16,16 dimethyl-trans-δ_2-PGE$_1$ methyl ester) or the antiprogestogen RU486. *Br J Obstet Gynaecol* 1988; 95:271–276.

Campbell WB: Vasectomy and arterial disease. *J R Soc Med* 1988; 81:682–695.

Cancer and Steroid Hormone Study of the Centers for Disease Control and the National Institute of Child Health and Human Development: Oral contraceptive use and the risk of breast cancer. *N Engl J Med* 1986; 315:405–411.

Cancer and Steroid Hormone Study of the Centers for Disease Control and the National Institute of Child Health and Human Development: Combination oral contraceptive use and the risk of endometrial cancer. *JAMA* 1987a; 257:796–800.

Cancer and Steroid Hormone Study of the Centers for Disease Control and the National Institute of Child Health and Human Development: The reduction in risk of ovarian cancer associated with oral contraceptive use. *N Engl J Med* 1987b; 316:650–655.

Carp HJ, Oelsner G, Serr DM, et al: Fertility after nonsurgical treatment of ectopic pregnancy. *J Reprod Med* 1986; 31:119–122.

Cates W Jr, Jordaan HVF: Sudden collapse and death of women obtaining abortions induced with prostaglandin F$_{2\alpha}$. *Am J Obstet Gynecol* 1979; 133:398–400.

Cates W Jr, Schulz KF, Grimes DA: The risks associated with teenage abortion. *N Engl J Med* 1983; 309:621–624.

Cates W Jr, Blackmore CA: Sexual assault and sexually transmitted disease, in Holmes KK, Mårdh P-A, Sparling PF, et al (eds): *Sexually Transmitted Diseases*. New York, McGraw-Hill Book Co, 1984, pp 119–125.

Cederqvist LL, Birnbaum SJ: Rupture of the uterus after midtrimester prostaglandin abortion. *J Reprod Med* 1980; 25:136–138.

Centers for Disease Control Cancer and Steroid Hormone Study: Long term oral contraceptive use and the risk of breast cancer. *JAMA* 1983a; 249:1591–1595.

Centers for Disease Control Cancer and Steroid Hormone Study: Oral contraceptive use and the risk of ovarian cancer. *JAMA* 1983b; 249:1596–1599.

Centers for Disease Control Cancer and Steroid Hormone Study: Oral contraceptive use and the risk of endometrial cancer. *JAMA* 1983c; 249:1600–1604.

Centers for Disease Control Epidemiologic Notes and Reports: Maternal deaths associated with barbiturate anesthetics—New York City. *MMWR* 1986; 35:579–587.

Chervenak FA, Farley MA, Walters L, et al: When is termination of pregnancy during the third trimester morally justifiable? *N Engl J Med* 1984; 310:501–504.

Clarke EA, Hatcher J, McKeown-Eyssen GE, et al: Cervical dysplasia: Association with sexual behavior, smoking, and oral contraceptive use? *Am J Obstet Gynecol* 1985; 151:612–616.

Connell EB: Oral contraceptives. The current risk-benefit ratio. *J Reprod Med* 1984; 29:513–523.

Cook CL, Lance JW, Kraft SL: Pregnancy prophylaxis: Parenteral postcoital estrogen. *Obstet Gynecol* 1986; 67:331–333.

Craft I, Foss GL, Warren RJ, et al: Effect of norgestrel administered intermittently on pituitary ovarian function. *Contraception* 1975; 12:589–598.

Cramer DW: Infertility in relation to the use of intrauterine devices. *Infect Dis Letters Obstet Gynecol*, 1989; 11:59–62.

Cramer DW, Goldman MB, Schiff I, et al: The relationship of tubal infertility to barrier method and oral contraceptive use. *JAMA* 1987; 257:2446–2450.

Cramer DW, Hutchinson GB, Welch WR, et al: Factors affecting the association of oral contraceptives and ovarian cancer. *N Engl J Med* 1982; 307:1047–1051.

Cramer DW, Schiff I, Schoenbaum SC, et al: Tubal infertility and intrauterine device. *N Engl J Med* 1985; 312:941–947.

Crooij MJ, de Nooyer CCA, Rao BR, et al: Termination of early pregnancy by the 3β-hydroxysteroid dehydrogenase inhibitor epostane. *N Engl J Med* 1988; 319:813–817.

Croxatto HB, Diaz S, Fuentealba B, et al: Studies on the duration of egg transport in the human oviduct: I. The time interval between ovulation and egg recovery from the uterus in normal women. *Fertil Steril* 1972; 23:447–458.

Daling JR, Weiss NS, Metch BJ, et al: Primary tubal infertility in relation to the use of an intrauterine device. *N Engl J Med* 1985; 312:937–941.

Darj E, Stralin EB, Nilsson S: The prophylactic effect of doxycycline on postoperative infection rate after first-trimester abortion. *Obstet Gynecol* 1988; 70:755–758.

Darney PD: Long-acting hormonal contraception. *Contemp Obstet Gynecol* 1988; 32:90–100.

Darney PD, Dorward K: Cervical dilation before

first-trimester elective abortion: a controlled comparison of meteneprost, laminaria, and hypan. *Obstet Gynecol* 1987; 70:397–400.

Dattel BJ, Landers DV, Coulter K, et al: Isolation of *Chlamydia trachomatis* from sexually abused female adolescents. *Obstet Gynecol* 1988; 72:240–242.

del Junco DJ, Annegers JF, Luthra HS: Do oral contraceptives prevent rheumatoid arthritis? *JAMA* 1985; 254:1938–1941.

Dericks-Tan JSE, Kock P, Taubert HD: Synthesis and release of gonadotropins: Effect of an oral contraceptive. *Obstet Gynecol* 1983; 62:687–690.

DeStefano F, Greenspan JR, Dicker RC, et al: Complications of interval laparoscopic tubal sterilization. *Obstet Gynecol* 1983; 61:153–158.

Diamond MP, Wentz AC, Cherrington AD: Alterations in carbohydrate metabolism as they apply to reproductive endocrinology. *Fertil Steril* 1988; 50:387–397.

Diaz S, Croxatto HB, Pavez M, et al: Ectopic pregnancies associated with low dose progestagen-releasing IUDs. *Contraception* 1980; 22:259.

Dingfelder JR, Black J, Brenner WE, et al: Intra-amniotic administration of 15(S)-15-methyl-prostaglandin $F_{2\alpha}$ for the induction of midtrimester abortion. *Am J Obstet Gynecol* 1976; 125:821–826.

Dixon GW, Schlesselman JJ, Ory HW, et al: Ethinyl estradiol and conjugated estrogens as postcoital contraceptives. *JAMA* 1980; 244:1336.

Duguid HLD, Parratt D, Traynor R: Actinomyces-like organisms in cervical smears from women using intrauterine contraceptive devices. *Br Med J (Clin Res)* 1980; 281:534–537.

Eaton CJ, Cohn F, Bollinger CC: Laminaria tent as a cervical dilator prior to aspiration type therapeutic abortion. *Obstet Gynecol* 1972; 39:533–536.

Elger W, Fahnrich M, Beier S, et al: Endometrial and myometrial effect of progesterone antagonists in pregnant guinea pigs. *Am J Obstet Gynecol* 1987; 157:1065–1074.

Ellis JW: Multiphasic oral contraceptives—efficacy and metabolic impact. *J Reprod Med* 1987; 32:28–36.

Engel HJ, Enge E, Lichtlen PR: Coronary atherosclerosis and myocardial infarction in young women—role of oral contraceptives. *Eur Heart J* 1983; 4:1–8.

Eyong E, Buchi K, Elstein M: Effects of 180 µg and 250 µg norgestimate on pituitary-ovarian function and cervical mucus. *Fertil Steril* 1988; 50:756–760.

Faich G, Pearson K, Fleming D, et al: Toxic shock syndrome and vaginal contraceptive sponge. *JAMA* 1986; 255:216–218.

Farabow WS, Fulton JW, Fletcher V Jr: Cervical pregnancy treated with methotrexate. *NC Med J* 1983; 44:91.

Farquharson D, Wittman B, Hansmann M, et al: Management of quintuplet pregnancy by selective embryocide. Paper presented at the 32nd Annual Convention of the American Institute of Ultrasound in Medicine, New Orleans, October 1987.

Fihn SD, Latham RH, Roberts P, et al: Association between diaphragm use and urinary tract infection. *JAMA* 1985; 254:240–245.

Franceschi S, LaVecchia C, Parazzini F, et al: Oral contraceptives and benign breast disease: A case-control study. *Am J Obstet Gynecol* 1984; 149:602–606.

Freie HMP: Sickle cell diseases and hormonal contraception. *Acta Obstet Gynecol Scand* 1983; 62:211–217.

Frigoletto FD, Pokoly TB: Electrolyte dynamics in hypertonic saline-induced abortions. *Obstet Gynecol* 1971; 38:647–652.

Fruzzetti F, Melis GB, Strigini F, et al: Use of sulprostone for induction of preoperative cervical dilation or uterine evacuation: A comparison among the effect of different treatment schedules. *Obstet Gynecol* 1988; 72:704–708.

Frydmann R, Taylor S, Ulmann A: Transplacental passage of mifespristone. *Lancet* 1985; 2:1252.

Fylling P, Fagerhol M: Experience with two different medicated intrauterine devices: A comparative study of the Progestasert and Nova-T. *Fertil Steril* 1979; 31:138–141.

Garzo VG, Liu J, Ulmann A, et al: Effects of an antiprogesterone (RU486) on the hypothalamic-hypophyseal-ovarian-endometrial axis during the luteal phase of the menstrual cycle. *J Clin Endocrinol Metab* 1988; 66:508–517.

Gaspard UJ: Metabolic effects of oral contraceptives. *Am J Obstet Gynecol* 1987; 157:1029–1041.

Ginsburg KA, Moghissi KS: Alternate delivery systems for contraceptive progestogens. *Fertil Steril* 1988; 49(suppl):16S–30S.

Goldacre MJ, Holford TR, Vessey MP: Cardiovascular disease and vasectomy. *N Engl J Med* 1983; 308:805–808.

Goldsmith MF: Pregnancy Dx? Rx may now include condoms. *JAMA* 1989; 261:678–679.

Goldzieher JW: Hormonal contraceptives, past,

present, future. *Horm Contracept* 1984; 75:75–86.

Goldzieher JW, Moses LE, Averkin E, et al: A placebo controlled double blind crossover investigation of the side effects attributed to oral contraceptives. *Fertil Steril* 1971; 22:609–623.

Goodlin RC, Kresch AD: Amniotic fluid osmolality following intra-amniotic injection of saline. *Am J Obstet Gynecol* 1968; 100:839–842.

Gordon T, Castelli WP, Njortland M: HDL as a protective factor against corony heart disease—the Framingham study. *Am J Med* 1977; 62:707–714.

Gore BZ, Caldwell BV, Speroff L: Estrogen-induced human luteolysis. *J Clin Endocrinol Metab* 1973; 36:615.

Gravanis A, Schaison G, George M, et al: Endometrial and pituitary responses to the steroidal antiprogestin RU486 in postmenopausal women. *J Clin Endocrinol Metab* 1985; 60:156–163.

Grimes DA, Mishell DR, Sharpe D, et al: Early abortion with a single dose of the antiprogestin RU-486. *Am J Obstet Gynecol* 1988; 158:1307–1312.

Grimes DA, Schulz KF: Morbidity and mortality from second-trimester abortions. *J Reprod Med* 1985; 30:505–514.

Grimes DA, Schulz KF, Cates W Jr, et al: Mid-trimester abortion by dilatation and evacuation: a safe and practical alternative. *N Engl J Med* 1977; 296:1131–1145.

Grimes DA, Schulz KF, Cates W Jr, et al: Local vs. general anesthesia: Which is safer for performing suction curettage abortions? *Am J Obstet Gynecol* 1979; 135:1030–1035.

Gupta PK, Woodruff JD: Actinomyces in vaginal smears. *JAMA* 1982; 247:1175–1176.

Hahn DW, Allen GE, McGuire J: The pharmacological profile of Norgestimate, a new orally active progestin. *Contraception* 1977; 16:541–553.

Halbert DR, Darnell-Jones DE: Medical management of the sexually assaulted woman. *J Reprod Med* 1978; 20:265–274.

Hale RW, Pion RJ: Laminaria: An underutilized clinical adjunct. *Clin Obstet Gynecol* 1972; 15:829–850.

Hankins GD, Berrymay GK, Scott RT Jr, et al: Maternal arterial desaturation with 15-methyl prostaglandin F_2 alpha for uterine atony. *Obstet Gynecol* 1988; 72:367–370.

Harlap S, Shiono PH, Ramcharan S: Congenital abnormalities in the offspring of women who used oral and other contraceptives around the time of conception. *Int J Fertil* 1985; 30:39–47.

Harrison DD, Cooke CW: An elucidation of factors influencing physicians' willingness to perform elective female sterilization. *Obstet Gynecol* 1988; 72:570.

Hasson HM: Open laparoscopy, in Zatuchni GI, Daly MJ, Sciarra JJ (eds): *Gynecology and Obstetrics*. Philadelphia, Harper & Row, Publishers, 1982, vol 6, Chapter 44, pp 1–8.

Hennekens CH, Speizer FE, Lipnick RJ, et al: A case-control study of oral contraceptive use and breast cancer. *J Natl Cancer Inst* 1984; 72:39–42.

Henry A, Rinehart W, Piotrow P: Reversing female sterilization. *Popul Rep Ser G* 1980; C8:97–123.

Hicks DJ: Rape: Sexual assault. *Am J Obstet Gynecol* 1980; 137:931–935.

Hirsh MP, Levy HM: The varied ultrasonographic appearance of laminaria. *J Ultrasound Med* 1988; 7:45–47.

Hogue CJR, Cates W Jr, Tietze C: The effects of induced abortion on subsequent reproduction. *Epidemiol Rev* 1982; 4:66–94.

Hong CY, Turner P: Influence of lipid solubility on the sperm immobilizing effect of β-adrenoceptor blocking drugs. *Br J Clin Pharmacol* 1982; 14:269–272.

Hornstein MD, Osathanondh R, Birnholz JC, et al: Ultrasound guidance for selected dilatation and evacuation procedures. *J Reprod Med* 1986; 31:947–950.

Hseih CC, Crosson AW, Walker AM, et al: Oral contraceptive use and fibrocystic breast disease of different histologic classifications. *J Natl Cancer Inst* 1984; 72:285–290.

Hulka BS, Chambless LE, Kaufman DG: Protection against endometrial carcinoma by combination-product oral contraceptives. *JAMA* 1982; 247:475–477.

Ingvardsen A, Eriksen T: Cervical rupture following prostaglandin-induced mid-trimester abortion. *Ugeskr Laeger* 1979; 141:3531–3532.

Irwin KL, Rosero-Bixby L, Oberle MW, et al: Oral contraceptives and cervical cancer risk in Costa Rica. *JAMA* 1988; 259:59–64.

Janerick DT, Polednak AP, Glebatis DM, et al: Breast cancer and oral contraceptive use: A case-control study. *J Chronic Dis* 1983; 36:639–646.

Jick H, Westerholm E, Vessey MP, et al: Venous thromboembolic disease and ABO blood type. *Lancet* 1969; 1:539–542.

Johansson EDB: Inhibition of the corpus luteum function in women taking large doses of diethylstilbestrol. *Contraception* 1973; 8:27–35.

Kafrissen ME, Schulz KF, Grimes DA, et al:

Midtrimester abortion. Intra-amniotic instillation of hyperosmolar urea and prostaglandin $F_{2\alpha}$ v. dilatation and evacuation. *JAMA* 1984; 251:916–919.

Kalache A, McPherson K, Barltrop K, et al: Oral contraceptives and breast cancer. *Br J Hosp Med* 1983; 30:278–283.

Karim SMM, Sivasamboo R: Termination of second trimester pregnancy with intra-amniotic 15(S)-15-methyl prostaglandin $F_{2\alpha}$—A two dose schedule study. *Prostaglandins* 1975; 9:487–494.

Kasdorf G, Kalkhoff RK: Prospective studies of insulin sensitivity in normal women receiving oral contraceptive agents. *J Clin Endocrinol Metab* 1988; 66:846–852.

Katz Z, Lancet M, Skornik J, et al: Teratogenicity of progestogens given during the first trimester of pregnancy. *Obstet Gynecol* 1985; 65:775–780.

Kaufman DW, Shapiro S, Slone D, et al: Decreased risk of endometrial cancer among oral contraceptive users. *Med Intellig* 1980; 303:1045–1047.

Kay CR: Progestogens and arterial disease—evidence from the Royal College of General Practitioner's study. *Am J Obstet Gynecol* 1982; 142:762–766.

Kelaghan J, Rubin GL, Ory HW, et al: Barrier method contraceptives and pelvic inflammatory disease. *JAMA* 1982; 248:184–187.

Kelly RW, Abel MH: Copper and zinc inhibit the metabolism of prostaglandin by the human uterus. *Biol Reprod* 1983; 28:883–983.

Kesseru E, Garmendia F, Westphal N, et al: The hormonal and peripheral effects of d-norgestrel in postcoital contraception. *Contraception* 1974; 10:411–424.

Koch JP: The Prentiff contraceptive cervical cap: A contemporary study of its clinical safety and effectiveness. *Contraception* 1982; 25:135–159.

Kohorn EI, McGinn RC, Gee JBL, et al: Pulmonary embolization of trophoblastic tissue in molar pregnancy. *Obstet Gynecol* 1978; 51:16s–20s.

Kubba AA, White JO, Guillebaud J, et al: The biochemistry of human endometrium after two regimens of postcoital contraception: A dl-norgestrel/ethinylestradiol combination or danazol. *Fertil Steril* 1986; 45:512–516.

Lahteenmaki P, Rapeli T, Kaariainen M, et al: Late postcoital treatment against pregnancy with antiprogesterone RU486. *Fertil Steril* 1988; 50:36–38.

Lammer EJ, Cordero JF: Exogenous sex hormone exposure and the risk for major malformations. *JAMA* 1986; 255:3128–3132.

Lawson JS, Yuliano SE, Pasquale SA, et al: Optimum dosage of an oral contraceptive. *Am J Obstet Gynecol* 1979; 134:315–320.

Leads from the MMWR (Centers for Disease Control, Atlanta): Oral contraceptive use and the risk of breast cancer in young women. *JAMA* 1984; 252:326–327.

Leads from the MMWR (Centers for Disease Control, Atlanta): Abortion surveillance: Preliminary analysis—United States, 1984, 1985. *JAMA* 1988; 260:3410–3412.

Lee NC, Rubin GL, Borucki R: The intrauterine device and pelvic inflammatory disease revisited: New results from the women's health study. *Obstet Gynecol* 1988; 72:1–6.

Levin AA, Schoenbaum SC, Monson RR, et al: Association of induced abortion with subsequent pregnancy loss. *JAMA* 1980; 243:2495–2499.

Lewis JH, Tice HL, Zimmerman HJ: Budd-Chiari syndrome associated with oral contraceptive steroids. *Dig Dis Sci* 1983; 28:673–683.

Lincoln R: The pill, breast and cervical cancer, and the role of progestogens in arterial disease. *Fam Plann Perspect* 1984; 16:55–63.

Linn S, Schoenbaum SC, Monson RR, et al: The relationship between induced abortion and outcome of subsequent pregnancies. *Am J Obstet Gynecol* 1983a; 146:135–140.

Linn S, Schoenbaum SC, Monson RR, et al: Lack of association between contraceptive usage and congenital malformation in offspring. *Am J Obstet Gynecol* 1983b; 147:923–928.

Linos A, Worthington JW, O'Fallon WM, et al: Case control study of rheumatoid arthritis and prior use of oral contraceptives. *Lancet* 1983; 1:1299–1300.

Lipnick RJ, Buring JE, Hennekens CH, et al: Oral contraceptives and breast cancer. *JAMA* 1986; 255:58–61.

Lippes J, Malik T, Tatum HJ: The post coital copper T. Paper presented at the 13th Annual Meeting of the Association of Planned Parenthood Physicians, Los Angeles, April 17, 1975.

Liskin L: IUDs: An appropriate contraceptive for many women. *Popul Rep Ser G* 1982; 10(B4):101–135.

Liskin L, Rinehart W: Minilaparotomy and laparoscopy: Safe, effective and widely used. *Popul Rep Ser G* 1985; C8:125–167.

Liskin LS: Long-acting progestins-promise and prospects, injectables and implants. *Popul Rep Ser G* 1983a; K11:17–55.

Liskin LS: Vasectomy—safe and simple. *Popul Rep Ser G* 1983b; D11:61–100.

Liskin LS, Blackburn R: Hormonal contraception: New long-acting methods, injectables and implants. *Popul Rep Ser G* 1987; 15:K57–K87.

Litvak O, Taswell HF, Banner EA, et al: Fetal erythrocytes in maternal circulation after spontaneous abortion. *JAMA* 1970; 214:531–534.

Longman SM, Buehring GC: Oral contraceptives and breast cancer: in vitro. Effect of contraceptive steroids on human mammary cell growth. *Cancer* 1987; 59:281–287.

Louik C, Mitchell AA, Werler MM, et al: Maternal exposure to spermicides in relation to certain birth defects. *N Engl J Med* 1987; 317:474–478.

Louv WC, Austin H, Perlman J, et al: Oral contraceptive use and the risk of chlamydial and gonococcal infections. *Am J Obstet Gynecol* 1989; 160:396–402.

Mall-Haefeli M, Werner-Zodrow I, Hubur P, et al: Klinische und biochemische Resultate bei de Behandlung mit Marvelon-einem neuen steroidalen Ovulationishemmer. *Geburtshilfe Frauenheilkd* 1982; 42:215–222.

Mammen EF: Oral contraceptives and blood coagulation: A critical review. *Am J Obstet Gynecol* 1982; 142:781–790.

Mann JI, Inman WGW: Oral contraceptives and death from myocardial infarction. *Br Med J (Clin Res)* 1975; 2:245–248.

Massey FJ, Bernstein GS, O'Fallon WM, et al: Vasectomy and health: Results from a large cohort study. *JAMA* 1984; 252:1023–1029.

Mattson RH, Cramer JA, Darney PD, et al: Use of oral contraceptives by women with epilepsy. *JAMA* 1986; 256:238–240.

McCann MR, Liskin LS, Piotrow PT, et al: Breast-feeding, fertility and family planning. *Popul Rep Ser G* 1981; J24:525–575.

McPherson K, Neil A, Vessey MP, et al: Breast cancer and oestrogen content of oral contraceptives. *Lancet* 1984; 1:223.

McPherson K, Vessey MP, Neil A, et al: Early oral contraceptive use and breast cancer: Results of another case-control study. *Br J Cancer* 1987; 56:653–660.

Meade TW, Greenberg G, Thompson SG: progestogens and cardiovascular reactions associated with oral contraceptives and a comparison of the safety of 50 and 30 mcg oestrogen preparations. *Br Med J* 1980; 1:1157–1161.

Meirik O, Lund E, Adami H-O, et al: Oral contraceptive use and breast cancer in young women: A joint national case-control study in Sweden and Norway. *Lancet* 1986; 2:650–653.

Mishell DR Jr: Contraception by intrauterine device. Bardin CW (ed): *Current Therapy in Endocrinology and Metabolism,* ed 3. Toronto, BC Decker, 1988a, pp 199–202.

Mishell DR Jr: Use of oral contraceptives in women of older reproductive age. *Am J Obstet Gynecol* 1988b; 158:1652–1657.

Mishell DR Jr, Bell JH, Good RG, et al: The intrauterine device: A bacteriologic study of the endometrial cavity. *Am J Obstet Gynecol* 1966; 96:119–126.

Monk JP, Clissold SP: Misoprostol, a preliminary review of its pharmacodynamic and pharmacokinetic properties and therapeutic efficacy in the treatment of peptic ulcer disease. *Drugs* 1987; 33:1–30.

Moore KL: The developing human: Clinically oriented embryology, in *The Fetal Period: The Eighth Week to Birth.* Philadelphia, WB Saunders Co, 1973, p 78.

Morris JM, van Wagenen G: Compounds interfering with ovum implantation and development: III. The role of estrogens. *Am J Obstet Gynecol* 1966; 96:804–815.

Morris JM, van Wagenen G: Post-coital oral contraception, in Hankinson RKB, Kleinman RL, Eckstein P, et al (eds): *Proceedings of the Eighth International Conference of the International Planned Parenthood Federation, Santiago, Chile, April 9–15, 1967.* London, International Planned Parenthood Federation, 1967, pp 256–259.

Morris JM, van Wagenen G: Interception: The use of postovulatory estrogens to prevent implantation. *Am J Obstet Gynecol* 1973; 115:101–106.

Nadelson CC, Notman MT, Zackson H, et al: A follow-up study of rape victims. *Am J Psychiatry* 1982; 139:1266–1270.

Neil JR, Hammond GT, Nobel AD, et al: Late complications of sterilization by laparoscopy and tubal ligation: A controlled study. *Lancet* 1975; 2:669–671.

Newton BW: Laminaria tent: Relic of the past or modern medical device? *Am J Obstet Gynecol* 1972; 113:442–448.

Newton JR (ed): Contraception update. *Clin Obstet Gynecol* 1984; 11:551–819.

Nilsson CG, Luukkainen T, Diaz J, et al: Intrauterine contraception with levonorgestrel: A comparative randomised clinical performance study. *Lancet* 1981; 1:577–580.

Noonan JT Jr: *Contraception, a History of its Treatment by the Catholic Theologians and Canonists.* Cambridge, Mass, Harvard University Press, 1986.

Orme ML, Back DS, Breckenridge AM: Clinical pharmacokinetics of oral contraceptive steroids. *Clin Pharm* 1983; 8:95–136.

Ory HW: Mortality associated with fertility and fertility control. *Fam Plan Perspect* 1983; 15:57–63.

Ory SJ: Nonsurgical treatment of ectopic pregnancy [editorial]. *Fertil Steril* 1986; 46:767–769.

Osathanondh V: Suprapubic mini-laparotomy, uterine elevation technique: Simple, inexpensive and outpatient procedure for interval female sterilization. *Contraception* 1974; 10:251–262.

Osathanondh R, Donnenfeld AE, Frigoletto FD Jr, et al: Induction of labor with anencephalic fetus. *Obstet Gynecol* 1980; 56:655–657.

Osathanondh R, Greene MF, Ravnikar VA, et al: Prostaglandins for cervical softening and dilatation: Recent experience with prostaglandins as dilators, in *Advances in Cervical Dilatation*. Paper presented at the Ninth Annual Meeting of National Abortion Federation, Boston, June 1985.

Osathanondh R, Stubblefield PG, Golub JR, et al: Coagulopathy associated with midtrimester D&E. *Adv Plan Parent* 1981; 16:30–33.

Osborne MP, Rosen PP, Lesser ML, et al: The relationship between family history, exposure to exogenous hormones, and estrogen receptor protein in breast cancer. *Cancer* 1983; 51:2134–2138.

Ostensen M, Husby G: Pregnancy-associated α-glycoprotein, oral contraceptives, and rheumatoid arthritis. *Lancet* 1983; 1:1391.

Oyer R, Tarakjian D, Lev-Toaff A, et al: Treatment of cervical pregnancy with methotrexate. *Obstet Gynecol* 1988; 71:469–471.

Park T-K, Flock M, Schulz KF, et al: Preventing febrile complications of suction curettage abortion. *Am J Obstet Gynecol* 1985; 152:252–255.

Pastides H, Kelsey JL, LiVolsi VA, et al: Oral contraceptive use and fibrocystic breast disease with special reference to its histopathology. *J Natl Cancer Inst* 1983; 71:5–9.

Patterson SP, White JH, Reaves EM: A maternal death associated with prostaglandin E_2. *Obstet Gynecol* 1979; 54:123–124.

Paul C, Skegg DCG, Spears GFS, et al: Oral contraceptives and breast cancer: A national study. *Br Med J (Clin Res)* 1986; 293:723–726.

Peterson HB, DeStefano F, Rubin GL, et al: Deaths attributable to tubal sterilization in the United States. *Am J Obstet Gynecol* 1983; 146:131–136.

Peterson RN, Freund M: Effects of (H^+), (Na^+), (K^+) and certain membrane-active drugs on glycolysis, motility, and ATP synthesis by human spermatozoa. *Biol Reprod* 1973; 8:350–357.

Petitti DB, Klatsky AL: Malignant hypertension in women aged 15–44 years and its relation to cigarette smoking and oral contraceptives. *Am J Cardiol* 1983; 52:297–298.

Petitti DB, Wingerd J, Pellegrin FA, et al: Risk of vascular disease in women: smoking, oral contraceptives, noncontraceptive estrogens, and other factors. *JAMA* 1979; 242:1150–1154.

Pike MC, Henderson BE, Krailo MD, et al: Breast cancer and oral contraceptives: Reply to critics. *Lancet* 1983a; 2:1414.

Pike MC, Henderson BE, Krailo MD, et al: Breast cancer in young women and use of oral contraceptives: Possible modifying effect of formulation and age at use. *Lancet* 1983b; 2:926–930.

Pike MC, Wynn V, Chilvers CED, et al: Oral contraceptives and breast cancer rates. *Lancet* 1984; 1:389.

Piot P, Plummer FA, Mhalu FS, et al: AIDS: An international perspective. *Science* 1988; 239:573–579.

Pituity Adenoma Study Group: Pituitary adenomas and oral contraceptives: A multi-center case-control study. *Fertil Steril* 1983; 39:753–760.

Pizarro E, Gomez-Rogers C, Rowe PJ: A comparative study of the effect of the Progestasert and Gravigard IUDs on dysmenorrhea. *Contraception* 1979; 20:455–66.

Porter JB, Hunter JR, Jick H, et al: Oral contraceptives and nonfatal vascular disease. *Obstet Gynecol* 1985; 66:1–8.

Porter JB, Jick H: Malignant liver tumor associated with oral contraceptive use. *Pharmacotherapy* 1981; 1:160.

Potts M, Diggory P: *Textbook of Contraceptive Practice*, ed 2. New York, Cambridge University Press. 1983.

Rabe T, Basse H, Thuro H, et al: Effect of the PGE_1 methyl analog misoprostol on the pregnant uterus in the first trimester. *Geburtshilfe Frauenheilkd* 1987; 47:324–331.

Rakhshani R, Grimes DA: Prostaglandin E_2 suppositories as a second-trimester abortifacient. *J Reprod Med* 1988; 33:817–820.

Ramahi A, Richardson DA: Urodynamic changes in women using diaphragms. Paper presented at the 36th Annual Clinical Meeting of the American College of Obstetricians and Gynecologists, Boston, May 1988.

Ramcharan S, Pellegrin FR, Ray RM, et al: The Walnut Creek contraceptive drug study. A prospective study of the side effects of oral contraceptives. *J Reprod Med* 1980; 25(suppl 6):345–372.

Ravenholt RT, Kessell E, Speidel JJ: Comparison of the side effects of three oral contraceptives: a double blind cross-over study of Ovral, Norinyl and Norlestrin. *Adv Plan Parent* 1987; 12:222–239.

Rice-Wray E, Correu S, Gorodovsk, J, et al: Return of ovulation after discontinuance of oral contraceptives. *Fertil Steril* 1967; 18:212–218.

Rock J, Pincus G, Garcia CR: Effects of certain 19-nor-steroids on the normal human menstrual cycle. *Science* 1956; 124:891–893.

Rojanasakul A, Chailurkit L, Sirimongkolkasem R, et al: Effects of combined desogestrel-ethinylestradiol treatment on lipid profiles in women with polycystic ovarian disease. *Fertil Steril* 1987; 48:581–585.

Romaguero C, Grimalt F: Contact dermatitis from a copper-containing intrauterine contraceptive device. *Contact Dermatitis* 1981; 73:163–164.

Rosenberg L, Miller DR, Kaufman DW, et al: Breast cancer and oral contraceptive use. *Am J Epidemiol* 1984; 119:167–176.

Rosenberg L, Shapiro S, Slone D, et al: Epithelial ovarian cancer and combination oral contraceptives. *JAMA* 1982; 247:3210–3212.

Rosenberg MJ, Rojanapithayakorn W, Feldblum PJ, et al: Effect of the contraceptive sponge on chlamydial infection, gonorrhea, and candidiasis. *JAMA* 1987; 257:2308–2312.

Rosenfield AG: Injectable long-acting progestogen contraception: A neglected modality. *Am J Obstet Gynecol* 1974; 120:537–548.

Rowlands S: Morning-after pills. *Br Med J* 285:322–323, 1982.

Roy S, Mishell DR: Current status of research and development of vaginal contraceptive rings as a fertility control method in the female. *Res Front Fertil Regul* 1983; 2:1–10.

Royal College of General Practitioners' Oral Contraception Study: Further analyses of mortality in oral contraceptive users. *Lancet* 1981; 1:541–546.

Royal College of General Practitioners' Oral Contraception Study: Oral contraceptives and gall bladder disease. *Lancet* 1982; 2:957–959.

Royal College of General Practitioners' Oral Contraception Study: Incidence of arterial disease among oral contraceptive users. *J R Coll Gen Pract* 1983; 33:75–82.

Rubin GL, Cates W Jr, Gold J, et al: Fatal ectopic pregnancy after attempted legally induced abortion. *JAMA* 1980; 244:1705–1708.

Rubin GL, Ory HW, Layde PM: Oral contraceptives and pelvic inflammatory disease. *Am J Obstet Gynecol* 1982; 144:630–635.

Salhanick HA: Basic studies on aminoglutethimide. *Cancer Res* 1982; 42(suppl):3315s–3321s.

Samsioe G: Comparative effects of the oral contraceptive combinations 0.150 mg desogestrel + 0.030 mg ethinylestradiol and 0.150 mg levonorgestrel + 0.030 mg estinyl estradiol on lipid and lipoprotein metabolism in healthy female volunteers. *Contraception* 1982; 25:487–504.

Sands RX, Burnhill MS, Hakim-Elahi E: Postabortal uterine atony. *Obstet Gynecol* 1974; 43:595–598.

Schaison G: RU486: Antiprogestin and antiglucocorticoid. in *New Concept I*. Paper presented at the 70th Annual Meeting of the Endocrine Society, New Orleans, June 1988.

Schaison G, George M, Lestrat N, et al: Effects of the antiprogesterone steroid RU486 during midluteal phase in normal women. *J Clin Endocrinol Metab* 1985; 61:484–489.

Schiff I, Naftolin F: Small bowel incarceration after uncomplicated laparoscopy. *Obstet Gynecol* 1974; 43:674–675.

Schlesselman JJ, Stadel BV, Murray P, et al: Breast cancer risk in relation to type of estrogen contained in oral contraceptives. *Contraception* 1987; 36:595–613.

Schlesselman JJ, Stadel BV, Murray P, et al: Breast cancer in relation to early use of oral contraceptives: No evidence of a latent effect. *JAMA* 1988; 259:1828–1833.

Schulz KF, Grimes DA, Cates W Jr: Measures to prevent cervical injury during suction curettage abortion. *Lancet* 1983; 1:1182–1184.

Scott LD, Katz AR, Duke JH: Oral contraceptives, pregnancy and focal nodular hyperplasia of the liver. *JAMA* 1984; 251:1461–1463.

Secreto G, Recchione C, Miraglia M, et al: Increased urinary androgen levels in patients with carcinoma in situ of the breast with onset while taking oral contraceptives. *Cancer Detect Prev* 1983; 6:439–442.

Segal SJ, Alvarez-Sanchez F, Adejuwon CA, et al: Absence of chorionic gonadotropin in sera of women who use intrauterine devices. *Fertil Steril* 1985; 44:214–218.

Seligsohn U, Zivelin A, Zwang E, et al: Factor VII in plasma of women taking oral contraceptives. *Transfusion* 1984; 24:171–172.

Settlage DS, Motoshima M, Tredway DR: Sperm transport from the external cervical os to the Fallopian tubes in women: A time and quantitation study. *Fertil Steril* 1973; 24:655–661.

Shapiro AG, Lasseter K, Cobiella A, et al: Intravaginal administration of 9-deoxo-9-methylene-16,16-dimethyl PGE_2 for cervical dilation prior to suction curettage. *Int J Gynaecol Obstet* 1982; 20:137–140.

Shar SR, Kew MC: Oral contraceptives and hepatocellular carcinoma. *Cancer* 1982; 49:407–410.

Sharpe RM, Wrixon W, Hobson BM, et al: Absence of hCG-like activity in the blood of women fitted with intra-uterine contraceptive devices. *J Clin Endocrinol Metab* 1977; 45:496–499.

Shearman RP: Post-coital contraception: A review. *Contraception* 1973; 7:459–476.

Shy KK, McTiernan AM, Daling JR, et al: Oral contraceptive use and occurrence of pituitary prolactinoma. *JAMA* 1983; 249:2204–2207.

Siegberg R, Nilsson CG, Stenman U, et al: Sex hormone profiles in oligomenorrheic adolescent girls and the effect of oral contraceptives. *Fertil Steril* 1984; 41:888–893.

Silva DA, Singh PP, Bauman J, et al: Acute hypertensive response to prostaglandin $F_{2\alpha}$ during anesthesia administration. *J Reprod Med* 1987; 32:700–702.

Sivin I, Tatum HJ: Four years of experience with the TCU 380A intrauterine contraceptive device. *Fertil Steril* 1981; 36:159–163.

Smythe AR II, Underwood PB Jr: Ectopic pregnancy after postcoital diethylstilbestrol. *Am J Obstet Gynecol* 1975; 121:284.

Sonne-Holmes S, Heisterberg L, Hebjorn S, et al: Prophylactic antibiotics in first trimester abortion: A clinical controlled trial. *Am J Obstet Gynecol* 1981; 139:693–696.

Spence MR, King TM, Burkman RT, et al: Cephalothin prophylaxis for midtrimester abortion. *Obstet Gynecol* 1982; 60:502–505.

Stadel BV: Oral contraceptives and cardiovascular disease. *N Engl J Med* 1981; 305:612–618, 672–677.

Stadel BV, Rubin GL, Webster LA, et al: Oral contraceptives and breast cancer in young women. *Lancet* 1985; 2:970–974.

Stampfer MJ, Willett WC, Colditz GA, et al: A prospective study of past use of oral contraceptive agents and risk of cardiovascular diseases. *N Engl J Med* 1988; 319:1313–1317.

Stevens RG, Lee JAH, Moolgavkar SH: No association between oral contraceptives and malignant melanomas. *N Engl J Med* 1980; 302:966.

Stockley IH: Methotrexate-NSAID interactions. *Drug Intell Clin Pharm* 1987; 21:546.

Stubblefield PG, Fuller AF, Foster SC: Ultrasound-guided intrauterine removal of intrauterine contraceptive devices in pregnancy. *Obstet Gynecol* 1988; 72:961–964.

Stubblefield PG, Monson RR, Schoenbaum SC, et al: Fertility after induced abortion: A prospective follow-up study. *Obstet Gynecol* 1984; 63:186–193.

Sturgis SH, Albright F: The mechanism of estrin therapy in the relief of dysmenorrhea. *Endocrinology* 1940; 26:68–72.

Sturtevant FM: Breast cancer and oral contraceptives. *Lancet* 1983; 2:1145.

Swann SH, Petitti DB: A review of problems of bias and confounding in epidemiologic studies of cervical neoplasia and oral contraceptive use. *Am J Epidemiol* 1982; 115:10–18.

Swyer GIM: Progestagen "potency" and breast cancer. *Lancet* 1983; 2:1416.

Szoka PR, Edgren RA: Drug interactions with oral contraceptives: Compilation and analysis of an adverse experience report database. *Fertil Steril* 1988; 49(suppl):31S–38S.

Tatum HJ, Connell-Tatum EB: Barrier contraception: A comprehensive overview. *Fertil Steril* 1981; 36:1–12.

Thayssen P, Secher NJ, Arnsbo P: Systolic time intervals and haemodynamic changes during intravenous infusion of prostaglandins $F_{2\alpha}$ and E_2. *Br Heart J* 1981; 45:447–456.

Thiersch JB: Therapeutic abortions with a folic acid antagonist 4-aminopteroylglutamic acid administered by the oral route. *Am J Obstet Gynecol* 1952; 63:1298–1304.

Thomas DB: Do hormones cause breast cancer? *Cancer* 1984; 53:595–604.

Tietze C: New estimates of mortality associated with fertility control. *Fam Plan Perspect* 1977; 9:74–76.

Tietze C, Lewit S: Life risks associated with reversible methods of fertility regulation. *Int J Gynaecol Obstet* 1979; 16:456–459.

Toppozada M: The clinical use of monthly injectable contraceptive preparations. *Obstet Gynecol Surv* 1977; 32:335–347.

Toth M., Witkin SS, Ledger W, et al: The role of infection in the etiology of preterm birth. *Obstet Gynecol* 1988; 71:723–726.

Trapido EJ: A prospective cohort study of oral contraceptives and cancer of the endometrium. *Int J Epidemiol* 1983; 12:297–300.

Umapathysivam K, Jones WR: Effects of contraceptive agents on the biochemical and protein composition of human endometrium. *Contraception* 1980; 22:425–440.

Umpierre SA, Hill JA, Anderson DJ: Effect of "Coke" on sperm motility. *N Engl J Med* 1985; 313:1351.

U.S. Health and Human Services: Oral contraceptives and cancer. *FDA Drug Bull* 1984; 14:2–3.

Valenzuela G, Hayashi RH, Lackritz RN, et al: Uterine rupture at term with vaginal prostaglandin E_2. *Am J Obstet Gynecol* 1980; 138:1223–1224.

Valicenti JF, Pappas AA, Graber CD, et al: Detection and prevalence of IUD-associated actinomyces colonization and related morbidity. *JAMA* 1982; 247:1149–1152.

Vandenbroucke JP: Oral contraceptives and rheumatoid arthritis. *Lancet* 1983; 2:228–229.

Vandenbroucke JP, Boersma JW, Festen JJM, et al: Oral contraceptives and rheumatoid arthritis: Further evidence for a preventive effect. *Lancet* 1982; 2:839–842.

Vandenbroucke JP, Witteman JC, Valkenburg HA, et al: Noncontraceptive hormones and rheumatoid arthritis in perimenopausal and postmenopausal women. *JAMA* 1986; 255:1299–1303.

van der Spuy ZM, Jones DL, Wright CSW, et al: Inhibition of 3-beta-hydroxy steroid dehydrogenase activity in first trimester human pregnancy with trilostane and WIN 32729. *Clin Endocrinol* 1983; 19:521–531.

Vergote I, Oeyen L, De Schrijver D, et al: Uterine rupture due to 15-methylprostaglandin $F_{2\alpha}$. *Lancet* 1982; 2:1402.

Vessey M, Baron J, Doll R, et al: Oral contraceptives and breast cancer: Final report of an epidemiological study. *Br J Cancer* 1983a; 47:455–462.

Vessey M, Lawless M, Yeates D: Efficacy of different contraceptive methods. *Lancet* 1982; 1:841–843.

Vessey MP, McPherson K, Johnson B: Mortality among women participating in the Oxford Family Planning Association Contraceptive Study. *Lancet* 1977; 2:731–733.

Vessey MP: Exogenous hormones in the aetiology of cancer in women. *J R Soc Med* 1984; 77:542–549.

Vessey MP, Lawless M: The Oxford–Family Planning Association contraceptive study. *Clin Obstet Gynecol* 1984; 11:743–757.

Vessey MP, Lawless M, McPherson K, et al: Neoplasia of the cervix uteri and contraception—a possible adverse effect of the pill. *Lancet* 1983b; 2:930–934.

von Kaulla E, Droegemueller W, Aoki N, et al: Antithrombin III depression and thrombin generation acceleration in women taking oral contraceptives. *Am J Obstet Gynecol* 1971; 109:868–873.

Warburton D, Negut RH, Lustenberger A, et al: Lack of association between spermicide use and trisomy. *N Engl J Med* 1987; 317:478–482.

Washington AE, Browner WS, Korenbrof CC: Cost-effectiveness of combined treatment for endocervical gonorrhea. *JAMA* 1987; 257:2056–2060.

Washington AE, Gove S, Schachter J, et al: Oral contraceptives, chlamydia trachomatis infection, and pelvic inflammatory disease. *JAMA* 1985; 253:2246–2250.

Weiss NS, Sayvetz TA: Incidence of endometrial cancer in relation to the use of oral contraceptives. *N Engl J Med* 1980; 302:551–554.

Wessler S, Gitel SN, Wan LS, et al: Estrogen-containing oral contraceptive agents: a basis for their thrombogenicity. *JAMA* 1976; 236:2179–2182.

Wheeless CR, Katayama KP: Laparoscopy and tubal sterilization, in Mattingly RF, Thompson JD (eds): *Te Linde's Operative Gynecology,* ed 6. Philadelphia, JB Lippincott Co, 1985, pp 411–428.

White PF, Coe V, Dworsky WA, et al: Disseminated intravascular coagulation following midtrimester abortions. *Anesthesiology* 1983; 58:99–101.

Wilcox AJ, Weinberg CR, Armstrong EG, et al: Urinary human chorionic gonadotropin among intrauterine device users.: Detection with a higly specific and sensitive assay. *Fertil Steril* 1987; 47:265–269.

Willett WC, Bain C, Hennekens CH, et al: Oral contraceptives and risk of ovarian cancer. *Cancer* 1981; 48:1684–1687.

World Health Organization: Collaborative study of neoplasia and steroid contraceptives. Invasive cervical cancer and combined oral contraceptives. *Br Med J (Clin Res)* 1985; 290:961–965.

World Health Organization: Mechanism of action, safety and efficacy of intrauterine devices. *Tech Rep Ser* 1987a; 753:91.

World Health Organization: Special Programme of Research, Development and Research Training in Human Reproduction and Special Programme on AIDS. Report of a meeting on contraceptive methods and HIV infections, Geneva, no 21, 1987b.

Wu D-F, Yu Y-W, Tang Z-M, et al: Pharmacokinetics of $(\pm)-$, $(+)-$, and $(-)-$ gossypol in humans and dogs. *Clin Pharmacol Ther* 1986; 39:613–618.

Wu YT: Suction in artificial abortion: 300 cases (Chinese). *Chin J Obstet Gynecol* 1958; 6:447–449.

Ye BL, Yamamoto K, Tyson JE: Functional and biochemical aspects of laminaria use in first-trimester pregnancy termination. *Am J Obstet Gynecol* 1982; 142:36–39.

Yuzpe AA, Smith RP, Rademaker AW: A Multicenter clinical investigation employing ethinyl estradiol combined with dl-norgestrel as a postcoital contraceptive agent. *Fertil Steril* 1982; 37:508–513.

Yuzpe AA, Thurlow HJ, Ramzy I, et al: Post coital contraception—a pilot study. *J Reprod Med* 1974; 13:53–58.

Zipper J, Wheeler RG, Potts DM, et al: Propanolol as a novel effective spermicide: Preliminary findings. *Br Med J (Clin Res)* 1983; 287:1245–1246.

Zipper JA, Tatum H, Pastene L, et al: Metallic copper as an intrauterine contraceptive adjunct to the "T" device. *Am J Obstet Gynecol* 1969; 105:1274–1278.

18   Medical Genetics

Wayne A. Miller, M.D., F.A.C.O.G.

Genetic problems are frequently encountered initially by the gynecologist as primary physician to women. During routine prenatal evaluation, the gynecologist may become aware of specific risk factors such as advanced maternal age, family history of serious genetic disorder, ethnic background, or exposure to deleterious agents. Patients frequently pose questions about the risks and nature of genetic and nongenetic birth defects. Subsequently the obstetrician is often the first to observe the presence of a serious congenital defect in the child, necessitating proper diagnosis, management, and interpretation to the parents. Thus, the gynecologist must be familiar with both the fundamental principles of medical genetics and those disorders of greatest relevance to maternal-fetal health and reproductive function.

This chapter addresses basic aspects of medical genetics, examples of genetic disorders that may present primarily with gynecologic complaints, and a genetically oriented approach to certain major gynecologic problems. For a more extensive treatment of the subjects presented in this chapter or for topics beyond the scope of this chapter, the reader is referred to Vogel and Motulsky (1979), Sutton (1980), Simpson et al. (1982), Emery and Rimoin (1985), Nyhan and Sakati (1987) and McKusick (1988).

BASIC PRINCIPLES

Mendel in the 1860s formulated many basic concepts of inheritance on which we depend today, but his work received little attention until it was rediscovered in the first decade of this century. At that time Garrod (Harris, 1963) proposed the term "inborn errors of metabolism" to unify his observations on alkaptonuria, albinism, cystinuria, and pentosuria, the four inherited disorders that he had studied in detail. The first identification of a molecular basis for a human genetic disease was in 1949 when Pauling noted the abnormal electrophoretic mobility of sickle hemoglobin. In 1957 Ingram showed that this altered mobility resulted from a changed amino acid sequence in the hemoglobin molecule. The deciphering of the genetic code, begun by Nirenberg in 1961, led to the recognition that the altered amino acid sequence of hemoglobin S resulted from a point mutation in the gene for the globin β-chain. The first specific enzyme defect in an inborn error of metabolism was identified in 1952 when Cori and Cori showed that glucose-6-phosphatase activity was deficient in glycogen storage disease, type II. The first mammalian gene, mouse globin, was cloned in 1977 (Tilghman et al., 1977), and the first *restriction fragment length polymorphism* (RFLP) was identified in 1978 (Wyman and White, 1978).

Chromosomes were described in the 1870s, but not until 1956 was it determined that the normal diploid number of chromosomes in the human *karyotype,* or chromosome complement, is 46. The specific etiologic basis of a human chromosome disorder was first identified in 1959 when Lejeune demonstrated the presence of an extra number 21 chromosome in a child with Down syndrome. The 46 chromosomes normally present occur in pairs, one member of the pair having been inherited from each parent. Twenty-two pairs are homologous and are designated the *autosomes*. The 23rd pair constitutes the *sex chromosomes,* the X and the Y. Although the chromosomes are always present in the nucleus of the cell, it is only immediately prior to cell division, namely, at metaphase, that they condense and assume their characteristic form. At metaphase, each chromosome has already divided, the two sister chromatids thus produced remaining attached at the centromere, resulting in the familiar x-shaped appearance (not to be confused with the X chromosome). As shown schematically in Figure 18–1, the chromosome pairs are classified into seven groups, designated A through G, primarily on the basis of length and the position of the centromere (Bergsma et al., 1972). Figure 18–2 shows karyotypes of a normal female (A) and a normal male (B) stained by what was, until the early 1970s, the standard method. With this staining, normal chromosomes could be classified into groups without difficulty, but some of the pairs of homologues could not be distinguished. Furthermore, structurally abnormal chromosomes often could not be precisely characterized. Some useful additional information could be provided through the use of laborious special techniques, such as differential labeling of the chromosomes with tritiated thymidine followed by autoradiography.

In 1970 Caspersson and associates demonstrated that exposure of chromosomes to certain fluorescent compounds such as quinacrine hydro-chloride or quinacrine mustard resulted in the appearance of bands, designated *Q bands,* by which each chromosome pair as well as the X and the Y could be distinguished. Subsequently, several alternative banding techniques have been introduced, yielding different banding patterns and greater detail about certain specific chromosomal regions. In Figure 18–3 the chromosomes were first exposed to a dilute solution of trypsin and then to Giemsa stain to give characteristic *G bands.* The locations and intensities of the G bands are quite similar to those of the Q bands except for four chromosome segments. In contrast to the fluorescent banding, however, G-banding technique gives permanent preparations and requires no special microscopy equipment for observing the bands, hence its widespread use. *Minor variants,* which are structural variations with no apparent functional significance, occur frequently, making it possible in many instances to distinguish the maternally derived from the paternally derived member within each pair of homologues (Miller et al., 1973; Hoehn, 1975).

By convention, the karyotype is described by noting first the total number of chromosomes,

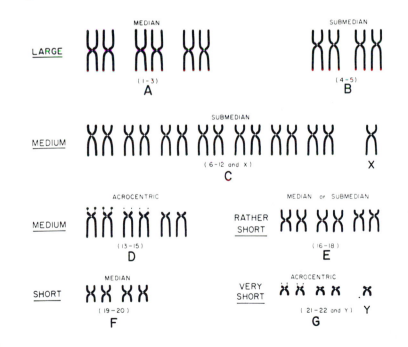

FIG 18–1.

Idiogram of a normal male with 22 pairs of autosomes and XY sex chromosome constitution. Chromosomes are arranged in seven groups, *A* through *G,* according to length and centromere position. Classification is a slight modification, after Patau, of the international system of nomenclature adopted in Denver. (From Sohval AR: *Fertil Steril* 1963; 14:180. Reproduced by permission.)

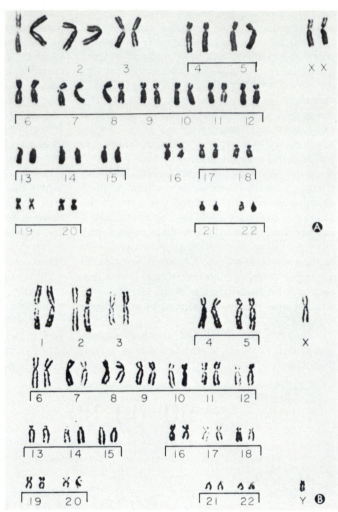

FIG 18–2.

A, normal female karyotype, and **B,** normal male karyotype stained with Giemsa. **B** From Hirschhorn K, Cooper LC: *Am J Med* 1961; 31:442. The chromosome pairs whose numbers are enclosed by *solid lines* cannot be distinguished using this staining technique.

followed by a designation of the sex chromosomes present, followed, in turn, by the description of any abnormality or variant (Bergsma et al., 1972). A normal female karyotype is designated 46,XX, and a normal male is 46,XY. A patient with Turner's syndrome (see the section on Turner's syndrome) might have a 45,X karyotype, whereas Klinefelter's syndrome is associated with 47,XXY. Additional chromosomes are indicated by a plus sign (+) followed by the identity of the extra chromosome. For example, a male with trisomy 21 Down syndrome is designated 47,XY + 21. When a plus sign follows the number of a specific chromosome, it indicates the presence of additional material on that chromosome as, for example, in 46,XY,14+. The *short arm* of a chromosome is designated *p*, and the long arm is *q*. An addition is designated +; a deletion is −.

Thus, the karyotype of a male with the *cri du chat syndrome,* which is due to a deletion of the short arm of chromosome 5, is represented 46,XY,5p−. Translocations of part or all of one chromosome to another have a complex, but specific, terminology and are discussed further in the section on meiosis.

The genotype or genetic constitution of an individual is encoded in the deoxyribonucleic acid (DNA) of the chromosomes (Watson, 1976; Stent, 1971). Four nucleotide bases make up each of the two strands of the DNA double helix. These nucleotide bases will pair only with a single complementary base on the opposite strand of the helix. When cell division occurs and the genetic material is duplicated, the two strands of DNA separate, and two complementary daughter strands are formed by the *replication enzymes,* ade-

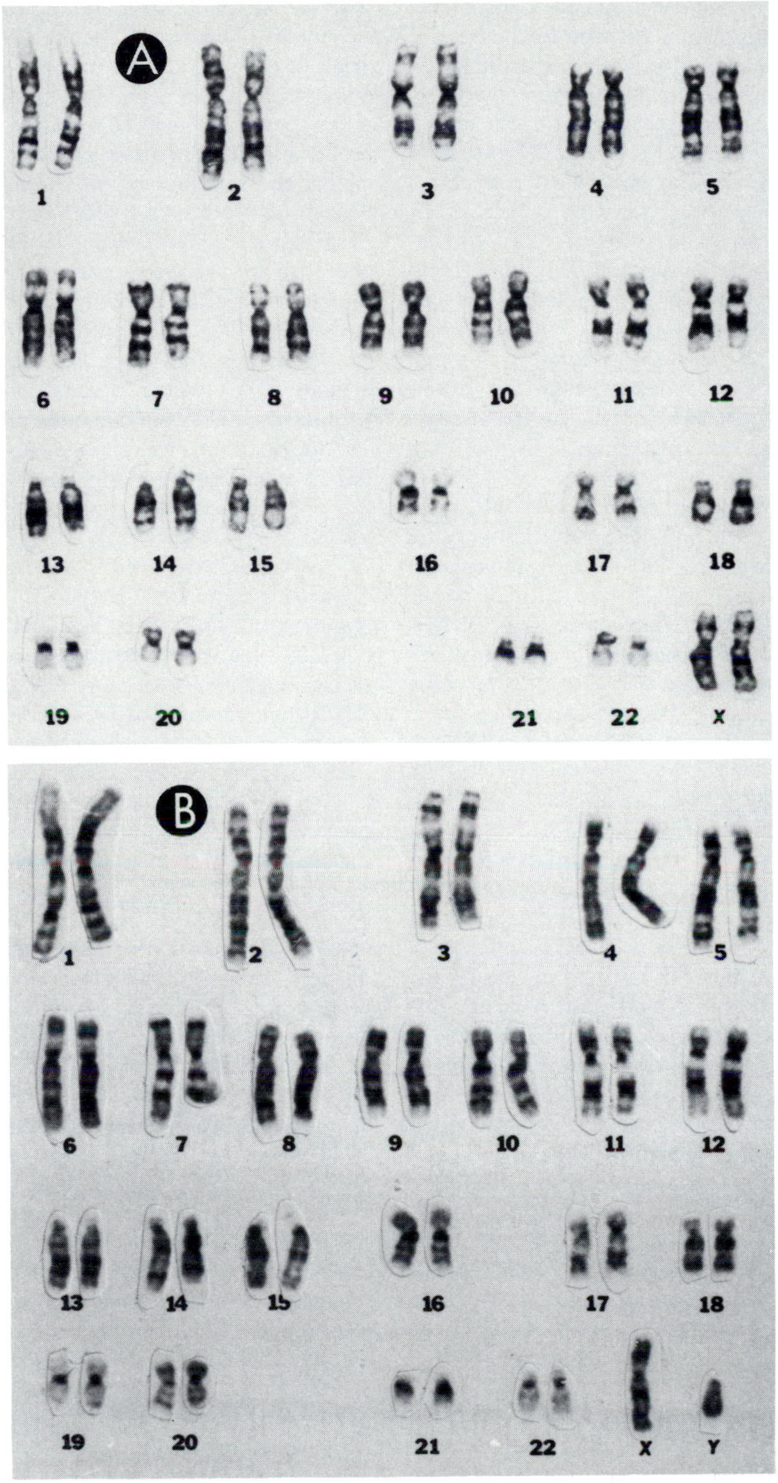

FIG 18–3.
A, normal female karyotype. **B,** normal male karyotype stained to reveal G bands. The characteristic patterns of light and dark bands allow for definitive recognition of each chromosome pair.

nine opposite thymine and guanine opposite cytosine. The information encoded in the gene is used to form a strand of ribonucleic acid (RNA) by the process designated *transcription*. The sequence of DNA bases is transcribed by the precise pairing of specific complementary RNA bases to the DNA template. The messenger RNA strand, in turn, interacts with ribosomes, transfer RNA and various proteins in a process called *translation*, leading to the production of specific amino acid sequences. Not only the zygote but each cell in the human body is thought to contain the entire genome (or genetic constitution), although the processes of differentiation allow the expression of certain portions of this genome in some cells and its repression in others, thus providing for specific cell types.

Recently developed recombinant DNA technologies hold great promise for medical genetics and have already produced much excitement. These technologies will be useful for diagnosis (especially prenatally) and for detecting carriers, as well as for fundamental studies of normal and pathologic gene action, and ultimately for gene therapy. Recombinant DNA studies rely on many concepts and techniques, only a few of which can be summarized here. More detailed reviews are available (Watkins, 1988, Landegren et al., 1988, Antonarakis, 1989). Most relevant to our presentation are the uses of recombinant DNA technologies in genetic diagnosis. These involve two basic approaches that will be described in some detail. The first approach is indirect and uses a nearby DNA marker not involved in causing the particular disorder to detect the presence of a disease-related gene or genes. Most often this linked, noncausal marker consists of an RFLP. In the second approach, the presence of the mutant gene is detected directly. Both approaches depend on the use of gene probes, restriction endonucleases, and gel electrophoresis. The DNA present in the nucleus of each cell in the body normally contains all of the genes of the individual. This DNA can be extracted from any convenient cell, such as a leukocyte or amniotic fluid cell. A consistent pattern of regular DNA fragments can be produced by incubation of this DNA with the enzymes restriction endonucleases, which cleave DNA at sequence-specific sites consisting of four, five, six, or seven DNA bases, the number and sequence depending on the specific restriction endonuclease used. The DNA restriction fragments can then be resolved by electrophoresis in agarose gels, which

separate the fragments according to their lengths as shown in Figure 18–4. Although all of the genes of the individual are present somewhere in this display of fragments, identifying the location of any particular gene requires the addition of a probe, a specially prepared segment of DNA containing the sequence of the gene being sought. Such probes are usually prepared from radioactively labeled, enzymatically labeled, or fluorophore-labeled precursors using various techniques to retrieve specific gene sequences from either messenger RNA or directly from DNA. After electrophoresis, the probe is added, its complementary DNA sequence causes it to hybridize with the fragment containing the gene of interest, and the location of this fragment and the gene can be identified by autoradiography, colorimetry, or fluorescent excitation as shown in Figure 18–4.

As noted previously, restriction endonucleases cleave the DNA at specific sequences. The fragment of DNA thus generated is that which normally connects two such sequence-specific cleavage sites. If one or more DNA bases within a cleavage site is changed by mutation, the restriction endonuclease no longer cleaves at that site, so the fragment of DNA containing that sequence is longer than it was before the mutation. We all carry a rather large number of mutations that change potential cleavage sites but do not seem to cause disease. In many cases the mutations have occurred in DNA sequences that do not normally code for proteins. These mutationally altered sequences found in individuals are inherited by progeny in a direct line of descent. Since these changes are relatively frequent in populations and are heritable, they are called RFLPs. The first application of recombinant DNA technology to the diagnosis of human genetic disease occurred in 1978 when Kan and Dozy (1978) developed a prenatal diagnostic test for sickle cell anemia using RFLPs. Their test took advantage of the concept of linkage, the fact that two markers that are close together on the same chromosome will assort nonrandomly, either both or neither being transmitted to the offspring of an individual. Kan and Dozy cleaved the DNA prior to electrophoresis using the restriction endonuclease *Hpa* I, which cleaves DNA at the sequence GTTAAC. After separating the fragments by electrophoresis and applying the radioactive globin-gene probe to locate the fragment containing the β-globin gene, the investigators found that the length of the

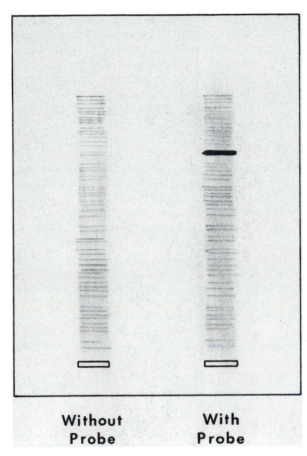

FIG 18–4.
Separation of restriction fragments by gel electrophoresis with and without gene-specific probe. Following digestion into fragments using a DNA sequence-specific restriction endonuclease, electrophoresis is used to separate the fragments according to their molecular lengths. Without hybridization with a gene-specific probe, it is not possible to distinguish the fragment bearing the gene of interest. After hybridization with a specific probe, however, the fragment containing the gene of interest is readily identified, usually by autoradiography.

Without Probe   **With Probe**

DNA fragment on which the β-globin gene was located differed for the different β-globin genotypes. In individuals in their test group who had normal hemoglobin A, the β-globin gene was present on a fragment that was either 7.6 kilobases (kb) (i.e., 7,600 DNA bases) or 7.0 kb long, whereas the β-globin gene in persons with hemoglobin S was located on a 13.0-kb fragment. The β-globin gene probe did not react differently to the β^A-gene than to the β^S-gene; it was not sensitive to the change in a single DNA base in the rather large globin gene. Diagnosis was made possible by the presence of a second, linked mutation, which altered a nearby DNA sequence so that the *Hpa* I restriction endonuclease no longer cleaved at the nearby site, thus making the β^S-globin gene part of a longer fragment defined by the next adjacent *Hpa* I cleavage site (Fig 18–5). Taking advantage of this linked RFLP, the β-globin genotype of any individual could be deduced from the analysis of DNA in leukocytes, amniotic fluid cells, or any other nucleated cells.

After incubation with *Hpa* I, electrophoresis of DNA from an individual with sickle cell trait and hemoglobin AS would have one band at 7.0/7.6 kb and a second band at 13.0 kb. In contrast, an individual with sickle cell anemia and hemoglobin SS would have a single band at 13.0 kb. This approach was successfully applied by Kan and Dozy (1978) to the prenatal diagnosis of a fetus at risk for sickle cell anemia, and the correctness of the diagnosis, which in this case was sickle cell trait, was confirmed in the child following her birth. An important point is that analysis of DNA from amniotic fluid cells, which usually do not express the globin gene, correctly predicted the hemoglobin genotype for the adult hemoglobin that would not become the major hemoglobin until much later in gestation.

Since this initial prenatal diagnosis of sickle cell anemia, other molecular diagnostic procedures using RFLPs have been developed. At present, more than 50 genetic diseases have been linked to RFLPs, including cystic fibrosis, Hun-

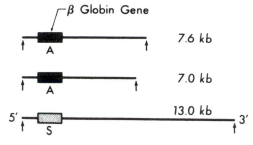

FIG 18–5.
Linkage of the globin gene to a restriction site polymorphism. *Hpa* I restriction endonuclease cleavage sites, indicated by *arrows*, to the left of the β-globin gene are constant, but those to the right differ depending on the specific globin gene present. These sites are closer in the case of the βA-globin gene, so that the total length of the restriction fragment bearing the βA-gene is either 7.6 or 7.0 kb in length. The mutation that produced the βS-gene, however, is linked to a mutation that eliminated the nearest *Hpa* I cleavage site to the right, resulting in a longer fragment that is 13.0 kb in length. Thus, the differences in the length of the restriction fragment bearing the βS-globin gene can be used to deduce the globin genotype of the individual whose DNA is being analyzed. (From Kan YW, Dozy AM: *Proc Natl Acad Sci USA* 1978; 75:5631–5635. Reproduced by permission.)

tington's disease, neurofibromatosis, thalassemia, hemophilia A and B, phenylketonuria, and Duchenne-type muscular dystrophy (Watkins, 1988). The techniques that use RFLPs are like all linkage analyses; they are essentially familial diagnoses and generally require the availability for analysis of samples from at least several family members. A single at-risk patient or fetus is insufficient for the application of this type of analysis.

The usefulness of the second approach, the direct detection of a mutant, disease-producing gene is also illustrated by sickle cell anemia. The direct detection of this disorder recently became possible through the use of the restriction endonuclease *Mst* II, which cleaves at the CCTNAGG sequence present in the βA-gene but not at the mutant sequence present in the βS-gene. This direct analysis requires a DNA sample from only one individual or a single fetus at risk. Other types of direct DNA analysis are also possible in approximately 45 genetic disorders in which the nature of the mutation is known (Landegren et al., 1988).

A new development in recombinant technology involves DNA amplification by polymerase

chain reaction (PCR). With this technique a specific segment of DNA can be amplified approximately 10^6-fold within a few hours by using oligonucleotide primers to direct synthesis of new complementary DNA strands. The large number of copies of the specific DNA sequence allow for analyses to be accomplished on smaller amounts of DNA, in situ, and using nonradioactive probes (Erlich et al., 1988; Kogan et al., 1987).

In view of the rapid pace of advances in recombinant DNA technology, the list of serious genetic disorders diagnosable through linkage analysis using RFLPs or directly is likely to grow rapidly in the coming years.

It is important to distinguish between two fundamentally different cell types. *Germ cells* are the gonadal cells that, through the process of meiosis, form the gametes. The genetic information carried by the germ cells can thus be transmitted to subsequent generations of individuals. *Somatic cells* make up the remainder of the body, replicate by mitosis, and transmit their genetic information to their somatic cell progeny but not between generations of whole individuals. Each cell has an ordered sequence of events in its life designated the *cell cycle*, shown in Figure 18–6. When two daughter cells are formed, each enters into a specific stage called the G_1 *period*, or first gap. During this time the chromosomes are present in the diploid number (2n) and are dispersed in the nucleus. The next stage of the cell cycle is the S period, which is defined as the time of DNA synthesis and duplication. At the end of this period the chromosome complement is doubled and the cell contains 4n chromosomes, twice the diploid number. The stage from the end of the S period to the initiation of mitosis is designated the G_2 *period*, or second gap. These three stages of the cell cycle are collectively called *interphase*. The final phase of the cell cycle is *mitosis* in somatic cells, whereas in germ cells during gametogenesis the final phase is *meiosis*. Each of these can be divided into prophase, metaphase, anaphase, and telophase (Swanson et al., 1967; Hamerton, 1971).

Meiosis

Meiosis is the process by which the chromosome constitution of cells destined to become gametes is reduced from the diploid number of 46, or 2n, to the haploid number of 23, or n. To accomplish this, these cells divide twice while replicating their chromosomes only once, as dia-

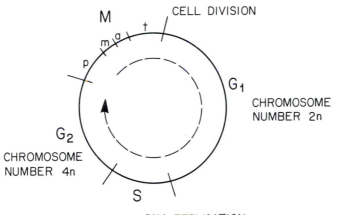

FIG 18−6.

The cell cycle. Newly formed daughter cells enter into the G_1 period, or first gap. At this stage, the chromosome number is diploid, or 2n. The S period begins with initiation of DNA synthesis and ends when DNA replication is complete, bringing the chromosome complement to 4n. The G_2 period ends with the initiation of mitosis. The four stages of mitosis are prophase (p), metaphase (m), anaphase (a), and telophase (t).

grammed in Figure 18−7. In the first meiotic division, or meiosis I, the dispersed interphase chromatin first condenses. In step *a*, it becomes apparent that the chromosomes have already replicated in the previous S phase, yielding the 4n number of chromosomes. These *sister chromatids,* each of which is one half of the replicated chromosome, next separate everywhere along their length except at the centromere. In step *b*, a feature unique to meiosis, homologous chromosomes attract each other and, by the process known as *synapsis,* pair lengthwise at the equatorial region of the nucleus. At this stage, homologous segments of the maternal and paternal chromosomes are exchanged in a process called *crossing over,* step *c*. Longer chromosomes generally exhibit more crossing over, but it occurs even in the small chromosomes. Crossing over is a normal process that increases the range of genetic diversity beyond the combinations produced by the random assortment of homologous chromosomes. At the time of cell division in meiosis I, the homologous paired chromosomes separate and move toward opposite poles of the nucleus in the process called *disjunction,* step *d*. As a result of this disjunction and because the maternal and paternal chromosomes were arranged in parallel, but at random, on the meiotic spindle, the products of the first meiotic division are two cells, each of which contains one member—maternal or pater-

nal—of each of the 23 pairs of chromosomes. Generally about one half of the chromosomes in each gametocyte will be of maternal origin and one half of paternal origin. Since the maternal and paternal chromosomes have been separated by the first meiotic division, this is referred to as a *reduction division*. It will be recalled, however, that chromosomal replication to the 4n state occurred prior to the beginning of meiosis I, and hence this reduction division still leaves the progeny cells with the 2n, or diploid, number of chromosomes. These paired chromatids that have remained joined at the centromere are identical except in those regions where crossing over has occurred with a chromatid of the homologous chromosome (McDermott, 1975).

Chromosome replication does not occur following meiosis I, and the gametogenic cells enter meiosis II with the 2n chromosome number. Meiosis II has been likened to a mitotic division because the chromatids align in the equatorial region, the spindle forms, the centromeres divide and one member of each chromatid pair moves to the opposite pole of the cell. Meiosis II differs from mitosis in that the progeny cells are haploid, with the n number of chromosomes, step *e*.

Although these features of meiosis apply to both males and females, oogenesis and spermatogenesis differ in important respects. Oogenesis begins early in the embryonic ovary. The primary

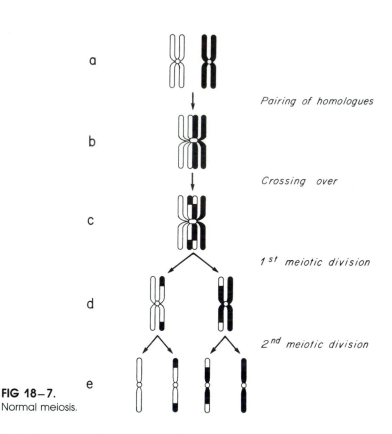

a

Pairing of homologues

b

Crossing over

c

1ˢᵗ meiotic division

d

2ⁿᵈ meiotic division

e

FIG 18–7.
Normal meiosis.

oocytes form during early fetal development and reach the late prophase of meiosis I by the fifth month of intrauterine life. The process of meiosis is arrested at what is termed the *dictyotene stage* of the meiosis I prophase. The meiotic processes resume 12 to 50 years later, after puberty, and only if that oocyte is to be activated in preparation for ovulation. This delay has been cited as a possible basis for certain of the chromosome anomalies shown to be due more often to errors in maternal than in paternal gametogenesis. When oogenesis resumes at metaphase in meiosis I, cell division results in two cells of very different sizes. The cell containing one half of the chromosome complement, but very little cytoplasm becomes the first polar body. The second meiotic division begins after the so-called pronucleus of the sperm has entered the large cell. Meiosis II in the oocyte is also highly asymmetric, yielding a small second polar body and an ovum that is nearly as large as the original primary oocyte. The male and female haploid pronuclei then unite to form the *zygote*.

Although development of testes proceeds much earlier in the embryo (Mittwoch, 1975), spermatogenesis is not initiated until puberty. In response to hormonal stimulation, primary spermatocytes are formed continuously by mitotic division and complete the first and second meiotic divisions. Each primary spermatocyte thus gives rise to four haploid sperm cells of equal size.

Nondisjunction, the failure of separation of paired chromosomes at metaphase—occurring during meiosis—leads to the formation of an aneuploid gamete, as shown in Figure 18–8. Instead of being diploid, the gamete will have an extra chromosome or will lack one chromosome. If these gametes are fertilized by normal gametes, the resulting zygote will be trisomic or monosomic, respectively. Monosomic cells can also be formed by *anaphase lag,* a process in which the migration of a chromosome is delayed, resulting in its exclusion from both daughter nuclei. Monosomies for the autosomes are lethal, whereas trisomies of many of the autosomes, though deleterious, are observed in live-born infants. Monosomy for the X chromosome results in Turner's syndrome, whereas monosomy with a Y chromosome but no X chromosome has not been observed. Trisomy of the X chromosome occurs and is associated with few, if any, serious abnormali-

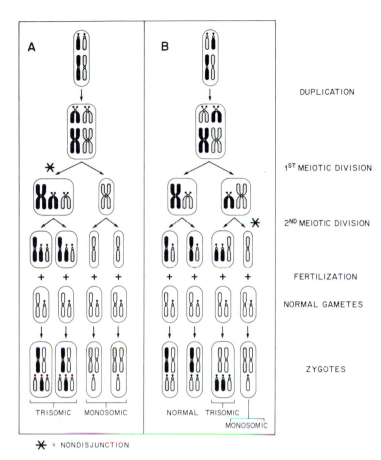

DUPLICATION

1ST MEIOTIC DIVISION

2ND MEIOTIC DIVISION

FERTILIZATION

NORMAL GAMETES

ZYGOTES

TRISOMIC MONOSOMIC NORMAL TRISOMIC MONOSOMIC

✱ = NONDISJUNCTION

FIG 18–8.
A, nondisjunction at first meiotic division, resulting in abnormal gametes having an extra homologous chromosome; and **B,** nondisjunction at second meiotic division, resulting in abnormal gametes having an extra sister chromosome.

ties. By definition, trisomy refers to the presence of three homologous chromosomes, and since the X and Y are not homologous, XXY and XYY individuals are classified simply as having sex chromosome aneuploidy. Since the homologous chromosomes and the sex chromosomes normally separate in meiosis I, whereas the sister chromatids separate in meiosis II, the consequences of nondisjunction at these steps will differ. Nondisjunction in meiosis I results in a gamete with an extra homologous autosome, or in the case of the sex chromosomes in the male, both an X and a Y. If nondisjunction occurs in meiosis II, however, the extra chromosome in the gamete will be a sister chromatid. Thus, for example, XYY must result from a second meiotic division nondisjunction in the male parent, whereas XXY could result from nondisjunction in meiosis I of the male or in ei-

ther meiosis I or meiosis II of the female parent. Occasionally nondisjunction occurs during both meiotic divisions, resulting in more complex aneuploidies, although survival is limited to those involving the sex chromosomes.

Nondisjunction can also occur during mitosis and may result in *mosaicism,* or the presence of two or more lines of cells differing in their genetic constitution but that have originated from single cells. Thus, mitotic nondisjunction early in embryonic life would be expected to yield two daughter cells, one trisomic and the other monosomic. If an autosome were involved, the monosomic cell would be inviable while the progeny of the trisomic cell would coexist with the remaining diploid cells. For example, mitotic nondisjunction involving chromosome 21 could result in an individual with a 46,XY/47,XY + 21 mosaicism.

Abnormalities in transfer of genetic information can also occur during meiosis if chromosomes are abnormal as the result of translocation. Chromosomes may become fragmented during either meiosis or mitosis, and the fragments may become joined to other chromosomes or fragments of chromosomes in a process called *translocation*. As shown in Figure 18–9, if breaks occur in two chromosomes and the chromosomal material is simply exchanged, the translocation is said to be *reciprocal*. When the breakage and rejoining occur at the centromeres of the two chromosomes, the translocation is classified as the *centric fusion*, or *Robertsonian* type. Translocations in which the sites of breakage and rejoining are not at the centromere are designated *non-Robertsonian*. Centric fusion translocations are far more common and usually involve the D and G group chromosomes, which have satellites, apparently because of the tendency of these chromosomes to be in close physical proximity ("satellite association") during mitotic metaphase. Translocations are designated with the symbol *t* followed in parentheses by a designation of the chromosomes involved. For example, a translocation of the long arm of a chromosome 21 to the long

arm of chromosome 14 is designated t(14q21q). If a sex chromosome is involved, it is listed first, such as t(X;2). Otherwise the chromosome having the lower number is specified first.

A reciprocal translocation with exchange of nonhomologous segments results in a rearrangement, but there is no loss of genetic material. The two new chromosomes will function well in mitotic division if each possesses a single centromere, although the minute chromosome produced in a centric fusion of acrocentric chromosomes is usually lost during subsequent divisions (see Fig 18–9). The individual with such a translocation is almost always phenotypically normal and is designated a *balanced translocation carrier*. Problems arise during meiosis when the homologous chromosome segments, rearranged by translocation, pair and then segregate in all possible combinations. As shown in Figures 18–10 and 18–11, the translocation carriers can form gametes having different chromosome contents, depending on the segregation patterns of segments and centromeres. A normal gamete can be produced and will result in a normal individual producing normal gametes and who therefore has no increased risk of a chromosome abnormality in his

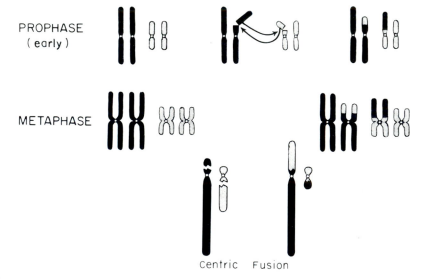

PROPHASE (early)

METAPHASE

Centric Fusion

FIG 18–9.

Mechanisms of translocation. *Top,* reciprocal translocation involving the exchange of parts of nonhomologous chromosomes early in prophase. *Center,* reciprocal translocation altering the structure of the individual chromosomes and the composition of the two pairs of homologous chromosomes at metaphase. *Bottom,* the mechanism of centric fusion, a special type of translocation involving acrocentric chromosomes. Breakage at or near the centromere occurs in both chromosomes. Of the two newly produced chromosomes, one is necessarily a minute fragment that is usually lost in a subsequent cell division. (From Sohval AR: *Am J Med* 1961; 31:397. Reproduced by permission.)

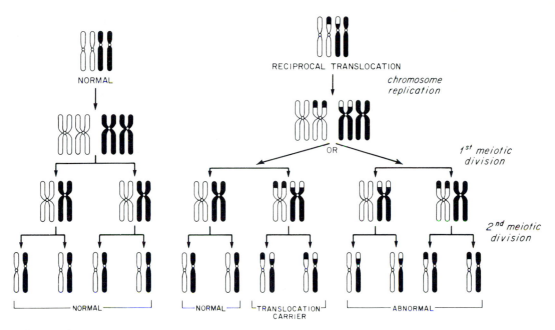

FIG 18–10.

Meiotic division of normal chromosomes and of chromosomes with reciprocal translocation. Shown here are two of the four possible abnormal chromo- some complements resulting from random segrega- tion of reciprocally translocated chromosomes.

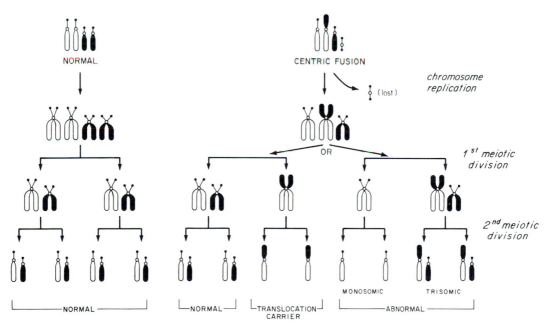

FIG 18–11.

Meiotic division of normal chromosomes and centric fusion of translocation chromosomes. As in Figure 18–10, two of the four possible abnormal chromo- some complements are illustrated.

or her offspring. Nevertheless, four of the gametes are unbalanced. In the case of reciprocal translocations, these contain two copies of a segment of one chromosome and lack a segment of another chromosome. In the case of centric fusion, they are either missing an entire chromosome or have an extra chromosome. Fertilization with a normal gamete will contribute an additional complete haploid set of chromosomes, and hence the zygotes will be chromosomally abnormal. Two of the possible gametes are balanced, containing a normal complement of structurally rearranged genetic information, and, on fertilization, will produce an individual who is phenotypically normal. This individual, however, is a balanced translocation carrier and will also produce both chromosomally normal and abnormal gametes.

Mitosis

With fertilization, the resulting zygote enters the mitotic cell cycle. During interphase, which includes G_1, S, and G_2 as previously noted, the chromosomes are dispersed within the nucleus and, with two exceptions, cannot be visualized. These exceptions are the Barr body, which, as discussed in detail in the following section, is an inactivated and condensed X chromosome, and the *Υ body,* a brightly fluorescent spot in the nuclei of male cells treated with quinacrine. Mitosis proper begins with prophase during which the chromosomes begin to condense and appear thin and threadlike. The chromosomes contract, revealing their distinctive morphologic features, and the sister chromatids become apparent, reflecting the fact that they have already replicated in the previous S period. In metaphase, the nuclear membrane disappears, the spindle appears, and the chromosomes align themselves along the midplane region of the cell. This alignment in mitosis occurs with individual chromosomes in contrast to the alignment of paired homologues that is characteristic of the first meiotic division. In anaphase, the centromeres separate, and the chromosomes migrate to opposite poles of the cell. Telophase begins when these chromosomes have reached the poles and begin to lose their distinct shapes. Formation of two new nuclear membranes and cell division complete telophase. Mitotic division thereafter occurs repetitively and, with rare exceptions, transmits the complete genome of the zygote to each successive progeny cell. The processes of differentiation result in selective expression and nonexpression of parts of the genome that determine specific cellular characteristics, including morphology, metabolic properties, and capacity to replicate.

Nondisjunction can occur during mitosis in a manner similar to that described for nondisjunction during meiosis II and results in monosomic and trisomic cells. Anaphase lag can occur in mitosis, producing a normal and a monosomic cell line. Depending on the stage of development during which the nondisjunction or anaphase lag occurs, some fraction of the cells in the body will contain aneuploid chromosome complements. As mentioned earlier, an individual with different cellular genotypes that originated from a single cell is termed mosaic, or *mixoploid.* In general, the earlier that the abnormal division occurs during development, the greater the proportion of aneuploid cells. There appear to be influences, however, that select against or for survival of certain cell lines. Hence, the final proportions of chromosomally normal and abnormal cells in a mosaic allow only a crude estimate of the timing of the nondisjunction or anaphase lag. The importance of mosaicism is that the expression of the abnormal complement may be modified by the normal cell line, producing individuals whose phenotype is intermediate between the normal and the full disease state.

Single-Active-X Hypothesis

The single-active-X, or Lyon, hypothesis (Fig 18–12) is essential for understanding both normal X-chromosome function and certain sex chromosome disorders. Proposed in 1961 by Lyon and by several others simultaneously, this principle states that in females, at an early stage of embryonic development, one of the two normal X chromosomes is functionally inactivated in all somatic cells. This inactivation is irreversible and applies to all functions except replication of that X chromosome. Whether it is the maternal or paternal X chromosome that is inactivated in a given cell is both random and mutually exclusive; that is, the identity of the inactivated X chromosome (maternal or paternal) does not affect, nor is it affected by the identity of the inactivated X chromosome in any other cell (Lyon, 1972, 1974). During interphase the inactive X is visible as a densely stained area adjacent to the nuclear membrane and is called the *nuclear chromatin,* or *Barr*

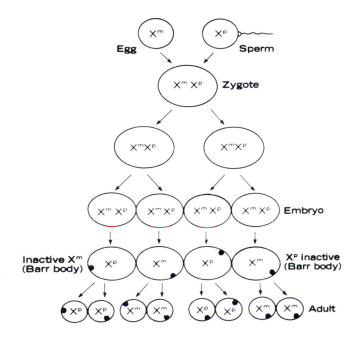

FIG 18–12.
Diagrammatic representation of X chromosome inactivation. (From Fralkow PJ: *N Engl J Med* 1974; 291:26. Reproduced by permission.)

body (Fig 18–13). The maximal number of Barr bodies is one less than the number of X chromosomes present. Thus, a normal male and a female with Turner's syndrome (45,X) have no Barr bodies. A normal female and a male with Klinefelter's syndrome (47,XXY) have one Barr body, and a triple-X (47,XXX) female has two Barr bodies. Sex chromatin status is usually evaluated by means of a buccal smear in which epithelial cells are scraped from the inner cheek and their DNA stained. One hundred or more cells are examined and their Barr body count tabulated to give the percentage that show Barr bodies. In normal females, at least 20% of buccal epithelial cells contain Barr bodies, whereas in normal males the cells showing clumped nuclear chromatin that meets the criteria for a Barr body are, at most, 1% to 2%. For diagnostic purposes a person having 5% or more cells with Barr bodies is *chromatin positive*. A person with no Barr bodies is *chromatin negative*.

Normal males have only a single X chromosome, namely, that which was inherited from the mother, and the genes on this X chromosome are expressed. Normal females, however, have two X chromosomes, one of which was inherited from each parent. As shown in Figure 18–12, during development one or the other X chromosome is inactivated in each somatic cell. On the average, in the adult female there will be about equal numbers of cells with active maternally and paternally derived X chromosomes. The inactivation, however, occurs early in embryonic life, apparently at about day 16, when there are a relatively small number of primordial somatic cells destined for certain tissues and functions. Thus, there is a finite probability that a deficiency encoded on one X chromosome will be expressed because of disproportional inactivation of the X with the normal gene. Correspondingly, some female carriers of X-linked recessive disorders cannot be detected by tests of function because of disproportionate inactivation of the X chromosome with the abnormal gene. Since X inactivation does not occur in oocytes, this will not affect the inheritance of the X chromosome.

SEXUAL DIFFERENTIATION

Normal sexual development depends on the normal function of genes both on the X chromosomes and on the autosomes, as well as, in the case of males, on the Y chromosome. It has long

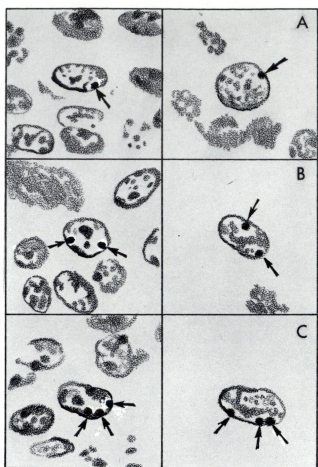

FIG 18–13.
Barr bodies in nuclei of cells from human skin *(left)* and buccal mucosa *(right)*. **A,** XX normal female. **B,** XXXY male with mental deficiency. **C,** XXXXY eunuch with micro-orchism and mental deficiency.

been recognized that the presence of a Y chromosome leads to male development. Furthermore, since the features of Turner's syndrome have been observed in individuals with one X chromosome and an isochromosome resulting from centric fusion of the long arms of the Y[46,Xi(Yq)], it seems likely that the short arm of the Y chromosome contains the gene or genes that determine male sex. The observation in highly inbred strains of mice that females reject skin grafts from males led to the identification of the *H-Y antigen*, a Y-linked plasma membrane transplantation antigen that has been highly conserved during mammalian evolution. A second and related, but not identical, antigen is called *serologically detectable male* (SDM) *antigen*. Several assays for H-Y type antigens have been developed, but each has its limitations. H-Y antigen has been claimed by some to be the testis-determining substance that directs the initial steps leading to differentiation

of the bipotential embryonic gonad as a testis. The presence of a testis nearly always signals the presence of H-Y antigen, but the presence of H-Y antigen may or may not be accompanied by testis development. Recent data, however, from clinical and laboratory studies in humans and mice indicate that neither H-Y transplantation antigen nor the SDM antigen is the primary cause of male gonadal determination (Silvers et al., 1982). Page and his co-workers (1987a, 1987b) have identified a Y-specific gene that has been named testis-determining factor (TDF), which appears to be present in most cases of XX males and absent in most cases of XY females. The TDF gene encodes for a zinc-finger protein. This class of proteins is associated with regulation of transcription. Therefore, it is reasonable to postulate that TDF controls differentiation of the indeterminate gonad. However, the TDF gene does not appear to be the complete answer since some XX males and all

XX true hermaphrodites lack TDF (Mittwoch, 1988; de la Chapelle, 1988). At this time, firm proof that any one gene or substance is the factor that determines human sex is lacking.

According to most current models, a gene usually present on the Y chromosome (most likely Yp) induces the bipotential embryonic gonad to differentiate into a testis. Once male gonadal sex has been determined, histologic as well as biochemical differentiation begins. A nonsteroidal substance secreted locally causes regression of the müllerian ducts. Androgens are produced by the fetal testis, but their uptake into cell cytoplasm and nucleus is dependent on the normal function of a specific androgen receptor that is encoded by the X chromosome and is present in probably all cells of both normal males and females. This androgen receptor is either completely absent or markedly defective (Amrhein et al., 1976) in complete testicular feminization, an X-linked recessive disorder (Meyer et al., 1975) analogous to the *Tfm* mutation well characterized in the mouse (Lyon and Hawkes, 1970). The clinical features of this and other relevant disorders of sexual development are described in a later section.

In normal males the synthesis of androgen stimulates development of the wolffian duct system. Even with a normal testis and wolffian system, proper differentiation of the male external genitalia requires the presence of the enzyme steroid 5α-reductase (Imperato-McGinley et al., 1979). This enzyme converts testosterone to dihydrotestosterone, is present normally in cells throughout the body, and is encoded by a locus on an autosomal chromosome. Deficiency of 5α-reductase results in a distinctive form of male pseudohermaphroditism characterized by ambiguous genitalia, a distinctly male puberty, and the absence of gynecomastia (Griffin and Wilson, 1980).

In the absence of the testis-determining factor, the bipotential gonad differentiates into an ovary, although normal ovarian development requires the presence of a second X chromosome. In the absence of androgen, the primitive wolffian system involutes, and the external genitalia become female. The müllerian system differentiates independent of the ovary, showing equally good development if no gonad is present.

When only a single X chromosome is present, as is the case in 45,X Turner's syndrome, the external genitalia and müllerian duct system are normal in the newborn, but ovarian develop-ment has been interrupted at a primitive stage. The resulting streak gonad is responsible for the sterility, primary amenorrhea, and failure to develop secondary sexual characteristics that are seen in these patients.

The exposure of a genetic female fetus to high levels of androgens, either from maternal sources or in a fetus having a masculinizing type of adrenogenital syndrome, results in female pseudohermaphroditism with varying degrees of virilization of the external genitalia but normal müllerian structures and ovaries and absent wolffian structures.

Characterization of normal and abnormal sexual development thus requires information regarding the genetic sex, the gonadal sex, and the phenotypic sex of individuals. Normal sexual development depends on the functions of gene loci on both the autosomes and sex chromosomes, as well as on a hormonally normal intrauterine environment. More extensive reviews can be found in Simpson (1976) and Saenger (1984).

GENETIC DISORDERS

Genetic disorders can be classified into three major groups: (1) chromosome disorders, (2) mendelian or single gene disorders, and (3) multifactorial disorders.

Chromosome Disorders

Chromosome disorders result from abnormalities in the number or makeup of chromosomes that can be visualized with the microscope. The commonest are aneuploid conditions, such as trisomies and monosomies, and chromosome rearrangements that result in deletions or additions of recognizable amounts of chromosome substance. Less often there are more complex defects, such as the formation of *ring chromosomes*, in which the normally free ends are joined, or *isochromosomes*, made up of two short arms or two long arms joined at a centromere, or *dicentric chromosomes*, having two centromeres. Any of these abnormalities can be present in all cells or as a mosaic in which two or occasionally more chromosomally distinct cell lines are present. The specific disorders involving individual autosomal chromosomes differ from the sex chromosome disorders in both frequency and severity. For both autosome and sex chromosome disorders, the frequencies of conception differ markedly from those at birth, since many are lethal in utero. As a group, however, chromosome disorders are recognized clinically by the malformations that they produce. In some individuals with major chromosome abnormalities detected in screening consecutive newborns, there are no accompanying physical features that would indicate the presence of the chromosome abnormality. The physician must consider obtaining a karyotype analysis in instances of unexplained fetal or neonatal demise, particularly when dysmorphic features are present, or when development is retarded, as manifested by small size, failure to thrive, or microcephaly. Many of the major chromosome abnormalities that are compatible with survival produce some degree of mental retardation.

Most of these disorders occur as sporadic cases, arising from an error in gametogenesis in one or the other parent. Although many are potentially heritable in classic mendelian patterns, few are actually transmitted because of the frequently reduced fertility resulting from decreased survival, physical abnormalities of both functional and cosmetic importance, mental retardation, or actual sterility. Thus, in most instances, risks of recurrence are calculated not according to mendelian principles but, instead, on a strictly empirical basis. Hence, it is essential that the physician be familiar with the incidence and recurrence risks for each specific chromosome disorder encountered.

Autosomal disorders are present in about 1 per 256 live births (Hook and Hamerton, 1977). The commonest type of autosomal abnormality results from nondisjunction in meiosis or, less often, in an early mitotic division. Such nondisjunction usually produces trisomic or monosomic (or both) cell lines. Although such nondisjunctional events are often lethal in utero (see the section on spontaneous abortion), certain trisomies account for a substantial proportion of congenital malformations. The frequency of autosomal trisomies in live-born infants is 1 per 704 (Hook and Hamerton, 1977).

Structural rearrangements are the commonest of the autosomal abnormalities in live-born children, occurring at the rate of 1 per 403. The majority of these, 1 per 515 live births, are present as balanced translocations, thereby providing a complete chromosome complement and producing no phenotypic abnormality. Unbalanced translocations with an abnormal chromosome complement and an observable disorder, however, are present in 1 per 1,852 live births (Hook and Hamerton, 1977).

Considering the fact that there are only 2 sex chromosomes but there are 44 autosomes, the incidence of sex chromosome disorders in live births (1 per 478) seems inordinately high. This is understandable in terms of differential survival. The defects produced by the sex chromosome abnormalities are less lethal and, in general, less damaging. Only monosomy Y (45,Y) appears to be incompatible with life. Although XO conceptions exhibit a high rate of fetal wastage, some 45 X individuals survive to birth and beyond.

Single Gene Disorders

Single gene defects result from submicroscopic changes in individual genes. Usually these changes involve only a single nucleotide base in the DNA, and occasionally several bases are deleted or inserted, but the changes are small relative to those in the chromosome disorders. The mode of inheritance depends on whether the mutant gene is located on an autosome or a sex chromosome and on whether it is dominant or recessive. The manifestations of a mutant gene on the X chromosome differ in males and females. If the mutant gene is on an autosome, it is present in males and females with equal frequency. A disorder is said to be *dominant* when it is manifest as a disease in the heterozygote, in other words, an individual having a normal gene on one chromosome and a mutant alternative form, or *allele,* of this gene on the other chromosome of the pair. *Recessive* disorders are those that are expressed only when they are unopposed by a normal gene, in other words, when both alleles specify a disorder in the case of the paired autosomal loci and in males whose single X chromosome bears a mutant gene. To date, 3,368 mendelian phenotypes have been described (McKusick, 1988). Of these, 1,827 are autosomal dominant, 1,298 are autosomal recessive, and 243 are X linked—almost all X-linked recessive. A complete family history is an essential part of the diagnostic evaluation and can be recorded in a pedigree using the symbols shown in Figure 18–14.

Autosomal dominant disorders often present a pattern of an affected parent having one or more affected children, as shown in Figure 18–15. The characteristics of autosomal dominant inheritance are (1) generation-to-generation

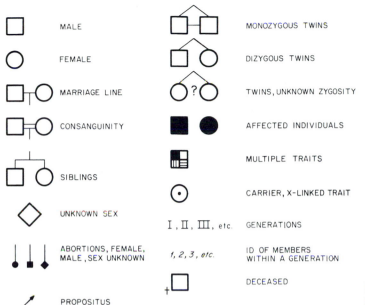

FIG 18—14.
Standard pedigree symbols.

MALE

FEMALE

MARRIAGE LINE

CONSANGUINITY

SIBLINGS

UNKNOWN SEX

ABORTIONS, FEMALE, MALE, SEX UNKNOWN

PROPOSITUS

MONOZYGOUS TWINS

DIZYGOUS TWINS

TWINS, UNKNOWN ZYGOSITY

AFFECTED INDIVIDUALS

MULTIPLE TRAITS

CARRIER, X-LINKED TRAIT

I, II, III, etc.   GENERATIONS

1, 2, 3, etc.   ID OF MEMBERS WITHIN A GENERATION

DECEASED

transmission without intervening unaffected individuals, (2) equal frequency in males and females, (3) an average of 50% of the offspring of an affected parent having the disorder, (4) transmission from either sex to either sex, and (5) no recurrence of the disorder in the offspring of individuals who have an affected parent but did not themselves inherit the gene. The role of spontaneous mutation is readily apparent since it results in the occurrence of autosomal dominant disorders in families in which there are no other similarly affected individuals. Such a new mutation presumably was present in one of the parental ga-

metes and therefore is present in all cells of the affected offspring. As a result, the offspring manifests the disorder, and since the abnormal gene is present in the gonads as well, this affected individual can transmit the gene to his or her offspring in characteristic autosomal dominant pattern. With very few exceptions there are no specific laboratory abnormalities in the autosomal dominant disorders, and hence the diagnosis relies heavily on clinical features, which often vary. The range of severity with which the characteristic features are manifest is termed *expressivity*. Some specific disorders show great variability of

A   ABNORMAL DOMINANT GENE

a   NORMAL GENE

NORMAL

AFFECTED

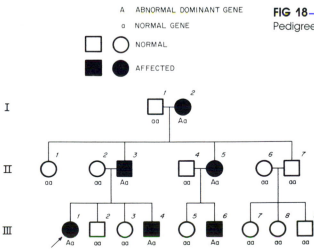

FIG 18—15.
Pedigree illustrating autosomal dominant inheritance.

expressivity, whereas in others the variations between affected individuals in the same family and even between affected individuals in different families are quite small. Occasionally an autosomal dominant disorder will appear to skip a generation, producing characteristic abnormalities in, for example, an individual and one of his or her grandparents but not in either parent. In this case the gene is said to be *nonpenetrant,* and the disorder to show *incomplete penetrance.* When complete examinations are carried out, however, the so-called unaffected parent frequently shows milder but definite evidence of the disorder. Incomplete penetrance is probably less common than is often supposed. Although the terms *expressivity* and *penetrance* are introduced here in conjunction with autosomal dominant disorders, they are entirely general concepts referring to alterations in the expression of the genome not only for any type of genetic disorder but for normal traits as well.

Autosomal recessive disorders occur when mutant disease-producing alleles are present at a locus on both chromosomes of the pair. Figure 18–16 shows a pedigree in which the affected child is the product of a first-cousin marriage. *Consanguinity,* or relatedness by blood, increases the probability that when an abnormal autosomal recessive gene is present a child will inherit one such gene from both parents and thus be an affected *homozygote.* The rarer an autosomal recessive gene for a disorder is, the greater will be the proportion of affected individuals who are the products of consanguineous matings. To produce a disorder, the mutant alleles need not be identical, as they are in the homozygote, but both must be abnormal. Thus, for example, an individual with hemoglobin SS disease (sickle cell anemia) is homozygous, having a β^S-gene at the globin β-chain locus on each member of the chromosome pair, whereas a person with hemoglobin SC disease has a β^S-gene on one chromosome and a β^C-gene on the other. Yet both have red blood cell sickling disorders. An individual with paired abnormal but nonidentical alleles at a locus is termed a *genetic compound.*

The characteristics of autosomal recessive inheritance are (1) pedigrees in which unaffected parents give birth to one or more affected offspring, (2) equal frequency in males and females, (3) an average of 25% of the offspring of carrier couples having the disorder, and (4) the presence of the carrier state in all offspring of couples in

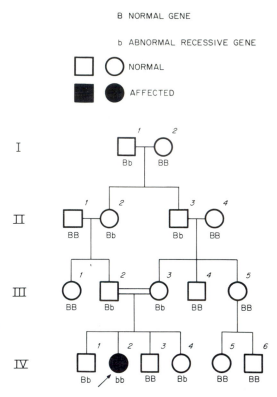

FIG 18–16.
Pedigree illustrating autosomal recessive inheritance. The double lines connecting individuals III-2 and III-3 indicate consanguinity, here a first-cousin mating.

which one person is affected and the other is homozygous normal. Specific biochemical defects have been identified in a number of autosomal recessive disorders so that precise laboratory diagnosis is often possible. In many of these disorders the carriers can also be identified by direct testing. New mutations producing abnormal autosomal recessive alleles certainly occur, but in practice this is rarely observed. Such a fresh mutation, occurring at a frequency of perhaps 1 per 10,000 genes per generation, would almost always occur in an individual who was previously normal and would thus produce only the carrier state. In turn, the carrier state would probably go unrecognized, since it seldom has any substantial effect on the health of the carrier. The birth of a child having an autosomal recessive disorder to parents in whom specific tests have shown that one but not the other is a carrier requires, after rigorous exclusion of laboratory error, that a distinction be made between nonpaternity, nonmaternity, and a new mutation.

For genes on the X chromosome, dominant and recessive patterns must again be distinguished, although nearly all the described X-linked disorders are recessive. The sine qua non of either type of X-linked inheritance is the absence of male-to-male transmission; in other words, affected males do not transmit the disorder to any of their sons. This is readily understandable, since when a male transmits his X chromosome via the sperm, the conception will be female. In contrast, to produce a son, the father must transmit his Y chromosome. Male relatives having X-linked disorders are always related to one another through an intervening female. Figure 18–17 shows the pedigree pattern of an X-linked dominant disorder, such as hypophosphatemic rickets or ornithine carbamoyltransferase deficiency. The characteristics of X-linked dominant inheritance are as follows: (1) male-to-male transmission is absent; (2) twice as many females are affected as males; (3) all female offspring of an affected male are themselves affected; (4) on the average, 50% of both male and female offspring of an affected female are themselves affected; and (5) the manifest severity of the disorder is greater in males than in females, since the latter have a normal gene on their second X chromosome, and this appears to ameliorate the abnormalities.

Correspondingly, since the male has only a single X chromosome, X-linked recessive disorders will be expressed in males who are said to be *hemizygous* for the X chromosome, whereas females will be carriers but will not (except in rare instances) manifest the signs and symptoms of the disorder. A typical pedigree is shown in Figure 18–18. The characteristics of X-linked recessive inheritance are as follows: (1) male-to-male transmission is absent; (2) there is a marked preponderance of affected males; (3) of the offspring of a carrier female, an average of 50% of the sons will be affected, and 50% of the daughters will be carriers; (4) all of the daughters of an affected male will be carriers; and (5) the disorder does not recur in the progeny of unaffected sons or noncarrier daughters. Occasionally females manifesting X-linked recessive disorders are encountered and in most instances are found by family studies to be either heterozygous but affected presumably because of disproportionate Lyon-type inactivation of the X chromosome with the normal gene or homozygous, the father being affected and the mother a carrier of the disorder. Less often such

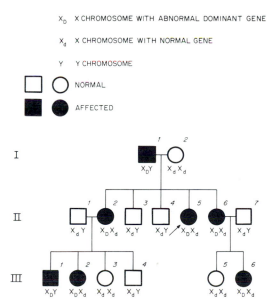

FIG 18–17.
Pedigree illustrating X-linked dominant inheritance.

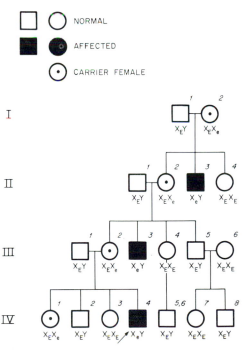

FIG 18–18.
Pedigree illustrating X-linked recessive inheritance.

an affected "female" will actually be 45 X or 46 XY with testicular feminization (see the section on single gene defects) and thus be hemizygous for the X chromosome.

The occurrence of new mutations is readily apparent in the X-linked disorders as, for example, in Duchenne-type muscular dystrophy. In this, the most severe type of muscular dystrophy, affected males show muscle weakness by about age 5 years, require a wheelchair or similar aids by their teens, and die by their early twenties. Since affected males never reproduce and, hence, never transmit the gene for Duchenne dystrophy, one might expect this disorder to decrease in frequency over the years and eventually disappear. Instead its frequency is thought to be nearly constant, with the genes that are lost each generation through the early death of affected males being replaced through mutation. The locus for Duchenne-type muscular dystrophy is on the X chromosome since the disorder follows an X-linked recessive pattern, and the mutation rate at that locus is about 1 per 10,000 per generation. This mutation rate applies to the Duchenne locus wherever the X chromosome is found, and since females have two X chromosomes and males have one, this new mutation is twice as likely to occur in females as in males. In this way the female becomes a heterozygous carrier of the gene for Duchenne-type muscular dystrophy and may have abnormally elevated levels of the muscle enzymes such as creatine phosphokinase or certain other laboratory abnormalities but will not have clinical manifestations. As noted in Figure 18–18, each of her sons has a 50% risk of being affected, and each of her daughters has a 50% risk of being a carrier.

When the diagnosis of Duchenne-type muscular dystrophy is established in a boy whose family history is negative, a new mutation is likely to be the basis. Accordingly, the chances that the mother is a carrier through new mutation are two thirds, and there is a one-third chance that the new mutation occurred in the affected son. Laboratory tests may or may not help in deciding whether the mother is a carrier. The birth of a second affected son means that the mother is surely a carrier since the alternative explanation, that of males affected through two separate mutations, would have a probability of $(1/10,000)^2$, or 1/100,000,000! It is in this and similar types of rather complex situations that a consultation with a medical geneticist can be particularly helpful.

Multifactorial Disorders

The group of multifactorial disorders encompasses a large number of quite heterogeneous abnormalities in which multiple genetic loci of smaller individual effects and environmental influences act together to produce defects. These disorders are sometimes referred to as *polygenic,* but though reflecting the multiplicity of gene loci involved, this term overlooks the great importance of environmental factors. The characteristics of multifactorial inheritance include (1) the simulation of mendelian pedigree patterns in individual families but a complex, nonmendelian pattern for the disorder when many affected families are compared; (2) a recurrence risk that is generally about 5%; (3) altered sex ratio (i.e., more males affected than females or vice versa); (4) increased recurrence rate with increased severity of the disorder; (5) a further increase in the recurrence rate with each affected offspring; (6) increased risk of occurrence in the offspring of an affected individual of the less likely sex (e.g., there are three times as many males with pyloric stenosis as females; the risk of pyloric stenosis in offspring of a parent with pyloric stenosis is much greater if the affected parent is female rather than male); and (7) the presence of the disease in microforms (i.e., states in which one or more of the characteristic manifestations of the disorder are present, but their expression is less severe). Examples of multifactorial disorders include anencephaly, meningomyelocele, cleft lip (alone or with cleft palate), pyloric stenosis, congenital dislocation of the hip, and various forms of congenital heart disease. The occurrence and recurrence risks are derived from empirical data about each specific disorder (Fraser and Hunter, 1975; Nora and Nora, 1976; Holmes et al., 1976) and a knowledge of the principles of multifactorial inheritance (Carter, 1968; Fraser, 1970).

GENETIC DISORDERS IN GYNECOLOGY

Abnormalities of Sexual Differentiation

Sex Chromosome Abnormalities

Turner's Syndrome.— Most often the Turner phenotype is associated with a 45,X chromosome constitution. Turner's syndrome occurs with a frequency of 1 per 2,500 live "female" births. The severity of this disorder is reflected in the fact that only about 1 in 64 conceptions that have a 45,X chromosome complement result in live births, the remainder being aborted spontaneously or stillborn. The diagnosis may be suspected at birth on the basis of small size and the presence of congenital lymphedema, which is usually transient but with slower disappearance of puffiness over the dorsal aspects of the toes and fingers. About 20% of patients have congenital cardiovascular malformations, the most frequent (about 70%) of which is coarctation of the aorta. Many patients are not diagnosed until later, often at puberty (Fig 18–19), based on the findings of short stature (the height rarely exceeding 152

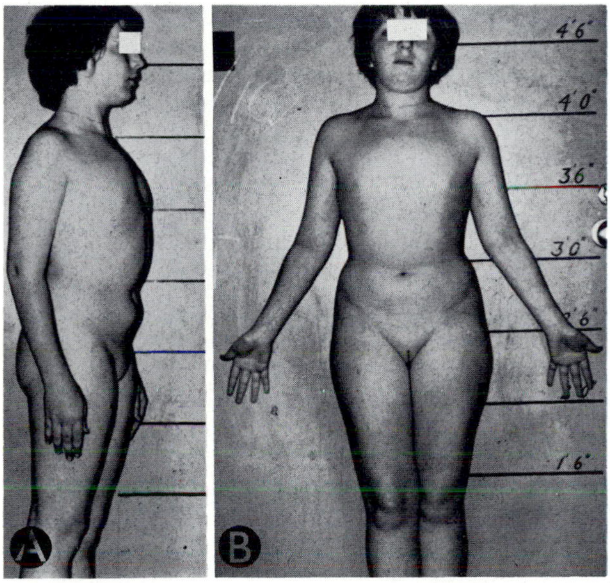

FIG 18–19.
A and **B,** Turner's syndrome in a 16-year-old apparent female with primary amenorrhea. 17-Ketosteroid and 17-hydroxysteroid values were normal, but the FSH was 105 mIU. Patient was chromatin negative, with castrate vaginal smear and absent pubic hair. There is mild cubitus valgus but no webbing of the neck. **C,** karyotype of patient with Turner's syndrome. There are 44 autosomes and a single X chromosome. (**A** and **B** from Kupperman HS: *Human Endocrinology.* Philadelphia, FA Davis Co, 1963. Reproduced by permission.)

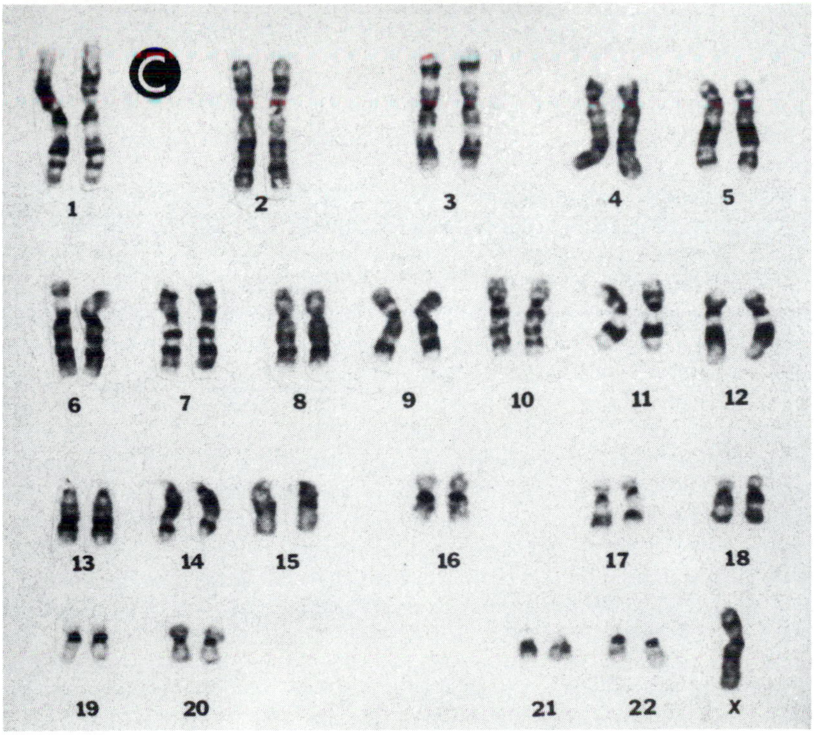

cm), primary amenorrhea, infantile but female genitalia, a shield-shaped chest with widely spaced nipples, hypoplastic nails, and signs of estrogen deficiency. About one half of the patients also show webbing of the posterolateral aspect of the neck, a short fourth metacarpal, and excessive numbers of pigmented cutaneous nevi. Intelligence is usually normal, mental retardation being present in about 10% of the cases. Urinary gonadotropin levels are markedly elevated. The ovaries consist of white streaks of gonadal tissue with absence or marked hypoplasia of germinal elements, and the patients are infertile (Smith, 1976). Most of the patients will have a 45,X karyotype and will be chromatin negative by buccal smear. About 30% of patients with Turner's syndrome stigmata, however, will be mosaics, most often 45,X/46,XX. These individuals are often chromatin positive. In general, the smaller the proportion of 45,X cells, the fewer the abnormalities. The karyotype of peripheral blood lymphocytes, however, may not always reflect precisely the proportions of normal and abnormal cells elsewhere. It has been postulated that some of the patients with Turner's syndrome who have been reported to be fertile are, in fact, X/XX mosaics who lack 46,XX cells in the karyotyped peripheral blood lymphocytes and the buccal epithelium. Mosaics with 45,X/46,XY are also seen, and these individuals may be masculinized to varying degrees. Dysgenetic gonads that contain a cell line with a Y chromosome are predisposed to gonadal malignancy, particularly gonadoblastoma (Scully, 1970a). Thus, when a cell line containing Y chromosome is identified in such a mosaic individual, prophylactic surgical removal of these dysgenetic gonads should be considered. Gonadal extirpation is not indicated for 45,X or 45,X/46,XX patients. These individuals can derive great psychological and social benefits from treatment with estrogens to promote the development of secondary sexual characteristics.

Other patients with features of Turner's syndrome have one normal X chromosome but are missing a portion of the second X chromosome, which has become abnormal by any of several possible mechanisms (Fig 18–20). Deletions resulting in the loss of parts of the X chromosome short arm, termed Xp, or long arm, Xq, produce phenotypic changes (Wyss et al., 1982). Patients with terminal Xp deletions have somatic traits characteristic of Turner's syndrome, but gonadal function is generally preserved. More extensive

Xp deletions, extending to the proximal portion of band p11, are associated in most cases with a complete Turner's syndrome phenotype, including gonadal dysgenesis. With regard to the long arm, a large deletion of Xq, with the breakpoint at or proximal to band q21, produces gonadal dysgenesis with primary amenorrhea and, in one half of the cases, somatic Turner's syndrome features. A terminal deletion of Xq, with the breakpoint distal to q22, is generally associated with pure gonadal dysgenesis. In these cases, in contrast to those with more extensive deletions, secondary amenorrhea is particularly characteristic.

These deletions can arise through nonreciprocal translocation or the formation of isochromosomes in which two X chromosomes break at the centromere and rejoin incorrectly, with the short arms or the long arms fused to one another. In both cases, the imbalance arises when one of the two rearranged chromosomes is subsequently lost, usually during meiosis (Lindsten, 1963; Böök et al., 1973; Yanagisawa and Yokoyama, 1975). Some or all of the features of Turner's syndrome are produced when a translocation involving the X chromosome and an autosome results in the loss of critical portions of the X chromosome (Dorus et al., 1979). Structural abnormalities of the X chromosome may produce a corresponding alteration in the Barr bodies. In general, when one X chromosome is normal and the other is structurally abnormal, it is the latter that is inactivated to form the Barr body, in marked contrast to the random choice for inactivation when two normal X chromosomes are present. Thus, a patient with an X deletion may show an unusually small Barr body, whereas one with additions to the X or with an isochromosome X may show large Barr bodies. These or any other abnormalities suspected from the results of a buccal smear must be confirmed by a complete karyotypic analysis (Polani et al., 1970).

Females with a 47,XXX chromosome constitution have been identified with a frequency of 1 per 1,100 live female births. These females appear normal at birth. Some later exhibit mild mental retardation, delayed neuromuscular maturation, learning and language disorders (Robinson et al., 1983), menstrual disturbances, and/or infertility (Puck et al., 1983).

Sex chromosome aneuploidies with still larger numbers of X chromosomes (48,XXXX, 49,XXXXX, etc.) are seen but are progressively rarer with increasing numbers of X chromosomes.

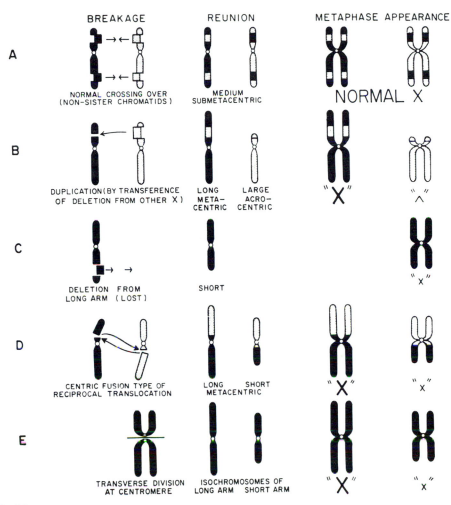

BREAKAGE   REUNION   METAPHASE APPEARANCE

A

NORMAL CROSSING OVER   MEDIUM   NORMAL X
(NON-SISTER CHROMATIDS)   SUBMETACENTRIC

B

DUPLICATION (BY TRANSFERENCE   LONG   LARGE   "X"   " ∧ "
OF DELETION FROM OTHER X)   META-   ACRO-
                                   CENTRIC   CENTRIC

C

DELETION FROM   SHORT   "x"
LONG ARM (LOST)

D

CENTRIC FUSION TYPE OF   LONG   SHORT   "X"   "x"
RECIPROCAL TRANSLOCATION   METACENTRIC

E

TRANSVERSE DIVISION   ISOCHROMOSOMES OF   "X"   "x"
AT CENTROMERE   LONG ARM   SHORT ARM

FIG 18–20.
Mechanisms of translocation producing structural abnormalities of X chromosome through improper reunion after breakage. Abnormally large metacentric X chromosomes are designated **"X."** Small Xs are represented as "x" or "∧", depending on location of centromere. Black chromosome is derived from one parent, light from the other. (From Sohval AR: *Fertil Steril* 1963; 14:180. Reproduced by permission.)

The frequency of mental retardation increases with the degree of aneuploidy, but other features are quite variable. Usually sexual development is normal, and these individuals are fertile. Although buccal smears show increased numbers of Barr bodies (the maximal number being one less than the total number of X chromosomes), only a small percentage of cells will show the maximal number, the remainder showing fewer. As before, although the smear is an appropriate screening test, a full karyotype is required if a chromosome abnormality is suspected (Gerald, 1976).

Klinefelter's Syndrome.—Klinefelter's syndrome is characterized by small, firm testes, azoospermia, gynecomastia, and elevated concentrations of plasma and urinary gonadotropins. The clinical phenotype is usually associated with a 47,XXY karyotype and occurs with a frequency of 1 per 900 live "male" births but at much higher frequencies of approximately 1 per 50 stillborn males and 1 per 10 azoospermic adult males, thus being the most prevalent of the major sex chromosome disorders and the most frequent disorder of sexual differentiation. Studies of chromosome markers have shown that in about 60% of these individuals the nondisjunction that led to the presence of the extra sex chromosome occurred in the maternal gametes, whereas in 40% of the cases the nondisjunction was paternal. Affected males usually appear normal until puberty, at which time they develop eunuchoid body proportions, gynecomastia, and sparse facial and body hair (Fig 18–21). Height may be increased, with the lower extremities being relatively long. Lower than average intelligence is common and may ac-

count for the behavioral abnormalities that are frequently described (Walzer and Gerald, 1975). At puberty the testes remain small, rarely being larger than 2 cm in greatest diameter, and produce neither sperm nor adequate amounts of testosterone. The testes are characterized by hyalinized and fibrotic seminiferous tubules, hypoplastic interstitial cells, and absent spermatogenesis. Levels of urinary gonadotropins are increased. A buccal smear for screening will be chromatin positive, and karyotype will usually show a 47,XXY chro-

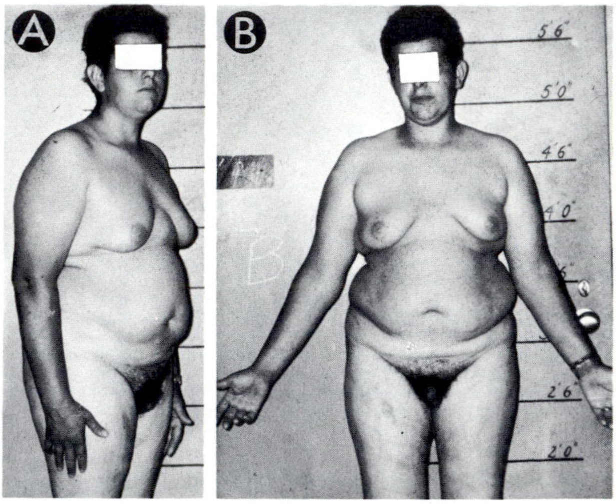

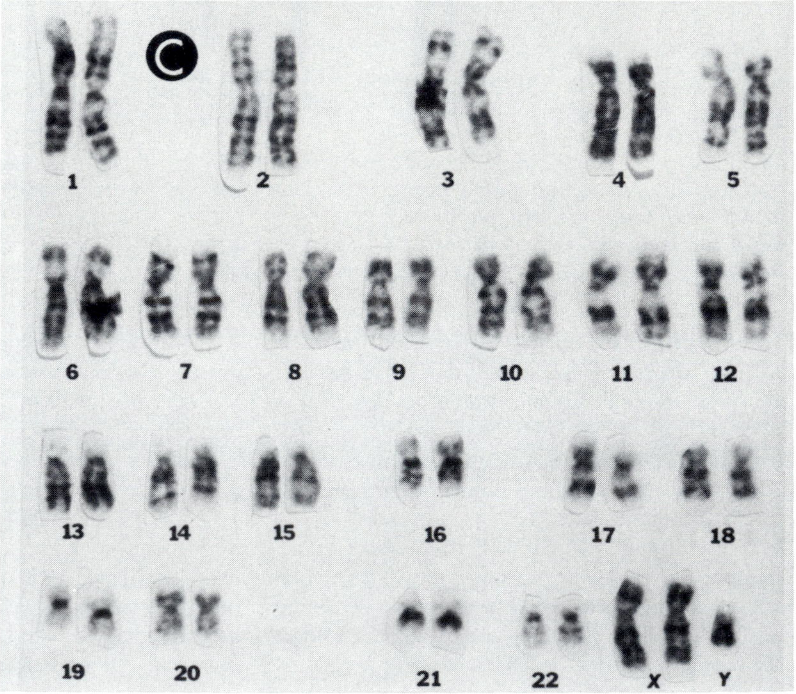

FIG 18–21.
A and **B,** Klinefelter's syndrome in 33-year-old chromatin-positive patient. Weight was 96.6 kg and height 171.5 cm. The small external genitalia and female fat distribution are typical. Note extreme gynecomastia and sparsity of body hair. **C,** karyotype of a patient with Klinefelter's syndrome, 47,XXY. **(A** and **B** from Kupperman HS: *Human Endocrinology.* Philadelphia, FA Davis Co 1963. Reproduced by permission.)

mosome constitution. Some individuals with the stigmata of Klinefelter's syndrome are found to be mosaics for XXY/XY or to have other karyotypic abnormalities such as 48,XXYY or 48,XXXY. Therapy with testosterone can produce virilization but does not affect the sterility.

Nondisjunction of the Y chromosomes at the paternal second meiotic division results in 47,XYY. The frequency of XYY is about 1 per 1,000 male births. The phenotypic manifestations, particularly regarding behavior, have been the subject of much public and scientific controversy. Increased height is a frequent feature, intelligence may be decreased, and nodulocystic acne at adolescence may be severe (Philip et al., 1976). These individuals are fully masculinized and fertile. Interestingly, there have been no reported instances of XYY in father and son, indicating that the risk of transmission is very low. Whether there is any increase in the frequencies of aggressive and criminal behavior is presently unresolved, but a recent study by Witken et al. (1976) of a large group of Danish males has shown that criminal behavior is no more frequent in XYY males than in other males having comparable reductions in intelligence.

Single Gene Defects

The single gene disorders discussed in this section are inherited in simple mendelian autosomal recessive patterns, with the exception of testicular feminization, which is inherited in an X-linked recessive pattern.

Familial gonadal dysgenesis, XX type, is a rare autosomal recessive disorder in which streak gonads are present in phenotypic females who have a 46,XX karyotype and usually lack the somatic stigmata of Turner's syndrome (Simpson et al., 1971; Perez-Ballester et al., 1970). Estrogens are deficient, and gonadotropins are elevated. There have also been a few reports of gonadal dysgenesis in phenotypic females with a 46,XY karyotype. Some of these have been familial in a pattern compatible with either X-linked recessive inheritance or autosomal dominant inheritance with expression only in males (Espiner et al., 1970; Chemke et al., 1970). Although the specific defects in these disorders are not known, they may prove to be developmental abnormalities in which the basic lesion is in the gonad and the associated abnormalities are secondary to hypogonadism.

5α-Reductase deficiency is a form of male pseudohermaphroditism that is inherited in an autosomal recessive pattern. It is an inborn error of steroid metabolism involving deficient conversion of testosterone to 5α-dihydrotestosterone. At birth only the external genitalia of affected males are abnormal. The phallus is small and the urethra opens on the perineum as part of a urogenital sinus. In most instances the urogenital sinus consists of an anterior urethral orifice with a blind vaginal pouch posteriorly. The scrotum is cleft and the testes, which are otherwise normal, may be in the inguinal canals, the abdomen, or labioscrotal folds. These clinical abnormalities led to the designation "pseudovaginal perineoscrotal hypospadias" prior to the recognition of the enzyme defect. Many of these children have been reared as females, with the error in sex assignment recognized only at puberty when masculinization occurs (Opitz et al., 1972; Imperato-McGinley et al., 1974; Imperato-McGinley et al., 1979). The penis enlarges to adult proportions, the cleft scrotum elongates, the testes enlarge, muscle mass increases, the voice deepens, and body hair growth follows a male pattern. In addition to a distinctly male puberty, the absence of gynecomastia is an important feature that distinguishes this disorder from other forms of male pseudohermaphroditism. Clearly it is exceedingly important to be aware of this disorder to avoid serious errors resulting from inappropriate management and incorrect sex assignment. The diagnosis should be suspected in any child with the genital ambiguities just noted and a male karyotype and can be established by identification in cultured skin fibroblasts of decreased conversion of testosterone to 5α-dihydrotestosterone. This decrease is due to deficiency of the enzyme steroid 5α-reductase. Androgen receptors that are normally present in all cells can bind both testosterone and dihydrotestosterone, but the affinity of the receptor for dihydrotestosterone is much greater. During fetal development and childhood, the circulating levels of testosterone are normally low, and the 5α-reductase deficiency in affected individuals interferes with its conversion to the more potent androgen, dihydrotestosterone, resulting in incomplete masculinization. This is overcome at puberty when testosterone increases to normal pubertal levels and sufficiently large amounts of testosterone, the weaker androgenic compound, enter the cells to produce essentially normal virilization. Parents carrying a gene for this autosomal recessive disorder show normal sexual development, but in most instances measurement of the appropriate urinary steroid indicates intermediate degrees of metabolic abnormality (Imperato-McGinley et al., 1979).

Testicular feminization includes one or more X-linked recessive disorders that produce a striking type of male pseudohermaphroditism. The external genitalia are female, as are the postpubertal secondary sex characteristics, except for the sparse or absent pubic and axillary hair (Fig 18–22). Internally, the urogenital sinus ends blindly, müllerian and wolffian structures are usually absent. The gonads consist of testes that have differentiated normally but show histologic changes resulting from the effects of cryptorchidism. Plasma androgen levels are in the normal male range. Serum LH level is increased, whereas the FSH level is usually normal (Kelch et al., 1972; Judd et al., 1972).

The syndrome of complete testicular feminization was in the past erroneously attributed to 5α-reductase deficiency. More recent studies on the basic defect have shown that in some families the affected siblings and individuals lack the cellular dihydrotestosterone-testosterone receptor and are therefore unable to initiate cytoplasmic effects and to transport androgen to its acceptor site in the nucleus where it normally interacts with chromatin to produce additional effects. This receptor-negative defect is analogous to that in the *Tfm* mutation in the mouse (Lyon and Hawkes, 1970). There are, however, presumably steps beyond those presently identified, since clinically indistinguishable patients in other families have shown normal androgen binding as well as nuclear uptake and retention (Amrhein et al., 1976). For the receptor-negative form, the defect has been shown to be located on the X chromosome and inherited in an X-linked recessive pattern (Meyer et al., 1975). As with other instances where gonadal tissue containing a Y chromosome is located intra-abdominally, gonadal extirpation should be considered to avoid the possibility of gonadal malignancy, although the magnitude of the risk of malignancy is presently controversial.

A variety of male pseudohermaphrodites, with what has been called *incomplete testicular feminization,* attributed to lesser degrees of androgen insensitivity, have been described. No specific defects have been identified to explain the clinical findings. In general, these individuals manifest some phallic enlargement, partial labioscrotal fusion, incomplete development of female secondary sexual characteristics at puberty, and pubertal hirsutism or even frank virilization.

In female pseudohermaphroditism, the karyotype is 46,XX, and the ovaries and müllerian structures are normally developed, but the external genitalia are virilized to some degree. *Congenital virilizing adrenal hyperplasia* is the commonest cause of female pseudohermaphroditism. In this group of autosomal, recessively inherited disorders, deficiencies of individual or, in rare instances, coupled adrenal enzymes interrupt normal steroid biosynthesis and decrease cortisol production (Fig 18–23). As a result, the anterior pituitary is derepressed and produces increased amounts of ACTH, leading morphologically to adrenal hyperplasia and biochemically to overproduction of other adrenal steroids, many of which are either themselves androgenic or become androgenic after conversion in nonadrenal tissues. In approximately one half of the patients, the site of the specific block interferes with the production of cortisol, corticosterone, and aldosterone, leading to a sodium-losing state that is often life threatening.

At birth, clinical features in females include some degree of clitoromegaly, labial fusion, and persistence of the urogenital sinus and, depending on the specific enzyme defect, dehydration, and hypotension. Immediate therapy for affected newborns includes the replacement of the deficient steroid products and correction of the electrolyte and fluid imbalances. The clinical features beyond the newborn period and the appropriate management depend on the specific deficiency and its severity. This information is clearly important in the diagnosis and management of such patients, and the reader is referred to Liddle (1974) for further details. Because these disorders can produce genital ambiguities in both genetic males and females, accurate sex assignment by karyotype analysis is essential prior to undertaking surgical or sex hormone therapy.

Other Endocrine Disorders

Familial isolated gonadotropin deficiency results in hypogonadism in both males and females because of deficiency of both FSH and LH. The levels of the other pituitary hormones are normal. No associated somatic abnormalities have been described. Inheritance is in an autosomal recessive pattern (Ewer, 1968; Spitz et al., 1974).

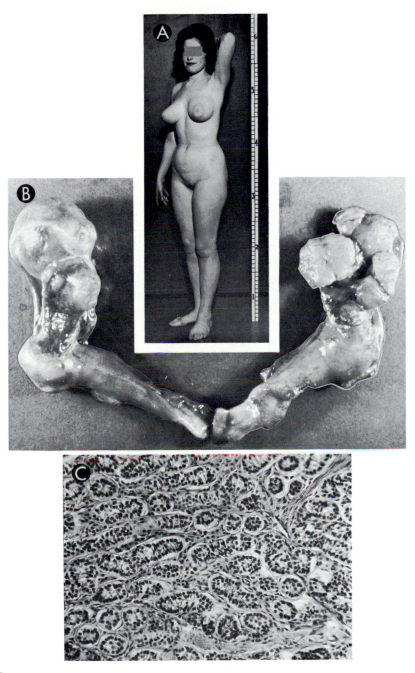

FIG 18–22.

Testicular feminization. **A,** 18-year-old apparent female with primary amenorrhea, minimal sexual hair, large breasts and areolae, but small nipples. FSH concentration before surgery: more than 13, less than 52 mIU; 17-ketosteroids, 21 mg/24 hours; 17-ketogenic steroids, 5.5 mg/24 hours; pregnanetriol, 1.2 mg/24 hours. **B,** gonads and rudimentary uterine structures removed from patient in **A.** Note nodular appearance of the gonad. **C,** photomicrograph of gonad. Immature testicular tubules are lined principally by primitive germ cells with some Sertoli's cells present. There is a marked resemblance to the fetal testis. (From Morris JM, Mahesh VB: *Am J Obstet Gynecol* 1963; 87:731. Reproduced by permission.)

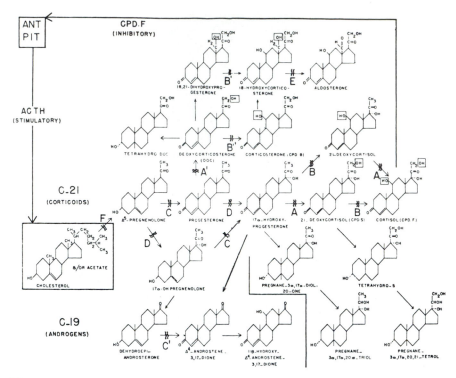

FIG 18–23.

Adrenal steroid pathways indicating sites of specific enzyme deficiencies: *A,* 21-hydroxylase; *B,* 11-hydroxylase; *C,* 3β-ol-dehydrogenase; *D,* 17-hydroxylase; *E,* 18-hydroxysteroid dehydrogenase; *F,* desmolase. (Courtesy of John F. Crigler, Jr., M.D., Harvard Medical School.)

The *Stein-Leventhal syndrome* is inherited in an autosomal dominant pattern with different manifestations in males and females and variable expressivity among members of each sex. The clinical features in females consist of oligomenorrhea, hirsutism, and polycystic ovaries, frequently with secondary amenorrhea and infertility. Males suspected of having inherited the gene occasionally manifest hirsutism. Laboratory abnormalities consist of elevated androstenedione and LH levels in affected females (Givens et al., 1971).

Müllerian Tract Anomalies

Congenital absence of the vagina has been described in a large number of patients, although its exact frequency is uncertain. Based on the analysis of more than 500 cases, Ross and Van de Wiele (1974) estimated that congenital absence of the vagina is second only to gonadal dysgenesis as a cause of primary amenorrhea. Absent vagina, however, can occur in association with several other types of malformations as an isolated abnormality or as part of several malformation syndromes (Buchta et al., 1973; Bryan et al., 1949). Most cases are thought to be sporadic, in other words, affected individuals are the only ones in their respective families to be affected. In many instances, however, the relatives have not been examined for specific müllerian tract, renal, skeletal, and other abnormalities. Hence, the ascertainment is incomplete, particularly in regard to more mildly affected individuals, and systems of classifications at present are necessarily only approximate, with many exceptions to be anticipated.

The *Rokitansky-Küster-Hauser syndrome* consists of congenital absence of the vagina and a rudimentary uterus composed of bicornuate muscular cords without or, less often, with a lumen. The ovaries, fallopian tubes, and associated ligaments are normal, as are the female secondary sexual characteristics, body proportions, endocrine functions, and karyotype. Autosomal recessive inheritance with the characteristic expression in females has been observed in some families. In many published reports the term *Rokitansky-Küster-Hauser syndrome* has been applied to patients having some of these features in association with various renal and skeletal abnormalities (Griffin et al., 1976). It seems likely that several and perhaps many different disorders are present within this broad spectrum, but their individual characteristics have not yet been resolved.

Some patients with müllerian tract malformations associated with the *Klippel-Feil anomaly,* involving varying degrees of vertebral fusion, most often in the cervical spine, have been described. Some of these patients also manifest deafness. No simple pattern of inheritance has been identified.

Absent vagina is to be distinguished from *transverse vaginal septum* or *hydrometrocolpos.* In this autosomal, recessively inherited disorder, a thick transverse membrane prevents the discharge of cervical secretions and menses. The remainder of the reproductive system is normal. Surgical removal of the septum allows full reproductive and sexual function.

Gynecologic Tumors

In the past 5 years, expression of specific genes only in association with certain malignant neoplasms has been described. These cancer-associated genes have been called *oncogenes.* In general, these genes are not foreign DNA inserted into the human genome but normal embryonic genes or growth-controlling genes that are usually turned off in differentiated cells that become derepressed or are being expressed in an unregulated manner. In cases of oncogenes that are of viral origin, there appears to always be a highly homologous human gene counterpart present in the genome (Weiss et al., 1984). Multiple mechanisms have been identified to date as causes for the reactivation of these genes. Rearrangement of chromosomal material leading to the loss of a repressor region or addition of a powerful promoter in close proximity to the embryonic gene appears to be the cause in many leukemias and lymphomas. Insertion of a viral genome containing an oncogene that is expressed during virus replication or insertion in close proximity to a normal embryonic gene leading to loss of repression or enhancement of expression are other confirmed causes. Viral genome insertion and replication can also lead to amplification or production of multiple copies of an oncogene, which in turn causes abnormal transcription or messenger RNA production. In still another model, viral insertion interferes with normal cellular growth control genes, thereby allowing undifferentiated, uncontrolled cellular growth. Other mutagenic agents such as radiation and certain chemicals may act in a similar manner to cause cancer. To date, oncogene transformation in humans has been identified for leukemias, lymphomas, carcinomas, and sarcomas (Krontiris, 1983; Kohl et al., 1984). Although the association of oncogenes and most gynecological malignancies has not been as common or as consistent, oncogene expression has been reported in ovarian cancer, cervical cancer, and uterine sarcomas (Slamon et al., 1984; Feig et al., 1984). It seems likely that the association of specific strains of papillomavirus with cervical cancer will be best explained by site-specific insertion of these viral genomes or the presence of specific oncogenes within the genome of the implicated strains (Josephs et al., 1984).

Benign cystic teratomas (or dermoid cysts) of the ovary are, by definition, composed of tissues that have differentiated from all three germ layers: the ectoderm, mesoderm, and endoderm. It has been known for years that these ovarian teratomas have a 46,XX chromosome constitution. Although theoretically these tumors could arise by any of four mechanisms during meiosis, recent studies have examined both the cytogenetic and biochemical features relating to individual chromosomes from several of the homologous pairs (Linder et al., 1975). Based on the findings that the ovarian teratomas were consistently homozygous for morphologic centromeric markers but often heterozygous for biochemical markers located at a distance from the centromeres, it was possible to demonstrate that these tumors arise from single oocytes after the first meiotic division but prior to completion of the second meiotic division. Either the second polar body is not formed or it is formed but recombines its haploid chromosome complement with that of the haploid oocyte to produce a diploid cell. In either case, this diploid cell then undergoes parthenogenic development into a benign cystic teratoma.

The *Peutz-Jeghers syndrome* is an autosomal dominant disorder consisting of multiple hamartomatous gastrointestinal polyps accompanied by abnormal melanotic pigmentation, most frequently in the buccal and perioral areas. About 5% of females with Peutz-Jeghers syndrome have primary tumors in one or both ovaries. Although various pathologic diagnoses have been assigned, Scully (1970b) has found that a substantial proportion of these show a highly distinctive architecture that he designates as a "sex cord tumor with annular tubules" and that appear to be a specific manifestation of the Peutz-Jeghers gene.

Autosomal Chromosome Disorders

Several autosomal chromosome disorders are encountered frequently enough by the gynecologists either directly or through questions from patients that they deserve mention.

Down syndrome is the commonest of the autosomal disorders, with an overall incidence of 1 per 800 live births. The clinical features include small size, hypotonia, microcephaly, characteristic facies, transverse palmar or simian creases, and cardiovascular malformations, of which ventricular septal defect is commonest. Karyotype analysis of patients indicates that in 95% of cases the abnormalities result from trisomy 21, the presence

of a third 21 chromosome in addition to the normal diploid complement, as shown in Figure 18–24. About 2% of Down syndrome patients are mosaics with both trisomy 21 and normal cell lines in blood and tissues. The remaining 3% of patients have translocation Down syndrome of the D/G or G/G type. These individuals are abnormal because they possess three copies of part or all of the long arm of a 21 chromosome, which has been translocated to a D group (numbers 13–15 chromosome), to a 22 chromosome, or to another 21 chromosome. In the case of D/G translocations, about one third of patients have a parent—more often the mother—who is a balanced D/G translocation carrier. Theoretically, random segregation of chromosomes during gametogenesis would result in one third of the viable zygotes having Down syndrome. In fact, the observed outcome is quite different and varies with the sex of the carrier parent. The frequency

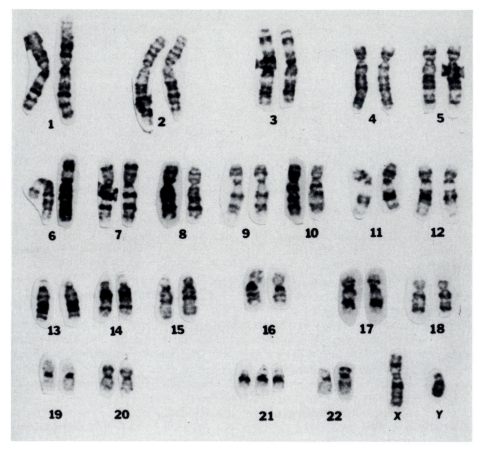

FIG 18–24.
G-banded karyotype of male with Down syndrome (47,XY,+21).

of Down syndrome of a female D/G translocation carrier is about 15%, whereas in offspring of a male translocation carrier the frequency is only about 3%. The unaffected offspring in both cases are equally divided between having normal chromosomes and being balanced translocation carriers.

Although the overall incidence of Down syndrome is 1 per 800 live births, the frequency of trisomy 21 (95% of cases of Down syndrome) increases from 1 per 2,300 live births for 20-year-old mothers to 1 per 40 live births at a maternal age of 45 years. This *maternal age effect,* the rise in frequency of meiotic nondisjunction with increasing maternal age, is seen not only in trisomy 21 but also in trisomy 18, trisomy 13, and Klinefelter's (47,XXY) syndrome. Despite this change in frequency, most children with these chromosome disorders are born to relatively young mothers because of the substantially greater total number of children born to younger age group.

The *trisomy 18 syndrome* (47,XX or XY,+18), previously called Edwards' syndrome, occurs in about 1 per 8,000 live births. It is characterized clinically by low birth weight, a clenched hand position, short sternum, and various other malformations. Affected females exceed males by a ratio of 3:1. Only about 10% of these patients survive the first year, and these show a uniform degree of severe mental retardation.

The *trisomy 13 syndrome* (47,XX or XY,+13), previously called Patau's syndrome, occurs with a frequency of about 1 per 20,000 live births. Clinical features include malformations of eye, nose, lip, and forebrain; polydactyly; and defects of the skin and posterior scalp. About 20% of these individuals survive the first year and are severely retarded.

Miscellaneous Genetic Disorders With Female Reproductive Tract Anomalies

In addition to the conditions just described, many other genetic disorders that involve genital abnormalities are encountered primarily by the gynecologist. Further details regarding these disorders are available in Smith (1976) and McKusick (1988).

Ambiguous or malformed external genitalia are often found in Robinow's syndrome, trisomy 18 syndrome, and 18q syndrome and are found less frequently in de Lange's syndrome, fetal alcohol syndrome, and popliteal web syndrome.

Müllerian tract abnormalities, including bicornuate uterus, double vagina, or both, are reported frequently in the cryptophthalmos syndrome, Johanson-Blizzard syndrome, and trisomy 13 and occasionally in Robert's syndrome and trisomy 18.

Hypogonadism is frequent in Down syndrome, Prader-Willi syndrome, myotonic dystrophy, De Sanctis–Cacchione syndrome, and Laurence-Moon-Biedl syndrome and occasionally in Noonan's syndrome, multiple lentigines syndrome, Albright's hereditary osteodystrophy, and Fanconi's anemia.

SPONTANEOUS ABORTION

Chromosome anomalies are present in a substantial proportion of abortuses. As reviewed by Carr (1971), most chromosomally abnormal conceptuses that are aborted spontaneously do so within the first trimester, 40% to 50% of such abortuses showing chromosome abnormalities. Most of these abnormalities are numerical, of which about 45% consist of trisomies, about 25% of polyploidy, and about 20% of 45,X. Retrospective and prospective karyotype analysis of 1,500 spontaneous abortions by Boue et al. (1975) have yielded useful epidemiologic information. The presence of a chromosomal abnormality in a spontaneously aborted first conception was associated with a definite increase in the risk of some chromosome abnormality in a subsequent conception, but there was no consistency in the specific type of abnormality. In couples previously having only full-term deliveries, the occurrence of a chromosomally abnormal abortus was associated with a favorable prognosis for subsequent pregnancies, but a normal karyotype in the abortus signaled a higher (24%–33%) risk of recurring abortion, postulated to reflect maternal causes such as incompetent cervix. The highest risk of recurring abortion (41.5%) was found in those couples who had already experienced one or more spontaneous abortions of a chromosomally abnormal fetus and where the mother was more than 30 years of age. Bove et al. (1975) found no effect of oral contraceptive use on the frequency of abortions or chromosome abnormalities. An increased frequency of chromosome abnormalities was observed after the use of ovulation-inducing drugs and after occupational exposure of the fathers to radiation. There were no changes in fertility rate or in the frequency of congenital malformations in births following the abortions.

Bauld, Sutherland, and Bain (1974) conducted chromosome studies of consecutive stillbirths and neonatal deaths, compiling results of 153 cases during a 1-year period. Chromosome abnormalities were found in 11 cases, giving a frequency of 7.2%. Most of the abnormalities were trisomies, of which trisomy 18 was most frequent. It should be noted that chromosome studies can often be carried out successfully if done hours or even several days after clinical death of the fetus by using material from the spleen, lung, or sterile skin from which fibroblasts can be grown.

In these studies of spontaneous abortions and perinatal deaths, the vast majority of the chromosome abnormalities observed were of types that would be expected to arise de novo during parental gametogenesis rather than being transmitted from a parent who carries a chromosome abnormality. This distinction was addressed directly by Kim et al. (1975), who obtained karyotypes using the new banding techniques on a consecutive series of 50 couples who had more than two early abortions, stillbirths, live births of infants with multiple congenital anomalies, or a combination of the latter two. Three women were found to be balanced reciprocal translocation carriers, but none of these translocations was detectable by chromosome analysis without banding. An additional woman was found to be a mosaic, and four parents (three females and one male) showed mitotic chromosome abnormalities. Kim et al. (1975) estimated that between 6% and 16% of fetal wastage so defined results from parental chromosome abnormalities and that such couples could benefit from prenatal monitoring to detect chromosome abnormalities in future pregnancies. Numerous studies have confirmed the finding of a high rate of translocation carriers in couples who have experienced repeated fetal loss (Portnoi et al., 1988, Sachs et al., 1985). Such monitoring done in the second trimester would detect fetal chromosome abnormalities that had not resulted in spontaneous abortion but that would produce perinatal death or serious birth defects in surviving offspring.

PRENATAL DIAGNOSIS

Second trimester amniocentesis for prenatal diagnosis is both a safe and an important means for preventing the birth of children with various genetic disorders. The National Institute of Child Health and Human Development Collaborative Amniocentesis Registry Project found no increase in fetal loss when 1,040 pregnancies in which amniocentesis was performed were compared with 992 controls. Similarly, there were no major maternal complications in the study group. There have been reports of fetal injury resulting from the amniocentesis needle, but fortunately these instances are rare.

Amniocentesis should be performed between 16 and 18 weeks of gestation and should routinely be preceded or accompanied by ultrasound studies. Ultrasound imaging allows localization of the placenta, detection of multiple fetuses (which would confuse the interpretation of results of many studies), and assessment of gestational age by measurement of the biparietal diameter of the fetal head. Approximately 20 ml of amniotic fluid is withdrawn, and after separation by centrifugation with precautions to preserve sterility, the supernatant fluid is analyzed for α-fetoprotein content, and the cells are placed in culture for later chromosome analysis, biochemical studies, or molecular analyses.

The current indications for prenatal genetic diagnosis are generally considered to consist of the following: (1) maternal age of 35 years or greater; (2) history of a previous child with trisomy 21 (Down syndrome); (3) pregnancy at risk for a mendelian disorder specifically diagnosable in utero; (4) presence of a balanced chromosome abnormality in either parent; (5) history of a previous child with anencephaly or meningomyelocele; and (6) elevated maternal serum α-fetoprotein concentration. When the fetus is at risk for having a severe X-linked recessive disorder that is not specifically diagnosable (e.g., Duchenne-type muscular dystrophy or severe hemophilia A), amniocentesis for identification of male sex by karyotyping is another possible indication. At a maternal age of 35 years, the risk of a chromosome abnormality is 1 per 200 live births and increases to 1 per 65 live births by age 40 years. The observed frequencies of chromosome abnormalities measured at 15 to 16 weeks of gestation have been higher than those found in newborn surveys. This apparent decrease in the frequencies of chromosome abnormalities between 15 and 16 weeks of gestation and birth has been attributed in part to the spontaneous abortion of some of these abnormal fetuses in the interim. The birth of a child with trisomy 21 appears to identify couples who are at higher risk for recurrence of this abnormality, although the reasons are not known. The risk of a second trisomy 21 for a woman less than age 35 years appears to be approximately 1% and is higher for older women, being about double the age-related occurrence risk. Although individuals differ in their perception of the importance of a 1% risk, in many instances the anxiety produced by the birth of the first affected child will prompt the couple to seek prenatal diagnosis. Analysis of the karyotype in cultured amniotic fluid cells will, of course, detect not only trisomy 21 but also any other major chromosome abnormality.

Although the list of mendelian disorders specifically diagnosable in utero by biochemical methods has increased steadily, it is still a minority of disorders that can be detected. Table 18−1 lists those disorders that have already been diagnosed prenatally or in which the possibility of doing so is very likely, based on detection of the defect in cultured skin fibroblasts. In addition, several forms of β-thalassemia, sickle cell anemia, and hemophilia have been diagnosed experimentally by analysis of fetal erythrocytes. All of the disorders listed in Table 18−1 are inherited in autosomal recessive or X-linked recessive patterns except for acute intermittent porphyria and familial hypercholesterolemia, which, along with myotonic dystrophy, are the only three autosomal dominant disorders of the more than 1,000 described that can be diagnosed in utero.

Anencephaly, encephalocele, meningomyelocele, and meningocele all appear to be part of a spectrum of neural tube disorders that manifest features of multifactorial inheritance. Couples who have given birth to a child with any of these disorders have a recurrence risk of about 2% for any of the disorders in this group. Thus, after the birth of an anencephalic child, the couple has about a 2% risk in the subsequent pregnancy of anencephaly, encephalocele, meningomyelocele, or meningocele. When the fetus is affected with any of these neural tube defects, the α-fetoprotein concentration will be elevated, and this can be detected by analysis of the level in fluid obtained by amniocentesis. False positive and false negative results have been reported, and there are other fetal disorders that can elevate the α-fetoprotein concentrations. Acetylcholinesterase isozyme assay by electrophoresis provides a qualitative technique that has proved to be extremely useful in differentiating between the various causes of elevations in α-fetoprotein concentration (Haddow et al., 1983; Goldfine et al., 1983). Anencephaly is usually detected during the ultrasound examination prior to amniocentesis (Haddow and Miller, 1982).

Now that the safety of early second trimester amniocentesis has been established, and as diagnostic capabilities expand, the gynecologist can expect a steady increase in requests for information about prenatal diagnosis.

Recently there has been renewed interest in a technique first described by Hahnemann and Mohr (1968) and Kullander and Sandahl (1973). Chorionic villus sampling (CVS) involves the transcervical or transabdominal sampling of placental tissue with guidance by ultrasound. Since it is usually performed between 9 and 11 weeks of gestation and the tissue can be analyzed directly for biochemical or DNA studies without the need for culture, prenatal diagnosis can be performed much earlier in pregnancy and the result provided to the patient after a much shorter wait following the procedure, both of which are powerful advantages. Cytogenetic studies can also be performed directly on uncultured tissue, but because of a number of technical limitations, most laboratories have chosen to use cultured chorionic tissue for chromosome analysis. This technique requires 5 to 14 days for completion of studies. To date, chorionic villi have been used for the cytogenetic, biochemical, and DNA analyses (Old and Ward, 1982; Simoni et al., 1983; Williamson et al., 1981). Since no amniotic fluid is obtained by this technique, α-fetoprotein and acetylcholinesterase assays to screen for neural tube defects, omphalocoele, gastroschisis, and congenital nephrosis cannot be performed. If necessary, the tissue obtained can be established in culture and the volume of cells expanded beyond the amount provided by the initial biopsy sample. The 10 to 40 mg of chorionic villi regularly obtained provides a far greater amount of viable tissue than is obtained by amniocentesis and is sufficient for most biochemical assays and as a source of DNA for recombinant DNA techniques without the need for culture.

TABLE 18–1.

Inborn Errors of Metabolism Diagnosable Prenatally by Biochemical Assay

Lipidoses
  Adrenoleukodystrophy
  Ceroid-lipofuscinosis
  Cholesterol ester storage disease
  Fabry's disease
  Farber disease
  Gaucher's disease, several forms
  GM$_1$ gangliosidosis, types 1 and 2
  GM$_2$ gangliosidosis
    Tay-Sachs disease
    Sandhoff disease
    AB variant
  Krabbe's disease
  Metachromatic leukodystrophy, several forms
  Multiple sulfatase deficiency
  Niemann-Pick disease, several forms
  Refsum disease
  Wolman disease
Mucopolysaccharidoses
  β-Glucuronidase deficiency
  Hurler-Scheie syndrome
  Hunter's syndrome
  I-cell disease
  Morquio syndrome, A and B
  Maroteaux-Lamy syndrome, several forms
  Sanfilippo's syndrome, A, B, C, and D
Carbohydrate and glycoprotein metabolism
  disorders
    Aspartylglucosaminuria
    Fucosidosis
    Galactosemia
    Glucose-6-phosphate dehydrogenase
      deficiency
    Glucose phosphate isomerase deficiency
    Glycogen storage disease, types II, III, IV, and
      VIII
    Mannosidosis
    Pyruvate decarboxylase deficiency
    Pyruvate dehydrogenase complex deficiency,
      several forms
Amino acid metabolism disorders
  Dihydropteridine reductase deficiency
  Hereditary tyrosinemia, type I
  Hyperprolinemia, type II
  Lysine disorders
    Hyperlysinemia
    Saccharopinuria
  Sulfur pathway disorders
    Cystathionine synthase deficiency
      (homocystinuria)
    Sulfite oxidase deficiency
  Urea cycle disorders
    Argininosuccinicaciduria
    Citrullinemia
    Ornithine carbamyltransferase deficiency

Organic acid disorders
  Glutaric aciduria
  3-Hydroxy-3-methylglutaryl-CoA lyase deficiency
  Isovaleric acidemia
  Maple syrup urine disease, several forms
  Methylmalonic acidemia, several forms
  Mevalonic aciduria
  Propionic acidemia
Vitamin metabolism disorders
  5,10-Methylenetetrahydrofolate reductase
    deficiency
  Methylmalonic acidemia
Collagen disorders
  Ehlers-Danlos syndrome, types IV, V, and VIII
  Hydroxylysine deficient collagen disease
Miscellaneous disorders
  Acatalasia, several forms
  Adenosine deaminase deficiency
  Agammaglobulinemia
  Chronic granulomatous disease
  Combined immunodeficiency due to adenosine
    deaminase or nucleoside phosphorylase
    deficiency
  Congenital adrenal hyperplasia, 21-hydroxylase
    deficiency
  Cytochrome oxidase C deficiency
  Cystinosis
  Hypercholesterolemia, several forms
  Lesch-Nyhan syndrome
  Lysosomal acid phosphatase deficiency
  Menkes disease
  Mucolipidosis, types II, III, and IV
  Orotic aciduria, types I and II
  Porphyria
    Acute intermittent porphyria
    Congenital erythropoietic porphyria
    Protoporphyria
  Prolidase deficiency
  Triosephosphate isomerase deficiency
  Wiskott-Aldrich syndrome
  X-linked ichthyosis
  Zellweger syndrome

The biopsy procedure itself requires both an experienced ultrasonographer and obstetrician-gynecologist. The ultrasonographer scans the uterus to determine the location of the placenta, the viability of the fetus by observing the fetal heart movements, and the gestation age by measuring crown-rump length. The obstetrician introduces the sampling instrument transabdominally or through the cervical canal and into the placenta under direct ultrasound guidance and takes the chorionic villus biopsy.

Although the potential advantages of first-trimester prenatal diagnosis by means of CVS appear to be enormous, the safety and accuracy of these diagnostic procedures have not been fully evaluated, and thus CVS cannot at present be regarded as an established method. Fetal risks are not clearly defined, although recent studies suggest a fetal loss rate of approximately 2%. This rate is somewhat difficult to evaluate, because data on spontaneous fetal loss rates after ultrasound proof of viability at 8 to 11 weeks of gestation are limited. Currently it is estimated that in experienced hands, the CVS technique is associated with at least a 0.7% greater pregnancy loss rate than amniocentesis performed at 15 to 18 weeks of gestation. Since most experienced operators report a loss rate of less than 0.2% associated with amniocentesis, CVS has an associated loss rate of 0.9%, or about five times greater than the amniocentesis-associated loss rate. Maternal risks likewise have yet to be fully evaluated. It is clear that the rates of vaginal bleeding and uterine cramping are much greater after CVS than after amniocentesis (Crane et al., 1988). Although serious maternal complications are rare, they do occur at a frequency greater than that reported for amniocentesis. Serious uterine infections leading to septic shock and in some cases surgical removal of the uterus have been reported (Barela et al., 1986; Black and Schulman, 1988). In addition, technical difficulties in the laboratory can lead to failure to provide a diagnosis or an inaccurate diagnosis. Maternal cell contamination, unexplained chromosomal mosaicism, and biochemical errors have been reported at a greater frequency than those reported for amniotic fluid cell cultures (Hunter, 1988; Callen et al., 1988; Canadian Collaborative CVS–Amniocentesis Clinical Trial Group, 1989).

Percutaneous umbilical blood sampling under ultrasound guidance is another new technique that has yet to be fully evaluated. At any stage after 18 weeks of gestation, fetal blood can be obtained by needle puncture of the umbilical vessels under ultrasound guidance. The advantages of this technique include the ability to sample a different fetal tissue type, rapidity of completion of chromosome studies, and the ability to test for certain hematologic disorders that are not expressed in other tissue types. Disadvantages include a higher associated fetal loss (approximately 1%–2%), maternal blood contamination, and inability to perform the procedure safely and accurately prior to 18 weeks' gestation.

Early amniocentesis is amniocentesis per-

formed prior to 15 weeks of gestation. Some individuals have reported performing amniocentesis as early as 9 weeks' gestation, although most of these procedures have been performed between 11 and 14 weeks of gestation (Benacerraf et al., 1988; Miller et al., 1987; Hanson et al., 1987). The technique is the same as that described for amniocentesis with the exception that less amniotic fluid is withdrawn. The accuracy and success of this technique appear to be equal to that reported for amniocentesis, whereas the fetal loss rate appears to be greater than that reported for amniocentesis but less than that reported for CVS. Preliminary reports on pregnancy outcome do not indicate a higher rate of prematurity, low birth weight, or fetal injury (Miller et al., 1988). Because of the lower volume of amniotic fluid obtained by this procedure, it is not usually applicable to biochemical or DNA studies requiring a large number of cells.

Chorionic villus sampling, percutaneous umbilical blood sampling, or early amniocentesis cannot be considered at present as alternatives to amniocentesis at 16 to 18 weeks' gestation, the safety and accuracy of which are well established. Instead, these techniques should be reserved for those pregnancies that are known to be at high risk for genetic defects, such as inborn errors of metabolism, X-linked disorders, and unbalanced chromosome translocation, so that the risk of the disorder is clearly higher than the likely risk of the new procedure.

GENETIC COUNSELING

The gynecologist as primary physician to women is in a key position to assess the risk of and to aid in preventing serious genetic disorders in the patients' offspring.

The first step in genetic counseling is accurate and precise diagnosis; all that follows depends on this. In various instances this may be by history, physical examination, or review of medical records regarding the patient, affected relatives, or both. Since genetic heterogeneity is the rule, many common and rare disorders that superficially appear quite similar are fundamentally different with regard to recurrence risks, means of diagnosis, and management. For example, from the discussion of congenital absence of the vagina, it will be recalled that this abnormality can be part of an autosomal recessive disorder with a 25% recurrence risk, or it may be an isolated developmental anomaly with a negligible recurrence risk. The family history and careful examination of the patient for associated anomalies, as well as complete examination of female relatives, may allow the physician to distinguish which of the possible etiologies applies in any given patient.

Once the diagnosis is established, the physician can provide information regarding the nature of the disorder, its mode of inheritance, the magnitude of the risk, the natural history of the disorder, and the prospects for treatment. Depending on the specific disorder in question and the potential burden that the family perceives would result from the birth of an affected child, the physician needs to discuss the relevant reproductive alternatives, including prenatal diagnosis, artificial insemination, and adoption of children. In addition to the informative aspects of counseling, the physician should also provide support for the emotional needs of the patient and often for those of the family as well. It may also be advisable to consult a medical geneticist not only for aid in diagnosis of rare disorders but also to make available additional educational and supportive resources.

REFERENCES

Amrhein JA, Meyer WJ, Jones HW, et al: Androgen insensitivity in man: Evidence for genetic heterogeneity. *Proc Natl Acad Sci USA* 1976; 73:891.

Antonarakis S: Diagnosis of genetic disorders at the DNA level. *N Engl J Med* 1989; 320:153.

Bardin CW, Bullock LP, Sherins RJ, et al: Androgen metabolism and mechanisms of action in male pseudohermaphroditism: A study of testicular feminization. *Recent Prog Horm Res* 1973; 29:65.

Barela AI, Kleinman GE, Golditch IM, et al: Septic shock with renal failure after chorionic villus sampling. *Am J Obstet Gynecol* 1986; 154:1100.

Bauld R, Sutherland GR, Bain AD: Chromosome studies in investigations of stillbirths and neonatal deaths. *Arch Dis Child* 1974; 49:782.

Benacerraf BR, Greene MF, Saltzman DH, et al: Early amniocentesis for prenatal cytogenetic evaluation. *Radiology* 1988; 169:709.

Bergsma D, Hamerton JL, Jacobs PA, et al (eds): Paris Conference (1971): Standardization in human cytogenetics. *Birth Defects* 1972; 8(7):2.

Black SH, Schulman JD: Prenatal sampling and bicornuate uterus. *Prenat Diagn* 1988; 8:476.

Böök JA, Eilon B, Halbrecht I, et al: Isochromosome Y (46,X,i(Yq)) and female phenotype. *Clin Genet* 1973; 4:410.

Boue J, Boue A: Chromosomal analysis of two consecutive abortions in each of 13 women. *Hum Genet* 1973; 19:275.

Boue J, Boue A, Lazar P: Retrospective and prospective epidemiological studies of 1500 karyotyped spontaneous human abortions. *Teratology* 1975; 12:11.

Bryan AL, Nigro JA, Counseller VS: 100 cases of congenital absence of the vagina. *Surg Gynecol Obstet* 1949; 88:79.

Buchta RM, Viseskul C, Gilbert EF, et al: Familial renal agenesis and hereditary renal adysplasia. *Eur J Pediatr* 1973; 115:111.

Callen DF, Korban G, Dawson G, et al: Extra embryonic/fetal karyotypic discordance during diagnostic chorionic villus sampling. *Prenat Diagn* 1988; 8:453.

Canadian Collaborative CVS–Amniocentesis Clinical Trial Group: Multicentre randomised clinical trial of chorion villus sampling and amniocentesis. *Lancet* 1989; 1:1.

Carr DH: Chromosomes and abortion. *Adv Hum Genet* 1971; 2:201.

Carter CO: Genetics of common disorders. *Br Med Bull* 1968; 25:52.

Chemke J, Carmichel R, Stewart JM, et al: Familial XY gonadal dysgenesis. *J Med Genet* 1970; 7:105.

Crane JP, Beaver HA, Cheung SW: First trimester chorionic villus sampling versus midtrimester genetic amniocentesis—preliminary results of a controlled prospective trial. *Prenat Diagn* 1988; 8:355.

de la Chapelle A: The complicated issue of human sex determination. *Am J Hum Genet* 1988; 43:1.

de la Chapelle A, Tippett PA, Wetterstrand G, et al: Genetic evidence of X-Y interchange in a human XX male. *Nature* 1984; 307:170.

Dorus E, Amarose AP, Tredway DR, et al: A reciprocal translocation (X;11) in a female with gonadal dysgenesis. *Clin Genet* 1979; 16:253.

Emery AEH, Rimoin DL: *Principles and Practice of Medical Genetics.* New York, Churchill Livingstone, 1985.

Erbe RW: Prenatal diagnosis of inherited disease in Altman PL, Katz DD (eds): *Human Health and Disease.* Bethesda, Md, Federation of American Societies for Experimental Biology, 1977, p 91.

Erickson RP, Gondas B: Alternative explanations of the differing behavior of ovarian and testicular teratomas. *Lancet* 1976; 1:410.

Erlich HA, Gelfand DH, Saik RK: Specific DNA amplification. *Nature* 1988; 331:461.

Espiner EA, Veale AM, Sands VE, et al: Familial syndrome of streak gonads and normal male karyotype in five phenotypic females. *N Engl J Med* 1970; 283:6.

Ewer RW: Familial monotropic pituitary gonadotropin insufficiency. *J Clin Endocrinol Metab* 1968; 28:783.

Feig LA, Bast RC, Knapp RC, et al: Somatic activation of ras^k gene in a human ovarian carcinoma. *Science* 1984; 223:698.

Ford EHR: *Human Chromosomes.* New York, Academic Press, 1973.

Fraser FC: The genetics of cleft lip and cleft palate. *Am J Hum Genet* 1970; 22:336.

Fraser FC, Hunter ADW: Etiologic relations among categories of congenital heart malformations. *Am J Cardiol* 1975; 36:793.

Gasser DL, Silvers WK: Genetics and immunology of sex-linked antigens. *Adv Immunol* 1972; 15:215.

Gerald PS: Sex chromosome disorders. *N Engl J Med* 1976; 294:706.

Givens JR, Wiser WL, Coleman SA, et al: Familial ovarian hyperthecosis: A study of two families. *Am J Obstet Gynecol* 1971; 110:959.

Goldfine C, Miller WA, Haddow JE: Amniotic fluid gel cholinesterase densities ratios in fetal open defects of the neural tube and ventral wall. *Br J Obstet Gynecol* 1983; 90:238.

Gordan JW, Ruddle FH: Mammalian gonadal determination and gametogenesis. *Science* 1981; 211:1265.

Griffin JE, Edwards C, Maddin JD, et al: Congenital absence of the vagina. *Ann Intern Med* 1976; 85:224.

Griffin JE, Wilson JD: The syndromes of androgen resistance. *N Engl J Med* 1980; 302:198.

Guellan G, Casanova M, Bishop C, et al: Human XX males with Y single-copy DNA fragments. *Nature* 1984; 307:172.

Haddow JE, Miller WA: Prenatal diagnosis of open neural tube defects. *Methods Cell Biol* 1982; 26:67.

Haddow JE, Morin ME, Holman MS, et al: Acetylcholinesterase and fetal malformations: Modified qualitative technique for diagnosis of neural tube defects. *Clin Chem* 1981; 27:61.

Hahnemann N, Mohr J: Genetic diagnosis in the embryo by means of biopsy from extraembryonic membrane. *Bull Eur Soc Hum Genet* 1968; 2:23.

Hamerton JL: *Human Cytogenetics.* New York, Academic Press, 1971, vol 1 and 2.

Hamerton JL, Canning N, Ray M, et al: A cytogenetic survey of 14,069 newborn infants: I. Incidence of chromosome abnormalities. *Clin Genet* 1975; 8:223.

Hanson FW, Zorn EM, Tennant FR, et al: Amniocentesis before 15 weeks gestation: Outcome, risks and technical problems. *Am J Obstet Gynecol* 1987; 156:1524.

Harris H: *Garrod's Inborn Errors of Metabolism.* New York, Oxford University Press, 1963.

Hoehn H: Functional implications of differential chromosome banding. *Am J Hum Genet* 1975; 27:676.

Holmes LB, Driscoll SG, Atkins L: Etiologic heterogeneity of neural tube defects. *N Engl J Med* 1976; 294:365.

Hook EB, Hamerton JL: Frequency of chromosome abnormalities detected in consecutive newborns—differences between studies, in Hook EB, Porter IH (eds): *Population Cytogenetics: Studies in Newborns.* New York, Academic Press, 1977.

Hook EB, Warburton D: The distribution of chromosomal genotypes associated with Turner's syndrome: Livebirth prevalence rates and evidence for diminished fetal mortality and severity in genotypes associated with structural X abnormalities or mosaicism. *Hum Genet* 1983; 64:24.

Hsu LY, Peterson RE: Male pseudohermaphroditism: The complexities of male phenotypic development. *Am J Med* 1976; 61:251.

Hsu LY, Shapiro LR, Gertner M, et al: Trisomy 22: A clinical entity. *J Pediatr* 1971; 79:12.

Hunter A: False-positive and false-negative findings on chorionic villus sampling. *Prenat Diagn* 1988; 8:475.

Imperato-McGinley J, Guerrero L, Gautier T, et al: Steroid 5α-reductase deficiency in man: An inherited form of male pseudohermaphroditism. *Science* 1974; 186:1213.

Imperato-McGinley J, Peterson RE, Gautier T, et al: Androgens and the evolution of male-gender identity among male pseudohermaphrodites with 5-α-reductase deficiency. *N Engl J Med* 1979; 300:1233.

Josephs SF, Ratner L, Clarke MF, et al: Cellular transformation by human papillomavirus DNA *in vitro.* Science 1984; 225:634.

Judd HL, Hamilton CR, Barlow JJ, et al: Androgen and gonadotropin dynamics in testicular feminization syndrome. *J Clin Endocrinol Metab* 1972; 34:229.

Kan YW, Dozy AM: Antenatal diagnosis of a sickle-cell anaemia by DNA analysis of amniotic-fluid cells. *Lancet* 1978; 2:910.

Keenan BS, Meyer WJ, Hadjian AJ, et al: Syndrome of androgen insensitivity in man: Absence of 5α-dihydrotestosterone binding protein in skin fibroblasts. *J Clin Endocrinol Metab* 1974; 38:1143.

Kelch RP, Jenner MR, Weinstein R, et al: Estradiol and testosterone secretion by human, simian, and canine testes, in males with hypogonadism and in male pseudohermaphrodites with the feminizing testes syndrome. *J Clin Invest* 1972; 51:824.

Kim HJ, Hsu LYF, Paciuc S, et al: Cytogenetics of fetal wastage. *N Engl J Med* 1975; 293:844.

Kogan SC, Doherty ABM, Gitschier J: An improved method for prenatal diagnosis of genetic diseases by analysis of amplified DNA sequences. *N Engl J Med* 1987; 317:985.

Kohl NE, Gee CE, Alt FE: Activated expression of the N-myc gene in human neuroblastomas and related tumors. *Science* 1984; 226:1335.

Krontiris TG: The emerging genetics of human cancer. *N Engl J Med* 1983; 309:404.

Kullander S, Sandahl B: Fetal chromosome analysis after transcervical placenta biopsies during early pregnancy. *Acta Obstet Gynecol Scand* 1973; 52:355.

Landegren U, Kaiser R, Caskey CT, et al: DNA diagnostics—molecular techniques and automation. *Science* 1988; 242:229.

Liddle GW: The adrenal cortex, in Williams RH (ed.): *Textbook of Endocrinology*, ed 5. Philadelphia, WB Saunders Co, 1974, pp 233–282.

Linder D, Kaiser-McCraw B, Hecht F: Parthenogenic origin of benign ovarian teratomas. *N Engl J Med* 1975; 292:63.

Lindsten J: *The Nature and Origin of X Chromosome Aberrations in Turner's Syndrome: A Cytogenetical and Clinical Study of 57 Patients.* Stockholm, Almqvist and Wiksell, 1963.

Lyon MF: X chromosome inactivation and developmental patterns in mammals. *Biol Rev* 1972; 47:1.

Lyon MF: Mechanisms and evolutionary origin of variable X chromosome activity in mammals. *Proc R Soc Lond Biol* 1974; 187:243.

Lyon MF: Hawkes SG: X-linked gene for testicular feminization in the mouse. *Nature* 1970; 227:1217.

McDermott A: *Cytogenetics of Man and Other Animals—Outline Studies in Biology.* New York, John Wiley & Sons, 1975.

McKusick VA: *Mendelian Inheritance in Man: Catalogs of Autosomal Dominant, Autosomal Recessive and X-linked Phenotypes,* ed 8. Baltimore, The Johns Hopkins University Press, 1988.

McKusick VA, Bauer RL, Koop CE, et al: Hydrometrocolpos as a simply inherited malformation. *JAMA* 1964; 189:813.

McKusick VA, Weilbaecher RG, Gragg GW: Recessive inheritance of a congenital malformation syndrome. *JAMA* 1968; 204:113.

Meyer WJ, Migeon BR, Migeon CJ: Locus on human X chromosome for dihydrotestosterone receptor and androgen insensitivity. *Proc Natl Acad Sci USA* 1975; 72:1469.

Miller OJ, Miller DA, Warburton D: Application of new staining techniques to the study of human chromosomes. *Prog Med Genet* 1973; 9:1.

Miller WA, Davies RM, Thayer BA, et al: Success, safety and accuracy of early amniocentesis [abstract]. *Am J Hum Genet* 1987; 41(suppl):A281.

Miller WA, Davies RM, Thayer BA, et al: First trimester amniocentesis [abstract]. *Am J Hum Genet* 1988; 43:A240.

Milunsky A: Prenatal diagnosis of genetic disorders. *N Engl J Med* 1976; 295:377.

Mittwoch U: Y chromosome and sex determination. *Lancet* 1988; 2:52.

Mittwoch U, Kirk D: Superior growth of the right gonad in human foetuses. *Nature* 1975; 257:791.

Nora JJ, Nora AH: Recurrence risks in children having one parent with a congenital heart disease. *Circulation* 1976; 53:701.

Nyhan WL, Sakati NO: *Diagnostic Recognition of Genetic Disease.* Philadelphia, Lea & Febiger, 1987.

Ohno S: Major regulatory genes for mammalian sexual development. *Cell* 1976; 7:315.

Old JM, Ward RHT, Petrcoum M, et al: First trimester diagnosis for haemoglobinopathies: Three cases. *Lancet* 1982; 2:1413.

Opitz JM, Simpson JL, Sarto GE, et al: Pseudovaginal perineoscrotal hypospadias. *Clin Genet* 1972; 3:1.

Page DC, Brown LG, de la Chapelle A: Exchange of terminal portions of X and Y chromosomal short arms in human XX males. *Nature* 1987a; 328:437.

Page DC, Mosher R, Simpson EM, et al: The sex-determining region of the human Y chromosome encodes a finger protein. *Cell* 1987b; 51:1091.

Perez-Ballester B, Greenblatt RB, Byrd JR: Familial gonadal dysgenesis. *Am J Obstet Gynecol* 1970; 107:1262.

Philip J, Lundsteen C, Owen D, et al: The frequency of chromosome aberrations in tall men with special reference to 47,XYY + 47,XXY. *Am J Hum Genet* 1976, 28:404.

Polani PE, Angell R, Giannelli F, et al: Evidence that the Xg locus is inactivated in structurally abnormal X chromosomes. *Nature* 1970; 227:613.

Portnoi M, Joye N, Van Den Akker J, et al: Karyotypes of 1142 couples with recurrent abortion. *Obstet Gynecol* 1988; 72:31.

Puck MH, Bender B, Borelli JB, et al: Parents' adaptation to early diagnosis of sex chromosome anomalies. *Am J Med Genet* 1983; 16:71.

Rimoin DL, Schimke RN: *Genetic Disorders of the Endocrine Glands*. St Louis, CV Mosby Co, 1971.

Robinson A, Bender B, Borelli J, et al: Sex chromosomal anomalies: Prospective studies in children. *Behav Genet* 1983; 13:321.

Ross GT, Van de Wiele RL: The ovaries, in Williams RH (ed): *Textbook of Endocrinology,* ed 5. Philadelphia, WB Saunders Co, 1974, pp 368–422.

Sachs ES, Jahoda MGJ, Van Homel JO, et al: Chromosome studies of 500 couples with two or more abortions. *Obstet Gynecol* 1985; 65:375.

Saenger P: Abnormal sex differentiation. *J Pediatr* 1984; 104:1–17.

Scully RE: Gonadoblastoma: A review of 74 cases. *Cancer* 1970a; 24:1340.

Scully RE: Sex cord tumor with annular tubules: A distinctive ovarian tumor of the Peutz-Jegher syndrome. *Cancer* 1970b; 25:1107.

Silvers WK, Gasser DL, Eicher EM: H-Y antigen, serologically detectable male antigen and sex determination. *Cell* 1982; 28:439.

Simpson JL: *Disorders of Sexual Differentiation*. New York, Academic Press, 1976.

Simpson JL: Repeated suboptimal pregnancy outcome. *Birth Defects* 1981; 17:113.

Simpson JL, Christakos AC, Horwith M, et al: Gonadal dysgenesis in individuals with apparently normal chromosome complements: Tabulation of cases and compilation of genetic data, in Bergsma D, McKusick VA (eds): *The Clinical Delineation of Birth Defects,* vol 10: *Endocrine System*. Baltimore, Williams & Wilkins Co, 1971.

Simpson JL, Golbus MS, Martin AO, et al: *Genetics in Obstetrics and Gynecology*. New York, Grune & Stratton, 1982.

Simoni G, Brambati B, Danesino C, et al: Efficient direct chromosome analysis and enzyme determination from chorionic villi samples in the first trimester of pregnancy. *Hum Genet* 1983; 63:349.

Slamon DJ, DeKernion JB, Verma IM, et al: Expression of cellular oncogenes in human malignancies. *Science* 1984; 224:256.

Smith DW: *Recognizable Patterns of Human Malformations,* ed 2. Philadelphia, WB Saunders Co, 1976.

Spitz IM, Diamant Y, Rosen E, et al: Isolated gonadotropin deficiency: A heterogeneous syndrome. *N Engl J Med* 1974; 290:10.

Stein Z: Early fetal loss. *Birth Defects* 1981; 17:95.

Stent GS: *Molecular Genetics*. San Francisco, WH Freeman & Co, Publishers, 1971.

Sutton EH: *An Introduction to Human Genetics,* ed 3. New York, Holt, Rinehart & Winston, 1980.

Swanson CP, Merz T, Young WJ: *Cytogenetics*. Englewood Cliffs, NJ, Prentice-Hall, 1967.

Tilghman SM, Tiemeier DC, Polsky F, et al: Cloning segments of the mammalian genome: Bacteriophage containing mouse globin and surrounding gene sequences. *Proc Natl Acad Sci USA* 1977; 77:4406.

Vogel F, Motulsky AG: *Human Genetics: Problems and Approaches*. New York, Springer-Verlag, New York, 1979.

Walzer S, Gerald PS: Social class and frequency of XYY + XXY. *Science* 1975; 190:1228.

Watkins PC: Restriction fragment length polymorphism (RFLP): Applications in human chromosome mapping and genetic disease research. *BioTechniques* 1988; 6:310.

Watson JD: *Molecular Biology of the Gene,* ed 3. New York, WA Benjamin, 1976.

Weiss RA, Marshall CJ: Oncogenes. *Lancet* 1984; 2:1138.

Williams RH: *Textbook of Endocrinology,* ed 5. Philadelphia, WB Saunders Co, 1974.

Williamson R, Eskdale J, Coleman DV, et al: Direct gene analysis of chorionic villi: A possible technique for first trimester antenatal diagnosis of haemoglobinopathies. *Lancet* 1981; 2:1125.

Wilson JD, George FW, Griffin JE: The hormonal control of sexual development. *Science* 1981; 211:1278.

Witkin HA, et al: Criminality in XYY and XXY men. *Science* 1976; 193:547.

Wyman A, White R: A highly polymorphic locus in human DNA. *Proc Natl Acad Sci USA* 1978; 77:6754.

Wyss D, DeLozier CD, Daniell J, et al: Structural anomalies of the X chromosome: Personal observation and review of non-mosaic cases. *Clin Genet* 1982; 21:145.

Yanagisawa S, Yokoyama H: Symptoms of Turner's syndrome and interstitial heterochromatin in i(Xq). *Clin Genet* 1975; 7:299.

19 Gynecological Infections

Ruth Tuomala, M.D.

In this chapter, infectious diseases that affect the female genital tract will be discussed, with emphasis on clinical diagnosis and management. The specific diseases that will be presented have been chosen on the basis of prevalence, importance of sequelae, or, in some cases, because they are considerations in the differential diagnosis of commoner entities.

PELVIC INFLAMMATORY DISEASE

Pelvic inflammatory disease (PID) is a disease of the upper genital tract that is characterized primarily by infection of the endosalpingeal cells lining the fallopian tubes. Infection may be confined to the tubes (salpingitis) or, in addition, involve the ovaries (salpingo-oophoritis). Occasionally, either the endometrium (endometritis) or ovary (oophoritis) may be the sole focus of infection. Infection involves disruption and destruction of normal architecture on a microscopic or macroscopic level. Even apparently mild disease can lead to functional impairment. Marked inflammation resulting in the involvement of contiguous intraperitoneal structures in inflammatory processes and massive suppuration leading to tubo-ovarian abscess (TOA) formation can totally destroy normal architecture as well as function.

Pelvic inflammatory disease is a disease of sexually active, menstruating women. It is rare during pregnancy and in premenarchal, postmenopausal, and celibate women, and when it does occur in these groups, it is often secondary to spread from other foci of intra-abdominal sepsis such as ruptured appendiceal abscesses. The exact incidence of PID in the United States is unknown, although it is estimated to account for 300,000 annual hospitalizations and 2.5 million annual outpatient visits. One million new cases of PID occur each year. The costs associated with diagnosing and treating PID and its sequelae will reach approximately $3.5 billion in the United States in 1990.

The majority of cases of PID are thought to be ascending infections, caused by microorganisms that ascend from the lower genital tract through the cervix, along the endometrium to the normally sterile tubes. Infection may also spread to the tubes and ovaries via the parametrium from cervical vessels and lymphatics. Pelvic inflammatory disease is a polymicrobial infection. Both organisms that are recognized to be sexually transmitted and organisms that are considered to be part of the normal, endogenous flora of the lower genital tract are participants in PID. Sexually transmitted organisms such as *Neisseria gonorrhoeae* and *Chlamydia trachomatis* may be found as sole pathogens in cases of PID or may be found along with other nonsexually transmitted organisms. Current estimates are that in the United States, 25% to 80% of cases of PID involve the gonococcus. The exact role of *C. trachomatis* in PID in the United States is being elucidated, and *Chlamydia* may be an important pathogen in 10% to 30% or more of cases of PID. *Mycoplasma* species have been recovered from sites of pelvic infection; their role as a major contributor in causing infection has not been demonstrated.

Multiple species of aerobic and anaerobic bacteria normally found in the lower genital tract of asymptomatic women can be found at the site of upper genital tract infection both in the presence of and in the absence of sexually transmitted organisms. Pelvic inflammatory disease may be a pure aerobic, pure anaerobic, or mixed aerobic-anaerobic infection. In approximately two thirds of cases, anaerobes are involved. Aerobic endogenous bacteria that are associated with PID include the Enterobacteriaceae, particularly *Escherichia coli*, staphylococcal species, and streptococcal species, including the enterococci. Anaerobes that are associated with PID include peptococci, peptostreptococci, anaerobic streptococci, and *Bacteroides* species, including *Bacteroides fragilis* and *Bacteroides melaninogenicus.*

It is likely that key organisms are responsible for initial invasion of the upper genital tract and that other organisms can become involved in infection under altered conditions and structure of the upper genital tract. The exact microbial and host factors responsible for tissue invasion and infection are currently the subject of much ongoing research.

The exact organisms involved in a particular infection can be ascertained only by direct culture of the infected site. In PID, this involves culture of tubal exudate or tubal biopsy specimens or cul-de-sac fluid obtained at the time of laparoscopy or laparotomy. Cultures of the lower genital tract do not accurately reflect the organisms that are present in upper genital tract infection. Contamination of peritoneal fluid cultures obtained by culdocentesis by lower genital tract flora render these unacceptable specimens. Although endometrial cultures also suffer from a high degree of lower genital tract contamination, particularly by low virulence pathogens, endometrial cultures specifically for *C. trachomatis* may be helpful. The presumed microbiology of individual infections is largely an estimation based on usual organism involvement and to some extent, differential clinical presentation.

Diagnosis

The clinical diagnosis of PID is inexact. There are multiple potential symptoms and signs ascribable to PID as predicted by areas of inflammatory involvement. No symptoms or signs are pathognomonic for PID.

Reports in which all clinical diagnoses of PID are confirmed by laparoscopy suggest that in one third of cases, the clinical diagnosis of PID is in error. Other conditions that may be diagnosed as PID include appendicitis, ectopic pregnancy, endometriosis, adhesions, and adnexal tumors, including ruptured or hemorrhagic functional ovarian cysts. In addition, some 10% to 15% of cases of PID initially are diagnosed as another process, such as those just listed.

For the majority of cases in which PID is erroneously diagnosed, no pelvic pathological features can be defined by laparoscopy. Without treatment for PID, symptoms in these women resolve, and long-term sequelae associated with PID do not ensue. A portion of disease in this group with normal visual findings may be infection confined to the lower genital tract or endometrium, and a portion may involve disease of other organ systems.

The largest such laparoscopy series has been conducted on an ongoing basis by Jacobson and Weström in Sweden, which was first reported in 1969. When these investigators compared the incidence of various symptoms and signs between women with PID and women with a laparoscopically normal pelvis, very few symptoms and signs were seen more frequently in the group of women with PID (Table 19–1). Although seen in a minority of cases, multiple signs and symptoms present in one person confer the greatest accuracy of clinical diagnosis.

Traditional laboratory studies do little to improve the accuracy of diagnosis of PID. The white blood cell (WBC) count is elevated in both women with PID and normal women. The ESR is often elevated in women with PID and may be helpful in judging response to therapy but is a nonspecific test, and the rate may also be elevated in a large number of women without PID. Ultrasound and computed tomographic (CT) scanning

TABLE 19–1.

Symptoms and Signs Seen Significantly More Often in Patients With Pelvic Inflammatory Disease Than in Those With Laparoscopically Normal Pelvic Findings*

	PID (%)	Visually Normal (%)
Symptoms		
Fever and chills	41.0	20.0
Proctitis	6.9	2.7
Signs		
Adnexal tenderness	92.0	87.0
Palpable mass or swelling	49.4	24.5
Erythrocyte sedimentation rate (ESR) >15 mm/hr	75.9	52.7
Abnormal discharge	63.2	40.2
Temperature >38° C	32.9	14.1

*From Jacobson L, Weström L: Objectivized diagnosis of acute pelvic inflammatory disease: Diagnostic and prognostic value of routine laparoscopy. *Am J Obstet Gynecol* 1969; 105:1088. Used by permission.

may be of aid in detecting the presence of and following resolution of TOAs but cannot accurately differentiate abscess formation from other causes of pelvic masses.

Virtually all women who have PID have WBCs present in lower genital tract discharge. If WBCs are not present in this discharge, the diagnosis of PID is unlikely. A Gram stain of cervical discharge that is positive for intracellular gram-negative diplococci supports but does not confirm and is not necessary for a diagnosis of gonococcal PID, although a positive Gram stain can be helpful in determining therapy.

Normal cul-de-sac fluid contains 1,500 WBCs/cu mm. The great majority of cul-de-sac samples taken by culdocentesis from women with PID contain 15,000 to 30,000 WBCs/cu mm. Though not often helpful for culture, culdocentesis can be helpful in establishing a clinical diagnosis of PID.

When the differential diagnosis of pelvic pain is between PID and a surgical condition and in cases of nonresponse or recurrent clinical disease not associated with an obvious precipitating cause, diagnostic laparoscopy should be performed. The use of laparoscopy in other cases should be individualized, although some investigators have suggested that extending the use of laparoscopy to all may prove to be cost effective. Laparoscopic criteria for the diagnosis of PID are listed in Table 19–2.

It is now apparent that endometritis may be seen in association with salpingitis in up to 70% to 85% of selected cases. In addition, women with signs and symptoms of PID without laparo-scopic evidence of PID may be found to have evidence of endometritis. It is assumed that endometritis in these cases is responsible for symptomatology. The overlap in symptoms between women with laparoscopically documented PID and those with endometritis is such that differential diagnosis by any specific clinical criteria is not possible. Endometritis is strongly associated with the presence of *C. trachomatis,* isolated from the cervix, both the cervix and the endometrium, or the endometrium alone, and to a lesser extent with *N. gonorrhoeae*. A large number of women with clinically apparent cervicitis may also have endometritis found on biopsy. The majority of cases show histopathological evidence of plasma cell endometritis, although severe endometritis including even microabscesses has been described. There is no correlation between the histopathological severity of endometritis described and the degree of tubal damage in cases of coincidental PID. The discovery of the association between cervicitis, endometritis, and PID and overlap in symptomatology has given support to the ascending theory of infection and has led some to propose endometrial biopsy as a justified diagnostic procedure in women with pelvic pain in whom a diagnosis of PID is entertained.

To establish at least minimal criteria for the diagnosis of PID and to better compare data between institutions, Hager et al. (1983) proposed baseline criteria for a clinical diagnosis of PID. These are listed in Table 19–3. In addition, classification of disease by severity may aid in establishing prognosis and developing comparative data bases.

Approximately 5% of women with PID will have an associated syndrome of perihepatitis called the *Fitz-Hugh–Curtis syndrome*. This is an inflammatory, fibrinous perihepatitis associated with right upper quadrant pain, tenderness, and mildly deranged liver function tests. Eventual scarring results in the classic fibrous "violin string" adhesions between the dome of the liver and the diaphragm. This process has been associated with both gonococcal and chlamydial PID. Laparoscopic assessment of women with either acute or chronic pelvic pain should include assessment of the right upper quadrant if a diagnosis of acute or past PID is entertained.

Some risk factors for the occurrence of PID have been delineated and should be considered when a history is taken from a woman who presents with pelvic pain. These risk factors include

TABLE 19–2.

Laparoscopic Criteria for Acute Pelvic Inflammatory Disease*

Minimum criteria
  Erythema of fallopian tubes
  Edema and swelling of fallopian tube
  Exudate from fimbria or on serosa of fallopian
    tube
Scoring
  Mild: minimum criteria, tubes freely movable and
    patent
  Moderate: more marked, tubes not freely
    movable, patency uncertain
  Severe: inflammatory mass

*From Jacobson L: Differential diagnosis of acute pelvic inflammatory disease. *Am J Obstet Gynecol* 1980; 138: 1006–1011. Used by permission.

TABLE 19–3.

Salpingitis: Clinical Criteria for Diagnosis*

Abdominal direct tenderness, with or without rebound tenderness Tenderness with motion of cervix and uterus Adnexal tenderness	All three necessary for diagnosis
	Plus
Gram stain of endocervix—positive for gram-negative, intracellular diplococci Temperature (38° C) Leukocytosis (>10,000/cu mm) Purulent material (WBCs present) from peritoneal cavity by culdocentesis or laparoscopy Pelvic abscess or inflammatory complex on bimanual examination or by sonography	One or more necessary for diagnosis

*Hager et al: *Obstet Gynecol* 1983; 61:114. Used by permission.

those related to sexual activity, age, and contraceptive practices.

A history of sexual activity is necessary to seriously consider the diagnosis of PID. Number of sexual partners and frequency of coitus increase the risk of development of PID. The risk is probably largely confined to women who are heterosexually active. Prior or concomitant documented sexually transmitted disease, including prior PID and gonorrhea, increase the risk of PID.

Age is an important risk factor for the occurrence of PID. Peak incidence of PID in the United States is the 15- to 24-year age group. After age 25 years, particularly after age 30 years, the incidence of PID declines markedly. It is unclear whether age-related risk is associated with sexual habits, the development of protective antibodies at the cervical level, or other factors.

Contraceptive practices influence the risk of PID, although exact risks may be skewed by the fact that the bulk of data is based on PID cases requiring hospitalization. Using oral contraceptives and barrier methods both decrease the risk of PID compared with using no contraceptive method. In addition, women with PID who use oral contraceptives appear to have milder disease. The presence of an intrauterine device (IUD) increases the risk of PID 1.5 to 4.0 times above that of women using no contraception. This risk is greatest for the Dalkon shield but is increased for all types of IUDs and does not appear to differ appreciably among all other types of IUDs. The risk of development of PID is most likely the greatest immediately after IUD insertion, but thereafter there is a risk of development of PID regardless of duration of IUD use, socioeconomic status, and parity. Nulliparous women may be at a greater risk for developing IUD-associated PID than multiparous women and also appear to be at greater risk for tubal factor infertility associated with the IUD.

It was formerly thought that unilateral TOA formation was highly associated with IUD use and presumably occurred because of parametrial spread of infection secondary to erosion of the endometrium by the IUD. More recent studies have documented that approximately 60% of all TOAs are unilateral and that this percentage is constant regardless of whether an IUD is present or not.

All invasive gynecological procedures are associated with a risk for upper genital tract infection. Such procedures include tubal lavage, hysterosalpingograms, endometrial biopsies, and dilatation and curettages (D&Cs) done for the purpose of either diagnosis or therapeutic abortion. Such iatrogenic infection may be associated with either endogenous flora or sexually transmitted organisms. It has been suggested that the presence of C. trachomatis in the cervix increases risk for postabortal PID. It is not clear whether prophylactic antibiotics prevent pelvic infections associated with gynecological procedures, whether antibiotics would be appropriate in these varied settings, or whether the widespread use of antimicrobial prophylaxis for such procedures is cost effective.

There may be differences in the clinical presentation of PID depending on the primary pathogens involved. Gonococcal PID tends to present acutely within 48 hours of onset of symptoms with multiple symptoms and signs, including high fevers, peritoneal signs, and purulent vaginal discharge. It often presents as an initial episode of PID. Abscess formation is less frequent with gonococcal PID, and therapeutic response is usually prompt. Chlamydial PID tends to present with more moderate symptoms and a more protracted course. Chronic, low-grade pelvic pain, irregular bleeding, subtle signs on physical examination but an elevated ESR, and more severe inflammatory changes by laparoscopic examination with a high percentage of tubal scarring may all be features of chlamydial infection. *Chlamydia* and *N. gonorrhoeae* are often found together in cases of PID, and a great deal of overlap in symptomatology exists. Therefore, treatment for both organisms is standard as opposed to relying on differential clinical features to guide therapy.

Nongonococcal, nonchlamydial PID is often recurrent and presents with a semiacute course. Unlike PID associated with either gonorrhea or *Chlamydia*, whose symptoms tend to begin within 7 days of the menses, symptoms occur more frequently more than 14 days after menses. Patients present after having symptoms for 5 to 7 days and do not look acutely ill. Fever and peritoneal signs are not prominent, but ESRs are often elevated, abscess formation is frequent, and response to therapy is often not dramatic. Anaerobic organisms, particularly *Bacteroides* species, are of particular concern in multiple recurrences, in women more than 30 years of age, and when abscesses are present.

There are four well-documented long-term consequences of PID: (1) disease recurrence, (2) pelvic pain, (3) infertility, and (4) ectopic pregnancy. Approximately one fourth of all women who have had PID will suffer from one or more of these sequelae. As previously mentioned, PID is a recurrent disease despite apparently adequate therapy. It remains to be seen whether aggressive attempts at elucidating and eradicating the microbiological pathogens and treatment of sexual partners will appreciably decrease rates of recurrence of upper genital tract infections.

Approximately 20% of all women who have had documented PID will have some type of chronic pelvic pain. This may be sporadic or cyclic or may be constant and debilitating. This sequela often eventuates in hysterectomy; PID and its sequelae are responsible for approximately 25% of abdominal hysterectomies performed in the United States each year.

Women who have had PID have an increased risk of infertility due to tubal obstruction. The risk of infertility is related to the number of episodes of infection and severity of episodes, and it may also be associated with the infecting organism and adequacy of therapy (Table 19–4). If pregnancy is achieved after PID, there is an increased incidence of ectopic pregnancies. Pelvic inflammatory disease is thought to increase the risk of ectopics up to 10 times and is a major fac-

TABLE 19–4.

Summary of Long-Term Sequelae Seen in 415 Cases of Laparoscopically Documented Pelvic Inflammatory Disease and in 100 Controls With Laparoscopically Normal Pelvic Findings*

Sequelae	Normal Pelvis	PID
Chronic abdominal pain >6 mo	5.0%	18.1%
Ectopic/intrauterine pregnancy	1/147	1/24
Involuntary infertility related to tubal factor	3.0%	17.3%

Infertility-Related Episodes of PID		Infertility Related to Severity of PID (First Episode Only)	
No. of Episodes	% Infertile	Severity of Episodes	% Infertile
1	12.8	Mild	2.6
2	35.5	Moderate	13.1
3+	75.0	Severe	28.6

*From Weström L: Effect of acute pelvic inflammatory disease on fertility. *Am J Obstet Gynecol* 1975; 121:707. Used by permission.

tor in the increasing incidence of ectopic pregnancies in the United States.

Treatment

Although it has not yet been proved, it is hoped that early, aggressive therapy of PID will decrease the incidence and severity of the long-term sequelae. To date, there have been no large-scale comparative trials that support any therapeutic regimen as being the most efficacious for the treatment of PID. Essential components of adequate therapy are frequent observation for response, thoughtful use of antibiotics, and contact tracing and treatment of sexual partners for the presence of gonorrhea and *Chlamydia*.

Currently suggested antibiotic treatment regimens as outlined by the Centers for Disease Control (CDC) are presented in Table 19–5. The efficacy and toxicity effects of these regimens are untested, but the microbiological rationale for their selection is sound. Most authorities support the need for multiple drug regimens for either inpatient or outpatient therapy of PID. Failure rates for single-drug therapy of 15% to 20% have been documented and are considered to be unacceptably high. The appropriate length of time necessary for adequate antimicrobial therapy, the need for protracted oral therapy in follow-up of parenteral therapy, and correlations between resolution of symptoms and length of therapy have not been determined.

Hospitalization for the treatment of PID with parenteral antibiotics and close observation is suggested for all patients with severe disease as defined by peritoneal signs or abscess formation. In addition, outpatients in whom the diagnosis is in doubt, who cannot take oral antibiotics for any reason, or in whom an initial course of oral therapy has failed should be hospitalized. An inability to maintain close observation as an outpatient for monitoring response is another indication for hospitalization. In addition, suspected pregnancy is an indication for hospitalization. Pelvic inflammatory disease during pregnancy is quite rare; however, when it does occur, it can be particularly virulent, resulting in severe morbidity and high rates of pregnancy loss, and requires close observation and aggressive antibiotic therapy. Many authorities believe that all adolescents with PID should be hospitalized because of concerns regarding compliance with medical care and the grave long-term consequences of such lack of compliance.

The best manner to treat IUD-associated PID has not been determined. The need for IUD removal to effect clinical cure has not been proved. However, the resolution of disease may be slower and less complete if an IUD is left in situ. Therefore, it is common practice to remove an IUD when associated PID is treated.

TABLE 19–5.

Examples of Combination Regimens With Broad Activity Against Major Pathogens in Pelvic Inflammatory Disease*

Inpatient treatment
  Regimen A
    Doxycycline, 100 mg intravenously twice daily, plus Cefoxitin, 2.0 g intravenously 4 times daily
      Continue drugs intravenously for at least 4 days and at least 48 hours after the patient improves. Then continue 100 mg of doxycycline by mouth twice daily to complete 10–14 days of total therapy.
  Regimen B
    Clindamycin, 600 mg intravenously 4 times daily, plus Gentamicin, 2.0 mg/kg intravenously, followed by 1.5 mg/kg 3 times daily in patients with normal renal function
      Continue drugs intravenously for at least 4 days and at least 48 hours after the patient improves. Then continue 450 mg of clindamycin by mouth 4 times daily to complete 10–14 days of total therapy.
Ambulatory treatment
  Recommended regimens
    Cefoxitin, 2.0 g intramuscularly; or amoxicillin, 3.0 g by mouth; or ampicillin, 3.5 gm by mouth; or aqueous procaine penicillin G, 4.8 million units intramuscularly at 2 sites; or ceftriaxone, 250 mg intramuscularly
      Each of these regimens except ceftriaxone is accompanied by 1.0 gm of probenecid by mouth.
  Followed by
    Doxycycline, 100 mg by mouth twice daily for 10–14 days
      Tetracycline hydrochloride, 500 mg 4 times daily, may be substituted for doxycycline but is less active against certain anaerobes and requires more frequent dosing; these are potentially important drawbacks in the treatment of PID.

*From Centers for Disease Control: Sexually transmitted diseases treatment guidelines. *MMWR* 1985; 34(suppl4):19–21.

Tubo-ovarian abscesses deserve a trial of medical therapy because 80% of cases may respond to antibiotic therapy. The majority of abscesses less than 8 cm will respond to medical therapy on an acute basis. Ruptured TOAs, TOAs that do not respond to medical therapy within 4 to 5 days, TOAs that result in chronic pain require surgical extirpation. While under observation, 3% of TOAs may rupture and require immediate surgical intervention. Rates of "late failures" requiring surgical intervention to cure persistent abscesses or to handle sequelae of persistent pain may be as high as 30%. Because successful pregnancy rates after TOA are in only the 4% to 15% range and the potential need for later surgery to deal with persistent symptoms, some advocate more aggressive surgical management of acute disease. There is no strong evidence that operative complication rates are dependent on the time between onset of medical therapy and surgical intervention. It is clear that decisions regarding medical and surgical management of TOA should be individualized.

The approach of total abdominal hysterectomy with bilateral salpingo-oophorectomy as the sole surgical therapy for TOA is now outmoded. Although necessary or desired in some cases, greater conservation is appropriate in the majority of patients. In particular, unilateral adnexectomy with continued medical management is an accepted surgical approach to treat unilateral TOA. Simple drainage of collections with aggressive medical therapy is advocated by some as the best way to maximize ovarian conservation for future reproduction. After cure of acute PID complicated by TOA, there is increasing justification for fertility surgery and treatment with procedures aimed at optimizing either natural or in vitro fertilization techniques.

Finally, evaluation and therapy of both symptomatic and asymptomatic male partners is an integral part of treatment of PID. Assessment of male partners should take into account the reservoir of asymptomatic males who harbor gonorrhea and *Chlamydia*, regardless of organisms isolated from their female partners with PID.

GONORRHEA

Gonorrhea is one of the most prevalent sexually transmitted diseases in the United States to-day. More than 1 to 1.5 million cases are reported each year. The peak age of occurrence of gonorrhea is in the 16 to 24 year age group, and gonorrhea is commoner in urban populations, lower socioeconomic groups, those who are unmarried, and prostitutes. After a steady decrease in new cases of gonorrhea reported in the United States from 1975 to 1984, this trend appears to have halted. The number of new cases of gonorrhea being reported are of concern particularly among heterosexuals and adolescents, indicating a particular need for effective control of disease among these populations.

Gonorrhea may present as localized infection of the lower genital tract, as invasive infection of the upper genital tract, or as disseminated disease with systemic manifestations, or it may be totally asymptomatic. The causative organism of gonorrhea is *N. gonorrhoeae,* a gram-negative aerobic diplococcus that grows best in carbon dioxide and is very sensitive to drying and extremes in temperature. The organism commonly infects columnar and transitional cells.

The majority of gonorrhea cases are transmitted through sexual activity. An infected male partner transmits infection through vaginal intercourse with approximately a 50% efficiency. The incubation period is approximately 3 to 5 days in those cases in which symptoms are recognizable. In women, *N. gonorrhoeae* is harbored chiefly in the endocervix. It is also found in the urethra, rectum, and oropharynx and occasionally may be found in one of these locations in the absence of cervical gonorrhea. Infection of multiple sites may occur in more than 20% of cases.

The manifestations of gonorrhea in women are most often subtle. Endocervical gonorrhea is associated with a purulent cervical discharge, which may or may not be noticed as being abnormal. Occasionally irregular vaginal bleeding may also be noted. Urethral gonorrhea or involvement of Skene's glands may be associated with symptoms of lower urinary tract infection, such as dysuria and frequency of urination. Rectal gonorrhea most often causes no symptoms. *Neisseria gonorrhoeae* present in the oropharynx may cause an acute pharyngitis; however, it is usually asymptomatic. Because colonization with *N. gonorrhoeae* in women produces either no symptoms or vague ones in 80% of cases, they do not seek medical attention and form a major reservoir of disease transmission. Interpretation of symptoms and diagnosis of gonorrhea may further be complicated by coinfection by other sexually transmitted diseases, in particular *C. trachomatis* and *Trichomonas vaginalis*.

Lower genital tract gonorrhea can lead to infection of the Bartholin's glands and the formation of Bartholin's abscesses. Bartholin's abscesses associated with gonorrhea are most often unilateral, acutely suppurative, and painful. They may drain spontaneously or require incision and drainage; they occasionally resolve spontaneously.

Ten percent to 20% of women with endocervical gonorrhea will develop acute salpingitis. *Neisseria gonorrhoeae* can invade and infect the upper genital tract as a solitary pathogen or may be part of a polymicrobial infection. Some strains of *N. gonorrhoeae* are more pathogenic for the upper genital tract than others. A lipopolysaccharide endotoxin is responsible for both local cytotoxicity and inflammation as well as fever and systemic toxicity. Furthermore, outer membrane pili proteins and IgA protease facilitate attachment of the gonococcus to host cells. In addition, certain risk factors in the host that predispose to the occurrence of salpingitis have been defined as previously outlined. The exact microbial and host factors that lead to invasion and infection of the upper genital tract by *N. gonorrhoeae* are incompletely understood. In the United States, estimates of the incidence of gonococcal salpingitis range from 25% to 80% of all cases of salpingitis.

Although 40% of rectal cultures obtained from women with gonorrhea may be positive, some of these cultures are positive because of perineal contamination and do not reflect true rectal colonization. Rectal colonization may produce symptoms of discharge, bleeding, pain, tenesmus, or constipation and signs such as exudate or mucosal bleeding. However, rectal gonorrhea is most frequently asymptomatic. Rectal gonorrhea is more likely to be ineffectively treated by tetracycline therapy. In addition, 30% of treatment failures in women are discovered only by posttreatment rectal culture, leading some to suggest that posttreatment cultures should always include a rectal culture.

Pharyngeal carriage of *N. gonorrhoeae* is most often asymptomatic. It can occasionally be associated with an acute, exudative pharyngitis. The etiology of pharyngeal gonorrhea is thought to be almost exclusively as a result of fellatio with an infected male partner. Largely asymptomatic, pharyngeal gonorrhea is not thought to be very contagious or to be a major reservoir of disease transmission. There is evidence that without treatment, spontaneous remission may occur over a 10- to 12-week period. However, there may be a greater tendency for pharyngeal gonorrhea to disseminate, because the number of cases of disseminated gonococcal infection (DGI) associated with pharyngeal gonorrhea appears to be disproportionately high. Also, pharyngeal gonorrhea is more resistant to therapy with the standard antimicrobial regimens.

The incidence of DGI in all persons with gonorrhea is approximately 5%. Exact risk factors for the occurrence of DGI are unknown, although pregnancy may predispose to DGI. Twenty-eight percent to 42% of cases of DGI in some series have been in pregnant women.

Disseminated gonococcal infection usually presents in one of two distinct forms. It may present as a systemic illness associated with chills, fever, malaise, asymmetric polyarthralgias, and painful skin lesions. The fingers, toes, hands, wrists, knees, and ankles are most frequently involved in what appears to be a tenosynovitis and, rarely, a frank, suppurative arthritis. Skin lesions classically appear as a slightly raised, erythematous base with a necrotic center but may be petechial, papular, pustular, hemorrhagic, and, occasionally, bullous. These lesions are lightly scattered about the body, usually fewer than 20, often on extremities. An average of 10% to 30%, though up to 50%, of acutely symptomatic patients with DGI may have positive blood cultures.

The second common clinical syndrome of DGI is that of a septic, monoarticular arthritis. *Neisseria gonorrhoeae* may be the commonest cause of septic arthritis in patients less than 30 years of age. Knees are most frequently involved; elbow, ankle, and wrist involvement are also seen. Joint effusion is exudative, often frankly purulent, with the gonococcus present by Gram stain or routine culture in approximately 50% of cases. Culture positivity is proportional to the WBC count in joint fluid. Blood cultures are not positive.

Disseminated *N. gonorrhoeae* may also rarely cause endocarditis, myocarditis, pericarditis, hepatitis, or meningitis.

People with DGI often lack more typical local symptoms of gonorrhea. If DGI is suspected, all common sites for gonococcal colonization should be cultured. The need for hospitalizing all with DGI is unclear; however, close observation for the first 48 hours of treatment to judge early therapeutic response and rule out serious complications seems prudent.

Diagnosis

The diagnosis of gonorrhea is most accurately made by a culture of the organism on selective media, such as modified Thayer-Martin agar, a chocolate-based agar modified by the addition of antibiotics to inhibit the growth of organisms from sites commonly contaminated by polymicrobial growth, such as the cervix or rectum. The specimen should be plated directly on warmed media and incubated in CO_2 without delay to minimize false-negative results due to improper handling. Growth decreases markedly with more than 3 hours away from proper environment.

Obtaining specimens from multiple sites increases the yield of culturing for suspected gonorrhea. The endocervix is the site that most frequently produces positive cultures in women and should always be sampled. Cultures from the urethra, rectum, and pharynx may be positive even with negative cervical cultures and should be performed when indicated by history, strong clinical suspicion of gonococcal disease, and in all cases of recurrent disease.

A Gram stain may be helpful in making a tentative diagnosis of gonorrhea in patients who are symptomatic or who have a history of contact with known gonorrhea. A Gram stain is considered to be positive if intracellular gram-negative diplococci are seen in a minimum of three polymorphonuclear leukocytes per high-power field (HPF). Sensitivity and specificity vary by site of isolation. Up to two thirds of women with endocervical gonorrhea will have suggestive Gram stains, but specificity in asymptomatic women may be as low as 40% to 70%.

Treatment

Treatment of gonorrhea in the United States has now been complicated somewhat by two factors: (2) the emergence of resistant strains of *N. gonorrhoeae* and (2) the need to provide concomitant treatment for *C. trachomatis* when gonorrhea is treated.

The majority of *N. gonorrhoeae* organisms in the United States are sensitive to high-dose peni-

cillin. However, penicillin resistance is rapidly becoming a factor in multiple communities. First recognized in 1976, a plasmid-mediated β-lactamase or penicillinase is responsible for most gonococcal resistance. Initially confined to defined urban areas, particularly in California, New York, and Florida, with most cases in other areas related to travel to high-risk areas, currently more than 75% of reported cases of penicillinase-producing *N. gonorrhoeae* (PPNG) are associated with endemic contact. Overall, 2% of reported cases of gonorrhea in the United States are PPNG strains. Two other forms of resistant *N. gonorrhoeae* are now emerging. A chromosomally mediated resistant *N. gonorrhoeae* strain that is resistant to penicillin, tetracycline, and other antibiotics is recognized but not yet widespread. A plasmid-mediated tetracycline-resistant *N. gonorrhoeae* has recently been reported. Spectinomycin is effective against virtually all PPNG strains, and ceftriaxone is effective against all resistant strains.

In women, *C. trachomatis* is isolated from 30% to 50% of those in whom the gonococcus has been isolated. Studies of single-drug therapy for gonorrhea have shown that rates of posttreatment isolation of *C. trachomatis* and occurrence of PID are high if a penicillin, penicillin-derivative, or cephalosporin are used but are low if a tetracycline is used. However, up to 10% of cases of gonorrhea are not cured if tetracycline is the sole treatment. Therefore, multiple drug therapies for treatment of gonorrhea, taking into account *Chlamydia* treatment, are now standard.

Proper treatment for gonorrhea factors in local rates of resistance and likely sites of infection. Penicillin is the treatment of choice if rates of resistance are less than 1%. Nonpenicillin alternatives are preferred if rates of resistant strains are more than 1%. Ampicillin and spectinomycin are less effective for pharyngeal gonorrhea. Spectinomycin is an excellent drug for rectal gonorrhea. Penicillin and probably most cephalosporins eradicate incubating syphilis; however, spectinomycin is ineffective for this indication. Current guidelines for treatment of gonorrhea are as outlined in Table 19–6.

It is important to reculture all pertinent sites for gonorrhea 3 to 7 days after therapy has been completed. If repeat cultures are positive, retreatment should be with a regimen as described for PPNG.

Most cases of positive gonorrhea cultures after therapy are due to reinfection from untreated

TABLE 19–6.

Current Approaches to Therapy for Uncomplicated Gonorrhea

Group A regimens*
  Amoxicillin, 3.0 gm, plus probenecid, 1.0 gm, both orally; or ampicillin, 3.5 gm, plus probenecid, 1.0 gm, both orally; or aqueous procaine penicillin G, 4.8 million units intramuscularly, plus probenecid, 1.0 gm orally (drug of choice only for pharyngeal infection or infection in homosexual men); or spectinomycin, 2.0 gm intramuscularly (recommended for patients allergic to penicillin or for whom penicillin failed)
Group B regimens
  Ceftriaxone, 250 mg intramuscularly; or cefotaxime, 1.0 gm intramuscularly, plus probenecid, 1.0 gm orally; or cefoxitin, 2.0 gm intramuscularly, plus probenecid, 1.0 gm orally; or spectinomycin, 2.0 gm intramuscularly

*For use in areas where gonococci have maintained chromosomal sensitivity to antimicrobial agents and PPNG strains comprise <1% of isolates. The addition of doxycycline, 100 mg orally twice daily for 7 days, to therapy for uncomplicated gonorrhea to treat possible *C. trachomatis* coinfection is recommended. Tetracycline hydrochloride, 500 mg orally 4 times daily, is cheaper and can be substituted when compliant patients are treated.

sexual partners. It is now recognized that the prevalence of asymptomatic gonorrhea in male partners may be as high as 20% to 30%. Adequate contact tracing remains an integral part of adequate therapy for gonorrhea, as does screening of all populations in which the prevalence of culture positivity is more than 1% to 1.5%.

CHLAMYDIA

Chlamydia trachomatis is an obligate intracellular parasite of columnar and transitional epithelial cells whose role as a pathogen for the genital tract was first recognized to be as the causative agent of lymphogranuloma venereum (LGV). Non-LGV serotypes of *C. trachomatis* have now been associated with asymptomatic carriage in a variety of infections of the female genital tract.

Chlamydia is now thought to be the most prevalent sexually transmitted disease in the United States, with an estimated 3 to 4 million cases yearly. The overall prevalence of *C. trachomatis* in the female genital tract varies by practice site, ranging from 2% to 35% in prenatal clinics and 5% to 23% in family planning clinics. It is most prevalent in those younger than 20 years, in nulliparas, in users of nonbarrier contraceptive methods, and in those with recent multiple or new sexual partners. *Chlamydia* is frequently associated with gonorrhea; approximately 30% to 50% of the time it may be cultured from the genital tract after successful therapy for gonorrhea, and the gonococcus may be found in 25% to 50% of women with *Chlamydia*. It is recognized to be a major pathogen in cases of postgonococcal and nongonococcal urethritis in the male, and female partners of males with these syndromes are at high risk for chlamydial colonization and disease.

Up to 70% of women colonized with *Chlamydia* are asymptomatic. *Chlamydia trachomatis* has been associated with cervicitis, which may or may not cause symptoms and urethritis. The presence of *C. trachomatis* in the cervix has been associated with a cervicitis characterized by a hypertrophic-appearing, friable central eversion or ectopy with mucopus. Endocervical mucus that appears yellow against the tip of cotton-tipped applicator (abnormal Q-tip test result) and microscopic examination that reveals the presence of WBCs signify mucopurulence, and if both are present, *Chlamydia* may be found in 85% of cases. Cervical erythema and friability have also been independently correlated with *Chlamydia*. If signs of cervicitis are seen in a woman with symptoms of PID, suspicion for *Chlamydia* should be high.

The female urethral syndrome of dysuria, pyuria greater than 10 WBCs/HPF, and negative bacterial culture has been associated with *C. trachomatis* in up to 50% of cases. Therapy with doxycycline will result in resolution of symptoms.

Chlamydia trachomatis has also been implicated as a cause of bartholinitis and late postpartum endometritis. It can also be transmitted to neonates at the time of birth through an infected birth canal and in neonates is associated with a distinctive conjunctivitis and pneumonitis.

Chlamydia may be associated with up to 30% to 50% of cases of PID, particularly in adolescents. The exact contribution of *Chlamydia* to morbidity and long-term sequelae associated with PID is unclear. If PID is treated with antibiotics, which are not effective against *Chlamydia*, acute symptoms subside, but recurrence of disease is common. Some cases of chlamydial PID are very subtle yet associated with unexpectedly severe disease by laparoscopy. In addition, *C. trachomatis* has been associated with unexplained "silent" tubal obstruction causing infertility.

In recognition of the rapidly increasing prevalence of *C. trachomatis* and of the potential reproductive tract sequelae caused by *Chlamydia,* strategies to monitor prevalence, control spread, and educate the public have been proposed. These strategies include screening of all groups at risk for disease, particularly adolescents and those with other STDs, evaluation of all with referable symptoms, signs, or exposures, and potential empiric treatment of all females at high risk for chlamydial disease.

Diagnosis

The presence of *C. trachomatis* is determined most accurately by demonstrating the intracellular organism in tissue culture. Direct fluorescent antibody slide staining and enzyme-linked immunosorbent assay (ELISA) techniques for rapid chlamydial antigen detection have been introduced. These tests can be expected to be more widely available and less expensive than the presently available culture techniques; however, sensitivity and specificity are less when used in low-prevalence populations and are best in the hands of experienced laboratories with demonstrated ongoing quality control. The use of rapid tests for assessment of cure is unproved.

Intensive study of cytological findings associated with *Chlamydia* by routine Papanicoloau smear techniques has revealed certain typical cytological changes. Inflammatory changes, particularly the presence of lymphocytes and histiocytes, plus mild cellular atypia such as reactive or atypical metaplasia or reactive endocervical cells have all been correlated with the presence of *Chlamydia*. However, specificity of these findings is 30% to 60% at best, and their presence should prompt no more than further assessment of individual cases. Sensitivity of cytology is too low for a screening technique.

Invasive infection with *C. trachomatis* does produce an immunogenic response, and chlamydial antibodies are measurable using complement fixation, microimmunofluorescence, and ELISA techniques. When a fourfold rise in IgG titer or the presence of specific IgM antibodies is documented, chlamydial disease may be diagnosed. The presence of preexisting antibody, cross-reactivity of various serotypes of *Chlamydia,* and the lack of antibody response to some chlamydial carriage limit serological analysis as a diagnostic tool.

Treatment

The drug of choice for the treatment of *Chlamydia* is tetracycline. The exact duration of therapy necessary to achieve cure is unknown. Tetracycline, 500 mg four times daily for 7 days appears to be adequate. Tetracycline, 250 mg four times daily for 14 to 21 days, is also curative. *Chlamydia* are also sensitive to erythromycin and some sulfa drugs. Cephalosporins and penicillins are not effective antichlamydial agents. Newer penicillin derivatives and clindamycin have some antichlamydial spectrum. Although treatment to eliminate *Chlamydia* should be based on culture documentation, when such culture facilities are not available or culture is impractical, presumptive therapy may be instituted for suspected carriage or disease in a high-risk population. Documentation of organism presence may aid effective education, compliance, and partner treatment.

Repeat cultures after therapy should be performed, at the earliest, 3 to 4 weeks after completion of antimicrobial therapy. All sexual partners must also be referred for evaluation and treatment.

ACTINOMYCOSIS

Infection by *Actinomyces israelii* is an infrequent cause of disease of the upper genital tract. *Actinomyces israelii* is a gram-positive, non–acid fast anaerobic bacterium with characteristic radially branching filamentous formation. It is most typically found in the oral cavity. Actinomycosis is a sporadic infection of soft tissues characterized by invasion of areas of trauma, with chronic, suppurative infection that results in tissue destruction, fibrosis, and the formation of draining sinuses. Active actinomycotic infection usually is polymicrobial, with other anaerobic organisms frequently being involved.

Actinomycosis is a rare cause of indolent pelvic infection secondary to seeding of the upper genital tract from other intra-abdominal sources or hematogenous dissemination of *Actinomyces*. In addition, the occurrence of ascending pelvic actinomycosis has been described in the presence of an IUD.

Colonization of the lower genital tract by *Actinomyces* is seen most frequently in IUD users. The prevalence of colonization increases with the duration of IUD use. A small percentage of women in whom colonization occurs will manifest upper genital tract infection with actinomycosis. This may be preceded by irregular vaginal bleeding and mild, chronic pelvic discomfort. By the time of presentation, the pelvic organs may be massively indurated and fibrotic, with near total destruction of anatomy and adherence to surrounding structures. At this stage, because of the limited chance of restoration of structure and function by medical therapy, the treatment is frequently surgical removal of affected organs.

Diagnosis

The diagnosis of actinomycosis can be suspected by a suggestive Gram stain. Histological sections of actinomycotic infections show necrotic debris and inflammation associated with "sulfur granules," which are central organisms with branching filaments that stain yellow with a silver stain. Diagnosis can be confirmed by culture using appropriate anaerobic media and techniques.

Treatment

When colonization is suspected by Papanicolaou smear, treatment with antibiotics has not been shown to effectively eliminate *Actinomyces* from the lower genital tract. Current recommendations are to remove IUDs in cases of suspected colonization and repeat Papanicolaou smears in a few months; if the smear is normal, the IUD may then be reinserted.

Actinomycosis is sensitive to penicillins, tetracycline, chloramphenicol, and clindamycin. Treatment of infection is with high-dose parenteral antibiotics, typically penicillin. The exact length of therapy necessary is not established, although the slow growth of these organisms and extensive involvement in cases of infection at other sites usually necessitate a minimum of 6 weeks of therapy. Treatment of actinomycotic pelvic infection should also include coverage for other organisms typically found in cases of upper genital tract infection, in particular, anaerobic organisms. Despite aggressive medical therapy, surgical intervention is commonly required.

GENITAL TRACT TUBERCULOSIS AS AN ETIOLOGIC AGENT FOR PELVIC INFLAMMATORY DISEASE

Tuberculosis is a rare cause of upper genital tract infection in developed countries. Today it most often presents in older women who were exposed to tuberculosis before the advent of effective chemoprophylaxis and in younger women who emigrate from countries where tuberculosis is endemic.

Genital tract tuberculosis is usually secondary to hematogenous spread from pulmonary or other nongenital tract foci. It can rarely spread to the genital tract from other intraperitoneal foci or from male sexual partners with tuberculous epididymitis.

The most frequent site of tuberculous involvement in the female genital tract is the fallopian tube. Central spread of infection will result in involvement of the uterus, cervix, vagina, and vulva, in order of decreasing frequency. Ovarian involvement in the tuberculous process varies from 5% to 30%.

Genital tract tuberculosis is an extremely indolent infection. Disease may not become manifest for more than 10 years after initial seeding of the genital tract. Presenting symptoms may be those of unusual vaginal bleeding patterns, including altered menses, amenorrhea, and postmenopausal bleeding. Approximately 25% to 35% of women with pelvic tuberculosis may complain of vague, chronic lower abdominal or pelvic pain. The chief presenting complaint of young women with genital tract tuberculosis is infertility. Occasionally, women with genital tract tuberculosis can present with tuberculous peritonitis and ascites, although this is more frequently secondary to direct hemotogenous seeding of the peritoneum.

The diagnosis of genital tract tuberculosis may be suspected from past medical history, travel history, and a chest roentgenogram with evidence of healed pulmonary tuberculosis. Except for debilitated, systemically ill patients, a skin test with a purified protein derivative of tuberculin will yield positive findings. Hysterosalpingogram may show characteristic changes suggestive of tuberculous infection, including beading, sacculation, sinus formation, and a rigid "pipestem" pattern.

Diagnosis can be confirmed by histological examination that reveals typical granulomas, or acid-fast stain and culture of surgical or endometrial biopsy specimens. Menstrual blood collected in a vaginal cup or cervical cap may also be submitted for culture.

The treatment of genital tract tuberculosis is primarily medical, with administration of two or three antituberculosis drugs for 18 to 24 months.

Surgery is indicated if symptoms or physical examination suggest persistence or increase in disease despite adequate therapy or if culture or biopsy results suggest resistant organisms. Surgical therapy most often consist of total abdominal hysterectomy and bilateral salpingo-oophorectomy.

GENITAL HERPES

Genital herpes is a sexually transmitted infection of increasing concern for all sexually active women. There are an estimated 270,000 to 600,000 new cases per year, with the peak incidence in the third decade. Symptomatic genital herpes is the most frequent cause of painful lesions of the lower genital tract of women in the United States. Herpes infection of the lower genital tract has been associated with cervical cancer, although a causative role remains unproven. In addition, contact with genital herpes during passage through the birth canal has been associated with systemic neonatal infection, which carries major risks of serious morbidity and a high mortality rate.

The exact prevalence of genital herpes infection is unknown, since not all people with active infections seek medical care. However, some consider that the incidence of herpes may be steadily increasing and that genital herpes may be one of the most frequent sexually transmitted diseases in the United States today.

Genital herpes is caused by the herpes simplex virus (HSV), a member of the DNA containing Herpesviridae family. There are two major types of HSV, types 1 (HSV-1) and 2 (HSV-2), which are closely related and are homologous for approximately 50% of antigens. Although the majority of genital herpes lesions are caused by HSV-2 infections and HSV-1 primarily cause oral-labial lesions, it is clear that there is significant overlap. Approximately 85% to 90% of genital infections are caused by HSV-2, whereas the remainder are caused by HSV-1. This proportion varies, and up to 50% of genital lesions were found to be due to HSV-1 in a survey that took place in England.

Genital herpes is a recurrent infection. Periods of active infection are separated by periods of latency during which the inactive virus resides in the dorsal root sacral ganglia. Under the stimulus of various endogenous and exogenous factors, the virus travels down the sensory nerve root to the lower genital area where virus replicates, outward manifestations of disease become apparent, and HSV can be identified by culture.

The lesions of genital herpes are typically painful lesions that begin as fluid-filled vesicles or papules, which progress to well-circumscribed, occasionally coalescent, shallow-based ulcers, and heal by reepithelialization of mucous membranes or by crusting over of epidermal surfaces. Virus is shed from active lesions until healing begins, and virus can be transmitted during the time of shedding. The clinical presentation and duration of active infection vary widely and are dependent on virus type, location of presentation, the preexistence of antibodies and on presentation as initial or recurrent disease.

Initial presentation of genital herpes infection occurs 1 to 45 days (mean 5.8 days) after exposure to the virus. Manifestations of initial HSV infection are more severe and last longer than those of recurrent disease. Multiple painful, usually bilateral, lesions occur on the external genitalia. Symptoms tend to peak within 8 to 10 days and gradually decrease over the next week. Crops of new lesions form over a mean of 10 days. Ulcers last 4 to 15 days, and the mean time from the onset of lesions to total healing is 20 to 21 days. Virus is shed from lesions up to the time of crusting over, with the average duration of shedding being 11 days. Most often, local lesions are accompanied by bilateral, tender lymphadenopathy of the inguinal and, sometimes, femoral and iliac regions. When adenopathy of the deep inguinal nodes is present, it can be responsible for severe lower pelvic pain. Adenopathy appears somewhat after the onset of lesions and often takes longer to resolve, lasting beyond the period of the lesions themselves.

Local involvement includes urethritis in the majority of cases, with 82% of urethral cultures being positive for virus. Urination may be problematic either because of periurethral and vulvar edema or because of intense dysuria due to urethral herpetic involvement.

Initial genital herpes infection involves the cervix in more than 80% of cases. Cervical involvement may be clinically apparent with friability of the cervix, ulcerative and occasionally necrotic lesions of the cervix, and a marked increase in cervical discharge. Both the exocervix and endocervix may be involved. In some cases, involvement of the cervix may not be clinically apparent, although virus can be cultured from the cervix.

Other genital tract sites may also be involved. Vaginal lesions are apparent in 4% of cases. Although HSV has been cultured from the fallopian tube, it is unclear how often the upper genital tract is involved during initial cases of genital herpes. At present, it is not believed to be a major clinical problem.

Women develop complications of initial HSV infection more commonly than men. Such complication may be due to local spread or to more distant effects of virus.

Coincident with initial symptomatic genital herpes infection, symptomatic pharyngitis has been reported to occur in approximately 10% of cases. The herpes simplex virus can be isolated from the pharynx of individuals with both symptomatic pharyngitis and from those without pharyngeal symptoms. Pharyngitis and pharyngeal viral shedding occur with genital infection with both HSV-1 and HSV-2.

Secondary spread of local lesions to other body sites occurs after the onset of lesions and before lesions have crusted over in approximately one fourth of cases. Extragenital involvement is most often of sites below the waist such as the buttocks and upper legs; however, involvement of the fingers and eyes has also been reported. Secondary spread of lesions to extragenital sites is thought to be primarily due to autoinoculation and most often occurs in the second week of disease.

In one half to two thirds of cases of initial genital herpes infection, systemic symptoms are apparent, usually early in the course of illness. Fever, malaise, headache, and myalgias are common. Other systemic complications can include hepatitis, aseptic meningitis, and autonomic nervous system dysfunction.

Hepatitis exhibits a picture typical for hepatocellular necrosis and presents after the onset of local genital lesions. This usually occurs within the first week of illness and is most often accompanied by other systemic symptoms.

Aseptic meningitis is seen much more frequently with HSV-2 than with HSV-1 infections. It has been reported to occur in up to 36% of initial genital herpes infections. The presentation is of headache, stiff neck, and photophobia, with or without fever. It is accompanied by a cerebrospinal fluid pleocytosis consisting largely of lymphocytes. Meningitis is self-limited, requires only supportive care, and resolves without permanent neu-

rological sequelae. Encephalitis is rarely a complication of genital herpes infection.

Sacral autonomic nervous system dysfunction is an uncommon complication of initial genital herpes infection. Typical symptoms include decrease in sensation along the sacral nerve route distribution, inability to void due to bladder dysfunction, and constipation due to bowel dysfunction. Nerve dysfunction can be confirmed through electromyography and may last up to 6 to 8 weeks. Occasionally, sensory involvement may take the form of hyperesthesia in a radicular pattern. A presentation of self-limited transverse myelitis with paralysis has also been reported.

Recurrent genital herpes infection is typically less severe, of shorter duration, and less frequently involves systemic manifestations than initial disease. One to 2 days to a few hours prior to the onset of recurrent lesions, prodromal symptoms may occur. This is typically described as a tingling sensation, itching, or hyperesthesia of the genital area where lesions will occur. The prodrome may also include a sacral dermatomal neuralgia with pain radiating to the buttocks and hips.

Recurrent genital lesions are fewer, smaller, and more often unilateral. Recurrent lesions may not have the typical ulcerative appearance and may be more similar in appearance to a fissure or excoriation. Recurrences are usually painful and tend to occur in the same location and have the same appearance from episode to episode. Symptoms of recurrent lesions last 4 to 8 days, and there are fewer crops of new lesions. The mean time to disappearance of recurrent lesions is 9 to 10 days, and the duration of viral shedding averages 5 days.

Both urethritis and cervicitis are less frequently seen with recurrent genital infection than with initial infection. Cervicitis is typically manifest solely as virus positivity. Tender local adenopathy may be present but is usually less severe and of shorter duration. Systemic manifestations are uncommon, and extragenital involvement is seen in less than 5% of cases.

The frequency of recurrent disease and the length of time between recurrences of active infection are highly variable. The average number of recurrences in women who have symptomatic recurrent genital herpes is 5 to 8 per year. There is some evidence that mean time to recurrence is greater from initial episode to first recurrence than between subsequent recurrences. Recurrences may be precipitated by an obvious endogenous stimulus, such as cyclic hormonal variation or stress, or recurrent infection may be precipitated by exposure to HSV through sexual contact with an infected partner. It is unclear whether contact with exogenous virus precipitates recurrent infection or whether this is actually reinfection with a different viral strain. Although it has been the general impression that frequency of recurrent disease decreases as time from initial infection increases, the frequency of recurrent disease may be independent of time for at least the first 3 to 4 years of disease.

It is now apparent that the clinical presentation of genital herpes does not always follow classic patterns. Asymptomatic infection as defined by culture-positive viral shedding in the absence of symptoms or lesions has been documented to occur from both the cervix and the vulva. The prevalence of asymptomatic shedding is unknown, as is the frequency or risk factors for shedding. It does appear that asymptomatic shedding is of brief duration and lasts for an average of 3 to 5 days per episode. Transmission of virus from one individual to another can occur during asymptomatic shedding, but how often this occurs is unknown.

Approximately 25% of initial genital herpes infections present in women who have preexisting antibody to HSV. These so-called nonprimary first episodes tend to be less severe with fewer systemic manifestations than true primary episodes in an antibody-negative individual. Some of these mild, nonprimary initial episodes may actually be recurrent infection in a person with previous asymptomatic HSV-2 infection. In up to 70% of other cases, the presence of antibody to HSV-1 of oral-labial origin may serve to ameliorate the clinical expression of genital infection.

Although initial presentation of genital herpes infection caused by HSV-1 cannot be distinguished from initial presentation of infection caused by HSV-2, HSV-1 is less likely to result in recurrent genital infection. Recurrences of infection after initial infection caused by HSV-1 are much less frequent and less severe. The reason for this difference in recurrence rates is unclear but probably is related to virus type and not antibody response.

Diagnosis

The diagnosis of genital herpes is often suggested by characteristic clinical presentation and appearance of lesions. The most accurate diagnostic test to confirm clinical impression is virus isolation by tissue culture. The virus may be isolated from both vesicle fluid and the base of a wet ulcer. If vesicles are present, the vesicles should be unroofed and the fluid cultured directly. A single virus culture done of an appropriate lesion will identify live virus in 85% of 90% of cases. Virus grown in culture can be typed. Less sensitive but helpful tests when viral cultures are not available rely on cytological methods to identify changes in cells typically produced by the HSV. Scrappings of viral lesions may be gathered for fluorescent staining for a Papanicolaou smear or for Tzanck preparation. Genital tract smears appear to be neither sensitive nor specific. A Tzanck smear stained with either Wright's or Giemsa stain is positive if multinucleated giant cells are identified, as may occur in up to 50% of cases. Antibody testing is generally of no value to the diagnosis of genital herpes infections. Forty percent to 60% of adults have antibodies to HSV-1, and 15% to 35% have antibodies to HSV-2, which represents past exposure that may have resulted in clinically apparent infection or asymptomatic infection. Although it is possible to distinguish antibodies to HSV-2 from antibodies to HSV-1, antibody response to type common antigens leads to a large crossover in identification and difficulty in detecting new antibody formation in a person with a previous type common antibody response. In these cases, the existence of antibody to HSV at the onset of an initial genital herpes infection may preclude identification of this episode as either primary infection in a previously antibody-negative host or recurrent infection in a previously asymptomatic host. In addition, the presence of antibody to HSV at the onset of a herpes genital lesion may identify past exposure to this virus but not, however, help identify the etiology of active lesions. Occasionally, if there is no antibody to HSV present at the onset of a suspected primary genital herpes infection and antibody is documented to develop during the course of illness, antibody testing can be of some value. It is obvious that due to the variety in expression of disease and the inherent inaccuracies in diagnosis by antibody assessment, timing and sources of specific infection may be difficult if not impossible to determine.

Treatment

There is no therapy that effectively prevents establishment of latency of genital herpes or eradicates infection. The currently available antiviral agent that most effectively alters the course of genital herpes infection is acyclovir. Acyclovir is available in three forms. Topical application of acyclovir every 4 hours has been demonstrated to decrease the duration of symptoms and the length of viral shedding for initial disease. Its use is sometimes limited by the side effect of local irritation. Topical acyclovir is not effective in altering the course of recurrent genital herpes infection. Intravenous acyclovir is used to treat disseminated herpetic infection in immunosuppressed individuals. In addition, both intravenous (IV) and oral acyclovir have been used to ameliorate the course of initial episodes of genital herpes. If given within 7 days of onset of a first episode, IV acyclovir decreases the duration of symptoms, lesions, viral shedding, systemic manifestations, and episodes of new vesicle formation. If given within 5 to 6 days of onset of a first episode, oral acyclovir decreases the duration of symptoms, lesions, viral shedding, and new vesicle formation. Both are more effective for primary than for nonprimary first episodes, and neither change the course of subsequent recurrences.

Oral acyclovir can be given either on a daily basis to suppress recurrent disease or on an episodic basis to ameliorate the effects of recurrent disease. When it is given as suppressive therapy, women on acyclovir therapy have fewer recurrences, and any recurrences are less severe and of shorter duration. A significant proportion will have no recurrences, although the proportion who remain totally recurrence free decreases with time. There is no evidence that suppression influences the long-term natural history of recurrent disease, and recurrences occur with previous frequency when suppression is discontinued. The length of time one can safely remain on suppressive therapy is unknown, although no cumulative toxicity is apparent with up to 2 years of use. The possibility of emergence of resistant virus remains a concern, however. It is currently suggested that those with more than six recurrences yearly, with complications associated with recurrent disease, and immunosuppressed individuals are candidates for suppressive therapy. Suppressive therapy should periodically be discontinued to assess the frequency of recurrences and need for further therapy. Episodic oral acyclovir, patient initiated at the earliest sign of a recurrence, decreases the duration of lesions, symptoms, viral shedding and formation of new lesions. It does not alter the time period between recurrences.

The mainstay of treatment of genital herpes infections remains care of local lesions and supportive care through any systemic illness. Local measures to decrease superinfections of lesions and to increase comfort are encouraged. Use of an indwelling bladder catheter may be necessary in severe cases of herpes urethritis. Hospitalization for observation and supportive care during episodes of aseptic meningitis may be necessary. Finally, appropriate counseling must be provided to handle the emotional and informational needs of patients in whom genital herpes infection has been diagnosed.

SYPHILIS

Syphilis occurs when the causative organism, the spirochete *Treponema pallidum,* is inoculated into mucous membranes. This occurs most frequently during sexual activity. In the United States, approximately 20,000 to 30,000 new cases of syphilis are reported each year, predominantly in the 15- to 40-year age group. In the late 1980s, the incidence of new cases of syphilis increased for the first time in a number of years. Syphilis exists in well-described stages defined by both clinical presentation and time course.

The incubation period from contact to the onset of lesions of primary syphilis ranges from 9 to 90 days, with an average time of 3 weeks. The lesion of primary syphilis is the chancre, a solitary, painless ulceration that forms at the site of inoculation. A chancre begins as a firm papule and breaks down to become a well-demarcated hard ulcer with raised, rolled borders and a finely granular, erythematous base. The average size of a chancre is 0.5 to 2.0 cm. Most frequently, they occur on the labia, posterior fourchette, cervix, or vagina, although pharyngeal and anal chancres also occur. Bilateral, firm, nontender regional adenopathy is common. Because chancres are not painful, they often go unnoticed and undetected. Spirochetes are found at the base of the ulcer, and chancres are infectious. If untreated, chancres heal spontaneously by 2 to 6 weeks.

Nine to 90 days after chancre formation, or an average of 6 to 12 weeks after exposure, hematogenous dissemination of spirochetes occurs, and the onset of symptoms of secondary syphilis takes place. The chancre of primary syphilis may still be present at this time. Secondary syphilis has mucocutaneous and systemic manifestations with multiorgan involvement. Various types of generalized skin lesions may occur. Usually only one type exists at a time, although lesions may evolve over time. Macular, maculopapular, or primarily papular generalized skin eruptions are typical. Facial sparing and involvement of the palms and soles is classic. Pustular and discoid lesions as well as alopecia and mucous membrane patches are well-described variants of the mucocutaneous lesions of secondary syphilis. Another classic lesion of secondary syphilis is the condyloma latum, which is a confluence of raised, moist, flat hypertrophic, exuberant granulomatous papular lesions occurring primarily in intertriginous or moist areas. These lesions are infectious.

Generalized, usually nontender, lymphadenopathy may commonly present along with the skin lesions of secondary syphilis. Influenza-type symptoms, with fever, malaise, headache, sore throat, arthralgias, leukocytosis, anemia, and occasional splenomegaly, typlify the systemic manifestations of secondary syphilis. Manifestations of involvement of other organ systems, such as hepatitis and meningitis, also occur.

Following resolution of signs of secondary syphilis, the infection enters a latent period. Formerly, latent syphilis was classifed as early latent syphilis for up to 4 years' duration, with syphilis of more than 4 years' duration being classified as late latent syphilis. Currently, all syphilis of less than 1 year's duration is classified as early syphilis with little distinction made for all latent syphilis of more than 1 year's duration. During early syphilis of less than 1 year's duration, there can be a recurrence of symptoms of secondary syphilis. Otherwise, latent syphilis is asymptomatic and not infectious.

Manifestations of late syphilis are thought to be largely a result of endothelial damage and ongoing chronic inflammation. Five to 20 years or more after initial disease, the consequences of late syphilis present as single-system or multisystem involvement.

Benign, mucocutaneous late disease presents with painless, indolent, destructive lesions. The classic skin lesion of late syphilis is the solitary gumma, a progressive, granulomatous, necrotic ulcer, but lesions may also be nodular and multiple. Gummas and destructive lesions of late syphilis may also involve visceral organs, long bones, and joints.

Two other distinct forms of late syphilis are cardiovascular syphilis and neurosyphilis. Cardiovascular syphilis most prominently involves the aorta, resulting in aortic insufficiency and thoracic aortic aneurysms. Neurosyphilis may be asymptomatic, may present as acute meningitis, or may be responsible for gradual deterioration of intellectual and motor capacity.

Syphilis can be transmitted to the fetus at any stage of pregnancy, resulting in deformities, acute neonatal illness, and late manifestations of disease. Congenital syphilis can be prevented or ameliorated by maternal treatment during pregnancy. For this reason, premarital and prenatal screening for syphilis are the rule.

Diagnosis

When an infectious lesion of syphilis such as a chancre is recognized, a dark-field examination should be performed on secretions from a cleaned lesion. If spirochetes are demonstrated, a diagnosis of syphilis may be made. False-negative results of dark-field examinations can occur, particularly when topical or systemic antimicrobial therapy suppresses the numbers of spirochetes.

The diagnosis of syphilis is most often made by serological methods. Serological tests for syphilis are of two types: the nontreponemal and the treponemal tests.

The nontreponemal tests most widely available are the Veneral Disease Research Laboratory slide tests and the rapid plasma reagin circle card test. These tests detect the presence of cardiolipin, a nonspecific antigen produced during syphilitic infection. These tests are quantitative, and serial titers may be used to judge therapeutic response. An abnormal nontreponemal test result is suggestive of, but not specific for, a diagnosis of syphilis. Positive nontreponemal test results for syphilis are also associated with a variety of conditions and disorders, including collagen-vascular diseases, lymphomas, drug abuse, sarcoidosis, and acute infections such as mononucleosis, *Mycoplasma* infections, and other febrile illnesses.

A definitive diagnosis of syphilis is made by testing for the presence of specific antitreponemal antibodies. The fluorescent treponemal antibody absorption test (FTA-ABS) is the treponemal test most widely used. This test will confirm a diagnosis of syphilis with a low false positive rate of 1% to 2%. Once positive, an FTA-ABS result will remain positive despite successful therapy.

A serological test for syphilis will be predictive of disease in about 75% of cases by the fourth week after exposure. By 6 weeks to 3 months, 99% to 100% of serological test results will be abnormal. Although a chancre may be present prior to seropositivity, secondary syphilis is almost always accompanied by an abnormal serological test result. If a serological test result for syphilis remains negative 3 months after suspected exposure, the diagnosis of syphilis can be excluded. In late stages of syphilis, nontreponemal test results for syphilis may become negative in up to 30% of cases; however, the treponemal test result will be positive in virtually 100% of cases.

When results of a screening serological test for syphilis are positive, the stage of disease is determined using historical guidelines. If the patient is presently asymptomatic and a result of a serological test for syphilis performed within the preceding year was negative or symptoms of primary or secondary syphilis were present within 1 year, early syphilis is diagnosed. If normal serological testing within 1 year cannot be documented and there is no documentation of symptoms of primary or secondary syphilis, syphilis of more than 1 year's duration is presumed. If latent syphilis of prolonged duration is suspected, a decision to perform a lumbar puncture to rule out neurosyphilis must be individualized. If no neurological or psychiatric abnormalities exist and the treatment is to be with penicillin, it may be reasonable to forego a lumbar puncture since standard penicillin therapy for syphilis of more than 1 year's duration is curative for the majority of cases of asymptomatic neurosyphilis.

Treatment

Treatment of syphilis will abort acute disease and prevent progression of disease but will not alter permanent changes produced by tissue destruction. Primary therapy of syphilis is with benzathine penicillin. Penicillin-allergic patients are treated with tetracycline. The length of therapy is determined by the stage of disease. Early syphilis is treated with 2.4 million units of benzathine penicillin G intramuscularly at a single session or 500 mg of tetracycline orally four times daily for 15 days. Syphilis of more than 1 year's duration is treated with the penicillin regimen just described once per week for 3 successive weeks or with tetracycline therapy for 30 days. Penicillin-allergic patients who are pregnant may need to be hospitalized for desensitization and treatment with

TABLE 19–7.

Treatment of Syphilis*

Early syphilis (primary, secondary, or latent syphilis of <1 yr's duration)
  Benzathine penicillin G, 2.4 million units, intramuscularly at a single session
  Penicillin-allergic patients:
    Tetracycline hydrochloride, 500 mg orally 4 times daily for 15 days; or erythromycin,† 500 mg orally 4 times daily for 15 days
Syphilis of 1 yr's duration (except neurosyphilis)
  Benzathine penicillin G, 2.4 million units intramuscularly once per week for 3 successive weeks (7.2 million units total)
  Penicillin-allergic patients:
    Tetracycline hydrochloride, 500 mg orally 4 times daily for 30 days; or erythromycin, 500 mg orally 4 times daily for 30 days
Neurosyphilis
  Aqueous crystalline penicillin G, 12–24 million units intravenously each day for 10 days, followed by benzathine penicillin G, 2.4 million units intramuscularly once per week for 3 doses; or aqueous procaine penicillin G, 2.4 million units intramuscularly each day, plus probenecid, 500 mg orally 4 times daily, both for 10 days, followed by benzathine penicillin G, 2.4 million units intramuscularly weekly for 3 doses; or benzathine penicillin G, 2.4 million units intramuscularly once per week for 3 doses
  Penicillin-allergic patients:
    Patients with histories of allergies to penicillin should have their allergy confirmed and managed in consultation with an expert.

*Adapted from Centers for Disease Control: Sexually transmitted diseases treatment guidelines 1982. *MMWR* 1982; 31(suppl):33–62.
†The efficacy of erythromycin has not been firmly established; therefore, complications and serological follow-up should be assured.

parenteral penicillin for optimal therapy to prevent congenital syphilis (Table 19–7).

After successful therapy, nontreponemal serological test results will revert to normal in a large percentage of cases, depending on the duration of disease. Within 1 year, 100% of patients with primary syphilis will be seronegative. Within 2 years, virtually all patients with secondary syphilis will have normal nontreponemal serological test results. Within 5 years, approximately 45% of patients with latent syphilis will be seronegative. Titers should be followed after therapy until they stabilize or disappear. If titers increase by fourfold, or if symptoms persist or recur, reinfection is presumed and retreatment indicated.

The Jarisch-Herxheimer reaction is a well-described phenomenon occurring in a variable number of patients treated for primary or secondary syphilis. Approximately 12 hours after therapy, skin lesions become more prominent, and pronounced systemic symptoms of fever, rigors, headache, myalgias, and arthralgias occur. This is presumed to be due to either release of treponemal toxins or formation of circulating antigen-antibody complexes. Symptoms are self-limited and do not recur, and no specific therapy is indicated.

CHANCROID

Chancroid is a sexually transmitted disease caused by *Hemophilus ducreyi,* a short, thick, gram-negative bacillus that is a facultative anaerobe. Chancroid is characterized by painful genital ulcers and suppurative inguinal lymphadenopathy with a lack of systemic signs or symptoms. Since 1981, multiple outbreaks of chancroid in the United States have been documented, with more than 3,000 cases documented in 1986. It is endemic in tropical and subtropical developing countries.

After an incubation period averaging 3 to 7 days, the genital lesions of chancroid begin as small papules or vesicles, which become pustular and rupture, forming an ulcer within 1 to 3 days of their onset. Ulcers are soft, not indurated, and have irregular, ragged borders with undermined edges. Surrounding the ulcer may be a rim of erythema. The base of the ulcer is granulomatous and friable, often covered with gray, adherent, sometimes necrotic, sometimes serosanguinous exudate. Ulcers are painful and tender. Ulcers may be single but are more often multiple. Contiguous spread results from autoinoculation. Ulcers vary from a few millimeters to 20 mm. Most often the labia, posterior fourchette, and the perianal region are involved, but the cervix, vagina, clitoris, and urethra may also be involved.

Regional lymph nodes are involved in more than 50% of cases. Bilateral involvement of inguinal nodes is common, although if genital lesions are unilateral, lymph node involvement will also be unilateral. Lymph nodes are tender, increase in size, and may become matted, suppurate, and fluctuant. Overlying skin becomes thinned and necrotic, leading to spontaneous rup-

ture and drainage. If lymph nodes are noted to be indurated and fluctuant, the lymph node may be aspirated and a large, chronic, draining sinus prevented.

Diagnosis

The diagnosis of chancroid can be made by scraping material from the edges of an ulcer or collecting material from a suppurating lymph node and culturing this on specific media. A Gram strain of this material reveals predominantly gram-negative coccobacillary forms. *Hemophilus ducreyi* may be one of many bacterial species present in a lesion of chancroid; the diagnosis in these cases may be more difficult to document. Experience is being gained with both immunofluorescent staining of lesion material and immunobinding serological testing. The diagnosis of chancroid is often made by clinical presentation and by exclusion of other causes of genital ulceration such as genital herpes, LGV, and syphilis.

Treatment

If untreated, ulcers may persist, increase in size, and form more extensive, erosive lesions. Occasionally, local lesions may run a self-limited course. Treatment has classically consisted of administration of sulfa or tetracycline. Tetracycline resistance is now widespread, however, and there are increasing reports of sulfa resistance. Currently recommended therapeutic options include erythromycin, trimethoprim-sulfamethoxazole, and ceftriazone. It is now apparent that short courses of therapy are curative for chancroid. *Hemophilus ducreyi* is rapidly eliminated from lesions and nodes, although healing takes longer, occasionally weeks. Successful therapy is heralded by subjective improvement in pain and tenderness within 2 to 3 days. Progression to fluctuance of lymph nodes can occur despite effective therapy; this should be handled by aspiration of fluctuance. Sexual partners should be treated whether or not they are symptomatic or have visible lesions.

LYMPHOGRANULOMA VENEREUM

Lymphogranuloma venereum is a sexually transmitted disease whose major clinical manifestations are due to infection of regional lymph nodes that drain sites of transient local infection. The causative organism of LGV is *C. trachomatis*, specifically immunotypes L-1, L-2, and L-3. Lymphogranuloma venereum is currently rare in North America and other industrialized countries. It is common in the tropical and semitropical areas, particularly in developing countries.

The transient mucosal or cutaneous lesion of LGV occurs at the site of inoculation 4 to 21 days after exposure. In women, lesions are usually singular, although they may be multiple. They occur predominantly on the posterior vulva, urethral meatus, and medial labia, although the vagina and cervix may be involved. Lesions are small, vesicular, papular, or pustular lesions, less than 6 mm, which progress to small, shallow ulcers with irregular borders and an erythematous base. Ulcers are usually not painful and often not recognized. After a short time, local lesions heal spontaneously, and after variable periods of latency, symptoms of local lymphadenitis become manifest.

The symptoms of adenitis vary according to the lymph chains that are involved and the chronicity of infection. The immediate course of lymph node involvement entails a 1- to 4-week period during which multiple nodes become inflamed and suppurate, become fixated to overlying skin, and spontaneously rupture and drain. Chronic inflammation of involved lymphatics may lead to obstruction with retrograde edema and occasional ulceration. Involved tissue is often totally replaced by fibrosis and constriction with scarring. Repeated episodes of spontaneous rupture and drainage may lead to chronically draining sinuses, fistula formation, and scarring.

Initial LGV lesions of the anterior vulva and lower portion of the vagina drain into femoral and inguinal lymphatics, resulting in the *inguinal syndrome*. Multiple nodes of both inguinal and femoral regions become firm, adherent to each other, and eventually form buboes, which are fluctuant and painful with skin fixation. If both the inguinal and femoral areas are involved, buboes are separated by the inguinal ligament forming the pathognomonic *groove sign*. Involvement most often is unilateral. If fluctuant nodes are aspirated through normal skin, this can prevent spontaneous rupture with chronic sinus formation. Chronic inflammation of inguinal lymph nodes can lead to fibrous constriction of the inguinal area, often accompanied by draining sinuses. Hypertrophy and edema of vulvar lymphatic tissues

can be marked. When this occurs, it is called *esthiomene* and is analogous to elephantiasis in men. Overlying vulvar skin may ulcerate. Chronic inflammation in the vaginal and periuretheral area can lead to stricture and fistula formation.

More often in women, the perirectal and pelvic lymph nodes are involved, leading to genitorectal manifestations of LGV. This presents as a proctocolitis with bloody diarrhea and perianal discharge. Fibrosis of edematous mucosa eventfully leads to stricture formation, and rectovaginal fistulas are common.

As opposed to chancroid, systemic symptoms may be present at the time of presentation of LGV. Approximately 50% of patients will have fever, malaise, headache, and anorexia at the time of initial lymphadenitis.

Diagnosis

The diagnosis of LGV is most frequently made by antibody testing. Complement fixation titers to *C. trachomatis* greater than or equal to 1:128 are suggestive of LGV. Antibody testing by microimmunofluorescence may show an increase in specific IgG titers or the presence of specific IgM antibody. Chlamydial organisms may occasionally be isolated from the exudate of fluctuant or draining buboes. Histological examination of involved nodes may show suggestive palisading aggregates of mononuclear cells surrounding granulomas or microabscesses but may be fairly nonspecific, and biopsy is not the primary mode of diagnosis.

Treatment

Treatment of LGV is usually with tetracycline given for at least 2 weeks after the remission of all systemic symptoms and local disease. Alternative therapies include sulfonamides and erythromycin.

DONOVANOSIS

Donovanosis, formerly termed *granuloma inguinale*, is a disease of the lower genital tract characterized by slowly progressive, hypertrophic ulceration with tissue destruction. Donovanosis is a sexually transmitted disease associated with the encapsulated gram-negative bacillus *Calymmatobacterium granulomatis*.

The incubation period of donovanosis may be up to 6 months, although it averages 2 to 4 months. The initial genital tract lesion is a painless, indurated, reddish brown papule, which, over a course of days to weeks, erodes and ulcerates. Ulcerations have well-defined borders and clean bases with exuberant velvety granulation tissue. Lesions are fairly superficial and spread by contact, autoinoculation, and lymphatic extension. They are not tender unless superinfected. Involved tissue undergoes repeated granulomatous proliferation, ulceration, and scarring with eventual extensive tissue destruction. Extension to the inguinal area is associated with subcutaneous induration, swelling, and eventual breakdown with pseudobubo formation. Lymph nodes may be slightly increased in size and occasionally tender, but they do not suppurate. Systemic signs are rare and, when they do occur, are related to extensive disease with secondary infection.

Donovanosis is currently rare in Europe and North America. It is commonest in tropical and subtropical countries.

Diagnosis

The diagnosis of donovanosis is established by demonstrating the presence of Donovan bodies in tissue preparations stained with Wright's or Giemsa stain. Donovan bodies are mononuclear cells containing large numbers of encapsulated bacilli. Scrappings of lesions, crush preparations of tissue, or biopsy samples taken from the edge of an ulcer all may reveal these characteristic formations.

Treatment

If untreated, lesions of donovanosis appear to undergo periods of spontaneous resolution or healing, with subsequent relapse of active disease. Active lesions resolve with antibiotic therapy and relapse less frequently. Occasionally, prolonged courses of antibiotics need to be administered to prevent "recurrent" disease. The antibiotic of choice is doxycycline or tetracycline; erythromycin and ampicillin have also been demonstrated to be effective.

GENITAL WARTS

Genital warts are caused by the human papillomavirus (HPV), a DNA virus structurally and probably antigenically related to the causative agent of common skin warts. Currently, more than 50 types of HPV have been defined. Genital warts are sexually transmitted with an incubation period ranging from 3 weeks to 8 months, averaging approximately 3 months. There is a 25% to 60% transmission rate for genital warts, and infectivity may be influenced by the number and age of lesions. Genital warts of longer duration tend to be less infectious.

Typical genital warts are exophytic growths that appear as papillary, pink to white frondlike lesions. These lesions are superficial, may be solitary, may occur in clusters, or may coalesce into large cauliflower-like masses. Some gross warts appear as discrete, flat-topped hyperkeratotic papules. The lesions are not usually painful, although they may be pruritic. When warts are exceptionally large, they may become necrotic and secondarily infected, with superficial bleeding, discharge, and fetid odor.

Any part of the vulva may be involved by HPV, but particularly the posterior fourchette. The mons, the perineum, and the perianal areas may be involved, as may be the vagina, cervix, and anal canal. If warts are present surrounding orifices, there may be internal involvement in 50% to 70% of cases. For this reason, all patients with vulvar warts should have speculum examination performed, and all patients with perianal warts should have a rectal examination and sometimes anoscopy. Visible warts that occur in the vagina and on the cervix usually appear as flat or papular lesions. The majority of cervical warts are flat and are visible only by acetic acid staining or colposcopy.

The growth of genital warts is stimulated by heat, moisture, and, probably, the number and age of lesions. Autoinoculation may be responsible for contiguous spread. In addition, some genital warts may grow remarkably during pregnancy, only to recede postpartum. It is unclear whether this is related to hormonal factors or to changes in local cellular immunity. There is a tendency for growth of warts to slow with time, and up to one third will undergo spontaneous remission within 6 to 12 months. Cellular immune mechanisms are thought to play a part in controlling HPV. Diabetic individuals, immunosuppressed individuals, and those with systemic illness affecting cellular immunity often have massive growth of warts that is difficult to control.

The prevalence of HPV genital disease is underestimated by documentation of gross disease only. By colposcopy, cytological assessment, and immunoperoxidase and DNA techniques, unapparent viral presence can be documented surrounding gross disease or in multicentric locations along with gross disease or may be found multifocally in the genital tract with no apparent visible foci.

Human papillomavirus has been associated with dysplasia and cancer of the lower genital tract, particularly the vulva and cervix. Among other evidence, there is a statistical association between cervical warts and cervical dysplasia, and HPV DNA has been detected in several types of genital malignancies. Of the multiple types of HPV, certain types more than others are associated with malignancy. For example, HPV types 6 and 11 are seen in most cases of typical genital warts or in association with mild dysplasia. Human papillomavirus types 16 and 18 are disproportionately associated with severe dysplasia and malignancy of both the cervix and the vulva.

Diagnosis

The diagnosis of genital warts is suggested by a typical gross appearance and the exclusion of other processes by biopsy. Colposcopic localization of lesions may be of value. Histological features of genital warts include papilomatosis, acanthosis, and parakeratosis with vacuolization of epithelial cells. In addition, cervical Papanicoloau smears may suggest the presence of HPV in up to 1% to 2% of all childbearing women by revealing characteristic koilocytotic changes.

Treatment

Genital warts are commonly treated with either local cytotoxic agents or ablative therapy. Local application of 20% to 25% podophyllin in benzoin is an antimitotic agent that is incorporated into the wart and will cause sloughing of the tissue within 3 to 4 days after application. This treatment is slightly less effective for hyperkeratotic warts and may need to be repeated at weekly intervals for resolution of larger warts. Trichloroacetic acid and bichloroacetic acid may also be used, with particular value for treatment of flat warts and warts on mucosal surfaces.

Cryocautery, laser therapy, and electrocautery have all been used for ablative therapy with success. With cryocautery, the lesions should be frozen to the base. Blistering and resolution of the lesion may take place with initial freezing or may require repeated freezings. Laser therapy and electrocautery both attempt to totally remove lesions at the time of initial therapy. Fewer recurrences occur after laser therapy if a margin of normal-appearing tissue is also treated. Occasionally, the large size of warts necessitates surgical removal. Both electrocautery and surgical removal can be associated with significant blood loss, particularly during pregnancy. Increasing experience with interferon therapy, either systemic, topical, or intralesional, suggests that this may be useful as adjunctive therapy in addition to ablative therapy for treatment of extensive lesions.

Any associated vaginal infections should be treated concomitantly. Any decrease in local moisture can be helpful in limiting growth of lesions that are present. Occasionally, small lesions may resolve spontaneously with such symptomatic therapy. After initial disappearance or removal of lesions, it is necessary to closely follow up patients and treat new or recurrent lesions promptly.

Patients with a history of genital warts or those with persistent or atypical genital warts should be followed for the possibility of dysplasia or malignancy, and biopsies of persistent or atypical lesions should be performed.

VAGINITIS

Vaginitis is characterized by abnormal discharge, vulvovaginal discomfort, or both. Many microorganisms, including those associated with vaginitis, can be cultured from the vagina of totally asymptomatic women. Unless symptoms are present, the diagnosis of vaginitis should not be made, and in the majority of cases treatment is not indicated.

An average of four to seven organisms per person can be found on routine culturing of the vagina. Both aerobic and anaerobic bacteria are present. Organisms such as gram-negative enteric rods, *Staphylococcus* species, streptococci (including enterococci), anaerobic gram-positive cocci, and *Bacteroides* species, which are potential pathogens of the upper genital tract, are considered to be normal flora of the vagina. In addition, nonpathogens such as lactobacilli and diphtheroids are also frequently found. The normal pH of the vagina is 3.5 to 4.5. The pH of the vagina is influenced by the organic acid by-products of metabolism, which are produced by the predominant species in the vaginal flora. Both vaginal pH and normal vaginal flora must be considered when vaginitis is diagnosed. In addition, it is important to consider cervical mucus and normal vaginal discharge when symptoms of vaginitis are interpreted.

There are three types of infectious vaginitis currently recognized (Table 19–8). These will be discussed in turn.

Candidiasis

The majority of candidiasis is caused by *Candida albicans*, an organism that can be found in the lower genital tract of 30% to 80% of women with minimal to no symptoms. A small number of fungal vaginal infections are caused by *Candida glabrata*.

The hallmark of candidiasis is itching, irritation, or both. Itching may be quite severe and noticed in either the vaginal or vulvar area. Irritation may be associated with dysuria and dyspareunia. When discharge is present, it is commonly described as cottage cheesy or thick, white, and clumpy. Discharge is not always present with symptomatic candidiasis, however, and occasion-

ally there may be only a thin watery discharge or no discharge.

Symptoms of candidiasis frequently have their onset just prior to the menses. In addition, a number of precipitating factors for the occurrence of symptomatic candidiasis have been delineated. *Candida* species may frequently be found in the vagina, and some of the precipitating factors for symptomatic candidiasis are those that foster overgrowth of the vagina by *Candida*. This may occur through depression of normal bacterial flora, depression of local cellular immunity, alterations in the metabolic and nutritional milieu of the vagina, and unknown mechanisms. Precipitating factors for symptomatic candidiasis include the use of systemic antibiotics, immunosuppressive therapy, diabetes mellitus, pregnancy, stress, and, potentially, oral contraceptive agents.

Candidiasis often presents as apparent vulvitis or vulvovaginitis. Examination reveals well-demarcated erythema of the vulva with occasional satellite lesions surrounding the major rim of erythema. The vulva can be notably edematous. The vagina may also be edematous and erythema-

TABLE 19–8.

Diagnosis of Vaginitis

	Typical Symptoms	Clinical Findings	Discharge	pH	Wet Preparation	Other
Candidiasis	Itching, irritation, dyspareunia	Erythema, edema	White and clumpy, occasionally watery and clumpy, may be none	< 4.5	Potassium hydroxide reveals hyphae, buds	Culture may be of value
Trichomoniasis	Discharge, pain, occasionally itching	Strawberry cervix or vagina	Copious, pooling, frothy gray-white to yellow-green	> 5.5	Saline reveals motile *Trichomonas*	> 10 WBCs/HPF
Bacterial vaginosis	Discharge, odor	No mucosal changes	Sticky, homogeneous	> 4.7	Saline reveals clue cells	Positive Whiff test result shows lack of WBCs and lactobacilli

tous, with erythema extending onto the squamous exocervix. It is not unusual for there to be excoriations and fissuring of the vulva and, occasionally, the vagina. Even if discharge has not been described by the patient, an adherent clumpy white discharge may be found in the upper portion of the vagina. The pH of this discharge is most often less than 4.5. When 1 drop of the discharge is mixed with 1 drop of 10% KOH, covered with a coverslip, and examined under the microscope, normal cellular elements will be lysed, and the branching hyphae and buds of the *Candida* will be visible. In up to 25% of cases of symptomatic candidiasis, the KOH wet preparation will be falsely negative. When candidiasis is suspected from the clinical presentation, diagnostic accuracy can be improved by use of the Gram stain or culture on specific media. Hyphae and buds are gram positive; buds are slightly larger than WBCs. Solid media that can be used for specific *Candida* cultures include Nickerson's media and Sabouraud agar.

Initial treatment of candidiasis is with local vaginal antifungal preparations. Nystatin suppositories or cream can be used twice daily for 14 days. Miconazole and clotrimazole cream or suppositories are used once daily for 7 days and have a slightly higher initial cure rate. It may be possible to use these preparations for shorter periods of time and achieve acceptable cure rates. Interest has developed in the use of boric acid (600–650 mg in a gel capsule used daily for 14 days) for the treatment of candidiasis. Initial results would indicate acceptable cure rates, and the lack of compounding chemicals makes this an attractive therapeutic alternative in patients who develop a hypersensitivity reaction to other local anti-infective agents. The use of gentian violet–impregnated tampons is messy and occasionally irritating but may prove useful in some patients.

Ketoconazole is a systemic oral antifungal agent that has been shown to be efficacious in the treatment of vulvovaginal candidiasis. It is not clear that this therapy is any more effective than local preparations. The exact duration of therapy to achieve highest cure rates is unknown; however, 1- to 2-week courses of therapy are probably effective in the majority of cases. With the use of more long-term ketoconazole, the most serious side effect is reversible but occasionally severe hepatotoxic reaction.

There are a number of approaches to recurrent candidiasis. Longer courses of therapy can be used. Since at least 10% of male sexual partners of women with candidiasis are found to have a candidal balanitis, it is reasonable to treat male sexual partners, particularly those who have displayed any symptoms. Gastrointestinal (GI) tract colonization by *Candida* is present in 50% of adults. For this reason, some advocate the simultaneous use of oral nystatin and local vaginal anti-infectives to decrease the GI tract colonization and prevent cross-contamination of the vagina by perirectal spread. The efficacy of this approach, however, remains unproved. It is occasionally necessary to remove all potential precipitating factors to achieve long-lasting cure. Long-term, low-dose suppressive ketoconazole has been shown to be effective in decreasing multiple recurrences of symptomatic candidiasis.

Some women develop chronic symptoms or multiply recurrent episodes of candidiasis. Such recurrent vulvovaginitis has been associated with transient suppression of cell-mediated immunity and, in some, with enhanced local allergic responses to *Candida* as well as other locally applied substances. Therapeutic responses to antiprostaglandin agents and antiallergenic agents are currently under investigation.

Trichomoniasis

Trichomoniasis is caused by the flagellated parasite *T. vaginalis*. Male partners of women with trichomoniasis may be found to harbor *Trichomonas*, and there is a high rate of reinfection of women whose male sexual partners are not treated concomitantly for *Trichomonas;* therefore, trichomoniasis is considered to be a sexually transmitted disease. It is often isolated along with other sexually transmitted organisms, in particular, *N. gonorrhoeae.*

The incubation period for trichomoniasis is approximately 20 days. Symptoms often peak just after the menses. Classic symptoms of trichomoniasis include the presence of a copious, frothy discharge, along with symptoms of local pain and irritation. Dysuria, dyspareunia, and dull lower abdominal pain may be present. Occasionally, itching is the predominant local symptom.

Examination of the vulva and vagina is usually most remarkable for a copious discharge. This discharge is most often white to greenish yellow and may be frothy. The pH of the discharge is greater than 6.0. A wet preparation made by mixing 1 drop of the discharge with 1 drop of normal saline will reveal motile trichomonads in the majority of cases of symptomatic trichomoniasis. These parasites are slightly larger than WBCs, ovoid, possess a central undulating membrane, and a terminal flagella. In addition, in the majority of cases, greater than 10 WBCs/HPF will be found on wet preparation. Diagnostic accuracy in suspected cases with normal findings from a wet preparation can be improved by culture in specific media such as Diamond medium or Tichosel broth.

Occasionally, the cervix and upper portion of the vagina will have an appearance of raised, punctuate erythema. This "strawberry" appearance is pathognomonic for trichomoniasis but is found in the minority of cases.

The most effective therapy for trichomoniasis currently available in the United States is oral metronidazole. Two dosage regimens have been shown to be effective. Single high-dose therapy with 2 gm of metronidazole has been shown to effectively eradicate *Trichomonas* in 90% of cases. Occasionally, severe nausea and vomiting, particularly when taken in association with other medications, will preclude effective use of this dose schedule. Lower-dose longer-term therapy with 250 mg three times daily for 7 to 10 days may also be used. There is a high rate of reinfection of females if male sexual partners are not treated concomitantly; therefore, it is common practice for even asymptomatic male partners to be treated. When metronidazole cannot be used, intravaginal clotrimazole or boric acid may provide relief from symptoms and may be curative in some cases.

Bacterial Vaginosis

Bacterial vaginosis, formerly called *Gardnerella-associated vaginitis* or *nonspecific vaginitis,* is a vaginitis characterized by excessive discharge and odor. Although for many years the exact microbiological etiology of this infection was unknown, it is now accepted that this infection is a result of synergism between various bacteria, including *Gardnerella vaginalis,* mobiluncus species, and vaginal anaerobes. *Gardnerella vaginalis* is commonly found as part of the vaginal flora in approximately one third of sexually active women. Without a critical concentration of other vaginal bacteria, in particular, anaerobes, this organism is not thought to be responsible for symptoms. The effect of bacterial synergy in causing symptoms has been most convincingly shown using gas-liquid chromatography on specimens from patients with symptomatic disease, which reveals organic acid metabolites of anaerobes and disappearance of symptoms that correlated with the appearance of metabolites produced by *Lactobacillus* and streptococcal species. The absence of lactobacilli is a characteristic feature of bacterial vaginosis (BV).

The onset of odor and discharge associated with BV is evenly distributed throughout the menstrual cycle, and local discomfort is rarely a problem. The diagnosis of BV is made with a high degree of certainty on examination of the patient and the discharge.

The discharge of BV is typically homogeneous, grayish white to yellow-white, and somewhat adherent to the vulvar and vaginal walls. Underlying edema or erythema of the vulva or vagina are not typical. The pH of this vaginal discharge is greater than 4.7. When 1 drop of KOH is added to 1 drop of discharge, an intense amine odor is elaborated, producing a positive whiff test result. The typical appearance of this discharge on normal saline wet preparation is of a paucity of WBCs and a predominance of "clue" cells. By wet preparation, clue cells are best identified by a stippled birefringence that so densely covers the epithelial cell that the normal borders and nuclei are obscured. By Gram stain, clue cells can be identified as epithelial cells almost totally covered by small, gram-negative rods. There is a paucity of other organisms seen in the background. Notably, there is an absence of lactobacilli. Culture on specific media and the use of gas-liquid chromatography are rarely of benefit clinically.

The most effective treatment for bacterial vaginosis is metronidazole at a dose of 500 mg twice daily or 250 mg three times daily for 7 days. The single high-dose therapy used for *Trichomonas* is not believed to be effective for *Gardnerella*-associated vaginitis. Metronidazole is thought to be efficacious for curing this infection because of its effect on the vaginal anaerobes. When metronidazole is contraindicated, alternative therapy of 500 mg of ampicillin four times daily for 7 days is effective in a smaller number of cases. The need to treat male sexual partners is controversial. Reinfection of women after treatment is common. Most would agree that in cases of recurrent BV, the male partner should also be treated. Condom use may discourage reinfection. The use of intravaginal sulfa creams or acidifying agents in the treatment of this infection may be effective in some cases, as may be promotion of the growth of normal vaginal lactobacilli.

Other Causes of Vaginitis Symptoms

Excessive vaginal discharge may be a manifestation of cervicitis. Organisms associated with cervicitis include *T. vaginalis, N. gonorrhoeae, C. trachomatis,* and herpes simplex virus. When diagnosed, they should be treated accordingly. In addition, excess vaginal discharge may be associated with cervical ectopy or eversion, with no apparent infectious etiology.

Discharge and odor are associated with the presence of foreign bodies in the vaginal vault. Although this is chiefly of concern in pediatric populations, forgotten tampons may also be a source of discharge.

In addition to vulvar dystrophies, dysplasias, and vulvar vestibulitis syndrome, vulvar discomfort may be due to hypersensitivity reactions. In particular, this should be considered in women who have received numerous courses of topical anti-infective therapy.

URINARY TRACT INFECTION

One in every 5 women will have a urinary tract infection (UTI) at some time during life, up to 25% of women will experience symptoms of acute dysuria each year, and 3 to 5 million visits to physicians yearly are for the evaluation of UTIs or related symptoms. Although not a gynecological infection, symptoms associated with UTI occur with various gynecological disorders, and women frequently present to a gynecologist for diagnosis of UTI.

The vast majority of symptomatic UTIs involve the lower urinary tract, commonly termed "cystitis". Urinary tract infections may also present as asymptomatic bacteriuria or acute pyelonephritis. Symptoms of lower UTIs are also seen with sexually transmitted diseases, various noninfectious urethral syndromes, and vaginitis.

Women with lower UTI present with acute symptoms of dysuria, frequency, and urgency. Gross hematuria, suprapubic pain, and flank or back discomfort are also seen. Both pyuria and bacteriuria are present in symptomatic lower UTI.

The previously held belief that "significant bacteriuria" necessary for diagnosis of UTI consisted of 100,000 or more organisms/ml is clearly erroneous when one is referring to lower UTI. Although 50% of women with lower UTI do have 100,000 or more organisms cultured from urine, approximately one third of women who present with symptoms of acute dysuria, frequency, and urgency have between 100 and 100,000 organisms by properly obtained culture and yet warrant a diagnosis of UTI. Studies using bladder urine specimens obtained by suprapubic aspiration or transurethral catheterization have demonstrated that smaller numbers of organisms in symptomatic women are associated with reproducible bladder bacteriuria, pyuria, and a predictable response to UTI therapy. The concept of significant bacteriuria or a single organism colony count of 100,000 or more organisms/ml is appropriate only when applied to asymptomatic bacteriuria or acute pyelonephritis.

More than 90% of UTIs in women are caused by two organisms, *E. coli* and *Staphylococcus saprophyticus,* with at least 80% caused by *E. coli.*

Approximately 20% of women with UTI will have recurrences of symptoms within variable periods of time. Recurrences are most often reinfections, as demonstrated by culture negativity between episodes and the isolation of different organisms by biotyping and sensitivity patterns with each different episode of symptoms. Such reinfections rarely represent serious morbidity or renal involvement. Recurrences develop in characteristic clusters of symptomatic UTI, often during 6- to 12-month time periods.

Less frequently, recurrent symptoms will be due to persistence of the same organism. Close intervals of 10 to 14 days between symptomatic recurrences in particular may indicate upper tract infection. Persistence of a single organism should always raise the concern of congenital or acquired structural or functional abnormalities of the urinary tract.

The occurrence of UTI is dependent on both host factors and properties of infecting organisms. Bacterial adherence to uroepithelial cells precedes infection. Flora, in particular coliforms, from the GI tract colonizes the vaginal introital and periurethral-meatal area, and this flora ascends into the bladder to cause both symptomatic and asymptomatic bacteriuria. Various bacterial adhesions, surface receptor sites, and attachment properties of bacteria have been identified. Women who are susceptible to UTIs have been demonstrated to have an increase in the incidence and density of colonization and more sites for bacterial attachment on uroepithelial surfaces compared with women without UTIs. The efficiency of bacterial adherence is probably influenced by genetic, hormonal, and other factors. Natural defenses against bacterial adherence to and ascent into the urinary tract may be genetically determined. These include various substances elaborated by the urinary tract, local immunoglobulin, competitive bacterial flora, and normal voiding patterns.

Among sexually active women, most lower UTI is associated with sexual intercourse. The largest proportion of susceptible women become symptomatic within a short period of time after intercourse. Intercourse is thought to introduce colonizing bacteria into the bladder and has been shown to transiently increase numbers of bacteria in the urine up to 10-fold.

An independent risk factor for UTI is diaphragm use. Diaphragm users have two to two and one-half times the increased risk for UTI and have an increase in vaginal colonization with coliforms. Other risk factors for UTI include a past history of UTI and failure to void following intercourse. Factors not associated with the occurrence of UTI include "perineal hygiene," the direction of wiping, tampons, and oral contraceptives.

Two percent to 10% of women have asymptomatic bacteriuria as defined by the presence of 100,000 or more of a single pathogen found on more than two midstream, clean voided specimens. Asymptomatic bacteriuria may be transient or intermittent, and it is not clear whether its natural, long-term course is influenced by treatment. In nonpregnant, nonimmunocompromised women with normal urinary tracts, it does not appear to be associated with UTI or long-term morbidity and does not have to be eradicated. In conditions that predispose to upper UTI, such as pregnancy, attempts at eradication are warranted.

Studies suggest early infection or colonization of the upper urinary tract in a proportion of women with lower UTI. It is unclear how many such women would go on to develop acute pyelonephritis if untreated. However, it does appear that the majority of women with lower UTI are not predisposed to the development of acute pyelonephritis. The occurrence of pyelonephritis is influenced by pathogenic properties of bacteria and factors in the host that affect bacterial adherence and ascent. Abnormalities of the urinary tract such as reflux, obstruction, or stones, abnormalities in host defenses as occur with diabetes and immunosuppression, and the introduction of virulent bacteria during catheterization or other instrumentation are all associated with pyelonephritis. Pyelonephritis presents with symptoms of dysuria, frequency, and urgency in 50% of cases. In addition, fever, chills, malaise, and flank or back (costovertebral angle) pain and tenderness are hallmarks. Pyelonephritis is a more morbid event than lower UTI, with a greater risk of bacteremia and long-term sequelae and the need for longer treatment.

Women who present with symptoms of dysuria, frequency and urgency may not have bacterial infection of the lower urinary tract. Urethritis caused by sexually transmitted diseases such as *C. trachomatis, N. gonorrhoeae, T. vaginalis,* and herpes simplex can cause identical symptoms. Epidemiological risk factors, sexual history or history of disease in sexual partners, and associated symptomatology may suggest these diagnoses. Symptoms of urethritis typically occur less acutely, and urinalysis reveals pyuria but rarely hematuria. In symptomatic women, pyuria with negative urine culture should raise a suspicion for urethritis. In particular, *Chlamydia* is the cause of symptoms in one third of women with dysuria, pyuria, and a negative urine culture.

Vaginitis may also cause symptoms of dysuria and urgency. Although classically vaginitis causes dysuria experienced "externally," and UTI dysuria is experienced "internally," this distinction is unreliable. If a urinalysis is properly obtained and bacteriuria and pyuria are not demonstrable, other symptoms and signs of vaginitis should become apparent by direct history and exam.

Diagnosis

The diagnosis of UTI is made by using urinalysis and urine culture.

The majority of women with symptomatic UTI later documented to have bacteriuria have pyuria, with more than 8 to 10 WBCs/ml in unspun urine and 2 to 5 WBCs/HPF in spun urine sediment. It has been suggested that the presence of pyuria be used as a screen to determine which urine specimens should be cultured and which women treated presumptively for UTI.

A midstream, clean voided urine sample cultured using quantitative techniques is appropriate for evaluation of asymptomatic bacteriuria, pyelonephritis, and the majority of cases of lower UTI. If lower UTI is associated with bacterial counts between 100 and 100,000 colonies/ml, contamination of specimens with other organisms may confuse the interpretation of culture results. Clarification by culture of suprapubic aspiration or catheterization specimens may occasionally be of value. Urine cultures that reveal 100,000 or more colonies/ml of a single pathogen support the diagnosis of UTI; cultures that reveal 100 or more colonies/ml of a single pathogen support the diagnosis of UTI in a symptomatic woman. Microbiology laboratories should be instructed to identify all bacterial species in cultures obtained from symptomatic women and, in particular, to quantify and appropriately identify all *E. coli* and staphylococcal species in cultures obtained from symptomatic women.

It should be determined if recurrences of infection are episodes of reinfection or persistent infection. Persistence of infection despite adequate antibiotic therapy or multiple episodes of reinfection, variably defined as more than three to six episodes in 1 year, warrant urological referral and evaluation for urinary tract abnormality. In addition, any episode of pyelonephritis in a nonpregnant woman or infection with an unusual organism such as *Proteus* or other "urea splitters" that may be associated with stone formation are indications for urological consultation.

The majority of symptomatic lower urinary tract reinfections are not associated with urinary tract abnormalities. Women can correctly predict the presence of UTI by symptoms in cases of reinfection with a 90% accuracy. With proper assurance of normalcy of the urinary tract and known patterns of previous cultures and infections, the institution of therapy without laboratory diagnosis has been suggested to be a cost-effective and appropriate alternative.

The proper diagnosis of lower UTI must take into account alternative diagnoses for symptoms of dysuria, frequency, and urgency. In addition to urinalysis and urine culture, pelvic examination, wet preparations, and sexually transmitted disease cultures may be warranted (Table 19–9).

Treatment

Single-dose antimicrobial therapy or standard dosage schedules of antibiotics for periods of 3, 5, 7, or 10 days have all been shown to be appropriate therapy for lower UTI. Without antibiotic therapy, UTI resolves spontaneously in up to 70% of women. However, treatment does eliminate symptoms more quickly, may treat unrecognized upper UTI, and may decrease recurrent, symptomatic infection.

Approximately 80% of lower UTI is cured with single-dose therapy. Appropriate single-dose

TABLE 19–9.
Differential Diagnosis of Symptoms of Dysuria, Frequency, and Urgency

	Onset	Urinalysis	Urine Culture	Causative Organisms
Lower UTI	Acute	pyuria hematuria	≥100 organisms/ml	*E. coli, S. saprophyticus*
Pyelonephritis	Subacute (up to 10 days)	pyuria hematuria casts	≥ 100,000 organisms/ml	*E. coli,* other gram-negative enterics, enterococci
Urethritis	Acute or subacute	pyuria	—	*C. trachomatis, T. vaginalis, N. gonorrhoeae,* herpes simplex
Vaginitis	Acute or subacute	—	—	*T. vaginalis, C. albicans*
Other lower urinary tract syndromes	Subacute	—	—	—

agents include trimethoprim-sulfamethoxazole, tri-methoprim, sulfasoxizole, and ampicillin or amoxi-cillin. Cephalosporins are not effective sin-gle-agent choices. Single-dose therapy should not be used for children, pregnant women, or women with underlying medical problems. Disappearance of symptoms often does not occur for 2 to 3 days, and persistence of symptoms to this point is not a demonstration of failure of single-dose therapy.

Standard antibiotic dosage regimens given for 3 to 5 days cure 80% to 90% of lower UTI and may have fewer early recurrences when com-pared with single-dose therapy. It is not clear whether 7- to 14-day courses of antibiotics pro-vide further benefit. Appropriate standard dosage regimen choices include nitrofurantoin, tri-methoprim-sulfamethoxazole, other sulphas, tri-methoprim, penicillins, ampicillin or ampicillin combinations, and cephalosporins. The use of the newer quinoline antibiotics should probably be reserved for infection with resistent gram-negative organisms.

Pyelonephritis should be treated with stan-dard antibiotic dosage regimens for at least 10 days. If hospitalization for IV therapy is chosen because of degree of illness or fever, IV therapy should continue for at least 24 hours of afebrility and a total course of 10 days completed with oral antibiotics.

The frequency of recurrent symptomatic lower UTI due to reinfection can be decreased by the use of low-dose antibiotics given prophylacti-cally either as a single night time dose or as a sin-gle postintercourse dose. Agents of demonstrable benefit for this purpose include nitrofurantoin and trimethoprim-sulfamethoxazole. Such therapy should be instituted only after cure of infection has been achieved and empirically continued for 6-month periods. The alternative of self-medication with short-course therapy at early signs of reinfection may be more cost effective and acceptable to patients than prophylaxis.

POSTOPERATIVE INFECTIONS

Virtually all major and minor surgical proce-dures of the lower genital tract may result in lo-calized postsurgical infection. The risk of opera-tive site infection is most strongly correlated with contamination of the operative site by potential pathogens. Procedures that expose the upper gen-ital tract, intra-abdominal cavity, or skin wounds to lower genital tract flora may result in signifi-cant postoperative infection.

To understand the microbiology of postoper-ative infection, we must discuss the microbiology of the lower genital tract. The vulva, vagina, and cervix are normally colonized with a wide variety of bacteria. The lower genital tract flora is poly-microbial and includes both aerobic and anaero-bic organisms. The exact composition of lower genital tract flora varies among individuals and appears to be influenced by age, hormonal status, sexual experience, and possibly immune status. Tissue type may also affect flora, possibly because of differences in bacterial adherence to cell sur-faces, and differences in cell turnover. Although the vulva, vagina, and cervix are colonized with similar species of organisms, the exact types and quantities of organisms present in each area may be distinct. Bacteriological surveys of lower geni-tal tract flora have been performed on varied pa-tient populations by several investigators.

The results of prevalence surveys of lower genital tract flora have been compared with infec-tion site cultures. Some species of bacteria are fre-quently found at sites of infection and are classi-fied as potential pathogens. Other organisms that are part of the normal lower genital tract flora do not commonly cause local or systemic infections and are considered to be of very low pathogenic potential. Certain bacterial species such as *E. coli* and *Bacteroides fragilis* appear to be under repre-sented in the lower genital tract in comparison with their occurrence at the site of infections. This may represent a propensity of organisms such as these to invade and cause infection. The presence of virulence factors in certain organisms may con-tribute to their pathogenicity; the presence of a polysaccharide capsular antigen that helps to resist phagocytosis and opsonization while enhancing tissue invasiveness is one such factor.

The pathogenic potential of the lower genital tract flora may also be determined by interactions between bacteria. There may be some organisms that are capable of initially invading tissue and causing an inflammatory reaction. Other organ-isms may be able to contribute to that inflamma-tory reaction and further the infectious process once initial tissue destruction has progressed and anaerobic conditions have been achieved. There-fore, the types and quantity of organisms present and the proportions of potential pathogens at an operative site may all be important determinants of postoperative infection.

The major aerobic pathogens of importance in postoperative infections are Enterobacteriaceae, including *E. coli*, streptococci, including *Streptococcus viridans* and enterococci, and staphylococci, in particular *Staphylococcus aureus. Staphylococcus aureus* and streptococcal species may be found as the sole pathogens at the site of wound infections, and other organisms may be found as sole pathogens at the site of postoperative infection; however, most often these organisms are seen in combination with other aerobic or anaerobic organisms. The most numerous anaerobic pathogens are the anaerobic gram-positive cocci, including anaerobic streptococci, peptococci, and peptostreptococci. *Bacteroides* species, including *B. fragilis* and *Bacteroides melaninogenicus,* are major anaerobic pathogens of wound and soft tissue infection. *Clostridium perfringens* and other anaerobic bacteria are less prevalent but need to be considered as potential pathogens.

Cultures of the lower genital tract may not accurately reflect the organisms that are present at the site of postoperative infection. Unless material from postoperative abscesses or wound infections is obtained for culture, treatment is most often based on knowledge of which species may be involved in infection. Aerobic organisms such as the streptococci and coliforms are of particular concern in acute illness. Anaerobes, in particular the *Bacteroides* species, are of concern, especially with abscess formation.

The risk of infection after hysterectomy ranges from 7% to 30%. After vaginal hysterectomy, major operative site infections are pelvic infections such as cuff cellulitis or pelvic abscess. After abdominal hysterectomy, there is the risk of both pelvic and abdominal wound infection. Posthysterectomy pelvic cellulitis presents as fever and lower pelvic pain that occurs between 2 to 5 days after surgery. The vaginal cuff is often indurated, warm, and exquisitely painful. Postoperative pelvic abscesses of the vaginal cuff, pelvic floor, and side walls, at the site of intra-abdominal blood collection, or in the adnexal structures usually present more than 5 days after hysterectomy. Pelvic cellulitis often responds to simple broad-spectrum antibiotic therapy, not including extensive coverage for *B. fragilis.* If there is a suggestion of early abscess formation, if response to initial therapy is not prompt, or if there is severe ill-

ness, antimicrobial coverage for gram-negative enteric bacilli, streptococci, anaerobic cocci, and *B. fragilis* must be provided. Drainage of the vaginal cuff can be a helpful adjunct to antibiotic therapy; surgical management of postoperative abscesses must be considered when the response to antibiotic therapy is not prompt and complete.

Postoperative wound infections may present acutely with fever and incisional pain along with erythema, induration, warmth, and tenderness. Group A β-hemolytic *Streptococcus* cause wound infection and high fevers within 24 to 48 hours of surgery. A less immediate onset of wound infection is more typical, however. Often a wound infection is the cause of spiking, low-grade fevers, whose source does not become obvious until a collection of pus is discovered through spontaneous drainage or by wound exploration. More than 20% of wound infections become apparent after hospitalization. *Staphylococcus aureus* and other skin organisms are common causes of postoperative wound infections. After genital tract surgery, mixed flora may also cause wound infections. Because of the somewhat unique exposure to mixed aerobic-anaerobic pathogens at the time of surgery, patients undergoing gynecological surgery are at risk for development of a distinct but uncommon *synergistic wound infection.* Synergistic wound infections occur when tissue planes are invaded by both aerobic and anaerobic organisms. It has been theorized that aerobic organisms cause initial tissue infection and damage and that anaerobic organisms then cause further tissue destruction in an atmosphere of decreased oxygen tension. Diabetes, debilitating disease, obesity, and prior radiation therapy are risk factors for the occurrence of synergistic infections.

Synergistic infections may be rapidly progressive with necrosis spreading along fascial lines or through the subcutaneous tissue in a matter of hours. This is termed *necrotizing fasciitis,* or *cellulitis.* In such cases, fever and signs of systemic sepsis are almost always present. Examination of skin and subcutaneous tissue reveals necrotic eschar formation and underlying crepitance. Cross-table lateral x-ray films may reveal a subcutaneous gas pattern. Necrotizing wound infection due to *Clostridium perfringens* may also cause a similar picture.

In other cases, synergistic wound infections have a more insidious onset with lack of systemic signs. Physical pain is often intense, and by the time the characteristic skin changes of central necrosis with surrounding erythema become apparent, the subcutaneous tissue necrosis is more advanced than one would suspect from outward appearance. This type of infection is sometimes called *progressive synergistic bacterial gangrene.*

A number of combinations of flora can cause synergistic wound infections. Original descriptions of these wound infections were of mixed aerobic staphylococcal and microaerophilic streptococcal infection. Combinations of *E. coli* and other gram-negative enteric bacilli or aerobic streptococci with anaerobic cocci and *Bacteroides* species can also be isolated from these types of wound infections. Antibiotic therapy in cases of suspected synergistic wound infections must provide broad-spectrum coverage for both aerobic and anaerobic organisms and must also include coverage for clostridial infections. It is rare, however, that antimicrobial therapy alone will be curative. Most often, wide debridement of all affected tissues is necessary. In cases of rapidly progressive disease, prompt debridement may be lifesaving. At the time of surgery, the infected tissue appears to undermine the skin and classically is described as gray, stringy, and devitalized with a purulent and fetid discharge. All such devitalized tissue must be totally resected to the point of healthy-appearing, bleeding tissue. Healing should be by secondary intention. Fascial grafting with synthetic grafts may be necessary.

The risk of pelvic infection after vaginal hysterectomy and the risk of pelvic and wound infection after abdominal hysterectomy is significantly reduced through the use perioperative antimicrobial prophylaxis. Parenteral antibiotics should be used for such prophylaxis, should be administered just prior to surgery, and should be continued postoperatively for less than 24 hours. There is no benefit to the use of either extended preoperative or postoperative antibiotics for preventing infection. The usual type of antibiotics used for prophylaxis during hysterectomy are broad-spectrum first-generation antimicrobials, such as cefazolin. There does not appear to be any additional benefit in terms of further decrease in postoperative infection through the use of more expensive and toxic regimens that provide additional coverage for anaerobes and resistent gram-negative enteric bacilli. In addition to expense and toxicity, the development of superinfection by resistant organ-

isms is a potential danger with use of more broad-spectrum antibiotic regimens.

The use of properly functioning, active intraperitoneal or subperitoneal drains does prevent some postoperative infection. It is not clear whether the use of such drains is as effective or is additive to the efficacy of perioperative antimicrobial prophylaxis. The efficacy of antimicrobial prophylaxis for other gynecological surgical procedures such as adnexal surgery or infertility surgery has not been proved.

TOXIC SHOCK SYNDROME

Toxic shock syndrome (TSS) is a multisystem illness caused by toxin-producing *Staphylococcus aureus* that is most prevalent in menstruating women. Although described as early as 1927, it was first characterized as a uniform syndrome occurring in a group of children by Todd et al. in 1978. In 1980, TSS was recognized as occurring in epidemic proportions in menstruating women. Subsequent case reporting and mobilization of the epidemiological and research communities lead to elucidation of pathophysiology and efforts aimed at disease control. These efforts were somewhat successful in halting the further spread of the epidemic. In 1980 to 1981, TSS occurred in 6 to 6.2 per 100,000 women. Currently the prevalence of this disease is 4 per 100,000.

Toxic shock syndrome is a dramatic illness that presents acutely and is most commonly associated with high fevers, characteristic skin changes, prominent GI manifestations, hypotension, and other systemic effects. The case fatality ratio is approximately 3%.

Menstrual TSS typically has its onset on the third or fourth day of the menses. The earliest manifestation is of high fever, with a temperature usually in excess of 38.9° C. Soon a diffusely erythematous, finely macular rash resembling a sunburn in appearance and often in sensation may be noticed, in particular on the upper trunk, face, or extremities. Profuse diarrhea occurs. Within 2 to 3 days, profound hypotension ensues. Virtually any other organ system may become involved, as evidenced by either symptoms, signs, or laboratory abnormalities. Of particular note is the almost universal muscle involvement leading to severe myalgias and tenderness to touch. A more distinctly macular rash may evolve, along with erythema and some edema of the palms and soles. Eventually, fine desquamation of areas of rash and, by days 8 to 12, sloughing of the skin from the palms and soles are characteristic. This desquamation heals by reepithelialization without scarring.

Full-blown TSS must fit a rigid case definition, as outlined in Table 19–10. Most authorities agree that similar but less dramatic presentations probably represent variations of TSS that occur by similar pathophysiological mechanisms.

The major long-term effect of TSS is that of recurrence. Toxic shock syndrome can recur during subsequent menses in approximately 30% of cases. Typically, recurrences are milder and may occur over a period of time. Recurrences with up to five subsequent menses have been reported.

A particular toxin-producing *S. aureus* has been associated with TSS. In one series, greater than 90% of women who had TSS had *S. aureus*

TABLE 19–10.

Case Definition of Toxic Shock Syndrome
___

Fever:
   Temperature, ≥38.9° C
Rash:
   Diffuse macular erythroderma
Desquamation:
   Palms and soles 1–2 weeks after onset
Hypotension:
   Systolic blood pressure <90 mm Hg or orthostatic
      drop in diastolic blood pressure >15 mm Hg or
      orthostatic dizziness
Multisystem involvement (three or more of the
   following):
   Gastrointestinal: Vomiting or diarrhea at onset
   Muscular: Myalgia or elevated creatine
      phosphokinase level
   Mucous membrane: Vaginal, or oropharyngeal or
      conjunctival hyperemia
   Renal: Elevated serum urea nitrogen or creatinine
      levels or aseptic pyuria
   Hepatic: Elevated serum bilirubin, serum glutamic
      oxaloacetic transaminase (AST), or serum
      glutamic pyruvic transaminase (ALT) levels
   Hematological: Platelets ≤100,000/mm^3
   Central nervous system: Disorientation or altered
      consciousness without focal neurological signs
Negative results for the following, if obtained:
   Blood (except *S. auresus*), throat, or cerebrospinal
      fluid cultures; rise in titer to Rocky Mountain
      spotted fever, leptospirosis, or rubeola
___

isolated from the genital tract. In other surveys, only approximately 9% of women may have *S. aureus* isolated from the vagina or cervix. A distinct toxin, TSS toxin-1 has been isolated from up to 90% strains of *S. aureus* associated with TSS. This toxin is presumed to be responsible for the typical systemic effects seen in TSS. However, it is recognized that some of the multisystem effects may also be secondary to the effects of profound hypotension.

The major factor epidemiologically associated with the occurrence of menstrual TSS is the use of tampons as opposed to sanitary pads. The absorbency of tampons is directly related to the risk for TSS.

Nonmenstrual TSS also occurs. It has been associated with a number of staphylococcal infections, including cutaneous and subcutaneous abscesses, osteomyelitis and other deep-seated infections, postsurgical wound infections, postpartum infections, and staphylococcal superinfections seen with influenza. In addition, TSS has been reported to occur with the use of diaphragms and contraceptive sponges.

Toxic shock syndrome is diagnosed by the characteristic clinical picture in the absence of documentation, by either culture or serology, of another cause for an acute febrile illness of similar nature. The differential diagnosis includes Kawasaki disease, Rocky Mountain spotted fever, streptococcal scarlet fever, and bacteremia. Although in TSS blood cultures are negative for *S. aureus*, supportive evidence for TSS should be sought by culturing the genital tract, oropharynx, urine, and any referable skin sites for *S. aureus*. Complete laboratory evaluation for multisystem involvement as indicated in Table 19–10 should be performed.

Initial treatment for TSS is supportive care, with particular attention to aggressive fluid, electrolyte, and blood product replacement. Any tampons, foreign bodies, or collections of purulence present at onset of symptoms should be removed. The administration of a β-lactamase-resistent antibiotic, such as oxacillin, a cephalosporin, or vancomycin, for 10 days has been shown to decrease recurrences. In addition, stopping use of tampons indefinitely has been shown to decrease recurrences.

Although not a common illness, the risk for TSS can be decreased by counseling women to use tampons intermittently as opposed to continually throughout menses and, if used, to use the least absorbent tampon that is reasonable.

HUMAN IMMUNODEFICIENCY VIRUS DISEASE, INCLUDING ACQUIRED IMMUNE DEFICIENCY SYNDROME

Acquired immune deficiency syndrome (AIDS) is the most advanced stage in a continuum of clinical syndromes caused by the human immunodeficiency virus (HIV-1). These syndromes are characterized by both the direct effect of this virus on organ systems and the sequelae of profound alterations in normal immune mechanisms that eventually lead to death.

Acquired immune deficiency syndrome was first described in United States populations in 1981, although this disease existed and was described in other countries, most notably in Africa and the Caribbean, prior to this time. Infection with HIV is now recognized to be a major, worldwide epidemic. Unique medical, societal, economical, legal, and other dilemmas are posed by this virus, whose long latency is in part responsible for an as of yet incompletely understood pathophysiology and natural history and whose cure remains elusive.

Current estimates are of greater than 1 million total cases of HIV infection in the United States alone. By 1992, 365,000 cases of AIDS are expected to have been reported to the CDC, with 263,000 deaths attributed to AIDS during the same time period. In the United States, this epidemic has occurred initially largely within the male homosexual and bisexual community. By 1988, reported cases of AIDS in women and the pediatric population accounted for approximately 7% of the total reported cases. However, this disease is increasing in the two populations, and by 1991, 10% of all reported AIDS cases are anticipated to be in women. Currently, HIV disease in women is a disease of minority, disadvantaged, and young women, with 70% of AIDS cases reported in black or Hispanic women and 80% in women of childbearing age.

Human immunodeficiency virus is a retrovirus that possesses a unique reverse transcriptase that allows its RNA to encode DNA within the infected cell, which then becomes irreversibly incorporated within the host DNA. Such intertwining of viral and host genetic structure leads to ma-

jor alterations in function and probable eventual destruction of host cells as well as provides a mechanism for further infection of target cells within the body. The HIV target cells are cells whose membranes contain a surface molecule, CD4 receptor, to which a CD4 envelope protein on the surface of the virus binds. Chief among the target cells for this virus are T_4-helper lymphocytes. It is the gradual alteration in function and eventual depletion of this subpopulation of T lymphocytes that lead to the profound effects on cellular immunity characteristic of HIV infection and the occurrence of associated life-threatening diseases characteristic of AIDS. Infection of macrophages and other monocytes is probably also central to HIV's pathogenicity. Human immunodeficiency virus has also been demonstrated within lymph nodes, bone marrow, spleen, lung, brain, and retinal tissue.

There is a spectrum of HIV disease whose categorization is still evolving. Shortly after initial infection, many people will experience a self-limited, nonspecific mononucleosis-like illness. Following this, HIV infection remains asymptomatic for variable periods of time. Eventually, illnesses associated with defects in cellular immunity or with HIV infection of target organs such as the GI tract or the central nervous system begin to occur. At any time during the asymptomatic stage or during early manifestations of illness, laboratory abnormalities associated with immune dysfunction, such as lymphopenia, thrombocytopenia, and T_4 cell depletion may evolve. Generalized lymphadenopathy, isolated or in conjunction with diffuse, constitutional symptoms, can occur at variable places along the time course of disease.

The last stage of HIV infection is AIDS. The current case definition of AIDS is achieved when one of a list of illnesses associated with immune suppression is diagnosed in a person with no underlying reason such as age, malignancy, or immunosuppressive medication. These illnesses include key infections such as *Pneumocystis carinii*, disseminated viral infections, unusual protozoal and helminthic infections, and atypical mycobacterial infections; typical malignancies such as Kaposi's sarcoma, non-Hodgkin's lymphoma, and primary brain lymphoma; and a number of other clinical findings or diseases indicative of a defect in cell-mediated immunity. In 1987, dementia and a "wasting syndrome" of inexorable weight loss, persistent, intractable diarrhea, and fever were added to this list. Despite maximal efforts at treatment, these associated diseases and conditions lead to death.

Because the HIV epidemic is of such relatively early onset, the time course for disease progression is not absolutely known. Forty percent of one group of individuals followed since the exact time of onset of infection progressed to AIDS within 8 years. It is assumed that all infected persons will eventually acquire AIDS and die from their disease should a permanent cure not be discovered. The interaction between disease progression and factors such as age, lifestyle, and other infections and illnesses is unknown.

Human immunodeficiency virus is known to be transmitted by three major routes: (1) direct blood contact, (2) sexual transmission, and (3) perinatal transmission from an infected woman to her fetus or child either through in utero exposure or at the time of birth. Specific activities and lifestyles clearly place one at risk for acquisition of this disease. Transmission through casual, household contact does not occur.

Intravenous drug abuse using shared needles is the major means by which blood contact leads to HIV infection in the United States. In areas of the country where HIV disease is particularly prevalent among IV drug abusers, most notably New York City and New Jersey, 50% to 60% of IV drug abusers are estimated to be HIV infected. Although medical transfusion of infected blood products accounts for a low level of AIDS cases currently reported, since 1985, screening of blood products has markedly reduced this mode of transmission of HIV.

Semen, cervical, and vaginal secretions can contain virus, and transmission of HIV during sexual activity has clearly been documented. Factors influencing rates of sexual transmission are incompletely understood. Heterosexual transmission both from male to female and female to male can occur. Male to female transmission may be more efficient. Anal receptive intercourse may be associated with the greatest risk of transmission, although vaginal intercourse can also apparently lead to infection. An exact risk of transmission associated with oral intercourse is unknown.

The majority of HIV disease in women is associated with either personal IV drug abuse or with heterosexual transmission, particularly from a drug-abusing partner. It is estimated that 30% of HIV disease in women is a result of such het-

erosexual exposure. A recent seroprevalence study suggested that 40% of women heterosexually infected by HIV were unaware of any risk of exposure to HIV.

Eighty percent of pediatric AIDS is associated with perinatal transmission. An HIV-infected woman transmits the infection perinatally to her child at a rate of approximately 30% to 50%. Such perinatal AIDS may be particularly virulent with a shorter latent period and earlier mortality. The effect of HIV disease on pregnancy outcome and the effect that pregnancy itself may have on affecting HIV disease expression in an infected woman remain to be determined.

Factors influencing transmissibility of HIV are poorly understood. Frequency of exposure to virus, underlying conditions in the exposed individual, and the "efficiency" of the infecting individual are all no doubt factors. It is likely that progressive immune suppression is associated with greater viral shedding, thus greater efficiency of transmission; however, all HIV-infected individuals must be considered to be potentially infectious. Recent attention has been directed to the probability that ulcerative genital diseases increase the likelihood of HIV transmission.

Diagnosis of HIV infection is typically made by testing for the presence of antibody to HIV. Virus can be inconstantly cultured from blood and various secretions of an infected individual, but the presence of virus is unpredictable, and cultures are time consuming, expensive, and not generally available.

Antibody testing is carried out by first performing an efficient, inexpensive, very sensitive ELISA test. If the results are positive for HIV, the test is repeated a second time to decrease the likelihood of false positive reactions, which may be as high as 4:1 on initial testing. If the results again are abnormal, a more specific assay that detects exact viral antigen patterns, typified by the Western Blot, must be performed for confirmation. The majority of serological conversions take place within 6 months of initial viral infection.

Although multifocal efforts based on understanding of the pathogenesis of HIV infection are being directed at finding a treatment that will eradicate this infection, currently there is no effective treatment for cure of HIV infection. It is assumed that treatment during asymptomatic infection will eventually be most effective. Medical efforts are now aimed at treating associated conditions and preventing associated illnesses. Major public health efforts are being directed at primary prevention of disease through educating people about disease transmission and modification of activities to avoid transmission. Success of such efforts is dependent on suppressing fear of disease, fostering acceptance by all segments of society of such efforts, and committing all possible financial and human resources toward these goals.

BIBLIOGRAPHY

Anonymous: Ketoconazole (Nizoral): A new antifungal agent. *Med Lett Drugs Ther* 1981; 23:85–87.

Anonymous: Criteria for diagnosis and grading of salpingitis [editorial]. *Obstet Gynecol* 1983; 61:113.

Anonymous: Interferon for treatment of genital warts. *Med Lett Drugs Ther* 1988a; 30:70–72.

Anonymous: Treatment of sexually transmitted diseases. *Med Lett Drug Ther* 1988b; 30:5–10.

Bartlett JG, Moon NE, Goldstein PR, et al: Cervical and vaginal bacterial flora: Ecological niches in the female lower genital tract. *Am J Obstet Gynecol* 1978; 130:658–661.

Bartlett JG, Onderdonk AB, Drude E, et al: Quantitative bacteriology of the vaginal flora. *J Infect Dis* 1977; 136:271–277.

Becker LE: Lymphogranuloma venereum. *Int J Dermatol* 1976; 15:26–33.

Bell TA, Grayston JT: Centers for Disease Control guidelines for prevention and control of *Chlamydia trachomatis* infections: Summary and commentary. *Ann Intern Med* 1986; 104:524–526.

Berkley SF, Hightower AW, Broome CV, et al: The relationship of tampon characteristics to menstrual toxic shock syndrome. *JAMA* 1987; 258:917–920.

Brown ST, Zaidi A, Larsen SA: Serologic response to syphilis treatment: A new analysis of old data. *JAMA* 1985; 253:1296–1299.

Brunham RB, Paavonen J, Stevens CE, et al: Mucopurulent cervicitis: The ignored counterpart of urethritis in the male. *N Engl J Med* 1984; 311:1–6.

Burkman R, Schlesselman S, McCaffrey L, et al: The relationship of genital tract actinomycetes and the development of pelvic inflammatory disease. *Am J Obstet Gynecol* 1982; 143:585–589.

Burkman RT and Women's Health Study: Association between intrauterine device and pelvic inflammatory disease. *Obstet Gynecol* 1981; 57:269–277.

Burnakis TG, Hildebrandt NB: Pelvic inflammatory disease: A review with emphasis on antimicrobial therapy. *Rev Infect Dis* 1986; 8:86–116.

Campion MJ: Clinical manifestations and natural history of genital human papilloma virus infection. *Obstet Gynecol Clin North Am* 1987; 14:363–388.

Caplan LR, Kleeman FJ, Berg S: Urinary retention probably secondary to herpes genitalis. *N Engl J Med* 1977; 297:920–921.

Centers for Disease Control: Toxic-shock syndrome—United States, 1970–1980. *MMWR* 1981; 30:25–33.

Centers for Disease Control: Sexually transmitted diseases treatment guidelines 1982. *MMWR* 1982; 31:33–62.

Centers for Disease Control: *Chlamydia trachomatis* infections. Policy guidelines for prevention and control. *MMWR* 1985; 34(suppl 35):1S–74S.

Centers for Disease Control: Additional recommendations to reduce sexual and drug abuse–related transmission of human T-lymphotropic virus type III/lymphadenopathy-associated virus. *MMWR* 1986; 35:152–155.

Centers for Disease Control: Antibiotic-resistant strains of *Neisseria gonorrhoeae*. Policy guidelines for detection, management, and control. *MMWR* 1987; 36(suppl 5):1S–18S.

Centers for Disease Control: Continuing increase in infectious syphilis—United States. *MMWR* 1988a; 37:35–38.

Centers for Disease Control: Syphilis and congenital syphilis—United States, 1985–1988. *MMWR* 1988b; 37:486–489.

Cooper T, Altman S, Baltimore D, et al: *Confronting AIDS: Update 1988*. Washington, DC, National Academy Press, 1988.

Corey L, Adams HG, Brown ZA, et al: Genital herpes simplex virus infections: Clinical manifestations course and complications. *Ann Intern Med* 1983; 98:958–972.

Corey L, Spear PG: Infections with herpes simplex viruses (2). *N Engl J Med* 1986; 314:749–757.

Corriere JN Jr: Avoiding "overkill" in diagnosis and treatment of lower urinary tract infections. *Urology* 1988; 32(2 suppl):17–21.

Dalaker K, Gjonnaess H, Kvile G, et al: *Chlamydia trachomatis* as a cause of acute perihepatitis associated with pelvic inflammatory disease. *Br J Vener Dis* 1981; 57:41–43.

Daly JW, King R, Monif GRG: Progressive necrotizing wound infection in postirradiated patients. *Obstet Gynecol* 1978; 52(suppl):5–8.

Davis JP, Chesney PJ, Wand PJ, et al: Toxic-shock syndrome. Epidemiologic features, recurrences, risk factors, and prevention. *N Engl J Med* 1980; 303:1429–1435.

Dorsky DI, Crumpacker CS: Drugs five years later: Acyclovir. *Ann Intern Med* 1987; 107:859–874.

Douglas JM, Critchlow C, Benedetti J, et al: A double-blind study of oral acyclovir for suppression of recurrences of genital herpes simplex virus infection. *N Engl J Med* 1984; 310:1551–1556.

Edelman DA, Berger GS: Contraceptive practice and tubo-ovarian abscess. *Am J Obstet Gynecol* 1980; 138:541–544.

Eschenbach DA: Vaginal infection. *Clin Obstet Gynecol* 1983; 26:186–202.

Eschenbach DA, Buchanan TM, Pollock HM, et al: Polymicrobial etiology of acute pelvic inflammatory disease. *N Engl J Med* 1975; 293:166–171.

Eschenbach DA, Harnisch JP, Holmes KK: Pathogenesis of acute pelvic inflammatory disease: Role of contraceptive and other risk factors. *Am J Obstet Gynecol* 1977; 128:838–850.

Eschenbach DA, Hillier S, Critchlow C, et al: Diagnosis and clinical manifestations of bacterial vaginosis. *Am J Obstet Gynecol* 1988; 158:819–828.

Eschenbach DA, Holmes KK: Acute pelvic inflammatory disease: Current concepts of pathogenesis, etiology and management. *Clin Obstet Gynecol* 1975; 18:35–50.

Ferenczy A, Mitao M, Nagai N, et al: Latent papillomavirus and recurring genital warts. *N Engl J Med* 1985; 313:784.

Fihn SD: Behavioral aspects of urinary tract infection. *Urology* 1988; 32(suppl 3):168.

Fihn SD, Lathan RH, Roberts P, et al: Association between diaphragm use and urinary tract infection. *JAMA* 1985; 254:240–245.

Fiumara NJ: Treatment of seropositive primary syphilis: An evaluation of 196 patients. *Sex Transm Dis* 1977a; 4:92–95.

Fiumara NJ: Treatment of secondary syphilis: An evaluation of 204 patients. *Sex Transm Dis* 1977b; 4:96–99.

Fiumara NJ: Reinfection primary, secondary, and latent syphilis: The serologic response after treatment. *Sex Transm Dis* 1980; 7:111–115.

Fischl MA, Dickinson GM, Scott GB, et al: Evaluation of heterosexual partners, children, and household contacts of adults with AIDS. *JAMA* 1987; 257:640–644.

Fonts AC, Kraus SJ: *Trichomonas* vaginalis: Re-evaluation of its clinical presentation and laboratory diagnosis. *J Infect Dis* 1980; 141:137–143.

Fowler JE Jr: Urinary tract infections in women. *Urol Clin North Am* 1986; 13:673–683.

Friedland GH, Klein RS: Transmission of the human immunodeficiency virus. *N Engl J Med* 1987; 317:1125–1135.

Galask RP, Larsen B, Ohm MJ: Vaginal flora and its role in disease entities. *Clin Obstet Gynecol* 1976; 19:61–81.

Gardner HL: *Haemophilus* vaginalis vaginitis after 25 years. *Am J Obstet Gynecol* 1980; 137:385–391.

Gilstrap LC, Herbert WNP, Cunningham EG, et al: Gonorrhea screening in male consorts of women with pelvic infection. *JAMA* 1977; 238:965–966.

Gjonnaess H, Dalaker K, Anestad G, et al: Pelvic inflammatory disease: Etiologic studies with emphasis on chlamydial infection. *Obstet Gynecol* 1982; 59:550–555.

Gloeb DJ, O'Sullivan MJ, Efantis J: Human immunodeficiency virus infection in women: I. The effects of human immunodeficiency virus on pregnancy. *Am J Obstet Gynecol* 1988; 159:756–761.

Golde SH, Israel R, Ledger WJ: Unilateral tuboovarian abscess: A distinct entity. *Am J Obstet Gynecol* 1977; 127:807–812.

Guinan ME: Oral acyclovir for treatment and suppression of genital herpes simplex virus infection. A review. *JAMA* 1986; 255:1747–1749.

Guinan ME, Hardy A: Epidemiology of AIDS in women in the United States. *JAMA* 1987; 257:2039–2042.

Guinan ME, MacCalman J, Kern ER, et al: The course of untreated recurrent genital herpes simplex infection in 27 women. *N Engl J Med* 1981; 304:759–763.

Hager WD, Brown ST, Kraus SJ, et al: Metronidazole for vaginal trichomoniasis: Seven-day v single-dose regimens. *JAMA* 1980; 224:1219–1220.

Handsfield HH, Jasman LL, Roberts PL, et al: Criteria for selective screening for chlamydia trachomatis infection in women attending family planning clinics. *JAMA* 1986; 255:1730–1734.

Haverkos HW, Edelman R: The epidemiology of acquired immunodeficiency syndrome among heterosexuals. *JAMA* 1988; 260:1922–1929.

Henry-Suchet J, Loffredo V: Chlamydial and *Mycoplasma* genital infection in salpingitis and tubal sterility. *Lancet* 1980; 1:539–543.

Holmes KK, Counts GW, Beaty HN: Disseminated gonococcal infection. *Ann Intern Med* 1971; 74:979–993.

Holmes KK, Mardh PA: *International Perspectives on Neglected Sexually Transmitted Diseases.* New York, Hemisphere Publishing Corp, 1983, pp 1–336.

Hook EW III, Holmes KK: Gonococcal infections. *Ann Intern Med* 1985; 102:229–243.

Hovelius B, Mårdh PA: *Staphylococcus saprophyticus* as a common cause of urinary tract infections. *Rev Infect Dis* 1984; 6:328–337.

Hunter CA, Long KR: Vaginal and cervical pH in normal women and in patients with vaginitis. *Am J Obstet Gynecol* 1958; 75:872–874.

Jacobson L, Weström L: Objectivized diagnosis of acute pelvic inflammatory disease: Diagnostic and prognostic value of routine laparoscopy. *Am J Obstet Gynecol* 1969; 105:1088–1098.

Jones RB, Mammel JB, Shepard MK, et al: Recovery of *Chlamydia trachomatis* from the endometrium of women at risk for chlamydial infection. *Am J Obstet Gynecol* 1986; 155:36.

Judson FN, Allaman J, Dans PE: Treatment of gonorrhea: Comparison of penicillin G. procaine, doxycycline, spectinomycin, and ampicillin. *JAMA* 1974; 230:705–708.

Kass EH: Chemotherapeutic and antibiotic drugs in the management of infections of the urinary tract. *Am J Med* 1955; 18:764–781.

Kass EH, Finland M: Asymptomatic infections of the urinary tract. *Trans Assoc Am Physicians* 1956; 69:56–64.

Kelaghan J, Rubin GL, Ory HW, et al: Barrier-method contraceptives and pelvic inflammatory disease. *JAMA* 1981; 248:184–187.

Komaroff AL: Acute dysuria in women. *N Engl J Med* 1984; 310:368–375.

Klein TA, Richmond JA, Mishcell DR Jr: Pelvis tuberculosis. *Obstet Gynecol* 1976; 48:99–105.

Lafferty WE, Coombs RW, Bennedetti J, et al: Recurrences after oral and genital herpes simplex virus infection. Influence of site of infection and viral type. *N Engl J Med* 1987; 316:1444–1449.

Landers DV, Sweet RL: Current trends in the diagnosis and treatment of tuboovarian abscess. *Am J Obstet Gynecol* 1985; 151:1098–1110.

Landesman S, Minkoff H, Holmans S, et al: Serosurvey of human immunodeficiency virus infection in parturients. *JAMA* 1987; 258:2701–2703.

Larsen B, Galask RP: Vaginal microbial flora: Practical and theoretic relevance. *Obstet Gynecol* 1980; 55(suppl):1005–1135.

Lee NC, Rubin GL, Ory HW, et al: Type of intrauterine device and the risk of pelvic inflammatory disease. *Obstet Gynecol* 1983; 62:1–6.

Lee TJ, Sparling F: Syphilis: An algorithm. *JAMA* 1979; 242:1187–1189.

Lightfoot TW, Gotschlich EC: Gonococcal disease. *Am J Med* 1974; 56:347–356.

Linder JGEM, Plantema FHF, Hoogkamp-Korstamje JAA: Quantitative studies of the vaginal flora of healthy women and of obstetric and gynaecological patients. *J Med Microbiol* 1978; 11:233–241.

Lynch PJ: Sexually transmitted diseases: Granuloma inguinale, lymphogranuloma venereum, chancroid and infectious syphilis. *Clin Obstet Gynecol* 1978; 31:1041–1052.

Lynch PJ: Condylomata acuminata. *Clin Obstet Gynecol* 1985; 28:142–151.

McCormack WM (ed): *Diagnosis and Treatment of Sexually Transmitted Diseases.* Littleton, Mass, John Wright PSG, 1983, pp 1–260.

McLellan R, Spence MR, Brockman M, et al: The clinical diagnosis of trichomoniasis. *Obstet Gynecol* 1982; 60:30–34.

Mårdh P-A, Ripa KT, Svensson L, et al: *Chlamydia trachomatis* infection in patients with acute salpingitis. *N Engl J Med* 1977; 296:1377–1379.

Mårdh P-A, Weström L: Tubal and cervical cultures in acute salpingitis with special reference to *Mycoplasma hominis* and T-strain mycoplasmas. *Br J Vener Dis* 1970; 46:179–186.

Mårdh P-A, Weström L: Adherence of bacteria to vaginal epithelial cells. *Infect Immunol* 1976; 13:661–666.

Mead PB: Cervical-vaginal flora of women with invasive cervical cancer. *Obstet Gynecol* 1978; 52:601–604.

Meisels A: Dysplasia and carcinoma of the uterine cervix: IV. A correlated cytologic and histologic study with special emphasis on vaginal microbiology. *Acta Cytol* 1969; 13:224–234.

Meleney FL: Bacterial synergism in disease processes. *Ann Surg* 1931; 94:961–981.

Meltzer RM: Necrotizing gasciitis and progressive bacterial synergistic gangrene of the vulva. *Obstet Gynecol* 1980; 61:757–760.

Mertz GJ, Eron L, Kaufman R, et al: Prolonged continuous versus intermittent oral acyclovir treatment in normal adults with frequently recurring genital herpes simplex virus infection. *Am J Med* 1988a; 85:14–19.

Mertz GJ, Jones CC, Mills J, et al: Long-term acyclovir suppression of frequently recurring genital herpes simplex virus infection. A multicenter double-blind trial. *JAMA* 1988b; 260:201–206.

Miles MR, Olsen L, Rogers A: Recurrent vaginal candidiasis: Importance of an intestinal reservoir. *JAMA* 1977; 238:1836–1837.

Minkoff HL: Care of pregnant women infected with human immunodeficiency virus. *JAMA* 1987; 258:2714–2717.

Monif GRG: *Infectious Diseases in Obstetrics and Gynecology*. New York, Harper & Row, Publishers, 1982, pp 1–671.

Muller-Schoop JW, Wang SP, Munzinger J, et al: *Chlamydia trachomatis* as possible cause of peritonitis and perihepatitis in young women. *Br Med J (Clin Res)* 1978; 1:1022–1024.

Nahmias AJ, Roizman B: Infection with herpes simplex viruses 1 and 2. *N Engl J Med* 1973; 289:667–674, 719–725, 781–789.

Nettleman MD, Jones RB: Cost-effectiveness of screening women at moderate risk for genital infections caused by chlamydia trachomatis. *JAMA* 1988; 260:207–213.

Oriel JD: Genital warts. *Sex Transm Dis* 1977; 4:153–159.

Oriel JD, Partridge BM, Denny MJ, et al: Genital yeast infections. *Br Med J (Clin Res)* 1972; 4:761–764.

Oriel JD, Ridgway GL: *Genital Infection With Chlamydia trachomatis*. New York, Elsevier North-Holland, 1982, pp 1–144.

Paavonen J, Kiviat N, Brunham RC, et al: Prevalence and manifestations of endometritis among women with cervicitis. *Am J Obstet Gynecol* 1985; 152:280–286.

Padian N, Marquis L, Francis DP, et al: Male-to-female transmission of human immunodeficiency virus. *JAMA* 1987; 258:788–790.

Parsons CL: Urinary tract infections. *Clin Obstet Gynecol* 1985; 12:487–496.

Parsons CL: Lower urinary tract infections in women. *Urol Clin North Am* 1987; 14:247–250.

Peterman TA, Cates W, Curran JW: The challenge of human immunodeficiency virus (HIV) and acquired immunodeficiency syndrome (AIDS) in women and children. *Fertil Steril* 1988; 49:571–578.

Pheifer TA, Forsyth PS, Durfee MA, et al: Nonspecific vaginitis: Role of *Haemophilus vaginalis* and treatment with metronidazole. *N Engl J Med* 1978; 298:1429–1434.

Phillips RS, Aronson MD, Taylor WC, et al: Should tests for *Chlamydia trachomatis* cervical infection be done during routine gynecologic visits? *Ann Intern Med* 1987; 107:188–194.

Polk BF: Antimicrobial prophylasis to prevent mixed bacterial infection. *J Antimicrob Chemother* 1981; 8:115–129.

Polk BF, Shapiro M, Goldstein P, et al: Randomised clinical trial of perioperative cefazolin in preventing infection after hysterectomy. *Lancet* 1980; 1:438–441.

Redfield RR, Markham PD, Salahuddin SZ: Heterosexual acquired HTLV-III/LAV disease (AIDS-related complex and AIDS). *JAMA* 1985; 254:2094–2096.

Reichman RC, Badger GJ, Mertz GJ, et al: Treatment of recurrent genital herpes simplex infections with oral acyclovir. A controlled trial. *JAMA* 1984; 251:2103–2107.

Reid G, Sobel JD: Bacterial adherence in the pathogenesis of urinary tract infection: A review. *Rev Infect Dis* 1987; 9:470–487.

Reid R, Greengerg M, Jenson AB, et al: Sexually transmitted papilloma viral infections: I. The anatomic distribution and pathologic grade of neoplastic lesions associated with different viral types. *Am J Obstet Gynecol* 1987; 156:212–222.

Rein MF: Current therapy of vulvovaginitis. *Sex Transm Dis* 1981; 8:316–370.

Rice RJ, Thompson SE: Treatment of uncomplicated infections due to neisseria gonorrhoeae. *JAMA* 1986; 255:1739.

Ronald AR, Plummer FA: Chancroid and *Haemophilus ducreyi*. *Ann Intern Med* 1985; 102:705–707.

Rubin GL, Ory HW, Layde PM: Oral contraceptives and pelvic inflammatory disease. *Am J Obstet Gynecol* 1982; 114:630–635.

Rudolph AH: Examination of the cerebrospinal fluid in syphilis. *Cutis* 1976; 17:749–752.

St John RK, Brown ST: International symposium on pelvic inflammatory disease. *Am J Obstet Gynecol* 1980; 138:845–1112.

Sanders LL Jr, Harrison HR, Washington AE: Treatment of sexually transmitted chlamydial infections. *JAMA* 1986; 255:1750–1756.

Scaling ST, Levinson CJ, Plavidal F, et al: The correlation of pelvic ultrasound and laparoscopy in the diagnosis and management of gynecologic disorders. *J Reprod Med* 1978; 21:53–58.

Schaeffer AJ: Recurrent urinary tract infection in the female patient. *Urology* 1988; 32(suppl 3):12–15.

Schacter J: Chlamydial infections. *N Engl J Med* 1978; 298:428–435, 490–495, 540–549.

Schiffer MA, Elguezabal A, Sultana M, et al: Actinomycosis infections associated with intrauterine contraceptive devices. *Obstet Gynecol* 1975; 45:67–71.

Schmid GP: The treatment of chancroid. *JAMA* 1986; 255:1757–1762.

Schmid GP, Sander LL Jr, Blount JH, et al: Chancroid in the United States. Reestablishment of an old disease. *JAMA* 1987; 258:3265–3268.

Scott WC: Pelvic abscess in association with intrauterine contraceptive devices. *Am J Obstet Gynecol* 1978; 131:149–156.

Shands KN, Schmid GP, Dan BB: Toxic-shock syndrome in menstruating women. Association with tampon use and *Staphylococcus aureus* and clinical features in 52 cases. *N Engl J Med* 1980; 303:1436–1442.

Sobel JD: Recurrent vulvovaginal candidiasis. A prospective study of the efficacy of maintenance ketoconazole therapy. *N Engl J Med* 1986; 315:1455–1458.

Souney P, Polk BF: Single-dose antimicrobial therapy for urinary tract infections in women. *Rev Infect Dis* 1982; 4:29–34.

Spaulding LB, Gelman SR, Wood SD, et al: The role of ultrasonography in the management of endometritis/salpingitis/peritonitis. *Obstet Gynecol* 1979; 53:442–446.

Speigel CA, Amsel R, Eschenbach D, et al: Anaerobic bacteria in nonspecific vaginitis. *N Engl J Med* 1980; 303:601–607.

Spence MR: The treatment of gonorrhea, syphilis, chancroid, lymphogranuloma venereum, and granuloma inguinale. *Clin Obstet Gynecol* 1988; 31:453–465.

Stamey TA: Recurrent urinary tract infection in female patients: An overview of management and treatment. *Rev Infect Dis* 1987; 9(suppl 2):S195–210.

Stamm WE: Diagnosis of *Chlamydia trachomatis* genitourinary infections. *Ann Intern Med* 1988a; 108:710–717.

Stamm WE: Protocol for diagnosis of urinary tract infection: Reconsidering the criterion for significant bacteriuria. *Urology* 1988b; 32(suppl 2):6–12.

Stamm WE, Counts GW, Running KR, et al: Diagnosis of coliform infection in acutely dysuric women. *N Engl J Med* 1982; 307:463–468.

Stamm WE, Guinan ME, Johnson C, et al: Effect of treatment regimens for *Neisseria gonorrhoeae* on simultaneous infection with *Chlamydia trachomatis*. *N Engl J Med* 1984; 310:545–549.

Stamm WE, Running K, McKevitt M, et al: Treatment of the acute urethral syndrome. *N Engl J Med* 1981; 304:956–958.

Stamm WE, Wagner KF, Amsel R, et al: Causes of the acute urethral syndrome in women. *N Engl J Med* 1980; 303:409–415.

Stone HH, Martin JD: Synergistic necrotizing cellulitis. *Ann Surg* 1972; 175:702–711.

Stone RL, Schlievert PM: Evidence for the involvement of endotoxin in toxic shock syndrome. *J Infect Dis* 1987; 155:682–689.

Straus SE, Takiff HE, Seidlin M, et al: Suppression of frequently recurring genital herpes. *N Engl J Med* 1984; 310:1545–1550.

Strom BL, Collins M, West SL, et al: Sexual activity, contraceptive use and other risk factors for symptomatic and asymptomatic bacteriuria. *Ann Intern Med* 1987; 107:816–823.

Sweet RL, Blankfort-Doyle M, Robbie MO, et al: The occurrence of chlamydial and gonococcal salpingitis during the menstrual cycle. *JAMA* 1986; 255:2062–2064.

Sweet RL, Mills J, Hadley KW, et al: Use of laparoscopy to determine the microbiologic etiology of acute salpingitis. *Am J Obstet Gynecol* 1979; 134:68–78.

Thompson SE, Brooks C, Eschenbach DA, et al: High failure rates in outpatient treatment of salpingitis with either tetracycline alone or penicillin/ampicillin combination. *Am J Obstet Gynecol* 1985; 152:635–641.

Thompson SE, Hager WD, Wong KH, et al: The microbiology and therapy of acute pelvic inflammatory disease in hospitalized patients. *Am J Obstet Gynecol* 1980; 36:179–186.

Todd J, Fishaut M, Kapral F, et al: Toxic-shock syndrome associated with phage-group-1 staphylococci. *Lancet* 1978; 2:1116.

Todd JK, Ressman M, Caston SA, et al: Corticosteroid therapy for patients with toxic shock syndrome. *JAMA* 1984; 252:3399–3402.

Tofte RW, Williams DN: Clinical and laboratory manifestations of toxic shock syndrome. *Ann Intern Med* 1982; 96:843–847.

Valicenti JE, Pappas AA, Graber CD, et al: Detection and prevalence of IUD-associated actinomyces colonization and related morbidity. *JAMA* 1982; 247:1149–1152.

Van Slyke KK, Michel VP, Rein MF: Treatment of vulvovaginal candidiasis with boric acid power. *Am J Obstet Gynecol* 1981; 141:145–148.

Wager GP: Toxic shock syndrome: A review. *Am J Obstet Gynecol* 1983; 146:93.

Washington AE, Arno PS, Brooks MA: The economic cost of pelvic inflammatory disease. *JAMA* 1986; 255:1735–1738.

Washington AE, Johnson RE, Sanders LL: *Chlamydia trachomatis* infections in the United States. What are they costing us? *JAMA* 1987; 257:2070–2072.

Wasserheit JN, Bell TA, Kiviat NB, et al: Microbial causes of proven pelvic inflammatory disease and efficacy of clindamycin and tobramycin. *Ann Intern Med* 1986; 104:187–193.

Weström L: Effect of acute pelvic inflammatory disease on fertility. *Am J Obstet Gynecol* 1975; 121:707–713.

Wiesner PJ, Thompson SE: Gonococcal diseases. *DM* 1980; 26:1–44.

Witkin SS: Immunology of recurrent vaginitis. *Am J Reprod Immunol Microbiol* 1987a; 15:34–37.

Witkin SS: Transient, Local immunosuppression in recurrent vaginitis. *Immunol Today* 1987b; 8:360.

Witkin SS, Jeremias J, Ledger WJ: A localized vaginal allergic response in women with recurrent vaginitis. *J Allergy Clin Immunol* 1988; 81:412–416.

Wofsy GB, Hauer LB, Michaelis BA, et al: Isolation of AIDS-associated retrovirus from genital secretions of women with antibodies to the virus. *Lancet* 1986; 1:527–529.

Wolner-Hanseen P, Mardh PA, Svensson L, et al: Laparoscopy in women with chlamydial infection and pelvic pain: A comparison of patients with and without salpingitis. *Obstet Gynecol* 1983; 61:299–303.

20 Pediatric and Adolescent Gynecology

Donald Peter Goldstein, M.D.

The gynecological treatment of the prepubertal and adolescent patient differs in many respects from the care of the adult woman. Unique problems are encountered in this population, especially in infants and young children, that are not usually seen by the practicing obstetrician-gynecologist. For this reason, it is appropriate that a chapter devoted to a discussion of the gynecological problems of this age group be included in a textbook of this scope. It is reassuring, however, that the evaluation and treatment of the commonest of the conditions that affect these patients requires a minimum of knowledge and technical skill beyond the capabilities of most gynecologists.

In older adolescents, the gynecological problems encountered are quite similar to those seen in adults. The distinction between these two groups lies in the emotional instability characteristic of the maturing individual. The psychological impact of the first gynecological examination should not be underestimated. The outcome of this experience may have a profound influence on the care that that patient seeks for the rest of her life. There is no doubt that providing gynecological treatment to adolescents is time consuming, and the physician with a busy practice may elect to avoid this population. Adolescents need to be seen by a sensitive person who has time to listen to them, give satisfactory explanations, and answer questions in a way that is appropriate to their comprehension. This is the key to winning their confidence and, what is more important, to improving their compliance.

In this area of the gynecological practice, the attitude of the treating physician is also an important consideration. Children and adolescents are very sensitive to adults' attitudes. The gynecologist must, therefore, feel comfortable in communicating with these patients and their parents and should have overcome his or her own reticence about performing an adequate pelvic examination on young children and adolescents. Maintaining a nonjudgmental attitude toward their emerging sexuality is also of utmost importance.

In this chapter, I will discuss the most commonly encountered gynecological problems in the pediatric and adolescent age group. For the most part, those conditions that are shared with the adult patient will be discussed in other chapters more comprehensively. The material is organized from the perspective of the four broad etiological categories that underlie all gynecological conditions—infection and trauma, congenital malformations, endocrine-related disorders, and tumors. Since the disease spectrum and clinical signs and symptoms of the prepubertal child may differ significantly from those of the menstruating female, these age groups are discussed separately.

HISTORY TAKING AND THE GYNECOLOGICAL EXAMINATION

Infants and young children are most often referred by their pediatricians for specific reasons. In this situation, a referral note describing the problem, the results of prior diagnostic studies, and prereferral treatment greatly facilitates the history taking. As in any field of pediatrics, information in this age group is usually obtained from the parents, although the older child should be questioned directly. It is helpful for the physician to take his or her own history because this provides an opportunity to establish rapport.

Vulvovaginitis and vaginal bleeding are by

far the commonest complaints that bring these youngsters to the gynecologist. A thorough inquiry about recent infectious disease and antibiotic therapy, hygiene, and use of irritants (bubble bath, perfumed soap, etc.) is essential. The possibility of sexual abuse should always be kept in mind. Vague gynecological complaints may be used as a pretext to consult for actual or suspected sexual abuse. On the other hand, parents may feel misjudged or threatened if the physician raises this possibility abruptly. It is, therefore, essential to approach this matter tactfully.

The older child should also be questioned personally about her symptoms and matters of hygiene. It is sometimes interesting to note how answers differ from those given by her parents.

The technique of interviewing the teenager is more critical. This first contact is decisive in establishing communication between the patient and her gynecologist. The adolescent is frequently under a tremendous amount of tension during her first examination. She should, therefore, be approached sensitively in a nonjudgmental fashion. It is vital that the physician assure the patient that her confidentiality will be respected and only those issues agreed on will be discussed with her parents. The use of her first name rather than of impersonal terms such as "honey" or "sweetheart" certainly makes her feel her complaints are being taken seriously.

A complete medical history should be obtained on the first visit. The gynecological questionnaire (Fig 20–1) includes a careful assessment of the chief complaint, details of pubertal development and menstrual cycles, and history of in utero diethylstilbestrol (DES) exposure. Straightforward questions about sexual activity and the need for contraception are more likely to result in honest answers than an inquiry conducted in a roundabout way. The adolescent who is not sexually active should, however, not be left with the impression that her abstinence represents abnormal behavior.

Though it is desirable to interview the teenager alone, it is not always possible. When the parents accompany the teenager, they may desire to be present while the history is being taken. It is, however, appropriate to ask the parents to leave the room during the physical examination. At this time the patient has the opportunity to express her own concerns, ask questions, and bring up subjects she did not want to discuss in the presence of her parents.

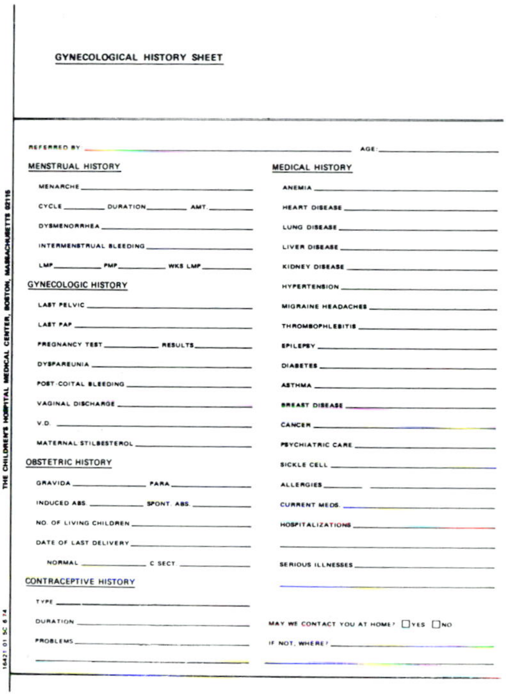
GYNECOLOGICAL HISTORY SHEET

REFERRED BY ______ AGE: ______

MENSTRUAL HISTORY
MENARCHE ______
CYCLE ______ DURATION ______ AMT. ______
DYSMENORRHEA ______
INTERMENSTRUAL BLEEDING ______
LMP ______ PMP ______ WKS LMP ______

GYNECOLOGIC HISTORY
LAST PELVIC ______
LAST PAP ______
PREGNANCY TEST ______ RESULTS ______
DYSPAREUNIA ______
POST-COITAL BLEEDING ______
VAGINAL DISCHARGE ______
V.D. ______
MATERNAL STILBESTEROL ______

OBSTETRIC HISTORY
GRAVIDA ______ PARA ______
INDUCED ABS. ______ SPONT. ABS. ______
NO. OF LIVING CHILDREN ______
DATE OF LAST DELIVERY ______
NORMAL ______ C SECT. ______

CONTRACEPTIVE HISTORY
TYPE ______
DURATION ______
PROBLEMS ______

MEDICAL HISTORY
ANEMIA ______
HEART DISEASE ______
LUNG DISEASE ______
LIVER DISEASE ______
KIDNEY DISEASE ______
HYPERTENSION ______
MIGRAINE HEADACHES ______
THROMBOPHLEBITIS ______
EPILEPSY ______
DIABETES ______
ASTHMA ______
BREAST DISEASE ______
CANCER ______
PSYCHIATRIC CARE ______
SICKLE CELL ______
ALLERGIES ______
CURRENT MEDS. ______
HOSPITALIZATIONS ______
SERIOUS ILLNESSES ______

MAY WE CONTACT YOU AT HOME? ☐ YES ☐ NO
IF NOT, WHERE? ______

THE CHILDREN'S HOSPITAL MEDICAL CENTER, BOSTON, MASSACHUSETTS 02115
16421 01 SC 6 74

FIG 20–1.
Gynecological history sheet used at the Gynecology Clinic, Children's Hospital, Boston.

Gynecological Examination of the Young Child

The gynecological examination should always be explained in advance to the mother and the patient. It is important to stress that a properly performed gynecological examination does not hurt the child and will not compromise the patient's virginity.

A general physical assessment of the child should be carried out, including examination of the head and neck, lungs, heart, breasts, and abdomen. Besides the importance of being thorough, this part of the examination allows the phyician to establish physical contact with the patient and gain her confidence. The physician should carry on a conversation with the child about her friends, family, and play so that rapport can be more readily established. A careful documentation of the patient's sexual development should always be made at this time to establish a baseline for future comparison.

The neonate and infant (birth to age 2 years) are best examined either on the table or on the parent's lap, in the so-called frog leg position, which is also used in some older children. A careful examination of the external genitalia is performed, looking for anatomical abnormalities, signs of infection or inflammation, and the presence of lesions, excoriations, or trauma. It is to be remembered that in young children, the clitoris seems disproportionately large compared to the remainder of the vulva. Attention should next be directed to the area of the urethral meatus, looking for urethral discharge or signs of an ectopic ureter or introital cyst. Hygiene can be assessed by noting the presence of debris and fecal remnants on the perineum. Good visualization of the vestibule and hymen is obtained by gently pulling the labia majora downward and outward, which causes the hymenal ring to gape open, thus allowing inspection of the distal posterior wall of the vagina (Fig 20–2). The presence of a hymenal septum, imperforation, or cyst should be noted. This maneuver should be avoided when labial adhesions are present because of the sharp pain produced when the labia are separated forcibly. The use of a moist urethral swab can facilitate this portion of the examination, particularly when one is looking for a small opening inferior to the urethral meatus in an otherwise imperforate-appearing hymen or if one is trying to determine the origin of a perihymenal cyst.

The young child (age 2–8 years) is best examined in the knee-chest position, exerting a gentle lateral and upward traction on the buttocks. This maneuver usually opens the hymen sufficiently to allow complete visualization of the posterior wall of the vagina and cervix without the necessity of any vaginal instrumentation, using an otoscope (without the speculum) for light and magnification (Fig 20–3). The vagina should be carefully inspected for the presence of discharge, bleeding, tumors, and foreign bodies. The physician should be aware that the vaginal epithelium in the young child is normally thin, reddened, and friable due to poor estrogenization. For the same reason, the cervix is a small reddish structure that barely protrudes from the surrounding vaginal mucosa. In our experience, a satisfactory visualization of the vagina and cervix can be obtained in most instances by examination in the knee-chest position. It is our belief that before the age of 8 years, invasive techniques should not be carried out in the awake patient. If the knee-chest position proves unsatisfactory, it is preferable to perform the examination under anesthesia or sedation.

When vaginal cultures or a wet preparation are indicated, they should be obtained at the end of the examination and collected from the deep vaginal fornix. Depending on the size of the hymenal opening, a moistened cotton-tipped application or a Calgiswab is introduced into the vagina while the child is asked to cough. When multiple specimens are required, an eyedropper attached to a 4- or 5-cm segment of intravenous (IV) tubing may be used to aspirate the vaginal contents. This system may be used for vaginal irrigation when the discharge is not abundant. Five to 10 ml of sterile, nonbacteriostatic saline is injected in the

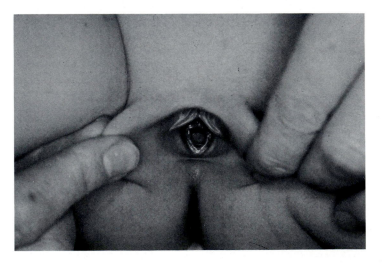

FIG 20–2.
Labial traction maneuver, ideal for use in newborns and infants to visualize introitus and lower vaginal vault.

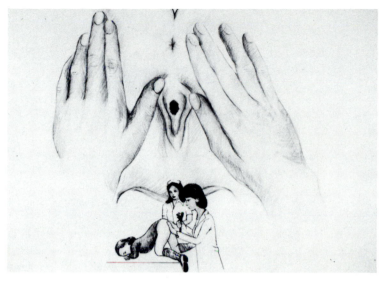

FIG 20–3.
Knee-chest position used for visualization of vagina with otoscope (without ear piece).

vagina and then aspirated. Once again, the child should be informed of what will happen, assured that the procedure will "tickle" but not hurt, and allowed to see and handle the material before cultures are taken.

After the examination in the knee-chest position is completed, the patient is then placed in the supine position, with her knees flexed and heels together, or the lithotomy position, and the pelvic organs are assessed by rectoabdominal examination. In these youngsters, the only palpable structure is the cervix, which feels like a small nodule behind the anterior wall of the rectum. The uterus and ovaries are not palpable in the prepubescent female except during the immediate postnatal period when the uterus is enlarged due to the influence of maternal estrogen. Any palpable pelvic structure should prompt a thorough investigation. While the rectal finger is withdrawn, gentle pressure should be applied against the anterior rectal wall so as to localize any tumor or foreign body and milk out any discharge. When indicated, the use of a colposcope is valuable for more careful scrutiny of the vulva and hymen and permits photographic documentation of visible lesions.

Gynecological Examination of the Older Child and Virginal Adolescent

The older premenarchal patient and the virginal adolescent are approached differently than the younger child since it is possible to have them participate more actively. We have found the use of a hand-held mirror to be of great value, since the patient can be distracted by a running commentary while visualizing her own external anatomy. Many patients in this age group come to their first gynecological examination already traumatized emotionally by "frightful stories about the torture of the gynecological examining room." It is, therefore, essential to explain the pelvic examination in detail. All instruments should be shown to the patient, and she should be assured that they are designed especially for young girls. The traditional dorsal lithotomy position using adjustable stirrups is used for the examination of these patients. The visualization of the vagina and cervix is best performed with a Huffman speculum (Fig 20–4). This instrument is narrow and long (1.3 by 10.8 cm) and conforms nicely to the virginal hymen and vagina. The morphology of the hymenal opening is first ascertained visually and then by gently introducing a lubricated finger in the vagina. In the presence of a microperforate or septate hymen, attempts to introduce a speculum result in an unsatisfactory examination and serve only to traumatize the patient physically and emotionally. When use of a speculum is made difficult by a rigid hymen or because of involuntary contraction, the postmenarchal patient should be taught how to use tampons and be given an appointment 3 months later if her problem does not require immediate examination. Otherwise, a pelvic examination under anesthesia and possibly a hymenot-

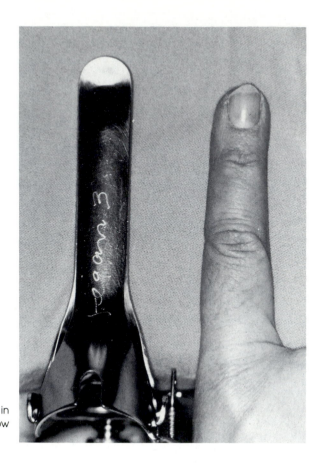

FIG 20–4.
Huffman speculum specially designed for use in virginal adolescents because of its narrow gauge and length.

omy to facilitate future examinations are in order.

When conditions are favorable for the use of a speculum, the perineal body is first relaxed by applying gentle pressure against the posterior vaginal wall. The finger is then slowly replaced by the warmed speculum. The vagina and cervix are inspected, and specimens for wet preparation, culture and Papanicolaou smears are obtained as indicated. Asking the patient to distinguish between the sensation of pressure and pain contributes to the success of this technique.

Internal genital structures are assessed by a rectovaginal examination. At the onset of puberty, the uterus becomes palpable secondary to estrogenization. In patients complaining of dysmenorrhea or pelvic pain, careful evaluation of the uterine size and shape is mandatory to detect the presence of genital tract malformations. The rectovaginal septum and cul-de-sac should also be examined to detect possible endometriosis. It is not unusual to palpate plump, tender ovaries during the premenarchal period. This finding corresponds to the exaggerated follicular activity taking place in the anovulatory ovary and most often regresses after menarche. Multicystic ovaries in this age group are a frequent cause of chronic pelvic pain.

After the gynecological examination is completed, it is a nice gesture to discuss the findings in an appropriate way with the patient and her parents, either separately or together, as the situation demands. Reassurance about both the examination and her condition is always appreciated. Treatment should also be discussed at that time.

GYNECOLOGICAL PROBLEMS IN YOUNG CHILDREN

Infection and Trauma

Vulvovaginitis

The vagina undergoes constant change from birth to old age. Consequently, the types and frequency of inflammatory conditions of the vagina and vulva are different at various ages. At birth, the mucous membranes of the uterus and vagina have an adult histological appearance because of stimulation by circulating maternal estrogens. The cervical, paraurethral, and Bartholin's glands are large and secrete mucus in the immediate neonatal period. The pH is 5 to 7. Within a few weeks, however, the vaginal lining has become a thin membrane.

Throughout childhood to the immediate premenarchal period, the child is especially vulnerable to vulvovaginitis because of poor estrogenization of the vaginal epithelium and unsupervised and inadequate perineal hygiene. It is also well known that compared with older females, these youngsters lack the protection provided by pubic hair and the fatty pads of the labia majora. Contaminants and irritants thus have free access to the sensitive vulvar and vaginal epithelium.

At puberty, estrogen stimulation changes the vaginal epithelium to a thick, stratified, squamous epithelium, and the establishment of the Döderlein's bacillus causes the pH to rise to the 6 to 8 range, which helps to maintain homeostasis and decrease infection.

The symptoms of vulvovaginitis are quite variable but most often consist of vaginal discharge that varies in quantity, color, and odor, vulvar pruritus or burning, and dysuria. Whatever the etiology of the problem, the examination usually reveals edema, redness, discharge, excoriations, and scratch lesions. The presence of fecal remnants and interlabial debris confirms poor hygiene.

Physiologic Leukorrhea.—Physiologic leukorrhea occurs at both extremes of childhood. During the neonatal period, maternal estrogens stimulate the newborn's endocervical glands and vaginal epithelium. The discharge is characteristically grayish, gelatinous, and sticky. On occasion in the neonate, a small amount of blood may be present due to hormonal withdrawal. This always provides the mother with some anxious moments, but a normal examination and lack of recurrence are reassuring.

During the 6 to 12 months preceding menarche, rising endogenous estrogen secretion is responsible for the appearance of a whitish discharge not associated with irritative symptoms. After appropriate evaluation, it is of great importance to explain to these young girls that this is part of the normal process of maturation. Usually breast development is also noted at this time, and the growth spurt is active. Unjustified prescrip-

tion of vaginal cream or antibiotics serves only to make the patient believe that any vaginal discharge is pathological and eventuates in multiple unnecessary consultations.

Nonspecific Vulvovaginitis.—Nonspecific or mixed vulvovaginitis accounts for a substantial proportion of vulvovaginal infection in this age group. The etiology can most often be traced to poor local hygiene and fecal contamination. Cultures usually grow predominantly *Escherichia coli* and other anal organisms such as enterococcus.

General hygienic measures are the first step of treatment. Sitz baths in warm plain water should be given two or three times daily and followed by thorough drying of the vulvar area with a hair dryer set at the lowest speed and heat. A small amount of unscented cornstarch-based powder helps keep the vulva dry. Only mild, nonperfumed soap should be used. Bubble bath should be avoided. Adequate counseling about clothing should also be provided (i.e., white 100% cotton underpants; avoidance of tight-fitting clothes, nonabsorbent fabrics, and wet bathing suits). The importance of front-to-back wiping with soft, white, unscented toilet tissue should also be stressed.

Specific Vulvovaginitis.—A variety of causes of vulvovaginitis are recognized. The differential diagnosis, symptoms, and treatment of the various types are summarized in Table 20–1.

The character of the discharge and other clinical features vary according to the organism responsible. Thus, the key to the correct diagnosis is identification of the offending organism. The commonest cause of vulvovaginitis is allergic, but bacterial or viral infections, parasitic infestation, and traumatic vulvovaginitis also occur.

Gonorrhea.—Gonococcal infection in the prepubertal child is usually manifested as a purulent vulvovaginitis rather than a cervicitis. The infection may also be asymptomatic or be evident as a thin mucoid discharge. Thus, a Gram stain and culture are important in the evaluation of vaginal discharge in a prepubertal girl. Although the Gram stain is helpful, *Neisseria meningitidis* rarely causes vaginitis; therefore, it is essential that the diagnosis be proved by cultures.

Once a diagnosis is made, the child should be interviewed by an experienced social worker, psychologist, or pediatrician to try to elicit a his-

TABLE 20–1.

Differential Diagnosis of Specific Vulvovaginitis in Infancy and Childhood

Etiology	Clinical Signs	Nature of Discharge	Other Characteristic Findings	Treatment
Dermatitis/allergy	Red, papular, pruritic vulvar rash	No discharge	Caused by bubble bath or laundry detergent	Discontinue bubble bath; symptomatic care with steroid or antihistaminic creams
Foreign body	Bloody discharge	Purulent, bloodtinged, foul smelling	Foreign body identified on pelvic examination	Removal of foreign body
Bacterial Gonococcal	Neonate and premenarchal: Bartholin's, Skene's, and cervical glands involved	May have only scant vaginal discharge	Conjunctivitis (neonate) upper genital tract involvement and systemic symptoms, gram-negative, intracellular diplococci in either type	Penicillin, bacterial sensitivities for resistant gonococcus
	Postmenarchal: Severe vulvar edema, purulent discharge	Profuse, yellow-green discharge, intense vulvovaginitis	Upper genital tract not involved	
Staphylococcus aureus	Labial abscesses	Thick, yellow	Abscesses present in other areas	Oxacillin
Streptococcus pyogenes, β-hemolytic, group A	Systemic symptoms and vulvar pruritus and redness	Purulent, thin, yellow	Occurs in presence of scarlet fever	Penicillin
Corynebacterium vaginale (Hemophilus vaginalis)	Mild pruritus and redness, nonspecific vaginitis	Thin, colorless, foul smelling	Rare prior to puberty; after puberty, "clue" cell is diagnostic	Ampicillin
Hemophilus influenzae, type B	May be associated with *H. influenzae* infections in more typical areas	Dark yellow, purulent, foul smelling	Rare in infancy and childhood	Ampicillin
Shigella	Reddened vulva, preceded by diarrhea	Severe, purulent vulvovaginitis	*Shigella* from stool and vaginal cultures	Ampicillin
E. coli (enteropathic)	Preceded by diarrhea	Thin, watery, foul smelling, copious	Culture *E. coli* from throat, stool, vagina	Intravaginal neomycin

(Continued.)

TABLE 20–1   (cont.)

Etiology	Clinical Signs	Nature of Discharge	Other Characteristic Findings	Treatment
Fungal *Candida albicans*	Beefy red vulvovaginitis	Profuse, foul smelling, curdy	Budding yeast on wet preparation or Gram stain; search for systemic disease (diabetes) in preadolescent; rare in childhood	1%–2% gentian violet or mystatin (Mycostatin) orally or intravaginally
Viral Herpes simplex, type II	Vulvovaginitis and herpetic stomatitis perineal edema, painful vulvar eruption	Thin, water	Tender, superficial labial ulcers; enlarged, tender inguinal lymph nodes; diagnosis by rising serum antibody titer or multinucleated giant cells on vaginal cytology; may be primary or recurrent	Symptomatic with douches and instillation of idoxuridine
Parasitic Pinworm	Severe pruritus	Thin, colorless	Usually associated with enteric infestation; diagnosis by seeing worms or ova on fresh smear	Piperazine citrate, pyrvinium pamoate
Trichomonas vaginalis	Moderate pruritus	Thin, malodorous	Rare prior to puberty	Metronidazole

tory of sexual abuse or misuse. Play therapy and repeated interviews may be necessary to establish the history, since in most cases of sexual abuse, the abuser is known to the child and is often a family member. All family members and caretakers of the child should be cultured. The source of infection is frequently found to be an older male relative or stepparent. Mothers and sisters are frequently infected. Although it is possible that *Neisseria gonorrhoeae* can be transmitted by sexual play between siblings and peers, the clinician should strongly suspect sexual abuse in most cases of prepubertal gonorrhea. Since sexual abuse often involves vulvar coitus or oral sex rather than penetration, a physical examination in many abused girls shows a normal hymen. Although contacts may be easier to culture and follow-up may be significantly improved if the child is hospitalized, an outpatient approach is used for most cases. Cases of suspected child sexual abuse must be reported to the mandated state agency.

Prior to treatment, rectal and pharyngeal cultures for *N. gonorrhoeae* should be obtained from the child with vaginal gonorrhea as well as vaginal culture for *Chlamydia trachomatis* and a serology for syphilis. For children who weigh more than 45 kg, adult schedules for treating cervicitis and urethritis are used. For children who weigh less than 45 kg, recommended regimens are 125 mg of ceftriaxone intramuscularly or 50 mg of amoxicillin/kg orally plus (for children more than 2 years old) 25 mg of probenecid/kg (maximum 1.0 gm). Children allergic to penicillins or cephalosporins are treated with 40 mg of spectinomycin/

kg intramuscularly. Coinfection with *C. trachomatis* should be treated with 50 mg of erythromycin/kg/day in four divided doses or in children older than 9 years with 40 mg of tetracycline/kg/day in four divided doses for 7 days.

Follow-up cultures of the throat, rectum, and vagina should be taken 7 to 14 days after treatment. Reinfection is likely if the source is not identified and treated. Persistent vaginal discharge in a girl who has been adequately treated and had negative cultures for gonorrhea may indicate a coinfection with *C. trachomatis* that was not adequately treated with single-dose therapy. The family may have been noncompliant with the 7-day course of tetracycline or erythromycin.

Only a few cases of salpingitis secondary to *N. gonorrhoeae* have been reported in prepubertal girls, and thus no data exist on the best form of treatment. Antibiotics with similar spectrum as used in adolescent and adult pelvic inflammatory disease (PID) are appropriate: 100 mg of ceftriaxone/kg/day intravenously in a single dose plus 40 mg of erythromycin/kg/day orally in four divided doses (or tetracycline for patients more than 9 years of age).

Candida albicans.—Monilial vulvovaginitis is infrequent in children and is usually associated with recent antibiotic therapy or diabetes mellitus. The clinical picture is quite characteristic and consists at the onset of erythematous vulva with oozing granulomatous lesions that later become crusted. Satellite lesions are frequently present. The cottage cheese appearance of the vaginal discharge is well known. Diagnosis is made by microscopic visualization of mycelia on potassium hydroxide preparation of vulvar exudate or vaginal discharge or by positive culture on appropriate medium.

Treatment consists of sitz baths three times daily, followed by vulvar application of an antifungal preparation. When symptoms persist after 2 weeks, intravaginal therapy or oral administration of ketoconazole compounds are indicated.

Trichomonas.—Although the nonestrogenized vaginal epithelium of the prepubertal child is unfavorable to the growth of *Trichomonas,* this parasite is occasionally responsible for vulvovaginitis. This infection is acquired by direct contact, and the possibility of sexual abuse should be considered, although nonsexual transmission is possible.

The vaginal discharge, characteristically greenish and malodorous, is associated with nonspecific signs of irritation. Treatment consists of oral administration of 10 to 30 mg of metronidazole/kg/day (maximum 125 mg three times daily) for 7 days or 1 gm in a single dose.

Pinworms.—*Enterobius vermicularis* (pinworms), which is a frequent intestinal parasite in children, may occasionally infect the vagina, giving rise to acute inflammatory symptoms and yellow mucopurulent discharge. Diagnosis for pinworms is suggested by perianal scratching lesions and confirmed by a positive Scotch tape test result, preferably done in the morning.

The parasite is usually eradicated by a single dose of 100 mg of mebendazole (Vermox). All members of the family should also be treated. Pinworm vulvovaginitis is frequently associated with infection by other anal contaminants, which is approached as discussed above.

Condylomata Acuminata.—Warty lesions associated with human papillomavirus infection are occasionally found in infants and young children. When present, the possibility of sexual molestation should be investigated. Treatment consists of application of 85% trichloroacetic acid or bichloracetic acid, or laser ablation, depending upon the degree of severity. Visualization of the urinary tract and anal canal is mandatory in cases where recurrence is a problem. A serological test for syphilis should be done to exclude condylomata lata (secondary syphilis).

Systemic Causes.—In children, vulvovaginitis often follows an episode of infection in another part of the body, especially the upper respiratory tract. β-Hemolytic *Streptococcus, Streptococcus pneumoniae, Staphylococcus,* and *N. meningitidis* should be treated according to the sensitivity of each organism.

Systemic diseases such as measles, chicken pox, and scarlet fever may have vulvovaginal manifestations. Symptoms usually follow the natural history of the primary disease. Due to scratching and fecal contamination, secondary bacterial infection may, however, occur.

Dermatological diseases such as herpes simplex and zoster, eczema, psoriasis, molluscum contagiosum, and poison ivy may also involve the vulvar skin.

Foreign Bodies.—The presence of an intravaginal foreign body is suggested by a greenish, bloody, and foul-smelling discharge. The most frequent finding is a small piece of toilet paper or stool. Cultures grow mixed flora. Any bloody or malodorous discharge should prompt a thorough vaginal examination, even if anesthesia or analgesia is required. Rarely, the patient complains of abdominal pain because of retrograde flow of infected vaginal secretions into the fallopian tubes, causing peritonitis.

A vaginal foreign body may be a perplexing problem for the clinician, since most are not visible on external examination. Reluctance to perform a pelvic examination in a child makes the diagnosis even more difficult. However, failure to diagnose and remove a foreign body can result in severe PID, peritonitis, and, on rare occasions, migration of the foreign body to another area.

Vaginal foreign bodies are most frequently seen between the ages of 3 and 7 years. Usually there is no history of insertion, and virtually any kind of object may be found within the vagina. A forgotten tampon may be the "foreign body" in a menarchal girl.

The foreign body can sometimes be washed out by vaginal irrigation with room temperature saline using IV tubing (Fig 20–5). When the object is felt on rectal examination, gentle attempts at milking it out may be successful. In girls less than 6 years of age, general anesthesia is most of-

ten necessary. Initially, a rectal examination should be done, which frequently reveals the presence of an intravaginal foreign body. Vaginoscopy may be performed with a Killian nasal speculum in the young child. Should vaginoscopy fail to reveal the foreign body, gentle probing of the vagina frequently reveals its presence. Once the object has been removed, the vaginal discharge ceases.

Although most foreign bodies are easily removed, on occasion the object erodes into the vaginal wall. An incision in the mucosa is then necessary to remove it. If a vaginal foreign body has been present for a long period of time, vaginal stenosis may occur.

Anatomical Causes.—In some instances, a microperforate hymen, especially when the opening lies high, near the urethral meatus, may be responsible for pooling of urine in the vagina. Constant maceration of vulvovaginal tissue causes irritation and often secondary infection. In these cases, hymenotomy is curative.

The discharge from ectopic ureters can masquerade as chronic vulvovaginitis. Oftentimes, these children are erroneously believed to be incontinent or to have enuresis. Workup should consist of pelvic ultrasound, IV pyelogram (IVP), and cystoscopy. The treatment is surgical and usually requires either high ligation or excision of the anomalous collecting system or nephrectomy.

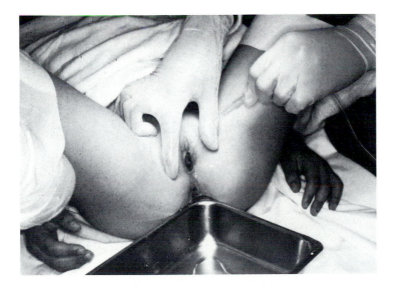

FIG 20–5.
Technique of vaginal irrigation used to wash out foreign bodies and debris. Also applicable in examining small children with perineal and labial tears to assess extent of injury.

Labial Adhesions.—Labial adhesions (synechiae vulvae), a complete or partial fusion of lower labia majora or labia minora in the midline, occur most commonly in girls 6 months to 6 years of age. The cause is unknown but may be related to low circulating estrogen levels and an irritation that erodes the vulvar epithelium, causing the labia to stick together. This concept is supported by the observations that synechia vulvae is not seen in neonates but is acquired within the first 2 years of life, when the level of circulating estrogen is extremely low, and by the fact that the use of estrogen creams causes synechiae to disappear. Occasionally, the vaginal orifice is completely covered, causing poor drainage of vaginal secretions and sequestering of urine in the vagina. Parents often become alarmed because the vagina appears "absent."

Diagnosis is made by simple observation. There is fusion of the labia minora. The hymen is not visible. The line of fusion is a thin, transparent membrane, which may involve the inner surfaces of the labia. In the most frequent form, the fusion ends several millimeters behind the clitoris but anterior to the external urethral meatus. There may be several perforations in the membrane, or the adhesions may be partial either anteriorly or posteriorly (Fig 20–6).

In mild cases, no treatment is necessary because the labia usually separate completely at puberty. If symptomatic, they should be treated.

In cases of complete synechia where vaginal or urinary drainage is impaired, or the child complains of pain, an estrogen-containing cream should be applied nightly for 3 weeks. Occasionally, a repeat course of therapy is necessary. Forceful separation without anesthesia is generally contraindicated because it is traumatic for the child and may cause the adhesions to form again. When estrogen therapy fails, separation is best performed under general anesthesia, followed by application of a bland ointment (e.g., Desitin or White's A and D) and gentle separation by the parent at regular intervals. Occasionally, separation can be accomplished in the examining room with application of 5% lidocaine gel and manipulation with a cotton swab.

Regardless of the method of treatment, 10% to 15% of synechiae recur.

Though spontaneous separation at puberty is the rule, we have seen patients in the midteens who were referred because of "hypoplastic labia." Once separation was accomplished under anesthesia, the vulva was found to be quite normal.

Vaginal Bleeding

Most girls have their first menstrual period sometime between the age of 9 and 16 years. Except for hormone withdrawal bleeding during the first or second week of life, genital bleeding before the age of 9 years is not normal and is most likely due to organic causes. Therefore, this sign should always be taken seriously and carefully assessed.

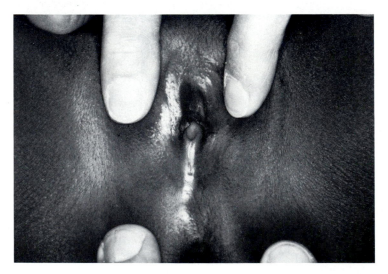

FIG 20–6.
Labial adhesions in a 4-year-old girl with only small opening at the level of urethra. Patient complained of recurrent pain and discharge due to sequestering of urine in vagina.

Classically, vaginal bleeding in childhood is divided into two types: (1) that associated with signs of isosexual precocity and (2) that not associated with signs of isosexual precocity. However, we find it more useful to classify the problem on the basis of etiological factors (Table 20–2).

Vulvovaginitis with or without the presence of a foreign body was the commonest cause of vaginal bleeding in 63 patients less than age 9 years who presented at our gynecology clinic between January 1974 and December 1983 (Table 20–3). When a young child presents with vaginal bleeding, it is mandatory to perform a thorough investigation to rule out the presence of malignancy, just as one would do in the postmenopausal age

TABLE 20–2.

Differential Diagnosis of Vaginal Bleeding in Children

Infection
  Primary
    Bacteria
    Fungal
    Parasitic
    Viral
  Secondary
    Foreign body
    Reflux of urine
    Pelvic abscess
    Fistula
Trauma
  Accidental
  Sexual
Endocrine abnormalities
  Newborn bleeding due to maternal estrogen
    withdrawal
  Isosexual precocity
  Exogenous hormone ingestion
  Hypothyroidism
Anatomical abnormalities
  Prolapse of urethral mucosa
  Vaginal and/or uterine prolapse
  Cervical ectropion
  Ectopic ureter
Idiopathic
  Vulvar dystrophy
  Vulvitis secondary to irritants
  Premature endometrial activity
  Self-induced
Neoplasms
  Benign
  Malignant
Blood dyscrasias
  Coagulopathy
  Hematologic neoplasms

TABLE 20–3.

Vaginal Bleeding in Children Less Than Age 9 Years, 1974–1983

Cause	No.	%
Infection	41	65
Trauma	10	16
Endocrine abnormalities	3	
Anatomical abnormalities	3	
Blood dyscrasias	3	19
Idiopathic	2	
Neoplasms	1	
TOTAL	63	100

group. It has been our policy to perform an anesthesia examination as part of the initial workup unless we were completely confident that full visualization of the cervix and vagina was possible during the outpatient examination. Since endometrial cancer does not occur in this age group, a dilation and curettage (D&C) is not required.

Hematological evaluation to rule out coagulation disorders should be performed preoperatively. Usually, however, patients with vaginal bleeding due to blood dyscrasias have other signs of bleeding such as epistaxis, petechiae, or hematomas.

Prolapse of the Urethra.—Occasionally, vaginal bleeding may be a sign of urethral prolapse. Examination reveals the characteristic friable red-blue (doughnut-like) annular mass (Fig 20–7). The patient may complain of dysuria, bleeding, and pain that developed after coughing or straining or, occasionally, following trauma. The diagnosis is made by the characteristic shape of the lesion and visualization of the vaginal orifice with the patient in the supine or knee-chest position. Urethral prolapse may resolve spontaneously with sitz baths, but some cases of prolapse require intervention. The CO_2 laser is ideally suited for this condition and appears to be less traumatic than cold knife excision.

Premature Menarche.—Cyclic vaginal bleeding without signs of pubertal development is rare. Although we have followed several girls with this problem, one of whom has a mother who had the same pattern of bleeding in her prepubertal years, full examination under anesthesia with endometrial biopsy is indicated to rule out endometrial pathology. Usually results of the biopsy show only early proliferative endometrium despite the

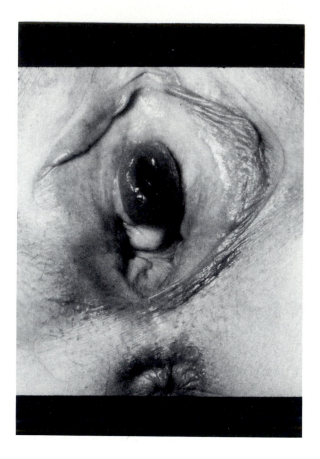

FIG 20–7.
Prolapse of urethral meatus in a 9-year-old girl who presented with bloody discharge and dysuria.

absence of sexual development. Although the etiology of precocious menarche is obscure, it probably results from the prolonged stimulation of unusually sensitive endometrium by weak extragonadal estrogens.

Lichen Sclerosus

Lichen sclerosus is an increasingly common disorder in prepubertal children. The reason for this is not certain, although the more prevalent use of synthetic fiber and clinical detergents may be unmasking latent cases in the prepubertal age group. Patients usually complain of itching, irritation, soreness, and dysuria and less commonly of constipation, vaginal discharge, and bleeding. The vulva characteristically has white, atrophic, parchment-like skin and evidence of chronic ulceration and inflammation from scratching. Often, the involvement of the perianal area along with the labia may give the affected area an hourglass con-

figuration. Secondary infection often occurs. The condition should be distinguished from vitiligo, which causes loss of pigmentation but not inflammation or atrophy.

The diagnosis of lichen sclerosus is made clinically and by examining a biopsy specimen (Fig 20–8). The treatment aims at elimination of local irritants and any vaginitis present and improved hygiene. Soaps should not be overused; the child should be encouraged to wear cotton underpants and loose-fitting pants or skirts to minimize local maceration and irritation. A short course of topical hydrocortisone ointment for a few weeks is currently used in an attempt to bring the condition under control. Oral medications such as hydroxyzine hydrochloride (Atarax) can be helpful for intense pruritus at bedtime.

The use of testosterone proprianate 2% to 5% in petrolatum gel applied one to three times daily has been advocated. We have used this med-

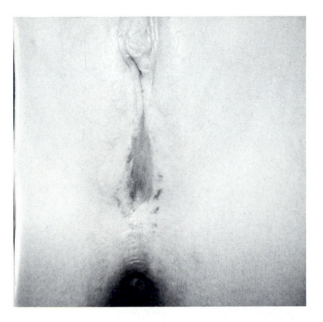

FIG 20–8.
Extensive lichen sclerosus in a prepubertal child with characteristic parchment-like skin, chronic ulceration, and inflammation.

ication and have seen an excellent response in some patients. However, the use of topical testosterone is limited by the development of clitoromegaly after 2 to 3 months of treatment.

Severe cases of lichen sclerosus, particularly when associated with extensive excoriation and debris, respond beautifully to superficial vaporization with the CO_2 laser (Fig 20–9). We have seen a number of rather dramatic results in patients who failed to respond to more conservative therapy. It may be that laser treatment interrupts the scratch-itch cycle and allows for healing. Most patients, but not all, will note improvement or regression of lesions with puberty.

Clitoral Infections

The clitoral hood may occasionally develop an infection with intense edema and erythema. Antibiotics such as dicloxicillin or cephalosporin should be given orally and warm soaks applied. Surgical incision and drainage are necessary if an abscess becomes fluctuant.

Recently a "clitoral tourniquet syndrome" in which a hair had become wrapped around the clitoris, resulting in edema and severe pain, has been described. After removal of the hair, the clitoris returned to normal size. This syndrome is similar to strangulation by hair of other parts of the body, such as fingers, toes, or penis.

Sexual Abuse: The Gynecologist's Role

Over the past 10 years we have experienced a marked increase in the number of young girls who are referred for examination because of suspected sexual abuse. Most cases of sexual abuse are dealt with most effectively by sexual abuse teams that include a pediatrician, clinical psychologist, social worker, and nurse practitioner. The gynecologist does, however, play a vital role in the assessment, documentation, and treatment of sexually induced infection and trauma.

Great care must be exercised by the physician who is asked to examine a child thought to have been sexually assaulted. Care must be taken in obtaining the history and in performing the physical examination, and appropriate specimens must be obtained for the forensic pathologist to evaluate.

The history of the assault is difficult to obtain from the very young child and must usually be obtained from relatives, police, or neighbors. These accounts are rarely accurate. A reliable history can usually be obtained directly from a child 4 to 5 years of age. However, the physician must first determine the words used by the child to de-

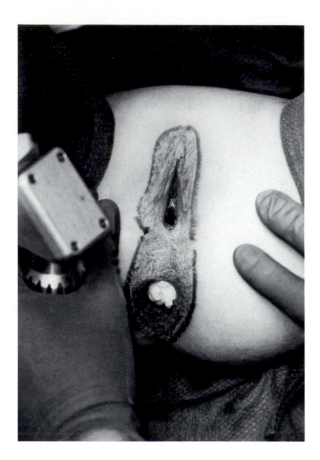

FIG 20–9.
Carbon dioxide laser debridement of extensive lichen sclerosus. The depth of the vaporization is carefully controlled to prevent scarring. Note moist pack
in anus to prevent explosion.

scribe the genitals. The information is usually
readily obtained from the child's parents.

The sex of the alleged assailant should
be determined. Rape refers to the forced act
of male penile penetration into the vagina without consent of the victim. However, penetration of the vagina can also be caused by a finger
and thus may involve either a male or female
assailant.

The assault may take the form of rape, but
just as frequently, the assault may be an excessive
form of punishment for such misbehavior as bed-
wetting or fouling of clothes. The term *pseudosex-
ual assault* should be applied here.

The examination of the victim requires
proper instrumentation, and in infants and children, general anesthesia is necessary. Table 20–4
outlines the examination of the pediatric patient
who has been sexually assaulted.

Colposcopic Evaluation of Hymen.—The
colposcope as a means of documentating sexual
trauma is becoming increasingly popular. The advantages of the colposcope are that the hymen
and vulva can be greatly magnified to detect small
changes not visible with the naked eye and that
photographs are easily taken at the time of the examination to provide future documentation. The
latter prevents the need for repeated examinations
when the presence of physical findings is disputed. The problem with the use of colposcopy
has been that until recently, normal genital anatomy in prepubertal girls has not been well defined. The problem has been compounded by the
difficulty in assessing the strength of the association between a history of sexual abuse and variations in the hymenal appearance in individual
cases, variations in the 50 states' statutory definition of sexual crimes, and misunderstanding

TABLE 20—4.

Examination of the Sexually Assaulted Child

1. Obtain consent to examination from parent or guardian, preferably written.
2. Obtain detailed general history: past illness, accidents, operations.
3. Obtain detailed specific history: details of alleged incident.
4. Observe: manner, dress.
5. Examine all clothing: remove with physician present; inspect each item separately; retain each item in clean bag; note damage to clothes, staining, soiling, ultraviolet light on underpants, etc.
6. Complete general clinical examination: examine entire body and record all findings; record all injuires, old and new, location, size, description.
7. Examine genitalia; swab vulva and vagina first without lubricant; note injury to labia, hymen, mucosa, thighs, signs of seminal fluid, blood, lubricant.
8. Obtain specimens: buccal swab; blood; saliva; hair; avulsed head hair, loose hairs, pubic hair combings; areas of soiling; fingernail scrapings, clippings; swabs from perineum; vaginal swabs from low, mid, high portions of the vagina; swabs of anal verge and anal canal.

among professionals providing examinations for victims of sexual abuse about the meaning of "penetration."

An atlas of photographs is being published by the North American Society for Pediatric and Adolescent Gynecology Task Force to aid physicians in assessing their own patients. The use of the colposcope has greatly increased the physician's knowledge of normal anatomy and fine-tuned visual skills. It is likely that knowledgeable physicians seeing a child for routine annual examination or assessing a genital problem will note changes suggestive of sexual abuse.

The value of the colposcopic examination in the determination of sexual abuse has been a subject of controversy. The percentage of children with a "normal" examination has varied from 16% to 85%, depending on the case mix and age of patients, the definition of normal vs. abnormal, and the examiners.

In a recent survey in our clinic, we compared children presenting with a history of sexual abuse with children seen for (1) routine examinations and (2) genital complaints. Girls with a history of sexual abuse were more likely to have scars, friability of the posterior forchette as the labia were separated, synechiae, and attenuated hymens than girls seen for routine examinations. Hymenal transections or tears, condylomata, and abrasions occurred among only the sexually abused girls. Girls with a history of genital complaints often had findings similar to those of girls with a history of sexual abuse. It is likely that vulvar erythema and friability of the posterior forchette may occur secondary to inflammation; scars are more likely the result of trauma. Since girls may take months to years to reveal a history of sexual abuse, it is probable that some of the girls evaluated for vaginitis may have been abused. The finding of a narrow thin posterior rim of the hymen in children with vaginitis may mean that these girls had been abused or that this particular anatomical variant may predispose a subset of girls to vaginal contamination and symptoms. In contrast, a narrow rim that has become rounded and scarred with attachment to the vagina likely has resulted from sexual abuse. The significance of a labial adhesion in a child with a history of sexual abuse is controversial because many normal children have adhesions, and yet it is possible that rubbing and irritation from abuse may also cause agglutination to occur. These adhesions have sometimes been mistaken for scars. The difference is usually evident with careful observation; if not, a short trial of estrogen-containing cream, which would lyse most labial adhesions but not scars, could be used. Another entity frequently confused with a scar in the posterior forchette is the white midline median raphe evident in some children. Conditions such as lichen sclerosus, failure of midline fusion from the anus to the posterior forchette, and ulcerating hemangioma have been confused with trauma from sexual abuse.

Children who have a history of sodomy frequently have no abnormal findings. Minor redness and hyperpigmentation and reflex anal dilatation are nonspecific findings that can have other etiologies. More specific findings include scars and distortion of the anus, although the latter can occur with inflammatory bowel disease. Fissures can result from abuse but also from constipation.

The significance of measurements of the diameter of the hymenal orifice is controversial. The transverse and anteroposterior measurements are influenced by age, relaxation of the child, method of examination and measurement, and type of hymen. The older the child and the more relaxed, the larger the opening. The opening is larger with retraction on the labia and in the knee-chest position than with gentle separation alone in the supine position. The orifice of a posterior rim hymen will appear larger than the opening of a redundant hymen. Because the hymen is distensible, vaginal penetration can have occurred even though the measurement is only 5 mm. In cases of sexual abuse, we measure both anteroposterior and transverse dimensions using a Tine test 5-cm ruler. Some colposcopes have the markings in the eyepiece, and direct measurement can be done during the examination. More data on normal children are needed, but our study of 3- to 6-year-old girls found a mean transverse measurement of 2.9 ± 1.3 mm (range 1–6 mm) and mean anteroposterior measurement of 3.3 ± 1.5 mm (range 1–7 mm). A good rule of thumb is 1 mm for each year of age as the upper limits of normal (e.g., 8 mm for an 8-year-old child), remembering all the caveats of changes with relaxation and position. The findings of a large hymenal orifice may be consistent with a history of sexual abuse but should be considered only a part of the evaluation, by no means the absolute criterion.

Repair of Sexual Trauma.—Another important role for the gynecologist in sexually abused children is the evaluation and repair of sexually induced trauma to the perineum. The extent of the genital injury depends on the nature and size of the penetrating object, the size of the pelvic outlet and vagina, and the force with which penetration is attempted. Thus, injury may run the gamut from a simple vulvar or hymeneal tear all the way to a full thickness laceration of the posterior forchette.

It is wise to postpone gynecological examination until all appropriate cultures and specimens are obtained. Photo documentation of all traumas is essential. If adequate examination is not possible in the office, clinic, or emergency room, the anesthesia examination is mandatory.

In general, the younger and smaller the child, the more widespread the injuries produced by penile penetration. The younger the child, the less able she is to resist assault.

The only form of resistance may be screaming, which may lead to attempts to silence her. The inner surfaces of the lips should be examined for abrasion or bruising from the lips being forced back against the teeth. Check for loose teeth and damage to the frenulum of the upper lip. Grasping injuries of the arms, thighs, wrists, legs, and ankles are common when the assailant is unknown to the child.

Anorectal injury must be evaluated by examination of the anal canal. Laxity of the anal sphincter and tears in the anorectum are evidence of anal penetration. Bruising and swelling of the anal verge are common findings.

Injuries to the female genitalia from assault are treated in the same manner as accidental injuries after appropriate evaluation.

Trauma to the External Genitalia

Female genital trauma is not an unusual occurrence. The injury may be localized and relatively minor or accompanied by other distant, life-threatening injuries.

The differences between the internal and external genitalia of the child and those of the adult make a perineal injury in a child potentially quite serious. The distance between the perineal skin and the peritoneal cavity is short in the young child. Thus, penetrating injuries can easily damage intraperitoneal organs. The bladder in the infant is an intraperitoneal organ and more easily injured. The urogenital diaphragm, which contains the pudendal nerves and vessels, is very superficial in infants and children, so a relatively superficial laceration can result in massive hemorrhage. Finally, the rectovaginal septum is thin, and the perineal body is small. Both can be easily torn.

Genital injuries may be accidental, self-induced, or the result of an assault. Straddle injury is responsible for 75% of genital injuries in girls. It may be blunt or penetrating. Other common causes are stabbing and automobile accidents. The commonest age of accidental genital trauma is between 4 and 12 years.

Examination of the perineum is often difficult in a bleeding, distraught child, so some sedation is advisable. The abdomen must be carefully examined for intra-abdominal injury. A urinalysis should be obtained and checked for blood. Flat abdominal radiographs that include the pelvis may show free air from a perforated viscus, or a pelvic fracture may be evident. If hematuria is present, an IVP and cystogram are indicated. No urine output may herald a urethral or bladder laceration.

Treatment.—Contusions of the perineum and vulva without laceration or bleeding are the commonest injury. They may range from a mild ecchymotic area to a large vulvar hematoma that may require surgical intervention. In general, however, we advocate a rather conservative approach in the management of these problems with application of ice packs, analgesia, and bed rest. Indwelling Foley catheter or suprapubic drainage may be required depending on the extent of the hematoma. Small lacerations of the labia and hymen usually require suturing. Bleeding can be profuse even though the laceration is small.

All lacerations require a thorough examination of the vulva and vagina. This can be accomplished by the use of saline irrigation using IV tubing (see Fig 20–5) directed toward the perineum and into the vagina. Irrigating fluid will wash out the vagina and permit injection of local anesthesia with epinephrine to decrease bleeding. An absorbable suture can then be taken on the spot. A laceration that does not extend through to the hymen usually does not invade the vagina.

More extensive lacerations always require general anesthesia for both evaluation and treatment. Thus, diagnosis and treatment often occur simultaneously. Endoscopic examination of the urethra, bladder, vagina, or rectum is indicated if injuries are nearby. Most lacerations can be closed primarily, even if extensive, unless fecal contamination is present due to rectal injury. In that event, delayed closure after appropriate antibiotic treatment and closure of the viscus is accomplished. Absorbable sutures should be used to avoid the need to remove sutures at a later date.

A particularly difficult injury occurs when the urogenital diaphragm is bluntly compressed against the pubic ramus. A tear in the periurethral structures bleeds profusely and requires a deep mattress suture. Lacerations near or into the urethra require catheterization for 7 to 10 days.

Lacerations into the vaginal fornix may require laparotomy for closure due to the small size of the child's introitus.

A laceration extending in the posterior direction from the introitus may be a sign of sexual abuse. A careful endoscopic search for rectovaginal tears must be carried out prior to closure. Laparotomy is indicated for intra-abdominal injury or for uncontrollable hemorrhage. Tetanus prophylaxis and antibiotic coverage are indicated.

The majority of properly diagnosed and treated genital injuries heal quickly. However, inadequate treatment of lacerations may result in infectious complications. Urethral and vaginal strictures may develop. An unrecognized rectovaginal tear results in a rectovaginal fistula.

Frequent examinations must be performed until complete healing has occurred. Infection, stricture formation, and delayed hemorrhage occur after adequate treatment in 11% to 25% of cases.

Congenital Malformations

A large proportion of congenital malformations of the female genital tract remain undiagnosed until adolescence, when reproductive function begins and symptoms develop. Those that are recognized in the infant and young child are external and usually noted either by a parent or the pediatrician.

Normal Female Embryology

By the ninth week of development, the embryo has both male (wolffian) and female (müllerian) genital ducts that extend from the mesonephros cranially to the cloaca caudally. A cloaca exists in the human embryo for only a brief period of time. It is divided into rectum and urogenital sinus by descent of the urorectal septum by 7 weeks. Normal female internal genitalia develop from the müllerian ductal system as the wolffian ducts regress.

The müllerian ducts develop from an invagination of the coelomic epithelium. These paired ducts are initially lateral but at the future pelvic brim turn in a medial direction to nearly touch in the midline before turning caudally to end on the posterior wall of the urogenital sinus, where the müllerian tubercle forms. Eventually the ducts fuse, forming the primitive uterovaginal canal. The first and second portions of the müllerian ducts eventually form the fimbria and the fallopian tubes, and the distal segment forms the uterus and part of the vagina.

After the müllerian tubercle is formed, two solid evaginations grow from its distal aspect. These are the sinovaginal bulbs, which are of urogenital sinus origin. Slightly proximal to the sinovaginal bulbs, growth from the müllerian ducts results in the solid vaginal plate. Growth of the plate and the bulbs changes the urogenital sinus from a long, narrow tube to a broad, flat vestibule, bringing the urethra down to the future perineum.

Canalization of the vaginal plate starts caudally and continues in a cranial direction. It is complete by the fifth month of intrauterine life. The distal-most portions of the sinovaginal bulbs coalesce to form the hymen. Shortly before birth, the central area of the hymen disintegrates, so that it is normally perforate at birth.

In summary, the uterus is of müllerian origin, as is the proximal four fifths of the vagina. The distal fifth of the vagina arises from the urogenital sinus. The vaginal epithelium arises from the urogenital sinus.

Introital Masses

The commonest abnormality seen in the neonate and young child is a cystic mass at the introitus. It is first observed in the delivery room by the obstetrician, during the neonatal examination by the pediatrician, or by the parent when changing diapers. The mass usually enlarges during crying spells. It is usually cystic, containing either clear or milky mucoid material. The differential diagnosis includes ectopic ureter, hymenal cyst, hymenal skin tag, periurethral cyst, vaginal cyst, or imperforate hymen with hydrocolpos.

The child should be examined in the frog-leg position, ideally with magnification, using a moistened Q-tip for retraction. The pull-down maneuver opens the introitus so that the origin of the cyst can be ascertained (see Fig 20–2).

Ectopic Ureter.—If the cyst appears to rise from the periurethral area or anterior vagina, ectopic ureter should be suspected and pelvic and renal ultrasound scans obtained. If this diagnosis is confirmed, consultation with a pediatric urologist is required. Usually, an IVP is obtained to determine the extent of the anomalous collecting system. High ligation of the ectopic ureter or partial nephrectomy is usually required.

Hymenal, Periurethral, and Vaginal Cysts.—Cysts arising from the hymen or periurethral area are usually of the epidermal inclusion variety. Spontaneous resolution is common. If regression does not occur within 3 months, simple marsupialization or electrofulguration is warranted. Before proceeding with surgery, however, one should perform urethroscopy to rule out the presence of a diverticulum of the distal urethra, which would require management by a urologist.

In the newborn period, vaginal cysts can be located posterior to the urethral meatus at the vaginal introitus, arising from the anterior or lateral wall of the vagina, and lined by squamous epithelium. Usually they do not cause pathological manifestations and can rupture spontaneously, or they disappear after surgical aspiration and removal of a milky white fluid. Occasionally, the cysts grow large enough to obstruct the urethra, causing urinary retention. Operative removal is indicated in such cases. Cysts in the caudal portion of the vagina probably are derived from the epithelium of the urogenital sinus and formed during the last months of gestation. In younger fetuses, multiple cysts can occur in proximal parts of the vagina. They have been considered derivatives of epithelia of the müllerian or wolffian ducts.

Imperforate Hymen and Hydrocolpos.— When the cystic structure appears to obstruct the vaginal opening and no perforation can be identified, an imperforate hymen with hydrocolpos is the most likely diagnosis. Hydrocolpos is due to distention of the vagina with retained secretions. The uterus is rarely involved because of the ability of the vagina to distend. The usual presenting symptoms of a massive hydrocolpos in the neonate are a midline lower abdominal mass, urinary retention due to bladder angulation, and, on occasion, respiratory distress. Bilateral hydroureter and hydronephrosis may be detected on an antenatal ultrasound examination. Compression of the ureters at the pelvic brim may also be present.

Respiratory distress may result from pressure on the diaphragm. Lower extremity edema may be caused by compression of the major abdominal veins. We have seen one patient in whom retrograde flow of secretion through the fallopian tubes caused intraperitoneal adhesions and partial bowel obstruction.

The treatment of hydrocolpos depends on its etiology. When hydrocolpos is diagnosed, surgery is indicated to avoid late complications of further fluid accumulation and reflux. Usually simple hymenectomy in the nursery using a Beaver blade is adequate when the hydrocolpos is small. No bleeding occurs, and sutures are not required. In the older child, hymenotomy and drainage of the fluid should be managed in the ambulatory operating room under general anesthesia.

We have encountered three patients who presented with a unilateral cystic mass. When drainage was carried out, a vaginal septum with unilateral obstruction and hydrocolpos was diagnosed. This müllerian abnormality usually is associated with duplication of the cervix and uterus (didelphys), which can be either partial or complete. Since this anomaly is frequently associated with urological malformations, investigation of the ureters and kidneys should be undertaken. The same problem is not encountered with simple imperforate hymen.

Other Hymenal Abnormalities.—Hymenal tags can be present at birth and appear as a fleshy mass protruding from the introitus. They frequently regress when the effects of maternal estrogen have diminished. If they are still present at 3 months, they can be removed by electrocautery or cold knife excision, because if large enough, they become inflamed and cause vaginal bleeding and discharge.

Inadequate perforation of the hymen, such as septation, microperforation, or cribriform fenestration, is generally asymptomatic in the young child and does not require intervention until puberty when it causes problems with tampon use and coitus. However, it should be operated on when it appears to be the cause of recurrent vulvovaginitis and urinary tract infections (UTIs) due to stagnation of urine within the partially obstructed vagina. Since most patients with this problem present between the ages of 3 and 6 years, either hymenectomy or hymenotomy and suturing the cut edges with absorbable sutures are satisfactory methods of treatment.

Perineal Fissures

Newborns may present with a deep fissure of the median raphe. This open area fails to heal spontaneously and remains open, granulating, with purulent drainage due to fecal soiling. The etiology is uncertain, although a perineorectal fistula must be ruled out. Initial treatment is conservative with topical antibiotic ointment, such as silver sulfadiazine (Silvadene Cream 1%), protective bland ointments, and silver nitrate applications. If healing does not occur in 2 to 3 months, laser vaporization or excision with primary closure is indicated.

Inguinal Ovary

Inguinal hernias in female infants are generally uncommon, with a male/female ratio of about 6:1. When a 1.5-cm firm mass is palpated in the groin or vulva, it usually indicates that the hernia is of the sliding type, where a portion of the wall of the sac is composed of a tube and ovary. It frequently cannot be reduced, but rarely is the blood supply compromised.

Rarely, a girl with a palpable gonad in the labia is actually a male with testicular feminization syndrome. This represents less than 1% of hernias in females. These patients can also be identified by the findings of a 46 XY karyotype and the operative findings of testicles. Early identification of these individuals is desirable, although there can be no gender changes made because the genitalia are female.

Cloacal Anomalies

A cloaca is a common channel into which the products of the gastrointestinal, urinary, and genital tracts empty. The pathogenesis of faulty cloacal division is unknown, but it could result from an arrest in the descent of the urorectal septum, preventing division of the cloaca into the rectum and urogenital sinus. It also stops approximation and fusion of the müllerian ducts, resulting in failure in the formation of the müllerian tubercle and a duplication of the uterus and proximal vagina. The sinovaginal bulbs do not form, and the vaginal plate does not enlarge. The urogenital sinus remains in its primitive state—a long, narrow tube—and the urethra empties into the urogenital sinus, high on its anterior wall. The hymen is absent.

A cloacal anomaly involves three major organ systems, with complete or partial obstruction of the urinary, genital, or gastrointestinal (GI) tracts. In the absence of other lethal anomalies, urinary tract sepsis due to obstruction accounts for the majority of deaths. The five major types of cloacal dysgenesis are as follows:

1. Type A has a single perineal orifice located between the labia minora. This orifice leads to a long, narrow tube, the cloaca, at the apex of which is an obstructed vagina. The urethral meatus enters the cloaca high on its anterior wall directly across from the posterior rectal fistula.
2. Type B is similar to type A, but the rectal fistula enters the vagina.
3. Type C has a short, broad cloaca.
4. Type D is similar to type A, but a distal vaginal atresia is present.

5. Type E has a high type of imperforate anus but no rectocloacal fistula.

Other major system anomalies are common, particularly in the cardiovascular, genitourinary, GI, central nervous, and respiratory systems. The commonest anomalies are those of müllerian origin: septate vagina, duplication of the uterus, and bicornuate uterus.

The pathognomonic physical finding in cloacal dysgenesis is a single perineal orifice between the labia minora. This opening is the entrance to the cloaca. If the hymen is present, cloacal dysgenesis is not. The urethral meatus and anus are not evident. Hydrometrocolpos is often present as an abdominal mass. Reconstruction is complex and best performed by a pediatric surgeon.

Ambiguous Genitalia in the Newborn

Although most clinicians will rarely see an infant with ambiguous genitalia at birth, the need to assess the situation as quickly as possible makes this subject essential for inclusion in this chapter. Any deviation from the normal appearance of male or female genitalia should prompt investigation, since apparent, but incomplete, male or female external genitals may be associated with the gonads and genotype of the opposite sex (e.g., the male with feminizing testicular syndrome and the markedly virilized female with congenital adrenal hyperplasia [CAH]). Even a slight doubt that arises in the initial newborn examination should be pursued systematically to prevent the possibility of later confusion. Bilateral cryptorchidism, unilateral cryptorchidism with incomplete scrotal fusion or hypospadias, labial fusion, or clitoromegaly require evaluation.

Determining Sex Assignment.—When the physician finds that an infant has ambiguous genitalia, the parents should be reassured that they have a healthy infant, but that because the external genital development is incomplete, tests are necessary to determine the sex. A straightforward explanation of the factors necessary for normal sexual development in utero may be helpful. Clearly, most parents will react with dismay and anxiety; they should be reassured that tests will show the cause of the problem and whether their baby is a girl or a boy. The possibility of an intersex disorder (hermaphroditism) should not be raised at this time. Speculation about possible sex assignment should be kept to a minimum. Within

a few days, or at most 1 to 2 weeks, a definite answer will be possible. The physician should examine the baby in the presence of the parents and explain the common genital anlage for boys and girls. The concept of an "underdeveloped" boy or "overdeveloped" girl helps parents accept their baby's condition.

Although a diagnosis of the patient's condition requires knowledge of the genotype, assignment of sex is based on other criteria as well. The first issue is fertility. The girl with CAH may be virilized at birth, yet with normal ovaries and uterus, she is potentially capable of bearing children. Thus, management, including surgery, must aim at female gender identity. When fertility is not possible, as with mixed gonadal dysgenesis (MGD) or male pseudohermaphroditism, decisions are based on surgical requirements for reconstruction of the external genitals. In general, surgical techniques are more suited to clitoral recession and, later, the creation of a vagina, than to the construction of a normal male phallus. Once the decision as to sex assignment is made, the physician should help the parents accept their infant as a normal boy or a normal girl. As long as attitudes toward the child's sex remain unequivocal, the child usually assumes his or her gender role without difficulty, regardless of the genotype.

The XX Newborn With Ambiguous Genitalia.—The differential diagnosis of XX patients with ambiguous genitalia includes (1) CAH; (2) female pseudohermaphroditism that is (a) due to drugs, (b) due to maternal CAH or a virilizing tumor, or (c) idiopathic; and (3) true hermaphroditism.

Congenital Adrenal Hyperplasia.—Congenital adrenal hyperplasia represents the commonest cause of ambiguous genitalia in the XX newborn. Because of the variability in enzymatic block, ambiguity may range from labial fusion with or without slight clitoromegaly to a "male phallus" with labial fusion and rugae on the labioscrotal folds. The enzyme most commonly involved is 21-hydroxylase. Because of inadequate cortisol synthesis, ACTH increases, with resultant increased adrenal androgen production. Salt losing is seen in about one half of patients with the 21-hydroxylase deficiency because of the severity of the deficiency with decreased aldosterone antagonists. Infants with more severe virilization tend to be salt losers. A deficiency of 11β-hydroxysteroid is usually associated with hypertension and moderately increased urinary excretion of pregnanetriol and the metabolites for 11-deoxycortisol and deoxycorticosterone (tetrahydro-S and tetrahydro-DOC). A rare form of CAH, 3β-hydroxysteroid dehydrogenase deficiency, results in severe adrenal insufficiency and increased ACTH levels; however, virilization is quite mild because the block is in the initial steps of hormone synthesis so that only the weak androgen (dehydroepiandrosterone) can be produced in excess.

The diagnosis of CAH should be made as soon as possible after birth because of the need to prevent dehydration, hyponatremia, and hyperkalemia with glucocorticoid and mineralocorticoid replacement.

It should be emphasized that XX persons with CAH are girls and are potentially fertile. Thus, regardless of the appearance of the external genitalia, the sex assignment should be female. Surgery may be undertaken later for (1) recession of the clitoris, (2) division of the labioscrotal folds, and (3) creation of an adequate vagina. Because the buried clitoris can respond with painful erections to high levels of androgens (which may occur with noncompliance during adolescence), recession is usually accompanied by partial corporectomy and preservation of the neurovascular bundle with reanastomosis of the glans. This procedure, along with a vaginoplasty in infants whose vagina enters distal to the external urethral sphincter, is usually carried out in the first 6 months of life. In patients with high entry of the vagina into the urethra, vaginoplasty is delayed until 2 years of age. A second vaginoplasty or the use of dilators may be needed during adolescence, the age determined by dialogue with the patient on her readiness to undertake operative and postoperative care. In cases in which surgical construction is necessary, postoperative use of dilators is usually necessary to keep the vagina patent until the patient has regular sexual relations.

Other Diagnoses of XX Neonates.—If an infant is XX and has no evidence of CAH, she either has a primary gonadal abnormality or has been exposed to exogenous hormones or a virilizing lesion in the mother. If the drug history is negative, the mother should have a careful physical examination and measurement of urinary and serum androgens. In the absence of a history of maternal virilization or hormone ingestion, the infant should have an evaluation of internal genital anatomy to determine the gonadal cause of the ambiguous genitalia: true hermaphroditism or idiopathic female pseudohermaphroditism.

The XY Newborn With Ambiguous Genitalia.—The differential diagnosis of the infant who is XY includes (1) male pseudohermaphroditism due to (a) defects of testicular differentiation, (b) deficient placental luteinizing hormone (LH) level (c) Leydig cell agenesis, (d) defects in testosterone synthesis, (e) 5α-reductase deficiency, and (f) receptor defects; and (2) hypogonadotrophic hypogonadism (Kallmann's syndrome).

Increased understanding of the differentiation of the fetal testis and the many steps involved in the development of the normal male has made it possible to diagnose more specifically the kind of syndrome seen in XY girls. The Y chromosome contains a testis-determining factor (TDF). If TDF is not present in spite of an XY karyotype, or if the receptors for the gene products are absent, the infant has a female phenotype.

The syndrome would be diagnosed during adolescence as pure gonadal dysgenesis or Swyer's syndrome (streak gonads, normal stature). If the first step occurs normally but the human chorionic gonadotropin (hCG) level is deficient because of a postulated placental insufficiency or inadequate LH level, stimulation of testosterone secretion would be insufficient for complete masculinization. If the testis is unresponsive to hCG or lacks normal Leydig cells (Leydig cell agenesis), the infant has abdominal testes, an elevated LH level, a female phenotype with short vagina, and absent uterus. Depending on when during fetal life the testicular regression occurred, patients will have phenotypes ranging from normal females to males with cryptorchidism.

A number of defects in testosterone synthesis have been described. They include deficiencies of 20,22-desmolase; 3β-hydroxy-Δ^5-steroid dehydrogenase; 17α-hydroxylase; 17,20-desmolase, and 17β-hydroxysteroid. The first three defects are also associated with adrenal insufficiency. Patients who have these deficiencies do not have müllerian structures, but the external genitalia are either female or ambiguous.

Failure to produce müllerian-inhibiting factor (MIF) or the lack of MIF receptors will cause persistence of müllerian structures and the presence of a uterus (hernia uteri inguinale) in a male who has unilateral or bilateral cryptorchidism.

The development of the wolffian ducts varies among individuals; males are fertile.

The enzyme 5α-reductase is responsible for the conversion of testosterone to dihydrotestosterone, which results in male differentiation of the external genitalia. Patients with 5α-reductase deficiency (so-called pseudovaginal perineoscrotal hypospadias), an autosomal recessive condition, have a cleft scrotum (hypospadias) and perineal invagination.

Ambiguous genitalia may also be caused by defects in receptor proteins or transcription mechanisms. Complete resistance to the action of testosterone results in the classic picture of testicular feminization; the infant appears as a phenotypic female, although occasionally testes are noted early in life. Partial androgen insensitivity results in a spectrum of ambiguous genitalia syndromes at birth and during adolescence; these include the Gilbert-Dreyfus, Reifenstein, Rosewater, and Lubs syndromes. These patients have partial wolffian development, some pubic hair, and partial labioscrotal fusion. Recent research in androgen insensitivity has delineated a number of different syndromes, some with absence of receptors, some with abnormal receptor structure, and some with presumed postreceptor defects. Errors in testosterone biosynthesis may give a similar phenotype. The pattern of X-linked inheritance coupled with a high LH and testosterone level (especially before and after hCG stimulation) suggests androgen insensitivity.

Cytogenetic studies may be helpful in distinguishing between patients who have structural defects or dysgenetic testes and those who have structurally normal testes. Many patients in the former group have abnormal sex chromosomes with mosaicism; the patients in the latter group have an XY karyotype. Biochemical studies can pinpoint a diagnosis. Retrograde contrast x-ray film studies, ultrasonography, magnetic resonance imaging, and possibly laparoscopy or laparotomy are necessary to establish the final diagnosis and determine the particular chromatin-negative syndrome present.

Choice of gender identity thus depends on the external genitalia and the possibility of future coital adequacy. When the sex assignment is definitively made, the gonads that conflict with the assignment should be electively removed. For example, the patient with MGD and XO/XY who is given a female sex assignment should have her testis removed to prevent virilization at puberty.

Intra-abdominal testes should be removed prophylactically in patients with male pseudohermaphroditism and MGD since there is a substantial risk of malignancy. In addition, it should be noted that all patients with genital abnormalities should have a careful search for associated anomalies, especially of the urinary tract.

Endocrine-Related Disorders

A thorough understanding of the normal progression of puberty is essential in the evaluation of patients with precocious puberty, premature thelarche, and premature adrenarche. It should be recalled that in normal adolescence, estrogen is responsible for breast development, maturation of the external genitalia, vagina, and uterus, and initiation of menses. An increase in adrenal androgens is associated with the appearance of pubic and axillary hair. Excess androgens of either ovarian or adrenal origin may cause acne, hirsutism, voice changes, increased muscle mass, and clitoromegaly. Thus, precocious puberty in girls can be divided into two categories: (1) isosexual precocity, in which the patient has normal pubertal development, including menses; and (2) heterosexual precocity, in which the patient has evidence of virilization with or without changes characteristic of a normal puberty.

Premature Thelarche

Premature thelarche is most commonly seen among young girls 1 to 4 years of age. Occasionally, neonatal breast hypertrophy fails to regress within 6 months after birth. This persistent breast development is also characterized as premature thelarche. The typical child with premature thelarche has bilateral breast buds of 2 to 4 cm with little or no change in the nipple or areola. The breast tissue feels granular and may be slightly tender. In some cases, development is quite asymmetric; one side may develop 6 to 12 months before the other. Growth is not accelerated, and the bone age is normal for height age. No other evidence of puberty appears; the labia remain prepubertal without obvious evidence of estrogen effect.

Although it was originally thought that premature thelarche was caused by an increased end-organ sensitivity to low levels of endogenous estrogen, the fact that there are at least transiently elevated serum estrogen levels suggests that small luteinized or cystic graafian follicles may be responsible in some cases. The usual clinical course of regression, or at least lack of progression, of breast development would then correlate with the waning of the estrogen levels as the follicles become atretic.

Treatment consists mainly of reassurance and careful follow-up to confirm that the breast development does not represent the first signs of precocious puberty.

Premature Adrenarche

Most patients with premature adrenarche have a slight increase in urinary 17-ketosteroid production and increased plasma dehydroepiandrosterone (DHEA) and dehydroepiandrosterone sulfate (DHEAS) levels, suggesting that hormone biosynthesis in the adrenal gland undergoes maturation prematurely to a pubertal pattern. Although production of these androgens is suppressible by dexamethasone and therefore dependent on ACTH, the mediator for the change at puberty and in premature adrenarche is unknown.

The assessment of the patient with premature adrenarche is similar to that for heterosexual precocious puberty. The important findings are the presence of pubic hair and the absence of breast development, estrogenization of the labia and vagina, and virilization.

The laboratory tests that should be obtained include an x-ray film of the wrist for bone age, vaginal smear, a 24-hour urine test for 17-ketosteroids and 17-hydroxysteroids, and serum DHEAS, estradiol, testosterone, and 17-hydroxyprogesterone. The differential diagnosis must exclude early precocious puberty, congenital adrenal hyperplasia, and an adrenal or ovarian tumor.

Treatment of premature adrenarche is reassurance and follow-up. The child should be examined every 6 months to confirm the original diagnostic impression. In general, pubertal development at adolescence can be expected to be normal.

Precocious Puberty

Puberty is considered precocious if secondary sexual characteristics occur prior to 8 years of age. This occurs in the general population in an incidence between 1 per 5,000 to 1 per 10,000. The female/male ratio is between 4:1 and 8:1. This is usually accomplished by accelerated linear growth (advanced bone age). Precocity may be due to constitutional or organic causes. The majority of cases of isosexual precocious puberty are of a constitutional or idiopathic form (85% of females), and it may be familial. It is, however, vital to distinguish these patients from those who have precocity based on lesions of the brain, ovary, or adrenal glands. Therefore, sexual precocity may be due to central or CNS causes (includes constitutional) or extrapituitary causes (ovarian tumors, adrenal tumors).

Isosexual Precocious Puberty.—In true isosexual precocity, the stimulus for development arises in the hypothalamus and pituitary gland. In response to rising LH and follicle-stimulating hormone (FSH) levels, the ovaries produce estrogen. The young girl develops breasts and pubic and axillary hair and begins menstruation, sometimes not in the usual sequence. With the establishment of the cyclic midcycle LH peak, the child becomes potentially fertile.

In isosexual pseudoprecocity, an ovarian tumor or cyst or adrenal adenoma produces estrogen autonomously. The fluctuating estrogen levels result in sexual development and anovulatory menses.

In more than 80% of patients with isosexual precocious puberty, the hypothalamic-pituitary axis is activated prematurely for unknown reasons. Interestingly, approximately 80% of patients with idiopathic precocious puberty have abnormal encephalograms, suggesting that a neuroendocrine dysfunction may contribute to precocious puberty.

Despite the relatively high incidence of constitutional or idiopathic precocious puberty, this diagnosis cannot be made without a thorough evaluation and exclusion of some of the following organic causes:

1. Cerebral disorders (5%–10% of cases)
2. Ovarian tumors (5% of cases)
3. Adrenal disorders (rare)
4. Gonadotropin-producing tumors (rare)
5. Hypothyroidism (rare)
6. Iatrogenic disorders (rare)

Patient assessment by the gynecologist prior to referral to the endocrinologist should include a careful history and physical examination as well as a family history. As previously noted, it is important to perform appropriate studies to rule out cerebral disorders and ovarian tumors, which are the two commonest organic causes of this condition.

The first crucial steps in an initial evaluation of precocious puberty are careful history taking (rule out exogenous steroid administration, history of encephalitis, and cerebral trauma) and meticulous physical examination. Blood pressure, accelerated development of thelarche, pubarche, gonadarche, and growth spurt are noted. Skin changes and any café au lait spots are documented. Pelvic and abdominal examination may indicate the presence of an ovarian or adrenal mass, which is further confirmed by ultrasound scanning. Bone x-ray films document accelerated linear growth and epiphyseal closure (and also exclude fibrous dysplasia). A skull x-ray film or computed tomography (CT) scan rules out intracranial pathologic lesions. Chemical precocity is indicated by adolescent levels of FSH, LH, and estradiol-17β. Thyroid function tests exclude hypothyroidism. Elevated urinary 17-ketosteroid excretion points to either possible late-onset CAH or an adrenal neoplasm (especially if documented by scan). In the latter condition, suppression does not occur with a dexamethasone suppression test, whereas suppression does occur in CAH. Increased urinary hCG level may indicate a rare trophoblastic tumor. Exogenous LH and releasing hormone (RH) administration can be used to discriminate between extrapituitary causes of precocity (ovarian tumors) and central causes. The latter will have a pubertal LH response after such stimulation, whereas the former will not. Finally, if the use of exogenous steroids, CNS disease, hypothyroidism, late-onset CAH, McCune-Albright syndrome, and adrenal or ovarian masses are excluded, idiopathic isosexual precocious puberty is the most likely diagnosis.

Treatment and follow-up depend on the diagnosis. Naturally, ovarian tumors and CNS tumors require surgical intervention. Idiopathic and CNS induced precocity can now be treated with LH-RH therapy, which is very effective.

Despite the diagnosis of idiopathic precocious puberty, follow-up must continue at least every 6 months to exclude the possibility of organic disease not originally evident. It should be remembered that children with sexual precocity do not automatically manifest intellectual or psychosocial precocity. In fact, the degree of psychological maturity of a young girl is more likely to be related to the life experiences she encounters and transacts.

Heterosexual Precocious Puberty.—Heterosexual precocity arises from excess androgen production from an adrenal or ovarian source, which results in acne, hirsutism, and virilization. The differential diagnosis includes (1) CAH; (2) Cushing's syndrome; (3) adrenal tumors; (4) ovarian tumors, such as arrhenoblastomas, lipoid cell, and Sertoli cell tumors; and (5) rarely, familial precocious puberty with isolated elevation of LH level.

As is true with isosexual precocity, patients should undergo careful history and physical examination. Laboratory tests should include determination of serum FSH, LH, estradiol, DHEA, DHEAS, testosterone, and androstenedione values. A 24-hour urine collection should be assayed for 17-ketosteroids, 17-hydroxycorticosteroids, and pregnanetriol values.

The treatment and follow-up of heterosexual precocious puberty is based on the diagnosis. Ovarian and adrenal tumors should be surgically excised, if possible. Patients with CAH should receive glucocorticoid replacement. Follow-up should include careful monitoring of urinary 17-ketosteroid levels, serum 17-hydroxyprogesterone levels, and growth every 3 months or so. If the bone age is not too advanced, breast development may regress with treatment of patients with CAH.

Tumors

Benign Tumors

Labial Masses.—Gynecological tumors are rare in childhood. They are usually benign and localized to the external genitalia. We have encountered a few patients with fibromas, lipomas, and myomas that should be surgically excised, generally on an outpatient basis.

Congenital Ovarian Cysts.—With the more widespread use of sonography in the third trimester, a number of newborn infants have been referred to our clinic for management of cystic masses in the pelvis. These are characteristically single, fluid-filled structures without septation or solid components. Most of these are functional cysts that usually resolve spontaneously within 2 to 3 months. They are generally palpable on rectal examination. If they are large and persistent, they may become palpable abdominally. Laparotomy may be indicated, although we have had success with aspiration under ultrasound guidance in one patient. Caution should be exercised in transabdominal or transvaginal aspiration because a cystic structure in the pelvis may be due to cysts of other organ systems, such as the urinary tract, mesentery, and paratubal or paraovarian structures.

Malignant Tumors

Sarcoma Botryoides.—The malignant tumor that involves the vagina, uterus, bladder, and urethra of young children most frequently is sarcoma botryoides. The symptoms include vaginal discharge, bleeding, abdominal pain or mass, or the passage of grapelike lesions. On examination, the tumors appear as prolapse of grapelike masses through the urethra or vagina. If a vaginal tag is seen on vaginal examination, it should never be assumed to be benign. Growth of the tumor is rapid and prognosis poor unless the diagnosis is made early and prompt radical surgical excision is performed. Whether there is additional treatment with radiotherapy and chemotherapy, or both, depends on the extent of disease.

GYNECOLOGICAL PROBLEMS IN THE ADOLESCENT

Infection and Trauma

Most gynecological infections in the adolescent are evaluated and treated in a manner similar to the adult patient, as discussed in Chapter 19. However, certain aspects of this problem are unique to the adolescent and are, therefore, included in this chapter as well.

Vulvovaginitis

In the adolescent, vaginitis represents a common gynecological problem despite the fact that the adolescent has developed a more resistant, estrogenized vaginal epithelium, pubic hair, and labial fat pads. The striking difference between prepubertal and adolescent vaginitis is the shift in etiology. Vulvovaginitis in the prepubertal child is often nonspecific and results from poor perineal hygiene, whereas vaginitis in the adolescent usually has a specific etiology, often related to sexual contact. A complaint of vaginal discharge may also be the presenting symptom of the adolescent with cervicitis secondary to *N. gonorrhoeae, C. trachomatis,* or herpes simplex. In addition to these true infections, physiological leukorrhea, a normal desquamation of epithelial cells secondary to estrogen effect, is probably the commonest cause of discharge in the pubescent girl.

The evaluation of vaginal discharge in the adolescent should include a history of symptoms (pruritus, odor, quantity), other illnesses (e.g., diabetes), recent medications (e.g., broad-spectrum antibiotics and birth control pills), and in utero exposure to DES. A history of broad-spectrum antibiotics or poorly controlled diabetes mellitus is frequently a clue to the diagnosis of *Candida* vaginitis. The patient should be questioned about recent sexual relations since treatment failure in an adolescent girl often occurs because of reexposure to an untreated contact. It should be remembered that several infections may coexist; a patient may be adequately treated for one infection and still have a second or third infection. For example, an adolescent may have *C. trachomatis* cervicitis, *Trichomonas* vaginitis, and vulvar condylomata. In addition, the use of oral broad-spectrum antibiotics for the treatment of the vaginitis may be followed by a second infection with *Candida*. Frequently in the evaluation of vaginitis, the patient is found to be in need of birth control as well. Although close family contact has been blamed for the spread of some infections, the clinician should assume that most, if not all, cases of *Trichomonas,* condyloma, and genital herpes in adolescents are sexually acquired either through consenting sexual relationships or through sexual abuse.

An adolescent may have symptoms for weeks or months before seeking medical help because of anxiety about a pelvic examination or because of guilt or trauma from a previous episode of rape, intercourse, touching, or sexual abuse. Therefore, it is important to explain carefully to the adolescent both the details of the pelvic examination and the possible causes of discharge.

Assessment of the adolescent usually includes a speculum examination to obtain specimens of the vaginal discharge for wet preparations, pH, and, in sexually active patients, endocervical cultures for *N. gonorrhoeae* and *C. trachomatis.*

A speculum examination may be omitted in the virginal adolescent 12 to 13 years old with a history of a whitish mucoid discharge, since samples for wet preparations obtained with a saline-moistened, cotton-tipped applicator or Calgiswab gently inserted through the hymenal ring are sufficient to confirm the diagnosis of leukorrhea. In the older adolescent with persistent discharge, a speculum examination should be done to assess the appearance of the cervix, since patients with cervicitis may complain of vaginal discharge.

Insertion of a speculum appropriate to the size of the hymenal ring should be preceded by a gentle one-finger digital examination of the vagina. A Huffman speculum can be used for most virginal adolescents. The slightly larger Pedersen speculum allows better visualization of the cervix in the virginal adolescent who has a wider hymenal opening and in the sexually active adolescent.

If a large ectropion is associated with any abnormality of the shape of the cervix or the presence of glandular cells extending into the anterior vaginal wall (adenosis), in utero exposure to DES should be strongly suspected in girls born before 1974.

Although not generally used for routine diagnosis of cervical and vaginal infections, the colposcope may also be helpful in making the diagnosis. In a study of patients with sexually transmitted disease, we found that endocervical mucopus was associated with *N. gonorrhoeae, C. trachomatis,* and herpes simplex; ulcers and necrotic areas and increased surface vascularity with herpes simplex; strawberry cervix (uniformly arranged red spots or stippling of a few millimeters, located on the squamous epithelium covering the ectocervix) with *Trichomonas;* hypertrophic cervicitis with *C. trachomatis;* and immature metaplasia with *C. trachomatis* and cytomegalovirus.

Vulvar Ulcers and Nevi

The diagnosis of vulvar ulcers is sometimes difficult. The commonest causes of ulcers in adolescents are herpes and syphilis. Syphilis is characterized by a nonpainful hard ulcer and a positive rapid plasma reagin (RPR) test by the seventh day of the ulcer. Genital herpes is characterized by painful, usually multiple, shallow ulcers that are positive on Tzanck preparation and culture. Inguinal lymph nodes are usually enlarged and tender. Rarely, Epstein-Barr virus infection with painful genital ulcers may occur with primary mononucleosis.

In the last 5 years, chancroid has reemerged as a potential etiology of genital ulcers. In 1986, 4,318 cases were reported by the CDC, the largest number since 1952. The disease typically presents as multiple purulent ulcers, often with ragged edges, and tender unilateral or bilateral inguinal adenopathy.

Diagnosis is made by excluding the diagnosis of genital herpes or syphilis. Culture of *H. ducreyi* is the only sure means of diagnosis, but special media and conditions are necessary, and thus detection from direct smears of the base of the genital lesion is the method used by most clinicians. The specimen is obtained from the ulcer base, which may involve peeling off the crust or wiping

away excess pus (but not extensive cleaning). The cotton swab is used to touch first the base and then the edges of the ulcer. The swab is then rolled onto a slide in a circle about the size of a dime, the slide is allowed to air dry and is Gram stained. The use of indirect immunofluorescence of ulcer smears using a monoclonal antibody directed against *H. ducreyi* and a dot-immunobinding serological test offer promise but require more studies to determine sensitivity and specificity. Thus, patients with ulcers without a history of blisters who do not have herpes or syphilis and have significant painful inguinal adenopathy should be suspected of having chancroid and treated with one of the following: 500 mg of erythromycin base orally four times daily for 7 days, with two tablets of trimethoprim-sulfamethoxazole (TMP-SMX) twice daily for 10 days (less reliable because of emerging resistance), 500 mg of amoxicillin with 125 mg of clavulanic acid three times daily for 7 days, or 250 mg of ceftriaxone intramuscularly. A clinical response should be evident within several days; patients should be seen in 7 days to make sure that ulcer healing is occurring and that adenopathy is less painful. Nodes may progress to fluctuation in spite of adequate medical therapy and require needle aspiration. If a response to therapy has not occurred by day 7, the diagnosis may be different (e.g., herpes and chancroid), the patient may be noncompliant with medication, or the organisms may be resistant to the antibiotic chosen. Sexual contacts should be examined and treated. Genital ulcers are of particular worry in the 1980s and 1990s because of the association of genital ulcers with acquired human immunodeficiency virus (HIV) infection.

Lymphogranuloma venereum (LGV) is caused by three serotypes (L-1, L-2, and L-3) of *C. trachomatis;* it is rare and commoner in men than women. The ulcer in LGV is the late sequela (enlarged inguinal nodes and rectal strictures). An LGV titer is used to make the diagnosis.

The diagnosis of carcinoma, pemphigus, or granuloma inguinale generally requires the taking of a biopsy specimen. Granuloma inguinale, a rare disease, causes painful ulcerations with red granulation tissue or keloid-like depigmented scars, elephantoid enlargement of the external genitalia, and fistulas.

Ulcers can also occur with chronic fistulas or Crohn's disease; local application of zinc oxide paste may help alleviate symptoms. A course of oral metronidazole (Flagyl) has proved beneficial in some patients with chronic fistulas. The mouth should always be examined in patients with vulvar ulcers. Behçet's disease is a multisystem disease characterized by recurrent oral and genital ulcers, often associated with uveitis, and, less commonly, arthritis, phlebitis, and rashes.

Although the disease usually does not appear until the third decade of life, rare cases in young children and adolescents have been reported. Therapy is unsatisfactory and includes high-estrogen oral contraceptives, corticosteroids, and immunosuppressive agents (e.g., azathioprine and chlorambucil).

Although most darkly pigmented lesions seen on the vulva of adolescent girls represent lentigo (a benign freckle-like lesion increase in the concentration of melanocytes in the basal layer of the epithelium) or a compound, junctional, or intradermal nevus, the rare occurrence of melanoma or other form of carcinoma makes it essential to perform an excisional biopsy to establish a benign diagnosis.

Dysuria

Dysuria is a common symptom in adolescent girls and is discussed in this section because vaginitis and vulvar lesions may produce symptoms usually associated with a UTI. The clinician needs to do a careful gynecological assessment of adolescents who complain of dysuria. Recent studies in adult women have revealed that only one half of the women with dysuria had bacteriuria with more than 100,000 organisms/ml. Vaginitis, vulvitis, infection with herpes, *N. gonorrhoeae, C. trachomatis,* and bacteriuria with fewer than 100,000 organisms/ml are responsible for most of the remaining group. A study of 53 adolescent girls (mean age 17.5 years) who came to our clinic because of dysuria is shown in Table 20–5. Pyuria on urinalysis was seen most frequently with UTI and *Trichomonas* vaginitis; however, the patients with gonococcal and mixed gonococcal-chlamydial infection (one case of each) also had pyuria. None of the patients who had acute urethral syndrome with unclear cause had pyuria.

When we assess an adolescent with dysuria, we take a history that asks specifically about onset of symptoms, sexual activity (recent and past), symptoms of urethritis in the boyfriend, previous UTIs, and internal dysuria (pain felt inside the body) vs. external dysuria (pain felt as urine

TABLE 20–5.

Etiology of Dysuria in Adolescent Girls

Diagnosis	Patients n	%
Vaginitis from	10	19
Candida	8	15
Trichomonas	2	4
Candida and *Trichomonas*	2	4
Bacterial UTI	9	17
Bacterial UTI and vaginitis	9	17
Other diagnoses		
Herpes progenitalis	2	4
N. gonorrhoeae	1	2
C. trachomatis	1	2
N. gonorrhoeae and *C. trachomatis*	1	2
Skene's gland abscess	1	2
Nonspecific vulvitis	2	4
Traumatic urethritis	1	2
Urethral syndrome of unclear etiology	4	8

passes over the inflamed labia). If the patient reports a clear-cut external dysuria and discharge, it is highly likely that the patient's symptoms are due to vaginitis or a vulvar cause. Although adult women who have internal dysuria and frequency usually have a UTI, many of the adolescent girls in our clinic had vaginitis either alone or in combination with a UTI. In contrast to older women, adolescents were less able to differentiate between internal and external dysuria.

The laboratory evaluation of the adolescent with dysuria should include urinalysis, two urine cultures, wet preparations of the vaginal secretions, and culture for gonorrhea (in sexually active patients). Incubating dip slides in the office is inexpensive. Inspection of the genitalia should be done to exclude urethral or vulvar pathology. Speculum examination should be done for sexually active patients. In virginal patients, samples for wet preparations can be obtained with a saline-moistened, cotton-tipped applicator gently inserted through the hymenal ring. A culture for *Candida* should be done in patients with itching or vulvar erythema in whom the KOH preparation does not reveal *Candida.*

The diagnosis is generally UTI or a specific infection. In patients who have undiagnosed dysuria and persistent pyuria on urinalysis, cultures for *Chlamydia* should be obtained. The patient should ask her partner again about symptoms of urethritis so that urethritis from *C. trachomatis* can be treated in the male at the same time. The patient with pyuria should then be treated with a course of antibiotics effective against low-count UTIs and *Chlamydia*.

Adolescents with uncomplicated cystitis may be treated with single-dose antibiotics or a 10-day course. The most well-studied single doses are 3 gm of amoxicillin or 320 and 1,600 mg, respectively, of TMP-SMX (four tablets), the cure rate with the latter being slightly higher than the former. The oral quinolones hold promise for effective single-dose therapy of gonorrhea and UTI; a longer course is necessary to eradicate *Chlamydia*. For example, in nonpregnant patients, 250 mg of ciprofloxacin twice daily for 10 days appears to be equally as efficacious as TMP-SMX for 10 days, with fewer adverse side effects.

Ultrasonography of the kidneys should be performed in adolescents with complicated UTIs, pyelonephritis, inadequate response to antibiotics, and possibly recurrent cystitis. The lack of response to a single dose of antibiotics can indicate a patient at higher risk of upper UTI, and, thus, this may be a good indicator of the need to evaluate the kidneys. In contrast to recommendations in children, a voiding cystourethrogram is generally reserved for patients with an abnormal ultrasound (or pyelonephritis) in adolescence.

Patients often have recurrent UTIs in relationship to coitus and especially diaphragm use. Other diaphragms or other methods of contraception may need to be considered. Coitus-related UTI can be treated with frequent voiding (every 2 hours during the day), voiding after intercourse, and suppressive antibiotics. Antibiotic regimens include 80 and 160 mg, respectively, of TMP-SMX (½ tablet) daily or ½ tablet three times per week, postcoital antibiotics, or single-dose therapy with each infection. The use of prophylactic antibiotics is considered cost effective when women experience more than two infections per year. Self-administration of antibiotics at the time of the UTI appears to be most useful in women who are accurate at self-diagnosis and have only one or two infections each year. One drawback to self-therapy is the failure to reduce the proportion of patients with enterobacterial colonization of the urethra and vagina.

Currently, the patient without pyuria or a diagnosis falls into a small category of patients with urethral syndrome of unclear etiology. Antibiotics do not benefit these patients. Studies in the future

are likely to shed light on the diagnosis and treatment of this group.

Toxic Shock Syndrome

Toxic shock syndrome (TSS) received much publicity in the early 1980s as a disease that was occurring in young women primarily in association with one type of tampon (Rely). Since that time there has been recognition of milder cases than the original Centers for Disease Control (CDC) definition as well as newer information on toxin production and risk factors.

Although the original description of toxic shock suggested a syndrome of boys and girls, it is now apparent that toxic shock is predominantly (70%–80%) a syndrome of young menstruating women who use tampons. The disease in menstruating young women is associated with the elaboration of an exotoxin, TSS toxin-1 (TSST-1) by *S. aureus*. *Staphylococcus aureus* has been cultured from the vagina of 98% of women with TSS vs. 7% of controls. It has a peak occurrence on the fourth day of the menses and has been associated with continuous tampon use.

Toxic shock syndrome continues to be reported, although the originally blamed tampon (Rely) was removed from the market in 1980. The incidence of TSS after 1980 has been reported to be 2 to 4 per 100,000 woman-years. Given the current information and the tremendous variability of absorbency with the current terminology of regular, super, and super-plus, mandatory labeling with standardized absorbency would allow the consumer to diminish her risk of TSS. Factors that appear to promote the recurrence of TSS are the neutral pH of the vagina during menstruation and the introduction of air into the vagina with the insertion of tampons. Cases of TSS do, however, occur during menses in women not using tampons.

Contraceptive sponge use and, to a lesser extent, diaphragm use have been associated with rare cases of TSS. The relative risk of nonmenstrual TSS associated with the sponge has been estimated to be 7.8 to 40. Although in vitro data suggest that *S. aureus* and TSST-1 production are inhibited by the sponge, clinicians should base their counseling on the rare possibility of TSS (the risk of death estimated at 0.1–0.6 per 100,000 women-years) and should discuss the symptoms with each patient using this method of contraception.

The toxin TSST-1 has been isolated in 90% to 100% of menstrual cases of TSS, whereas this toxin has been reported in only 62% of nonmenstrual cases, suggesting that other toxins are involved in the pathogenesis of nonmenstrual TSS. Most individuals develop antibody to TSST-1 by age 20 years. Toxic shock occurs predominantly in the population that lacks antibody either because of a genetic factor or lack of exposure. Young patients, especially adolescents, would be expected to be at increased risk of TSS. This toxin appears to block β-lymphocytes from making antibody. Women who have not made antibody to TSST-1 at follow-up are at high risk of recurrence with future menses and tampon usage.

Milder cases of TSS have also been described. Physicians and patients need to be aware of more minor symptomatology occurring with tampon (or sponge) use to intervene effectively. The criteria set up by the CDC to study the epidemiology of TSS are for the more severe manifestations of the syndrome. These criteria are as follows:

I. Fever (temperature more than 38.9° C)
II. Rash (diffuse macular erythroderma that looks like sunburn)
III. Desquamation 1 to 2 weeks after the onset of the illness, particularly of palms and soles
IV. Hypotension (systolic blood pressure less than 90 mm Hg for adults, or orthostatic syncope)
V. Involvement of three or more of the following organ systems:
   A. Gastrointestinal (vomiting or diarrhea)
   B. Muscular (severe myalgia or creatinine phosphokinase level more than two times the upper limits of normal)
   C. Mucous membranes (vaginal, oropharyngeal, or conjunctival hyperemia)
   D. Renal (blood urea nitrogen or creatinine level more than two times the upper limit of normal or more than five white blood cells/high-power field in the absence of UTI)
   E. Hepatic (total bilirubin, serum glutamic oxaloacetic transaminase, and serum glutamic pyruvic transaminase values more than two times the upper limit of normal)
   F. Hematological (platelet count less than 100,000/cu mm)
   G. Central nervous system (disorientation or alterations in consciousness when fever and hypotension are absent)
VI. Negative test results (if obtained) for:
   A. Blood, throat, or cerebrospinal fluid cultures
   B. Serological tests for Rocky Mountain spotted fever, leptospirosis, or measles

Adolescents with any of these symptoms or with vomiting, diarrhea, and rash during menstruation should be instructed to remove the tampon (or diaphragm) and go to the emergency room. Patients with TSS should be managed in the same way as those suffering from other forms of shock, including the administration of fluid. A vaginal examination should be done along with removal of the tampon (if still in place). Gram stain of the vaginal pool should be done. Cultures of blood, rectum, vagina, oropharynx, anterior nares, and urine should be obtained. Penicillinase-resistant antistaphylococcal antibiotics should be administered. Although evidence is lacking, most clinicians favor irrigating the vagina with saline, povidone-iodine (Betadine) solution, or vancomycin or gentamicin solution.

In patients with deep abscesses in which eradication of toxin-producing staphylococci is unlikely to occur rapidly, steroids and immunoglobulin therapy (which has high levels of antibody to TSST-1) are thought to improve outcome.

Because there is an approximately 30% risk of recurrence, patients should be warned to avoid tampons for at least 8 months. The presence of high levels of antibody to TSST-1 at follow-up in a patient with no antibody at presentation is reassuring. Serial cultures of the vagina may be difficult to interpret since other strains may be present. Testing for TSST-1-producing strains requires a specialized laboratory.

The use of all tampons in the United States fell initially in response to the publicity about TSS in the early 1980s. A significant number of young women desire to continue tampon use. There is insufficient knowledge to give absolute guidelines to patients, but I suggest (1) avoiding superabsorbent tampons (this should be easier with mandatory labeling); (2) using tampons intermittently by using pads at night; (3) changing tampons every 4 to 6 hours; and especially (4) removing tampons and calling a physician if vomiting, diarrhea, rash, or fever occurs. The recommendation about frequency of changing tampons has not been subjected to critical review.

Sexual Assault

In contrast to the pattern of sexual abuse in prepubertal children, sexual abuse during adolescence is more likely to be a one-time assault by a stranger and to involve vaginal intercourse. However, even among adolescents, the rape may involve an acquaintance or someone the teenager had seen in her neighborhood or school and who was assumed to be a safe individual. In these cases, the adolescent may accept a ride with that individual and then later be forced into a sexual relationship, often involving intercourse. In other cases, the developmental changes that take place during adolescence may make a long-standing incestuous relationship intolerable; the adolescent may then respond with a sudden disclosure, may seek medical care for somatic symptoms such as abdominal pain or headache, or may become involved in impulsive behavior such as running away. A pregnancy may be the first sign of a previous rape or chronic sexual abuse. It is, therefore, important to ask adolescents not only whether they have ever had sexual relations but also whether they have ever been forced into a sexual relationship.

In recording the history of the adolescent with alleged sexual assault, it is important to record the date of the visit, sources of the history, who brought in the patient, and who knows of the current situation. The date, time, and place of the sexual assault or assaults should be recorded. In acute situations, the patient should be asked if she has bathed, douched, or urinated since the assault. Menstrual and contraceptive history should be obtained. The physician should not try to decide whether rape or seduction has occurred on the basis of the patient's emotional response to the trauma; some patients will be tearful, tense, and hysterical, and others will appear controlled or subdued. Questions should focus on what happened and whether vaginal, rectal, or oral penetration occurred (terms understood by the patient should be used). These questions may need to be repeated during the examination when the adolescent is more familiar with the anatomical terms. The patient should be asked if she is aware of any other injuries or symptoms following the attack. A rape protocol should be used to collect evidence. It is extremely helpful if a nurse, preferably an experienced rape victim counselor, can be assigned to the adolescent throughout the 2- to 4-hour stay in the emergency ward and can be present during the history taking and physical examination and be an ally to the patient. A number of general hospitals now have a rotating system of nurses who have had special training in rape counseling and who are available on an on-call basis to provide such support for the victim. The police officer should not be present during the medical evaluation.

After the history is obtained, the patient should be told of the need for a thorough physical examination to assess injury and to collect laboratory specimens. The assessment that follows applies to the acute sexual assault. When there is a history of an ongoing incestuous relationship in which intercourse has occurred longer ago than 5 days before the physical examination, the search for motile sperm is omitted. The physical examination should include the following seven steps:

1. A description should be recorded of the patient's general appearance, emotional state, and especially the condition of the clothing. Any clothing that might provide evidence in a legal case should be included in the rape-evidence clothing bag.
2. A general physical examination should note any evidence of bruises, scratches, or lacerations. As noted in the assessment of the prepubertal child, debris and dried secretions should be properly collected. The Tanner stage of sexual development should be noted. If history indicates any attempt of the patient to scratch or fight the assailant, fingernail scrapings should be obtained with a wooden applicator stick and saved in an envelope.
3. The pelvic examination should include a careful inspection of the perineum, noting any evidence of bleeding or lacerations. A slightly moistened gauze pad should be used to swab any dried secretions, and the location of the dried secretions should be marked on a sketch. A collection paper should be placed under the buttocks of the patient and the pubic hair combed toward the paper to collect any debris. The comb and debris should be placed in the collection envelope. If any foreign hairs are noted, 6 to 12 pu-

bic hairs of the patient should be included and marked. The pubic hair can be cut near the surface to avoid discomfort. The size of the hymenal ring should be noted (e.g., Q-tip size, one-finger breadth, or two-finger breadths). Any evidence of a hymenal tear should be recorded. In most patients, a gentle vaginal examination can be done with a water-moistened narrow (Huffman) speculum. If the hymen is tight, samples may be obtained from the vagina with a saline-moistened cotton-tipped applicator or long eyedropper. It is extremely important to examine the teenager gently so that the examination does not represent a further trauma. The vagina is inspected for injury and the presence of semen or vaginal discharge. An endocervical culture should be obtained for gonorrhea. If a speculum examination is not done, a vaginal culture for gonorrhea can be obtained by inserting a moistened Q-tip well into the vagina. A Q-tip should be swabbed into the posterior vaginal pool, and wet preparations should be done to look for the presence of motile sperm, ducrells, and trichomonads. Another swab from the vaginal pool should be smeared onto two dry slides (frosted at one end so that the patient's name and date can be recorded) and allowed to air dry. The swab is then protected in a test tube and saved for examination by a police forensic laboratory. If cervical smears are also taken to check for motile sperm, the wet and dry slides should be appropriately marked. A police laboratory can test for acid phosphatase and the blood group antigens of semen and can examine the dry slides for the presence of nonmotile sperm. The anus should be inspected and a culture for gonorrhea obtained. Specimens for sperm and acid-phosphatase determinations should be obtained if there is a history of rectal assault. Anoscopy should be done if rectal bleeding is present or the rectal examination reveals Hematest-positive stool. A bimanual rectal-vaginal-abdominal examination should be done gently to make sure there is no tenderness and no enlargement of the uterus to suggest a pre-existing pregnancy. Rectal sphincter tone should be assessed, since patients subjected to chronic rectal abuse may have reflex relaxation.

4. If oral-genital contact has occurred, specimens from the girl's mouth should be obtained. A throat swab should be plated in modified Thayer-Martin-Jembec media.
5. Blood should be drawn for a serological test for syphilis (RPR or VDRL) and serum frozen to do future testing for HIV and hepatitis B, if indicated.
6. A sensitive urine pregnancy test such as ICON should be done to detect preexisting pregnancy (especially if the menses are late or irregular or the patient has had previous sexual exposure).
7. If the patient was unconscious, samples should be obtained from vagina, rectum, and mouth.

All laboratory specimens for the pathology laboratory or the police should be delivered personally by the physician or nurse involved in the case, and properly signed receipts should be obtained. Use of a rape evidence kit or rape protocol does not imply that the family or patient must push for prosecution; however, reporting the rape and using a protocol to collect the evidence ensures that the evidence has been appropriately handled and will be admissible in court if prosecution is to occur. Under the stress of the crisis, many families may have difficulty deciding whether prosecution will be sought; it therefore behooves the physician to obtain evidence that is medically and legally appropriate.

In cases of acute rape, the decision to prescribe antibiotics should be individualized and based on the risks. The benefits of prophylactic treatment for syphilis, gonorrhea, and *Chlamydia* should be discussed with the patient. In asymptomatic adolescents with long-standing incestuous relationships, the physician should wait for the cultures and blood tests before initiating treatment (unless the perpetrator is known to be infected). Because of the discomfort involved in intramuscular injection, the physician should use oral ampicillin or amoxicillin for gonococcal prophylaxis rather than intramuscular penicillin or ceftriaxone in areas with a low risk of penicillinase-producing *N. gonorrhoeae*. The single-dose therapy should be followed by 7 days of tetracycline, doxycycline, or erythromycin. If the initial RPR test result is normal, a follow-up serological test for syphilis is necessary if spectinomycin is chosen for gonococcal prophylaxis or no prophylaxis is given. Tetanus toxoid should be given following standard pediatric guidelines for injuries.

"Morning-after" estrogen therapy should be offered to the postpubertal adolescent who was raped less than 72 hours (preferably less than 48 hours) before being treated. It is important that the patient understand that the medicine should not be used if there is the possibility of a preexisting pregnancy; she should feel ready to have an abortion if she discovers several weeks later that she was, in fact, pregnant at the time of the estrogen administration. A sensitive pregnancy test should be done before medication is given.

A follow-up appointment should be given for 2 weeks later. A repeat pelvic examination is done to assess healing of injuries. The patient should be reassured that her genital anatomy is normal. Patients greatly benefit from drawings to show them the range of hymenal size. The virginal adolescent who has had a forced episode of sexual intercourse may feel considerably relieved to understand that her introitus is not different from some adolescents who have not had intercourse. She needs to be reassured that the assault in no way changes her ability to have normal sexual intercourse in the future or to have normal, healthy children. We have seen older teenagers who had unprotected intercourse because they believed that a rape that occurred when they were 12 or 13 years old markedly diminished their reproductive potential.

The extent of the counseling in the aftermath of a sexual assault depends on the initial encounter. For example, in the situation of an isolated episode of exhibitionism or nonforceful genital fondling by a stranger or neighbor, counseling should help integrate the event with a strongly positive view of the future. A case of a longstanding incestuous relationship requires proper reporting to the Children's Protective Services and a long-term treatment program. If the young adolescent has been trained to be a sexual object and to give and receive sexual pleasure to get approval, the outcome is often poor; such girls are often provocative in foster home settings. Cases of acute sexual assault during adolescence require that the physician discuss the possibility of prosecution and suggest the need for long-term counseling.

The availability of counseling should be stressed to the teenager. Even if she seems nonverbal or appears to be coping well, the counselor can often play an educational and supportive role in the initial interviews. The patient needs reassurance about her intactness and her femininity. She may need the opportunity to tell and retell her story to a caring, sympathetic person. Ideally, an experienced counselor should be available at the time the rape is reported and should be willing to follow up the patient by telephone or home visits. It is not unusual for a patient to have somatic reactions in the first several weeks following a rape, including muscle soreness, headache, fatigue, stomach pain, dysuria, sleep disturbances, and nightmares. Most rape victims express an extreme fear of physical violence and death. Many older women move and change their telephone numbers.

In the course of counseling, it is important to acknowledge to the patient that she may feel vulnerable and helpless and that the rape incident may interfere with her ability to form trusting relationships in the future.

Congenital Malformations

A large proportion of congenital abnormalities of the female genital tract remain undiscovered until adolescence. These are usually diagnosed when symptoms occur, especially menstrual disorders and coital difficulties, or simply because most patients undergo their first pelvic examination at this time.

Although some congenital malformations become obvious at first glance, the diagnosis of many of these defects requires a high index of suspicion. A thorough understanding of the nature of these anomalies is essential to gynecologists who deal with the teenage group. Early diagnosis, adequate treatment, and appropriate psychological support and counseling assure the preservation of reproductive function when feasible and allow these adolescents to develop a serene attitude toward their sexuality.

Vulva

Labia Minora Hypertrophy or Asymmetry.—In some instances, one or both labia minora are unusually large, and the patient consults because she notices the anomaly or because of symptoms of irritation associated with exercise. In most of these cases, simple reassurance is necessary. Comparison with asymmetry or hypertrophy of other parts of the body may help the patient to accept this peculiarity. Hygiene counseling and avoidance of tight clothes are usually sufficient to relieve discomfort. When these measures prove to be ineffective, or in the presence of a troublesome cosmetic problem, surgical reduction is in order. This can be accomplished in the ambulatory operating room by simply resecting the redundant labia so that they are symmetrical. Closure of the excised area is best accomplished with a running locking stitch of 3-0 chromic suture. The results are usually excellent, and the patients are generally quite pleased (Fig 20–10).

Labial Ahesions.—In adolescents, labial adhesions secondary to hypoestrogenism are quite infrequent. When it occurs, the problem is approached as for younger children. During adolescence, the most commonly encountered type of labial adhesion is an epithelial bridge between either the labia majora or minora, which may be congenital or due to trauma. Since these interlabial adhesions may be easily torn, surgical incision is advisable.

Congenital Adrenal Hyperplasia.—In female pseudohermaphrodism due to CAH, the external genitalia can be variously affected. The external urinary meatus is found most often at the base of the phallus, but sometimes it is extended to its end, where a glans penis and a prepuce are present, as in the male. There is a median perineal raphe, formed by scrotolabial folds in which no gonads can be felt. A vaginal opening is not always found externally, but cystoscopy reveals an opening on the floor of the urethra several centimeters from the vesical orifice, representing the distal end of the vagina. The vaginal size and length differ. The common urethrovaginal canal opening onto the perineum represents a urogenital sinus. If prenatal virilization is less progressed, there are separate urethral and vaginal openings. Similar external genital changes may exist in female pseudohermaphrodites without adrenal disorders. Uterus, tubes, and ovaries are normally formed. The vagina may be absent in female pseudohermaphrodites who are masculinized by a maternal virilizing tumor or by androgens or progestins administered to the mother during pregnancy. The internal genitalia are female in such children, and there are no renal anomalies. The nature of the reconstructive surgery required varies with the anomaly but usually includes clitoral recession and perioneoplasty with exteriorization of the vagina.

Hymen

Imperforate Hymen With Hematocolpos (or Hydrocolpos).—Although the diagnosis of an imperforate hymen should be made long before adolescence during routine neonatal and pediatric examinations, it is not infrequent to see a teenager present with the typical picture of pri-

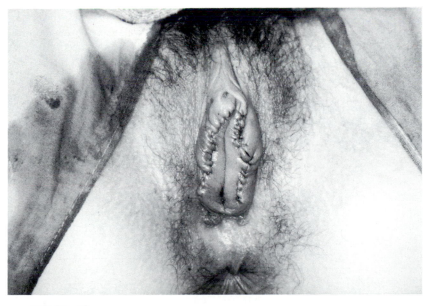

FIG 20–10.
Labial reduction surgery in a patient with symptomatic hypertrophic labia.

mary amenorrhea, cyclic or acyclic pelvic pain, bulging hymen, and hematocolpos. Hematometra does not usually develop with simple imperforate hymen because the vagina has great distensibility and can accommodate a large amount of blood. It is, however, quite commonly seen with high transverse septa.

Imperforate hymen occurs because of failure of degeneration of central epithelial cells of the hymenal membrane. If the vagina and the uterus are not distended by estrogen-induced secretions at the time of birth, the imperforate hymen may remain asymptomatic until puberty, when collection of menstrual material results in enlargement of the vaginal tract, causing pelvic or abdominal pain. It is of historical interest that this condition was known to Aristole and mentioned in his treatise on the "Generation of Animals.":

> We know of instances of women in whom the "os uteri" was grown together and continued so until the time arrived for the menstrual discharge to begin and pain come on; in some the passage burst open of its own accord, in others, it was separated by physicians; and in some cases, where the opening either was forcibly made or could not be made at all, the patients succumbed.

Approximately two thirds of the cases become manifest before the age of 15 years. A cystic mass is formed by enlargement of the vagina and uterus that can extend above the symphysis and into the abdominal cavity. Abdominal pain is a regular symptom, and urinary difficulties may develop. Many patients who are inadequately examined undergo extensive radiological evaluation before the diagnosis is finally made. Examination of the external genitalia reveals a mass protruding between the labia majora. The bulging mass is variable in size, is bluish red, and is continuous with the pelvic mass (Fig 20–11). Constipation results in some cases because of pressure on the rectum from the distended vagina.

The surgical therapy consists of hymenotomy, which often reveals a large accumulation of blood or secretion. Excision of the central part of the hymen should also be carried out to allow further unobstructed menstrual flow. We have found that the use of the needle-tip electrocautery facilitates hemostasis on the hymenal edge. It avoids the need for multiple sutures and minimizes the likelihood of secondary retraction. The use of a suction tip inserted high into the vagina or

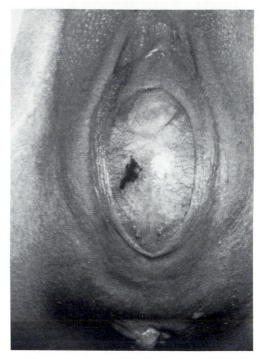

FIG 20–11.
Imperforate hymen in postpubertal patient who presented with abdominal pain and large pelvic mass; 850 ml of old blood was received from the vagina following hymenotomy.

through the dilated cervix into the uterus facilitates evacuation. At times the wall suction becomes plugged, and a high-speed suction evacuator is required. Infection is rare once drainage is established, and prophylactic antibody therapy is not required.

Microperforate, Cribriform, and Septate Hymen.—Incomplete fenestration of the hymenal opening is most often asymptomatic. These patients seek gynecological treatment because of unsuccessful attempts at inserting tampons or coital difficulties. With a microperforate hymen, the adolescent may also complain of postmenstrual vaginal spotting or malodorous discharge secondary to incomplete obstruction and poor drainage. Hymenectomy should be performed in all cases.

When the diagnosis is made fortuitously, the patient should be told about this anatomical variant and be informed of the necessity of surgical correction. Performing the procedure during the early teens allows the adolescent to use tampons without problems and may avoid later embarrassment when the patient desires to become sexually active.

Vagina

Vaginal Agenesis.—Vaginal agenesis in any of its forms is rare. There are three types: (1) total agenesis (the Rokitansky-Küster-Hauser syndrome), (2) proximal atresia, and (3) distal atresia. Only proximal vaginal atresia results in hydrometrocolpos. Total vaginal agenesis results from failure of the müllerian ducts to reach the urogenital sinus. Other müllerian derivatives, the uterus and fallopian tubes, are frequently absent or represented only by rudimentary structures. Proximal vaginal atresia results from failure of fusion of the müllerian ducts at their tips so that the vaginal plate does not form. The cervix is absent, but the uterus and tubes are present. Distal vaginal atresia results from failure of the sinovaginal bulbs to proliferate. The proximal vagina, cervix, uterus, and tubes are intact. The urogenital sinus remains as a long, narrow tubular structure distal to the atresia, and thus the urethra is located within the urogenital sinus high on its anterior wall.

Vaginal agenesis is rarely diagnosed in the newborn girl. Usually it is identified after the expected time of menarche when menstruation does not occur. Since the ovaries are present, development of secondary sexual characteristics occurs. Cyclic pain and an abdominal mass are indicative of hematocolpos. Absence of menses and lack of cyclic pain indicate agenesis of both vagina and uterus.

Proximal vaginal atresia may present in the newborn period as an abdominal mass but most often is identified after the expected time of menarche due to cyclic abdominal pain, an abdominal mass, and lack of menstruation. Distal vaginal atresia most often presents in the newborn period with an abdominal mass due to hydrometrocolpos. It may be a genetic disorder, inherited as a simple recessive trait.

In complete vaginal agenesis, the labia are underdeveloped, and there is a single opening between them. The normal vaginal introitus is absent. The patient with proximal vaginal atresia has a normal female perineum. The uterus is palpable on rectal examination. Vaginoscopy reveals a blind-ending vagina without a uterine cervix.

Plain roentgenograms of the chest, abdomen, and pelvis should be obtained first to identify associated pulmonary, cardiac, or bony anomalies. An excretory urogram or sonogram should be obtained in all patients with vaginal atresia. Injection of contrast media into any abnormal orifice also helps to clarify the complex anatomy.

Cystoscopy should be performed under anesthesia at the time of definitive treatment. The urethral meatus is found on the anterior wall of the urogenital sinus in the patient with distal atresia but is in the normal position in the patient having proximal vaginal atresia.

The pelvic examination of these patients reveals an absent vagina, and a particular feature is the small space separating the urethral meatus from the anus. The outer part of the vagina may be present as a blind vaginal canal of variable depth. This finding is more likely to be associated with testicular feminization syndrome. The presence or absence of a uterus is ascertained by rectoabdominal examination. External genitalia are usually of normal appearance. In cases of testicular feminization, characteristic stigmata can usually be observed.

The minimal workup should consist of pelvic ultrasound to confirm the presence or absence of a uterus, renal echography or IVP to detect urinary tract anomalies found in approximately one third of patients with müllerian agenesis, plasma testosterone level, which will be in the male range in cases of tesicular feminization syndrome, and a karyotype.

Associated anomalies are common in about one third of the patients; pelvic kidneys, solitary kidneys, fused kidney, duplication of ureter or renal pelvis, and other anomalies are noted. Spina bifida, hemivertebrae, and irregularities of the ribs are occasional findings. Rarely, absence of the vagina is combined with normal internal genitalia, resulting in blockage of menstrual discharge, hematometra, and hematosalpinx. Amenorrhea is considered a manifestation of absence or deficiency of the uterus.

The important point is that this syndrome seems to be part of a complex of congenital malformations occurring in females with 46 XX karyotype. Single kidney, bifid ureter, scoliosis, pectus excavatum, syndactyly, and situs inversus are associated anomalies. It has long been known that renal anomalies are frequent in women with vaginal agenesis. Pelvic kidney, solitary kidney, horseshoe kidney, and ureteric and pelvic duplications have been observed.

Treatment.—Therapy of vaginal agenesis aims at creating a vaginal canal to allow satisfactory sexual function and to establish adequate menstrual drainage when a functioning uterus is present. Management should be individualized for each patient.

When obstruction to menstrual flow is not a concern, therapy is best delayed until the patient has acquired enough maturity to comply with the demanding postoperative care that is the key to a successful outcome. In patients who already have a vaginal depth of 3 cm or more, treatment is not always needed since coital activity may be sufficient to induce vaginal deepening. When a rudimentary vagina is present, the nonsurgical Frank method, which consists of progressive vaginal dilation using dilators, should be attempted first.

The first attempt at vaginal reconstruction for vaginal agenesis was by Dupuytren in 1817. Since that time, numerous reports have appeared on vaginal reconstruction using a multitude of materials, including intestine, both small and large, peritoneum, amniotic membrane, hernial sacs, and bladder, as well as nonsurgical stretching procedures.

The timing of vaginal reconstruction is important. In the newborn infant with vaginal atresia and hydrometrocolpos or cloacal dysgenesis, immediate separation of genital and urinary tracts is necessary, so vaginal reconstruction is a logical and desirable part of the operation. However, if there is total vaginal agenesis, reconstruction is easier and more satisfactory if done at maturity. Patients who are first diagnosed as having atresia at menarche should have their vaginas reconstructed at that time. There is no advantage in waiting until the patient is "ready" for sexual activity. In fact, the patient's self-image may be irreversibly damaged should the situation be allowed to exist for a prolonged period once physical maturity has been reached.

The most commonly used technique in adolescents is that described by McIndoe (1950) in which a neovagina is constructed by the use of split thickness skin graft placed in a space created between the urethra and the rectum. A split thickness skin graft (0.015–0.018 inch) is taken from the lower abdomen or buttocks and sutured in a spiral fashion to an acrylic or pliable silicone mold with absorbable sutures, so that the epidermis is in contact with the mold. Using a transverse incision, two parallel tunnels are created on either side of the urethra, deepened 8 to 12 cm, and

united in the midline behind the urethra. Care must be taken to avoid entering either the urethra or the rectum. During the dissection, absolute hemostasis is mandatory. The epidermis-covered mold is then inserted into the tunnel, where it remains for 7 to 8 days (Fig 20–12). The patient is kept at bed rest for this period, and on the eighth day the mold is removed, the neovagina is cleansed, and the mold is reinserted. It is important that the mold be worn for at least 3 months postoperatively, until the contracture phase of the skin graft has ended. There are many modifications of this procedure.

The Williams vulvovaginoplasty is an acceptable therapeutic alternative (Fig 20–13). This technique offers the following advantages: (1) operative time is shorter, (2) it does not necessitate a skin graft, and (3) there is less risk of permanent stenosis if the patient does not comply with postoperative dilation. The Williams procedure is most often performed to lengthen a preexisting rudimentary vagina or when the McIndoe procedure result is not satisfactory.

When a functioning uterus and cervix are present, treatment cannot be delayed because of obstruction to menstrual flow. In these cases, the principal problem is the young age at which surgical correction is necessary. Creation of a neovagina using a centrally opened stent allowing drainage of menstrual blood is left in place for 4 to 6 months and decreases the likelihood of irreversible stenosis.

Vaginal Septum.—A vaginal septum is a relatively uncommon anomaly. Septa can be either congenital or acquired, can occur in various positions, and can be multiple. Transverse septa can occur at any level from above the hymenal ring to the junction of the vagina and cervix. Vertical septa can be oriented in an anteroposterior plan (sagittal septum) or in the lateral plane (coronal septum). Finally, septa can be complete or partial, and perforate or imperforate.

Transverse vaginal septa occur from lack of complete canalization of the solid primitive vaginal plate or sinovaginal bulbs. Vertical vaginal septa occur in two ways. Failure of the müllerian ducts to fuse results in a duplication of the uterus and vagina. What appears to be a vertical vaginal septum is, in fact, a duplicated vagina. Two vaginal openings are found. In others, incomplete canalization of the vaginal plate in a longitudinal direction results in a septum that may be oriented

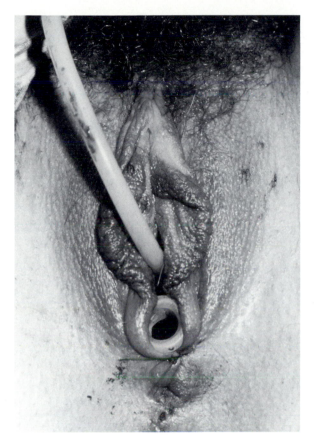

FIG 20–12.
Counseller's stent in place following neovagina reconstruction in 17-year-old patient with vaginal agenesis.

in either the anteroposterior or the lateral plane. The symptoms produced by vaginal septa depend on the age of the patient, the degree of vaginal obstruction, and the amount of stimulation of the cervical mucous glands by circulating estrogen. The neonate with a completely obstructed vagina due to a transverse septum may present with hydrometrocolpos. However, a transverse vaginal septum may not be recognized until the patient reaches menarche, when hematocolpos develops. The neonate or older child with a complete vertical septum may present with a unilateral hydrocolpos or hematocolpos, whereas an older patient with an incomplete vertical septum may seek help for dyspareunia or, if pregnant, for difficulty in delivery.

Transverse Septum.—Symptoms depend on the width as well as the location of the anomaly. A narrow annular septum usually is a fortuitous

finding of no clinical significance and does not require any treatment. On the other hand, primary amenorrhea and early symptoms of obstruction occur in cases of complete septum, and surgical excision is then imperative. When the upper and lower vaginal vaults communicate only by a small fistulous tract through the septum, the clinical picture is sometimes quite puzzling. These patients may present with dysmenorrhea, irregular vaginal spotting, or purulent discharge because of partial obstruction and accumulation of blood above the defect. Secondary PID due to anaerobic infection may also be the initial mode of presentation. A septum lying low in the vagina is frequently the cause of dyspareunia. Infertility and soft tissue dystocia are unusual presentations of this malformation in the adolescent group.

Surgical correction consists of complete excision of the septum and anastomosis of the upper vaginal vault to the lower vaginal vault. The use

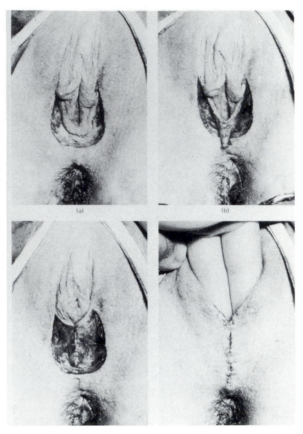

FIG 20–13.
Steps required to develop perineal pouch in Williams vulvovaginoplasty.

of a stent may be necessary when the septum involves a long vaginal segment and primary anastomosis is impossible. Care must be taken not to injure the urethra or rectum.

Postoperatively, periodic vaginal examinations at 6-week intervals should be performed with dilations as necessary. Recurrence is rare if the septum is entirely excised. Postoperatively, stricture is rarely encountered. In some patients, however, the fallopian tubes will have developed some degree of fibrosis because of pyocolpos with backflow prior to treatment.

Longitudinal Septum.—Longitudinal vaginal septa most often occur in association with abnormalities of uterine fusion but may sometimes be an isolated malformation. Such septa divide the vagina sagittally in two equal or unequal parts for its entire length or partially. Surgical excision is indicated when dyspareunia becomes a problem or when childbearing is anticipated.

In some instances, the septum fuses with the lateral vaginal wall and creates a blind vaginal pouch, giving rise to obstructive symptoms. This entity will be discussed together with obstructing uterine fusion anomalies.

Uterus and Cervix

As early as 1859, Kussmaul divided uterine malformations into two main groups: (1) deficiencies (agenesis or degeneration) and (2) duplications. Since then, many modifications of his detailed classification have been suggested, but the principal subdivisions still hold in morphological description. The relationship of these malformations to genetic, chromosomal, or exogenous teratogenic factors is still not clear in most cases, although some progress has been made in etiological classification.

Cervical Agenesis.—Congenital absence of the cervix can occur in association with vaginal agenesis or with a normal vagina. This rarity causes early obstructive signs and symptoms characterized by hematometra, tubal regurgitation of menstrual blood, and secondary endometriosis.

Attempts to preserve fertility by creation of a fistulous tract between the endometrial cavity and the vagina have been very disappointing. A conservative surgical approach usually leads to multiple repeated operations, and only two successful pregnancies are reported in the literature. Furthermore, death due to sepsis has been reported following conservative surgery. The recommended therapy of cervical agenesis, therefore, remains hysterectomy with ovarian conservation, when possible.

Uterine Agenesis.—Absence of the uterus is noted in some apparently female patients who have the syndrome of male pseudohermaphrodism with testicular feminization. Such persons are genetic males, have negative sex chromatin, and XY karyotype. They do not menstruate and cannot bear children, but their external genitalia are normal female, and they feminize at puberty, with good breast development. In rare cases, rudimentary tubes and uteri can be present. There are intra-abdominal or inguinal testes with nests of Leydig's cells.

The uterus is absent also in the majority of male pseudohermaphrodites with ambiguous genitalia. They may have testes situated intra-abdominally, in the inguinal canal, or in the scrotum. The vagina can be of differing size and length, often communicating with a hypospadic urethra. A minority of male pseudohermaphrodites with ambiguous external genitalia have a uterus and tubes. This can be of practical importance, if, at laparotomy, gonads at the site of ovaries are seen in a child with tubes, uterus, and vagina. Such gonads can be testes.

Uterine Duplication With Obstruction.—Abnormalities of uterovaginal fusion that are diagnosed during adolescent years are primarily those of the obstructing type. These anomalies can be divided into three categories according to the site of obstruction. Our experience at the Children's Hospital with 28 cases of uterine or vaginal (or both) obstructing duplications revealed that the most commonly encountered anomaly is a didelphic uterus with unilateral vaginal obstruction secondary to a blind vagina. Unicornuate uterus with a contralateral blind horn, either rudimentary or of normal size, is second in frequency. Finally, a small number of patients present with cervical obstruction of one horn of a bicornuate uterus associated with an ipsilateral blind vaginal pouch. Fistulous tracts of various types may connect the blind vagina to a septate cervix, to the main vaginal cavity, or to both. Intercervical fistulas have also been discovered.

Signs and symptoms depend on the type of abnormality. Since, in these cases, the obstruction is present only on one side, primary amenorrhea is not a feature. By far the commonest presenting complaint is pelvic pain, either cyclic or acyclic, which is the consequence of unilaterally obstructed menstrual flow and secondary endometriosis. Other frequent symptoms include abnormal vaginal bleeding and purulent discharge, usually associated with a fistulous tract connecting the obstructed to the unobstructed side. In the presence of a blind vagina, distention with menstrual blood may give rise to vaginal pain or the sensation of pressure. On physical examination, masses corresponding to distended pelvic structures, abnormal uterine shape, and discharge from possible fistulas can usually be visualized or palpated.

The minimal workup of these patients should include a combined pelvic and renal sonogram and an IVP. In our experience, unilateral renal agenesis is found in 75% of the patients. Associated vesicoureteral reflux has also been reported. Laparoscopy and hysterosalpingography should also be performed to determine the exact nature of the anomaly.

Therapy aims to preserve reproductive function. In the presence of a unilaterally blind double vagina, the only treatment needed is a vaginal septectomy. In cases of a blind uterine horn, the type of surgery depends on the size of the obstructed horn and consists of either unification metroplasty or hemihysterectomy. When one is dealing with combined cervical obstruction, blind vaginal pouch, and fistulous tracts, vaginal septectomy should be performed. Furthermore, due to the cervical obstruction, a unification procedure with complete removal of the cervical septum should also be performed. Associated endometriosis should be treated adequately when necessary.

Gynecological Abnormalities of Bladder Exstrophy

Fortunately, exstrophy of the urinary bladder is an uncommon anomaly. To the parents of such an afflicted newborn infant, the condition is distressing, frightening, and repulsive. The term exstrophy comes from two Greek words: The prefix *exo-* means outside of, and the verb *strophe* means to twist or turn about. The distraught parents see this condition as a twisted, inside-out urinary bladder accompanied by abnormal genitalia.

Girls always have a bifid clitoris. Several series report a high incidence of myelomeningocele, which is of significance in terms of sphincter incontinence. The distance from umbilicus to anus is foreshortened. Often the umbilicus is just cephalad to the exstrophic bladder, and some are associated with an omphalocele. The anal aperture is often close to the vagina.

Characteristically, the girl with bladder exstrophy presents to the gynecologist following puberty because of abnormalities of the lower abdominal and vulvar area that result from her urological reconstruction. Examination reveals scaring and deformity of the mons pubis, asymmetry of the labia, a bifid clitoris, and introital stenosis. The upper urinary tract is usually normal. Bladder exstrophy is one of the conditions that also lead to congenital prolapse of the uterus, myelodysplasia and spinal bifida being the other two. From the psychological standpoint, these patients are quite distraught because of their strange appearance and frequently shun their emerging female sexuality. It is quite important, therefore, to reassure them that total reconstruction can be accomplished.

We have performed a number of these operations in which a monsplasty, Williams vulvovaginoplasty, and a Manchester procedure are performed in a one-stage operation. The results are usually excellent, and full function is restored. Pregnancy can occur, but delivery should be cesarean.

Endocrine-Related Disorders

Puberty

The prerequisites for the development of normal reproductive function in the female are (1) normal ovaries capable of secreting steroids (estrogen and progesterone) in response to pituitary gonadotropins (LH and FSH), (2) normal hypothalamus capable of responding to elevated levels of steroids by appropriate pulsatile secretion of LH-RH, and (3) a normal pituitary that is sensitive to LH-RH and estrogen (or progesterone) and contains a pool of releasable LH large enough to provide an LH surge. The harmony of the menstrual cycle is a product of an elaborate pubertal process in which the hypothalamic-pituitary-ovarian axis develops concomitant to noted physical changes in the female. It is after the completion of the pubertal process that an individual is fully mature and able to reproduce. The onset of the pubertal event in each individual is variable and influenced profoundly by genetic and environmental factors (chronic disease and nutrition). In fact, as previously mentioned, the average onset of puberty in the United States is between ages 8 and 13 years. It is earlier than the average worldwide because of better nutrition. Also, since there is wide variation in the age at the onset of puberty among individuals (8–18 years), bone age correlates best with pubertal age. Therefore, when an individual with delayed or advanced puberty is evaluated, it is more important to match the bone age with other somatic pubertal changes.

To understand the hormone changes during puberty, we should review the changes in LH and FSH secretion from the time in utero to puberty. It is now speculated that the gonadarche and adrenarche are separate events. Puberty is believed to be controlled by an LH-RH sensitivity threshold in the hypothalamus that decreases with increased maturity of the hypothalamic-pituitary axis. Therefore, the CNS appears to control the onset of puberty and, thus, the secretion of steroid hormones. However, after normal pubertal development has been accomplished, the hypothalamic-pituitary axis becomes subservient to the positive and negative feedback signals from the ovary. The pituitary control of adrenarche is not completely understood. Adrenarche causes pubic and axillary hair growth. It precedes the growth spurt by 2 years and involves an acceleration in size of the zona reticularis. There is subsequent increased secretion of androgens (DHEA and DHEAS).

There is a temporary increase in LH and FSH levels to about 2 to 4 years of age. Pituitary secretion of gonadotropins decreases again from about age 4 to 11 years. This is believed to be due to the development of an intrinsic CNS inhibitory mechanism that suppresses pulsatile LH-RH release. Chronologically, the onset of puberty is thus heralded by a decrease in the CNS inhibitory restraint and a decrease in the negative feedback effect. There is then an increase in LH-RH secretion and pituitary responsiveness.

This responsiveness is demonstrated by the LH response to exogenous LH-RH administration. Prepubertal children show a minimal response to LH-RH, secreting a small but significant LH peak. Pubertal children and adults have a much greater LH response to LH-RH administration. This increase in pituitary reserve and secretion of LH is the hallmark of puberty, and it is elicited prior to any physical evidence of secondary sexual development. Another maturational change seen in puberty is sleep-associated pulsatile LH secretion.

The final phase of the maturational changes that take place is the development of cyclic release of LH due to the positive feedback of estradiol. This elicits the midcycle surge in gonadotropins seen after puberty in the normal female menstrual cycle. A typical cyclic adult pattern, however is not achieved until luteal progesterone concentrations are adequate (greater than 10 ng/ml).

Concomitant with these changes are also differences in adrenocortical functioning, with an increase in adrenal androgen, namely, DHEAS (adrenarche). Adrenal maturation, however, is a separate event. In agonadal children, a decrease in basal gonadotropins also occurs at ages 4 to 11 years, attesting to the isolated importance of a maturing CNS inhibitory influence during this period. Premature adrenarche (before 8 years) is not consonant with premature gonadarche. Adrenarche also occurs in patients with both hypergonadotropic and hypogonadotropic hypogonadism (not hypopituitarism).

"Minimum" weight is another criterion that appears to control normal menstrual function. Losses of weight of 10% to 15% of body weight affect the menstrual cycle. Therefore, a relative degree of fatness plays a role in determining sexual maturation.

Abnormalities of the pubertal process involve isosexual or heterosexual precocity or delayed puberty. There also may be variations in the pubertal process, with premature thelarche and premature adrenarche occurring in isolated form.

Delayed Menarche

The term delayed menarche indicates the absence of menses in females by age 18 years. This may be classified into three groups: (1) constitutional delay, (2) hypogonadotrophic hypogonadism, and (3) hypergonadotrophic hypogonadism.

The majority of patients with delayed adolescent development manifest no demonstrable organic pathological conditions. The developmental retardation in these individuals represents a nor-

mal variation in endocrine function that will usually be rectified by time alone. For this reason, a most perplexing problem is when to commence a diagnostic program. The answer lies in the individualization of each case, taking into account the history, findings of physical examination, and the emotional attitudes of the patient and her family. The practice of initiating therapy to promote sexual development, however, is to be deplored, unless adequate diagnostic studies have been undertaken.

The endocrine defect in delayed adolescent development and delayed menarche is the lack of proper estrogenic stimulation necessary for maturation of the accessory sex organs and initiation of uterine bleeding. The secretion of estrogen is dependent on the elaboration of gonadotropin hormones from the adenohypophysis. The secretion of gonadotropins may be diminished or entirely lacking. In these individuals, for reasons unknown, it is assumed that both FSH and LH are held in abeyance.

Malnutrition due to starvation or chronic wasting disease may be contributory. Similarly, emotional or psychosomatic factors are known causes of secondary amenorrhea and may act to delay the onset of the puberty. Imbalances of other endocrine organs, such as the thyroid or adrenal glands, may also delay adolescent development and the menarche.

Clinical evaluation of the patients manifesting delayed adolescent development should begin with a complete and thorough history and physical examination. Careful scrutiny of the accessory sex organs and the genitalia is mandatory. The internal genitalia may be examined rectally; negligible mental trauma and physical discomfort ensue if the examiner is reassuring and careful. Bone x-ray films document bone age. Neurological and ophthalmological examinations are indicated if suspicious signs or symptoms such as headaches, scotomata, or diplopia are manifested.

The importance of a thorough rectovaginal examination is emphasized by the fact that delayed menarche may on occasion be due to a congenital mechanical obstruction in the vagina or cervix. Most commonly this is an imperforate hymen, and rectal examination reveals accumulated menstrual discharge in the vagina. Normal menses will immediately follow incision into the hymen and relief of the obstruction.

Assay of gonadotropins will distinguish between pituitary and ovarian failure. An elevated serum gonadotropin titer suggests ovarian failure (hypergonadotropic hypogonadism). Diminished titers focus attention on pituitary dysfunction (hypogonadotropic hypogonadism). Plasma FSH levels appear to be the single most reliable assay for the presence or absence of ovarian failure. Estrogens measured in urine or blood are in the range of the prepubertal or postmenopausal female. Yet the function of the endometrium is not altered, since uterine bleeding may be induced by the administration of estrogens alone or estrogens followed by progesterone. As previously stated, the majority of patients with delayed adolescent development manifest no discernible pathological condition. The prognosis for normal sexual development and reproductive function is excellent. In the absence of proved lesions or hormonal deficiencies, the use of endocrine preparations is deemed advisable. Reassurance, explanation, and passage of time constitute the desired therapeutic regimen. Systemic abnormalities such as obesity, cachexia, infection, and diabetes should be appropriately treated. Adequate psychiatric therapy, if indicated, should be initiated.

Amenorrhea

Primary Amenorrhea.—The term primary amenorrhea denotes menarche that has not occurred by age 18 years. Primary amenorrhea is associated with normal pubertal development in vaginal or müllerian aplasia. Patients who have complete androgen insensitivity may also have normal thelarche but do not have normal hair development and are amenorrheic. In deciphering the cause of primary amenorrhea, one should look at the patient's secondary sex characteristics. If there is good sexual development, then testicular feminization, müllerian agenesis, vaginal atresia, and polycystic ovarian disease are possibilities. If there is poor or little sexual development, then gonadal dysgenesis, anorexia nervosa, or prepubertal athleticism are possibilities.

The majority of patients with primary amenorrhea will have hypogonadotropic hypogonadism or gonadal dysgenesis. Another group will be detected by elevated plasma testosterone levels, which indicate some form of polycystic ovary syndrome. The remaining patients with normal breast and uterine development will have prolactin elevation. If the patient is normoprolactinemic, a progesterone intramuscular challenge test discerns estrogen status. If the latter is adequate, withdrawal bleeding occurs, and further LH measurements discriminate between patients with polycystic ovarian disease and hypothalamic dysfunction. If results of the progesterone withdrawal test are negative, further FSH level testing rules out ovarian failure. This final diagnostic category is not primarily associated with primary amenorrhea but, rather, with secondary amenorrhea. It will be discussed further. The systemic approach, however, is very valuable in the diagnostic evaluation of primary amenorrhea.

Secondary amenorrhea denotes loss of menses for more than a 6-month period in a woman who has had previously normal cycles. Oligomenorrhea denotes irregular but consistent periods occurring at intervals of 2 to 5 months. Chronic anovulation usually accompanies secondary amenorrhea or oligomenorrhea. The commonest causes for secondary amenorrhea or oligomenorrhea are (1) hypothalamic dysfunction, (2) hyperprolactinemia, and (3) excess androgen production.

Anorexia nervosa, or excessive weight loss (or both), malnutrition, stress, sustained systemic illness, and certain levels of exercise activity are all possible causes for hypogonadism. This diagnosis is reached through exclusion, since pituitary, ovarian, and adrenal dysfunction must first be eliminated. Most patients with hypothalamic amenorrhea have normal puberty. With the onset of amenorrhea, gonadotropins and estrogen levels decrease. Depending on the length of their disorders and whether or not they have secondary amenorrhea, they may be normoestrogenic or hypoestrogenic. Physical examination also serves as a bioassay of estrogen status, since well-cornified, rugated vaginal epithelium denotes normal estrogen status. Poorly cornified vaginal epithelium with scant cervical mucus denotes a low estrogen state. The progesterone challenge test produces withdrawal bleeding if there is a normal estrogen state.

The three important factors to exclude are pregnancy, a pituitary tumor, or premature menopause. This is done by β-hCG precluding pregnancy; LH, FSH, and prolactin level assays and a CT scan of the pituitary, if necessary, exclude hyperprolactinemia or hypergonadotropism. Other pathological processes are therefore ruled out, and hypothalamic amenorrhea is indicated. Patients should be encouraged to gain weight or decrease exercise activity if these are thought to be causative factors. Hormonal supplementation should be suggested to prevent osteoporosis.

Patients with hypothalamic amenorrhea

should be counseled as to the possible causes of their dysfunction. Patients suffering from effects of excessive dietary restriction, specifically anorectics, and bulemics should receive appropriate psychiatric referral. The care of such individuals is founded on a multidisciplinary approach. There is no long-term effect on the uterus and ovaries in such individuals. This is important, since many worry that they will not be able to carry a child if they have had prolonged amenorrhea due to exercise or anorexia. However, they should be made aware of the long-term skeletal effects producing osteoporosis and resulting from prolonged amenorrhea. Adequate diet, reasonable exercise, and exogenous calcium supplementation help decrease premature onset of osteoporosis.

If amenorrhea or oligomenorrhea is due to hyperprolactinemia, a careful evaluation of pituitary sellar contents is mandatory. If a large pituitary adenoma exists, it is best removed transsphenoidally by an experienced neurosurgeon. The incidence of recurrent hyperprolactinemia is great, and patients should be made aware of this. If there is a microadenoma or if no tumor is visible on sellar CT scan, medical therapy with bromocriptine (Parlodel) is indicated. Therapy should be initiated at the lowest level possible and titrated against serum prolactin levels until the latter are brought into the normal range. Rarely is a dose of 7.5 mg of bromocriptine/day or greater necessary to bring the serum prolactin level down to the normal range. Yearly CT scans should be performed to rule out suprasellar enlargement of the pituitary. All hyperprolactinemic patients, even if they are not interested in fertility, should be treated since there is an association between osteoporosis and hypoestrogenemia due to elevated prolactin levels.

Patients with diagnoses of polycystic ovarian disease should have intermittent withdrawal of menses with a progestin because of the high incidence of endometrial hyperplasia in this disorder. If there is hirsutism, birth control pills should be used to decrease endogenous testosterone.

Menstrual Disorders

Acute Adolescent Menorrhagia.—Abnormal menstrual bleeding is one of the commonest reasons for gynecological consultation in adolescents. The spectrum of complaints ranges from minor deviations from the average menstrual pattern to life-threatening hemorrhage. Whatever the seriousness of symptoms, it is usually a subject of great concern for both the patient and her parents, and it deserves attentive consideration.

Acute menorrhagia usually occurs quite dramatically and requires prompt management. The classical picture is that of a pale, anxious teenager who presents at the emergency room with heavy bleeding of several days' or weeks' duration.

Since dysfunctional uterine bleeding, by definition, occurs on the basis of anovulatory cycles, the teenager in the first years of her menstrual life is the most susceptible candidate.

The differential diagnosis of acute adolescent vaginal hemorrhage is summarized in Table 20–6. Although dysfunctional (anovulatory) uterine bleeding accounts for the largest number of these cases, other etiologies of abnormal genital bleeding should be systematically ruled out.

Pregnancy-related complications are common in adolescents and should be excluded, even in a supposedly virginal patient. These include spontaneous abortions, complications of elective pregnancy termination procedures, ectopic pregnancy, and gestational trophoblastic disease. Occasionally, young patients present with third trimester bleeding in a previously undiagnosed pregnancy.

Though rare, benign and malignant condi-

TABLE 20–6.

Differential Diagnosis of Adolescent Menorrhagia

I. Anovulatory uterine bleeding (dysfunctional uterine bleeding)
II. Pregnancy-related complications
    A. Spontaneous abortion
    B. Complications of pregnancy termination procedures
    C. Ectopic pregnancy
    D. Gestational trophoblastic diseases
    E. Bleeding of the third trimester of pregnancy
III. Local genital tract conditions
    A. Benign and malignant tumors (vagina, cervix, uterus, or ovary)
    B. Infection
    C. Intrauterine contraceptive devices
    D. Trauma
    E. Intravaginal foreign bodies
IV. Systemic causes
    A. Coagulation disorders
    B. Thyroid dysfunction
    C. Diabetes mellitus
    D. Nutritional disorders, iron deficiency
    E. Hepatic diseases
    F. Renal diseases
V. Causes of anovulation

tions of the genital tract may be responsible for severe hemorrhage. Sarcoma botryoides, which most often occurs in the young child, will rarely present during adolescent years. Bleeding vaginal adenosis, clear cell adenocarcinoma, extensive ectropion, and cervical or vaginal polyps or hemangiomas may be found on pelvic examination. Other uterine neoplasms and endometrial polyps are rarely encountered in this age group. Estrogen-secreting ovarian tumors can also cause endometrial hyperplasia, which leads to heavy bleeding, as it can in the perimenopausal age group. Pelvic inflammatory disease with associated endometritis and intrauterine contraceptive devices may induce heavy vaginal bleeding. Traumatic conditions, either postcoital or self-imposed, and intravaginal foreign bodies should also be considered.

Coagulation disorders are probably the commonest systemic condition associated with acute menorrhagia, including idiopathic thrombocytopenia purpura, von Willebrand's disease, Glanzmann's disease, thalassemia major, and Fanconi's anemia. Leukemia, effects of radiation and chemotherapy, and some drugs (e.g., anticoagulants, aspirin, and hepatotoxic drugs) are possible causes of deficient coagulation mechanisms.

Other systemic conditions possibly associated with menorrhagia include thyroid dysfunction, diabetes mellitus, nutritional disorders, and hepatic and renal diseases.

Patients who present with acute menstrual hemorrhage in their late adolescence should be investigated for other causes of chronic anovulation.

A complete history should be obtained, insisting on the description of recent events as well as premenarchal development. In such cases, it may be difficult to assess the amount of blood loss because a frightened patient or overanxious patient may be too anxious to be objective. Questions about the number of perineal pads or tampons used, degree of saturation, the quantity and size of blood clots, and the presence of orthostatic symptoms facilitate estimation of blood loss. The normal volume of menstrual bleeding averages 30 to 40 ml and corresponds to 10 to 15 moderately soaked pads or tampons. Information pertinent to all possible causes of vaginal hemorrhage should also be obtained.

A complete physical examination should be performed. Special attention must be paid to signs of hypovolemia and anemia, namely, pallor, low blood pressure and orthostatic hypotension, tachycardia, and a functional heart murmur. The abdomen should be carefully palpated for the presence of a mass, localized pain, and peritoneal signs. A speculum examination is mandatory to evaluate the amount of bleeding, and rule out any vaginal abnormality, and visualize the cervix. In the presence of a tight hymen, blood clots may accumulate and distend the vagina. The finding of as much as 500 mg of coagulated blood in the vagina is not unusual. This retrograde accumulation of clots may also account for cervical dilatation, which can be erroneously attributed to a spontaneous abortion. Internal genital structures are assessed by rectovaginal examination, looking for the presence of uterine enlargement and adnexal masses or tenderness.

The laboratory workup should consist of hemoglobin and hematocrit values, platelet count, blood type and cross match, and basic clotting studies, including prothrombin time, partial thromboplastin time, and bleeding time. Blood specimens should be drawn before the institution of any hormonal therapy or transfusion. Serum β-hCG or another highly sensitive pregnancy test and a cervical culture for gonorrhea and *Chlamydia* should be obtained in every patient. Determination of blood glucose levels, thyroid function tests, and urinalysis are also recommended but not essential before treatment is instituted. In certain instances, a pelvic sonogram may be indicated for evaluation of an enlarged uterus or adnexal mass. The need for additional diagnostic studies depends on the clinical assessment of each patient.

The aims of the therapy of acute adolescent menorrhagia are to control bleeding, restore adequate intravascular volume and correct anemia, treat underlying conditions when present, and prevent recurrence. Method and intensity of therapy obviously depend on the severity of hemorrhage. The adolescent in whom the bleeding is mild to moderate without signs of hypovolemia can be treated on an outpatient basis, provided close follow-up and good compliance are assured. These patients often present with moderate anemia due to prolonged bleeding. In the presence of severe hemorrhage or anemia (hemoglobin level less than 8 gm/dl) or when the patient is hypovolemic, admission is mandatory.

The initial treatment is medical rather than surgical in most patients. Since the primary cause of bleeding is due to unstable endometrium because of fluctuating estrogen levels, the rationale of therapy is to stop the hemorrhage by administering estrogen and stabilize the endometrium with progestogens. We have used birth control pills containing 1 mg of norethindrone and 50 µg of ethinyl estradiol (Ortho-Novum 1/50, Norinyl 1+50) very effectively in this situation. These are administered at the rate of one pill every 4 hours until the bleeding subsides. If bleeding does not stop within 24 to 36 hours, other causes of bleeding should be seriously considered. In the presence of acute, severe hemorrhage, IV conjugated estrogens (e.g., Premarin) administered at a dosage of 25 mg every 4 hours for not more than four doses may be used in addition to the oral progestogens. The major side effect of oral progestogen and IV estrogen is nausea and vomiting, for which we use antinausea medications prophylactically. Blood replacement is used when necessary.

Once the bleeding has stopped or decreased appreciably, oral contraceptives are tapered gradually over 7 days and then continued at a rate of one pill a day for 21 days. Withdrawal bleeding will follow the discontinuation of treatment. The patient should be informed that this may be heavy but self-limited.

Dilatation and curettage is reserved for those cases where medical treatment fails to control the bleeding within 24 to 36 hours. Approximately 20% of patients require surgical intervention to control bleeding. In most instances where medical management has failed, endometrial hyperplasia or a polyp is present. Occasionally, curettings will be scant due to a complete endometrial slough.

We have encountered two patients who did not respond to D & C. In both instances, bleeding was controlled by uterine packing. This was carried out using an Iodoform gauze that was left in place for 24 hours and then withdrawn slowly. Prophylactic antibiotic coverage should be given in this unusual situation. The only patient who required hysterectomy was a 20-year-old woman with artificial heart valves who was anticoagulated.

Close follow-up of these patients is essential to prevent recurrence and provide adequate emotional support. After the initial phase of therapy, the patient may remain anovulatory. It is therefore advisable to continue these patients on low-dose birth control pills for at least 3 months. The adolescent in need of birth control can be continued on low-dose oral contraceptives. When the risk of unwanted pregnancy is not a concern, the best approach is to have the patient use basal body temperature charts and to administer oral progestogens cyclically if the temperature curve is monophasic. A rational regimen is to induce withdrawal bleeding every 6 weeks with a 10-day course of 10 mg of medroxyprogesterone acetate (Provera) daily. This treatment is usually adequate to prevent endometrial hyperproliferation. Since it does not suppress the hypothalamic-pituitary-ovarian axis, it allows the teenager to develop regular, ovulatory cycles on her own. When this occurs, the patient may menstruate spontaneously between medroxyprogesterone acetate courses.

Long-term follow-up includes correction of anemia with iron supplements, nutritional counseling, and surveillance for spontaneous occurrence of ovulatory cycles. Those patients presenting with acute menorrhagia during the perimenarchal period are at greater risk of chronic anovulation, infertility, and endometrial carcinoma.

The emotional aspects of this problem should not be underestimated. For these youngsters, a hemorrhagic event of this type is a very sad way to begin their active reproductive life. Adequate explanation, reassurance, and psychological support during the acute episode and over the subsequent months will serve to guide these teenagers through their menstrual problems optimistically.

Persistent Hypermenorrhea.—Cyclic heavy menses is also a frequent complaint in adolescents. These patients usually present with more or less regular menstrual cycles, ranging from 4 to 6 weeks, but characterized by excessive bleeding, either in amount or duration.

Although anovulation is the leading etiology of recurrent hypermenorrhea in this population, other causes such as uterine pathologies, coagulation defects, and systemic diseases must be considered.

Besides a thorough history and physical examination, the basic workup of these teenagers should consist of hemoglobin, hematocrit, serum iron, and platelet count determinations, screening clotting studies, and thyroid function tests.

Therapy depends on the degree of the bleeding abnormality. Patients with mildly increased menstrual flow in whom there is no secondary anemia can be managed expectantly. Anemia and low serum iron should be treated adequately.

Prostaglandin inhibitors may also be used to decrease the amount of bleeding. Adolescents in need of birth control obviously benefit from oral contraception. When treatment is required because of the degree of the flow or associated anemia, medroxyprogesterone acetate is prescribed to regularize cycles and induce a progestational effect on the endometrium. In this situation, 10 mg of medroxyprogesterone acetate daily is administered from the 15th to the 25th day of each cycle. For most of these young patients, a calendar month schedule (treatment for the first 10 days of each month) is understood more easily. After 3 to 6 months, therapy is discontinued, and the patient is observed for spontaneous occurrence of ovulatory cycles. Failure of hormonal therapy is an indication for D & C.

Persistent Polymenorrhea.—The complaint of too frequent periods is also common among this age group. Anovulation, once again, is the most frequent cause of polymenorrhea in adolescents. In some patients, this menstrual abnormality may also originate from a short follicular phase or corpus luteum dysfunction, which usually is self-limiting until such time as the hypothalamic-pituitary-ovarian axis matures.

The physician should, however, be aware of the fact that very often this complaint is unjustified. A thorough history frequently brings to light that the patient calculates her intermenstrual interval from the last day of a period to the first day of the next one. The recording of a menstrual calendar and information about normal physiology are usually sufficient to reassure these adolescents.

When cycles are shorter than 21 days, therapy with medroxyprogesterone acetate administered as described earlier is indicated. With very short intermenstrual intervals, it may be necessary to start the treatment on the 10th day of the cycle for a period of 15 days.

Premenstrual Symptoms.—Premenstrual symptoms are commonly reported by adolescents and adult women and include bloating, weight gain, breast soreness, hunger, thirst, fatigue, acne, constipation, hot flashes and chills, difficulty with concentration, and mood change (irritability or mood change) in the luteal phase of the cycle. Girls with migraine headaches may suffer an increase in headaches premenstrually and with menses; similarly, girls with epilepsy may note an increase in seizure severity or frequency premenstrually or with the onset of menses. Mentally handicapped girls may have behavior outbursts that are difficult for their caretakers, and psychotic patients may exhibit more uncontrollable actions. Although most adolescents are aware of some premenstrual symptoms, reassurance and a few suggestions about diet and exercise are usually all that is needed. Adolescents who experience severe symptoms often are under stress and have other psychosocial issues that need to be addressed, not just with medical evaluation of the premenstrual symptoms but also with psychological counseling. About 20% to 40% of adult women of reproductive age have sufficiently bothersome symptoms to cause a temporary deterioration in interpersonal relationships or job effectiveness; less than 5% of adult women have severe symptoms.

The cause of premenstrual syndrome has been variously attributed to estrogen and progesterone levels because of the occurrence of these symptoms in the luteal phase of the cycle and the disappearance when ovulation is inhibited with the use of gonadotropin-releasing hormone (GnRH) agonists. Since weight may not increase in spite of bloating, changes that the patient notes may occur because of local fluid shifts and bowel wall edema. The release of the opiates may also increase appetite and result in unusual food cravings as well as fatigue, depression, and emotional lability. Later in the cycle, the shift toward anxiety and irritability, vague abdominal cramps with loose bowel movements or diarrhea, headaches, and chills and sweats may result from withdrawal of endogenous opiates as hormone levels fall. In sensitive women, cyclic exposure to, and subsequent withdrawal from, the central effects of the neuropeptides may result in a cascade of neuroendocrine changes and cause clinical symptoms.

In the next decade, therpaeutic approaches to premenstrual syndrome may be improved by increased understanding of the pathophysiology. Alteration of the ovulatory menstrual cycle can alleviate symptoms. The GnRH agonists can prevent the cyclic progesterone and estrogen production; however, this approach may be more useful as a probe in defining the etiology of the problem than as a long-term treatment because of the potential for osteoporosis in estrogen-deficient patients. Preventing ovulation but allowing some estrogen secretion might protect the bones from osteoporosis but would potentially place the endometrium at risk of unopposed estrogen and carcinoma. Danazol may inhibit ovulation but may have undesirable side effects in adolescents. Although oral contraceptives have given variable results in adult women with premenstrual syndrome, many adolescents, especially those with premenstrual exacerbation of seizures or headaches, show striking improvement on pills low in estrogen and progestin.

For most adolescents, premenstrual symptoms are mild, and the recognition that they are a real entity can be reassuring. For those troubled by their symptoms, the cyclic occurrence should be established by recording symptoms on a special calendar for two to three cycles. Otherwise, mood alterations and depression occurring throughout the cycle may be attributed to "premenstrual syndrome" and adequate psychological intervention not undertaken. A calendar is also useful in deciding which symptoms are most troubling to the patient. Although no controlled studies have demonstrated benefit from changes in diet or exercise, most centers start with this approach because the lifestyle changes are healthy and undoubtedly give the adolescent a sense of control over her life. Patients are instructed to avoid salty foods, alcohol, caffeine, chocolate, and concentrated sweets and to eat four to six smaller meals per day during the premenstrual period. A written sheet with foods to avoid (e.g., cola, coffee, hot dogs, canned foods, and chips) and to add to the diet (e.g., unsalted popcorn, raw vegetables and fruits, skim milk, complex carbohydrates, high-fiber foods, and low-fat meats) is helpful to the young woman. A program of aerobic exercise should be strongly encouraged, and areas of stress should be identified. Many patients experience an increased sense of well-being and control with this type of program.

In adolescents with specific symptoms, drug therapy may be considered after a period of intervention with diet and exercise and stress reduction. For indications such as edema and weight gain from fluid retention, a mild diuretic such as 250 to 500 mg of hydrochlorothiazide once or twice daily during the last week of the cycle (plus supplemental potassium by diet) or spironolactone can be prescribed. Starting on day 18 of the cycle, 250 mg of mefenamic acid (Ponstel) every 8 hours, increased to 500 mg on day 19 of the cycle, has been shown to improve fatigue, headache, and general aches and pains; this medication may be especially useful in those patients with severe dysmenorrhea as well. Other nonsteroidal anti-inflammatory drugs (NSAIDs) used in treating dys-

menorrhea may be similarly useful; none of these should be prescribed to the adolescent at risk of pregnancy. Oral contraceptives may be effective in adolescent girls and are especially useful if birth control is also needed.

A variety of other drugs have been used in adult women, but none of the studies have focused on adolescents. For example, low-dose danazol (200 mg/day) has appeared beneficial. Alprazolam (0.25 mg three times daily from day 20 until the second day of menstruation and then tapered by one tablet daily) relieved anxiety, but concern about patients becoming dependent on this drug and having withdrawal symptoms has made us reluctant to use this group of drugs in adolescents. Severe depressive reaction may be treated with fluoxetine (Prozac), 20 mg, one to three times daily. Bromocriptine has been used in adult women to alleviate breast soreness, but this symptom is rarely a major complaint of adolescents. In adolescents with breast soreness, we prefer to suggest reducing caffeine consumption and prescribing a small dose of NSAIDs. None of these medications should be prescribed to adolescents at risk of having unprotected intercourse. In addition, adolescents need to be questioned about whether they are taking over the counter medications. Vitaming B_6 has been popular with some self-help groups. In view of concern about the toxic potential of this vitamin even in low doses to cause sensory neuropathy, patients need to be cautioned about this indication.

Pelvic Pain

Dysmenorrhea.—Dysmenorrhea is probably the commonest gynecological complaint of adolescents. Most dysmenorrhea in adolescents is primary (or functional); however, it can be secondary to endometriosis, obstructing müllerian anomalies, and other pelvic pathology.

In typical histories, the 14- or 15-year-old teenager, 1 to 3 years after menarche, begins to develop crampy lower abdominal pain with each menstrual period. Usually the pains start within 1 to 4 hours of the onset of the menses and last for 24 to 28 hours. In some cases, the pain may start 1 to 2 days before the menses and continue for 2 to 4 days into the menses. Nausea or vomiting (or both), diarrhea, lower backache, thigh pain, headache, fatigue, nervousness, dizziness, or, rarely, syncope may accompany the cramps. Although dysmenorrhea is usually associated with the onset of ovulatory menses, some adolescents may experience cramps from the first few cycles (which are often anovulatory) or with episodes of anovulatory dysfunctional bleeding associated with heavy menses and clots.

In the uterus, phospholipids from the dead cell membranes are converted to arachidonic acid, which can be metabolized by at least two enzymes: lipoxygenase, which begins the production of leukotrienes, and cyclo-oxygenase, which leads to cyclic endoperoxides (prostaglandin G and prostaglandin H). The cyclic endoperoxides are then converted by specific enzymes to prostacyclin, thromboxanes, and the prostaglandins D_2, E_2 (PGE_2), and F_2 (PGF_2). Prostaglandin F_2 mediates pain sensation and stimulates smooth muscle contraction, whereas prostaglandin E potentiates platelet disaggregation and vasodilation. Exogenously administered PGE_2 and PGF_2 can produce uterine contractions as well as systemic symptoms such as vomiting, diarrhea, and dizziness. Although plasma levels of prostaglandin are normal in dysmenorrheic women, increased sensitivity or generalized overproduction of prostaglandins may occur.

The prostaglandin hypothesis has been further strengthened by the observation that drugs that inhibit prostaglandin synthesis could relieve dysmenorrhea and the associated symptoms. A number of clinical studies have found that NSAIDs are effective in the relief of pain. The NSAID agents are divided into two classes: carboxylic acids and enolic acids. Enolic acid agents include phenylbutazone and piroxicam and act by inhibition of the isomerase-reductase step in the production of PGE_2 and PGF_2. Phenylbutazone is not prescribed in dysmenorrhea because of side effects, and piroxicam requires further studies to delineate its role in the therapy of this problem. The carboxylates, most frequently used in the treatment of dysmenorrhea, can be divided into four categories: (1) salicylic acids and esters (e.g., aspirin and diflunisal), (2) acetic acids (e.g., indomethacin, sulindac, and tometin), (3) propionic acids (e.g., ibuprofen, naproxen, fenoprofen, ketoprofen, and flurbiprofen), and (4) fenamates (e.g., mefenamic acid, meclofenamate, tolfenamic acid, and flufenamic acid). The salicylic acids and esters appear to inhibit cyclo-oxygenase, but aspirin has little potency compared with some of the other NSAIDs in reducing prostaglandin synthesis and may increase menstrual flow. Thus, aspirin is used less often than previously in the treatment of dysmenorrhea. Indomethacin is the best

known drug of the acetic acid group for treating dysmenorrhea, but side effects have prevented its use for most, if not all, patients. Thus, the clinician selects chiefly from the two last groups, propionic acids and fenamates, for clinical treatment.

Ibuprofen and naproxen have been most widely studied for the relief of pain in dysmenorrhea. Numerous clinical studies have found these agents to be effective in both adults and adolescent women, with pain relief in 67% to 86% of patients. The sodium salt of naproxen (Anaprox) has a more rapid absorption than naproxen and can give very rapid relief of symptoms. The newly released prostaglandin inhibitor flurbiprofen (an NSAID), at doses of 50 mg every 6 hours or 100 mg every 12 hours, also appears to be very effective in the relief of dysmenorrhea.

The fenamates are potent inhibitors of prostaglandin synthesis and, in addition, can antagonize the action of already formed prostaglandins. This increased activity may give this class of drugs a theoretical advantage in treatment, although comparative controlled drug trials are not available for reaching a conclusion. A trial of mefenamic acid (Ponstel) is useful when propionic acids are ineffective in the individual patient.

Oral contraceptives lessen dysmenorrhea, probably in part related to their antiovulatory actions as well as their ability to produce endometrial hypoplasia, less menstrual flow, and subsequently, less prostaglandins.

In assessing the adolescent with dysmenorrhea, the physician needs to know the patient's menstrual history, timing of the cramps, and premenstrual symptoms, as well as her response to the cramps. Key questions would be: Is she missing school? If so, how many days? Does she miss other activities? A party? Does she have nausea and vomiting, diarrhea or dizziness? What medications has she used before? What is the nature of the mother-daughter interaction? Did the mother or sister have cramps? Is there a family history of endometriosis? The question about previous medications is particularly crucial because with the availability of ibuprofen over the counter, many adolescents have tried this medication, in subtherapeutic doses, and have subsequently discarded the usefulness of ibuprofen.

For the virginal girl of 13 or 14 years who has mild cramps on the first day of her menses, a normal physical examination, including inspection of the genitalia to exclude an abnormality of the hymen, is reassuring. It is not necessary to do a speculum examination. Treatment includes a careful explanation to the patient of the nature of the problem and a chance for her to ask questions regarding her anatomy. Mild analgesics, such as aspirin, acetaminophen, and especially over-the-counter ibuprofen (200–400 mg), usually give symptomatic relief.

Adolescent girls with moderate or severe dysmenorrhea should have a careful pelvic examination. In the majority of adolescents who are carefully prepared, a vaginal examination is atraumatic. In some patients, a rectoabdominal examination in the lithotomy position is all that is possible, but even this will exclude adnexal tenderness and masses. The uterosacral ligaments should be palpated carefully for tenderness or the presence of nodules, which would suggest endometriosis. Ultrasonography is useful in defining uterine and vaginal anomalies with obstruction.

If the examination is normal, treatment should be directed at symptomatic relief. The commonest approach is to prescribe one of the NSAID compounds: 550 mg of naproxen sodium (Anaprox) given immediately and then 275 mg every 6 hours, 550 mg of naproxen sodium double strength (Anaprox DS) twice daily, 250 to 375 mg of naproxen (Naprosyn) twice to three times daily, 400 mg of ibuprofen every 4 to 6 hours to 800 mg three times daily (with a loading dose of 800–1,200 mg), or 500 mg of mefenamic acid (Ponstel) given immediately and then 250 mg every 6 hours. As previously noted, flurbiprofen (50 mg every 6 hours or 100 mg two or three times daily) and meclofenamate (100 mg initially, followed by 50–100 mg every 6 hours) are also promising.

For most patients, effective relief can be obtained by starting the antiprostaglandin medicine at the onset of the menses and continuing it for the first 1 to 2 days of the cycle (or for the usual duration of cramps). The patient should be told to start as soon as she knows her menses are coming, that is, "at the first sign of cramps or bleeding." A loading dose is important in patients with symptoms that are severe and occur rapidly. In this situation, a rapidly absorbed drug such as naproxen sodium would be preferable to naproxen. Generally, giving the medication at the onset of the menses prevents the inadvertent administration of the drug to a pregnant women. However, a nonsexually active patient with severe cramps may sometimes benefit from starting the drug 1 or 2 days before the onset of her menses.

A patients may respond to one of these drugs and not another, and thus each should be tried in increasing doses before changing to another drug. In addition, since life stresses may lessen the effectiveness in an individual patient, the dosage should be based on the response in more than one cycle. Usually medication is prescribed for two to three cycles before changing. In addition, the patient may have taken inadequate doses of a medicine previously, particularly ibuprofen, to obtain relief.

The NSAID compounds should be avoided in patients with known or suspected ulcer disease, GI bleeding, clotting disorders (because of effects on platelet aggregation), renal disease, in preoperative patients, in those with allergies to aspirin or NSAIDs, and in those with aspirin-induced asthma. All of these drugs should be taken with food, even though some patients prefer liquids on the first day of the cycle. The side effects of these drugs appear minimal in short-term use, but the possibility of allergy and GI irritation and bleeding should be explained to the patient. Some patients complain of fluid retention or fatigue with these agents.

In some patients, NSAIDs are contraindicated or produce undesirable side effects. In these girls, acetaminophen can be prescribed, often combined with 15 to 30 mg of codeine. Usually only a few pills are needed each month. However, adolescents frequently complain of dizziness and nausea with codeine-containing medications.

The adolescent should be seen initially every 3 or 4 months to evaluate the effectiveness of the medication. Such visits also facilitate the physician-patient rapport that is essential in the treatment of this problem. Although a few adolescents will use cramps as an excuse to stay out of school or to gain sympathy from parents, patients should not be made to feel emotionally unstable because they complain of cramps. Some girls can continue to exercise during their menses; others find the discomfort may be too great on the first day. It is likely that girls who are involved in competitive sports and have fewer ovulatory menses have less dysmenorrhea.

If the patient fails to respond to the antiprostaglandin drugs and continues to have severe pain or vomiting or at initial evaluation needs birth control, a course of oral contraceptives (e.g., Norinyl 1+35, Ortho-Novum 1/35, Triphasil, TriLevelen, Tri-Norinyl, or Ortho Novum 7/7/7) should be tried. A pelvic examination is necessary before this medication is prescribed. Cramps are usually substantially, if not completely, relieved with the anovulatory cycles and scantier flow. If severe cramps persist despite three to four cycles of ovulation suppression therapy or the examination reveals tenderness or nodularity, laparoscopy is indicated to exclude endometriosis or other organic causes.

If dysmenorrhea is relieved by oral contraceptive pills, medication is usually prescribed for 3 to 6 months and then discontinued (frequently during the summer when school attendance will not be disrupted). Often the patient will continue to have relief from cramps for several additional (commonly anovulatory) cycles before the more severe dysmenorrhea recurs. When the cramps recur, a trial of other antiprostaglandin drugs should again be attempted before oral contraceptives are reinstituted. The sexually active adolescent with severe dysmenorrhea usually prefers to continue long term on oral contraceptives. The return of increasingly severe dysmenorrhea in spite of the use of oral contraceptives raises the possibility of organic disease such as endometriosis and calls for a reevaluation and consideration of laparoscopy for diagnosis.

Acute Pelvic Pain.—Acute pelvic pain necessitates aggressive management because of the intensity of symptoms and the possibility that a potentially life-threatening condition may exist.

The differential diagnosis of acute pelvic pain in adolescents is summarized in Table 20–7. The gynecological causes can be divided into three categories: (1) infection, (2) rupture, and (3) torsion. In general, symptoms associated with infection usually develop progressively over a few days. In cases of rupture or torsion, pain occurs suddenly, and the patient can most often tell precisely at what time symptoms began. Nongynecological etiologies involve primarily the digestive or urinary tract.

The history should define, as exactly as possible, the sequence of events, the pain location and its radiation, and associated GI tract, urinary tract, and systemic symptoms. A careful menstrual, contraceptive, and sexual history is also mandatory.

A complete physical examination should, of course, be performed. Special attention is paid to the abdomen to localize the pain and define the presence of and identify peritoneal signs and evi-

TABLE 20–7.

Differential Diagnosis of Acute Pelvic Pain in Adolescent Girls

---

I. Gynecological causes
  A. Infection
    1. Pelvic inflammatory disease
  B. Rupture
    1. Follicular cyst
    2. Corpus luteum cyst
    3. Endometrioma
    4. Tumor
  C. Torsion
    1. Ovarian cyst
    2. Tube
    3. Hydatid of Morgagni
II. Nongynecological causes
  A. Gastrointestinal
    1. Appendicitis
    2. Meckel's diverticulitis
    3. Gastroenteritis
    4. Mesenteric adenitis
    5. Intestinal obstruction
  B. Urinary
    1. Cystitis
    2. Pyelonephritis
    3. Calculi

---

dence of bowel obstruction. A pelvic examination must be performed on every patient to determine the uterine size, shape, and symmetry, to determine the presence of adnexal or cervical tenderness, and to identify adnexal masses or thickening.

The basic laboratory workup should include a complete blood cell count with differential, an erythrocyte sedimentation rate (ESR), a complete urinalysis, a urine culture, a pregnancy test, and a cervical culture for gonococcus and *Chlamydia*.

The finding of a high white blood cell count or high ESR suggests the presence of either an infectious or inflammatory process or ischemia, usually secondary to adnexal torsion or bowel obstruction. Hemoglobin and hematocrit values are usually poor indicators of bleeding, since in acute hemorrhage hemodilution may not have occurred. Depending on the type of pregnancy test used, it should be remembered that a negative result does not always rule out early intrauterine or an ectopic pregnancy.

A pelvic ultrasound may be valuable to confirm the presence of a mass when the pelvic examination is not completely satisfactory, to identify the presence of free fluid in the cul-de-sac, and to localize a suspected pregnancy.

After these first steps have been taken, all patients fall into one of the following categories:

1. There is a definite surgical emergency that necessitates immediate attention. In this situation, the suspected diagnosis is usually an acute hemoperitoneum, torsion of the adnexa, a ruptured tubo-ovarian abscess, acute appendicitis or ruptured appendix, or some other GI surgical emergency.
2. The patient is suffering from a medical condition, and adequate treatment is started (e.g., UTI, gastroenteritis, or PID).
3. The problem needs further investigation (e.g., urinary calculi).
4. The condition remains undiagnosed, and the question usually is, "Does this patient have a PID, an ectopic pregnancy, appendicitis, or a rupture or torsive ovarian cyst?"

At this point, laparoscopy becomes an invaluable diagnostic tool. The potential risk of a surgical diagnostic procedure remains a concern for many physicians. In fact, a laparoscopy provides an immediate diagnosis that allows for appropriate medical or surgical treatment. It is also more cost effective to perform an immediate laparoscopy than to subject the patient to a long period of inpatient observation during which a surgical catastrophe, such as a ruptured appendix or ectopic pregnancy, remains a possibility. In cases of ruptured ovarian cysts or hemorrhagic corpus luteum, in which there is no more active bleeding, it is possible to aspirate free blood and clots and ensure hemostasis by fulguration of bleeders. This technique may save the patient several days of agonizing pain and usually allows her to be discharged within 12 hours of the procedure.

In my judgment, the advantages of laparoscopy certainly outweigh the minimal surgical risk in these generally healthy teenagers, particularly where appendicitis is a real possibility.

Table 20–8 summarizes the principal laparoscopic diagnosis in 121 patients ages 11 to 17 years who presented at Boston Children's Hospital with acute abdominal pain between 1980 and 1986. In general, the commonest cause of pain was due to some complication of an ovarian cyst. It is of interest that the causes of acute abdominal pain in the adolescent do not appear to be age related (Table 20–9).

Chronic Pelvic Pain

Chronic pelvic pain (CPP) in adolescents is a frequent complaint and a source of frustration for the patient, her parents, and her physician. It can be defined as 3 months or more of constant or intermittent, cyclic or acyclic pelvic pain, which has necessitated at least three separate visits to a physician without a definite diagnosis. Symptoms can be characterized by dull or severe pain, dysmenorrhea, dyspareunia, or vaginal pain. Very often these teenagers have been absent from school frequently, have seen a number of physicians, have undergone a number of radiological examinations, and have tried a variety of analgesics without success. Many have already been referred for psychological or psychiatric evaluation.

The CPP patient, after having been told, often more than once, that nothing is wrong with her, may come to you with a considerable amount of anger, frustration, or desperation. It is, therefore, important to assure her that all efforts will be made to sort out her problem and that she will not be abandoned or her symptoms dismissed as merely psychosomatic.

Table 20–10 summarizes the differential diagnosis of CPP in adolescent girls. It includes many organ systems that can be responsible for pelvic symptoms either directly or by referred pain, as well as symptoms of functional or psychogenic etiology.

An efficient approach to the problem depends on taking a thorough history and perform-

TABLE 20–8.

Principal Laparoscopic Diagnoses in 121 Adolescent Girls 11 to 17 Years Old With Acute Pelvic Pain, Children's Hospital, Boston, 1980–1986

Diagnosis	Patients	
	n	%
Ovarian cyst	47	39
Acute PID	21	17
Adnexal torsion	9	8
Endometriosis	6	5
Ectopic pregnancy	4	3
Appendicitis	13	11
No pathology	21	17

TABLE 20–9.

Age-Related Prevalence of Principal Laparoscopic Findings in 121 Adolescent Girls 11 to 17 Years Old With Acute Pelvic Pain, Children's Hospital, Boston, 1980–1986

	Age 11–13 yr	Age 14–15 yr	Age 16–17 yr
	No. of Patients (%)	No. of Patients (%)	No. of Patients (%)
Ovarian cyst	12 (50)	16 (35)	19 (37)
Acute PID	4 (17)	7 (16)	10 (19)
Adnexal torsion	0 (0)	7 (16)	2 (4)
Endometriosis	0 (0)	2 (4)	4 (7)
Ectopic pregnancy	0 (0)	3 (7)	1 (2)
Appendicitis	3 (13)	4 (9)	6 (12)
No pathology	5 (20)	6 (13)	10 (19)
TOTAL	24 (20)	45 (37)	52 (43)

ing an adequate physical examination as well as using diagnostic studies judiciously.

It is essential to review the complete history of the problem, including description, location, and radiation of the pain, exacerbating and relieving factors, association with the menstrual cycle,

TABLE 20–10.

Differential Diagnosis of Chronic Pelvic Pain in Adolescent Girls

I. Gynecological causes
  A. Dysmenorrhea (primary, secondary)
  B. Mittelschmerz
  C. Endometriosis
  D. Chronic pelvic inflammatory disease
  E. Ovarian cyst
  F. Genital tract malformations
  G. Pelvic congestion
  H. Pelvic serositis
II. Gastrointestinal causes
  A. Constipation, bowel spasms
  B. Appendiceal fecaliths
  C. Bowel inflammatory diseases
  D. Dietary intolerance (lactose)
III. Urinary causes
  A. Urinary tract infection
  B. Hydronephrosis
  C. Urethral stricture
  D. Urethral caruncle
  E. Urinary retention
IV. Orthopedic causes
  A. Lordosis, kyphosis, scoliosis
  B. Herniation of intervertebral disk
V. Adhesions
  A. Postoperative
  B. Post pelvic infection
VI. Psychogenic

and GI, urinary, and musculoskeletal symptoms. The past medical and surgical history may also provide a clue. All prior diagnostic procedures and trials of treatment should be recorded and, when possible, old medical records obtained. The familial and social history, as well as the association of the pain episodes with stressful events, should be detailed.

A complete physical examination should be performed, the abdomen being carefully palpated in search of any masses, tender areas, and organomegaly. Special care should be taken to differentiate deep pain from abdominal wall tenderness, especially in patients who have undergone prior surgeries, in whom adhesions to the abdominal wall scar may be present. A skeletal assessment to identify any orthopedic abnormality that may be the cause of referred pelvic pain or associated with a congenital reproductive tract anomaly is also of great importance. A speculum examination should be performed to identify any vaginal or cervical anomaly and obtain culture and cytology specimens. The bimanual rectovaginal-abdominal palpation evaluates the pelvic structures and localizes tender areas. The posterior cul-de-sac should also be assessed for tenderness and nodularity.

The minimal laboratory workup in these patients consists of a complete blood cell count with differential and ESR, a urine analysis and culture, and cervical cultures for gonococcus and *Chlamydia*. Other hematological and biochemical studies are ordered depending on clinical indications.

Pelvic ultrasonography may be useful to define a mass, provide information about a suspected genital tract malformation, and to screen patients in whom a satisfactory pelvic examination is impossible. Routine sonography in every patient is probably not advisable. It is not uncommon to see patients who have a pelvic mass detected by ultrasound or CT scan for which there is no evidence of on laparoscopy.

No specific rules can be given regarding radiological examination. It is certainly not advisable to submit all of these teenagers to pelvic radiation without clinical indications. Gastrointestinal, urological, and orthopedic studies should be ordered on the basis of the diagnostic impression after a thorough history and physical and laboratory workup are completed.

Laparoscopy is an invaluable tool in the diagnosis of CPP. It can be used to diagnose or confirm the presence of organic disease that cannot be demonstrated by physical, radiological, and sonographic examination. It allows one to obtain appropriate biopsies and to perform some primary therapy such as fulguration of endometriosis, lysis of adhesions, and aspiration of ovarian cysts. Normal findings at laparoscopy may be equally valuable in reassuring the patient that no organic disease is present and help her accept the idea that she might have a functional problem that requires medical or emotional treatment.

Indications for laparoscopy in the evaluation of adolescents with CPP can be summarized as follows:

1. Dysmenorrhea unresponsive to the usual therapy with prostaglandin inhibitors or ovulation suppression
2. Confirmation or exclusion of clinically suspected endometriosis, chronic PID, pelvic adhesions, appendiceal fecaliths, ovarian cyst, and pelvic serositis
3. Evaluation of undiagnosed pain after appropriate workup

At our clinic, experience with laparoscopy in the diagnosis of CPP in adolescent girls revealed that between July 1974 and December 1983, 282 patients ranging in age from 9 to 21 years underwent a diagnostic laparoscopy because of chronic pelvic symptoms. Most of these adolescents have been referred to our gynecology service after normal GI and urinary tract workup or because of dysmenorrhea unresponsive to the usual therapy with prostaglandin inhibitors or oral contraceptives. Many of these patients had undergone psychiatric evaluation because of persistent and undi-

agnosed pain. Cases of chronic PID were not included in the data because this condition is usually suspected on the basis of the past history and the finding of an elevated ESR. In these patients, a laparoscopy is usually performed to confirm the diagnosis and evaluate its severity rather than to establish the etiology of CPP.

All laparoscopies were performed under general endotracheal anesthesia on either an inpatient or ambulatory basis. A uterine mobilizer was attached to the cervix to permit mobilization of the uterus. Approximately 2 L of CO_2 was used to create a pneumoperitoneum, and a 7-mm Wolf or Stortz laparoscope was introduced through an infraumbilical incision. A second trocar site was established in the suprapubic area to allow the use of a probe or biopsy forceps.

Table 20–11 summarizes the postoperative diagnoses in these patients. Three fourths of the patients were found to have intrapelvic pathology. Endometriosis was the most frequent finding, being diagnosed in 45% of cases. In most instances, the disease was mild to moderate, with implants located in the posterior cul-de-sac, on the ovaries, and on the lateral pelvic side walls. The next commonest finding was postoperative adhesions, present in 13% of patients and, for the most part, secondary to appendectomy or ovarian cystectomy.

One of the most puzzling laparoscopic findings was the present of pelvic serositis in 5% of the patients, characterized by hyperemia and granuloma-like lesions of the pelvic peritoneum and uterine serosa. Peritoneal biopsy specimens revealed the presence of mesothelial hyperplasia with hemosiderin deposits. Peritoneal culture and

TABLE 20–11.

Postoperative Diagnoses in 282 Adolescent Girls With Chronic Pelvic Pain, Children's Hospital, Boston, 1974–1983

	Patients	
	n	%
Endometriosis	126	45
Postoperative adhesions	37	13
Serositis	15	5
Ovarian cyst	14	5
Uterine malformation	15	5
Others*	4	2
No pathology	71	25

*Ileitis, infarcted hydatid of Morgagni, or pelvic congestion.

cytology findings were normal. The significance of these changes remains unclear. Is it the appearance of very early endometriosis, a reaction to repeated hemoperitoneum secondary to leaking corpus luteum or hemoperitoneum, a viral infection, or an incidental finding? These patients are very difficult to treat. Due to the small number of cases, no uniform therapy has emerged. Some patients respond to therapy with long-term prostaglandin inhibitors, others to ovulation suppression, and others to steroid. Long-term follow-up will hopefully better define this entity. A few patients with this finding have since developed endometriosis, confirmed at subsequent laparoscopy.

Other findings included ovarian cysts, uterine malformations of the obstructive types, and cases of ileitis, infarcted hydatid of Morgagni, and pelvic congestion.

No organic disease was documented in 25% of the patients. In this group, pain was attributed to functional bowel disease or to psychogenic factors. Despite apparently normal bowel function, many teenagers with CPP improve when placed on a regimen of stool softeners and increased dietary fiber and fluid intake. The value of a normal laparoscopy should not be underestimated. In many instances, the assurance that their pelvic structures are normal is sufficient to improve the symptoms in these adolescents. A significant number of these patients were symptomatically improved after a normal laparoscopy. In a small number of these teenagers, adjunctive psychological or behavioral modification therapy is necessary.

For the years 1980 to 1983, the results were broken down into age groups (Table 20–12). It is interesting to note that the incidence of endometriosis among adolescents complaining of CPP increased progressively with age, from 12% in the 11- to 13-year-old group to 54% in patients aged 20 to 21 years. Pelvic serositis, on the other hand, was encountered in primarily the 11- to 15-year-old group. Other findings remained fairly constant in all age groups.

Acute and chronic pelvic pain in the adolescent patient needs to be taken seriously. In a vast majority of cases, an underlying cause can be identified. Under no circumstances should the label of psychogenic pain be offered on these teenagers without prior normal laparoscopy. Adequate diagnosis and early therapy are essential to improve the quality of life and preserve the reproductive prognosis in these young patients.

Tumors and Related Disorders

In Utero Exposure to Diethylstilbestrol

During the 1950s and early 1960s, DES and other nonsteroidal estrogens were given to pregnant women with the aim of preventing miscarriages. In 1971, Herbst et al. reported an association between maternal DES and the later development of clear cell adenocarcinoma of the vagina and cervix in female offspring. Somewhat later, the presence of glandular (columnar) epithelium of müllerian origin in the vaginal wall (normally stratified squamous epithelium), was described in 36% to 90% of exposed young women. Although adenosis is a benign lesion, the proximity of areas of adenosis to adenocarcinoma in several patients has necessitated the follow-up of all patients with DES exposure.

The number of exposed young women is es-

TABLE 20–12.

Age-Related Incidence of Laparoscopic Findings in 129 Adolescent Girls With Chronic Pelvic Pain, Children's Hospital, Boston, 1980–1983

	Age 11–13 yr	Age 14–15 yr	Age 16–17 yr	Age 18–19 yr	Age 20–21 yr
	No. of Patients (%)	No. of Patients (%)	No. of Patients (%)	No. of Patients (%)	No. of Patients (%)
Endometriosis	2 (12)	9 (28)	21 (40)	17 (45)	7 (54)
Postoperative adhesions	1 (6)	4 (13)	7 (13)	5 (13)	2 (15)
Serositis	5 (29)	4 (13)	0 (0)	2 (5)	0 (0)
Ovarian cyst	2 (12)	2 (6)	3 (5)	2 (5)	0 (8)
Uterine malformation	1 (6)	0 (0)	1 (2)	0 (0)	1 (0)
Others	0 (0)	1 (3)	2 (4)	1 (3)	0 (0)
No pathology	6 (35)	12 (37)	19 (36)	11 (29)	6 (23)

timated to range from at least several hundred thousands to perhaps several million. Reliable histories are often difficult to obtain, and thus all patients (prepubertal and postpubertal) who have abnormal bleeding should have a vaginal examination regardless of history. What should the general physician do?

1. Determine the maternal drug history of all patients.
2. Refer for gynecological examination at menarche or age 14 years all patients with a known maternal history of any amount of DES or other nonsteroidal estrogen.
3. Be available for counseling and discussion of the importance of gynecological follow-up.

The last point is particularly important because it is not unusual for mothers to feel extremely guilty about having taken the medication. Some desire to have their daughters checked under some other pretext. The adolescent girl may express great anger toward her mother in making her body imperfect. However, in general, it is much less destructive to a teenager to deal with these issues openly rather than allowing the physician and mother to have a "secret." Although mothers and daughters are usually seeking reassurance that the vagina is "clean," the high frequency of adenosis indicates that this is not possible. Although the carcinoma risk is minimal (probably less than 4 per 1,000) the long-term risk of the presence of adenosis is unknown.

What constitutes the gynecological examination of the teenager exposed in utero to DES?

1. Careful palpation of the vagina
2. Speculum examination with Papanicolaou smear and Schiller's stain of the vagina
3. Biopsies as indicated by the Schiller's stain

If colposcopy is available, follow-up is greatly facilitated. Colposcopy allows the whole spectrum of atypia, dysplasia, and carcinoma to be identified. Photos should be taken and then reviewed at subsequent visits. Colposcopy detects more cases of adenosis (80%–90%) than visual examination (less than 30%) or Schiller's stains (40%–80%).

Clear Cell Carcinoma.—Although sporadic cases of clear cell adenocarcinoma of the cervix and less commonly vagina had been reported prior to the 1960s, the incidence has dramatically risen since 1966 and correlates well with use of DES therapy for problem pregnancies. In all cases, nonsteroidal estrogens were started prior to the 18th week of pregnancy.

At the time of diagnosis, patients present most commonly with bleeding or discharge, but some are asymptomatic. Several of these asymptomatic patients are found to have cancer on routine examination done solely because of a positive maternal history; all of these patients are now living.

The average age at diagnosis was late teens. Occasional cases have occurred in prepubertal girls, but all had symptoms of bleeding for weeks to months prior to the diagnosis.

The current recommendation for therapy of stage I and II tumors is radical hysterectomy. Metastatic disease is common and implies a poor prognosis.

Benign Adenosis.—In contrast to the rare occurrence of adenocarcinoma, adenosis is a common finding in young women exposed in utero to DES, reported in 36% to 90% of patients. Adenosis is the presence of glandular epithelium of müllerian origin (similar to endocervix and endometrium) in the vaginal wall. Exposure to DES appears to have interfered with normal differentiation and development of the cervix and vagina. Several typical gross lesions have been described, including (1) vaginal hood, a circular fold that partially covers the cervix; (2) cockscomb appearance of the cervix, an irregular peak on the anterior border of the cervix; and (3) erythroplakia, reddish areas that may give the cervix or vagina a strawberry appearance.

The observation that adenosis is commonly found adjacent to foci of clear cell adenocarcinoma necessitates careful follow-up of this lesion. No form of treatment for adenosis has been determined, although there is good evidence that spontaneous healing occurs. At this time the most prudent course is follow-up examinations every 6 to 12 months.

Adnexal Masses

Over the past decade, gynecologists have been consulted more frequently for the problem with ovarian masses during childhood and adolescence. The true incidence of this condition has probably not changed, but the increasing use of ultrasound by pediatricians and family practitioners has led to the detection of many functional cysts previously undetected. Even though most of these masses are functional and require only reassurance, it is imperative that true ovarian neoplasms receive immediate attention and therapy. It is, therefore, important that gynecologists feel comfortable in the evaluation of a child or teenager with an adnexal mass.

The differential diagnosis of adnexal masses includes enlargement of other reproductive structures as well as masses of extragenital origin.

All types of ovarian tumors seen in the adult can also be encountered in children and adolescents. The relative incidence of each entity is quite different, however. For example, functional masses are much more frequent in the adolescent because of the high incidence of anovulatory cycles. In this age group, neoplastic tumors are more likely to be of germinal than epithelial origin.

Fortunately, in children and adolescents, only 1 in 10 ovarian tumors is malignant. It is difficult to obtain accurate statistics regarding the frequency of functional cyscts because most studies are based on surgical reviews. Since a large number of patients with functional adnexal enlargement are treated expectantly and never undergo surgery, they are not included in pubished series.

Studies at our clinic of 242 children and adolescents operated on for ovarian masses revealed that 31% were found to have a tumor-like condition, including follicle, corpus luteum, and simple and endometriotic cysts (Table 20–13). Of the 166 cases of primary ovarian tumors, there were 118 (71%) germ cell tumors, of which 78 (66%) consisted of benign mature teratoma. Of 27 epithelial tumors, 85% were benign. Twenty one (13%) of the patients had sex cord–stromal tumors, which are generally considered low-grade malignancies. These results are comparable to other similar reports.

A considerable number of ovarian tumors are asymptomatic and are discovered fortuitously during a routine pelvic examination. Since most young patients do not consult for periodic pelvic examinations, ovarian masses are often picked up when they become large enough to cause symptoms or to be felt by abdominal palpation. Smaller ovarian enlargements are frequently incidental ultrasonographic findings at the time of an examination performed for unrelated symptoms

such as pain. This accounts for a large number of consultations for masses that prove to be physiological.

Symptoms are usually related to the size of the mass or to mechanical accidents such as rupture, torsion, or hemorrhage. In the young prepubertal girl, pain is abdominal because of the reduced pelvic capacity and the fairly high position of the ovaries. In the older patient, symptoms are more often pelvic. Bladder and ureteral compression may also be encountered with larger masses. Malignant tumors that infiltrate the surrounding tissue may induce bowel obstruction. In cases of mechanical accidents, symptoms develop acutely and are usually characterized by severe pain and peritoneal signs, including nausea and vomiting. In hormone-producing tumors, precocious puberty, menstrual irregularities, or virilization may lead to the diagnosis.

On pelvic examination, the mass can usually be palpated by rectoabdominal examination with the patient in the lithotomy position. As men-

TABLE 20–13.

Pathological Diagnoses of 242 Ovarian Tumors Treated Surgically at Children's Hospital, Boston, 1928–1982*

	No. (%)
Tumor-like enlargements	76 (31)
Primary ovarian tumors	166 (69)
Germ cell tumors	
Mature teratoma	78
Immature teratoma	17
Endodermal sinus tumor	14
Dysgerminoma	8
Choriocarcinoma	1
Total	118 (71)
Epithelial tumors	
Serous	14
Mucinous	12
Mixed	1
Total	27 (16)
Sex cord–stromal tumors	
Granulosa	10
Sertoli-Leydig	7
Thecoma	2
Fibroma	1
Unclassified	1
Total	21 (13)
TOTAL	166 (69)

*Adapted from Lack EE, Goldstein DP: Primary ovarian tumors in childhood and adolescence. *Curr Probl Obstet Gynecol,* vol 7, no. 10, June 1984.

tioned previously, ovarian tumors in children are often intra-abdominal rather than pelvic and should be considered in the differential diagnosis of abdominal masses. Other physical findings depend on the degree of invasion of the tumor and its hormonal activity.

Ultrasound is an invaluable tool in the diagnosis of ovarian masses. It provides information about the size and location and consistency of the tumor (i.e., whether it is cystic, solid or complex). Ultrasound is also useful to determine the presence of free peritoneal fluid and ascites. A flat plate of the abdomen reveals the presence of calcifications, which suggest a diagnosis of dermoid cyst. This information can, however, also be obtained by ultrasonography.

The remainder of the workup depends on the clinical picture. In the presence of a solid or hormonally active tumor, blood should be drawn for hCG, α-fetoprotein, CA-125, and estradiol values. Follicle-stimulating hormone and LH levels may help to differentiate a true precocious puberty responsible for a functional cyst from an estrogen-secreting tumor inducing a pseudoprecocious puberty. When hirsutism or signs of virilization are present, a testosterone level should be obtained. When malignancy is suspected, a preoperative metastatic workup, including chest x-ray film, CT scan of brain, chest, and abdomen, and liver function tests, should be done.

In the postmenarchal patient, ovarian masses are approached quite similarly as in the young adult. On the finding of an ovarian mass, ultrasound should be obtained to confirm the diagnosis and further define the tumor's characteristics. Due to the high incidence of functional masses, an asymptomatic, purely cystic tumor with a diameter of 6 cm or less is observed for two or three cycles for spontaneous regression. In these patients, the use of oral contraceptives to inhibit ovarian function may accelerate regression and prevent the appearance of new functional enlargement. Cystic masses that do not decrease in size over a period of 3 months, enlarge, or are larger than 6 cm initially, should be operated on. A laparoscopy may be performed prior to laparotomy to confirm the diagnosis. When the cyst appears to be functional and is less than 6 cm in diameter, puncture-aspiration may be performed. All fluid obtained should be sent for cytological examination.

Solid and complex tumors should be removed without delay. A laparoscopy may be performed as the initial procedure to establish the diagnosis, help to decide on the optimal incision, and in cases of unexpected malignancy, allow the surgeon to discuss the extensiveness of the proposed surgery with the parents.

Laparotomy should be performed through an incision large enough to allow excision of the tumor without rupture and according to the principles of ovarian surgery (i.e., peritoneal lavage, complete abdominal exploration, frozen section, and periaortic node dissection when indicated).

Breast Masses

The majority of adolescents who present to the physician's office with a complaint of a "breast lump" have normal physiological breast tissue or fibrocystic changes. Adolescents typically have very dense breast tissue. Fibrocystic "changes" are characterized by diffuse cordlike thickening and lumps that may become tender and enlarged prior to menses each month. Physical findings tend to change each month, so that suspected cysts can often be followed clinically.

In contrast to the finding that most breast

TABLE 20–14.

Pathological Diagnoses of 100 Breast Biopsy Specimens

	No. (%)
Fibroadenoma	
Adult	58
Juvenile	19
Giant	2
Cellular	2
Papillary	1
Fibroadenoma with mixed stroma	1
TOTAL	83 (83)
Fibrocystic mastopathy	
Fibrocystic disease	4
Simple cyst	2
Fibrocystic mastopathy	1
Stromal sclerosis	1
TOTAL	8 (8)
Other	
Chronic mastitis	2
Epidermal inclusion cyst	1
Adenomatous hyperplasia	1
Intraductal hyperplasia with focal secretion	1
Capillary hemangioma	1
Fat necrosis	1
Normal fat and breast tissue	1
TOTAL	9 (9)

lumps seen in the office setting in adolescents are normal or simply fibrocystic changes, most breast masses that are excised in this age group are fibroadenomas (Table 20–14). These lesions are typically firm or rubbery, mobile, and usually have a clearly defined edge. They tend to be eccentric in position and occur more frequently in the lateral breast quadrants than the medial quadrant. The breast mass may remain unchanged or may increase in size with subsequent menstrual cycles. Recurrent or multiple fibroadenomas may occur. Giant fibroadenomas may replace most of the breast tissue and, in fact, are often mistaken initially for normal tissue.

Cancer of the breast is extremely rare in children and adolescents. Primary lymphoma may also present as a breast mass in adolescents. Patients with previous radiation therapy to the chest have an increased risk of developing cancer of the breast at a young age and, therefore, require careful ongoing surveillance. Cystosarcoma phylloides is a rare primary tumor that is sometimes malignant.

A new entity, juvenile papillomatosis, is a rare breast tumor of young women first described in 1980. The tumor features atypical papillary duct hyperplasia and multiple cysts. The mean age of the patient is 23 years, with a range of 12 to 48 years. The localized tumor is often initially mistaken for a fibroadenoma. Twenty-eight percent of the patients have a relative with breast cancer, and 7% have a first-degree relative with breast cancer. A small number of patients have breast cancer diagnosed concurrently with juvenile papillomatosis, and several patients develop cancer at follow-up. Bilateral juvenile papillomatosis may especially increase the risk of later developing cancer. Thus, careful surveillance is indicated in patients with this diagnosis found on excisional biopsy. Papillary hyperplasia without the cystic component of juvenile papillomatosis appears to be a more benign condition in young patients.

If the adolescent presents with the complaint of a breast mass, palpation may make the diagnosis evident in cases such as fibrocystic changes or tenderness with overlying erythema consistent with a breast infection. Trauma may cause a breast mass, but examination immediately following a contusion may locate a preexisting lesion. If the differential diagnosis is a cyst or fibroadenoma, the lesion can be measured and the patient

instructed to return after her next menstrual period. If the lesion has disappeared, a cyst was probably present. If the lesion is still present and the patient is cooperative, a needle aspiration of the mass can be performed in the office using a 23-gauge needle on a 3-ml syringe. (A small amount of lidocaine (Xylocaine] can be used to infiltrate the skin with a 25-gauge needle.) A cyst can be aspirated, whereas a fibroadenoma gives a characteristic gritty, solid sensation. Any material obtained (even if just on the tip of the needle) should be smeared on a ground glass slide and sent in Papanicolaou fixative for cytology examination. If the mass collapses after aspiration, it is assumed to be a cyst, and the mass is reevaluated in 3 months. Ultrasound of the breast tissue can also be helpful in delineating a fibroadenoma from a cyst and can be used in localizing an abscess. Mammography should not be used to evaluate breast masses in the adolescent age group since the breast tissue is very dense, the risk of the patient having carcinoma is negligible, and radiographic features have not influenced clinical management.

When aspiration of a persistent, discrete mass is not feasible or is nonproductive, or when masses are nonmobile and hard, enlarging, tender, or a source of considerable anxiety, the patient should have an excisional biopsy done. Unless there are underlying medical conditions, such as cardiac or pulmonary disease, an excisional biopsy can be done in an ambulatory setting under general or local anesthesia, depending on technical considerations and the patient's preference and ability to cooperate. Since breast scars can be cosmetically deforming, the optimal incision for a lesion near the center of the breast is a radial incision, in terms of wound healing and cosmetic results. Periareolar ectopic lobules (Montgomery's cysts), which often have clear or dark discharge from the areola (not the nipple), can be excised with a circumareolar incision.

Contusion.—A contusion to the breast may result in a poorly defined, tender mass that resolves over several weeks. A mass from severe trauma may take several months to resolve, and, occasionally, scar tissue remains palpable indefinitely. Fat necrosis may also result from trauma, although the patient may not notice the growing lesion until several months later. Biopsy is frequently indicated in such circumstances. It should be remembered that the examination immediately following trauma to the breast may locate a preexisting lesion. A sharply delineated, nontender mass is probably unrelated to the recent injury.

BIBLIOGRAPHY

Boley SJ: Lesions of the breast, in Holder TW, Ashcroft KW (eds): *Pediatric Surgery.* Philadelphia, WB Saunders Co, 1980, pp 1080–1087.

Bongiovanni AM (ed): *Adolescent Gynecology: A Guide for Clinicians.* New York, Plenum Publishing Corp, 1982.

Cali RW, Pratt JH: Congenital absence of the vagina. *Am J Obstet Gynecol* 1968; 100:752.

Capraro VJ, Dillon WP, Gallego MB: Microperforate hymen; a distinct clinical entity. *Obstet Gynecol* 1974; 44:903.

Capraro VJ: Gynecologic examination in children and adolescents. *Pediatr Clin North Am* 1972; 19:511.

Carson SA: Gynecologic problems of adolescence and puberty, in Sciarra JJ (ed): *Gynecology and Obstetrics.* Philadelphia, JB Lippincott Co, 1984, vol 1, Chapter 43.

Chisholm TC: Exstrophy of the urinary bladder, in Holder TW, Ashcroft KW (ed): *Pediatric Surgery.* Philadelphia, WB Saunders Co, 1980, pp 738–751.

Christensen EH, Oster J: Adhesions of labia minora (synechia vulvae) in childhood; a review and report of fourteen cases. *Acta Paediatr Scand* 1971; 60:709.

Claessons EA, Cowell CA: Acute adolescent menorrhagia. *Am Obstet Gynecol* 1981; 193:377.

Counseller VS, Davis CE: Atresia of the vagina. *Obstet Gynecol* 1968; 32:528.

Dewhurst CJ: *Practical Pediatric and Adolescent Gynecology.* New York, Marcel Dekker, 1980.

Donahue PK, Hendren WH: Intersex abnormalities in the newborn infant, in Holder TM, Ashcroft KW (Eds): *Pediatric Surgery.* Philadelphia, WB Saunders Co, 1980, pp 858–890.

Emans SJH, Goldstein DP: *Pediatric and Adolescent Gynecology,* ed 2. Boston, Little, Brown & Co, 1982.

Gantt PA, McDonough PG: Dysfunctional bleeding in adolescents, in Barwin BN, Belish S (eds): *Adolescent Gynecology and Sexuality.* New York, Masson, 1982, p 59.

Goldstein DP: Female genital tract, in Welch KJ (ed): *Complications of Pediatric Surgery.* Philadelphia, WB Saunders Co, 1982, pp 372–384.

Goldstein DP, DeCholnoky C, Emans SJ, et al: Laparoscopy in the diagnosis and management of pelvic pain in adolescents. *J Reprod Med* 1980; 24:251.

Heald FP (ed): *Adolescent Gynecology.* Baltimore, Williams & Wilkins Co, 1966.

Hebeler JR: The abused child, in Holder TW, Ashcroft KW (eds): *Pediatric Surgery.* Philadelphia, WB Saunders Co, 1980, pp 738–751.

Hein K, Dell R, Caten M: Self-detection of a breast mass in adolescent females. *J Adolesc Health Care* 1982; 3:15.

Herbst A: Clear cell adenocarcinoma of the vagina and cervix: Analysis of 170 registry cases. *Am J Obstet Gynecol* 1974; 119:713.

Herbst A: A prospective comparison of exposed female offspring with unexposed controls. *N Engl J Med* 1975; 292:334.

Herbst A, Ulfelder HJ, Poskanzer CP: Adenocarcinoma of the vagina. *N Engl J Med* 1971; 284:878.

Huffman JW, Dewhurst CJ, Capraro VJ: *The Gynecology of Childhood and Adolescence,* ed 2. Philadelphia, WB Saunders Co, 1981.

Jirasek JE: Normal sex differentiation, in Sciarra JJ (ed): *Gynecology and Obstetrics.* Philadelphia, JB Lippincott Co, 198 , vol 5, p 770.

Jones HW Jr, Hellen RH: *Pediatric and Adolescent Gynecology.* Baltimore, Williams & Wilkins Co, 1966.

Kreutner AKK, Hollingsworth DR: *Adolescent Obstetrics and Gynecology.* Chicago, Year Book Medical Publishers, 1978.

Koff AK: Development of the vagina in the human fetus. *Contrib Embryol* 1933; 24:59.

Lack EE, Goldstein DP: Primary ovarian tumors in childhood and adolescence. *Curr Probl Obstet Gynecol,* vol 7, no. 4, June 1984.

McGregor JA: Toxic shock syndrome, in Sciarra JJ (ed): *Gynecology and Obstetrics.* Philadelphia, JB Lippincott Co, 1988, vol 1, Chapter 43.

McIndoe A: Treatment of congenital absences and obliterative conditions of the vagina. *Br J Plast Surg* 1950; 2:254.

Muckle CW: Developmental abnormalities of the female reproductive organs, in Sciarra JJ (ed): *Gynecology and Obstetrics,* Philadelphia, JB Lippincott Co, 1988, vol 1, p 4.

Oberman HA: Breast lesions in the adolescent female. *Pathol Annu* 1979; 14:175.

Ramenofsky ML: Vaginal lesions, in Holder TM, Ashcroft KW (eds): *Pediatric Surgery.* Philadelphia, WB Saunders Co, 1980, pp 94–101.

Ravnikar VA: Endocrine disorders, in Kistner RW (ed): *Gynecology—Principles and Practice,* ed 4. Chicago, Year Book Medical Publishers, 1985, pp 525–549.

Reindollar RH, Byrd JR, McDonough PC: Delayed sexual development: A study of 252 patients. *Am J Obstet Gynecol* 1981; 140:371–380.

Rock JA: Surgical correction of uterovaginal anomalies, in Sciarra JJ (ed): *Gynecology and Obstetrics*. Philadelphia, JB Lippincott Co, 1984, vol 1, Chapter 70.

Stone SC: Physiology of puberty, in Sciarra JJ (ed): *Gynecology and Obstetrics*. Philadelphia, JB Lippincott Co, 1984, vol 5, Chapter 9.

21 _____ Pelvic Sonography

Beryl R. Benacerraf, M.D.

During the past several years, pelvic sonography has become an important factor in the armamentarium of gynecologists in evaluating the female pelvis. Sonography is commonly the first test ordered for assessing a wide variety of clinical problems, and the commonest indications for gynecologic ultrasound include (1) pelvic pain, (2) abnormal vaginal bleeding, (3) palpable mass, (4) infertility, (5) possible ectopic pregnancy, and (6) follow-up study on known fibroids or adnexal pathology. Recently, technological advances have improved pelvic sonography, and increasing resolution has made the diagnoses more reliable. In addition, the advent of the transvaginal probe has further enhanced our ability to detect pelvic pathology noninvasively. Sonography remains superior to any other radiologic modality for the evaluation of a gynecologic patient.

PREPARATION OF THE PATIENT

Sonography is a tomographic technique that visualizes thin slices of anatomy in a given imaging plane, depending on where the transducer is aimed. Multiple sections of the pelvis are needed, therefore, both transversely and longitudinally, for a complete examination. A full bladder is necessary so that gas-filled bowel can be displaced away from the pelvis, since ultrasound cannot penetrate air. Furthermore, the bladder is then juxtaposed against the pelvic organs, creating the best visibility since the fluid-filled bladder enhances sound transmission.

It is possible, however, to overfill the bladder and compress the uterus and ovaries too much. One can, therefore, manipulate the bladder so that if it is too full, it can be partially emptied or, if not full enough, it can be filled.

Even in some situations the pelvis can be better examined with only a small amount of fluid in the bladder; this is helpful in the examination of the endometrial echo or the localization of an intrauterine device (IUD) in an anteverted uterus (Carroll and Gombergh, 1987).

The use of the vaginal probe requires that the bladder be empty so that the pelvic organs can descend in close proximity to the probe. The probe can then be rotated side to side to evaluate the entire lower pelvis tomographically.

THE UTERUS

Normal Anatomy

The uterus should be the first organ identified in a pelvic sonogram and is usually centrally located (Fig 21–1). It appears as a pear-shaped structure on longitudinal scan, just behind the urinary bladder, and contains a midline echogenic stripe depicting the endometrial cavity (Fig 21–2). In transverse section, the uterus is round, homogeneous in texture, and contains a central echogenic dot, which is the endometrial cavity in cross section. The cervix is seen as the lowest extent and narrowest portion of the uterus inferiorly, and the endocervical canal often contains echolucent material representing mucus. The anteverted uterus is most easily seen transabdominally, even with only a partially full bladder; however, the retroverted uterus can be very difficult to see since it extends away from the ultrasound beam (Fig 21–3). The fundus of the uterus may have a hypoechoic texture when the uterus is retroverted due to lack of penetration of sound deep in the pelvis. Transvaginal sonography is extremely useful for the evaluation of the retroverted uterus, since fibroids can inadvertently be

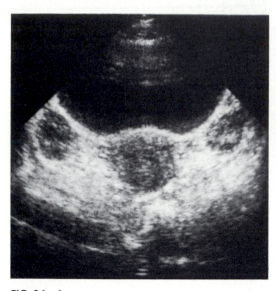

FIG 21−1.
Transverse view through a normal pelvis showing the uterus centrally located and both ovaries in cross section on either side.

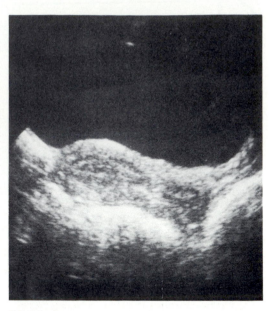

FIG 21−2.
Long axis view of the uterus showing the echogenic lines representing the endometrium in the center.

diagnosed when the retroverted uterus is seen transabdominally due to this hypoechoic echo pattern. The fundus of such a uterus should be examined transvaginally for optimal viewing of the myometrium if uterine fibroids are suspected.

Identifying the central uterine cavity echo is a useful sign for demonstrating that the uterus is empty, therefore excluding intrauterine pregnancy, submucous fibroids, and so forth. The demonstration of this echo is also helpful in identifying the uterus itself when confusing pelvic pathology such as dense adnexal masses or uterine fibroids is present (Callen et al., 1979). The width

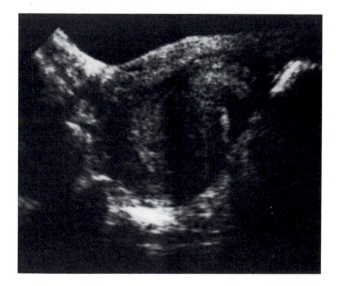

FIG 21−3.
Long axis view of a retroverted uterus. It is possible to follow the increased echogenicity of the endo-metrium as it extends posteriorly in the retroverted fundus.

of the endometrial echo changes during the cycle from a thin triple-line configuration in the proliferative phase to a markedly hyperechoic functional layer in the secretory phase (Forrest et al., 1988). In the postmenopausal patient not receiving hormone replacement, however, an endometrial echo greater than 5 mm wide is considered abnormal, a finding discussed later in this section (Fleischer et al., 1986).

Recently, the vaginal probe has proved very helpful in evaluation of the uterus and endometrial abnormalities. A recent study comparing transvaginal and transabdominal scanning in 29 patients showed that in 23% of the cases, transvaginal scanning provided additional diagnostic information not available with the transabdominal technique. In the other 77%, adequate diagnostic information was obtainable by either transabdominal or transvaginal techniques, but in 63% of these cases, the quality of the transvaginal image was judged to be superior to that obtained transabdominally (Mendelson et al., 1988a).

Congenital Abnormalities

Major congenital abnormalities of the uterus are easily detected by both transabdominal and transvaginal sonography. The easiest abnormality to identify is the double uterus, or uterus didel-phys, where two entirely separate uterine bodies and fundi are seen (Fig 21–4). It is important not to mistake one of the uterine fundi for an adnexal mass or an intrauterine for an ectopic pregnancy when the empty second uterus is visualized.

The bicornuate uterus is identifiable by locating the endometrial echo in transverse section and noting that it separates into two discrete portions at the fundus, each surrounded by myometrium (Fig 21–5). Normally, the endometrial echo at the fundus should extend in a line parallel to the bladder in transverse section, with no disruption of this line by myometrium in the center. A septated uterus can have an appearance similar to the bicornuate uterus, although a small septum may not be detectable sonographically. The examination of the shape of the intrauterine cavity, however, is better accomplished by hysterosalpingography, particularly for smaller defects. It is important to remember, however, that abnormalities of the müllerian ducts are associated with other genitourinary malformations, and the kidneys should be imaged when a uterine malformation is identified (Malini et al., 1984; Gilsanz et al., 1982; Shenker and Brickman, 1979).

Hydrocolpos and hydrometrocolpos result in a large pelvic fluid collection secondary to obstruction of the vagina or uterus. The commonest

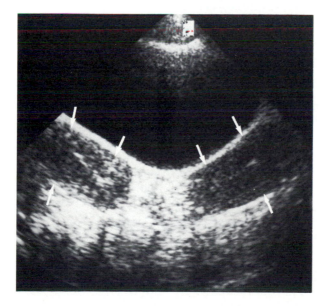

FIG 21–4.
Transverse view through the pelvis of a patient with a double uterus. The two separate uteri are shown by *arrows*.

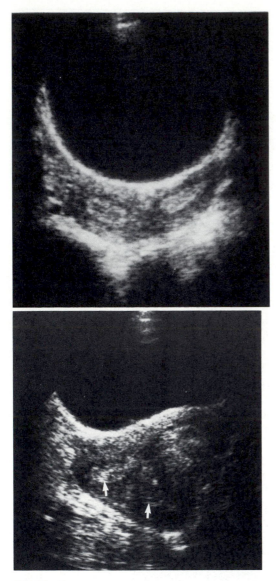

FIG 21–5.
A, transverse view through the pelvis of a patient with a bicornuate uterus. Note that the myometrium extends all the way around two separate islands of increased echogenicity representing the two portions of the endometrial cavity at the fundus. **B,** oblique view of a retroverted bicornuate uterus. The *arrows* indicate the two portions of the endometrial cavity at the fundus.

congenital abnormality causing hydrocolpos or hematocolpos is imperforate hymen.

Sonographically, the fluid collection is usually large and contains low-level echoes, indicating nonclotted blood or hemosiderin (an appear-

ance similar in texture to an endometrioma). When a hydrocolpos or hematocolpos is present, the fluid collection will be posterior to the bladder and underneath the uterus, in the characteristic location of the vagina (Fig 21–6). Hydrometrocolpos may be more difficult to diagnose, since it can be confused with an adnexal mass or cyst. The fluid-filled uterus can have a very thin wall and be difficult to recognize as the uterus. In addition, this fluid collection may also contain low-level echoes or material within it representing blood or blood clots in hematometrocolpos. It is crucial to search for the uterus and to consider this diagnosis if a normal uterus cannot be otherwise located (Wilson et al., 1978).

Primary amenorrhea is an indication for sonography, and a variety of congenital abnormalities can be diagnosed with this method. Patients with Mayer-Rokitansky-Küster-Hauser syndrome with vaginal atresia should be evaluated by sonography to determine the extent of malformations of the internal pelvic organs and kidneys (Rosenberg et al., 1986). A spectrum of malformations, including complete absence of the uterus with pelvic kidneys as the most severe, can be diagnosed definitively by ultrasound. Patients with Turner's syndrome have a characteristic appearance of the pelvis with a very tiny uterus, both longitudinally and transversely, and with unidentifiable ovaries (Shawker et al., 1986).

Uterine Tumors

The commonest intrauterine tumor is the fibroid. Leiomyomas can be detected by several sonographic features: (1) the uterine contour is often irregular and lobular, (2) there is often enlargement of the uterus, and (3) the echo pattern of the fibroid itself is most commonly hypoechoic (Gross et al., 1983). There are sometimes minimal contour irregularities of the uterus that may represent a subtle diagnostic sign of a leiomyoma, but with current high-resolution equipment and particularly transvaginal sonography, the contour and exact limits of the fibroids can often be recognized (Fig 21–7). Transvaginal sonography has helped to determine whether a fibroid is submucous or intramural. Although most fibroids are hypoechoic (but not cystic), some fibroids may be hyperechoic and may also contain calcification. Fibroids can calcify with small specks or clumps of calcium. Alternatively, the rim of the fibroid may calcify, similar to the appearance of a fetal head.

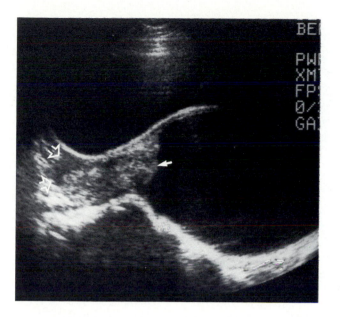

FIG 21–6.
Longitudinal view of the pelvis in a patient with a hematocolpos. *Open arrows* indicate the fundus of the uterus and the *closed arrow* the cervix. Directly beneath the cervix is a large fluid collection in the vagina, representing the hematocolpos.

Pedunculated fibroids may be difficult to diagnose if they occur laterally in the region of the broad ligament. The normal ovary on that side must be identified to be sure that the solid mass is, indeed, simply a fibroid. Unless the ovary can

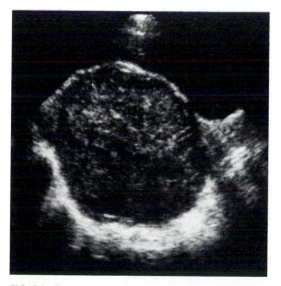

FIG 21–7.
Transverse view through the pelvis showing a uterine fibroid. Note that the appearance is solid, however, heterogeneous.

be identified with confidence, it will not be possible to exclude the possibility of an ovarian mass. Differentiation between an intramural and a submucosal fibroid depends on the appearance of the endometrial echo (Fig 21–8). A submucous fibroid will distort this echo and be located adjacent to it. Rarely, a submucous fibroid will prolapse through the cervix into the vagina, giving the appearance of a solid vaginal mass (Fig 21–9) (Walzer et al., 1983).

Occasionally, fibroids may degenerate, and irregular cystic areas can appear centrally within the fibroid (Fig 21–10). This commonly occurs during pregnancy and may be associated with severe pain. A cystic uterine mass in a nonpregnant patient is a more difficult diagnostic dilemma, however, and should not be assumed to be a degenerating fibroid by sonography alone. Ovarian tumors can invade the myometrium, or, rarely, fibroids can become sarcomatous, giving rise to abnormal uterine fluid collections. Further evaluation is therefore necessary if a cystic fibroid is identified in a nonpregnant patient (Nyberg et al., 1983).

Posterior fibroids are difficult to characterize sonographically, since, similar to the retroverted uterus, there is decreased penetration of sound in the cul-de-sac. The etiology of a hypoechoic mass in the cul-de-sac may be confusing, particularly if

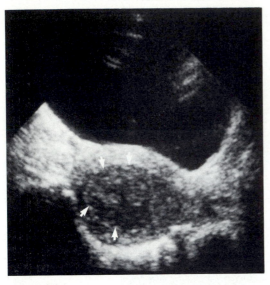

FIG 21–8.
Longitudinal view of the pelvis showing an enlarged uterus. The area of decreased echogenicity *(arrows)* represents a submucous fibroid. Note that a normal endometrial echo line is not visualized.

both ovaries cannot be definitively identified. Here again, transvaginal scanning has been extremely helpful as a diagnostic modality for the posterior pelvic compartment.

Other rare uterine benign tumors usually have a peculiar sonographic appearance and appear largely cystic rather than solid. An intrauterine mass can be differentiated from an adnexal mass since a uterine mass will lie within the confines of the uterine wall and be surrounded by serosa rather than being located outside the boundaries of the myometrium.

Adenomyosis is a difficult sonographic diagnosis to make. Adenomyosis can be suspected if the uterus is diffusely enlarged but the myometrial texture and contour appear normal. The myometrial texture can also have a heterogeneous appearance with small echolucent lakes (Fig 21–11). A recent study showed that ultrasound was able to suggest adenomyosis with a sensitivity of 63%, a specificity of 97% and a positive predictive value of 71% (Siedler et al., 1987). Diagnostic errors included three cases of adenomyosis diagnosed as leiomyomas due to the presence of contour and focal uterine abnormalities. Adenomyosis can certainly mimic leiomyomas, particularly when focal, and therefore a definitive sonographic diagnosis is very difficult. An occasional patient will have an intrauterine fluid collection and a thickened endometrial echo as a manifestation of adenomyosis, although further evaluation of such sonographic findings are necessary to rule out endometrial carcinoma (Lister et al., 1988).

Although an occasional intrauterine fluid collection and abnormal endometrial echoes can be

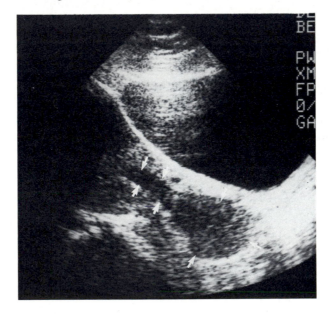

FIG 21–9.
Longitudinal view of the uterus and cervix. The arrows indicate a prolapsed submucous pedunculated fibroid. The largest portion of the fibroid is located in the vagina, whereas the stalk is seen coming through the cervix *(arrows)*.

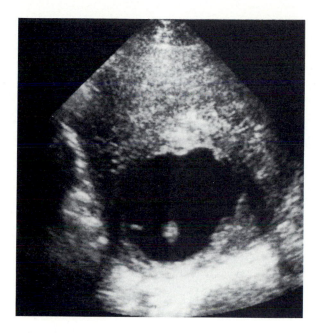

FIG 21–10.
Transverse view through an enlarged uterus showing an irregular cystic area with some solid material within it. This represents a degenerating fibroid.

secondary to adenomyosis, further evaluation of the patient is necessary since there is a spectrum of endometrial pathology that can be associated with abnormal endometrial echoes and fluid collections. McCarthy et al. (1986) studied postmenopausal endometrial fluid collections and found that although malignancy must always be excluded, benign causes of uterine fluid collections were commoner than previously reported. Seventy-five percent of these postmenopausal patients had benign processes such as endometrial polyp, chronic inflammation of the cervix and endometrium, and inflammatory processes. This is controversial, however, since Breckenridge et al.

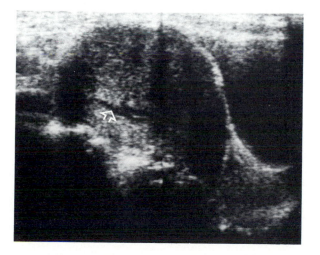

FIG 21–11.
Longitudinal view of an enlarged uterus. The *arrow* demonstrates the endometrial cavity and shows that the anterior myometrium is disproportionately wider than normal. Also note the heterogeneity of the appearance of the myometrium, representing adenomyosis.

(1982) showed widely differing results in a group of 17 postmenopausal patients, 94% of whom had uterine fluid collections associated with active carcinoma of the uterus or cervix (Figs 21–12 and 21–13). Occasionally, the uterus can remain obstructed either by carcinoma of the uterus or cervix or secondary to radiation therapy, causing a hematometrocolpos. The uterus takes on the appearance of a large thin-walled fluid collection, easily confused with a mass of ovarian origin. Just as in hematometrocolpos of the patient with a congenital uterine abnormality, it is important to think of this diagnosis particularly when a normal uterus cannot be otherwise identified (Scott et al., 1981).

Abnormal thickening of the endometrial echoes has been studied in 12 patients in whom the endometrial cavity echoes were wider than expected (Johnson et al., 1982). Eighty-three percent of these patients had endometrial pathology, including carcinoma in 33% and normal findings in 17%. As previously stated, the width of the endometrial echo should not exceed 5 mm in the postmenopausal patient, and in menstruating patients, it should be wide and echogenic only in the secretory portion of the cycle. Although the thickened endometrial echo is a useful sign for the presumptive diagnosis of endometrial pathology

such as carcinoma, many patients with endometrial carcinoma will have a normal uterus by ultrasound. In 10 of 15 cases of proved uterine malignancy, pelvic sonographic studies predicted the diagnosis. This reveals a 67% rate of success for the value of a normal sonogram and an 83% rate of success with an abnormal sonogram (Chambers et al., 1986). Chambers et al. (1986) suggests that although pelvic sonography is not a screening test for uterine malignancy, abnormal findings should prompt surgical investigation.

Detection of Intrauterine Contraceptive Devices

Inability to visualize the string of an IUD is an indication for sonography to determine whether the IUD has perforated, has been expulsed, or has become associated with an intrauterine or ectopic pregnancy. If pregnancy is suspected, a pregnancy test is crucial prior to the sonogram for optimal interpretation. Intrauterine devices have a particular type-specific morphology that was recognizable in 94% of patients with Lippe's Loop and in 81% of patients with Copper-7 devices in 1980 (Figs 21–14 and 21–15; Callen et al., 1980). With definite improvement in technique and operator ability since that time,

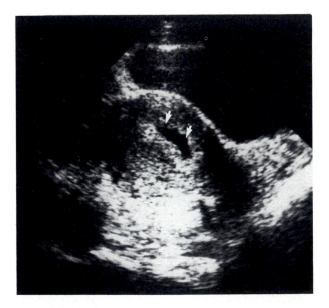

FIG 21–12.
Longitudinal view of the uterus showing a fluid collection in the endometrial cavity *(arrows)*. Also note the thickened endometrium shown by the increased echogenicity surrounding the fluid collection. This patient had endometrial carcinoma.

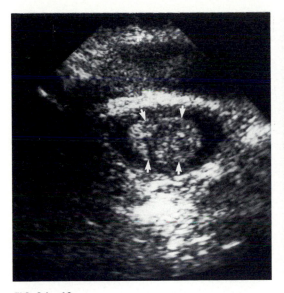

FIG 21–13.
Transverse view of the uterus showing markedly increased echogenicity centrally *(arrows)*. This patient was postmenopausal and had endometrial carcinoma.

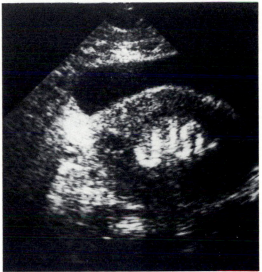

FIG 21–14.
Image of the uterus showing Lippe's Loop in normal position.

the type-specific morphology is probably more accurately determined today. A Lippe's Loop is characteristic when the uterus is viewed in longitudinal section and is identified by four or five small echogenic dots along the endometrial echo,

representing the loop cut in cross section at multiple points. The Copper-7, on the other hand, will have the appearance of a single echogenic line along the same projection as the endometrial echo and extending the length of the body of the uterus to the fundus. If the fundus is then viewed

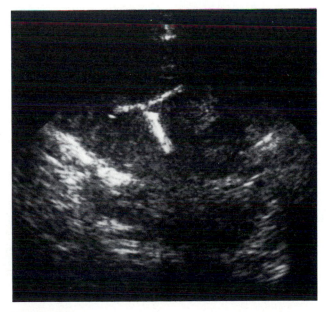

FIG 21–15.
Image of the uterus showing Copper-T in normal position.

transversely, a shorter line (the upper bar of the 7) will be viewed across the fundus of the uterus. Other types of unusual IUDs are encountered in clinical practice and are identifiable by their echogenic rounded or geometric shape. One can at least determine its location, even if the morphology itself is not easily recognized.

A patient is often sent for localization of IUD directly after her physician has probed the uterus in an attempt to locate it clinically. In doing so, air can be introduced into the intrauterine cavity, thus simulating a foreign body or IUD (Fig 21–16). It is contraindicated to probe the intrauterine cavity if the patient is to be sent for a sonogram for localization of an IUD, since instrumenting the uterus may confuse the issue.

The IUD is not the only echogenic structure that can be seen within the uterine cavity. Retention of a laminaria or fetal bones after a therapeutic abortion may have a very similar appearance and should be kept in mind when an intrauterine echogenic foreign body is seen, so as not to mistake a pathologic foreign body for an IUD (Chervenak et al., 1982; Hirsh and Levy, 1988; Bourgouin et al., 1985). Uterine perforation by the

IUD is readily noticeable when the IUD is traversing the myometrium between the endometrial cavity and the serosa. Occasionally, if it has perforated completely, it can be visualized in the cul-de-sac, although the increased echogenicity of bowel and bowel gas is likely to obscure an IUD located totally outside the uterus. If complete perforation is suspected and the IUD cannot be visualized sonographically, a pelvic x-ray film is helpful to determine whether the IUD has been completely expulsed or whether it is still within the pelvis. Imbedding of the IUD is more difficult to diagnose sonographically, since the IUD would still be located in the vicinity of the endometrial echo. Hysterosalpingography is better able to demonstrate imbedding than ultrasound (Rosenblatt et al., 1985). Transvaginal sonography may eventually be able to improve the ability of sonography to diagnose imbedding of the IUD.

If results of the pregnancy test are positive, and if the pregnancy is at least 5 weeks in gestation, the gestational sac must be located in the uterus sonographically to confidently exclude an ectopic pregnancy (see discussion on ectopic pregnancy later in the chapter). If the pregnancy is intrauterine, ultrasound is helpful in determining the relationship between the position of the gestational sac and the IUD (Fig 21–17). If the IUD is located in the lower segment, it can easily

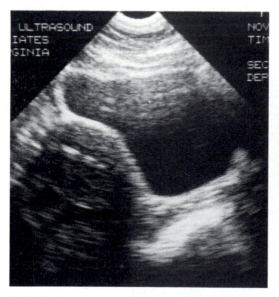

FIG 21–16.
Longitudinal view of the uterus a few hours after a D&C. Note that within the uterus is a linear echogenic streak that could be mistaken for an IUD. This actually represents air introduced by the D&C and demonstrates why imaging the uterus after instrumentation may be confusing when searching for an IUD.

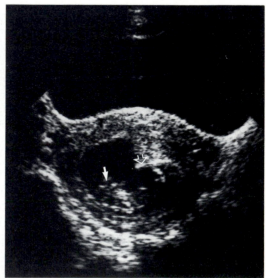

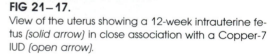

FIG 21–17.
View of the uterus showing a 12-week intrauterine fetus *(solid arrow)* in close association with a Copper-7 IUD *(open arrow)*.

be removed. Removal of IUDs located in very close proximity to the gestational sac or above it is much more hazardous and creates a greater chance of interrupting the pregnancy. Occasionally, IUDs can be removed under sonographic guidance.

Vaginal Masses

Cystic vaginal masses are characteristic in their location in that they elevate the floor of the bladder and the uterus still remains intact. Fluid in the vagina can be secondary to hydrocolpos, and when seen in the pediatric patient, this can be due to an imperforate hymen or other obstructive lesion of the vagina, as discussed earlier in this chapter (Schaffer et al., 1983). It is also possible for a patient to have a double vagina, one of which is obstructed. Sonographic evaluation of the uterus in these patients is crucial since congenital abnormalities of the uterine horns are likely. Gartner's duct cyst is a fairly common vaginal cyst usually found as an incidental finding during pelvic sonography. It can be single or multiple, along the anterolateral aspect of the vaginal wall, and is known to arise in caudal remnants of the mesonephric duct (Fig 21–18). Solid vaginal lesions are very rare and, even if they are present, would be difficult to identify by sonography un-

less they became large. A prolapsing fibromyoma, however, is easily seen and can be confirmed by physical examination (see Fig 21–9). The presence of a menstrual tampon is characteristic, since it contains air and creates an acoustic shadow (McCarthy and Taylor, 1983). Small cysts in the region of the cervix usually represent retention cysts or nabothian cysts. These are usually incidental findings during pelvic sonography, and such a cyst can vary between 6 and 20 mm (Fogel and Slasky, 1982). The vagina is normally collapsed and seen as a linear streak of tissue under the floor of the bladder during a pelvic sonogram. Occasionally, however, it can be filled with fluid after douching or secondary to reflux from voiding, mimicking a hematocolpos.

THE ADNEXA

The normal ovaries are usually located between the uterus and lateral side walls (see Fig 21–1). Ovarian volumes can vary between 2 and 6 cm³ in postpubertal patients and less than 0.1 cm³ in prepubertal patients (Sample et al., 1977). Tiny follicles less than 1 cm can be identified routinely on the ovaries and are not necessarily considered abnormal unless they are multiple. The fallopian tubes are rarely visualized unless patho-

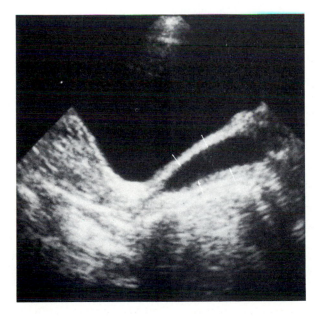

FIG 21–18.
Longitudinal view of the uterus and vagina showing a fluid collection in the region of the vagina *(arrows)*. This represents a Gartner's duct cyst.

logical or unless there is pelvic ascites (Fig 21–19). The use of the transvaginal probe has greatly improved our ability to visualize fallopian tubes, and even the ovaries are seen with better detail transvaginally (Fig 21–20) (Vilaro et al., 1987; Grandberg and Wikland, 1987). Studies have shown that transvaginal scanning offered additional information in 55% of patients than was obtainable transabdominally (Vilaro et al., 1987). Lande et al. (1988) studied 67 patients and concluded that transvaginal sonography added diagnostically useful information in 25 of 28 patients with cystic pathological changes in the adnexae and that transvaginal sonography was particularly useful in all patients with diseases of the cul-de-sac or fallopian tubes. In further studies done with the transvaginal probe, the transvaginal image quality was superior to the transabdominal image in 79% to 87% of cases, whereas the transabdominal image was better in 3% to 5% of scans. Both techniques provided equivalent diagnostic information in 60% to 84% of cases; however, individual organs and fine structures were better seen transvaginally (Mendelson et al., 1988b). Imaging of the fallopian tubes was particularly helpful using transvaginal scanning and a fluid-filled tube; tubo-ovarian inflammatory processes and ectopic pregnancy have been diagnosed

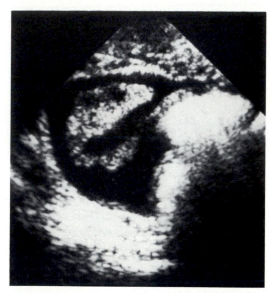

FIG 21–20.
Transvaginal view of the right fallopian tube seen well because it is surrounded by fluid in a patient with a small amount of pelvic ascites.

with better accuracy transvaginally (Timor-Tritsch and Rottem, 1987).

In addition to imaging the normal adnexae, knowledge of the time of the cycle is helpful. Small amounts of free pelvic fluid can be present during midcycle to late-cycle scans. Developing follicles up to 2 cm may be seen midcycle and should not be confused with ovarian cysts (Hall et al., 1979; Davis and Gosink, 1986). It is sometimes difficult to identify the ovaries sonographically, particularly when they are located in the cul-de-sac, possibly behind a bowel loop, or high up above the level of the distended bladder. Following the broad ligament from the lateral aspect of the uterus usually leads to the ovaries, and this is often very helpful for hard-to-find ovaries.

Ovarian Cysts

A typical ovarian cyst by sonography is completely anechoic with a thin wall and good through transmission, a characteristic of sound as it propagates through water. When such an ovarian cyst is encountered sonographically, it is wise to reexamine the patient 1 month later since these often represent functional cysts. Hemorrhagic cysts, on the other hand, have a variable appearance. Baltarowich et al. (1987) have described 76

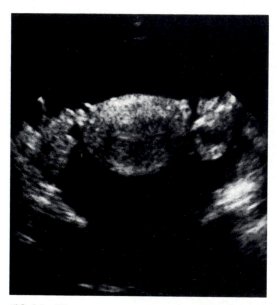

FIG 21–19.
Transverse view of the uterus and adnexae in a patient with a large amount of ascites. Note that the tubes are well seen due to the surrounding fluid.

hemorrhagic ovarian cysts, the overwhelming majority of which had good through transmission signifying the basic cystic nature of the lesion. The remainder of the sonographic features were variable, however, and most commonly consisted of a heterogeneous mass (83%), predominantly anechoic but with hypoechoic material within it. Seventeen percent of hemorrhagic cysts were completely homogeneous, either hypoechoic or hyperechoic (Fig 21–21; Baltarowich et al., 1987). Some hemorrhagic ovarian cysts can have thick and irregular walls; 87% of them can have internal echoes, and some can even have a few septations (Reynolds et al., 1986). These features are difficult to differentiate from endometriomas, tubo-ovarian abscesses, and even, in some cases, ovarian tumors. Percutaneous ovarian cyst aspiration has been performed using transvaginal sonography, with successful drainage of the cyst (Schwimer et al., 1985).

The simple adnexal cyst in the postmenopausal woman has always been more worrisome due to the usual quiescence of the postmenopausal ovary. Most of the simple clear adnexal cysts in postmenopausal women are benign, and in a series of 13 patients, only 1 patient had a borderline malignancy (Hall and McCarthy, 1986; Andolf and Jorgensen, 1988). Occasionally, cysts will be identified in the adnexa adjacent to a normal-appearing ovary, representing a paratubal or a paraovarian cyst. Paraovarian cysts are known to arise from the tissues of the broad ligament and may be symptomatic due to their potentially large size (Atheny and Cooper, 1985).

Not all pelvic cysts are ovarian, and indeed, inflammatory cysts of the peritoneum can occur in the pelvis, particularly in patients who have had previous surgery. These are usually multiloculated cysts, but their origin is difficult to diagnose sonographically, since often the ovaries cannot be visualized and the patients have had multiple surgical procedures (Fig 21–22; Lees et al., 1978). Other nongynecologic cystic masses occurring in the pelvis include hydroureters, bladder diverticula, pelvic kidneys, ectopic ureteroceles, urachal cysts, fixed loops of bowel, iliac artery aneurysms, lymphomas, and so forth (Fig 21–23; Rifkin et al., 1984). Occasionally, the posterior pelvic compartment or cul-de-sac is difficult to evaluate, and in the past, a water enema has been used to delineate the rectum and to attempt to map out loops of colon that may represent pseudotumors (Kurtz et al., 1979). The use of the transvaginal probe, however, has made the water enema virtually obsolete since it provides a new window to the posterior cul-de-sac not previously available.

Polycystic ovarian disease has a wide sonographic spectrum that includes enlargement of the ovaries bilaterally and symmetrically. The cysts can be discretely resolvable and multiple, less than 1 cm each, or the ovary can have a hypoechoic pattern suggesting that the cysts are too tiny to resolve sonographically (Fig 21–24). Approximately 30% of cases of polycystic ovarian disease have normal-size ovaries sonographically, and, therefore, a normal sonogram cannot exclude this diagnosis (el Tabbakh et al., 1986; Hann et al., 1984; Yeh et al., 1987). It is possible to mistake small pelvic varicosities for cystic ovaries, and if this is in question, Doppler may be helpful (Willard, 1988).

Adnexal Masses

In 1977, the accuracy of gray-scale sonography in determining the existence, size, and location of a pelvic mass was approximately 91% in 251 cases (Lawson and Albarelli, 1977). Since then, many studies have evaluated the accuracy of sonography for the detection and tissue diagnosis of pelvic masses. In 1979, Walsh et al. (1979b)

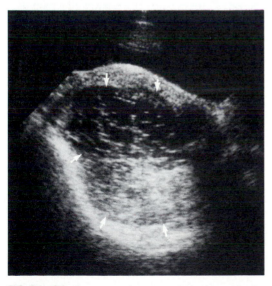

FIG 21–21.
The *arrows* demonstrate a large cystic mass containing stranding and echoes within it in a patient taking clomiphene. This represented a hemorrhagic cyst.

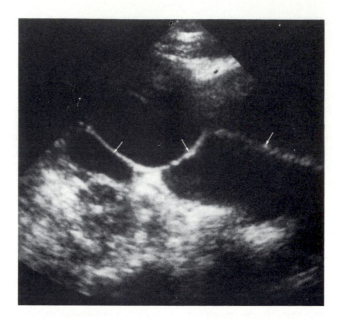

FIG 21–22.
Oblique view of the pelvis showing multiple cystic areas separated by septations *(arrows)*. This patient had undergone many pelvic surgical procedures, and these fluid collections represented peritoneal inclusion cysts.

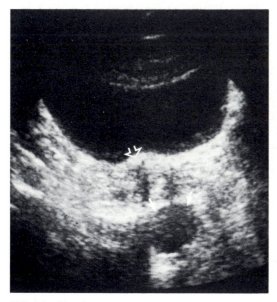

FIG 21–23.
Transverse view of the pelvis showing the uterus *(open arrow)*. Behind the uterus in the cul-de-sac is a hypoechoic mass indicated by the closed arrows. This represented a retroperitoneal lipoma.

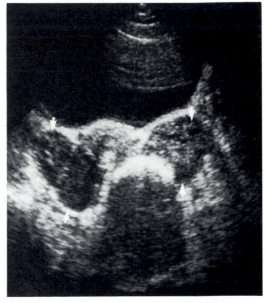

FIG 21–24.
Transverse view of the pelvis in a patient with typical Stein-Leventhal syndrome, or polycystic ovaries. The uterus is centrally located and both ovaries *(arrows)* are hypoechoic and enlarged.

examined 182 women and found that ultrasound provided information leading to the correct diagnosis in 56% of cases and contributory data in 23% of patients. This study differed from the O'Brien et al. (1984) study that claimed that the overall performance of sonography was inferior to clinical examination and made the correct diagnosis only 42% of the time. Wade et al. (1985) studied 900 patients and demonstrated that sonography established the correct diagnosis in 59% of the cases. Today, most investigators will agree that there has been an improvement in the sonographic diagnosis of pelvic masses. Requard et al. (1981) reported that sonography was 97% accurate in the detection and 84% correct in the characterization of pelvic masses. In this study, 87% of these tumors were malignant by sonographic criteria (Requard et al., 1981). More recently, Herrmann et al. (1987) reported a positive predictive value of sonography for the detection of malignancy at 73%, whereas benign tumors were predicted correctly in 95% of cases. Ultrasound was compared to computed tomography in the evaluation of patients suspected of pelvic masses, and both imaging techniques depicted similar pathology and used similar diagnostic criteria (Walsh et al., 1978). Computed tomography did not appear to be superior to ultrasound in the evaluation of pelvic masses; therefore, sonography is preferred due to the ease and relatively low cost of the technique.

Various criteria have been used in trying to differentiate types of pelvic masses and making tissue diagnoses, with variable success. In general, anechoic lesions have a high likelihood of being benign tumors, usually cystadenomas, and as the percentage of echogenic material increases, the likelihood of malignancy also increases (Moyle et al., 1983). Exceptions include benign teratomas, which are characteristically highly echogenic and reflective (Moyle et al., 1983; Sandler et al., 1979). Fleischer et al. (1978) devised criteria that have become helpful in the differential diagnosis of pelvic masses. Ovarian cystadenomas were predominantly cystic and septated (Fig 21–25). Tubo-ovarian abscesses were usually complex and predominantly cystic. Dermoid cysts had a characteristic echogenic focus (Fig 21–26); physiologic ovarian cysts, serous adenomas, and hydrosalpinx were predominantly cystic. Recently, we have further refined criteria for defining benignancy or malignancy of pelvic masses (Benacerraf et al., in press). The most likely lesions to be be-

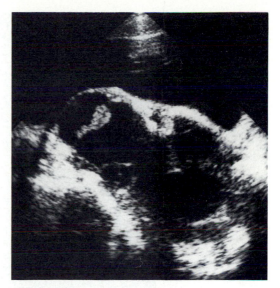

FIG 21–25.
Large multicystic adnexal mass showing septations, nodular solid material, and a thickened irregular wall. This patient had a cystadenocarcinoma of the ovary.

nign include a clear ovarian cyst with smooth borders, tubular cysts such as a hydrosalpinx, or a solid mass with a separate normal-appearing ovary, such as a fibroid. A clear cyst with slightly irregular borders or a cyst with smooth walls having faint low-level echoes is more likely to represent an endometrioma (see the next section). There is a group of cystic masses that are nonspecific in appearance but are usually largely cystic, with irregular and thickened walls, although lacking nodularity. These masses can contain solid material within them, and an accurate prediction of tissue diagnosis is extremely difficult without a good history. The differential diagnoses for such masses would include an endometrioma, a tubo-ovarian abscess, a benign or malignant tumor of the ovary or fallopian tube, or a hemorrhagic cyst, among others. Lesions that are cystic with irregular borders and nodularity are most likely to represent ovarian carcinomas (see Fig 21–25). Solid ovarian enlargement is also suspicious for ovarian tumors, such as dysgerminomas (Fig 21–27). An irregular cystic mass with ascites is virtually diagnostic of an ovarian malignancy. In our recent study evaluating pelvic masses in 100 patients undergoing laparotomy, the correct tissue diagnosis was made in 68% of cases based on the sonographic appearance as previously described. In ad-

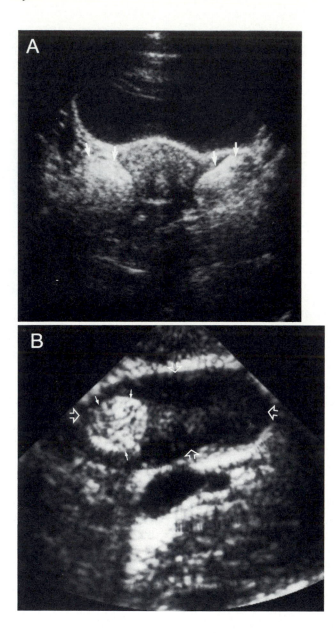

FIG 21–26.

A, transverse view through the pelvis showing a centrally located uterus. Both adnexae contain markedly echogenic solid masses with well-defined anterior walls and poorly defined posterior walls. These masses are indicated by *arrows* and represented bi- lateral dermoids. **B,** transvaginal image of a slightly enlarged ovary *(open arrows)* that contains a small, 1.2-cm dermoid *(small arrows)*. This image demonstrates the superior quality of imaging of the ovary possible with transvaginal scanning.

dition, sonography correctly identified a benign condition in 17% of cases without, however, arriving at an exact tissue diagnosis. Sonography was frankly misleading in 15% of cases. The identification of an ovarian malignancy was correct in 24 of 30 patients (80%), and the specificity for correctly diagnosing a benign condition was 87%. The positive predictive value of sonography for the diagnosis of an adnexal malignancy was 73%, and the negative predictive value for excluding a malignancy by sonography was 91% (Benacerraf et al., in press).

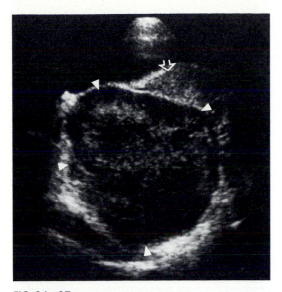

FIG 21–27.
Large solid mass *(closed arrowheads)* adjacent to the uterus *(open arrow)*. This mass is clearly separate from the uterus and different in texture. The pathology revealed dysgerminoma.

The sonographic appearance of carcinoma of the fallopian tube is entirely nonspecific and has been described as a complex mass with predominantly cystic components, echoes within it, and wall thickening. These findings could be confused with those of an ovarian tumor, hydrosalpinx, an inflammatory process, or endometriosis of the pelvis, among others (Meyer et al., 1987; Subramanyam et al., 1984). Fibromas and thecomas of the ovary also display a broad spectrum of sonographic features, anywhere from hypoechoic masses with posterior shadowing to cystic-appearing masses with good through transmission, as well as echogenic or calcified masses with mixed echogenicity (Athey and Malone, 1987). Krukenberg tumors, which are usually bilateral metastases to the ovaries from a primary neoplasm in the gastrointestinal tract, can become very large and usually appear as solid masses containing variable amounts of fluid, mimicking the appearance of a cystadenocarcinoma of the ovary (Athey and Butters, 1984). The bilaterality of these masses, however, should raise the question of metastases rather than ovarian primaries. Abdominal ultrasound has been very helpful not only in the examination of the malignant ovarian tumor itself but also in the staging process, since the entire pelvis can be scanned quickly and efficiently, giv-

ing valuable results. Sonography can uncover even small amounts of ascites, liver metastases, peritoneal implants, pleural effusions, hydronephrosis, abnormal omentum, and so forth (Paling and Shawker, 1981). The tumor itself, in a series of 57 patients, was usually either solid or mixed solid and cystic but in no case was the primary malignancy exclusively cystic (Paling and Shawker, 1981).

Sonographically, the postmenopausal ovaries are usually small, less than 2.5 cm^3. In a series of 30 postmenopausal women examined sonographically, both ovaries were visualized in 19 patients (Hall et al., 1986). One ovary was seen in three patients, and neither ovary could be identified in eight patients. When an ovarian mass is identified in the postmenopausal woman, however, further workup is indicated; however, the likelihood of malignancy seems to vary with the size of the mass. Only 1 of 32 masses less than 5 cm was malignant (Rulin and Preston, 1987). Of 55 masses 5 to 10 mm, 6 were malignant. Forty of the 63 tumors larger than 10 cm were malignant. The proportion of malignancies also increased with age (Rulin and Preston, 1987).

Endometriosis

Endometriosis is a common gynecological problem of women in their reproductive years, which is defined as growth of endometrial tissue outside the uterus, and is often responsible for infertility and pelvic pain. Its sonographic manifestations are varied. In a study of 25 patients with 31 lesions characterized at ultrasound, 17 were described as cystic, 4 as polycystic, 5 as mixed, and 4 as solid (Walsh et al., 1979a). Other authors have also experienced difficulty in defining the sonographic characteristics of endometriosis (Coleman et al., 1979; Friedman et al., 1985; Sandler and Karo, 1978). More recently, however, endometriomas have been described as being predominantly cystic but containing homogeneous and faint low-level echoes, which is fairly characteristic of a chocolate cyst (Figs 21–28 and 21–29; Birnholz, 1983). These chocolate cysts can contain echogenic material consistent with clots and a thickened wall and even sometimes some septations, which may make them difficult to differentiate from an ovarian tumor (Fig 21–30). Obtaining clinical history may be helpful in those cases. Unless the endometriosis is in the form of an endometrioma, sonography may not

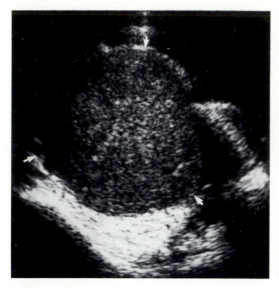

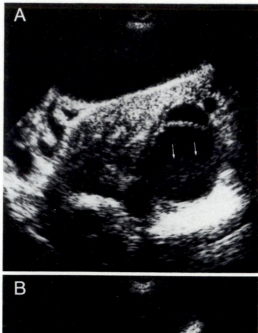

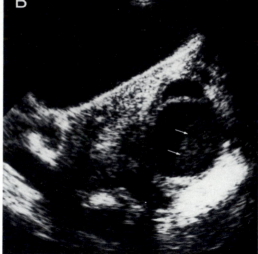

FIG 21–28.
Large homogeneous mass *(arrows)* that, although it appears solid in texture, is actually cystic, as shown by the increased through transmission of sound beyond it. (Note the increased brightness of the background beyond the back wall of the mass.) This is a typical appearance of an endometrioma.

be reliable in its detection. Tiny endometrial implants or deposits are too small to be visualized by ultrasound. In some cases, however, small irregular fluid collections in the cul-de-sac can actually represent endometrial implants (Fig 21–31).

Pelvic Inflammatory Disease

Early signs of pelvic inflammatory disease are difficult, if not impossible, to identify sonographically. Mild dilation of the fallopian tube is difficult to see, and, occasionally, a small amount of free fluid in the cul-de-sac may indicate early pelvic infection. A hydrosalpinx is a tubular fluid-filled structure sonographically, which can have a thick or thin wall. It often has a multicystic appearance because it is folded on itself and seen in cross section (Fig 21–32).

A late manifestation of pelvic inflammatory disease is a tubo-ovarian abscess, which is easily imaged by ultrasound as a complex multicystic loculated mass containing both cystic and solid areas and sometimes a small amount of gas with acoustic shadowing behind it (Fig 21–33). Although the appearance of a tubo-ovarian abscess

FIG 21–29.
A, transverse view of the pelvis showing a left-sided endometrioma. There is a fluid-debris or clot level *(arrows)* within the endometrioma. **B,** same patient as in **A,** but in decubitus position. The fluid or clot level has shifted *(arrows).*

may not be specific, a mass, together with lower abdominal pain, leukocytosis, fever, and vaginal discharge, can prompt the correct diagnosis (Landers and Sweet, 1985). The accuracy of the diagnosis of pelvic abscess is excellent, as reported by Taylor et al. (1978). They studied 220 patients with pelvic abscess and showed that 36 of 40 abdominal and 32 of 33 pelvic abscesses were cor-

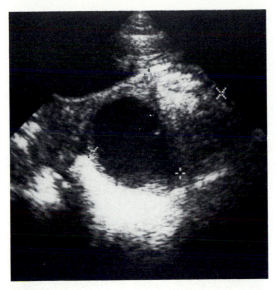

FIG 21–30.
Large left-sided pelvic mass *(calipers)*. One side is largely cystic, although there are faint low-level echoes seen, typical of an endometrioma. The other side of the mass is brightly echogenic, reminiscent of a dermoid. This ovary, indeed, contained both an endometrioma and a dermoid pathologically.

rectly identified. They correctly ruled out 112 of 113 possible abdominal and 33 of 34 possible pelvic abscesses.

The typical tubo-ovarian abscess has shaggy borders and walls that are indistinct, a feature of inflammatory processes. In addition, the pelvis can fill with pus, giving a hypoechoic masslike effect, in the cul-de-sac and adnexa and surrounding the uterus. A similar appearance can result from a blood clot and pelvic hematoperitoneum, which is occasionally seen with a ruptured ectopic pregnancy (Jeffrey and Laing, 1982). An organizing clot, however, is usually more echogenic than the lobulated hypoechoic appearance of pus. Tubo-ovarian abscesses can successfully be drained both percutaneously and transvaginally (Nosher et al., 1987; Worthen and Gunning, 1986).

POSTOPERATIVE COMPLICATIONS

One of the uses of pelvic sonography is to evaluate postoperative patients with surgical complications. Sonography has been helpful in the past in evaluating possible uterine perforation following a dilatation and curettage (D&C). Cunat

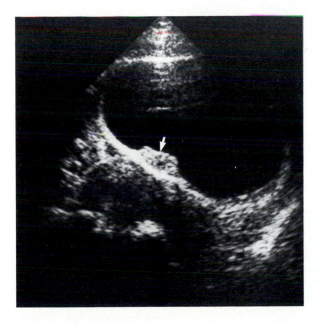

FIG 21–31.
Longitudinal view of the uterus showing the distended bladder and the uterus behind it. The *arrow* demonstrates an irregular mucosal lesion of the bladder that represented endometriosis of the bladder.

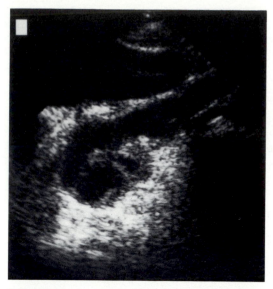

FIG 21–32.
View of the left side of the pelvis demonstrating an irregular tubular fluid collection that is serpiginous and represents a hydrosalpinx.

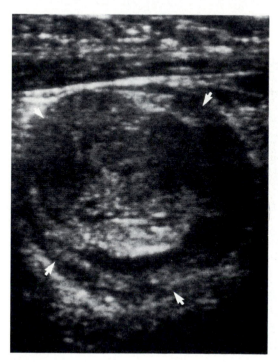

FIG 21–33.
The *arrows* indicate a large mass that is mostly solid but with a small cystic rim. Although it appears nonspecific, this patient had a tubo-ovarian abscess.

et al. (1984) report a case in which ultrasound demonstrated a loop of small bowel within the intrauterine cavity after a D&C. A loop of ileum had entered the uterine fundus through a laceration, and the ultrasound appearance prompted immediate operative repair. A pelvic abscess or infected hematoma in posthysterectomy patients can be either solid or cystic depending on how organized the hematoma has become and whether it contains loculations or pockets of pus. Occasionally, a hematoma can have a completely solid, echogenic, and lobulated appearance, not dissimilar to that of a fibroid uterus (Fig 21–34,A). A posthysterectomy abscess can be drained under direct ultrasound guidance (McArdle, 1984). Ultrasound enables the surgeon to visualize adequately and drain any loculation as well as ensure good positioning of the draining catheter. The ultrasound guidance is done transabdominally so as not to contaminate the surgical field.

Complications after cesarean section include a bladder flap hematoma, which is usually hypoechoic with low-level echoes and a thickened wall. It is located between the lower uterine segment and the bladder at the level of the incision (Baker et al., 1985; Winsett et al., 1986). Although it is difficult to differentiate a hematoma from an abscess, the presence of gas within the mass would signify infection. A subfascial hematoma after cesarean delivery results from extraperitoneal hemorrhage within the prevesicular space posterior to the rectus muscles but anterior to the peritoneum (Fig 21–34,B). Again, the sonographic appearance is predominantly cystic or possibly complex. Subfascial hematomas can often occur in association with bladder flap hematomas, although the distinction between these two types of complications must be made if a drainage procedure is contemplated (Wiener et al., 1987).

ULTRASOUND IN OVULATION INDUCTION

Sonography is an ideal method for visualizing developing follicles and timing ovulation induction with the use of human chorionic gonadotropin (hCG) administration for ovulation. In addition, in a series of 210 patients undergoing sonography for ovulation induction, baseline sonograms demonstrated adnexal abnormalities in 10.7% of cases, a useful adjunct to this technique (Hann et al., 1987). Although traditionally the

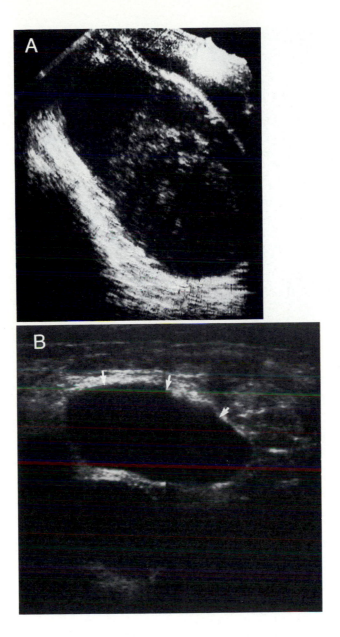

FIG 21–34.
A, large solid mass filling the pelvis in a patient who recently had a hysterectomy. The mass is heterogeneous, containing both solid and cystic areas, and represented an infected hematoma. **B,** wide field of view image of the pelvis after a cesarean section, demonstrating a superficial large cystic area *(arrows)*. This represents a rectus sheath hematoma.

ovaries have been evaluated transabdominally through a full bladder, transvaginal technique represents a vast improvement in the visualization of the developing follicles (Fig 21–35). It is also better accepted by patients being scanned frequently who want to avoid the repeated discom-

forts of a full bladder and inconvenience of drinking fluids as well as delays waiting for bladder filling.

Ultrasound is used (1) to distinguish between the presence of one or more mature follicles; (2) to suggest the possibility of multiple

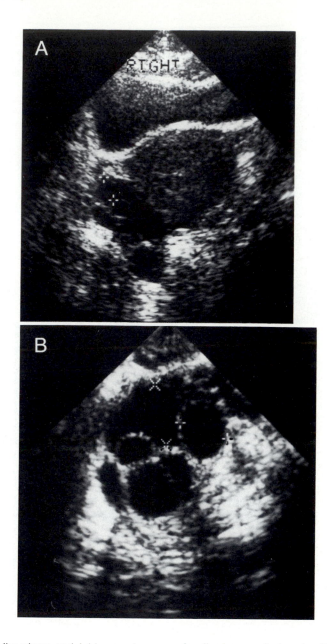

FIG 21–35.

A, transverse view of the uterus and right ovary showing an attempt at measuring follicular size *(calipers)*
in an obese patient. **B,** calipers indicated the same
follicles as were being measured in **A** but now seen
using the transvaginal probe. Note the markedly improved image of this patient's ovary compared with
the transabdominal approach.

ovulations, risking hyperstimulation and multiple
gestations; (3) to indicate optimal timing for the
use of hCG administration, allowing ovulation;
(4) to allow detection and confirmation of normal
follicular rupture and ovulation; (5) to indicate
optimal timing for oocyte retrieval in in vitro fertilization programs; and (6) to assess possible
pathologic pelvic conditions such as endometriosis or pelvic inflammatory disease (Mendelson et
al., 1985; Ritchie, 1986).

Patients undergoing treatment with clomiphene (Clomid) or menotropins (Pergonal) are

scanned every other day or daily around midcycle so as to time the administration of hCG.

Follicles are measured in at least two of their greatest dimensions to obtain an average size. The follicle should be larger than 15 mm and preferably between 18 and 20 mm before hCG should be administered to optimize ovulation (McArdle et al., 1983; O'Herlihy et al., 1982). When hCG was given at a mean follicular diameter of 18 mm, 92% of cycles were ovulatory, and 67% of patients conceived within six ovulatory treatment cycles (O'Herlihy et al., 1982). Five of the 7 patients who did not conceive were found to have endometriosis at laparoscopy (O'Herlihy et al., 1982). It has been difficult to predict when ovulation will occur, and follicles can grow at variable rates, between 1 and 3 mm/day. Sonographic signs of imminent ovulation, however, include a line of decreased reflectivity around the follicle in a crenation pattern within the follicle (Picker et al., 1983). These findings have been helpful when artificial insemination or in vitro fertilization is planned. Some investigators have tried to use the appearance of the endometrial echo in the prediction of fertility. Thickman et al. (1986) concluded that endometrial thickness was not a useful predictor of patients who would conceive. Brandt et al. (1985), on the other hand, believe that endometrial echo abnormalities may be a recognizable cause of infertility. This is a controversial issue, and more work needs to be done in this area. A risk of using clomiphene or mentropins is in creating ovarian hyperstimulation, which, in turn, can lead to ovarian torsion, electrolyte imbalance, ascites, as well as multiple pregnancy. Ovarian enlargement to greater than 5 cm is considered mild hyperstimulation, and ultrasound is used in screening patients who are at risk for this syndrome (Fig 21–36). When ovaries grow to large sizes with multiple mature follicles, hCG may be withheld to avoid ovulation, thereby minimizing the risk of multiple pregnancy or worsening hyperstimulation syndrome (McArdle and Sacks, 1980; McArdle et al., 1983; Rankin and Hutton, 1981).

Some patients undergoing ovulation induction remain unsuccessful in obtaining a pregnancy. Ovulation can be confirmed sonographically by acute deflation of the follicle with spillage of the follicular fluid into the cul-de-sac. Free fluid in the cul-de-sac with marked diminution of the follicular size indicates ovulation. When this does not take place, luteinizing of the unruptured

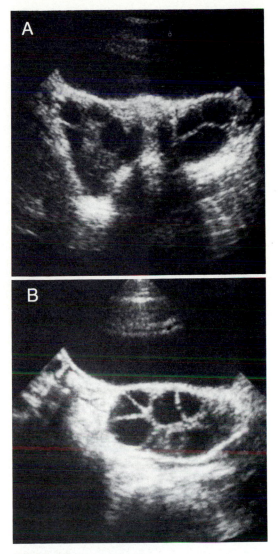

FIG 21–36.
Transverse **(A)** and longitudinal **(B)** views of the pelvis showing mild hyperstimulation of the ovaries. Note that each ovary contains multiple enlarged follicles.

follicle occurs. The follicle becomes hazy and filled with echoes; however, it does not decrease in size, and no free fluid appears in the cul-de-sac (Coulam et al., 1982).

Ultrasound has been used extensively in in vitro fertilization (IVF) programs not only for determining the time when oocyte retrieval should be undertaken but also recently as a means of retrieving the oocytes. Outpatient in vitro fertilization can be done using transvaginal ultrasound-guided oocyte retrieval with excellent results. In

61 patients who had oocyte retrievals performed with ultrasound-guided transvaginal aspiration of ovarian follicles, 10 patients conceived (Schulman, 1987). This is also an excellent technique for patients who have adhesions and whose ovaries may not be accessible via laparoscopy (Taylor et al., 1986).

An additional use of sonography to evaluate the infertile patient has been determination of the fallopian tube patency by injecting fluid into the uterus transcervically and identifying the fluid collecting in the cul-de-sac (Fig 21–37; Richman et al., 1984). Although this technique has been useful in the past and avoids x-ray exposure, it is inferior to hysterosalpingography for evaluating the shape of the intrauterine cavity and tubes. Furthermore, the patency of both tubes or one tube only will have the same sonographic appearance since only one tube need be patent for fluid to reach the cul-de-sac.

In summary, sonography has permitted dramatic advances in the treatment of infertility. The ability to visualize follicles in different phases of maturation has made it possible to treat problems of ovulation dysfunction and even retrieve mature follicles for in vitro procedures without laparoscopy. Sonography is also capable of identifying other explanations for lack of fertility, such as endometriosis, hydrosalpinx, and fibroids. More research may even uncover ways in which the appearance of the endometrium may help predict fertility.

EARLY PREGNANCY

One of the most frequent indications for pelvic sonography is the evaluation of early pregnancy. A gestational sac can be identified by the fifth week of amenorrhea and the embryo by 5 to 6 weeks. Cardiac motion should be visible at the time the fetal pole appears. In years past, repeated scanning was necessary to determine a viable from nonviable gestational sac, since prior to 7 weeks, the fetal pole and heartbeat could not normally be visualized. Although a good trophoblastic reaction was encouraging and a sac 2 to 2.5 cm in diameter without a fetal pole was a poor prognostic sign, many times follow-up scans were necessary to reliably diagnose a blighted ovum (Bernard and Cooperberg, 1985; Nyberg et al., 1986). More recently, transvaginal scanning has made the sonographic evaluation of early pregnancy more efficient by providing better resolution and permitting more reliable and better criteria for the diagnosis of a nonviable pregnancy (Fig 21–38). Levi et al. (1988) studied 62 patients and demonstrated that when gestational sacs were 8 mm or larger, the absence of a yoke sac predicted a nonviable pregnancy with a sensitivity of 67% and a specificity of 100%. When gestational sacs were larger than 16 mm, the absence of an embryo predicted a nonviable pregnancy with a sensitivity of 50% and a specificity of 100%. If, in addition, no cardiac activity could be identified, the sensitivity and specificity for this latter group was 100%. Indeed, transvaginal sonography has proved to be superior to transabdominal scanning for the evaluation of early pregnancy. The correct diagnoses (living embryos, missed abortions, blighted ovums, etc.) were correctly predicted in 32 patients who had had inconclusive transabdominal sonograms, and the transvaginal images were clearer with better resolution, providing diagnoses with more confidence than their transabdominal counterparts (Pennell et al., 1987).

When a pregnancy is scanned transabdominally, an overdistended bladder may compress the uterine cavity and diminish our ability to visualize the gestational sac (Baker et al., 1985).

Bleeding is the commonest indication for

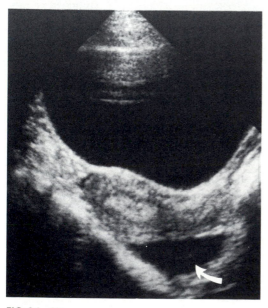

FIG 21–37.
Longitudinal view of the pelvis in a patient with a moderate amount of free fluid in the cul-de-sac *(arrow).*

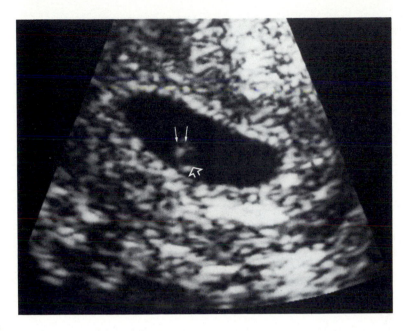

FIG 21–38.
Transvaginal view of a 6-week intrauterine pregnancy. In this magnified image, the yolk sac is indicated by the *open arrow*, and the two *small arrows* indicate the crown-rump length of the embryo (3 mm).

pelvic sonography in the early pregnant patient. Besides determining the viability of the pregnancy, other abnormalities to look for include a blighted twin or a subchorionic collection (Fig 21–39; Finberg and Birnholz, 1979; Goldstein et al., 1983). It is often difficult to tell these two abnormalities apart, since in both cases, an echolucent fluid collection will be present adjacent to the gestational sac, indicating some bleeding. To diagnose a blighted twin, however, the fluid collection adjacent to the viable gestational sac must itself be saclike and rounded, since many crescentic fluid collections partly surrounding gestational sacs have been mistaken for blighted twins and actually represent subchorionic bleeding. The diagnosis of a blighted twin carries a good prognosis for carrying the singleton to term. Goldstein et al. (1983) report a positive outcome of 80% associated with the presence of subchorionic bleeding. Sonographic follow-up is helpful in these cases. When a viable pregnancy is established by visualizing a fetal pole with a heartbeat, studies have shown that the risk of spontaneous abortion before 20 weeks is 2% (Cashner et al., 1987).

Sonologists are frequently asked to rule out an ectopic pregnancy. A sonogram, however, cannot be properly interpreted without results of the β-hCG test since a negative test result for β-hCG essentially rules out any pregnancy. When the pregnancy test result is positive, sonography is most useful for establishing the presence of an intrauterine pregnancy. The mere presence of an intrauterine fluid collection does not necessarily establish the pregnancy, however, since as many as 20% of ectopic pregnancies can be associated with irregular intrauterine fluid collections such as blood or debris, mimicking a gestational sac (Benacerraf et al., 1984; Marks et al., 1979; Nelson et al., 1983). It is often not practical to wait for the appearance of the fetal pole to be sure that the pregnancy is in the uterus. Recently, the *double decidual sac sign* has been established as one of the most important criteria for the presence of an intrauterine pregnancy. The double sac consists of two concentric rings partway around the fluid collection, one representing the decidua parietalis or decidua vera and the other the decidua capsularis. This enables the sonologist to discriminate between the actual gestational sac and the uterine cavity itself, which is separate and where a pseudogestational sac would reside (Bradley et al., 1982; Filly, 1987; Nyberg et al., 1983). The presence of the double sac sign correlated with an

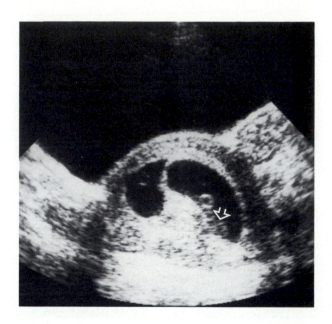

FIG 21–39.
Transverse view of the uterus showing two different gestational sacs. The *arrow* indicates the live embryo just behind the yoke sac. Note that the other gesta-tional sac has a faintly seen yolk sac but no embryo and represented a blighted twin.

intrauterine pregnancy in 98.3% of patients, and of 68 patients who lacked the double sac appearance, only 4 had a normal intrauterine pregnancy (Vilaro et al., 1987).

When no intrauterine gestational sac can be identified and results of the pregnancy test are positive, other signs of ectopic pregnancy must be sought. Rarely, the actual ectopic gestation, embryo, and heartbeat will be identified, and a definite diagnosis can be made (Fig 21–40). Nonspecific findings suggesting ectopic pregnancy include an adnexal mass, a fluid collection in the cul-de-sac, or echogenic mass indicating a clot in the cul-de-sac (Brown et al., 1978; Filly, 1987). Brown et al. (1978) found that 73% of patients with a positive pregnancy test result and no intrauterine gestational sac had an ectopic pregnancy. An adnexal ring is also a significant indicator of ectopic pregnancy (Fig 21–41; Brown et al., 1978). It is possible, however, that despite the presence of an ectopic pregnancy, the sonogram can be entirely normal, showing no evidence of adnexal mass. If the patient has a positive pregnancy test result, but no intrauterine pregnancy and no adnexal masses are identified, an ectopic pregnancy cannot be excluded by imaging alone (Lawson, 1978; Brown et al., 1978).

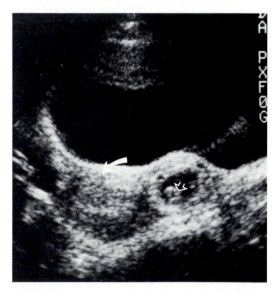

FIG 21–40.
Transverse view of the pelvis showing an ectopic gestation *(open arrow)*. The *curved arrow* indicates the empty uterus. This diagnosis was definitive since extrauterine cardiac motion of the fetus was identified.

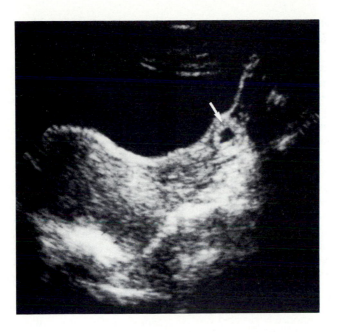

FIG 21–41.
Transverse view of the left adnexa showing a ring sign *(arrow)* directly above the left ovary. This represents an ectopic pregnancy.

In an attempt to improve our ability to diagnose ectopic pregnancy, the discriminatory β-hCG zone was established at 6,000 to 6,500 mIU/ml. If the β-hCG is above this level, the absence of an intrauterine gestational sac is virtually diagnostic of an ectopic pregnancy (Kadar et al., 1981; Romero et al., 1985). Since that time, better resolution of sonographic equipment and more experience have led to using a lower number (1,800 mIU/ml) for establishing the presence of an intrauterine pregnancy. Nyberg et al. (1987a) studied 150 women, of whom 76 had intrauterine pregnancy and 55 had a β-hCG level exceeding 1,800 mIU/ml. In each of these 55 patients, the gestational sac was identified. In comparison, 35 of the 74 patients with ectopic pregnancy had β-hCG levels of 1,800 mIU/ml or more and had no demonstrable intrauterine gestational sac. This is a more useful number in clinical practice, since ectopic pregnancies tend to have rather low β-hCG levels. With the advent of transvaginal scanning, it is clear that the level of β-hCG needed to visualize the gestational sac is lower, and Nyberg et al. (1988) again studied 84 women with early pregnancies, comparing the transvaginal sonogram to the β-hCG level. Four of 5 (80%) of these patients with a β-hCG level between 500 and 1,000 mIU/ml and all of the 17 patients with levels above 1,000 mIU/ml had sonograms demonstrating an intrauterine gestational sac. In comparison, none of the patients with ectopic pregnancy had intrauterine gestational sacs, including 17 of 26 women with ectopic pregnancy who had β-hCG levels above 1,000 mIU/ml. These data indicate that a gestational sac should be visualized in the uterus using transvaginal scanning when the β-hCG level exceeds 1,000 mIU/ml, and when the gestational sac is not seen, the patient has a high likelihood of ectopic pregnancy. Other studies have compared transvaginal with transabdominal sonography in the evaluation of ectopic pregnancy, and as expected, transvaginal scanning provided additional information in 60% of cases and less information in 4% of cases compared with transabdominal sonography (Nyberg et al., 1987b). It was possible to establish the presence of an extrauterine gestational sac not observed on transabdominal images in 10 cases and the extrauterine embryo in 2 cases (Nyberg et al., 1987b).

The presence of an intrauterine pregnancy is the most valuable criterion for excluding an ectopic pregnancy sonographically. Simultaneous ectopic and intrauterine pregnancy, however, can occur, although rarely, and this possibility must not be completely forgotten (Benacerraf et al., 1985). With the advent of fertility medication, the incidence of simultaneous ectopic and intrauterine pregnancy is higher than before, and this must be considered when an adnexal mass or free fluid is present in the cul-de-sac, even in the presence of an intrauterine gestational sac. Pregnancies can also implant in other ectopic locations such as the cervix, which may lead to large amounts of bleeding, sometimes life threatening (Werber et al., 1983). It is important to recognize the cervical gestational sac sonographically to avoid excess bleeding and maternal morbidity.

Ultrasound is the most definitive method for diagnosis of trophoblastic disease. The classic mole has no associated fetus, and the uterus is entirely filled with heterogeneous mass composed of tiny fluid collections in an echogenic matrix (Fig 21–42). The uterus is often large for dates in a patient with a disproportionately elevated β-hCG level. Occasionally, fibroid tumors can masquerade as hydatidiform moles, and correlation with the β-hCG is crucial in those cases. Partial moles

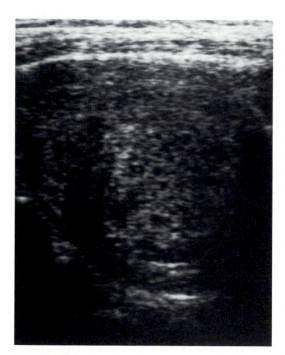

FIG 21–42.
Markedly enlarged uterus filled with heterogeneous material containing a multitude of very tiny cystic areas. This was a complete mole.

can have the appearance of a blighted ovum in early pregnancy but with a thickened or hydropic echogenic rim. Later in the first trimester, there may be a viable but usually abnormal fetus that is most often associated with triploidy. The placenta tends to be large, be thickened, and contain many small echolucencies.

CONCLUSION

Over the past few years, the resolution of sonographic equipment has vastly improved, and sonologists have acquired more experience. In addition, the development of the transvaginal probe has enhanced our diagnostic capability not only because the transducers can come closer to the pelvic organs but also because higher frequency transducers with better resolution can be used. Transvaginal sonography has been most important in the field of infertility, enabling the IVF patients to undergo easier outpatient egg retrievals. It has also been a major factor in improving diagnostic confidence for the evaluation of early or ectopic pregnancy. Transvaginal scanning has opened a diagnostic window to the posterior cul-de-sac not previously available and has increased the sensitivity and specificity for the diagnosis of pelvic masses. A complete gynecological scan still requires a full bladder, however, and the transabdominal component of the scan for visualizing the upper pelvis remains an important part of the pelvic sonogram. Transvaginal sonography does enable us to bypass the full bladder in certain situations, particularly in the evaluation of the emergency patient who cannot drink fluids or for whom awaiting bladder filling would delay urgent care.

REFERENCES

Andolf E, Jorgensen C: Simple adnexal cysts diagnosed by ultrasound in postmenopausal women. *J Clin Ultrasound* 1988; 16:301–303.

Athey PA, Butters HE: Sonographic and CT appearance of Krukenberg tumors. *J Clin Ultrasound* 1984; 12:205–210.

Athey PA, Cooper NB: Sonographic features of parovarian cysts. *AJR* 1985; 144:83–86.

Athey PA, Malone RS: Sonography of ovarian fibromas/thecomas. *J Ultrasound Med* 1987; 6:431–436.

Baker ME, Bowie JD, Killam AP: Sonography of post-cesarean-section bladder-flap hematoma. *AJR* 1985; 144:757–759.

Baker ME, Mahony BS, Bowie JD: Adverse effect of an overdistended bladder on first-trimester sonography. *AJR* 1985; 145:597–599.

Baltarowich OH, Kurtz AB, Pasto ME, et al: The spectrum of sonographic findings in hemorrhagic ovarian cysts. *AJR* 1987; 148:901–905.

Benacerraf BR, Finkler NJ, Wojciechowski C, et al: Sonographic accuracy in the diagnosis of ovarian masses. *J Reprod Med*, in press.

Benacerraf B, Parker-Jones K, Schiff I: Decidual cast mimicking an intrauterine gestational sac and fetal pole in a patient with ectopic pregnancy: A case report. *J Reprod Med* 1984; 29:498–500.

Benacerraf BR, Rinehart JS, Schiff I: Sonographic diagnosis of simultaneous intrauterine and ectopic pregnancy. *J Ultrasound Med* 1985; 4:321–322.

Bernard KG, Cooperberg PL: Sonographic differentiation between blighted ovum and early viable pregnancy. *AJR* 1985; 144:597–602.

Birnholz JC: Endometriosis and inflammatory disease. *Semin Ultrasound* 1983; 4:184–192.

Bourgouin P, Dubuc G, Vauclair R, et al: Sonographic demonstration of post-abortion intrauterine osseous tissue. *J Ultrasound Med* 1985; 4:507–509.

Bradley WG, Fiske CE, Filly RA: The double sac sign of early intrauterine pregnancy: Use in exclusion of ectopic pregnancy. *Radiology* 1982; 143:223–226.

Brandt TD, Levy EB, Grant TH, et al: Endometrial echo and its significance in female infertility. *Radiology* 1985; 157:225–229.

Breckenridge JW, Kurtz AB, Ritchie WGM, et al: Postmenopausal uterine fluid collection: Indicator of carcinoma. *AJR* 1982; 139:529–534.

Brown TW, Filly RA, Laing FC, et al: Analysis of ultrasonographic criteria in the evaluation for ectopic pregnancy. *AJR* 1978; 131:967–971.

Callen PW, DeMartini WJ, Filly RA: The central uterine cavity echo: A useful anatomic sign in the ultrasonographic evaluation of the female pelvis. *Radiology* 1979; 131:187–190.

Callen PW, Filly RA, Munyer TP: Intrauterine contraceptive devices: Evaluation by sonography. *AJR* 1980; 135:797–800.

Carroll R, Gombergh R: Empty-bladder (hysterographic) view on US for evaluation of intrauterine devices. *Radiology* 1987; 163:822–823.

Cashner KA, Christopher CR, Dysert GA: Spontaneous fetal loss after demonstration of a live fetus in the first trimester. *Obstet Gynecol* 1987; 70:827–830.

Chambers CB, Unis JS: Ultrasonographic evidence of uterine malignancy in the postmenopausal uterus. *Am J Obstet Gynecol* 1986; 154:1194–1199.

Chervenak FA, Amin HK, Neuwirth RS: Symptomatic intrauterine retention of fetal bones. *Obstet Gynecol* 1982; 59:58S–61S.

Coleman BG, Arger PH, Mulhern CB Jr: Endometriosis: Clinical and ultrasonic correlation. *AJR* 1979; 132:747–749.

Coulam CB, Hill LM, Breckle R: Ultrasonic evidence for luteinization of unruptured preovulatory follicles. *Fertil Steril* 1982; 37:524–529.

Cunat JS, Dunne MG, Butler M: Sonographic diagnosis of uterine perforation following suction curettage. *J Clin Ultrasound* 1984; 12:108–109.

Davis JA, Gosink BB: Fluid in the female pelvis: Cyclic patterns. *J Ultrasound Med* 1986; 5:75–79.

el Tabbakh GH, Lotfy I, Azab I, et al: Correlation of the ultrasonic appearance of the ovaries in polycystic ovarian disease and the clinical, hormonal, and laparoscopic findings. *Am J Obstet Gynecol* 1986; 154:892–895.

Filly RA: Ectopic pregnancy: The role of sonography. *Radiology* 1987; 162:661–668.

Finberg HJ, Birnholz JC: Ultrasound observations in multiple gestation with first trimester bleeding: The blighted twin. *Radiology* 1979; 132:137–142.

Fleischer AC, James AE Jr, Millis JB, et al: Differential diagnosis of pelvic masses by gray scale sonography. *AJR* 1978; 131:469–476.

Fleischer AC, Kalemeris GC, Machin JE, et al: Sonographic depiction of normal and abnormal endometrium with histopathologic correlation. *J Ultrasound Med* 1986; 5:445–452.

Fogel SR, Slasky BS: Sonography of nabothian cysts. *AJR* 1982; 138:927–930.

Forrest TS, Elyaderani MK, Muilenburg MI, et al: Cyclic endometrial changes: US assessment with histologic correlation. *Radiology* 1988; 167:233–237.

Friedman H, Vogelzang RL, Mendelson EB, et al: Endometriosis detection by US with laparoscopic correlation. *Radiology* 1985; 157:217–220.

Gilsanz V, Cleveland RH, Reid BS: Duplication of the Mullerian ducts and genitourinary malformations. *Radiology* 1982; 144:797–801.

Goldstein SR, Subramanyam BR, Raghavendra

BN, et al: Subchorionic bleeding in threatened abortion: Sonographic findings and significance. *AJR* 1983; 141:975–978.

Granberg S, Wikland M: Comparison between endovaginal and transabdominal transducers for measuring ovarian volume. *J Ultrasound Med* 1987; 6:649–653.

Gross BH, Silver TM, Jaffe MH: Sonographic features of uterine leiomyomas: Analysis of 41 proven cases. *J Ultrasound Med* 1983; 2:401–406.

Hall DA, Hann LE, Ferrucci JT Jr, et al: Sonographic morphology of the normal menstrual cycle. *Radiology* 1979; 133:185–188.

Hall DA, McCarthy KA: The significance of the postmenopausal simple adnexal cyst. *J Ultrasound Med* 1986; 5:503–505.

Hall DA, McCarthy KA, Kopans DB: Sonographic visualization of the normal postmenopausal ovary. *J Ultrasound Med* 1986; 5:9–11.

Hann LE, Crivello M, McArdle C, et al: In vitro fertilization: Sonographic perspective. *Radiology* 1987; 163:665–668.

Hann LE, Hall DA, McArdle CR, et al: Polycystic ovarian disease: Sonographic spectrum. *Radiology* 1984; 150:531–534.

Herrmann UJ Jr, Locher GW, Goldhirsch A: Sonographic patterns of ovarian tumors: Prediction of malignancy. *Obstet Gynecol* 1987; 69:777–781.

Hirsh MP, Levy HM: The varied ultrasonographic appearance of laminaria. *J Ultrasound Med* 1988; 7:45–47.

Jeffrey RB, Laing FC: Echogenic clot: A useful sign of pelvic hemoperitoneum. *Radiology* 1982; 145:139–141.

Johnson MA, Graham MF, Cooperberg PL: Abnormal endometrial echoes: Sonographic spectrum of endometrial pathology. *J Ultrasound Med* 1982; 1:161–166.

Kadar N, DeVore G, Romero R: Discriminatory hCG zone: Its use in the sonographic evaluation for ectopic pregnancy. *Obstet Gynecol* 1981; 58:156–161.

Kurtz AB, Rubin CS, Kramer FL, et al: Ultrasound evaluation of the posterior pelvic compartment. *Radiology* 1979; 132:677–682.

Lande IM, Hill MC, Cosco FE, et al: Adnexal and cul-de-sac abnormalities: Transvaginal sonography. *Radiology* 1988; 166:325–332.

Landers DV, Sweet RL: Current trends in the diagnosis and treatment of tuboovarian abscess. *Am J Obstet Gynecol* 1985; 151:1098–1110.

Lawson TL: Ectopic pregnancy: Criteria and accuracy of ultrasonic diagnosis. *AJR* 1978; 131:153–156.

Lawson TL, Albarelli JN: Diagnosis of gynecologic pelvic masses by gray scale ultrasonography: Analysis of specificity and accuracy. *AJR* 1977; 128:1003–1006.

Lees RF, Feldman PS, Brenbridge ANAG, et al: Inflammatory cysts of the pelvic peritoneum. *AJR* 1978; 131:633–636.

Levi CS, Lyons EA, Lindsay DJ: Early diagnosis of nonviable pregnancy with endovaginal US. *Radiology* 1988; 167:383–385.

Lister JE, Kane JG, Erhmann R, et al: Ultrasound appearance of adenomyosis mimicking adenocarcinoma in a postmenopausal woman. *J Clin Ultrasound* 1988; 16:519–521.

Malini S, Valdes C, Malinak LR: Sonographic diagnosis and classification of anomalies of the female genital tract. *J Ultrasound Med* 1984; 3:397–404.

Marks WM, Filly RA, Callen PW, et al: The decidual cast of ectopic pregnancy: A confusing ultrasonographic appearance. *Radiology* 1979; 133:451–454.

McArdle CR, Sacks BA: Ovarian hyperstimulation syndrome. *AJR* 1980; 135:835–836.

McArdle C, Seibel M, Hann LE, et al: The diagnosis of ovarian hyperstimulation (OHS): The impact of ultrasound. *Fertil Steril* 1983; 39:464–467.

McArdle CR, Seibel M, Weinstein F, et al: Induction of ovulation monitored by ultrasound. *Radiology* 1983; 148:809–812.

McArdle CR, Simon L, Kiejna C: Vaginal drainage of posthysterectomy abscess under direct ultrasonic guidance. *Obstet Gynecol* 1984; 63:90S–92S.

McCarthy KA, Hall DA, Kopans DB, et al: Postmenopausal endometrial fluid collections: Always an indicator of malignancy? *J Ultrasound Med* 1986; 5:647–649.

McCarthy S, Taylor KJW: Sonography of vaginal masses. *AJR* 1983; 140:1005–1008.

Mendelson EB, Bohm-Velez M, Joseph N, et al: Endometrial abnormalities: Evaluation with transvaginal sonography. *AJR* 1988a; 150:139–142.

Mendelson EB, Bohm-Velez M, Joseph N, et al: Gynecologic imaging: Comparison of transabdominal and transvaginal sonography. *Radiology* 1988b; 166:321–324.

Mendelson EB, Friedman H, Neiman HL, et al: The role of imaging in infertility management. *AJR* 1985; 144:415–420.

Meyer JS, Kim CS, Price HM, et al: Ultrasound presentation of primary carcinoma of the fallopian tube. *J Clin Ultrasound* 1987; 15:132–134.

Moyle JW, Rochester D, Sider L, et al: Sonography of ovarian tumors: Predictability of tumor type. *AJR* 1983; 141:985–991.

Nelson P, Bowie JD, Rosenberg ER: Early intrauterine pregnancy or decidual cast: An anatomic-sonographic approach. *J Ultrasound Med* 1983; 2:543–547.

Nocera RM, Fagan CJ, Hernandez JC: Cystic parametrial fibroids mimicking ovarian cystadenoma. *J Ultrasound Med* 1984; 3:183–187.

Nosher JL, Winchman HK, Needell GS: Transvaginal pelvic abscess drainage with US guidance. *Radiology* 1987; 165:872–873.

Nyberg DA, Filly RA, Laing FC, et al: Ectopic pregnancy: Diagnosis by sonography correlated with quantitative HCG levels. *J Ultrasound Med* 1987a; 6:145–150.

Nyberg DA, Laing FC, Filly RA: Threatened abortion: Sonographic distinction of normal and abnormal gestation sacs. *Radiology* 1986; 158:397–400.

Nyberg DA, Laing FC, Filly RA, et al: Ultrasonographic differentiation of the gestational sac of early intrauterine pregnancy from the pseudogestational sac of ectopic pregnancy. *Radiology* 1983; 146:755–759.

Nyberg DA, Mack LA, Jeffrey RB Jr, et al: Endovaginal sonographic evaluation of ectopic pregnancy: A prospective study. *AJR* 1987b; 149:1181–1186.

Nyberg DA, Mack LA, Laing FC, et al: Early pregnancy complications: Endovaginal sonographic findings correlated with human chorionic gonadotropin levels. *Radiology* 1988; 167:619–622.

O'Brien WF, Buck DR, Nash JD: Evaluation of sonography in the initial assessment of the gynecologic patient. *Am J Obstet Gynecol* 1984; 149:598–602.

O'Herlihy C, Pepperell RJ, Robinson HP: Ultrasound timing of human chorionic gonadotropin administration in clomiphene-stimulated cycles. *Obstet Gynecol* 1982; 59:40–45.

Paling MR, Shawker TH: Abdominal ultrasound in advanced ovarian carcinoma. *J Clin Ultrasound* 1981; 9:435–441.

Pennell RG, Baltarowich OH, Kurtz AB, et al: Complicated first-trimester pregnancies: Evaluation with endovaginal US versus transabdominal technique. *Radiology* 1987; 165:79–83.

Picker RH, Smith DH, Tucker MH, et al: Ultrasonic signs of imminent ovulation. *J Clin Ultrasound* 1983; 11:1–2.

Rankin RN, Hutton LC: Ultrasound in the ovarian hyperstimulation syndrome. *J Clin Ultrasound* 1981; 9:473–476.

Requard CK, Mettler FA Jr, Wicks JD: Preoperative sonography of malignant ovarian neoplasms. *AJR* 1981; 137:79–82.

Reynolds T, Hill MC, Glassman LM: Sonography of hemorrhagic ovarian cysts. *J Clin Ultrasound* 1986; 14:449–453.

Richman TS, Viscomi GN, deCherney A, et al: Fallopian tubal patency assessed by ultrasound following fluid injection. *Radiology* 1984; 152:507–510.

Rifkin MD, Needleman L, Kurtz AB, et al: Sonography of nongynecologic cystic masses of the pelvis. *AJR* 1984; 142:1169–1174.

Ritchie WGM: Sonographic evaluation of normal and induced ovulation. *Radiology* 1986; 161:1–10.

Romero R, Kadar N, Jeanty P, et al: Diagnosis of ectopic pregnancy: Value of the discriminatory human chorionic gonadotropin zone. *Obstet Gynecol* 1985; 66:357–360.

Rosenberg HK, Sherman NH, Tarry WF, et al: Mayer-Rokitansky-Kuster-Hauser syndrome: US aid to diagnosis. *Radiology* 1986; 161:815–819.

Rosenblatt R, Zakin D, Stern WZ, et al: Uterine perforation and embedding by intrauterine device: Evaluation by US and hysterography. *Radiology* 1985; 157:765–770.

Rulin MC, Preston AL: Adnexal masses in postmenopausal women. *Obstet Gynecol* 1987; 70:578–581.

Sample WF, Lippe BM, Gyepes MT: Gray-scale ultrasonography of the normal female pelvis. *Radiology* 1977; 125:477–483.

Sandler MA, Karo JJ: The spectrum of ultrasonic findings in endometriosis. *Radiology* 1978; 127:229–231.

Sandler MA, Silver TM, Karo JJ: Gray-scale ultrasonic features of ovarian teratomas. *Radiology* 1979; 131:705–709.

Schaffer RM, Taylor C, Haller JO, et al: Nonobstructive hydrocolpos: Sonographic appearance and differential diagnosis. *Radiology* 1983; 149:273–278.

Schulman JD, Dorfmann AD, Jones SL, et al: Outpatient in vitro fertilization using transvaginal ultrasound-guided oocyte retrieval. *Obstet Gynecol* 1987; 69:665–668.

Schwimer SR, Marik J, Lebovic J: Percutaneous ovarian cyst aspiration using continuous transvaginal ultrasonographic monitoring. *J Ultrasound Med* 1985; 4:259–260.

Scott WW, Rosenshein NB, Siegelman SS, et al: The obstructed uterus. *Radiology* 1981; 141:767–770.

Shawker TH, Garra BS, Loriaux DL, et al: Ultrasonography of Turner's syndrome. *J Ultrasound Med* 1986; 5:125–129.

Shenker L, Brickman FE: Bicornuate uterus with incomplete vaginal septum and unilateral renal agenesis. *Radiology* 1979; 133:455–457.

Siedler D, Laing FC, Jeffrey RB Jr, et al: Uterine adenomyosis: A difficult sonographic diagnosis. *J Ultrasound Med* 1987; 6:345–349.

Subramanyam BR, Raghavendra BN, Whalen CA, et al: Ultrasonic features of fallopian tube carcinoma. *J Ultrasound Med* 1984; 3:391–393.

Taylor KJW, DeGraaft MCI, Wasson JF, et al: Accuracy of grey-scale ultrasound diagnosis of abdominal and pelvic abscesses in 220 patients. *Lancet* 1978; 1:83.

Taylor PJ, Wiseman D, Mahadevan M, et al: "Ultrasound rescue": A successful alternative form of oocyte recovery in patients with periovarian adhesions. *Am J Obstet Gynecol* 1986; 154:240–244.

Thickman D, Arger P, Tureck R, et al: Sonographic assessment of the endometrium in patients undergoing in vitro fertilization. *J Ultrasound Med* 1986; 5:197–201.

Timor-Tritsch IE, Rottem S: Transvaginal ultrasonographic study of the fallopian tube. *Obstet Gynecol* 1987; 70:424–428.

Vilaro MM, Rifkin MD, Pennell RG, et al: Endovaginal ultrasound: A technique for evaluation of nonfollicular pelvic masses. *J Ultrasound Med* 1987; 6:697–701.

Wade RV, Smythe AR, Watt GW, et al: Reliability of gynecologic sonographic diagnosis, 1978–1984. *Am J Obstet Gynecol* 1985; 153:186–190.

Walsh JW, Rosenfield AT, Jaffe CC, et al: Prospective comparison of ultrasound and computed tomography in the evaluation of gynecologic pelvic masses. *AJR* 1978; 131:955–960.

Walsh JW, Taylor KJW, Rosenfield AT: Gray scale ultrasonography in the diagnosis of endometriosis and adenomyosis. *AJR* 1979a; 132:87–90.

Walsh JW, Taylor KJW, Wasson JFMcI, et al: Gray-scale ultrasound in 204 proved gynecologic masses: Accuracy and specific diagnostic criteria. *Radiology* 1979b; 130:391–397.

Walzer A, Flynn E, Koenigsberg M: Sonographic appearance of a prolapsing submucous leiomyoma. *J Clin Ultrasound* 1983; 11:101–102.

Werber J, Prasadarao PR, Harris VJ: Cervical pregnancy diagnosed by ultrasound. *Radiology* 1983; 149:279–280.

Wiener MD, Bowie JD, Baker ME, et al: Sonography of subfascial hematoma after cesarean delivery. *AJR* 1987; 148:907–910.

Willard DA: Pelvic varices: Sonographic and surgical recognition. *J Clin Ultrasound* 1988; 16:265–267.

Wilson DA, Stacy TM, Smith EI: Ultrasound diagnosis of hydrocolpos and hydrometrocolpos. *Radiology* 1978; 128:451–454.

Winsett MZ, Fagan CJ, Bedi DG: Sonographic demonstration of bladder-flap hematoma. *J Ultrasound Med* 1986; 5:483–487.

Worthen NJ, Gunning JE: Percutaneous drainage of pelvic abscesses: Management of the tubo-ovarian abscess. *J Ultrasound Med* 1986; 5:551–556.

Yeh HC, Futterweit W, Thornton JC: Polycystic ovarian disease: US features in 104 patients. *Radiology* 1987; 163:111–116.

22   Laparoscopy, Hysteroscopy, and Laser Surgery

Andrew J. Friedman, M.D.

LAPAROSCOPY

Laparoscopy, or peritoneoscopy, is an endoscopic procedure that enables the surgeon to directly visualize pelvic and abdominal contents. It is one of the most frequently performed surgical procedures and has become an essential tool in the gynecologist's armamentarium for the diagnosis and treatment of numerous gynecologic conditions. The development of operative laparoscopic equipment and techniques has enabled the pelvic and reproductive surgeon to perform a wide variety of extensive procedures, previously performed via laparotomy, as outpatient surgery.

History

The first recorded endoscopic procedure was performed by Bozzini in 1805 who attempted to visualize the urethral mucosa using a simple square-windowed tube and candlelight directed by a concave mirror. Bozzini (1807) met with disapproval and was censured by the Medical Faculty of Vienna for "undue curiosity." The first recorded human laparoscopy was by Jacobaeus of Sweden in 1910 (Gomel et al., 1986). He created a pneumoperitoneum using a trocar and cannula and was able to visualize the pelvis with a Nitze cystoscope (Germany, 1877) through the same cannula.

In 1911, Berheim reported on peritoneal cystoscopy performed for the first time in the United States (Steptoe, 1967). Ruddock, in 1937, reported on 500 laparoscopic cases with a mortality of 0.2% and utilized electrocautery with biopsy forceps (Steptoe, 1967). In 1944, Decker first introduced a pneumoperitoneum by creating negative intraabdominal pressure with the knee-chest position (Steptoe, 1967). "Gaseous distention" of the abdomen was first reported by Palmer in 1946 (Steptoe, 1967). In 1947, fiber optics were introduced by Hopkins and Kampany of England (Gomel et al., 1986). Laparoscopic sterilization by unipolar electrocoagulation was first reported in 1962 by Palmer. Since the early 1970s, numerous advances in equipment and technique have expanded the role of laparoscopy from primarily a diagnostic procedure to one with numerous operative capabilities.

Equipment

The basic equipment needed for laparoscopy includes a Verres needle, a primary trocar and cannula, a laparoscope, an insufflator, and a light source (Fig 22–1). Laparoscopes range from 5 to 13 mm in diameter. The smaller-caliber laparoscopes are adequate for diagnostic cases. Many surgeons prefer larger-diameter (8–13 mm) laparoscopes for operative laparoscopy. These larger instruments may have twin fiber bundles for better illumination, visualization, and often, photodocumentation; large laparoscopes may also have an operative channel for laser, mechanical, or electrocautery instruments. Larger laparoscopes require big primary trocars that have wider tips and require more force to penetrate the abdomen than smaller trocars, increasing the depth of penetration and increasing the risk of visceral injury (Gomel et al., 1986).

Different insufflation rates of carbon dioxide (CO_2) gas may be used to create the pneumoperitoneum. Most surgeons insufflate at 1 L/minute initially until an adequate pneumoperitoneum is obtained. Laparoscopy units equipped with "high" or "fast flow" modes are able to insufflate at 3 L/minute. This rapid insufflation rate is helpful to maintain an adequate pneumoperitoneum

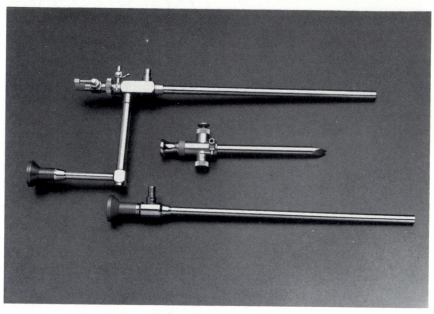

FIG 22–1.
Operative laparoscope, primary trocar, and diagnostic laparoscope. (Courtesy of Edward Weck, Inc., Princeton, N.J.)

in operative laparoscopic cases where instruments are changed frequently and in cases where laser plume may be evacuated at intervals. At a given flow rate, insufflators may deliver CO_2 by either a pressure-dependent or independent mode. The "manual" insufflation mode is pressure independent, insufflates at a constant flow rate, and is used for establishment of the pneumoperitoneum. The "automatic" mode is pressure dependent, maintains constant intraperitoneal pressure, and is used once pneumoperitoneum is established.

The light source is a fiber optic cable that transmits cool but intense light from the external source, through the laparoscope, and into the peritoneal cavity. The brightness of the light is a function of both the power of the external source and the diameter of the cable that contains the fiber bundles. Twin fiber bundles produce maximal illumination facilitating photodocumentation, video recording, or both.

Often, secondary and even tertiary or quaternary puncture sites are utilized for diagnostic or operative laparoscopy. Each additional site requires a separate trocar and cannula sleeve. Ancillary instruments can then be used through these additional sites for stabilization and surgical manipulation of pelvic and abdominal structures (Fig 22–2). The most commonly used ancillary instrument is a calibrated probe. The probe may be marked in centimeters, allowing measurement of internal structures that appear magnified through the laparoscopic lens. Probes may be used to stabilize or immobilize pelvic structures or to perform blunt dissection of filmy adhesions. Insulated probes with a metal tip may also be used to carry unipolar current for coagulation.

Various forceps may also be used in ancillary puncture sites. Atraumatic forceps allow for delicate handling of tissue, whereas traumatic forceps may be used for stabilization of "hard" tissue that is ultimately destroyed or removed from the peritoneal cavity. Biopsy forceps may also be used to aid in diagnosis. It is important not to use electrocautery when a biopsy for tissue is performed because it will make the pathologist unable to render an accurate diagnosis. Bipolar forceps have been especially useful for sterilization procedures and in coagulating bleeding sites and endometriotic lesions.

Many types of scissors (i.e., hooked, serrated, "micro") may be used with or without unipolar electrocautery. Cautery should be used when dividing vascular structures only when the operating surgeon has a clear view of the operative field and surrounding tissues to minimize inadvertent electrical injury to vulnerable viscera.

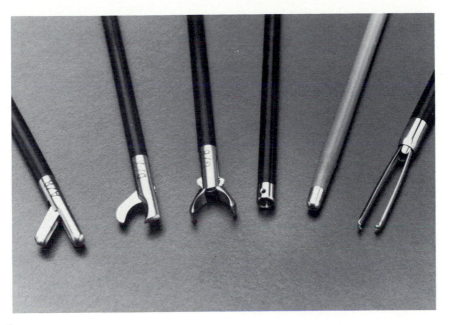

FIG 22–2.
Ancillary laparoscopic instruments including (from *left* to *right*) punch biopsy forceps, hook scissors, atraumatic grasping forceps, suction-irrigation probe, unipolar cautery probe, traumatic forceps. (Courtesy of Edward Weck, Inc., Princeton, N.J.)

Aspirating cannulas come with either blunt ends or pointed "needle" tips. Blunted aspiration cannulas may be used for irrigation or aspiration. A dual channel combined irrigation-aspiration instrument is especially useful to facilitate localization of bleeding sites. Needle tip aspirators with beveled tips have been used for laparoscopic oocyte harvesting in in vitro fertilization (IVF) procedures as well as for drainage of ovarian, paraovarian, or paratubal cysts or injection of saline or vasopressin (Pitressin) solutions into pelvic structures (i.e., mesosalpinx, leiomyomas, and uterine septa).

Most electrosurgical units contain both unipolar and bipolar modes. In unipolar electrocautery circuitry, the current passes from the generator through the instrument to a ground plate and then back to the generator. Unipolar electrocautery often causes a greater degree of thermal damage than the surface area of the distal coagulating tip of the instrument. In addition, it is possible to generate electrical sparks that may potentially induce thermal injury in adjacent bowel or other tissues. For these reasons, one must use extreme care when using unipolar cautery. In the bipolar system, current is passed from the generator into one insulated jaw of a forceps through the

grasped tissue into the second insulated forceps jaw and back to the generator. The passage of current heats and coagulates the grasped tissue in a controlled fashion.

Endocoagulation or thermocoagulation was developed by Semm in 1962 (Semm and Mettler, 1980). In this technique, hemostasis is achieved by heating the tissue from 100°C to 140°C. Endocoagulation may also be used to destroy endometriotic implants or to evert serosal edges in a newly created distal salpingostomy.

Endoscopic laser technology is rapidly evolving, providing new methods of coagulating, cutting, and vaporizing tissue. The four types of lasers used in gynecologic surgery include CO_2, argon, potassium titanyl phosphate (KTP), and the neodymium–yttrium aluminum garnet (Nd:YAG or YAG) lasers. These lasers are discussed in a later section. Lasers may be utilized through an operative channel in the laparoscope or through hollow ancillary instruments.

Endoscopic suturing may be used for certain advanced operative laparoscopic procedures. A Roeder loop (Ethbinder, Ethicon, Somerville, N.J.) is a Semm modification of the loop developed by Roeder in the early 1900s for tonsillectomy in children (Semm, 1978). The Roeder loop may be used for ligation of bleeding sites or for ligation of tissue (tube, ovary, tube and ovary, pedunculated myoma) prior to excision.

Removal of tissue from the abdomen may be accomplished with forceps. Large or hard pieces of tissue may be morcellated by a 10-mm diameter tissue punch instrument that stores pieces of tissue in its sheath (Semm, 1984).

Indications

As experience with operative laparoscopy increases, so does the list of indications to perform laparoscopy (Table 22–1). It cannot be overemphasized how valuable laparoscopy is for timely, accurate diagnosis and, often, as a therapeutic modality.

Contraindications

As more experience with laparoscopy accumulates, the list of contraindications to this procedure has diminished. However, it is essential that the gynecologic surgeon be familiar with these contraindications to maximize patient safety and decrease procedure-related morbidity. Although no uniform agreement regarding all contraindications for laparoscopy exists, a generally accepted list appears in Table 22–2. Some experts consider the past history of pelvic or abdominal surgery or any condition that predisposes the patient to extensive adhesions to be a relative contraindication to laparoscopy. These cases must be individualized according to the experience of the surgeon and the perceived likelihood of causing visceral injury. In some cases, open laparoscopy may be performed to minimize operative risks (Hasson, 1971).

Anesthesia

General endotracheal anesthesia is considered the ideal anesthesia by most experts for laparoscopic procedures. It is safe, provides excellent analgesia and muscle relaxation, and is ideally suited for prolonged operative cases or in cases where extensive manipulation of pelvic or abdominal structures is performed. Local anesthesia has been used successfully for laparoscopic tubal sterilization (Peterson et al., 1987) and may be reserved for the well-prepared patient undergoing short procedures with minimal intraperitoneal manipulation of tissue.

TABLE 22–1.

Indications for Laparoscopy

I. Infertility
  A. Diagnostic
    1. Unexplained etiology after thorough evaluation
    2. Past history of pelvic inflammatory disease (PID), previous pelvic surgery (including appendectomy), endometriosis
    3. Abnormal hysterosalpingogram
    4. Pelvic mass (or masses) and/or pain on examination
    5. Failure to achieve pregnancy after 6 mo. of "appropriate" therapy
    6. Possibly second-look laparoscopy after extensive surgery
  B. Operative
    1. In vitro fertilization, gamete intrafallopian transfer
    2. Reconstructive tubal surgery
      a. Neosalpingostomy
      b. Fimbrioplasty
      c. Salpingo-ovariolysis
    3. Uterine suspension
II. Pelvic pain
  A. Acute: Rule out appendicitis, ruptured cyst, ectopic pregnancy, adnexal torsion, PID, etc.
  B. Chronic: Rule out endometriosis, pelvic adhesions, etc.
  C. Uterosacral ligament ablation (Lichten and Bombard, 1987)
III. Tubal sterilization
IV. Pelvic mass
  A. Diagnostic laparoscopy
  B. Operative laparoscopy
    1. Ectopic pregnancy
    2. Ovarian cyst
    3. Endometriosis
    4. Lysis of adhesions
    5. Rule out neoplasia
    6. Myomectomy
    7. Oophorectomy, salpingectomy, adnexectomy
  C. Foreign body retrieval

Technique

After adequate anesthesia is induced, the patient is placed in dorsal lithotomy position with buttocks protruding slightly from the table, prepped, and draped, and the bladder is emptied. For procedures that may potentially last longer than 1 hour, it is recommended to insert an indwelling Foley catheter that may be removed at the completion of the case. A rigid cannula (e.g.,

TABLE 22–2.

Contraindications to Laparoscopy

I. Contraindications to general anesthesia
  A. Severe cardiopulmonary disease
II. Hypovolemic shock
III. Contraindications to pneumoperitoneum
  A. Severe cardiopulmonary disease
  B. Large (symptomatic) hiatal hernia
IV. Unacceptably high risk of visceral injury
  A. Severe ileus
  B. Bowel obstruction
  C. Generalized peritonitis with ileus
  D. Advanced pregnancy ($\geq$16 wk)
  E. Large ($>$10 cm) intra-abdominal mass
  F. Extreme thinness*
V. Extreme obesity*
VI. Inexperienced surgeon

*Relative contraindications

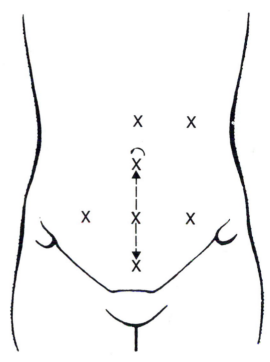

FIG 22–3.
Possible incision sites for the Verres needle (see text).

Cohen-Eder cannula) placed in the endocervix and affixed to a single-toothed tenaculum applied to the anterior cervix will aid in chromopertubation or uterine manipulation (or both) during the procedure.

A small (5- to 13-mm) vertical or transverse incision is made in the midline in the subumbilical fold. The incision should be only large enough to accommodate the laparoscope and still be occlusive. Alternative incision sites may be chosen if there is a high risk of adhesion formation in the region under the umbilicus (Fig 22–3). The Verres needle or cannula is inserted through this incision into the abdomen at approximately a 45-degree angle pointing toward the most dependent portion of the pelvis (i.e., hollow of the sacrum) to minimize the risk of injury. The spring-loaded Verres needle ensures penetration of the abdominal wall while decreasing the risk of visceral injury. To ascertain that the Verres needle is in the peritoneal cavity, one may attach a syringe with 5 ml of saline and observe free flow of saline into the abdomen with minimal force. Insufflation of 2 to 4 L of CO_2 is usually adequate to create a pneumoperitoneum prior to trocar insertion. The "opening pressure" at the start of insufflation should be no higher than 20 mm Hg at a flow rate of 1 L/minute. Higher pressures may indicate extraperitoneal Verres needle placement or partial occlusion of the distal tip of the needle by an intra-abdominal structure. During insufflation, confirmation of intraperitoneal Verres needle place-

ment may be obtained by noting the loss of percussed liver dullness after 1 L has been insufflated.

Once insufflation is complete, the Verres needle is withdrawn and the laparoscopic trocar and its sheath are introduced into the peritoneal cavity through the same subumbilical incision with a back and forth twisting motion aiming the trocar toward the hollow of the sacrum. The trocar is then removed, the laparoscope is placed into its sheath, and the light cable and insufflation tubing are connected to the laparoscope and its sheath, respectively. At this point, the surgeon will be able to observe directly whether or not the laparoscope is in the peritoneal cavity.

Ancillary puncture site (or sites) may then be utilized, if necessary, through separate incisions (Fig 22–4). Transillumination of the abdominal wall with the distal tip of the laparoscope may localize large vessels prior to choosing an ancillary puncture site. When choosing lateral ancillary trocar sites, one must be familiar with the anatomy of the inferior epigastric vessels to avoid vascular injury. Hypotensive collapse following inferior epigastric artery trauma has been reporeted (Pring, 1983). Secondary trocars and cannulas

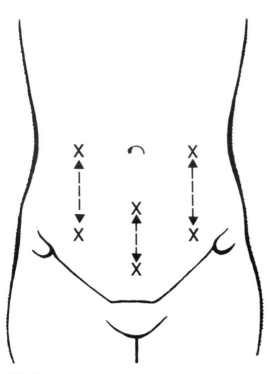

FIG 22–4.
Possible incision sites for ancillary laparoscopic instruments.

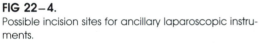

must be inserted under direct laparoscopic visualization to avoid intraperitoneal injury.

Diagnostic Laparoscopy

For diagnostic laparoscopic procedures, an orderly and organized survey of the pelvic anatomy will minimize the possibility of missing a subtle but significant finding. Although it is tempting to abandon this organized approach when obvious pelvic findings exist, the importance of a disciplined inspection of the pelvis cannot be understated.

Infertility

A major use of diagnostic laparoscopy is in the evaluation of infertility. Indications for laparoscopy in this setting include (1) abnormal hysterosalpingogram, (2) infertility without an etiology after a thorough evaluation (i.e., determination of ovulation, semen analysis, postcoital test, and hysterosalpingogram), (3) no conception following 6 months of "appropriate" infertility ther-

apy, (4) history of pelvic inflammatory disease, (5) history of abdominal or pelvic surgery, and (6) presence of a pelvic mass. In general, laparoscopy should be the final procedure performed in the basic infertility workup because it is the most invasive examination.

In several series of women undergoing diagnostic laparoscopies for primary infertility, no pathology was found in 51% to 52% of patients, endometriosis was found in 22% to 39%, and tubal or peritoneal factors were found in 9% to 27% (Musich and Behrman, 1982). In laparoscopies performed on women with secondary infertility, no pathology was found in 42% to 65%, endometriosis was found in 10% to 25%, and tubal or peritoneal factors were found in 10% to 42% (Musich and Behrman, 1982). In women with infertility without an etiology after a thorough evaluation, several series have yielded abnormal pelvic findings in 44% to 75% of patients undergoing laparoscopy (Drake et al., 1977; Elminawi et al., 1978; Goldenberg and Magendantz, 1976; Musich and Behrman, 1982; Peterson and Behrman, 1970; Wood, 1983). This underscores the dictum that laparoscopy is essential to the complete evaluation of the infertile woman.

The positive correlation of hysterosalpingographic and laparoscopic findings ranges from 46% to 84% in various studies (Cummings and Taylor, 1979; Drake et al., 1977; Gabos, 1976; Gomel, 1978; Hutchins, 1977; Musich and Behrman, 1982; Snowden et al., 1984). The majority of misdiagnoses were cornual or proximal tubal occlusion seen on hysterosalpingography. Despite the relatively high rate of inaccurate assessment of tubal status by radiographic methods, diagnostic laparoscopy is recommended shortly after a hysterosalpingogram is performed when abnormal findings are noted.

Pelvic Inflammatory Disease and Chronic Pelvic Pain

Laparoscopy is also a useful diagnostic tool in the evaluation of suspected PID and chronic pelvic pain. The clinical diagnosis of PID is associated with an average accuracy rate of 65% when preoperative impressions are confirmed or rejected by laparoscopy (Method et al., 1987). In a series of 100 women with chronic pelvic pain who underwent laparoscopy, 83% had associated pelvic pathology with the most frequent findings being pelvic adhesions (38%) and endometriosis (32%) (Kresch et al., 1984). In contrast, only

29% of asymptomatic women undergoing tubal ligation had abnormal findings at laparoscopy.

Operative Laparoscopy

The surgical techniques for various operative laparoscopic procedures are beyond the scope of this chapter and are reviewed elsewhere (Gromel et al., 1986; Leventhal, 1986; Murphy, 1987).

Table 22–3 lists surgical procedures performed via laparoscopy. With rapidly advancing technology and development of equipment, this list will continue to expand. In the remainder of this section, clinical experience with some of these procedures will be reviewed.

Tubal Sterilization

Laparoscopic tubal sterilization procedures have dramatically increased in popularity over the past 10 years. Laparoscopic techniques have lower pelvic and incision infection rates and shorter hospitalization and convalescent times than do procedures performed via laparotomy (Brenner, 1981). In addition, laparoscopic procedures have significantly lower pelvic infection rates compared with procedures performed by culdoscopy and culdotomy.

In 1985, a membership survey of the American Association of Gynecologic Laparoscopists revealed recent trends in laparoscopic tubal sterilization procedures (Hulka et al., 1987). Bipolar coagulation was the commonest method of sterilization in 1985, accounting for 57% of laparoscopic procedures; in 1976, only 20% of laparoscopic sterilization procedures were performed by this method. Unipolar coagulation, which accounted for 63% of laparoscopic sterilizations in 1976, was used in only 6% of cases in 1985. Mechanical methods of tubal occlusion such as the ring (29%) and the clip (8%) have increased in popularity in recent years because of their relative ease of application, safety, and easier reversibility when compared with electrocautery methods.

Complications requiring laparotomy following sterilization procedures occurred in 1.6 per 1,000 procedures compared with 3.1 per 1,000 diagnostic laparoscopic procedures. The most commonly encountered complication was hemorrhage (Uribe-Ramirez et al., 1977). In a review of more than 10,000 cases, Bhiwandiwala and coworkers (1983) found very few women who experienced menstrual changes subsequent to sterilization. When changes were experienced, equal proportions of women noted beneficial and adverse changes. The true failure rate of laparoscopic sterilization is similar to that reported for nonlaparoscopic techniques and ranges from 0.9 to 6.0 per 1,000 sterilizations, depending on the technique used (Loffer and Pent, 1980). When pregnancies occur following laparoscopic sterilization, the incidence of ectopic pregnancy is higher after coagulation procedures (29%–61% of all pregnancies) compared with mechanical occlusive techniques (19–33% of all pregnancies). In addition, the risk of ectopic pregnancy is highest dur-

TABLE 22–3.

Operative Laparoscopic Procedures

 I. Tubal sterilization
   A. Electrocautery
     1. Bipolar
     2. Unipolar
   B. Ring
   C. Clip
 II. Treatment of ectopic pregnancy
   A. Salpingostomy
   B. Segmental resection
   C. Salpingectomy
 III. Treatment of endometriosis
   A. Coagulation and vaporization of implants
   B. Excision of implants
   C. Endometrioma
     1. Drainage
     2. Cystectomy
 IV. Lysis of adhesions
   A. Filmy
   B. Vascular
 V. Tubal reconstruction
   A. Fimbrioplasty
   B. Terminal salpingostomy
 VI. Oocyte harvesting
   A. In vitro fertilization
   B. Gamete intrafallopian transfer
 VII. Second-look laparoscopy
   A. Ovarian carcinoma
   B. Tubal reconstructive surgery
 VIII. Ovarian biopsy for tissue diagnosis, karyotype, or both
 IX. Ovarian cysts
   A. Drainage
   B. Cystectomy
 X. Pelvic inflammatory disease
   A. Abscess drainage
 XI. Myomectomy
 XII. Oophorectomy, salpingectomy, adnexectomy
 XIII. Uterine suspension
 XIV. Uterosacral ligament ablation
 XV. Removal of foreign body

ing the first 2 years following tubal sterilization (DeStefano et al., 1982).

Ectopic Pregnancy

Numerous series demonstrating the efficacy of operative laparoscopy in the treatment of ectopic pregnancies have been published. Generally accepted guidelines for cases of unruptured ectopic pregnancy amenable to a laparoscopic approach include the following criteria: (1) hemodynamic stability; (2) ectopic gestation 3 cm or less in diameter; (3) adequate pelvic access for laparoscopic visualization and treatment; and (4) patient agreeable to close postoperative follow-up, including serial β-human chorionic gonadotropin (β-hCG) determinations (DeCherney and Diamond, 1987). Linear salpingostomy may be performed for unruptured ampullary ectopic pregnancies, whereas segmental resection is reserved for isthmic gestations (Fig 22–5). Salpingectomy, salpingo-oophorectomy, or coagulation of the entire gestation may also be performed. Complications following salpingostomy are relatively infrequent and include bleeding requiring laparotomy (2.5%), infection (1.3%), and slowly falling serum β-hCG levels (12.6%) (DeCherney and Diamond, 1987). In the largest reported series of laparoscopically treated ectopic pregnancies, Pouly et al. (1986) performed 321 conservative laparoscopic procedures on 295 patients. Fifteen patients (4.8%) required either a second laparoscopic procedure or a subsequent laparoscopy for retained trophoblastic tissue. In this series, 76 (64%) of 118 patients desiring a subsequent pregnancy had an intrauterine pregnancy, whereas 26 (22%) had a second ectopic pregnancy.

In most large series, fertility rates following laparoscopic treatment of ectopic pregnancy are approximately 50% to 60%, with repeat ectopic pregnancies occurring in 10% to 20% of pregnancies. These rates are comparable to those reported for procedures utilizing laparotomy (Bukowsky et al., 1979; DeCherney et al., 1981; Stromme, 1973; Timonen and Nieminen, 1967). In addition, a comparison between laparoscopy and laparotomy for the treatment of ectopic pregnancy demonstrated significantly shorter hospital stays (1.3 vs. 3.9 days), less operating time (78 vs. 104 minutes), shorter convalescence (8.7 vs. 25.7 days), and reduced postoperative analgesia requirements (0.8 vs. 4.6 doses) in the laparoscopy-treated group (Brumsted et al., 1988).

Endometriosis

Endometriosis is another major indication for operative laparoscopy. Surgical procedures may be performed during the initial diagnostic laparoscopy with little increase in the morbidity of the procedure. Unipolar or bipolar coagulation or laser vaporization may be employed for small implants. For endometriomas, drainage, puncture, and excision of the cyst wall with drainage and aspiration of its contents, coagulation or vaporization of the cyst base, or oophorectomy or adnexectomy may be performed (Fig 22–6; Reich and McGlynn, 1986). Electrocoagulation (Hasson, 1979) or laser vaporization (Keye et al., 1987) of pelvic endometriotic lesions appears to be successful in relieving pain in the majority of patients with chronic pelvic pain.

Many series evaluating the efficacy of laparoscopic treatment of endometriosis in infertile women have been published. The majority of these studies suffer from having small patient populations, short follow-up intervals, inconsistent evaluation of secondary diagnoses, and no randomization, making comparisons between lap-

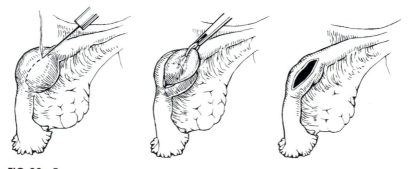

FIG 22–5.
Laparoscopic linear salpingostomy for unruptured ampullary ectopic pregnancy.

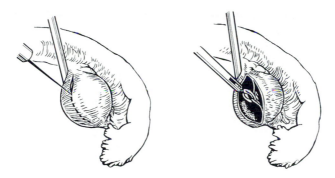

FIG 22–6.
Laparoscopic removal of endometrioma.

aroscopic treatment, conservative surgery by laparotomy, and medical therapy difficult to interpret. However, the pregnancy rates with laparoscopic surgery in stage I and II endometriosis compared favorably with those for danazol therapy alone (Barbieri et al., 1982) and conservative surgery (Buttram, 1979). In combined series totaling 348 patients treated with laparoscopic electrocautery and followed for 7 months to 7 years, 162 patients (47%) conceived (Martin and Diamond, 1986). Many of these studies failed to control for secondary diagnoses and the stage of endometriosis. In collected series totaling 374 patients evaluating CO_2 laser laparoscopy in the treatment of infertility due to endometriosis as an isolated factor, pregnancy was achieved in 73% of patients with stage I disease, 66% of patients with stage II, and 60% of patients with stage III and IV endometriosis (Martin and Diamond, 1986). One can conclude that laparoscopic treatment of pain, infertility, and pelvic masses due to endometriosis is an acceptable alternative to medical therapy or conservative laparotomy (or both) in

many cases. The role of preoperative and postoperative medical therapy in combination with laparoscopic surgery needs further study.

Lysis of Adhesions

One of the earliest reports of fertility enhancing laparoscopic surgery was in 1975 by Gomel, who performed salpingolysis and salpingostomy by laparoscopy. Pelvic adhesions may be characterized as thin and filmy or dense and vascular. The former type of adhesion is easily lysed laparoscopically; the latter kind of adhesion may require cauterization prior to lysis. It is essential to identify all structures prior to cutting, coagulating, or vaporizing (Gomel et al., 1986). There must be sufficient space between structures prior to lysis of adjoining adhesions, especially when coagulation is used, because thermal spread extends beyond visual tissue destruction (Fig 22–7). The importance of these and other safety measures cannot be overemphasized.

Several published series have demonstrated comparable efficacy between laparoscopic tech-

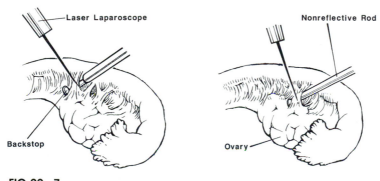

Laser Laparoscope

Nonreflective Rod

Backstop

Ovary

FIG 22–7.
Laparoscopic lysis of tubo-ovarian adhesions using laser.

niques used for adhesiolysis and conventional laparotomies in infertile women (Fayez, 1983; Gomel, 1983; Gomel et al., 1986; Jones and Rock, 1983). Gomel (1983) reported on laparoscopic lysis of moderate to dense periadnexal adhesions in 92 women, of whom 57 (62%) achieved at least one intrauterine pregnancy, 54 (59%) had one or more viable births, and 5 (5%) had ectopic pregnancy. Fayez (1983) reported pregnancy rates of 72%, 67%, and 50% for laparoscopic ovariolysis, salpingolysis, and salpingo-ovariolysis, respectively. Pregnancy rates for laparoscopic fimbrioplasty have ranged from 31% to 48% (Fayez, 1983; Gomel et al., 1986; Mettler et al., 1979). Laparoscopic terminal salpingostomies may also be performed on hydrosalpinges with either laser, electrocautery, or endocoagulation. Tubal patency rates for this procedure have ranged from 31% to 75%, with pregnancy rates of 10% to 44% (Daniell and Herbert, 1984; Gomel, 1977). The low rate of success with this procedure is similar to that reported for conventional laparotomy salpingostomies (Bateman et al., 1987). Many of these patients may benefit from in vitro fertilization (IVF).

Second-Look Laparoscopy

Infertility.—Following infertility surgery with either electrocautery or laser, a significant percentage of patients will have recurrence of adhesions, which may account for some surgical failures (Diamond et al., 1984). Some investigators (Diamond et al., 1984; Raj and Hulka, 1982; Surrey and Friedman, 1982; Trimbos-Kemper et al., 1985) have recommended performing early second-look laparoscopies for lysis of newly formed adhesions from 8 days to 12 weeks following the initial operation. Although some investigators have reported significantly fewer ectopic pregnancies following salpingostomy in those patients undergoing second-look laparoscopies compared with those who did not, there was no difference in viable birth rates (Trimbos-Kemper et al., 1985). No unanimity exists on the efficacy of second-look laparoscopy for infertility surgery, and some reproductive surgeons have abandoned its practice after discovering no difference in pregnancy rates (Gomel et al., 1986).

Oncology.—Second-look laparoscopy has also been used in patients with ovarian carcinoma to assess their response to chemotherapy (Berek et al., 1981; Lele and Piver, 1986; Piver et al.,

1980; Qu et al., 1984; Smith et al., 1977; Xygakis et al., 1984). In each of these studies, the majority of patients with recurrent ovarian carcinoma had positive findings at laparoscopy, sparing these women a more extensive traditional second-look laparotomy. However, a negative laparoscopy is not necessarily predictive of the absence of disease. It should be noted, however, that laparoscopy in this setting carries a high complication rate. Berek et al. (1981) found that 14% of patients had major complications requiring laparotomy. The most frequently observed laparoscopic complication was bowel perforation.

Advantages

Patient acceptance of operative laparoscopy is high. Some advantages of operative laparoscopy over traditional laparotomies are listed in Table 22–4.

In an analysis of the economic impact of laparoscopic surgery, Levine (1985) found a reduction of 69% in the length of postoperative stay for operative laparoscopy (0.5–2 days average) when compared to laparotomy (5–5.7 days). In addition, women were able to return to full activity 7 to 10 days following laparoscopic surgery compared with 4 to 6 weeks after traditional laparotomy. A decrease of 49% in overall hospital costs was observed in the operative laparoscopy group. Operative time for laparoscopic procedures was also equivalent to or shorter than that for infertility laparotomies. The one important question that remains to be answered is whether or not the results of surgery are as good with laparoscopy as with conventional laparotomy.

Risks and Complications of Laparoscopy

Early reports on the safety of laparoscopy estimated the incidence of complications to be 3% to 4%, with the need for laparotomy in 0.73% of

TABLE 22–4.

Advantages of Operative Laparoscopy Compared With Laparotomy

---

1. Higher patient acceptance
2. Decreased operative time
3. Decreased morbidity
4. Decreased length of postoperative stay in hospital
5. Decreased cost
6. Decreased recovery time
7. Comparable risk and complication profile

---

cases (Phillips et al., 1975, 1976). The commonest serious complications in these studies were hemorrhagic episodes, occurring in 0.66% of cases (Phillips et al., 1975), and penetrating injuries, especially of the gastrointestinal (GI) tract, resulting from the blind insertion of the Verres needle or trocar, in 0.1% to 0.54% of cases (Chamberlain and Beown, 1978). Another investigator has noted more than 100 cases of major blood vessel injury (Penfield, 1978). In one case report, penetration of the aorta resulted from Verres needle insertion, requiring a transfusion of 22 units of blood and an aortic patch (Corson, 1977).

Other risks include mechanical trauma, electrical, heat-, or laser-induced injury. Abdominal wall hemorrhage may occur when ancillary puncture sites are placed outside the midline. Occasionally, bleeding from the inferior epigastric vessels may lead to hypotensive collapse (Pring, 1983). Burns from noninsulated portions of unipolar and bipolar cautery may occur in any pelvic structure (i.e., bladder, small and large intestine, ureter, blood vessels). Large bowel perforation or full thickness burns will require bowel resection and colostomy.

With increasing experience, the incidence of complications has dramatically decreased. Semm (1984) reported an overall complication rate of 0.28% in 8,943 laparoscopies, 6,114 of which were operative cases. Of these, 13 (0.14%) were vascular injuries, 9 (0.1%) were gastric or bowel perforations, 1 (0.01%) was a ureteral injury, and 2 (0.02%) included cardiac arrest. In 10 instances (0.11%), laparotomy was required to treat the complications. No deaths were reported in this series. Daniell (1985) estimates the incidence of injury in operative laparoscopy cases using CO_2 laser to be less than 0.5%. A list of potential complications resulting from laparoscopy is shown in Table 22–5.

Summary

Both diagnostic and operative laparoscopy are safe procedures when guidelines are observed and the surgeon is aware of the limitations of the techniques.

HYSTEROSCOPY

Hysteroscopy is an endoscopic procedure that enables the surgeon to directly visualize the

TABLE 22–5.

Complications of Laparoscopy

  I. Induction of pneumoperitoneum
   A. Extraperitoneal insufflation
   B. Pneumo-omentum
   C. Penetration of a hollow viscus
   D. Vascular injury
   E. Gas embolism
   F. Subcutaneous emphysema
   G. Mediastinal emphysema
 II. Trocar insertion
   A. Vascular injury
     1. Abdominal wall (inferior epigastric vessels)
     2. Aorta
     3. Iliac vessels
     4. Mesenteric vessels
     5. Omental vessels
   B. Injury or penetration of a hollow viscus
   C. Incisional hernia
III. Operative laparoscopy
   A. Bleeding
   B. Mechanical trauma
   C. Electrosurgical injury
   D. Laser injury
   E. Infection
IV. Anesthesia
   A. Cardiac arrhythmias
   B. Aspiration

endocervical canal and uterine cavity. Although not as popular as laparoscopy, it facilitates accurate diagnosis and, often, treatment of numerous gynecologic disorders. This section will introduce the reader to some of the principles and applications of hysteroscopy.

History

Hysteroscopy was first described in 1869 when Pantaleoni (1869), using a 12-mm diameter Desormeaux cystoscope, evaluated a 60-year-old woman with abnormal uterine bleeding. Using reflected candlelight from a concave mirror, he was able to visualize endometrial polyps and cauterize them with silver nitrate. In 1879, Nitze, in collaboration with Leiter, a Viennese instrument maker, added optical lenses to a cystoscope, which increased illumination and field of vision (Nitze, 1879). The Nitze principle of endoscopy was not adopted for hysteroscopy until 1908 when David demonstrated the usefulness of hysteroscopy in the diagnosis of uterine disorders. Heineberg (1914) first described a water irrigation system in 1908, and Rubin (1925) first reported on CO_2 distention of the uterine cavity. Over the next 60 years, improvements in instruments and development of fiber optic light sources and ancillary equipment have facilitated the development of hysteroscopy.

Indications

As with laparoscopy, the list of indications for hysteroscopy is increasing. Table 22−6 lists some present-day indications for hysteroscopy. Indications that are still under investigation (i.e., sterilization procedures, salpingoscopy) are not included in this table.

Contraindications

Very few contraindications for hysteroscopy exist. Standard contraindications for this procedure are listed in Table 22−7.

Equipment

The basic equipment needed for hysteroscopy includes a hysteroscope, cervical dilators, a

TABLE 22−6.

Indications for Hysteroscopy

I. Diagnostic
  A. Abnormal uterine bleeding
    1. Premenopausal women
    2. Postmenopausal women
  B. Localization of foreign body (e.g., intrauterine device)
  C. Infertility
    1. Abnormal hysterosalpingogram
    2. Previous uterine manipulation or surgery
    3. In utero diethylstilbestrol exposure
  D. Recurrent pregnancy losses
    1. Abnormal hysterosalpingogram
  E. Secondary amenorrhea with failure of estrogen plus progestin withdrawal bleed
  F. Evaluation of failed first-trimester elective abortions
II. Operative
  A. Division of uterine septum (metroplasty)
  B. Myomectomy
  C. Removal of endometrial polyp
  D. Directed biopsy of intrauterine lesion
  E. Retrieval of foreign body
  F. Division and excision of intrauterine adhesions (Asherman's syndrome)
  G. Cauterization of active bleeding site
  H. Ablation of endometrium for menorrhagia.

TABLE 22−7.

Contraindications to Hysteroscopy

I. Pelvic inflammatory disease
  A. Salpingitis
  B. Endometritis
II. Untreated cervical infection
  A. Neisseria gonorrhea
  B. Chlamydia trachomatis
III. Contraindications to local or general anesthesia
IV. Pregnancy
V. Invasive carcinoma of the cervix
VI. Inexperienced surgeon
VII. Menstruation*

*Relative contraindication

light source, and a distending medium (Fig 22−8). There are several different types of hysteroscopes that may be used. Panoramic hysteroscopy requires a distending medium and a light source, whereas neither of these are required in contact hysteroscopy. The contact hysteroscope collects, traps, and transmits room or directed light through the previously dilated cervical canal (Parent et al., 1976). Only surfaces in contact with the tip of the hysteroscope are visible. Vision is not obstructed by blood or other fluids. Hysteroscopes range from 1 mm in diameter (needle hysteroscope) to an 8-mm operative hysteroscope. Operative hysteroscopes have an operative channel through which ancillary instruments or laser fibers may be placed. Hysteroscopes 5 mm or less in diameter usually require no cervical dilation in premenopausal women.

The optics of a hysteroscope consist of a system of lenses transmitting the image and fiberglass that conducts "cold" light. Most sources of cold light are fitted with halogen or xenon lamps with power ranging from 100 to 300 W. The light is transmitted to the hysteroscope by a fiberglass, loses its heat component entirely, and keeps its intensity. As in the laparoscope, a loss of light occurs at the site of connection of the conduction cord and the hysteroscope.

Either gas (CO_2) or liquid (32% dextran 70 and 5% dextrose) is used to distend the uterine cavity. Carbon dioxide is the only gas currently used in hysteroscopy and is popular in Europe. It requires a special insufflator that limits the flow of gas to 100 ml/min for safety reasons. In experiments on German shepherds to evaluate the effect of insufflated CO_2 on acid-base status, Lindemann et al. (1976) found no changes in pH,

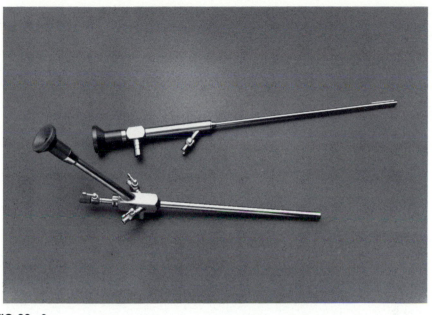

FIG 22–8.
Diagnostic and operative hysteroscopes. (Courtesy of Edward Weck, Inc., Princeton, N.J.)

P_{CO_2}, or P_{O_2} after direct insufflation of 200 ml/min into the femoral vein. When CO_2 was insufflated at 400 ml/min, tachypnea and cardiac arrhythmias occurred with no changes in pH, P_{CO_2}, or P_{O_2}. A lethal dosage was established at 1,000 ml/min after 60 seconds. The maximal intrauterine pressure must never exceed 200 mm Hg. The insufflator used for laparoscopy should never be used for hysteroscopy. Advantages of CO_2 as a distending medium are its perfect transmission of the image, its availability, its long history of safety in tubal patency tests (Rubin, 1947), and its rapid absorption. Some disadvantages of CO_2 include the need for a complicated, expensive insufflating apparatus, the need for a perfect cervical occlusion with the instrument, extreme care to avoid provoking bleeding or bubbles, and maintaining uterine distention with easy escape of CO_2 through patent tubes.

Dextran 70 (Hyskon) is a colorless liquid of 70,000 molecular weight with high viscosity and excellent optical qualities (Neuwirth, 1975). It is the most popular distention medium in the United States and Japan. Dextran is instilled via a 50-ml plastic syringe connected to the hysteroscope with a 25-cm piece of tubing with Luer-Lok connections. Manual pressure is maintained to ensure continuous flow with adequate uterine distention. Recently, a dextran pump controlled by a foot pedal switch operated by the surgeon has been described (Lavy et al., 1987). Less than 100 ml generally suffices for diagnostic procedures, although more may be necessary for prolonged operative hysteroscopy. The advantages of dextran 70 are that the transmission of light is excellent, only a simple apparatus is required for instillation, and it is immiscible with blood, allowing protracted visibility. Disadvantages of dextran 70 are that it is very viscous, necessitating immediate and thorough washing of instruments to prevent bonding; the rate of absorption in the abdominal cavity is not known; and it may transiently prolong bleeding time, and cause plasma volume expansion and occasional allergic reactions, including anaphylaxis. Hysteroscopy with dextran 70 is probably the easiest technique to master and gives the most reproducible results.

Five percent dextrose can also be used for uterine distention. It is delivered by inflating a pressure cuff around the bag of fluid, forcing the dextrose solution through connecting tubing and into the uterine cavity. The view is initially clear, but the field clouds rapidly, necessitating frequent rinsing. Advantages of 5% dextrose are that it is readily available, inexpensive, and rapidly absorbed through the peritoneal cavity, and the delivery system is simple. Disadvantages include the need for frequent rinsing to maintain a clear image and the use of large amounts of fluids to maintain adequate uterine distention.

Ancillary instruments used in operative hysteroscopy include grasping forceps, biopsy forceps, scissors, coagulating probes and loops, and laser-carrying quartz fibers (Fig 22–9). With the exception of laser-carrying fibers, most ancillary instruments may be rigid or flexible. For major operative procedures, rigid instruments are preferable. Flexible instruments can be used through a smaller operating shaft even under local anesthesia.

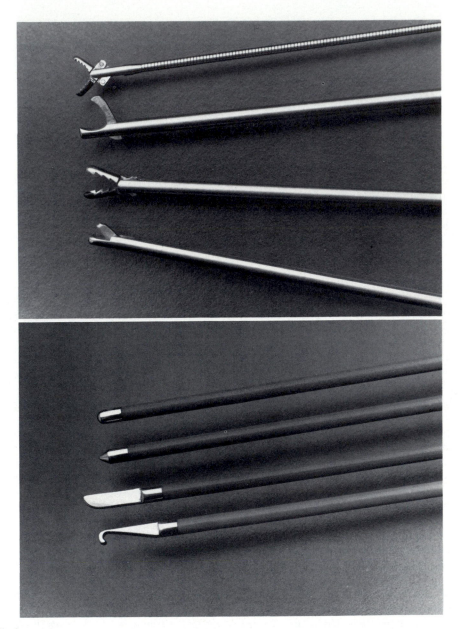

FIG 22–9.
Ancillary hysteroscopic instruments including (from *top* to *bottom*) grasping forceps, hook scissors, grasping forceps, punch biopsy forceps, unipolar cautery probe, unipolar cautery cone-tipped probe, knife electrode, hook electrode. (Courtesy of Edward Weck, Inc., Princeton, N.J.)

Technique

Prior to starting hysteroscopy, the patient should be placed in the dorsal lithotomy position, buttocks slightly protruding from the end of the table and elevated about 5 degrees. The speculum should have an opening on one lateral aspect to enable greater manipulation of the hysteroscope. After adequate anesthesia is given (see later discussion), a single-toothed tenaculum is placed on the anterior lip of the cervix, and cervical dilation with Hegar's dilators may be performed when using a hysteroscope greater than 5 mm in diameter or when performing hysteroscopy on a postmenopausal woman. It is important not to overdilate the cervix because a good seal between the cervical canal and hysteroscope is essential to maintain adequate uterine distention for panoramic hysteroscopy, especially when CO_2 is used as a distending medium. A cervical adapter is used when CO_2 is used to prevent CO_2 loss during operative hysteroscopy. The fiber optic light projector is then adjusted, and the tip of the hysteroscope is gently inserted into the cervical canal as the surgeon observes its entrance through the ocular. After exploring the cervical canal, some resistance is encountered just before the uterine cavity is entered.

Just as in laparoscopy, the surgeon must systematically explore the fundus, both horns and ostia, and the lateral, anterior, and posterior walls of the uterine cavity (Fig 22–10). Hysteroscopy is best performed in the postmenstrual or midproliferative phase to avoid encountering heaped up endometrium, which may obscure intracavitary viewing and make operative procedures more difficult. During the proliferative phase, the endometrium appears reddish yellow and assumes a more yellowish hue at ovulation. Throughout the secretory phase the endometrium is reddish purple, swollen, with wispy projections of tissue into the cavity.

Contact hysteroscopy (Marleschki, 1971) and microhysteroscopy (Hamou, 1981), with its ability to magnify up to 150 times during contact, may be used to view endocervical and endometrial vascular patterns and histology. These techniques are especially useful in the diagnosis of

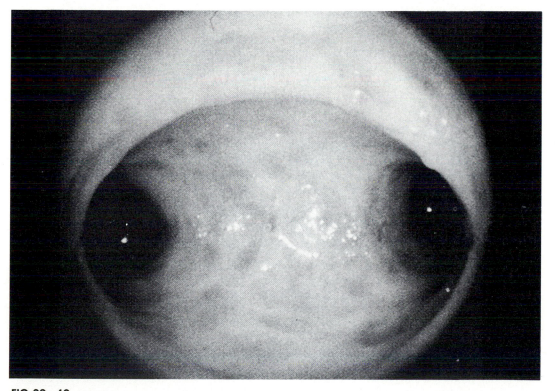

FIG 22–10.
Panoramic hysteroscopic view of normal uterine cavity.

premalignant or malignant lesions. No distention medium is needed for these techniques.

Anesthesia

Local anesthesia alone or in combination with systemic analgesia is sufficient and preferable for most hysteroscopic examinations (Andersen et al., 1981; Barbot et al., 1980). General anesthesia is necessary if concurrent laparoscopy is performed. Some surgeons perform hysteroscopy without any anesthesia (Barbot et al., 1980), whereas others use analgesia and sedation only. In a series of 1,000 patients undergoing microhysteroscopy, 949 (94.9%) required no anesthesia, 12 (1.2%) required local anesthesia, and 41 (4.1%) received general anesthesia, 13 of whom had an associated surgical procedure done at the time of hysteroscopy (Sugimoto, 1978). For conventional hysteroscopy, a paracervical block provides adequate anesthesia in 92% to 96% of patients (Lindemann, 1979; March et al., 1978; Parent et al., 1976; Sciarra and Valle, 1977; Siegler et al., 1976). Gentleness of technique and adequate patient education and preparation will increase the acceptance of local anesthesia, making hysteroscopy an ideal ambulatory procedure. The discomfort experienced by patients is often comparable to that experienced during hysterosalpingography.

Diagnostic Hysteroscopy

Abnormal Uterine Bleeding

Hysteroscopy is not a substitute for tissue diagnosis. However, hysteroscopic findings will increase the information available to the gynecologist in various clinical situations. Abnormal uterine bleeding in the perimenopausal and postmenopausal woman is a common gynecologic disorder in which hysteroscopy will often provide information that will add greatly in diagnosis and treatment. Dilatation and curettage has long been the diagnostic gold standard for abnormal uterine bleeding. However, even a trained gynecologist curettes at best 70% to 80% of the endometrium (Deutschmann and Lueken, 1984). Failure rates in making tissue diagnosis may occur in 36% to 50% in some patient populations (Englund et al., 1957; Surrey and Aronberg, 1984). Polyps and submucous fibroids are frequently undetected by curettage alone (Burnett, 1964; Englund et al., 1957; Siegler et al., 1976; Ward et al., 1958).

Hysteroscopic findings correlate highly with histologic results, and hysteroscopy should be considered a basic diagnostic procedure in the diagnosis of abnormal uterine bleeding.

In a series of 853 hysteroscopies performed for abnormal uterine bleeding in perimenopausal (age 45–55 years, $n = 516$) and postmenopausal women (age more than 55 years, $n = 337$), normal findings were noted in 557 patients (65%) (Deutschmann and Lueken, 1984). Women in the perimenopausal age group demonstrated normal endometrial architecture in 78% of cases, whereas 45% of postmenopausal women had no pathology. Uterine polyps were noted in 204 (25%) of all cases or in 10% and 45% of perimenopausal and postmenopausal women, respectively. Submucous fibroids were noted in 67 (8%) patients and comprised 11% of the diagnoses in the perimenopausal age group and 3% of the postmenopausal women. Carcinoma was present in only 1 (0.2%) perimenopausal woman compared with 24 (7%) postmenopausal women. Hysteroscopy, combined with the traditional dilatation and curettage, can be viewed as a perfected curettage by enabling the surgeon to directly visualize the endometrial cavity.

Infertility

Hysteroscopy may also be useful in the diagnosis of uterine causes of infertility and recurrent pregnancy losses. Several studies have demonstrated the increased accuracy of hysteroscopy over hysterosalpingography in this setting (Taylor, 1977; Taylor and Cumming, 1979; Valle, 1980). Coupled with laparoscopy, a thorough anatomic evaluation of the woman of an infertile partnership is possible (Cumming and Taylor, 1980). In studies comparing hysteroscopy to hysterosalpingography, an accuracy rate of 50% to 62% for the latter has been noted (Valle, 1980). False negative diagnoses are uncommon in hysterography, and this method may therefore be used as a screening test for women in the infertility evaluation.

Intrauterine Synechiae

Asherman's syndrome, the presence of intrauterine synechiae or scar tissue, is most frequently observed following curettage in a pregnant or recently pregnant uterus (Fig 22–11; Asherman, 1948). The commonest symptoms include amenorrhea, hypomenorrhea, dysmenorrhea, recurrent abortions, and infertility. Al-

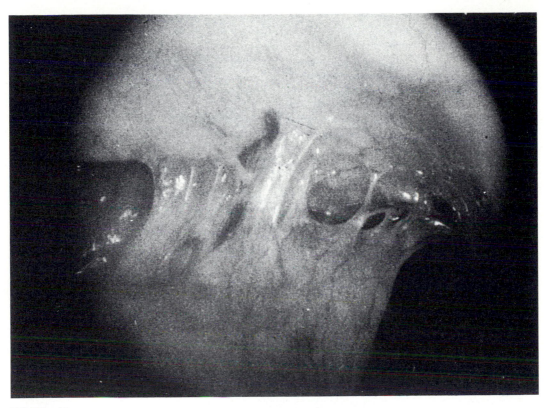

FIG 22–11.
Hysteroscopic view of intrauterine synechiae. (From Salat-Baroux J, Hamou JE, Uzan S, et al: Postabortal hysteroscopy, in Siegler AM, Lindemann HJ (eds): *Hys-* *teroscopy: Principles and Practice,* Philadelphia, JB Lippincott Co/New York, Harper & Row, 1984. Reproduced by permission.)

though cavitary filling defects noted on hysterography have been used to make the diagnosis, several studies have demonstrated the superiority of hysteroscopy over hysterography in the evaluation of Asherman's syndrome (March et al., 1978; Sugimoto, 1978). Asherman (1950) had the foresight to recognize the potential value of hysteroscopy in the treatment of intrauterine adhesions, as he wrote:

> Hysteroscopy, which has so often been mentioned in the literature and just as often discarded, may be of use for this purpose. If it were possible to see the adhesions and to loosen them instrumentally, using the eye as the guide, the ideal method will have been found. We have the intention of trying out the practical application of this theoretical hypothesis.

Today, hysteroscopy is the accepted method for evaluating and treating intrauterine adhesions (Sugimoto, 1978; Valle, 1980; Valle and Sciarra, 1979).

Operative Hysteroscopy

Intrauterine Synechiae

When hysteroscopy is used to divide thick intrauterine adhesions, a surgical assistant should perform concurrent laparoscopy to move bowel away from the uterus and to observe for potential uterine perforation. Hysteroscopic scissors, probes, or the unipolar cautery resectoscope can be used to divide adhesions. Postoperative therapy often includes placement of an intrauterine stent (e.g., intrauterine device, Foley catheter) to keep the cavity walls separated, high-dose estrogen treatment for 1 to 2 months, and antibiotics. In a review of the literature, Schenker and Margalioth (1982) reported a return of normal menses in 73% to 92% of hysteroscopically treated patients compared with 78% of patients treated by hysterotomy. Conception rate ranged from 47% to 55% in hysteroscopy-treated patients, with 48% to 78% of these patients delivering viable infants. These numbers compared favorably with a 52% conception rate and 76% viable birth rate in those patients treated by hysterotomy. Thus, hysteroscopy is the method of choice in the treatment of the vast majority of cases of intrauterine synechiae.

Myomectomy

Neuwirth (1983) has reported on hysteroscopic myomectomy in patients with submucous fibroids and menorrhagia (Fig 22–12). Following resection of fibroids, he inserted into the uterine cavity and inflated a Silastic balloon to tamponade the raw surface. The balloon was left in place for 24 hours. In his series of 28 patients, 19 (68%) had no recurrence of symptoms following the procedure, and 2 (7%) required a second hys-

teroscopic myomectomy. Five women (18%) required hysterectomy 2 weeks to 3 years following hysteroscopic fibroid resection for persistent bleeding. Thus, hysteroscopic myomectomy may be successful in a large proportion of well-chosen patients.

Metroplasty

Hysteroscopic metroplasty may be performed in patients with a uterine septum with a history of recurrent miscarriage or poor obstetrical outcome (Fig 22–13). In many instances, this approach can replace the more traditional Tompkins or Jones metroplasties. A cystoscopic resectoscope (DeCherney et al., 1986) or hysteroscopic scissors (Daly et al., 1983; Fayez, 1986) may be used to divide the septum. Laparoscopy is essential to distinguish between a septate and bicornuate uterus prior to operative hysteroscopy. In a comparative study between abdominal and hysteroscopic metroplasty, Fayez (1986) performed

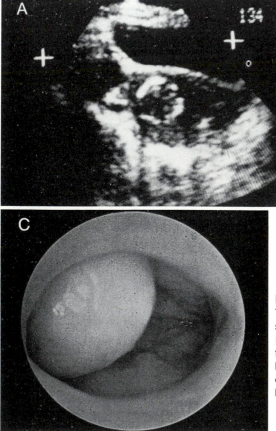

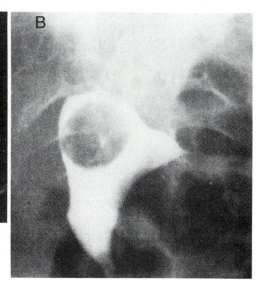

FIG 22–12.
Three views of a submucous leiomyoma. **A,** ultrasound. **B,** hysterosalpingogram. **C,** hysteroscopy. (From Gamerre M, Porto R, Serment H: Hysteroscopy for diagnosis and therapy, in Siegler AM, Lindemann HJ (eds): *Hysteroscopy: Principles and Practice*, Philadelphia, JB Lippincott Co/New York, Harper & Row, Philadelphia, 1984. Reproduced by permission.)

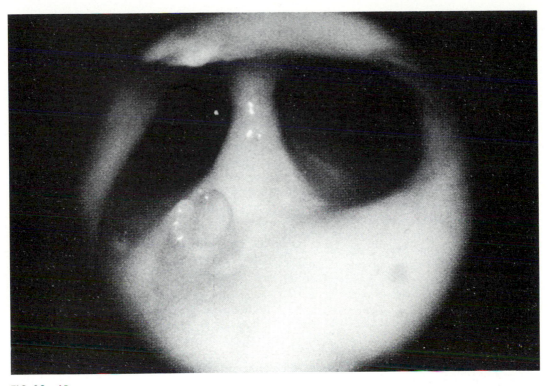

FIG 22–13.
Hysteroscopic view of uterine septum.

postoperative hysterosalpingography in 33 patients. Of 14 patients treated by Tompkins metroplasty, 72% had normal uterine cavities, 14% demonstrated incomplete septum excision, and 14% had intrauterine filling defects. The corresponding percentages in the hysteroscopically treated group were 88% normal cavities, 12% incomplete excision, and 0% filling defects. Most experts believe that hysteroscopic metroplasty is equal or superior to a transabdominal approach except, possibly, in cases with thick septa.

Endometrial Ablation

Hysteroscopy may also be used for endometrial ablation in cases of menorrhagia or intractable uterine bleeding secondary to coagulopathies. Early studies have reported success rates (i.e., amenorrhea or hypomenorrhea) of greater than 90% (DeCherney et al., 1987; Loffer, 1987). The two methods employed are the Nd:YAG laser using a nontouch technique (Loffer, 1987) and the cystoscopic resectoscope (DeCherney et al., 1987). Long-term follow-up is needed to assess the efficacy of this procedure.

Risks and Complications of Hysteroscopy

Hysteroscopy has a very low rate of complications. In several large series totaling more than 800 patients undergoing hysteroscopy, no complications were reported (Esposito, 1968; Marleschki, 1968; Schroeder, 1934). Faulty technique and poor patient selection account for most complications.

Cervical lacerations may result from tenaculum placement, especially with vigorous manipulation. Cervical or endometrial bleeding may result from forceful cervical dilation. Uterine perforation may also occur, rarely, during cervical dilation or intrauterine placement of the hysteroscope. Lindemann (1980) reported only 6 fundal perforations in 5,220 hysteroscopic examinations.

Intravasation of CO_2 and liquid media may occur. With imperfect gas flow monitors using excessive CO_2 insufflation rates, changes in pH, P_{CO_2}, P_{O_2}, and ECG may occur. In the most extreme cases, a CO_2 embolus may result in death of the patient. In all cases of CO_2 embolus and death, gas flow rates exceeded 350 ml/minute.

Following guidelines listed earlier (i.e., flow rate 100 ml or less of CO_2/minute; peak intrauterine pressure of 200 mm Hg or less), the risk of gas embolism approaches zero (Bartisch and Dillon, 1976). The risks of intravasation of high molecular weight dextran are proportionate to the amount of dextran 70 used. Maddi and colleagues (1969) described seven cases of anaphylaxis in patients receiving intravenous high molecular weight dextran. Leake and co-workers (1987) reported two cases of noncardiogenic pulmonary edema after operative hysteroscopy with 32% dextran 70. Another reported rare but serious complication is bleeding diathesis.

Infection may result following hysteroscopy. The first reported infection after hysteroscopy was reported by Bumm in 1895. Hysteroscopy may exacerbate latent salpingitis, especially in patients with active cervical infections or a history of salpingitis. Table 22–8 summarizes the complications of hysteroscopy.

Summary

With proper training, good equipment and rigid adherence to safety standards, hysteroscopy can be an invaluable aid in the diagnosis and treatment of numerous gynecologic disorders. With development of new equipment and techniques, experimental procedures (i.e., steriliza-tion, embryoscopy, salpingoscopy) will be perfected and added to the growing list of hysteroscopic applications.

LASER SURGERY

Since the invention of the laser almost 30 years ago, laser technology has continued to evolve rapidly, having a significant impact on almost every medical and surgical subspecialty. It is essential for the clinician to have an understanding of the basics of laser-tissue interaction and safety principles to use these tools properly and effectively.

Laser Physics

Light is energy with a dual nature described both by wave and particle theory. According to wave theory, light may be characterized by wavelength (λ), frequency (f), and amplitude. The parameters of wavelength and frequency are inversely related, determine the energy level of light, and determine where it falls on the electromagnetic spectrum. Light characterized by long wavelengths (i.e., low frequency) has low energy and falls into the infrared, microwave, or radiowave zone. Conversely, light characterized by short wavelengths (i.e., high frequency) has high energy and includes ultraviolet light, x-rays, and gamma rays.

According to particle theory, light is considered to be a stream of particles of negligible mass called photons, each carrying a quantity (quantum) of energy associated with a specific wavelength of light. When excited by an external energy source, electrons from each element or molecule will jump to a higher energy orbit. Following excitation, electrons fall from high- to low-energy orbits, emitting a photon at a wavelength characteristic for that specific element or molecule. Thus, the wavelengths of light emitted are a function of the type of atom or molecule excited and not a function of the wavelength of light or energy originally used to excite the atom or molecule. If the wavelength of emitted light happens to be within the narrow range of wavelengths of visible light within the electromagnetic spectrum, the emitted light of a specific atom will have a characteristic color.

The word laser is an acronym for light amplification by the stimulated emission of radiation,

TABLE 22–8.

Complications of Hysteroscopy

I. Cervical laceration
II. Cervical or uterine bleeding
III. Uterine perforation
   A. Visceral trauma
IV. Intravasation of distending medium
   A. Carbon dioxide
      1. Acidosis
      2. ECG changes
      3. Cardiac arrest
      4. Death
   B. High molecular weight dextran
      1. Anaphylaxis
      2. Bleeding diathesis
      3. Pulmonary edema
      4. Intravascular volume overload
   C. 5% dextrose
      1. Intravascular volume overload
      2. Pulmonary edema
V. Infection
   A. Salpingitis

which is the process by which such a beam is created. Laser light differs from other kinds of light because of three unique properties: (1) it is monochromatic (i.e., the waves are all one wavelength), (2) it is coherent (i.e., all waves are in phase), and (3) it is collimated (i.e., all waves are parallel). Because of these three properties, laser light is able to maintain an intense focused energy over long distances.

Laser light is created by stimulating a medium of a single pure element or compound and emitting photons simultaneously. This creates a light source that is both monochromatic and coherent. A collimated beam is created by reflecting the light in a resonator tube with reflective mirrors at each end (Fig 22–14). One mirror is 100% reflective, whereas the other is partially reflective, allowing the laser beam to exit as a series of parallel waves. These waves remain parallel for long distances with only minimal divergence.

Lasing media may be either gas, liquid, or solid. Most lasing media used for gynecologic indications are gas; only the Nd:YAG crystal is solid (Table 22–9).

Laser Unit

The laser unit consists of a few essential components. The laser head contains the lasing medium, an excitation source, and an aiming beam. For gas lasing media, direct (DC) electrical current is often used as the excitation source. For solid lasing media, incoherent optical flash lamps (i.e., krypton or xenon arc lamps) may be used.

An aiming beam is necessary for lasers with wavelengths outside of the visible spectrum (e.g., CO_2, Nd:YAG). The most commonly used aiming beam is a low-power He-Ne laser that emits

TABLE 22–9.

Properties of Gynecologic Lasers

Medium	Phase	Wavelength(s) (nm)	Color
CO_2	Gas	10,600	Infrared
He-Ne	Gas	632	Red
Nd:YAG	Solid	1,320	Infrared
		1,064	Infrared
Argon	Gas	515	Green
		488	Blue
KTP	Gas	532	Green

light at a wavelength of 632 nm and appears red. The He-Ne beam may be projected coaxially with the surgical laser, giving important information about the integrity of the fiber and delivery system as well as the spot size of the beam at the target tissue. Since the He-Ne wavelength is different from the wavelength of the surgical laser, it will give only an approximation of the characteristics of the surgical beam. When large differences in wavelength exist between the aiming and surgical beams (e.g., CO_2 and He-Ne beams), the aiming beam does a poorer job in approximating the characteristics of the surgical beam.

The bulkiness of most laser units is due to several supporting elements such as a power amplifier, a cooling system, and a delivery system. Because the process of generating a coherent light beam from an incoherent energy source is inefficient, the electrical current used to excite the lasing medium must be amplified many times. This is accomplished with a high-voltage electrical amplifier.

The inefficiency of creating the laser beam causes tremendous dissipation of heat. Most laser units use a water or air-cooling system to absorb

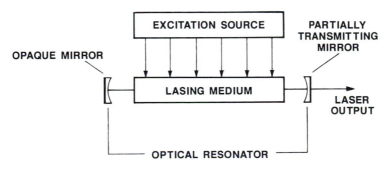

FIG 22–14.
Schematic of the creation of a laser beam.

heat and prevent damage of internal components. High-powered and inefficient lasers (e.g., argon) require high volumes of water for cooling, whereas low-powered lasers may be air cooled.

A delivery system is needed to transmit the laser beam from the laser head to the target tissue. Some lasers (e.g., argon, KTP, Nd:YAG) may be transmitted by flexible 0.2- to 1-mm diameter flexible quartz optical fibers. Fibers are typically surrounded by tight Teflon sleeves. The main advantage of fiber optic transmission is its flexibility, allowing the surgeon to reach areas of the body otherwise accessible only through open surgery. A disadvantage of fiber optic transmission is that 20% of the generated power is lost through multiple internal reflections along the inner walls of the fiber. In addition, fiber-transmitted laser beams exit the fiber tip with a 10- to 12-degree divergence, decreasing the precision.

A second type of delivery system uses a rigid system of articulated jointed arms with mirrors. This system is used when the laser wavelength (e.g., CO_2) is absorbed by the optical fiber, making fiber optic transmission impossible. The mirrors in the articulated arms are made of zinc and selenium and have an added reflective coating, because regular glass mirrors would absorb the CO_2 wavelength. Although much bulkier than the fiber optic delivery system, one advantage of transmission via articulated arms is that the laser still emerges as a collimated beam, allowing it to be focused with greater precision than an uncollimated beam emerging from an optical fiber. As precision of focus of the surgical laser increases, the spot size of the laser decreases, increasing the power density of the delivered beam. Thus, a smaller spot size increases the predictability, control, and effectiveness of the laser beam.

Laser-Tissue Interaction of Gynecologic Lasers

Carbon Dioxide Laser

The CO_2 laser is the most frequently used laser in gynecologic surgery and has been used for virtually all indications. It has a wavelength of 10,600 nm, which is almost totally absorbed by water (McKenzie, 1984) and is not color dependent. In effect, 98% of a CO_2 beam is absorbed within the first 10 μm of tissue (i.e., depth of a few cells), and 99.9% is absorbed within 100 μm (Fisher, 1985). By instantaneously boiling intracellular water, the CO_2 laser "explodes" cells and removes tissue by vaporization (Fig 22–15). Coagulation due to penetration of the CO_2 laser is limited to 100 to 200 μm (Fig 22–16; Martin

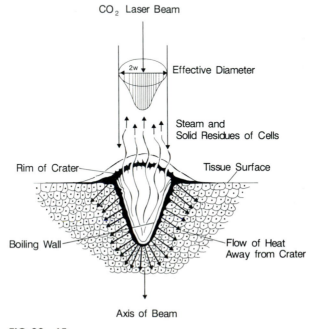

FIG 22–15.
Vaporization of tissue by the CO_2 laser.

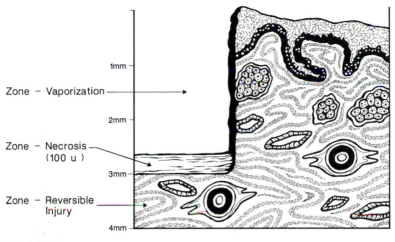

FIG 22–16.
Zones of vaporization, necrosis, and reversible injury by the CO_2 laser.

and Diamond, 1986). Thermal penetration ranges from 200 to 700 µm, depending on the speed at which the operating surgeon guides the laser beam over tissue. Because of its shallow penetration of tissue, the CO_2 laser is characterized by high precision but poor hemostasis. It is able to seal vessels with a diameter of 0.5 mm when focused and 1.0 mm when the spot is defocused (Fischer, 1985). Other characteristics of the CO_2 laser are that there is minimal scattering of energy from the target site, it is absorbed by plastic and glass and reflected by most metals, and the conversion of radiant energy to heat has not been shown to cause genetic mutations of cells (Fischer, 1985). The CO_2 laser requires an He-Ne aiming beam, is delivered by a system of articulated arms and mirrors, and may be used in continuous or pulsed modes. Characteristics of the CO_2, argon, KTP, and Nd:YAG lasers are summarized in Table 22–10.

Argon and KTP Lasers

Argon and KTP lasers have wavelengths that are preferentially absorbed by reddish pigments (e.g., heme, melanin) and pass through water. The depth of penetration for both the argon and KTP lasers is 2 mm, and their qualities of precision cutting and coagulation are intermediate between those of the CO_2 and Nd:YAG lasers. Because of their preferential absorption by red pigments, these lasers cause coagulation of blood within the vessel, not the vessel wall itself. The specificity of their absorption properties has made these lasers ideally suited for the treatment of en-

dometriosis (Daniell et al., 1986; Keye and Dixon, 1983; Keye et al., 1983). Other investigators (Daniell et al., 1986; Diamond et al., 1986) have used these lasers for laparoscopic neosalpingostomies, fimbrioplasties, adhesiolysis, and transection of the uterosacral ligaments for pain control. These lasers are delivered via fibers and have a green-blue color so that no aiming beam is necessary.

Neodymium:Yttrium-Aluminum-Garnet Laser

The Nd:YAG laser is only minimally absorbed by water, plastic, or glass. It is absorbed by protein of opaque tissue, with darker tissues showing preferential absorption. The Nd:YAG laser has a deep penetration of 4 to 6 mm of tissue (Hunter and Dixon, 1985), with significant scat-

TABLE 22–10.

Characteristics of Gynecologic Lasers

	CO_2	Argon/KTP	Nd:YAG
Aiming beam	He-Ne	Argon/KTP	He-NE
Delivery system	Articulated, rigid mirrors	Fiber	Fiber
Absorption	Water, glass, plastic	Heme, melanin	Proteins
Penetration	0.1 mm	2.0 mm	4–6 mm
Maximum power	100 W	20 W	100 W
Precision cut	+++	+	+
Coagulation	+	++	+++

ter to adjacent tissues, estimated at up to 25% of the incident energy (Frank et al., 1981). The Nd:YAG laser creates a uniform well-defined zone of tissue necrosis with a sharp boundary (Keiditsch et al., 1981). It has a more predictable depth of penetration and distribution within tissue than does electrocoagulation since it does not follow the paths of least electrical resistance within the different tissue types (Keiditsch et al., 1981). It will cause thermal necrosis but not vaporization of tissue. Because of its deeper penetrating ability, the Nd:YAG laser is capable of coagulating vessels up to 4 mm in diameter (Fischer, 1985).

The Nd:YAG laser is delivered by a fiber and requires an He-Ne aiming beam. Its main application in gynecology is for hysteroscopic endometrial ablation (Loffer, 1987), although it has been used in the laparoscopic treatment of endometriosis (Lomano, 1983, 1985).

Laser Safety

It is essential that surgeons and assisting personnel working with lasers take formal courses to learn about laser operation, applications, and safety. The major aspects of laser safety will be reviewed in this section.

Lasers with wavelengths greater than 319 mm (i.e., all lasers used in gynecologic practice) emit photoradiation and not ionizing radiation (Fischer, 1985). Gynecologic lasers are therefore not mutagenic, and there have been no reports of carcinoma developing in treated tissue or in health care workers handling the equipment (Fischer, 1985). Some of the materials used to make the laser may themselves be toxic, such as the thallium bromide in experimental CO_2 fibers (Fuller, 1984). However, gynecologic lasers currently marketed do not contain toxic materials.

Laser destruction of tissue creates plume (especially the CO_2 laser), contains chemicals and cell fragments that may be mutagenic or cause irritation of pulmonary mucosa, which may lead to chronic bronchitis if inhaled (Mihashi et al., 1981). Most investigators believe there is only minimal or no risk from viable cancer cells released into the laser plume with the CO_2 laser (Osterhuis, 1977). However, more studies need to be performed with the argon, KTP, and Nd:YAG lasers, which are less efficient at vaporization. It is therefore advisable to use good ventilation and smoke evacuators with all laser surgery to reduce these potential risks.

Since the collimated laser beam does not lose much power over distance, it is important to fire the laser only when it is aimed at an appropriate target. One must also make certain that there are no shiny surfaces near the operating field that may reflect the beam toward an unplanned target. Carbon dioxide lasers have the highest risk of reflection, and it is recommended to use anodized instruments with a rough matte finish to further decrease this risk.

Eye safety is probably the most important aspect of laser safety. With some lasers, eye injury could result in instantaneous and permanent blindness. The He-Ne aiming beam is the safest of all medical lasers with its low intensity (2–5 mW). It is recommended that protective glasses be used with this beam because it may be hazardous with prolonged direct viewing, but glasses are not required.

A CO_2 laser is absorbed immediately by the superficial corneal layers and never reaches the retina (Winburn, 1985). If a CO_2 laser beam strikes the retina, it will produce a painful corneal burn, which usually heals spontaneously. Glasses (but not contact lenses) or goggles with side shields are therefore necessary when this laser is used.

Lasers with wavelengths between 350 and 1,400 nm (i.e., argon, KTP, and Nd:YAG lasers) are not stopped by the superficial layers of the cornea and lens and may produce painless but permanent retinal damage (Winburn, 1985). Special goggles marked according to which wavelengths they are designed to block must therefore always be used when working with the argon, KTP, or Nd:YAG lasers. The goggle lens will also be marked with an optical density according to the degree of protection it will afford from a given wavelength. Goggles are primarily designed to protect the eye from scattered radiation and to afford a short margin of protection from a direct beam exposure.

These protective goggles will also reduce the transmission of visible light by 25% to 40% (Rockwell, 1985). This property, in addition to the color of the goggles (i.e., Nd:YAG goggles are green; argon/KTP goggles are tinted amber), may decrease visual acuity of the operative field. In addition to the surgeon and nurses, anesthesiologists and patients must also wear protective goggles.

The laser unit should be placed in a restricted location, clearly marked, and accessible only by trained personnel. Only trained personnel should manage the laser unit because the high-power voltage amplifier may be a potential electrical hazard. All medical lasers, especially the CO_2 laser, have the potential to ignite flammable objects. For this reason, all lap pads, towels, and gauze pads must be kept moistened, and flammable gases and prepping materials must not be used. Polyvinyl chloride endotracheal tubes are especially flammable, and several patients have died of severe pulmonary burns when tubes ignited (Lipow, 1986). The importance of proper safety protocols for operative laser cases cannot be overstated.

Laser Applications

The actual surgical techniques for the gynecologic indications listed in the following sections will not be covered. For a description of these techniques, the reader is referred to a thorough review of operative techniques (Baggish, 1985).

Vulvar Intraepithelial Neoplasia

The stratified squamous epithelium of the vulva is less than 1 mm thick, with the deepest rete peg rarely extending more than 1 mm into the underlying dermis. Vaporization with the CO_2 laser should therefore be performed to a depth of 3 mm only. Because vulvar intraepithelial neoplasia (VIN) is often a multifocal disease, it may be necessary to treat some patients in stages, waiting 2 weeks in between treatments. Several studies (Baggish and Dorsey, 1981; Townsend et al., 1982b) have demonstrated remarkable efficacy of CO_2 laser therapy for VIN, with greater than 90% cure rates noted by 12-year follow-up.

Condyloma Acuminatum

Condyloma acuminatum is caused by the human papillomavirus, which has been linked to the genesis of lower genital tract neoplasia (Aurelian et al., 1987). The virus proliferates in the prickle and basal cell layers of the epidermis (Laverty, 1979) so that the CO_2 laser may eliminate condylomatous lesions to a depth of 1 mm. Because these lesions may be multifocal and have microwarty epithelial changes, colposcopy may aid in the localization and treatment of condylomata. Warts may be vaporized or excised, and this can be accomplished safely in pregnant patients (except for cervical lesions) up to 34 weeks of gestation. In addition, because treatment is limited to the epidermis, there is minimal blood loss and

rarely significant scarring. It is important to treat several millimeters of surrounding normal tissue because the papillomavirus often exists in normal tissue around the proliferative lesion. Several series totaling 428 patients (Baggish, 1980, 1982; Caulkins et al., 1982) have demonstrated greater than 90% cure rates in patients with condylomatous lesions, many of whom had failed multiple courses of medical therapy. For vaginal condylomata, a special nonreflective vaginal speculum must be used.

Vaginal Intraepithelial Neoplasia

Vaginal intraepithelial neoplasia (VAIN) is a relatively uncommon preinvasive neoplastic process that is associated with cervical intraepithelial neoplasia (CIN; Graham and Meigs, 1962), radiation therapy (Novak and Woodruff, 1959), chemotherapy, and immunosuppressive therapy. It is usually an asymptomatic lesion that is brought to the attention of the physician by an abnormal Papanicolaou smear and investigated with the aid of colposcopy. Lesions may be surgically excised, treated with topical 5-fluorouracil (Woodruff et al., 1975), or, in the postmenopausal patient, treated with intravaginal estrogens. Stafl et al. first reported on the successful treatment of VAIN with CO_2 laser therapy in 1977. Since then, other groups have reported success rates of 84% to 90% with either focal laser therapy or total laser ablation of the vaginal mucosa (Jobson and Homesley, 1983; Townsend et al., 1982b). It is recommended that a 2-mm border of normal tissue be vaporized down to a depth of approximately 2 mm to treat VAIN.

Cervical Intraepithelial Neoplasia

Laser vaporization of ectocervical intraepithelial neoplasia was one of the first gynecologic applications of the CO_2 laser. In cases of persistently abnormal Papanicolaou smears with inconsistent colposcopic findings, endocervical involvement, or when the transformation zone cannot be fully visualized on colposcopic examination, cervical conization may be performed with the CO_2 laser (Dorsey, 1982).

In the treatment of ectocervical intraepithelial neoplasia, it is recommended to have a margin extending at least 3 to 4 mm beyond the lesion and transformation zone. Vaporization of the entire transformation zone, including the area of pathology, must be performed with colposcopic guidance to a minimum depth of 6 mm to ensure eradication of CIN lesions extending into cervical crypts. In a series of 514 patients with ectocervical intraepithelial neoplasia (CIN I, II, and III) Wright (1985) reported a cure rate of 95.5% after one laser treatment and 99.6% after two vaporization procedures. In a series of 138 laser excisional conizations, Dorsey (1985) reported a cure rate of 96%, a mean blood loss of 2 ml, and 6 patients (4.3%) requiring emergency visits for delayed heavy vaginal bleeding.

Currently, the CO_2 and Nd:YAG lasers are under investigation for the treatment of some invasive gynecologic cancers. However, these modalities are not recommended for treatment of these diseases at this time.

Infertility and Endometriosis

Laser techniques have been used extensively in female reconstructive pelvic surgery, including salpingo-ovariolysis, fimbrioplasty, terminal salpingostomy, vaporization and excision of endometriosis, myomectomy, metroplasty, and ovarian wedge resection. The CO_2 laser has been used far more frequently than other types of lasers for these indications. However, most reports have been anecdotal and uncontrolled with small numbers of subjects, making interpretation of true efficacy difficult. This section will provide a brief overview of the use of lasers in female reconstructive pelvic surgery.

Critical aspects in the success of pelvic reconstructive surgery for infertility are degree of postoperative adhesion formation and the extent of tissue injury. When the CO_2 laser was first used for abdominal reconstructive surgery in 1974 (Bellina, 1974), much enthusiasm was generated as laser surgery was touted as potentially superior to conventional surgery (i.e., scalpel, electrocautery) because of its no-touch technique, precision, and minimal tissue injury adjacent to the surgical site. However, in several animal studies comparing the degree of postoperative adhesion formation in laser-treated vs. electrocautery-treated animals, no clear advantage has been proved. Some studies have concluded that there is no significant difference in postoperative adhesion formation when CO_2 laser or electrocautery is used (Luciano et al., 1987; Pittaway et al., 1983). Other studies report that the CO_2 laser is superior to electrocautery in reducing postoperative adhesion formation (Bellina et al., 1984; Choe et al., 1983; Filmar et al., 1986).

Postoperative adhesion formation after CO_2 laser infertility surgery was evaluated in a prospec-

tive multicenter study utilizing early second-look laparoscopy (Diamond et al., 1984). These investigators found postoperative adhesions in 86% of patients (91 of 106) and concluded that the CO_2 laser was not a panacea for the treatment of tuboperitoneal causes of infertility.

In human studies, both laser and electromicrocautery techniques appear to have comparable efficacy. Tulandi (1986) reported pregnancy rates of 53% and 52% in laser ($n = 30$) and electrocautery ($n = 33$) salpingo-ovariolysis procedures, respectively, after a 2-year follow-up period. In this study there was a tendency toward a shorter surgery-to-conception interval in laser-treated patients (laser, 9.9 months; electrosurgery, 13.1 months), although the difference was not statistically significant.

In another comparative study, Tulandi and Vilos (1985) reported on the efficacy of laser surgery vs. electrosurgery for bilateral hydrosalpinges. Terminal salpingostomies were performed on 67 women, with an intrauterine pregnancy rate of 24% in the laser group ($n = 37$) and 20% in the electrocautery group after a 2-year follow-up period, demonstrating no statistical difference. As in the salpingo-ovariolysis study, the surgery-to-conception interval tended to be shorter in the laser group (8.3 months vs. 12.1 months), but no statistical difference was reached. Tulandi and Vilos (1985) concluded that the CO_2 laser did not offer a distinct advantage over conventional surgery in the treatment of infertility due to pelvic adhesions or distal tubal occlusion.

Endometriosis is a relatively frequent finding in women with infertility, pelvic pain, or both. Several studies have demonstrated the efficacy of conventional infertility surgery by laparotomy and laparoscopic surgery using electrocautery techniques (Buttram, 1979; Martin and Diamond, 1986). Although no comparative studies have been performed, CO_2 laser treatment of endometriosis appears to yield results that are similar to or better than for these other techniques. In combined series of 374 infertile patients whose diagnostic evaluations demonstrated only endometriosis, 69% conceived following CO_2 laser laparoscopy (Martin and Diamond, 1986). The complication rate for CO_2 laser laparoscopy is less than 0.5%, suggesting that it is quite safe in skilled hands (Daniell, 1985). The KTP, argon, and Nd:YAG lasers have also been used in the treatment of endometriosis, and preliminary results suggest that these may be safe alternative modes of therapy in selected patients. (Daniell et al., 1986; Keye and Dixon, 1983; Keye et al., 1987; Lomano, 1983, 1985). Uterosacral ligament ablation, performed by the CO_2 or KTP laser, may also be utilized for pain relief in patients with endometriosis (Daniell et al., 1986).

Summary

The present role of laser surgery remains undefined in gynecologic surgery. Although laser therapy has demonstrated efficacy in lower reproductive tract preinvasive neoplasia, condyloma acuminatum, pelvic reconstructive surgery, and endometriosis, it is unknown whether laser surgery is superior to more traditional surgical modalities. The advantages of less bleeding, decreased tissue handling, and less tissue injury are counterbalanced by the added equipment expense and the need for extra training for surgeons and supporting personnel. Laser surgery does offer an alternative approach in the treatment of many gynecologic disorders, and the evolving laser technology will no doubt add to the present surgical armamentarium.

REFERENCES

Andersen PK, Stokke DB, Hole P: Carbon dioxide tension in manually ventilated, prone patients. *Anaesthesist* 1981; 12:610–613.

Asherman JG: Amenorrhoea traumatica (atretica). *J Obstet Gynaecol Br Emp* 1948; 55:23–25.

Asherman JG: Traumatic intrauterine adhesions. *J Obstet Gynaecol Br Emp* 1950; 57:892–895.

Aurelian L, Kessler I, Rosenshein NB: Viruses and gynecologic cancers. *Cancer* 1987; 48:455–463.

Baggish MS: Carbon dioxide laser treatment for condylomata acuminata venereal infections. *Obstet Gynecol* 1980; 55:711–715.

Baggish MS: Treating viral venereal infections with the CO_2 laser. *J Reprod Med* 1982; 27:737–741.

Baggish MS: *Basic and Advanced Laser Surgery in Gynecology*. New York, Appleton-Century-Crofts, 1985.

Baggish MS, Dorsey JH: CO_2 laser for the treatment of vulvar carcinoma in situ. *Obstet Gynecol* 1981; 57:371–374.

Barbieri RL, Evans S, Kistner RW: Danazol in the treatment of endometriosis: Analysis of 100 cases with a 4-year follow-up. *Fertil Steril* 1982; 37:737–742.

Barbot J, Parent B, Dubuisson JB: Contact hysteroscopy: Another method of endoscopic examination. *Am J Obstet Gynecol* 1980; 136:721–726.

Bartisch EG, Dillon TF: Carbon dioxide hysteroscopy. *Am J Obstet Gynecol* 1976; 124:756–761.

Bateman BG, Nunley WC Jr, Kitchin JD III: Surgical management of distal tubal obstruction. Are we making progress? *Fertil Steril* 1987; 48:523–542.

Bellina JH: Gynecology and the laser. *Contemp Obstet Gynecol* 1974; 4:24–33.

Bellina JH, Hemmings R, Voras JI, et al: Carbon dioxide laser and electrosurgical wound study with an animal model: A comparison of tissue damage and healing patterns in peritoneal tissue. *Am J Obstet Gynecol* 1984; 148:327–331.

Berek JS, Griffiths CT, Leventhal JM: Laparoscopy for second-look evaluation in ovarian cancer. *Obstet Gynecol* 1981; 58:192–198.

Bhiwandiwala PP, Mumford SD, Feldblum PJ: Menstrual pattern changes following laparoscopic sterilization with different occlusion techniques: A review of 10,004 cases. *Am J Obstet Gynecol* 1983; 145:684–694.

Bozzini P: Der Lichtleiter oder Beschreibung einer einfachen Vorrichtung und ihrer Anwendung zur Erleuchtung innerer Hohlen und Zwischenraume des lebenden animalischen Korpers. Weimar, Landes-Industrie-Comptoir, 1807.

Brenner WE: Evaluation of contemporary female sterilization methods. *J Reprod Med* 1981; 26:439–453.

Brumsted J, Kessler C, Gibson C, et al: A comparison of laparoscopy and laparotomy for the treatment of ectopic pregnancy. *Obstet Gynecol* 1988; 71:889–892.

Bukowsky I, Lauger K, Herman A: Conservative surgery for tubal pregnancy. *Obstet Gynecol* 1979; 53:709–713.

Bumm E: Diskussion uber die Endometriosis, in Chrobak R, Pfannenstiel J (eds): *Verhandlungen der Deutschen Gesellschaft fur Gynakologie Kongress (Wien)*. Leipzig, Breitkopf and Hartel, 1895, p 524.

Burnett JE Jr: Hysteroscopy-controlled curettage for endometrial polyps. *Obstet Gynecol* 1964; 24:621–623.

Buttram VC Jr: Conservative surgery for endometriosis in the infertile female: A study of 206 patients with implications for both medical and surgical therapy. *Fertil Steril* 1979; 31:117–122.

Caulkins JW, Masterson BJ, Magrina JF, et al: Management of condylomata acuminata with the carbon dioxide laser. *Obstet Gynecol* 1982; 59:105–109.

Chamberlain G, Beown JC: The report of the working party of the confidential enquiry into gynecological laparoscopy, in *Gynecological Laparoscopy.* Royal College of Obstetricians and Gynecologists, London, 1978.

Choe JK, Dawood MY, Andrews AH: Conventional versus laser reanastomosis of rabbit ligated uterine horns. *Obstet Gynecol* 1983; 61:689–692.

Corson SL: Operating room preparations and basic techniques, in Phillips JM (ed): *Laparoscopy.* Baltimore, Williams & Wilkins Co, 1977.

Cumming DC, Taylor PJ: Historical predictability of abnormal laparoscopic findings in infertile women. *J Reprod Med* 1979; 23:295–300.

Cumming DC, Taylor PJ: Combined laparoscopy and hysteroscopy in the investigation of the ovulatory infertile female. *Fertil Steril* 1980; 33:475–478.

Daly DC, Walters CA, Soto-Albers CE, et al: Hysteroscopic metroplasty: Surgical technique and obstetric outcome. *Fertil Steril* 1983; 39:623–628.

Daniell J: Operative laparoscopy for endometriosis. *Semin Reprod Endocrinol* 1985; 3:353–359.

Daniell JF, Herbert CM: Laparoscopic salpingostomy utilizing the CO_2 laser. *Fertil Steril* 1984; 41:558–562.

Daniell JF, Miller W, Tosh R: Initial evaluation of the use of the potassium-titanyl-phosphate (KTP/532) laser in gynecologic laparoscopy. *Fertil Steril* 1986; 46:373–377.

David C: L'Endoscopie uterine (hysteroscopie). Applications au diagnostic et au traitement des affections intrauterines. Master's thesis, University of Paris, G Jacques, Paris, 1908.

DeCherney AH, Diamond MP: Laparoscopic salpingostomy for ectopic pregnancy. *Obstet Gynecol* 1987; 70:948–950.

DeCherney AH, Diamond MP, Lavy G, et al: Endometrial ablation for intractable uterine bleeding: Hysteroscopic resection. *Obstet Gynecol* 1987; 70:668–670.

DeCherney AH, Romero R, Naftolin F: Surgical management of unruptured ectopic pregnancy. *Fertil Steril* 1981; 35:21–24.

DeCherney AH, Russell JB, Graebe RA, et al: Resectoscopic management of mullerian fusion defects. *Fertil Steril* 1986; 45:726–728.

DeStefano F, Peterson HB, Layde PM, et al: Risk of ectopic pregnancy following tubal sterilization. *Obstet Gynecol* 1982; 60:326–330.

Deutschmann C, Lueken RP: Hysteroscopic findings in postmenopausal bleeding, in Siegler AM, Lindemann HJ (eds): *Hysteroscopy:*

Principles and Practice. Philadelphia, JB Lippincott Co, 1984.

Diamond MP, Daniell JF, Martin DC, et al: Tubal patency and pelvic adhesions at early second-look laparoscopy following intra-abdominal use of the carbon dioxide laser: Initial report of the intra-abdominal laser study group. *Fertil Steril* 1984; 42:717–723.

Diamond MP, DeCherney AH, Polan ML: Laparoscopic use of the argon laser in nonendometriotic reproductive pelvic surgery. *J Reprod Med* 1986; 31:1011–1013.

Dorsey JH: Excisional conization of the cervix, in Andrews AH, Polanyi TG (eds): *Microscopic and Endoscopic Surgery With the CO_2 Laser.* Boston, John Wright, 1982, p 231.

Dorsey JH: Excisional conization of the cervix, in Baggish MS (ed): *Basic and Advanced Laser Surgery in Gynecology.* Norwalk, CT, Appleton-Century-Crofts, 1985, pp 229–240.

Drake TS, Tredway D, Buchanan G, et al: Unexplained infertility—a reappraisal. *Obstet Gynecol* 1977; 50:644–649.

El-minawi MF, Abdel-hadi M, Ibrahim AA, et al: Comparative evaluation of laparoscopy and hysterosalpingography in infertile patients. *Obstet Gynecol* 1978; 51:29–34.

Englund F, Ingelman-Sundberg A, Westin B: Hysteroscopy in diagnosis and treatment of uterine bleeding. *Gynaecologia* 1957; 143:217–220.

Esposito A: Une exploration gynecologique trop negligee: L'hysteroscopie. *Gynecol Pract* 1968; 19:165–169.

Fayez JA: An assessment of the role of operative laparoscopy in tuboplasty. *Fertil Steril* 1983; 39:476–480.

Fayez JA: Comparison between abdominal and hysteroscopic metroplasty. *Obstet Gynecol* 1986; 68:399–403.

Filmar S, Gomel V, McComb P: The effectiveness of CO_2 laser and electromicrosurgery in adhesiolysis: A comparative study. *Fertil Steril* 1986; 45:407–410.

Fischer JC: Principles of safety in laser surgery and therapy, in Baggish MS (ed): *Basic and Advanced Laser Surgery in Gynecology.* New York, Appleton-Century-Crofts, 1985.

Frank F, Hofstetter A, Keiditsch E: Experimental investigations and new instrumentation for Nd:YAG laser treatment in urology, in Bellina JH (ed): *Gynecologic Laser Surgery.* New York, Plenum Publishing Corp, 1981.

Fuller TA: From source to patient: The surgical laser delivery system. *Lasers Surg Med* 1984; 3:349–355.

Gabos P: A comparison of hysterosalpingography and endoscopy in examination of tubal function in infertile women. *Fertil Steril* 1976; 27:238–241.

Goldenberg RL, Magendantz HG: Laparoscopy and the infertility evaluation. *Obstet Gynecol* 1976; 47:410–416.

Gomel V: Laparoscopic tubal surgery in infertility. *Obstet Gynecol* 1975; 46:47–55.

Gomel V: Salpingostomy by laparoscopy. *J Reprod Med* 1977; 18:265–269.

Gomel V: Salpingostomy by microsurgery. *Fertil Steril* 1978; 29:380–384.

Gomel V: *Microsurgery in Female Infertility.* Boston, Little, Brown & Co, 1983, p 80.

Gomel V, Taylor PJ, Yuzpe AA, et al (eds): *Laparoscopy and Hysteroscopy in Gynecologic Practice.* Chicago, Year Book Medical Publishers, 1986.

Graham JF, Meigs JV: Recurrence of tumor after total hysterectomy for carcinoma in situ. *Am J Obstet Gynecol* 1962; 64:1159–1164.

Hamou J: Hysteroscopy and microhysteroscopy with a new instrument: The microhysteroscope. *Acta Eur Fertil* 1981; 12:29–35.

Hasson HM: A modified instrument and method for laparoscopy. *Am J Obstet Gynecol* 1971; 110:886–889.

Hasson HM: Electrocoagulation of pelvic endometriotic lesions with laparoscopic control. *Am J Obstet Gynecol* 1979; 135:115–121.

Heineberg A: Uterine endoscopy, an aid to precision in the diagnosis of intrauterine disease. *Surg Gynecol Obstet* 1914; 18:513–520.

Hulka JF, Peterson HB, Surrey M, et al: American Association of Gynecologic Laparoscopists' 1985 Membership Survey. *J Reprod Med* 1987; 32:732–735.

Hunter JG, Dixon JA: Lasers in cardiovascular surgery: Current status. *West J Med* 1985; 142:506–510.

Hutchins CJ: Laparoscopy and hysterosalpingography in the assessment of tubal patency. *Obstet Gynecol* 1977; 49:325–328.

Jobson VW, Homesley HD: Treatment of vaginal intraepithelial neoplasia with carbon dioxide laser. *Obstet Gynecol* 1983; 62:90–94.

Jones HW Jr, Rock JA: *Reparative and Constructive Surgery of the Female Genital Tract.* Baltimore, Williams & Wilkins Co, 1983, p 72.

Keiditsch E, Hofstetter A, Rothenberger K: Comparative morphological investigations of the effects of the neodymium-YAG laser and electrocoagulation in experimental animal research, in Bellina JH (ed): *Gynecologic Laser Surgery.* New York, Plenum Publishing Corp, 1981.

Keye WR, Dixon J: Photocoagulation of endometriosis with the argon laser through the laparoscope. *Obstet Gynecol* 1983; 62:383–387.

Keye WR, Hansen LW, Astin M, et al: Argon laser therapy of endometriosis: A review of 92 consecutive patients. *Fertil Steril* 1987; 47:208–212.

Keye WR Jr, Matson GA, Dixon J: The use of the argon laser in the treatment of experimental endometriosis. *Fertil Steril* 1983; 39:26–30.

Kresch AJ, Seifer DB, Sachs LB, et al: Laparoscopy in 100 women with chronic pelvic pain. *Obstet Gynecol* 1984; 64:672–674.

Laverty C: Noncondylomatous wart virus infection of the cervix: Cytologic, histologic and electron microscopic features. *Obstet Gynecol Surv* 1979; 34:820–829.

Lavy G, Diamond MP, Shapiro B, et al: A new device to facilitate intrauterine instillation of dextran 70 for hysteroscopy. *Obstet Gynecol* 1987; 70:955–957.

Leake JF, Murphy AA, Zacur HA: Noncardiogenic pulmonary edema: A complication of operative hysteroscopy. *Fertil Steril* 1987; 48:497–499.

Lele SB, Piver MS: Interval laparoscopy as predictor of response to chemotherapy in ovarian carcinoma. *Obstet Gynecol* 1986; 68:345–347.

Leventhal JM: Laparoscopy in female infertility. *Curr Probl Obstet Gynecol Fertil* 1986; 9:174–224.

Levine RL: Economic impact of pelviscopic surgery. *J Reprod Med* 1985; 30:655–661.

Lichten EM, Bombard J: Surgical treatment of primary dysmenorrhea with laparoscopic uterine nerve ablation. *J Reprod Med* 1987; 32:37–41.

Lindemann HJ: CO_2 hysteroscopy today. *Endoscopy* 1979; 11:94–102.

Lindemann HJ: *Atlas der Hysteroskopie.* Stuttgart, FRG, Gustav Fischer, 1980.

Lindemann HJ, Mohr J, Gallinat: Der Einfluss von CO_2-Gas wahrend der Hysteroskopie. *Geburthshilfe Frauenheilkd* 1976; 36:153–157.

Lipow M: Laser physics made simple. *Curr Probl Obstet Gynecol Fertil* 1986; 9:442–493.

Loffer FD: Hysteroscopic endometrial ablation with the Nd:YAG laser using a nontouch technique. *Obstet Gynecol* 1987; 69:679–682.

Loffer FD, Pent D: Pregnancy after laparoscopic sterilization. *Obstet Gynecol* 1980; 55:643–648.

Lomano JM: Laparoscopic ablation of endometriosis with the YAG laser. *Lasers Surg Med* 1983; 3:179–183.

Lomano JM: Photocoagulation of early pelvic endometriosis with Nd:YAG laser through the laparoscope. *J Reprod Med* 1985; 30:77–81.

Luciano AA, Whitman G, Maier DB, et al: A comparison of thermal injury, healing patterns, and postoperative adhesion formation following CO_2 laser and electromicrosurgery. *Fertil Steril* 1987; 48:1025–1029.

Maddi VI, Wyso EM, Zinner EN: Dextran anaphylaxis. *Angiology* 1969; 20:243–246.

March CM, Israel R, March AD: Hysteroscopic management of intrauterine adhesions. *Am J Obstet Gynecol* 1978; 130:633–637.

Marleschki V: Hysteroskopische Feststellung der spontanen perfusionsschwankungen am menschlichen Endometrium. *Zentralbl Gynaekol* 1968; 90:1094–1098.

Marleschki V: Geburtserleichterung unter Kontrolle. *Urania* 1971; 11:34–38.

Martin DC, Diamond MP: Operative laparoscopy: Comparisons of lasers with other techniques. *Curr Probl Obstet Gynecol Fertil* 1986; 9:564–617.

McKenzie AL: Lasers in surgery and medicine. *Phys Med Biol* 1984; 29:619–641.

Method MW, Urnes PD, Neahring R, et al: Economic considerations in the use of laparoscopy for diagnosing pelvic inflammatory disease. *J Reprod Med* 1987; 32:759–764.

Mettler L, Giesel H, Semm K: Treatment of female infertility due to tubal obstruction by operative laparoscopy. *Fertil Steril* 1979; 32:384–389.

Mihashi S, Veda S, Hirano M: Some problems about condensates induced by CO_2 laser irradiation, in Atsumi K (ed): *Transactions, 4th Congress of the International Society for Laser Surgery.* Tokyo, Intergroup Corp, 1981.

Murphy AA: Operative laparoscopy. *Fertil Steril* 1987; 47:1–18.

Musich JR, Behrman SJ: Infertility laparoscopy in perspective: Review of five hundred cases. *Am J Obstet Gynecol* 1982; 143:293–303.

Neuwirth RS: Hysteroscopy, in Friedman EA (ed): *Major Problems in Obstetrics and Gynecology.* Philadelphia, WB Saunders Co, 1975, vol 8.

Neuwirth RS: Hysteroscopic management of symptomatic submucous fibroids. *Obstet Gynecol* 1983; 62:509–511.

Nitze M: Uber eine neue Beleuchtungsmethode der Hohlen des menschlichen Korpers. *Wien Med Presse* 1879; 20:851–857.

Novak ER, Woodruff JD: Postirradiation malignancies of the pelvic organs. *Am J Obstet Gynecol* 1959; 77:667–672.

Osterhuis JW: *Tumor Surgery With the CO_2 Laser: Studies with the Cloudman S-91 Mouse Melanoma.* Groningen, Netherlands, Veenstra-Visser, 1977.

Pantaleoni D: On endoscopic examination of the cavity of the womb. *Med Press Circ* 1869; 8:26–32.

Parent B, Barbot B, Doeufleu B: *Hysteroscopie de contact. Documentation scientifique.* Paris, Laboratories Roland Marie SA, 1976.

Penfield AJ: Vascular injuries and their management, in Phillips JM (ed): *Endoscopy in Gynecology.* Downey, Calif, American Association of Gynecologic Laparoscopists, 1978.

Peterson EP, Behrman SJ: Laparoscopy of the infertile patient. *Am J Obstet Gynecol* 1970; 36:363–368.

Peterson HB, Hulka JF, Spielman FJ, et al: Local versus general anesthesia for laparoscopic sterilization: A randomized study. *Obstet Gynecol* 1987; 70:903–908.

Phillips J, Keith D, Hulka B: Gynecologic laparoscopy in 1975. *J Reprod Med* 1976; 16:104–111.

Phillips J, Keith D, Keith L: Survey of gynecologic laparoscopy for 1974. *J Reprod Med* 1975; 15:45–51.

Pittaway DE, Maxson WS, Daniell JF: A comparison of the CO_2 laser and electrocautery on postoperative intraperitoneal adhesion formation in rabbits. *Fertil Steril* 1983; 40:366–370.

Piver MS, Lele SB, Barlow JJ, et al: Second-look laparoscopy prior to proposed second-look laparotomy. *Obstet Gynecol* 1980; 55:571–573.

Pouly JL, Mahnes H, Mage G, et al: Conservative laparoscopic treatment of 321 ectopic pregnancies. *Fertil Steril* 1986; 46:1093–1097.

Pring DW: Inferior epigastric haemorrhage, an avoidable complication of laparoscopic clip sterilization. *Br J Obstet Gynaecol* 1983; 90:480–482.

Qu JY, Sun AD, Lien LC: Laparoscopy in the diagnosis and management of ovarian cancer. *J Reprod Med* 1984; 29:483–488.

Raj SG, Hulka JF: Second-look laparoscopy in infertility surgery: Therapeutic and prognostic value. *Fertil Steril* 1982; 38:325–328.

Reich H, McGlynn F: Treatment of ovarian endometriomas using laparoscopic surgical techniques. *J Reprod Med* 1986; 31:577–583.

Rockwell RJ: Laser safety and training: Reviewing risks and safety protocols, in Breedlove B (ed): *Clinical Lasers: Expert Strategies for Practical and Profitable Management.* Atlanta, American Health Consultants, 1985.

Rubin IC: Uterine endoscopy, endometroscopy with the aid of uterine insufflation. *Am J Obstet Gynecol* 1925; 10:313–318.

Rubin IC: *Uterotubal Insufflation.* St Louis, CV Mosby Co, 1947.

Schenker JG, Margalioth EJ: Intrauterine adhesions: An updated appraisal. *Fertil Steril* 1982; 37:593–610.

Schroeder C: Uber den Ausbau und die Leistungen der Hysteroskopie. *Arch Gynaekol* 1934; 156:407–413.

Sciarra JJ, Valle RF: Hysteroscopy: A clinical experience with 320 patients. *Am J Obstet Gynecol* 1977; 127:340–345.

Semm K: Tissue-puncher and loop ligation: New aids for surgical-therapeutic pelviscopy. *Endoscopy* 1978; 10:119–125.

Semm K: *Endoscopic Intraabdominal Surgery*. Kiel, Christina-Albrechts-Universität, 1984, p 4.

Semm K, Mettler L: Technical progress in pelvic surgery via operative laparoscopy. *Am J Obstet Gynecol* 1980; 138:121–126.

Siegler AM, Kemmann EK, Gentile GP: Hysteroscopic procedures in 257 patients. *Fertil Steril* 1976; 25:1267–1271.

Smith WG, Day TG Jr, Smith JP: The use of laparoscopy to determine the results of chemotherapy for ovarian cancer. *J Reprod Med* 1977; 18:257–260.

Snowden EU, Jarret JC II, Dawood MY: Comparison of diagnostic accuracy of laparoscopy, hysteroscopy, and hysterosalpingography in evaluation of female infertility. *Fertil Steril* 1984; 41:709–713.

Stafl A, Wilkinson EJ, Mattingly RF: Laser treatment of cervical and vaginal neoplasia. *Am J Obstet Gynecol* 1977; 128:128–132.

Steptoe PC: *Laparoscopy in Gynecology*. Edinburgh, E & S Livingstone, 1967.

Stromme WB: Conservative surgery for ectopic pregnancy. *Obstet Gynecol* 1973; 41:215–220.

Sugimoto O: Diagnostic and therapeutic hysteroscopy for traumatic intrauterine adhesions. *Am J Obstet Gynecol* 1978; 131:539–544.

Surrey MW, Aronberg S: Hysteroscopic diagnosis of abnormal uterine bleeding: A clinical study, in Siegler AM, Lindemann HJ (eds): *Hysteroscopy: Principles and Practice*. Philadelphia, JB Lippincott Co, 1984.

Surrey MW, Friedman S: Second-look laparoscopy after reconstructive pelvic surgery for infertility. *J Reprod Med* 1982; 27:658–663.

Taylor PJ: Correlations in infertility: Symptomatology, hysterosalpingography, laparoscopy and hysteroscopy. *J Reprod Med* 1977; 8:339–344.

Taylor PJ, Cumming DC: Laparoscopy in the infertile female. *Curr Probl Obstet Gynecol* 1979; 2:3–32.

Timonen S, Nieminen V: Tubal pregnancy: Choice of operative method of treatment. *Acta Obstet Gynecol Scand* 1967; 46:327–331.

Townsend DE, Levine RU, Crum CP, et al: Treatment of vaginal carcinoma in situ with the carbon dioxide laser. *Am J Obstet Gynecol* 1982a; 143:101–105.

Townsend DE, Levine RU, Richart RM: Management of vulvar intraepithelial neoplasia by carbon dioxide laser. *Obstet Gynecol* 1982b; 60:97–102.

Trimbos-Kemper TCM, Trimbos JB, van Hall EV: Adhesion formation after tubal surgery: Results of eighth-day laparoscopy in 188 patients. *Fertil Steril* 1985; 43:395–399.

Tulandi T: Salpingo-ovariolysis: A comparison between laser surgery and electrosurgery. *Fertil Steril* 1986; 45:489–491.

Tulandi T, Vilos GA: A comparison between laser surgery and electrosurgery for bilateral hydrosalpinx: A 2-year follow-up. *Fertil Steril* 1985; 44:846–847.

Uribe-Ramirez LC, Camerena R, Hernandez F, et al: Outpatient laparoscopic sterilization: A review of complications in 2,000 cases. *J Reprod Med* 1977; 18:103–108.

Valle RF: Hysteroscopy in the evaluation of female infertility. *Am J Obstet Gynecol* 1980; 137:425–431.

Valle RF, Sciarra JJ: Current status of hysteroscopy in gynecologic practice. *Fertil Steril* 1979; 32:619–623.

Winburn DC: *Practical Laser Safety*. New York, Marcel Dekker, 1985.

Wood GP: Laparoscopic examination of the normal infertile woman. *Obstet Gynecol* 1983; 62:642–643.

Woodruff JD, Parmley TH, Julian CG: Topical 5-fluorouracil in the treatment of vaginal carcinoma in situ. *Gynecol Oncol* 1975; 3:124–128.

Word B, Gravlee LC, Wideman GL: The fallacy of simple uterine curettage. *Obstet Gynecol* 1958; 12:642–645.

Wright VC: Laser vaporization of the cervix for the management of cervical intraepithelial neoplasia, in Baggish MS (ed): *Basic and Advanced Laser Surgery in Gynecology*. New York, Appleton-Century-Crofts, 1985, pp 207–215.

Xygakis AM, Politis GS, Michalas SP, et al: Second-look laparoscopy in ovarian cancer. *J Reprod Med* 1984; 29:583–585.

Index